DIETARY GUIDELINES FOR AMERICANS, 2010

Key Recommendations for Each Area of the Guidelines:

Balancing Calories to Manage Weight

a. Prevent and/or reduce overweight and obesity through improved eating and physical activity behaviors.

b. Control total Calorie intake to manage body weight; for people who are overweight or obese, this means consuming fewer Calories from foods and beverages.

c. Increase physical activity and reduce time spent in sedentary behaviors.

d. Maintain appropriate Calorie balance during each stage of life—childhood, adolescence, adulthood, pregnancy and breastfeeding, and older age.

Foods and Food Components to Reduce

a. Reduce daily sodium intake to less than 2,300 mg and further reduce intake to 1,500 mg among those who are 51 years of age and older, and those of any age (including adolescents and children) who are African American or have hypertension, diabetes, or chronic kidney disease.

b. Consume less than 10 percent of Calories from saturated fatty acids by replacing them with monounsaturated and polyunsaturated fatty acids.

c. Consume less than 300 mg per day of dietary cholesterol.

d. Keep *trans* fatty acid consumption as low as possible, especially by limiting foods containing synthetic sources of *trans* fats—such as partially hydrogenated oils—and by limiting other solid fats.

e. Reduce the intake of Calories from solid fats and added sugars.

f. Limit the consumption of foods containing refined grains, especially refined grain foods with solid fats, added sugars, and sodium.

g. If alcohol is consumed, it should be in moderation—up to one drink per day for women, and two drinks per day for men—and only by adults of legal drinking age.

Foods and Nutrients to Increase

a. Individuals should meet the following recommendations as part of a healthy eating pattern and while staying within their Calorie needs.

b. Increase vegetable and fruit intake.

c. Eat a variety of vegetables, especially dark green, red, and orange vegetables, and beans and peas.

d. Consume at least half of all grains as whole grains; increase whole-grain intake by replacing refined grains with whole grains.

e. Increase intake of fat-free or low-fat milk and milk products, such as milk, yogurt, cheese, or fortified soy beverages.

f. Choose a variety of protein foods, which include seafood, lean meat and poultry, eggs, beans and peas, soy products, and unsalted nuts and seeds.

g. Increase the amount and variety of seafood consumed by choosing seafood in place of some meat and poultry.

h. Replace protein foods that are higher in solid fats with ones that are lower in solid fats and Calories and/or are sources of oils.

i. Use oils to replace solid fats where possible.

j. Choose foods that provide more potassium, dietary fiber, calcium, and vitamin D, which are nutrients of concern in American diets.

Building Healthy Eating Patterns

a. Select an eating pattern that meets nutrient needs over time at an appropriate Calorie level.

b. Account for all foods and beverages consumed and assess how they fit within a total healthy eating pattern.

c. Follow food safety recommendations when preparing and eating foods to reduce the risk of foodborne illnesses.

(There are additional key recommendations for specific population groups, including women capable of becoming pregnant, women who are pregnant or breastfeeding, and people 50 years of age and older. Go to www.dietaryguidelines.gov for more information.)

Data from the U.S. Departments of Agriculture (USDA) and Health and Human Services (HHS). *Dietary Guidelines for Americans 2010*. 7th Edition, Washington, DC: U.S. Government Printing Office, December 2010.

Tolerable Upper Intake Levels (ULs[*])

	Vitamins							
Life Stage Group	Vitamin A (μg/d)[a]	Vitamin C (mg/d)	Vitamin D (μg/d)	Vitamin E (mg/d)[b,c]	Niacin (mg/d)[c]	Vitamin B₆ (mg/d)	Folate (μg/d)[c]	Choline (g/d)
Infants								
0–6 mo	600	ND[d]	25	ND	ND	ND	ND	ND
6–12 mo	600	ND	38	ND	ND	ND	ND	ND
Children								
1–3 y	600	400	63	200	10	30	300	1.0
4–8 y	900	650	75	300	15	40	400	1.0
Males								
9–13 y	1,700	1,200	100	600	20	60	600	2.0
14–18 y	2,800	1,800	100	800	30	80	800	3.0
19–30 y	3,000	2,000	100	1,000	35	100	1,000	3.5
31–50 y	3,000	2,000	100	1,000	35	100	1,000	3.5
51–70 y	3,000	2,000	100	1,000	35	100	1,000	3.5
>70 y	3,000	2,000	100	1,000	35	100	1,000	3.5
Females								
9–13 y	1,700	1,200	100	600	20	60	600	2.0
14–18 y	2,800	1,800	100	800	30	80	800	3.0
19–30 y	3,000	2,000	100	1,000	35	100	1,000	3.5
31–50 y	3,000	2,000	100	1,000	35	100	1,000	3.5
51–70 y	3,000	2,000	100	1,000	35	100	1,000	3.5
>70 y	3,000	2,000	100	1,000	35	100	1,000	3.5
Pregnancy								
≤18 y	2,800	1,800	100	800	30	80	800	3.0
19–50 y	3,000	2,000	100	1,000	35	100	1,000	3.5
Lactation								
≤18 y	2,800	1,800	100	800	30	80	800	3.0
19–50 y	3,000	2,000	100	1,000	35	100	1,000	3.5

Data from: Reprinted with permission from the Dietary Reference Intakes series. Copyright 1997, 1998, 2000, 2001, 2005, 2011 by the National Academies of Sciences, courtesy of the National Academies Press, Washington, D.C. These reports may be accessed via www.nap.edu.

[a] As preformed vitamin A only.

[b] As α-tocopherol; applies to any form of supplemental α-tocopherol.

[c] The ULs for vitamin E, niacin, and folate apply to synthetic forms obtained from supplements, fortified foods, or a combination of the two.

[d] ND = Not determinable due to lack of data of adverse effects in this age group and concern with regard to lack of ability to handle excess amounts. Source of intake should be from food only to prevent high levels of intake.

[*]Note: A Tolerable Upper Intake Level (UL) is the highest level of daily nutrient intake that is likely to pose no risk of adverse health effects to almost all individuals in the general population. Unless otherwise specified, the UL represents total intake from food, water, and supplements. Due to a lack of suitable data, ULs could not be established for vitamin K, thiamin, riboflavin, vitamin B₁₂, pantothenic acid, biotin, and carotenoids. In the absence of a UL, extra caution may be warranted in consuming levels above recommended intakes. Members of the general population should be advised not to routinely exceed the UL. The UL is not meant to apply to individuals who are treated with the nutrient under medical supervision or to individuals with predisposing conditions that modify their sensitivity to the nutrient.

Tolerable Upper Intake Levels (ULs[*])

Life Stage Group	Boron (mg/d)	Calcium (mg/d)	Copper (µg/d)	Fluoride (mg/d)	Iodine (µg/d)	Iron (mg/d)	Magnesium (mg/d)[e]	Manganese (mg/d)	Molybdenum (µg/d)	Nickel (mg/d)	Phosphorus (g/d)	Selenium (µg/d)	Vanadium (mg/d)[f]	Zinc (mg/d)	Sodium (g/d)	Chloride (g/d)
Infants																
0–6 mo	ND[d]	1,000	ND	0.7	ND	40	ND	ND	ND	ND	ND	45	ND	4	ND	ND
6–12 mo	ND	1,500	ND	0.9	ND	40	ND	ND	ND	ND	ND	60	ND	5	ND	ND
Children																
1–3 y	3	2,500	1,000	1.3	200	40	65	2	300	0.2	3	90	ND	7	1.5	2.3
4–8 y	6	2,500	3,000	2.2	300	40	110	3	600	0.3	3	150	ND	12	1.9	2.9
Males																
9–13 y	11	3,000	5,000	10	600	40	350	6	1,100	0.6	4	280	ND	23	2.2	3.4
14–18 y	17	3,000	8,000	10	900	45	350	9	1,700	1.0	4	400	ND	34	2.3	3.6
19–30 y	20	2,500	10,000	10	1,100	45	350	11	2,000	1.0	4	400	1.8	40	2.3	3.6
31–50 y	20	2,500	10,000	10	1,100	45	350	11	2,000	1.0	4	400	1.8	40	2.3	3.6
51–70 y	20	2,000	10,000	10	1,100	45	350	11	2,000	1.0	4	400	1.8	40	2.3	3.6
>70 y	20	2,000	10,000	10	1,100	45	350	11	2,000	1.0	3	400	1.8	40	2.3	3.6
Females																
9–13 y	11	3,000	5,000	10	600	40	350	6	1,100	0.6	4	280	ND	23	2.2	3.4
14–18 y	17	3,000	8,000	10	900	45	350	9	1,700	1.0	4	400	ND	34	2.3	3.6
19–30 y	20	2,500	10,000	10	1,100	45	350	11	2,000	1.0	4	400	1.8	40	2.3	3.6
31–50 y	20	2,500	10,000	10	1,100	45	350	11	2,000	1.0	4	400	1.8	40	2.3	3.6
51–70 y	20	2,000	10,000	10	1,100	45	350	11	2,000	1.0	4	400	1.8	40	2.3	3.6
>70 y	20	2,000	10,000	10	1,100	45	350	11	2,000	1.0	3	400	1.8	40	2.3	3.6
Pregnancy																
≤18 y	17	3,000	8,000	10	900	45	350	9	1,700	1.0	3.5	400	ND	34	2.3	3.6
19–50 y	20	2,500	10,000	10	1,100	45	350	11	2,000	1.0	3.5	400	ND	40	2.3	3.6
Lactation																
≤18 y	17	3,000	8,000	10	900	45	350	9	1,700	1.0	4	400	ND	34	2.3	3.6
19–50 y	20	2,500	10,000	10	1,100	45	350	11	2,000	1.0	4	400	ND	40	2.3	3.6

[d] ND = Not determinable due to lack of data of adverse effects in this age group and concern with regard to lack of ability to handle excess amounts. Source of intake should be from food only to prevent high levels of intake.

[e] The ULs for magnesium represent intake from a pharmacological agent only and do not include intake from food and water.

[f] Although vanadium in food has not been shown to cause adverse effects in humans, there is no justification for adding vanadium to food, and vanadium supplements should be used with caution. The UL is based on adverse effects in laboratory animals, and this data could be used to set a UL for adults but not children and adolescents.

[*]Note: A Tolerable Upper Intake Level (UL) is the highest level of daily nutrient intake that is likely to pose no risk of adverse health effects to almost all individuals in the general population. Unless otherwise specified, the UL represents total intake from food, water, and supplements. Due to a lack of suitable data, ULs could not be established for vitamin K, thiamin, riboflavin, vitamin B_{12}, pantothenic acid, biotin, and carotenoids. In the absence of a UL, extra caution may be warranted in consuming levels above recommended intakes. Members of the general population should be advised not to routinely exceed the UL. The UL is not meant to apply to individuals who are treated with the nutrient under medical supervision or to individuals with predisposing conditions that modify their sensitivity to the nutrient.

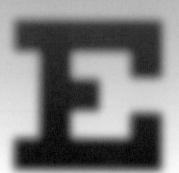
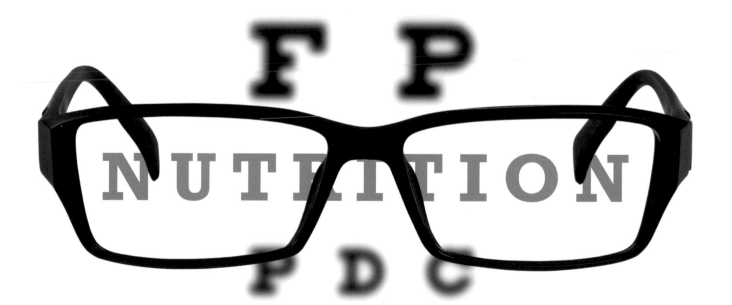

Bring your nutrition course

INTO FOCUS

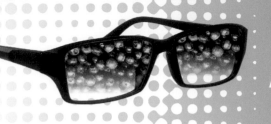

An approach that focuses

The Science of Nutrition, **Third Edition** offers the best combination of text and media resources to help students master the toughest nutrition course concepts, while providing the richest support to save instructors time. This nutrition text is uniquely organized around the highly-regarded functional/applied approach, located primarily in the organization of the micronutrient chapters. The functional approach— pioneered by this author team—avoids the need for rote memorization by presenting micronutrients based on their functions within the body.

Reviewers say *The Science of Nutrition* serves up a great nutrition course

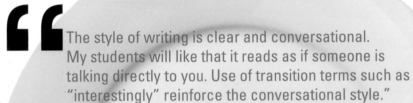

"The style of writing is clear and conversational. My students will like that it reads as if someone is talking directly to you. Use of transition terms such as "interestingly" reinforce the conversational style."

—Deborah Myers, Ed.D., R.D., L.D., *Bluffton University*

"You Do the Math" is the most valuable feature. Students always have a problem with math calculations, so any math examples you can provide throughout the text are valuable."

—Lori Zienkewicz, Ed.D., R.D., *Mesa Community College*

"I like the special features. I particularly like the Highlight with practical advice for starting a first kitchen in Chapter 17. The Nutri-Case really hits home with many of my students.

—Renee M. Romig, Ph.D., *Western Iowa Community College*

on **student learning**

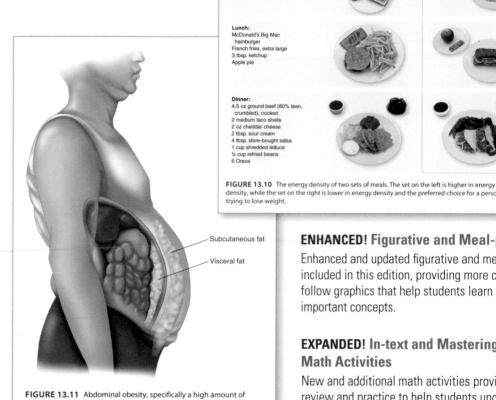

About 3,300 Calories (kcal)/day	About 1,700 Calories (kcal)/day
Breakfast: 1½ cups Fruit Loops cereal 1 cup 2% milk 1 cup orange juice 2 slices white toast 1 tbsp. butter (on toast)	**Breakfast:** 1½ cups Cheerios cereal 1 cup skim milk ½ fresh pink grapefruit
Lunch: McDonald's Big Mac hamburger French fries, extra large 3 tbsp. ketchup Apple pie	**Lunch:** Subway cold-cut trio 6" sandwich Granola bar, hard, with chocolate chips, 1 bar (24 g) 1 fresh medium apple
Dinner: 4.5 oz ground beef (80% lean, crumbled), cooked 2 medium taco shells 2 oz cheddar cheese 2 tbsp. sour cream 4 tbsp. store-bought salsa 1 cup shredded lettuce ½ cup refried beans 6 Oreos	**Dinner:** 5 oz ground turkey, cooked 2 soft corn tortillas 3 oz low-fat cheddar cheese 4 tbsp. store-bought salsa 1 cup shredded lettuce 1 cup cooked mixed veggies 3 Oreos

FIGURE 13.10 The energy density of two sets of meals. The set on the left is higher in energy density, while the set on the right is lower in energy density and the preferred choice for a person trying to lose weight.

Subcutaneous fat

Visceral fat

FIGURE 13.11 Abdominal obesity, specifically a high amount of visceral fat stored deep within the abdomen, is one of the risk factors for metabolic syndrome.

ENHANCED! Figurative and Meal-planning Art

Enhanced and updated figurative and meal-planning art is included in this edition, providing more colorful and easy-to-follow graphics that help students learn and integrate these important concepts.

EXPANDED! In-text and MasteringNutrition™ Math Activities

New and additional math activities provide hands-on math review and practice to help students understand and apply the material. Features include in-text sample problems, expanded and new You Do the Math feature boxes, and practice calculations in the new end-of-chapter Math Review questions.

 YOU Do the **Math**

Calculating Your Body Mass Index

Calculate your personal BMI value based on your height and weight. Let's use Theo's values as an example:

BMI = weight (kg)/height (m)^2

1. Theo's weight is 200 lb. To convert his weight to kilograms, divide his weight in pounds by 2.2 lb per kg:

200 lb/2.2 lb per kg = 90.91 kg

2. Theo's height is 6 feet 8 inches, or 80 inches. To convert his height to meters, multiply his height in inches by 0.0254 meters/inch:

80 in. × 0.0254 m/in. = 2.03 m

3. Find the square of his height in meters:

2.03 m × 2.03 m = 4.13 m^2

4. Then, divide his weight in kilograms by his height in square meters to get his BMI value:

90.91 kg/4.13 m^2 = 22.01 kg/m^2

Is Theo underweight according to this BMI value? As you can see in Figure 13.1, this value shows that he is maintaining a normal, healthful weight!

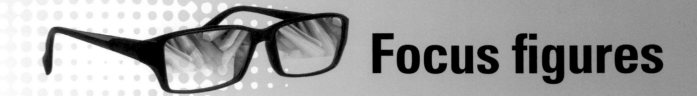

Focus figures

NEW! Focus Figures teach students key concepts in nutrition. These colorful, full-page figures highlight key topic areas through visually oriented displays that are bold, clear, and detailed. These dynamic new figures also have corresponding tutorials in MasteringNutrition.™

NEW! Third Edition

Focus Figures are presented with **introductory text** that explains how the figure is key to other concepts students will learn in this chapter and future chapters.

Students get **clear direction with stepped out art** that guide the eye through complex processes, breaking them down into clear, manageable pieces that make concepts easier to teach and understand.

Pairing of dynamic art and actual photographs provide students with the visual reinforcement needed for concepts to come alive.

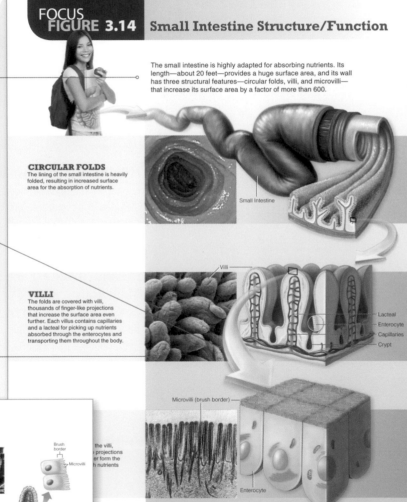

FOCUS FIGURE 3.14 **Small Intestine Structure/Function**

The small intestine is highly adapted for absorbing nutrients. Its length—about 20 feet—provides a huge surface area, and its wall has three structural features—circular folds, villi, and microvilli—that increase its surface area by a factor of more than 600.

CIRCULAR FOLDS
The lining of the small intestine is heavily folded, resulting in increased surface area for the absorption of nutrients.

Small Intestine

VILLI
The folds are covered with villi, thousands of finger-like projections that increase the surface area even further. Each villus contains capillaries and a lacteal for picking up nutrients absorbed through the enterocytes and transporting them throughout the body.

Villi

Lacteal
Enterocyte
Capillaries
Crypt

Microvilli (brush border)

Enterocyte

Second Edition

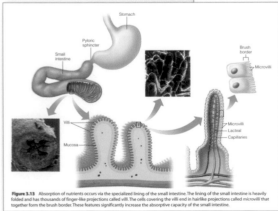

Figure 3.13 Absorption of nutrients occurs via the specialized lining of the small intestine. The lining of the small intestine is heavily folded and has thousands of finger-like projections called villi. The cells covering the villi end in hairlike projections called microvilli that together form the brush border. These features significantly increase the absorptive capacity of the small intestine.

p. 90

p. 95

bring clarity to tough topics

NEW! Third Edition

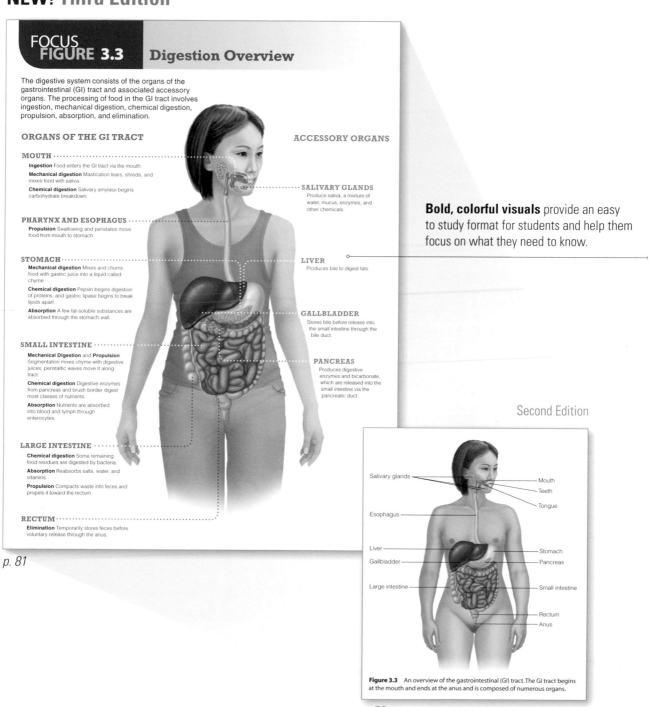

FOCUS FIGURE 3.3 — Digestion Overview

The digestive system consists of the organs of the gastrointestinal (GI) tract and associated accessory organs. The processing of food in the GI tract involves ingestion, mechanical digestion, chemical digestion, propulsion, absorption, and elimination.

ORGANS OF THE GI TRACT

MOUTH
- **Ingestion** Food enters the GI tract via the mouth.
- **Mechanical digestion** Mastication tears, shreds, and mixes food with saliva.
- **Chemical digestion** Salivary amylase begins carbohydrate breakdown.

PHARYNX AND ESOPHAGUS
- **Propulsion** Swallowing and peristalsis move food from mouth to stomach.

STOMACH
- **Mechanical digestion** Mixes and churns food with gastric juice into a liquid called chyme.
- **Chemical digestion** Pepsin begins digestion of proteins, and gastric lipase begins to break lipids apart.
- **Absorption** A few fat-soluble substances are absorbed through the stomach wall.

SMALL INTESTINE
- **Mechanical Digestion** and **Propulsion** Segmentation mixes chyme with digestive juices; peristaltic waves move it along tract.
- **Chemical digestion** Digestive enzymes from pancreas and brush border digest most classes of nutrients.
- **Absorption** Nutrients are absorbed into blood and lymph through enterocytes.

LARGE INTESTINE
- **Chemical digestion** Some remaining food residues are digested by bacteria.
- **Absorption** Reabsorbs salts, water, and vitamins.
- **Propulsion** Compacts waste into feces and propels it toward the rectum.

RECTUM
- **Elimination** Temporarily stores feces before voluntary release through the anus.

ACCESSORY ORGANS

SALIVARY GLANDS
Produce saliva, a mixture of water, mucus, enzymes, and other chemicals.

LIVER
Produces bile to digest fats.

GALLBLADDER
Stores bile before release into the small intestine through the bile duct.

PANCREAS
Produces digestive enzymes and bicarbonate, which are released into the small intestine via the pancreatic duct.

p. 81

Bold, colorful visuals provide an easy to study format for students and help them focus on what they need to know.

Second Edition

Salivary glands · Mouth · Teeth · Tongue · Esophagus · Liver · Stomach · Gallbladder · Pancreas · Large intestine · Small intestine · Rectum · Anus

Figure 3.3 An overview of the gastrointestinal (GI) tract. The GI tract begins at the mouth and ends at the anus and is composed of numerous organs.

p. 79

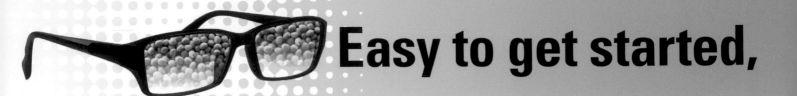

MasteringNutrition™

www.masteringnutrition.pearson.com
www.pearsonmylabandmastering.com

For Students

Proven, assignable, and automatically graded nutrition activities reinforce course learning objectives.

Mastering is the most effective and widely used online homework, tutorial, and assessment system for the sciences. It delivers self-paced tutorials that focus on your course objectives, provide individualized coaching, and respond to each student's progress.

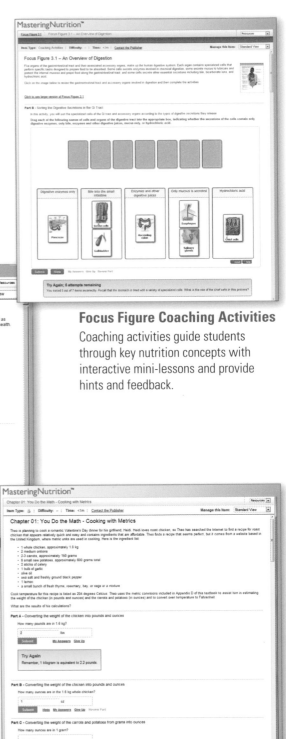

Focus Figure Coaching Activities

Coaching activities guide students through key nutrition concepts with interactive mini-lessons and provide hints and feedback.

NutriTools Coaching Activities

These unique activities allow students to combine and experiment with different food options and learn firsthand how to build healthier meals.

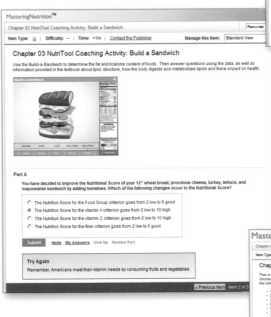

Math Activity

End-of-chapter math activities provide hands-on math review and practice to help students understand and apply the material, with helpful wrong-answer feedback.

Other automatically graded nutrition activities, with wrong answer feedback that act like a "Virtual TA" to help students learn include:

- MyDietAnalysis Case Study Coaching Activities
- Reading Quizzes
- *ABC News* Videos
- MP3 Case Studies
- Animations
- Math and Chemistry primer

use, and make your own

For Instructors

Mastering helps instructors maximize class time with easy-to-assign, customizable, and automatically graded assessments that motivate students to learn outside of class and arrive prepared for lecture or lab. Single sign on to MyDietAnalysis is automatic within MasteringNutrition.™

Calendar Feature for Instructors and Students

The Course Home default page features a Calendar View displaying upcoming assignments and due dates.

- Instructors can schedule assignments by dragging and dropping the assignment onto a date in the calendar.
- The calendar view lets students see at a glance when an assignment is due, and resembles a syllabus.

Customize Publisher-provided Problems or Quickly Add Your Own

MasteringNutrition makes it easy to edit any questions or answers, import your own questions, and quickly add images or links to further enhance the student experience.

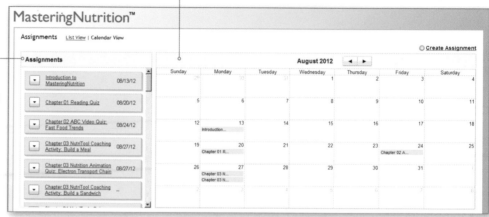

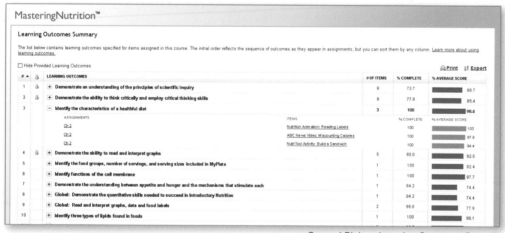

General Biology Learning Outcomes Example

Learning Outcomes

Tagged to book content and tied to Bloom's Taxonomy, Learning Outcomes are designed to let Mastering do the work in tracking student performance against your learning outcomes. Mastering offers a data supported measure to quantify students' learning gains and to share those results quickly and easily:

- Add your own or use the publisher-provided learning outcomes
- View class performance against the specified learning outcomes
- Export results to a spreadsheet

Bring focus to your course
with **dynamic supplements**

For Instructors

Instructor's Resource and Support Manual
978-0-3218-63010 | 0-321-86301-1

This resource enables instructors to create engaging lectures and course activities with chapter summaries; learning objectives; lecture outlines; key terms; discussion questions; web resources; and in-class activity ideas, including diet analysis and Nutrition Debate activities for each chapter.

Printed Test Bank
978-0-3218-6300-3 | 0-321-86300-3

The Test Bank, available in both print and computerized formats, provides multiple-choice, true/false, and essay questions for material from each text chapter. In this edition, the test bank is enhanced through the inclusion of links to chapter Learning Objectives and Bloom's Taxonomy indicators.

Great Ideas: Active Ways to Teach Nutrition
978 -0-321-59646-8 | 0-321-59646-3

This updated, revised booklet compiles the best ideas from nutrition instructors across the country on innovative ways to teach nutrition topics with an emphasis on active learning.

Instructor's Resource DVD (IR-DVD)
978-0-321-86299-0 | 0-321-86299-6

This valuable teaching resource offers everything you need to create lecture presentations and course materials, including JPEG and PowerPoint® files of all the art, tables, and selected photos from the text, including "stepped-out" art for selected figures from the text, as well as animations for the majors nutrition course.
The IR-DVD allows for "click and play" in the classroom—no downloading required, and also includes:

- PowerPoint® lecture outlines with embedded links to animations and *ABC News* Lecture Launcher Videos
- Jeopardy-type quiz show questions
- Test Bank Microsoft® Word files
- Computerized TestGen® Test Bank
- Questions for Classroom Response Systems (CRS) in PowerPoint format, allowing you to import the questions into your own CRS

MyDiet Analysis

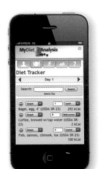

www.mydietanalysis.com

MyDietAnalysis was developed by the nutrition database experts at ESHA Research, Inc. and is tailored for use in college nutrition courses. It offers an accurate, reliable, and easy-to-use program for your students' diet analysis needs. MyDietAnalysis features a database of nearly 20,000 foods and multiple reports. MyDietAnalysis is also available as a single sign-on to MasteringNutrition.

NEW FOR SPRING 2013! For online users, a new mobile website version of MyDietAnalysis is available. Students can track their diet and activity intake accurately, anytime and anywhere, from their mobile device.

Food Composition Table

978-0-321-66793-9 | 0-321-66793-X

In the Third Edition, the USDA Nutrient Database for Standard Reference is provided as a stand-alone practice supplement, offering the current nutritional values of over 1,500 separate foods in an easy-to-follow format.

For Students

Food Composition Table
978-0-321-66793-9 | 0-321-66793-X

See "For Instructors" for full description.

NEW! MasteringNutrition with MyDietAnalysis and Pearson eText Student Access Code Card
978-0-321-73390-0 | 0-321-73390-8

See "For Instructors" for full description.

THE SCIENCE OF
NUTRITION

THIRD EDITION

Janice L. Thompson, PhD, FACSM
University of Birmingham | University of New Mexico

Melinda M. Manore, PhD, RD, CSSD, FACSM
Oregon State University

Linda A. Vaughan, PhD, RD
Arizona State University

PEARSON

Boston   Columbus   Indianapolis   New York   San Francisco   Upper Saddle River
Amsterdam   Cape Town   Dubai   London   Madrid   Milan   Munich   Paris   Montréal   Toronto
Delhi   Mexico City   São Paulo   Sydney   Hong Kong   Seoul   Singapore   Taipei   Tokyo

Executive Editor: Sandra Lindelof
Project Editor: Susan Scharf
Development Manager: Barbara Yien
Editorial Assistant: Briana Verdugo
Development Editor: Laura Bonazzoli
Art Development Editor: Jay McElroy
Media Producers: Joe Mochnick, Lee Ann Doctor
Managing Editor: Deborah Cogan
Production Project Manager: Megan Power
Production Management and Composition:
    S4Carlisle Publishing Services

Interior Design: Elise Lansdon
Cover Design: Jodi Notowitz
Image Management: Donna Kalal
Manufacturing Buyer: Stacey Weinberger
Executive Marketing Manager: Neena Bali
Text Printer: R.R. Donnelley
Cover Printer: Lehigh Phoenix Color
Cover Photo Credit: FOODCOLLECTION/
    AGE Fotostock

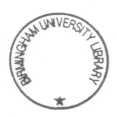

ISBN 10:   0-321-88365-9 (International Edition)
ISBN 13: 978-0-321-88365-0 (International Edition)

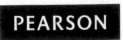

1 2 3 4 5 6 7 8 9 10 11 12—DOW—17 16 15 14 13

Dedication

This book is dedicated to my amazing family, friends, and colleagues—you provide constant support, encouragement, and unconditional love. It is also dedicated to my students and the communities with which I work—you continue to inspire me, challenge me, and teach me. —**JLT**

This book is dedicated to my wonderful colleagues, friends, and family—your guidance, support, and understanding have allowed this book to happen. —**MMM**

This book is dedicated to my strong circle of family, friends, and colleagues. Year after year, your support and encouragement sustain me. —**LAV**

About the Authors

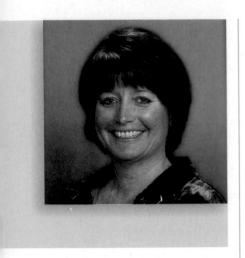

Janice L. Thompson, PhD, FACSM
University of Birmingham | University of New Mexico

Janice Thompson earned a doctorate in exercise physiology and nutrition at Arizona State University. She is currently Professor of Public Health Nutrition and Exercise at the University of Birmingham in the School of Sport and Exercise Sciences. Her research focuses on designing and assessing the impact of nutrition and physical activity interventions to reduce the risks for obesity, cardiovascular disease, and type 2 diabetes in high-risk populations. She also teaches nutrition and research methods courses, and mentors graduate research students.

Janice is a Fellow of the American College of Sports Medicine (ACSM), a member of the Scientific Committee of the European College of Sports Science, and a member of the American Society for Nutrition (ASN), the British Association of Sport and Exercise Science (BASES), and the Nutrition Society. Janice won an undergraduate teaching award while at the University of North Carolina, Charlotte, and a Community Engagement Award while at the University of Bristol. In addition to *The Science of Nutrition,* Janice coauthored the Pearson textbooks *Nutrition: An Applied Approach* and *Nutrition for Life* with Melinda Manore.

Janice loves hiking, yoga, traveling, and cooking and eating delicious food. She likes almost every vegetable except fennel and believes chocolate should be listed as a food group.

Melinda M. Manore, PhD, RD, CSSD, FACSM
Oregon State University

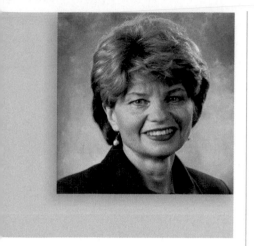

Melinda Manore earned a doctorate in human nutrition with minors in exercise physiology and health at Oregon State University (OSU). She is the past chair of the Department of Nutrition and Food Management, and is currently a professor of nutrition, at OSU. Prior to her move there, she was a professor at Arizona State University. Melinda's area of expertise is nutrition and exercise, particularly the role of diet and exercise in health and prevention of chronic disease, exercise performance, and weight control. She has a special focus on the energy and nutritional needs of active women and girls across the life cycle.

Melinda is an active member of the Academy of Nutrition and Dietetics (AND) and the American College of Sports Medicine (ACSM). She is the past chair of the AND Research Dietetic Practice Group, served on the AND Obesity Steering Committee and is an active member of the Sports, Cardiovascular and Wellness Nutrition Practice Group. She is a Fellow of ACSM and has served as Vice-President and on the Board of Trustees.

Melinda is also a member of the American Society of Nutrition (ASN) and the North American Association for the Study of Obesity (NAASO). She is the past chair of the USDA Nutrition and Health Committee for Program Guidance and Planning and currently is Chair of the USDA, ACSM, AND Expert Panel Meeting, *Energy Balance at the Crossroads: Translating Science into Action*. She serves on the editorial board of numerous research journals, and has won awards for excellence in research and teaching. Melinda also coauthored the Pearson textbooks *Nutrition: An Applied Approach* and *Nutrition for Life* with Janice Thompson.

Melinda is an avid walker, hiker and former runner who loves to garden, cook and eat great food. She is also an amateur birder.

Linda A. Vaughan, PhD, RD
Arizona State University

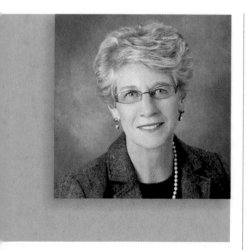

Linda Vaughan is a professor and the Director of the School of Nutrition and Health Promotion at Arizona State University. Linda earned a doctorate in agricultural biochemistry and nutrition at the University of Arizona. She currently teaches, advises graduate students, and remains involved in research as time permits. Her area of specialization is older adults and life cycle nutrition.

Linda is an active member of the Academy of Nutrition and Dietetics (AND), the American Society of Nutrition (ASN), and the Arizona Dietetic Association. She has served as chair of the Research and Dietetic Educators of Practitioners practice groups of the AND. Linda has received numerous awards, including the Arizona Dietetic Association Outstanding Educator Award (1997) and the Arizona State University Supervisor of the Year award (2004). In addition to being a coauthor of *The Science of Nutrition*, Linda is also a key contributor to the Pearson textbooks *Nutrition: An Applied Approach* and *Nutrition for Life* by Janice Thompson and Melinda Manore.

Linda enjoys swimming, cycling, and baking bread in her free time.

Welcome to *The Science of Nutrition,* Third Edition!

As nutrition researchers and educators, we know that the science of nutrition is constantly evolving. Our goal as authors is to provide students and instructors with the most recent and scientifically accurate nutrition information available.

Learning to Avoid Nutrition Confusion

What should I eat? In this age of information saturation, many different answers to that question are available 24 hours a day, from multiple sources: via the Internet, social media, television, and radio; in books, newspapers, and magazines; and on billboards, posters, and the sides of vending machines—even food packages offer nutrition advice. From research studies with contradictory findings to marketing claims for competing products, potential sources of confusion abound.

You're probably not fooled by the ads for diets and supplements in your e-mail inbox, but what kinds of nutrition messages *can* you trust? Which claims are backed up by scientific evidence, and of those, which are relevant to you? How can you evaluate the various sources of nutrition information and find out whether the advice they provide is accurate and reliable? How can you navigate the Internet to find reliable nutrition facts and avoid nutrition myths? How can you develop a way of eating that's right for you—one that supports your physical activity, allows you to maintain a healthful weight, and helps you avoid chronic disease? And if you're pursuing a career in nutrition or another healthcare field, how can you continue to obtain the most current and valid information about food and physical activity as you work with individual clients?

Why We Wrote This Book

The Science of Nutrition began with the conviction that both students and instructors would benefit from an accurate, clear, and engaging textbook that links nutrients with their functional benefits. As instructors, we recognized that students have a natural interest in their bodies, their health, their weight, and their success in sports and other activities. We developed this text to demonstrate how nutrition relates to these interests. *The Science of Nutrition* empowers you to reach your personal health and fitness goals while teaching you about the scientific evidence linking nutrition with disease. This information will be vital to your success as you build a career in nutrition or another health-related discipline.

You'll also learn how to debunk nutrition myths and how to distinguish nutrition fact from fiction. Throughout the chapters, material is presented in lively narrative that is scientifically sound and that continually links the evidence with these goals. Information on current events, and recent and ongoing research, keeps the inquisitive spark alive, illustrating how nutrition is very much a "living" science and a source of spirited ongoing debate.

The content of this text is designed for nutrition and other science and healthcare majors, but is also applicable and accessible to students in the liberal arts. We present the *science* of nutrition in a conversational style with engaging features that encourage you to apply the material to your own life and to the lives of your future clients, patients, or students. To support visual learning, the writing is supplemented by illustrations and photos that are attractive, effective, and level-appropriate. As teachers, we are familiar with the myriad challenges of presenting nutrition information in the classroom. We have therefore developed an exceptional ancillary package with a variety of tools to assist instructors in successfully meeting these challenges. We hope to contribute to the excitement of teaching and learning about nutrition: a subject that affects every one of us, a subject so important and relevant that correct and timely information can make the difference between health and disease.

Hallmark Text Features

A multitude of popular features have been updated throughout this new edition, challenging you to think about how the recommendations of different nutritional experts (and others who may be less than expert, such as some media sources) apply to your unique health issues, activity level, energy requirements, food preferences, and lifestyle. **Nutrition Myth or Fact?** boxes explore the science supporting or challenging common beliefs about foods, while the **Highlight** boxes explore research across a range of important, specific nutritional issues. **Nutrition Label Activity** feature boxes help you understand how to interpret food label information, so that you can make better nutritional choices.

Four visually vibrant **In Depth** "mini chapters" still cover the key areas of alcohol, vitamins and minerals, phytochemicals, and disordered eating, and offer instructors flexibility in incorporating them into their course. The Vitamins and Minerals In Depth specifically provides an overview of micronutrient basics prior to the first functional chapter.

New or revised **Nutrition Debates,** with follow-up Critical Thinking questions, encourage you to be better-informed and discriminating consumers of nutrition information. **Key content areas** feature updated text and references reflecting current research and recommendations, enhancing the text's relevance and clarity. Enhanced **figurative art** throughout the book helps you better visualize important processes in the body. Updated **food source diagrams** provide vivid images of the best food sources for each nutrient, so that they are more easily identifiable.

In providing these features, in addition to the new features listed below, we hope that by the time you finish this book you'll feel more confident and engaged in making decisions about your diet and physical activity.

Nutri-Case | You Play the Expert!

In addition to the features mentioned above, our Nutri-Case scenarios provide you with the opportunity to evaluate the nutrition-related beliefs and behaviors of five people representing a range of backgrounds and nutritional challenges. As you encounter them, keep in mind that these case scenarios are for instructional purposes, not intended to suggest that students using this text are qualified to offer nutritional advice to others. In the real world, only properly trained and licensed health professionals are qualified to provide nutritional counseling. Take a moment to get acquainted with our Nutri-Case characters here.

Hannah

Hi, I'm Hannah. I'm 18 years old and in my first year at Valley Community College. I'm 5'6" and right now I weigh 171 lbs. I haven't made up my mind yet about my major. All I know for sure is that I don't want to work in a hospital like my mom! I got good grades in high school, but I'm a little freaked out by college so far. There's so much homework, plus one of my courses has a lab, plus I have to work part-time because my mom doesn't have the money to put me through school . . . Sometimes I feel like I just can't handle it all. And when I get stressed out, I eat. I've already gained 10 pounds and I haven't even finished my first semester!

Theo

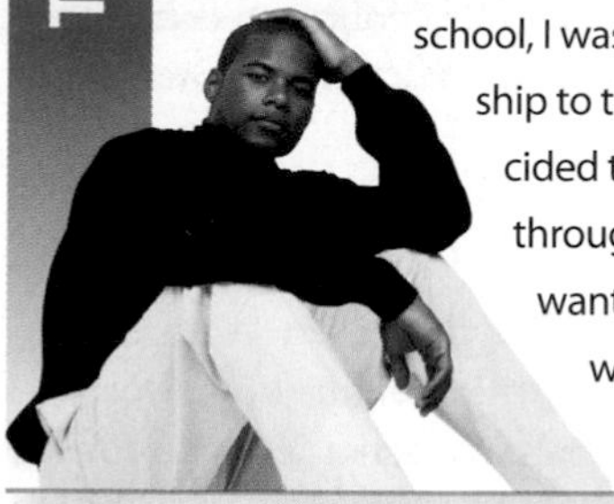

Hi, I'm Theo. Let's see, I'm 21, and my parents moved to the Midwest from Nigeria 11 years ago. I'm 6'8" tall and weigh in at 200 lbs. The first time I ever played basketball, in middle school, I was hooked. I won lots of awards in high school and then got a full scholarship to the state university, where I'm a junior studying political science. I decided to take a nutrition course because, last year, I had a hard time making it through the playing season, plus keeping up with my classes and homework. I want to have more energy, so I thought maybe I'm not eating right. Anyway, I want to figure out this food thing before basketball season starts again.

Liz

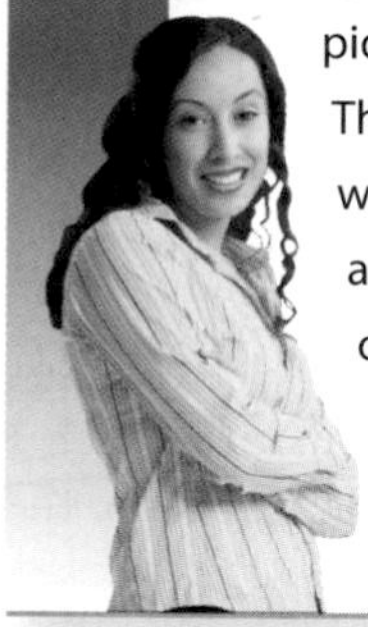

I'm Liz, I'm 20, and I'm a dance major at the School for Performing Arts. I'm 5'4" and currently weigh about 103 lbs. Last year, two other dancers from my class and I won a state championship and got to dance in the New Year's Eve celebration at the governor's mansion. This spring, I'm going to audition for the City Ballet, so I have to be in top condition. I wish I had time to take a nutrition course, but I'm too busy with dance classes, rehearsals, and teaching a dance class for kids. But it's okay, because I get lots of tips from other dancers and from the Internet. Like last week, I found a website especially for dancers that explained how to get rid of bloating before an audition. I'm going to try it for my audition with the City Ballet!

Judy

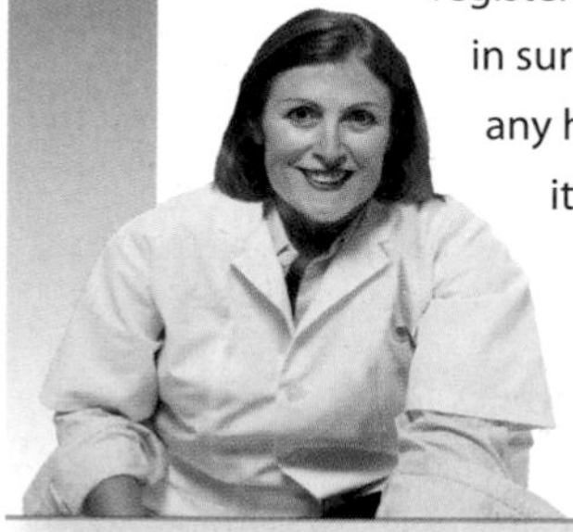

I'm Judy, Hannah's mother. I'm 38 years old and a nurse's aide at Valley Hospital. I'm 5'5" and weigh 200 lbs. Back when Hannah was a baby, I dreamed of going to college so I could be a registered nurse. But then my ex and I split up, and Hannah and me, we've been in survival mode ever since. I'm proud to have raised my daughter without any handouts, and I do good work, but the pay never goes far enough and it's exhausting. I guess that's partly because I'm out of shape, and my blood sugar's high. Most nights, I'm so tired at the end of my shift that I just pick up some fast food for supper. I know I should be making home-cooked meals, but like I said, I'm in survival mode.

Gustavo

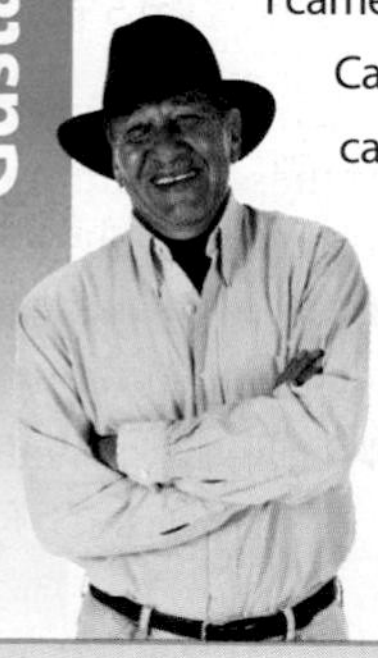

Hello. My name is Gustavo. I'm 69 years young at the moment, but when I was 13 years old I came to the United States from Mexico with my parents and three sisters to pick crops in California. Now I manage a large vineyard. They ask me when I'm going to retire, but I can still work as hard as a man half my age. Health problems? None. Well, maybe my doctor tells me my blood pressure is high, but that's normal for my age! I guess what keeps me going is thinking about how my father died 6 months after he retired. He had colon cancer, but he never knew it until it was too late. Anyway, I watch the nightly news and read the papers, so I keep up on what's good for me, "Eat less salt" and all that stuff. I'm doing great! I'm 5'5" tall and weigh 166 lbs.

Throughout this text, you'll read about these five characters as they grapple with various nutrition-related challenges in their lives. As you do, you might find that they remind you of people you know, and you may discover you have something in common with one or more of them. Our hope is that by applying the information you learn in this course to their situations, you will deepen your understanding of the importance of nutrition in your own life.

New in the Third Edition

This Third Edition of *The Science of Nutrition* includes a wealth of dynamic new features and innovations. Key among these is the addition of the **MasteringNutrition** online homework, tutorial, and assessment system, which delivers self-paced tutorials and activities that provide individualized coaching, focus on course objectives, and tools enabling instructors to respond individually to each student's progress. The proven Mastering system provides instructors with customizable, easy-to-assign, automatically graded assessments that motivate students to learn outside of class and arrive prepared for lecture. Key MasteringNutrition features include:

- Focus Figure Coaching Activities that guide students through key nutrition concepts with interactive mini-lessons.
- MyDietAnalysis Case Study Activities which provide students with hands-on diet analysis practice that can be automatically graded.
- Reading Quizzes (20 questions per chapter) that ensure students have completed the assigned reading before class.
- 28 *ABC News* Videos with up-to-date topics that arise in the nutrition field, including multiple choice questions that provide wrong-answer feedback to redirect students to the correct answers.
- 40 animations that provide an overview of the most difficult topics in nutrition, including questions with wrong-answer feedback addressing common misconceptions.
- NutriTool Coaching Activities that allow students to combine and experiment with different food options and learn firsthand how to build healthier meals.
- MP3s related to chapter content, with multiple choice questions that provide wrong-answer feedback.
- Access to *Get Ready for Nutrition*, providing students with extra math and chemistry study assistance.
- A Study Area which is broken down into learning areas and includes videos, animations, MP3s, and other resources.

New **Focus Figure** displays illuminate some of the toughest topics for students to learn and understand. These dramatic, visual full-page figures are unmatched in their integrated treatment of key aspects in digestion, metabolism, and chemical processes in addition to bold, clear, and detailed information displays. Focus Figures also double as MasteringNutrition tutorial topics, with hints and wrong answer feedback, that can be assigned and graded.

The prior **In Depth mini-chapter** on "Phytochemicals and Functional Foods" has been substantially revised and is now comprised of just phytochemicals content, with the functional foods information shifting more logically to Chapter 15.

Expanded **Math Activities,** both in-text and as part of MasteringNutrition, provide helpful hands-on math review and practice to help with student preparedness, including expanded and new You Do the Math feature boxes, and where applicable, new Math Review questions following the end-of-chapter Review questions.

Significantly **updated content** includes material on digestion, metabolism, and bone health feature updated content reflecting current research and recommendations, enhancing the text's relevance and clarity.

Enhanced figurative art and meal-planning art is included in this edition, providing more colorful and easy-to-follow graphics with greater detail and clarity.

Chapter 15, previously Food Safety and Technology: Impact on Consumers, has been re-titled and significantly revised to more fully address a range of consumer issues, including expanded treatment of food trends and movements, and more emphasis on the positive aspects of food safety information. Food safety content has been streamlined and revised to more effectively address areas of student interest.

Chapter 19 on Global Nutrition has undergone a thorough update and revision by a highly regarded field expert, providing more expansive and up-to-the-moment content.

Nutri-Case scenarios, which now number one per chapter, include height and weight (in addition to age) information for each character at the front of the text, which reviewers asked for and which align well with our enhanced overall math coverage.

This edition adds **new in-text URLs** that cover a wide range of important linked areas that are identified throughout the text. In addition, **box references** appear with citations within each box, for easier reference and access, and all **In Depth mini chapters** are now numbered for easier reference.

The visual overview at the front of the book provides additional information on the new features in the Third Edition. Specific changes to each chapter, in addition to the updates and features described above, includethe following:

Chapter 1

- Updated all numbered Figures 1.1 through 1.12, and select photos.
- Revised title of chapter to more accurately reflect its content and purpose.
- Revised text throughout the chapter to reflect the increasing use of the Internet for nutrition research and information.
- Added new information on conflict of interest within the section on evaluating media reports.
- Inserted a bulleted section on how to determine if a website is reliable.
- Added new Nutrition Online links.
- Included additional websites in the end-of-chapter Web Links.
- Added two new end-of-chapter Math Review questions.
- Added a You Do the Math feature box focusing on converting a recipe from metric units to imperial units.
- Added a Nutrition Milestone about the calorimeter.
- Added expanded and updated content on reliable sources of nutrition information and students responding to spam.
- Updated the Nutrition Debate on Nutrigenomics, including references.
- Updated the chapter opener to reflect increased use of the internet to access nutrition information.
- Updated the section on Healthy People 2020.
- Updated all applicable references.

Chapter 2

- Updated Figures 2.1, 2.2, 2.4, 2.5, 2.6, 2.7, 2.9, 2.10, and 2.11, and select photos.
- Added new Nutrition Online links.
- Added an end-of-chapter Math Review question.

- Added a new You Do the Math on determining the healthiest food choices when eating out at a fast food restaurant.
- Updated and revised sections on 2010 Dietary Guidelines for Americans and MyPlate (now Figure 2.5).
- Added a Nutrition Milestone on the evolution of food guides.
- Included a revised figure on Food Groups of the USDA Food Patterns (now Figure 2.6).
- Deleted the figure on MyPyramid Tracker, and replaced with a Nutrition Online link to MyPlate SuperTracker.
- Included a new Nutrition Debate on whether revising MyPyramid will promote America's health.
- Deleted old Table 2.5 on tips for eating out from the American Diabetes Association—replaced with bulleted list within the text and a Nutrition Online link to a video on how to make healthier choices when eating out.
- Updated all applicable references.

Chapter 3

- Updated Figures 3.1, 3.2, 3.4, 3.5, 3.6, 3.7, 3.8, 3.9, 3.10, 3.11, 3.12, 3.15, 3.16, 3.17, 3.18, 3.19, and select photos.
- Tightened discussion of how environmental cues affect appetite.
- Converted and updated previous See for Yourself feature into a Highlight box, Do You Eat in Response to External or Internal Cues?
- Added new Focus Figure (3.3) of the GI tract and its functions.
- Added new Nutrition Online links.
- Reorganized discussion of the functions and secretions of the stomach.
- Added a new You Do the Math box, Negative Logarithms and the pH Scale.
- Added a Nutrition Milestone on bile as soap.
- Expanded the discussion of the portal venous system and included a new figure (Figure 3.13).
- Added with new Focus Figure (3.14) of absorption within the small intestine.
- Added a Nutrition Label Activity feature box, Recognizing Common Allergens in Foods.
- Added content on new pharmaceutical and food product development efforts to help people with celiac disease.
- Added a new section on acute vomiting and cyclic vomiting syndrome.
- Revised the Highlight feature box on traveler's diarrhea.
- Added a new end-of-chapter Math review question.
- Updated all applicable references.

Chapter 4

- Updated Figures 4.2, 4.3, 4.4, 4.5, 4.7, 4.9, 4.20, 4.11, 4.12, 4.15, 4.16, and 4.18, and select photos.
- Revised the section on fiber, adding additional narrative on what makes a whole grain whole—also included a new figure on structure of a whole grain (now Figure 4.14).
- Expanded bulleted list on how to increase fiber intake.
- Expanded and updated the section on diabetes to include more detail on complications.
- Added a new end-of-chapter Math Review question.

- Enhanced the Nutrition Label Activity to incorporate more math and revised style to allow students to fill in the blanks.
- Expanded previous Figure 4.6 on carbohydrate digestion and absorption into a Focus Figure.
- Expanded previous Figure 4.8 on blood glucose regulation into a Focus Figure.
- Edited and updated the Highlight box on "Living with Diabetes".
- Revised chapter opener on diagnosis of type 2 diabetes in younger people.
- Added new Nutrition Online links.
- Deleted the figures on fiber content of bread and alternative sweeteners—added in photo of the toe amputation.
- Added Nutrition Milestone on discovery of treatment of type 1 diabetes with insulin.
- Updated Nutrition Debate on High Fructose Corn Syrup.
- Updated all applicable references.

Chapter 4.5 In Depth: Alcohol

- Updated Figures 2, 3, and 5, and select photos.
- Included recommendations on alcohol consumption from the 2010 Dietary Guidelines for Americans.
- Expanded the discussion of Fetal Alcohol Syndrome to describe the whole range of alcohol-related birth defects.
- Updated all applicable references.

Chapter 5

- Updated Figures 5.1, 5.2, 5.3, 5.4, 5.5, 5.6, 5.7, 5.9, 5.10, 5.11, 5.13, 5.16, and 5.18, and select photos.
- Added new Figure 5.15.
- Added new Nutrition Myth or Fact Box, Is Margarine More Healthful Than Butter?
- Expanded section on the roles of fat in satiation and satiety.
- Expanded section on how to eat more beneficial fats and the foods that contain these fats.
- Revised and updated information on the links between nutrition and cardiovascular disease.
- Added Nutrition Milestones.
- Added two new Focus Figures; Figure 5.8 on Lipid Digestion Overview, and Figure 5.18 on Lipoprotein Transport and Distribution.
- Added Nutrition Online links.
- Updated all applicable references.

Chapter 6

- Updated Figures 6.1, 6.2, 6.3, 6.4, 6.5, 6.7, 6.8, 6.10, 6.12, 6.13, 6.14, 6.16, and 6.17, and select photos.
- Deleted box on Mad Cow Disease (now included in Chapter 15).
- Added a section on how proteins are used to make other biological compounds such as neurotransmitters and blood clotting.
- Added new Focus Figure (Figure 6.6) on Protein Synthesis Overview.
- Figure on protein digestion and absorption now expanded into new Focus Figure (now Figure 6.11).
- Updated and added information on the role of protein in cardiovascular disease.

- Added a new end-of-chapter Math Review question.
- Added a new figure on urea excretion (now Figure 6.15).
- Added Nutrition Milestone on discovery of, and treatment for, PKU.
- Revised, updated and expanded section on food sources of protein, now referred to as Protein: Much More Than Meat!
- Added more tips on how to add legumes to your daily diet.
- Added narrative on the use and effects of amino acid supplements.
- Inserted new Highlight box on What's So Great About Soy?
- Updated Nutrition Debate on Tofu to the Rescue.
- Added new Nutrition Online links.
- Updated chapter opener.
- Updated all applicable references.

Chapter 7

- Updated all the chapter's numbered Figures, 7.1 through 7.25, and select photos.
- Added new Nutrition Debate on lifestyle factors that impact metabolic rate and/or total energy expenditure.
- Added two new Focus Figures: Figure 7.26a on the metabolic responses to feeding, and Figure 7.26b on the metabolic responses to short- and long-term fasting.
- Updated discussion on the potential value of carnitine supplements as "fat burners".
- Added a new Nutrition Milestone on the historical roots and metabolic consequences of re-feeding syndrome.
- Added an end-of-chapter Math Review question to tie metabolism in with daily food choices.
- Updated calcium and vitamin D RDA and UL values.
- Added Nutrition Online links that illustrate the functioning of cells and various metabolic pathways.
- Updated all applicable references.

Chapter 7.5 In Depth: Vitamins and Minerals: Micronutrients with Macro Powers

- Updated select photos.
- Added a new section on how to best retain the vitamins and minerals in healthful foods.
- Updated calcium and vitamin D RDA and UL values.
- Updated all applicable references.

Chapter 8

- Updated Figures 8.1, 8.2, 8.4, 8.5, 8.6, 8.8, 8.10, 8.11, 8.13, 8.15, 8.16, 8.18, 8.21, and 8.22, and select photos.
- Added sections on folate and Vitamin B_{12} to complete the overview of B-vitamins. The role of folate and B_{12} in blood health is still covered in Chapter 12.
- Revised and updated content on the role of vitamin B_6 and folic acid and for the treatment of PMS.
- Added a Nutrition Milestone on the discovery of the cause of beriberi a thiamin deficiency disease.
- Revised and updated the 'Nutrition Myth or Fact? Can Chromium Supplementation Enhance Body composition?

- Added new Nutrition Online links.
- Updated all applicable references.

Chapter 9

- Updated Figures 9.1, 9.2, 9.3, 9.4, 9.5, 9.6, 9.7, 9.8, 9.9, and 9.10, and select photos.
- Converted prior Table 9.4 into new full Figure 9.12 on the DASH diet plan.
- Added new chapter opening scenario on fluid overload.
- Expanded discussion of beverage options within U.S. diet.
- Expanded Nutrition Debate on sports beverages to address their use with children and adolescents.
- Added tips on how to increase potassium intake.
- Expanded discussion on diseases related to fluid/electrolyte imbalances.
- Added new section on regulation of acid/base balance.
- Revised You Do The Math box.
- Added Nutrition Milestone on the discovery of electrolytes.
- Added Nutrition Online links.
- Updated all applicable references.

Chapter 10

- Updated Figures 10.1, 10.2, 10.3, 10.5, 10.7, 10.8, 10.10, 10.11, 10.12, 10.14, 10.15, 10.16, and 10.17, and select photos.
- Revised chapter title to reflect primary function of vitamin A.
- Added a You Do the Math box on Vitamin A Conversions from Food and Supplement Sources.
- Added an end-of-chapter Math Review question on Vitamin E unit conversions.
- Deleted the Myth versus Fact box on beta-carotene supplements, and revised the text on beta-carotene to report newest findings on this topic.
- Deleted the Highlight box on Nutritional Factors that Influence Cancer Risk and incorporated this information into the section on cancer.
- Revised and updated section on vitamin A to reflect current evidence on primary functions.
- Added more food sources for vitamins E, C, and beta-carotene within text.
- Moved content on age-related eye diseases to Chapter 18.
- Added information on acne in section on vitamin A.
- Added Nutrition Milestone on discovery of vitamin E as antioxidant.
- Added new Nutrition Online links.
- Updated and expanded Nutrition Debate on vitamin and mineral supplements.
- Updated all applicable references.

Chapter 10.5 In Depth: Phytochemicals

- Updated Figure 1 and select photos.
- The prior content on functional foods has been moved to Chapter 15 on consumer food safety, production, and environmental impact issues.
- Updated and expanded content in the Highlight feature box, Will a PB&J Keep the Doctor Away?
- Updated and expanded content on the basic mechanisms of phytochemicals' protective effects.

■ Added a short discussion of the new research into the role of phytochemicals in increasing the effectiveness of traditional medications used to treat disease.

■ Included a Nutri-Case feature, using Hannah, which challenges students to think about the influence of socioeconomic factors on an individual's access to fresh fruits and veggies.

■ Updated all applicable references.

Chapter 11

■ Updated Figures 11.2, 11.3, 11.6, 11.7, 11.8, 11.10, 11.13, 11.14, and 11.18, and select photos.

■ Revised two Test Yourself questions.

■ Updated and revised the chapter opening scenario.

■ Added a You Do the Math box on vitamin D unit conversions from foods and supplements.

■ Added additional tips for increasing calcium intake.

■ Updated and revised section on osteoporosis.

■ Updated and revised Nutrition Debate to reflect current issues related to vitamin D recommendations.

■ Added Nutrition Milestone on vitamin D and rickets.

■ Added a math question to end of chapter related to calcium availability in various foods.

■ Added new Nutrition Online links.

■ Updated all applicable references.

Chapter 12

■ Updated Figures 12.1, 12.2, 12.3, 12.4, 12.6, 12.7, and 12.8, and select photos.

■ Added new Figure 12.9 on spina bifida.

■ Revised and updated the Nutrition Debate on the efficacy of zinc lozenges in fighting colds.

■ Added a new You do the Math feature box on Calculating Daily Iron Intake.

■ Added a new Nutrition Milestone on the role of zinc in blood health and normal reproductive health box.

■ Updated the Highlight box, "Iron Deficiency Around the world."

■ Moved content and corresponding figures on folate, folic acid, and vitamin B_{12} to Chapter 8.

■ Added Nutrition Online links illustrating the role of vitamin K in blood clotting.

■ Updated all applicable references.

Chapter 13

■ Updated Figures 13.1, 13.2, 13.3, 13.6, 13.9, 13.10, and 13.11, and select photos.

■ Deleted Highlight box on genetic influences on body weight gain and overfeeding—included this information as narrative within the text.

■ Inserted new Nutrition Online links.

■ Revised organization and content in section on evaluating body weight.

■ Included additional information on portion size awareness.

■ Added additional narrative and bulleted tip list on increasing physical activity to help in weight loss and maintenance of weight loss.

- Updated and revised chapter opener to focus on singer, Adele.
- Added new Nutrition Milestone on research examining effect on social networks on risk for obesity.
- Included new Nutrition Debate on whether high-carbohydrate, moderate-fat diets have been oversold.
- Updated Table 13.2 with revised data on energy costs of various physical activities.
- Added two end-of-chapter Math Review questions.
- Added new figure on abdominal obesity (now Figure 13.11).
- Revised, updated and expanded content on the dynamics of energy balance, differences in individual weight loss and gain, and the energy balance equation.
- Added an additional math activity focusing on how consuming 3500 extra kcal results in a gain of one pound of body fat—included within section on energy intake.
- Added new section on metabolic factors that influence weight loss and gain.
- Updated and expanded content on how to achieve and maintain a healthful body weight.
- Updated all applicable references.

Chapter 13.5 In Depth: Disordered Eating

- Updated Figure 3 and select photos.
- Updated content regarding eating disorder behaviors.
- Updated content on the Female Athlete Triad and the components of the Traid.
- Added Nutrition Online links.
- Updated all applicable references.

Chapter 14

- Updated Figures 14.1, 14.2, 14.4, 14.5, 14.6, 14.9, 14.10, and 14.11, and select photos.
- Revised and restructured content on how physical activity increases fitness to enhance clarity.
- Added Nutrition Milestone on Dr. Jerry Morris (father of physical activity epidemiology).
- Included a new section describing how much physical activity is enough, highlighting details and controversies surrounding recent physical activity recommendations and guidelines.
- Expanded and updated content on the influence of intrinsic and extrinsic motivation on physical activity related behavior.
- Added the factor of Time to the FITT principle.
- Revised Figure 14.2 on the FITT principle to be consistent with the 2008 Physical Activity Guidelines for Americans.
- Provided many specific examples of types of activities of varying intensity levels.
- Deleted the figure on RPE; in place of this, emphasised the more recent CDC guidance on calculating training heart rate ranges for activities of varying intensities.
- Expanded the You Do the Math feature box by providing the student with an additional scenario in which to calculate training heart rate range.
- Added more examples of how to add physical activity to one's daily life.
- Added a section explaining how the utilization of fat and expenditure of energy differs between situations of performing low-intensity exercise versus high-intensity exercise of various durations.

- Deleted prior Table 14.5 on protein needs of athletes and active people (as this information is now presented in Chapter 6), and updated this section to include the latest research on how protein needs of athletes may be higher than previously suggested.
- Revised Figure 14.9 to include both meals and snacks.
- Added an end-of-chapter Math Review question.
- Added a new Nutrition Debate topic focusing on ergogenic aids.
- Added Nutrition Online links, including topics such as tools used to assess physical activity levels and bodybuilding among people eating a vegan diet.
- Updated all applicable references.

Chapter 15

- Updated Figures 15.1, 15.3, 15.5, 15.9, 15.10, 15.12, and 15.13, and select photos.
- Added new Nutrition Online links.
- Added new Nutrition Milestone on pasteurization.
- Expanded content on food toxins.
- Updated and condensed food safety information according to latest CDC and USDA guidelines.
- Replaced prior "Thermy" chart with a link to most current cooking temps.
- Moved boxed essay on mad cow disease (vCJD) from Chapter 6 to this chapter, and updated to summer, 2012 statistics.
- Removed prior Highlight box on Typhoid Mary.
- Revised and condensed content on preservation methods.
- Added a list of "Dirty Dozen" and "Clean Fifteen" shopping guides for organically grown foods.
- Added new closing section on the food movement, covering issues of sustainability, food diversity, public health, and fair trade.
- Revised and updated all other chapter topics, including the safety of sushi and the Nutrition Debate on GMOs.
- Updated all applicable references.

Chapter 16

- Updated Figures 16.1, 16.2, 16.3, 16.4, 16.6, and 16.9, and select photos.
- Added new Highlight box on pica.
- Expanded content on cleft lip and cleft palate and added new Figure 16.13.
- Added Nutrition Milestone on developments in infant formula production over time.
- Added Nutrition Online links.
- Updated all applicable references.

Chapter 17

- Updated Figure 17.5 and select photos.
- Added a new Nutrition Debate on Bariatric Surgery for Adolescents.
- Added a new Nutrition:Myth or Fact feature box, Is Breakfast the Most Important Meal of the Day?
- Added a new Nutrition Milestone on the History of the Federal School Lunch Program.

- Expanded the discussion on alcohol, tobacco, and illegal drugs.
- Added "Inadequate Calcium Intake" as a nutrition-related concern for children.
- Expanded the discussion on the seeds of pediatric obesity.
- Added Nutrition Online links.
- Updated all applicable references.

Chapter 18

- Updated Figure 18.1 and select photos.
- Added a new opening scenario reflecting the many options now available to older adults.
- Expanded discussions on drug/nutrient interaction; age-related disorders of the eye.
- Added new Nutrition Milestone on "Screening for Geriatric Malnutrition".
- Expanded and updated the Nutrition Debate on caloric restriction as a means of extending longevity.
- Updated calcium and vitamin D discussions to reflect new RDAs for older adults.
- Added a new discussion on gut microbes in older adults.
- Replaced the priior Food Pyramid visuals with MyPlate-based images.
- Updated the roster of community food resource programs available to low income seniors.
- Added new Figure 18.2 on MyPlate for older adults.
- Added Nutrition Online links.
- Updated all applicable references.

Chapter 19

- Updated Figures 19.1 and 19.2, and select photos.
- Added new Figure 19.4 on the prevalence of food insecurity and very-low food insecurity from 1998 to 2010.
- Revised and expanded content on global undernutrition and the impact on preventable diseases.
- Moved sections on overnutrition and overweight, and revised and expanded content.
- Revised and expanded content on solutions to malnutrition, and on the potential for technological solutions.
- Added Nutrition Milestone on the growth and impact of diabetes worldwide.
- Added Nutrition Online links.
- Updated all applicable references.

Appendices, Front Matter, and Back Matter

- Updated the Dietary Guidelines for Americans to the 2010 version.
- Added new Appendix A on the USDA Food Guide Evolution.
- Updated the figures in Appendices B, C, and D.
- Updated contact information and URLs in Appendix I, Organizations and Resources.
- Revised and/or updated, as needed, all applicable information in the RDI and Upper Intake Levels charts.

Supplemental Resources for Instructors and Students

For the Instructor

Exam Copy

978-0-321-88746-7 / 0-321-88746-8

Instructor Resource and Support Manual

978-0-321-86301-0 / 0-321-86301-1

This popular and adaptable resource enables instructors to create engaging lectures and additional activities via chapter summaries; learning objectives; chapter outlines; key terms; in-class discussion questions; and activity ideas, including a diet analysis activity and a Nutrition Debate activity for each chapter, in addition to a list of all web resources, by chapter.

Instructor Resource DVD (IR-DVD)

978-0-321-86299-0 / 0-321-86299-6

This rich teaching resource offers everything you need to create lecture presentations and course materials, including JPEG and PowerPoint® files of the art, tables, and selected photos from the text, and "stepped-out" art for selected figures from the text, as well as animations for the majors nutrition course.

The IR-DVD allows for "click and play" in the classroom—no downloading required, and includes:

- PowerPoint lecture outlines with embedded links to nutrition animations and ABC News Lecture Launcher Videos.
- Jeopardy-type Quiz Show questions.
- Test Bank Microsoft® Word files and Computerized TestGen® Test Bank.
- Questions for Classroom Response Systems (CRS) in PowerPoint format, allowing you to import the questions into your own CRS.

Printed Test Bank

978-0-321-86300-3 / 0-321-86300-3

The Test Bank, available in both print and computerized formats, provides multiple-choice, true/false, and essay questions for content from each chapter, in addition to new Bloom's Taxonomy levels and correlations to the start-of-chapter Learning Objectives. A computerized test bank version is provided within the IR-DVD (see below).

Great Ideas: Active Ways to Teach Nutrition

978-0-321-59646-8 / 0-321-59646-3

This updated, revised booklet compiles the best ideas from nutrition instructors across the country on innovative ways to teach nutrition topics with an emphasis on active learning. Broken into useful pedagogic areas including targeted and general classroom activities, and an overview of active learning principles, this booklet provides creative ideas for teaching nutrition concepts, along with tips and suggestions for classroom activities that can be used to teach almost any topic.

TestGen® Computerized Test Bank

0321862988 / 978-0-321-86298-3 / 0-321-86298-8

The computerized Test Bank, provided within the IR-DVD, provides short answer, multiple-choice, true/false, matching, and essay questions for material from each text chapter, in addition to new Bloom's Taxonomy levels and correlations to the start-of-chapter Learning Objectives.

MyDietAnalysis Website

www.mydietanalysis.com
ISBN: Value Pack ISBN
ISBN: Standalone Student Access Code Card
0321667697: CD-ROM

MyDietAnalysis was developed by the nutrition database experts at ESHA Research, Inc. and is tailored for use in college nutrition courses. It offers an accurate, reliable, and easy-to-use program for your students' diet analysis needs. MyDietAnalysis features a database of nearly 20,000 foods and multiple reports. Available on CD-ROM or online, the program allows students to track their diet and activity, and generate and submit reports electronically. MyDietAnalysis is also available as a single sign-on to MasteringNutrition.

For online users, a new mobile website version of MyDietAnalysis is available, so students can track their diet and activity intake accurately, anytime and anywhere, from their mobile device.

Food Composition Table

978-0-321-66793-9 / 0-321-66793-X

In the Third Edition, the USDA Nutrient Database for Standard Reference is provided as a practice supplement, offering the nutritional values of over 1,500 separate foods in an easy-to-follow format.

Course Management Options for Instructors
MasteringNutrition™

www.masteringnutrition.pearson.com/www.pearsonmylabandmastering.com
MasteringNutrition™
The MasteringNutrition online homework, tutorial, and assessment system delivers self-paced tutorials and activities that provide individualized coaching, focus on your course objectives, and are responsive to each student's progress. The Mastering system helps instructors maximize class time with customizable, easy-to-assign, and automatically graded assessments that motivate students to learn outside of class and arrive prepared for lecture.

For the Student
Food Composition Table

978-0-321-66793-9 / 0-321-66793-X

In the Third Edition, the USDA Nutrient Database for Standard Reference is provided as a practice supplement, offering the nutritional values of over 1,500 separate foods in an easy-to-follow format.

MyDietAnalysis Website

www.mydietanalysis.com
MyDietAnalysis was developed by the nutrition database experts at ESHA Research, Inc. and is tailored for use in college nutrition courses. It offers an accurate, reliable, and easy-to-use program for your students' diet analysis needs. MyDietAnalysis features a database of nearly 20,000 foods and multiple reports. Available on CD-ROM or online, the program allows students to track their diet and activity, and generate and submit reports electronically. MyDietAnalysis is also available as a single sign-on to MyNutritionLab.

For online users, a new mobile website version of MyDietAnalysis is available, so students can track their diet and activity intake accurately, anytime and anywhere, from their mobile device.

MasteringNutrition™

**www.masteringnutrition.pearson.com/www.pearsonmylabandmastering.com
MasteringNutrition™**
The MasteringNutrition online homework, tutorial, and assessment system delivers self-paced tutorials and activities that provide individualized coaching, focus on your course objectives, and are responsive to each student's progress. The Mastering system helps instructors maximize class time with customizable, easy-to-assign, and automatically graded assessments that motivate students to learn outside of class and arrive prepared for lecture.

Eat Right! Healthy Eating in College and Beyond
978-0-805-38288-4 / 0-805-38288-7

This handy, full-color, eighty-page booklet provides students with practical guidelines, tips, shopper's guides, and recipes, so that they can start putting healthy eating guidelines into action. Written specifically for students, topics include healthy eating in the cafeteria, dorm room, and fast-food restaurants; eating on a budget; weight-management tips; vegetarian alternatives; and guidelines on alcohol and health.

Acknowledgments

It is eye-opening to write a textbook and to realize that the work of so many people contributes to the final product. There are numerous people to thank, and we'd like to begin by extending our thanks to the fabulous staff at Pearson for their incredible support and dedication to this book. Publisher Frank Ruggirello continues to commit extensive resources to ensure the quality of each new edition of this text, and his ongoing support and enthusiasm help us maintain the momentum we need to complete this project. Our executive editor, Sandy Lindelof, provided unwavering vision, support, and guidance throughout the process of writing and publishing this book. We could never have completed this text without the exceptional writing and organizational skills of Laura Bonazzoli, our developmental editor and co-writer. Laura's energy, enthusiasm, and creativity significantly enhanced the quality of this textbook. We also express our sincere gratitude to our project editor, Susan Scharf. We know that managing all the aspects of a textbook is a bit like herding cats. Susan works tirelessly to improve the text and steer us on our course, and keeps us sane with her patience, sense of humor, and excellent editorial instincts. We are also indebted to art development editor Jay McElroy, who contributed to the art enhancements in this edition. Briana Verdugo, editorial assistant extraordinaire, provided superior editorial and administrative support that we would have been lost without. Our thanks also to Marie Beaugureau, Laura Southworth, and Deirdre Espinoza, for their support and guidance in previous editions.

Multiple talented players helped build this book in the production and design process as well. Megan Power, our talented production supervisor, and the resourceful Tiffany Rupp and her colleagues at S4Carlisle Publishing Services kept manuscripts moving throughout the process and expertly tracked the many important details in this complex project. We'd also like to thank Debbie Cogan, senior managing editor, for her guidance and assistance; Derek Bacchus, design manager, who developed the elegant interior for this edition; and Donna Kalal, senior art and photo coordinator, who supervised the photo program. Under the steady guidance of Marilyn Perry, designer Elise Lansdon created a stunning cover and guided us in the beautiful chapter-opening photos. Stephen Merland conducted the research for most of the photos that appear in and enhance this edition.

We can't go without thanking the marketing and sales teams who have been working so hard to get this book out to those who will benefit most from it, especially executive marketing manager Neena Bali and the excellent Pearson marketing and market development teams for their enthusiastic support and innovative ideas.

We want to express our thanks to Barry Bogin, Ph.D., Professor of Biological Anthropology at Loughborough University, UK, for his contributions in this edition to the revision of Chapter 19, Global Nutrition. Also, our goal of meeting instructor and student needs could not have been realized without the team of educators and editorial staff who worked on the substantial supplements package for *The Science of Nutrition*. Joe Mochnick, media producer, expertly supervised all aspects of the media program, and Lee Ann Doctor coordinated the complex new MasteringNutrition aspects. Miriam Adrianowicz expertly guided every aspect of the IR-DVD, and Dorothy Cox was our production editor for the Instructor Support Manual. Thanks to our supplements authors and contributors, with special appreciation to Patricia Longoria for the extensive Test Bank revisions, and Linda Fleming for her contributions to the Instructor Support Manual. Our gratitude to all for their valuable contributions to this edition.

We would also like to thank the many colleagues, friends, and family members who helped us along the way. Janice would specifically like to thank her supportive and hard-working colleagues at the University of Birmingham. "Their encouragement and enthusiasm keep me going through seemingly endless deadlines. My family and friends have been so incredibly wonderful throughout my career. Mom, Dianne, Pam, Steve, Aunt Judy, and cousin Julie are always there for me to offer a sympathetic ear, a shoulder to cry on, and endless encouragement. Although my Dad is no longer with us, his unwavering love and faith in my abilities inspired me to become who I am. I am always amazed that my friends and family actually read my books to learn more about nutrition—thanks for your never-ending support! You are incredible people who keep me sane and healthy and help me to remember the most important things in life."

Melinda would specifically like to thank her husband, Steve Carroll, for the patience and understanding he has shown through this process—once again. He has learned that there is always another chapter due! Melinda would also like to thank her family, friends, and professional colleagues for their support and listening ear through this whole process. They have all helped make life a little easier during this incredibly busy time.

Linda would like to acknowledge the unwavering support of her family and friends, a solid network of love and understanding that keeps her afloat. She would also like to thank Janice and Melinda for providing the opportunity to learn and grow through the process of writing this book.

Janice L. Thompson

Melinda M. Manore

Linda A. Vaughan

Reviewers

We extend our sincere gratitude to the following reviewers for their invaluable assistance in guiding the revision of and improvements in this text.

Shiu-Ming Kuo
University at Buffalo

Monica Meadows
University of Texas at Austin

Deborah Myers
Bluffton University

Renee M. Romig
Western Iowa Tech Community College

Janet M. Sass
Northern Virginia Community College

Shannon Smith
Mesa Community College

Cindy Sullivan
Oakland Community College

Daryle Wane
Pasco-Hernando Community College

Chris Wendtland
Monroe Community College

Lori Zienkewicz
Mesa Community College

Brief Contents

Contents

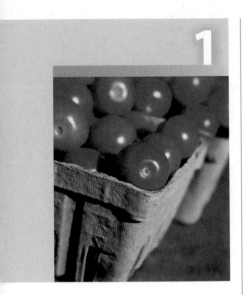

Designing a Healthful Diet 42

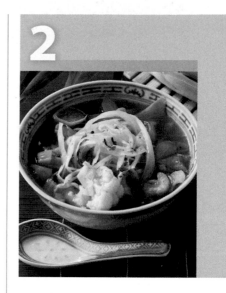

The Human Body: Are We Really What We Eat? 74

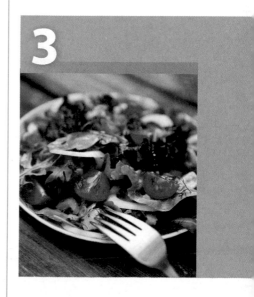

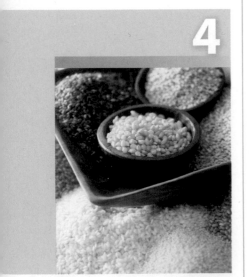

Carbohydrates: Plant-Derived Energy Nutrients 116

Alcohol 160

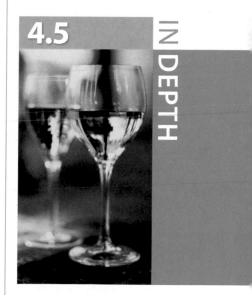

4.5 IN DEPTH

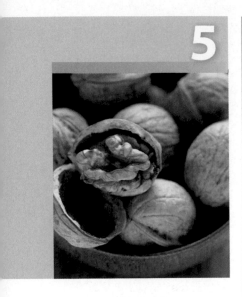

5 Lipids: Essential Energy-Supplying Nutrients 172

Proteins: Crucial Components of All Body Tissues 216

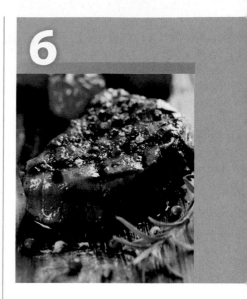

6

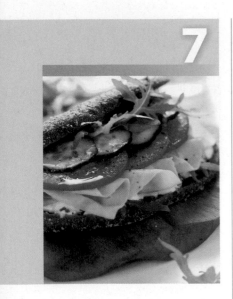

Metabolism: From Food to Life 258

Vitamins and Minerals: Micronutrients with Macro Powers 300

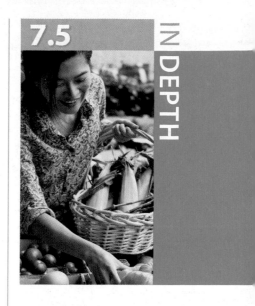

7.5 IN DEPTH

Nutrients Involved in Energy Metabolism 310

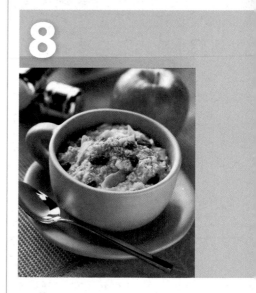

8

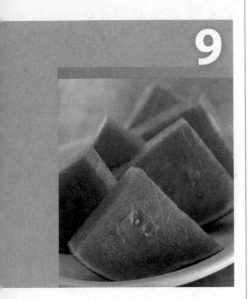

Nutrients Involved in Fluid and Electrolyte Balance 346

Nutrients Involved in Antioxidant Function and Vision 386

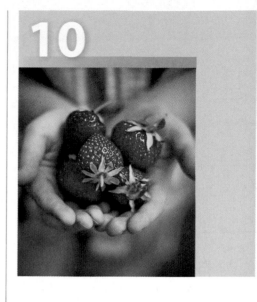

Phytochemicals 426

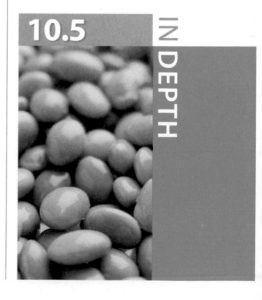

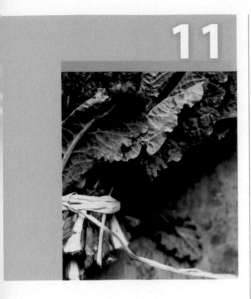

Nutrients Involved in Bone Health 432

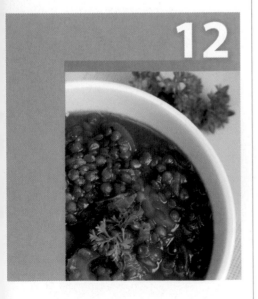

Nutrients Involved in Blood Health and Immunity 470

Achieving and Maintaining a Healthful Body Weight 504

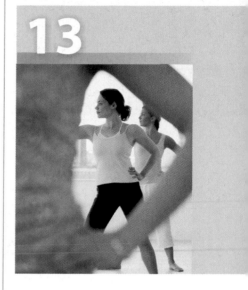

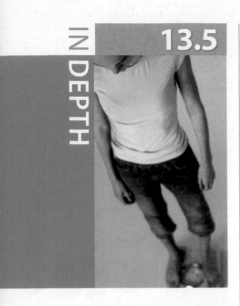

IN DEPTH

13.5

Disordered Eating 548

Nutrition and Physical Activity: Keys to Good Health 560

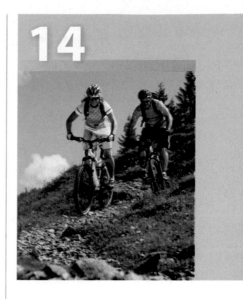

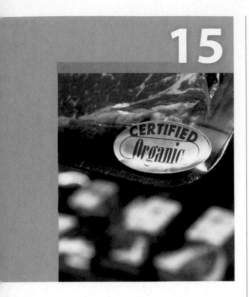

Consumer Issues: Food Safety, Production, and Impact on the Environment 596

Nutrition Through the Life Cycle: Pregnancy and the First Year of Life 634

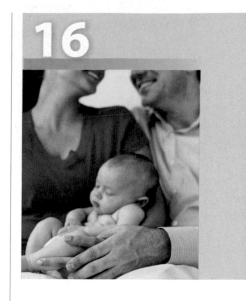

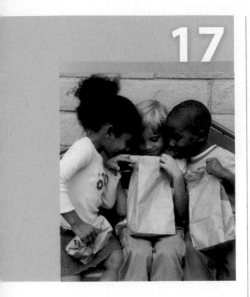

17 Nutrition Through the Life Cycle: Childhood and Adolescence 686

Nutrition Through the Life Cycle: The Later Years 722

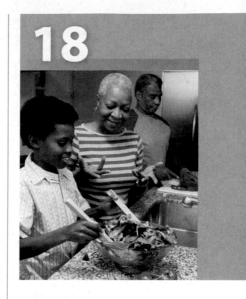

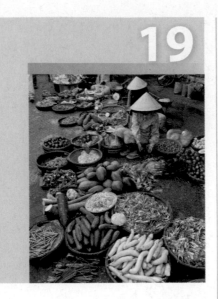

19

Global Nutrition 754

Appendices

THE SCIENCE OF
NUTRITION

THIRD EDITION

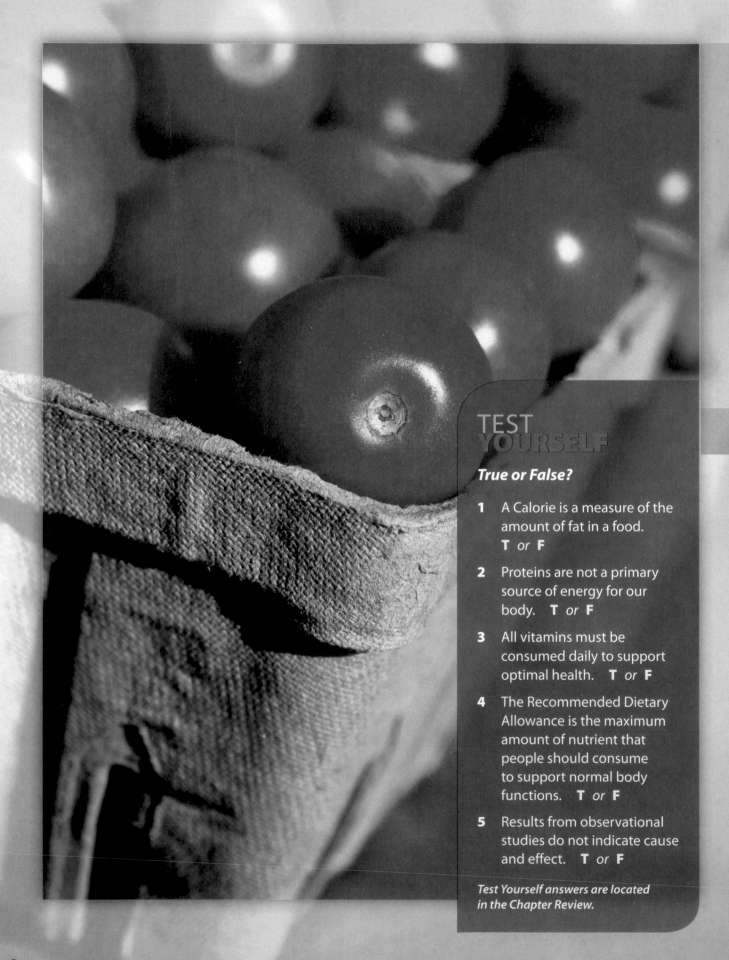

TEST YOURSELF

True or False?

1   A Calorie is a measure of the amount of fat in a food. **T** *or* **F**

2   Proteins are not a primary source of energy for our body. **T** *or* **F**

3   All vitamins must be consumed daily to support optimal health. **T** *or* **F**

4   The Recommended Dietary Allowance is the maximum amount of nutrient that people should consume to support normal body functions. **T** *or* **F**

5   Results from observational studies do not indicate cause and effect. **T** *or* **F**

Test Yourself answers are located in the Chapter Review.

1

The Science of Nutrition: Linking Food, Function, and Health

Learning Objectives

After studying this chapter, you should be able to:

1. Define the term *nutrition* and describe the history of nutritional science, *pp. 4–5*.

2. Discuss why nutrition is important to health, *pp. 5–9*.

3. Identify the six classes of nutrients essential for health and describe their functions, *pp. 9–16*.

4. Identify the Dietary Reference Intakes for nutrients and their roles in promoting wellness, *pp. 16–19*.

5. Describe the processes nutritional professionals use for assessing an individual's nutritional status, *pp. 19–22*.

6. Discuss the four steps of the scientific method and the types of research studies used in establishing nutritional guidelines, *pp. 23–27*.

7. Describe various approaches consumers can use to evaluate the truth and reliability of media reports and other sources of nutritional information, *pp. 27–30*.

8. List at least four sources of reliable and accurate nutrition information and state why they are trustworthy, *pp. 30–33*.

MasteringNutrition™

M arilyn is 58 years old and works as a clerk at a small gift shop. During the last year, she has noticed that she is becoming increasingly tired at work and feels short of breath when performing tasks that she used to do easily, such as stocking shelves. This morning, she had her blood pressure checked for free at a local market and was told by the woman conducting the test that the reading was well above average. Assuming the woman's white lab coat meant that she was a healthcare professional, Marilyn asked her whether or not high blood pressure could explain her fatigue. The woman replied that fatigue was certainly a symptom and advised Marilyn to see her physician. When Marilyn explained that she had no health insurance and little expendable income, the woman said, "Well, I'm not a physician, but I *am* a nutritionist, and I can certainly tell you that the best thing you can do to reduce your high blood pressure is to lose weight. We're running a special all month on Fiber Lunch, our most popular weight-loss supplement. You take it 30 minutes after your midday meal and it cleans out your digestive tract, keeping you from absorbing a lot of the food you eat. I can personally recommend it, because it helped me lose 30 pounds."

Marilyn wasn't convinced that she needed to lose weight. Sure, she was stocky, but she'd been that way all her life, and her fatigue had only started in the past year. But then she remembered that lately she'd been having trouble getting her rings on and off and that her shoes were feeling tight. So maybe the nutritionist was right and she should lose a few pounds. And hadn't she seen an ad for Fiber Lunch in her favorite women's magazine, or maybe on their website? Noticing Marilyn wavering, the nutritionist added, "A few weeks after I started taking Fiber Lunch, my blood pressure went from sky-high to perfectly normal." She certainly looked slender and healthy, and her personal testimonial convinced Marilyn to spend $12 of her weekly grocery budget on the smallest bottle of the supplements.

What do you think of the advice Marilyn received? Was the nutritionist's assessment of her nutritional status adequate? Was the treatment plan sound? Just what is a "nutritionist," anyway? In this chapter, we'll begin to answer these questions as we explore the role of nutrition in human health, identify the six classes of nutrients, and describe what constitutes a professional assessment of a person's nutritional status. You'll also learn how to evaluate nutrition-related research studies, as well as how to distinguish science from scams. But first, let's take a quick look at the evolution of nutrition as a distinct scientific discipline.

What Is the Science of Nutrition and How Did It Evolve?

Although many people think that *food* and *nutrition* mean the same thing, they don't. **Food** refers to the plants and animals we consume. It contains the energy and nutrients our body needs to maintain life and support growth and health. **Nutrition,** in contrast, is a science. Specifically, it is the science that studies food and how food nourishes our body and influences our health. It identifies the processes by which we consume, digest, metabolize, and store the nutrients in foods and how these nutrients affect our body. Nutrition also involves studying the factors that influence our eating patterns, making recommendations about the amount we should eat of each type of food, maintaining food safety, and addressing issues related to the global food supply.

When compared with other scientific disciplines, such as chemistry, biology, and physics, nutrition is a relative newcomer. The cultivation, preservation, and preparation of food have played a critical role in the lives of humans for millennia, but in the West, the recognition of nutrition as an important contributor to health has developed slowly only during the past 400 years.

It started when researchers began to make the link between diet and illness. For instance, in the mid-1700s, long before vitamin C itself had been identified, researchers

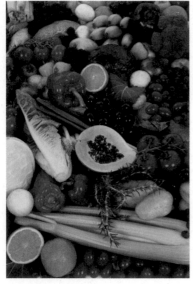

The study of nutrition encompasses everything about food.

food The plants and animals we consume.

nutrition The scientific study of food and how it nourishes the body and influences health.

discovered that the vitamin C–deficiency disease *scurvy* can be prevented by consuming citrus fruits. By the mid-1800s, the three energy-providing nutrients—carbohydrates, lipids, and proteins—had been identified, as well as a number of essential minerals. Nutrition was coming into its own as a developing scientific discipline.

Still, vitamins were entirely unrecognized, and some fatal diseases that we now know to be due to vitamin deficiency were then thought to be due to infection. For instance, when Dutch physician Christian Eijkman began studying the fatal nerve disease *beriberi* in the 1880s, he conducted experiments designed to ferret out the causative bacterium. Finally, Eijkman discovered that replacing the polished white rice in a patient's diet with whole-grain brown rice cures the disease. Still, he surmised that something in the brown rice confers resistance to the beriberi "germ." It was not until the 20th century that the substance missing in polished rice—the B-vitamin *thiamin*—was identified and beriberi was definitively classified as a deficiency disease.[1] Another B-vitamin, niacin, was discovered through the work of Dr. Joseph Goldberger in the early 1900s. The accompanying **Highlight** box describes Dr. Goldberger's daring work.

Nutrition research continued to focus on identifying and preventing deficiency diseases through the first half of the 20th century. Then, as the higher standard of living after World War II led to an improvement in the American diet, nutrition research began pursuing a new objective: supporting wellness and preventing and treating **chronic diseases**—that is, diseases that come on slowly and can persist for years, often despite treatment. Chronic diseases of particular interest to nutrition researchers include obesity, cardiovascular disease, type 2 diabetes, and various cancers. This new research has raised as many questions as it has answered, and we still have a great deal to learn about the relationship between nutrition and chronic disease.

In the closing decades of the 20th century, an exciting new area of nutrition research began to emerge. Reflecting our growing understanding of genetics, *nutrigenomics* seeks to uncover links among our genes, our environment, and our diet. The **Nutrition Debate** (pages 38–41) describes this new field of research in detail.

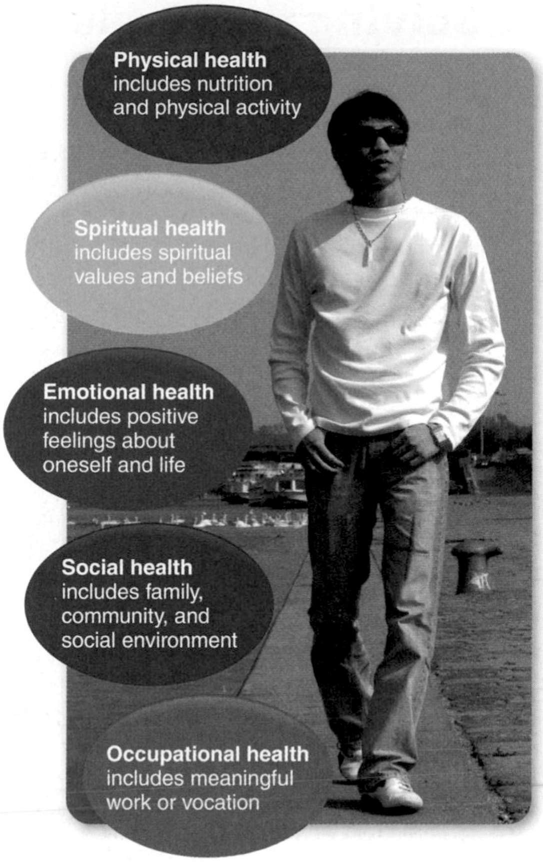

FIGURE 1.1 Many factors contribute to an individual's wellness. Primary among these are a nutritious diet and regular physical activity.

How Does Nutrition Contribute to Health?

Proper nutrition can help us improve our health, prevent certain diseases, achieve and maintain a desirable weight, and maintain our energy and vitality. When you consider that most people eat on average three meals per day, this results in almost 11,000 opportunities during a 10-year period to affect our health through nutrition. The following section provides more detail on how nutrition supports health and wellness.

Nutrition Is One of Several Factors Supporting Wellness

Traditionally, **wellness** was defined simply as the absence of disease. However, as we have learned more about our health and what it means to live a healthful lifestyle, our definition has expanded. Wellness is now considered to be a multidimensional process, one that includes physical, emotional, and spiritual health (**Figure 1.1**). Wellness is not an end point in our lives but rather is an active process we work with every day.

In this book, we focus on two critical aspects of wellness: nutrition and physical activity. These two are so closely related that you can think of them as two sides of the same coin: our overall state of nutrition is influenced by how much energy we expend doing daily activities, and our level of physical activity has a major impact on how we use the nutrients in

chronic disease A disease characterized by a gradual onset and long duration, with signs and symptoms that are difficult to interpret and that respond poorly to medical treatment.

wellness A multidimensional, lifelong process that includes physical, emotional, and spiritual health.

Solving the Mystery of Pellagra

In the first few years of the 20th century, Dr. Joseph Goldberger successfully controlled outbreaks of several fatal infectious diseases, from yellow fever in Louisiana to typhus in Mexico. So it wasn't surprising that, in 1914, the Surgeon General of the United States chose him to tackle another disease thought to be infectious that was raging throughout the South. Called pellagra, the disease was characterized by a skin rash, diarrhea, and mental impairment. At the time, it afflicted more than 50,000 people each year, and in about 10% of cases it resulted in death.

Goldberger began studying the disease by carefully observing its occurrence in groups of people. He asked, if it is infectious, then why would it strike children in orphanages and prison inmates yet leave their nurses and guards unaffected? Why did it overwhelmingly affect impoverished mill workers and share croppers while leaving their affluent (and well-fed) neighbors healthy? Could a dietary deficiency cause pellagra? To confirm his hunch, he conducted a series of trials in which he fed afflicted orphans and prisoners, who had been consuming a limited, corn-based diet, a variety of nutrient-rich

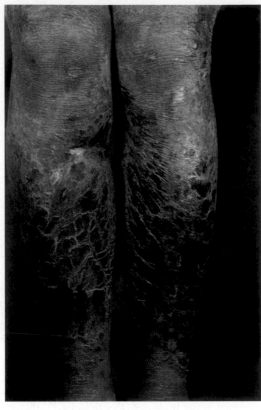

Pellagra is often characterized by a scaly skin rash.

foods, including meats. They recovered. Moreover, orphans and inmates who did not have pellagra and ate the new diet did not develop the disease. Finally, Goldberger recruited eleven healthy prison inmates, who in return for a pardon of their sentence agreed to consume a corn-based diet. After 5 months, six of the eleven developed pellagra.

Still, many skeptics were unable to give up the idea that pellagra was an infectious disease. So to prove that pellagra was not spread by germs, Goldberger and his colleagues deliberately injected and ingested patients' scabs, nasal secretions, and other bodily fluids. He and his team remained healthy.

Although Goldberger could not identify the precise component in the new diet that cured pellagra, he eventually found an inexpensive and widely available substance, brewer's yeast, that when added to the diet prevented or reversed the disease. Shortly after Goldberger's death in 1937, scientists identified the precise nutrient that was deficient in the diet of pellagra patients: niacin, one of the B-vitamins, which is plentiful in brewer's yeast.

Sources: Kraut, A. *Dr. Joseph Goldberger and the War on Pellagra.* National Institutes of Health, Office of NIH History. http://history.nih.gov/exhibits/goldberger; and Markel, H. 2003. The New Yorker who changed the diet of the South. *New York Times,* August 12, 2003.

our food. We can perform more strenuous activities for longer periods of time when we eat a nutritious diet, whereas an inadequate or excessive food intake can make us lethargic. A poor diet, inadequate or excessive physical activity, or a combination of these also can lead to serious health problems. Finally, several studies have suggested that healthful nutrition and regular physical activity can increase feelings of well-being and reduce feelings of anxiety and depression. In other words, wholesome food and physical activity just plain feel good!

A Healthful Diet Can Prevent Some Diseases and Reduce Your Risk for Others

Nutrition appears to play a role—from a direct cause to a mild influence—in the development of many diseases (**Figure 1.2**). As we noted earlier, poor nutrition is a direct cause of deficiency diseases, such as scurvy and pellagra. Thus, early nutrition research focused on identifying the causes of nutrient-deficiency diseases and means to prevent them.

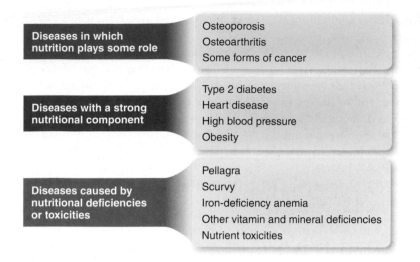

FIGURE 1.2 The relationship between nutrition and human disease. Notice that, whereas nutritional factors are only marginally implicated in the diseases of the top row, they are strongly linked to the development of the diseases in the middle row and truly causative of those in the bottom row.

These discoveries led nutrition experts to develop guidelines for nutrient intakes that are high enough to prevent deficiency diseases, and to lobby for the fortification of foods with nutrients of concern. These measures, along with a more abundant and reliable food supply, have ensured that most nutrient-deficiency diseases are no longer of concern in developed countries. However, they are still major problems in many developing nations (see Chapter 19, Global Nutrition).

In addition to directly causing disease, poor nutrition can have a more subtle influence on our health. For instance, it can contribute to the development of brittle bones, a disease called *osteoporosis,* as well as to the progression of some forms of cancer. These associations are considered mild; however, poor nutrition is also strongly associated with three chronic diseases that are among the top ten causes of death in the United States (**Figure 1.3**). These are heart disease, stroke, and diabetes. In one study following more

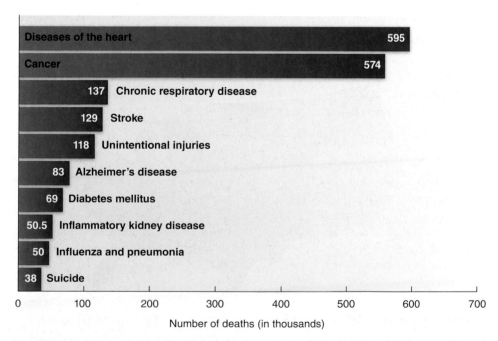

FIGURE 1.3 Of the ten leading causes of death in the United States in 2010, three—heart disease, stroke, and diabetes—are strongly associated with poor nutrition. In addition, nutrition plays a limited role in the development of some forms of cancer. (*Source:* Based on "FastStats: Deaths and Mortality" from the Centers for Disease Control and Prevention website, October 17, 2012.)

Want to see how the prevalence of obesity has changed in the United States year-by-year for the past 25 years? Watch the changing obesity maps at www.cdc.gov/obesity/data/trends.html.

than 100,000 participants for a minimum of 20 years, poor diet was associated with a 23% increased risk of death.[2]

It probably won't surprise you to learn that the primary link between poor nutrition and mortality is obesity. That is, obesity is fundamentally a consequence of consuming more energy than is expended. At the same time, obesity is a well-established risk factor for heart disease, stroke, type 2 diabetes, and some forms of cancer. Unfortunately, the prevalence of obesity has dramatically increased throughout the United States during the past 25 years (**Figure 1.4**). Throughout this text, we will discuss in detail how nutrition and physical activity affect the development of obesity and other chronic diseases.

Healthy People 2020 Identifies Nutrition-Related Goals for the United States

Because of its importance to the wellness of all Americans, nutrition has been included in the national health promotion and disease prevention plan of the United States. Revised every decade, the *Healthy People* plan promotes optimal health and disease prevention

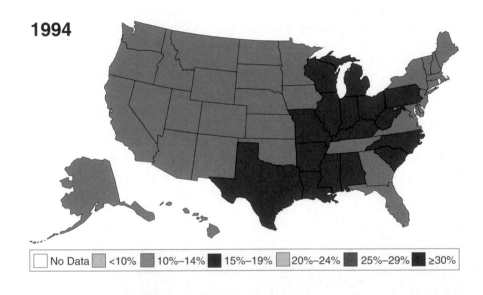

1994

No Data | <10% | 10%–14% | 15%–19% | 20%–24% | 25%–29% | ≥30%

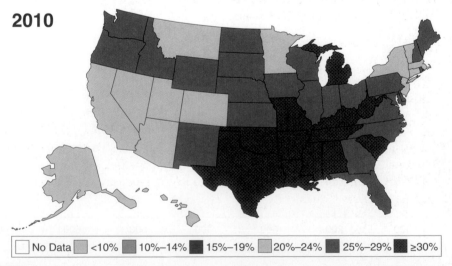

2010

No Data | <10% | 10%–14% | 15%–19% | 20%–24% | 25%–29% | ≥30%

FIGURE 1.4 These diagrams illustrate the increase in obesity rates across the United States from 1994 to 2010. Obesity is defined as a body mass index greater than or equal to 30, or approximately 30 lb overweight for a 5'4" woman. (*Source:* Graphics from Centers for Disease Control and Prevention, US Obesity Trends 1985 to 2010.)

TABLE 1.1 Nutrition and Physical Activity Objectives from *Healthy People 2020*

Topic	Objective Number and Description
Weight status	NWS-8. Increase the proportion of adults who are at a healthy weight from 30.8% to 33.9%. NWS-9. Reduce the proportion of adults who are obese from 34.0% to 30.6%. NWS-10.2. Reduce the proportion of children aged 6 to 11 years who are considered obese from 17.4% to 15.7%.
Food and nutrient composition	NWS-14. Increase the contribution of fruits to the diets of the population aged 2 years and older. NWS-15. Increase the variety and contribution of vegetables to the diets of the population aged 2 years and older.
Physical activity	PA–1. Reduce the proportion of adults who engage in no leisure-time physical activity from 36.2% to 32.6%. PA–2.1. Increase the proportion of adults who engage in aerobic physical activity of at least moderate intensity for at least 150 minutes per week, or 75 minutes per week of vigorous intensity, or an equivalent combination from 43.5% to 47.9%. PA–2.3. Increase the proportion of adults who perform muscle-strengthening activities on 2 or more days of the week from 21.9% to 24.1%.

Data from: US Department of Health and Human Services. 2012.

across the United States. *Healthy People 2020*, launched in January 2010, identifies a set of goals and objectives (as an agenda) that we hope to reach as a nation by the year 2020.[3] This agenda was developed by a team of experts from a variety of federal agencies under the direction of the Department of Health and Human Services. Input was gathered from a large number of individuals and organizations, including hundreds of national and state health organizations, and the general public was asked to share its ideas.

The four overarching goals of *Healthy People* are to (1) attain high-quality, longer lives free of preventable disease, disability, injury, and premature death; (2) achieve health equity, eliminate disparities, and improve the health of all groups; (3) create social and physical environments that promote good health for all; and (4) promote quality of life, healthy development, and healthy behaviors across all life stages. These goals are supported by hundreds of more specific goals and objectives. The importance of nutrition is underscored by the number of nutrition-related objectives in the agenda. Other objectives address physical activity and the problem with overweight and obesity, both of which are, of course, influenced by nutrition. **Table 1.1** identifies some of the specific goals and objectives related to nutrition and physical activity from *Healthy People 2020*.

RECAP

Food refers to the plants and animals we consume, whereas *nutrition* is the scientific study of food and how food affects our body and our health. Nutrition is an important component of wellness and is strongly associated with physical activity. In the past, nutrition research focused on the prevention of nutrient-deficiency diseases, such as scurvy and pellagra; currently, a great deal of nutrition research is dedicated to identifying dietary patterns that can lower the risk for chronic diseases, such as type 2 diabetes and heart disease. *Healthy People 2020* is a health promotion and disease prevention plan for the United States. ■

What Are Nutrients?

We enjoy eating food because of its taste, its smell, and the pleasure and comfort it gives us. However, we rarely stop to think about what our food actually contains. Foods are composed of many chemical substances, some of which are not useful to the body and others of which are critical to human growth and function. These latter chemicals are referred

SIX GROUPS OF ESSENTIAL NUTRIENTS

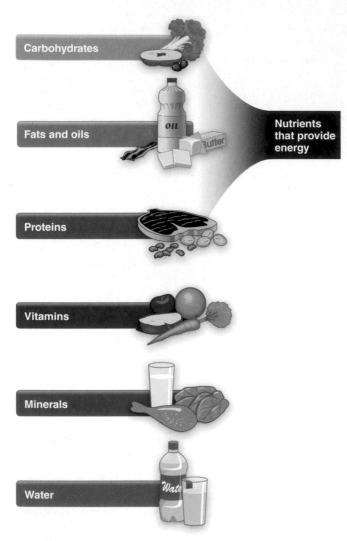

FIGURE 1.5 The six groups of nutrients found in the foods we consume.

to as **nutrients.** The six groups of nutrients found in foods are (**Figure 1.5**)

- Carbohydrates
- Lipids (including fats and oils)
- Proteins
- Vitamins
- Minerals
- Water

As you may know, the term *organic* is commonly used to describe foods that are grown with little or no use of chemicals. But when scientists describe individual nutrients as **organic,** they mean that these nutrients contain the elements *carbon* and *hydrogen*, which are essential components of all living organisms. Carbohydrates, lipids, proteins, and vitamins are organic. Minerals and water are **inorganic.** Both organic and inorganic nutrients are equally important for sustaining life but differ in their structures, functions, and basic chemistry. You will learn more about the details of these nutrients in subsequent chapters; a brief review is provided here.

Carbohydrates, Lipids, and Proteins Provide Energy

Carbohydrates, lipids, and proteins are the only nutrients in foods that provide energy. By this we mean that these nutrients break down and reassemble into a fuel that the body uses to support physical activity and basic physiologic functioning. Although taking a multivitamin and a glass of water might be beneficial in some ways, it will not provide you with the energy you need to do your 20 minutes on the stair-climber! The energy nutrients are also referred to as **macronutrients.** *Macro* means "large"; thus, macronutrients are those nutrients needed in relatively large amounts to support normal function and health.

Alcohol is found in certain beverages and foods, and it provides energy—but it is not considered a nutrient. This is because it does not support the regulation of body functions or the building or repairing of tissues. In fact, alcohol is considered to be both a drug and a toxin. (Details about alcohol are provided in Chapter 4, In Depth, pages 160–171).

Within the world of nutrition science, metric units are commonly used in addition to non-metric units. Thus, it is important for anyone learning about nutrition to learn how to express and calculate both metric and non-metric units. Refer to the **You Do the Math** box "Cooking with Metrics" to see how to cook a delicious meal using new skills. And for help converting between customary and metric measures, see Appendix D.

We express energy in metric units called *kilocalories* (*kcal*). Check the **Highlight** box "What Is a Kilocalorie?" (page 12) for a definition of this term. Both carbohydrates and proteins provide 4 kcal per gram, alcohol provides 7 kcal per gram, and lipids provide 9 kcal per gram. Thus, for every gram of lipids we consume, we obtain more than twice the energy as compared with a gram of carbohydrate or protein.

Carbohydrates Are a Primary Fuel Source

Carbohydrates are the primary source of fuel for the human body, particularly for neurologic functioning and physical exercise (**Figure 1.6**). A close look at the word *carbohydrate* reveals the chemical structure of this nutrient. *Carbo-* refers to carbon, and *-hydrate* refers

nutrients   Chemicals found in foods that are critical to human growth and function.

organic   A substance or nutrient that contains the elements carbon and hydrogen.

inorganic   A substance or nutrient that does not contain carbon and hydrogen.

macronutrients   Nutrients that the body requires in relatively large amounts to support normal function and health. Carbohydrates, lipids, and proteins are macronutrients.

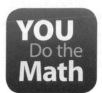

Cooking with Metrics

Theo is planning to cook a romantic Valentine's Day dinner for his girlfriend, Heidi. Heidi loves roast chicken, so Theo has searched the Internet to find a recipe for roast chicken that appears relatively quick and easy and contains ingredients that are affordable. Theo finds a recipe that seems perfect, but it comes from a website based in the United Kingdom, where metric units are used in cooking. Here is the ingredient list:

- 1 whole chicken, approximately 1.6 kg
- 2 medium onions
- 2–3 carrots, approximately 150 grams
- 8 small new potatoes, approximately 600 grams total
- 2 sticks of celery
- 1 bulb of garlic
- olive oil
- sea salt and freshly ground black pepper
- 1 lemon
- a small bunch of fresh thyme, rosemary, bay, or sage or a mixture

Cooking temperature for this recipe is listed as 240°C. Theo uses the metric conversions included in Appendix E of this textbook to assist him in estimating the weight of the chicken (in pounds and ounces) and the carrots and potatoes (in ounces) and to convert oven temperature to Fahrenheit. Here are the results of his calculations:

1. Converting the weight of the chicken into pounds and ounces:
   a. One kg is equivalent to 2.2 pounds. By multiplying the weight of the chicken in kg by 2.2, Theo will get the weight of the chicken in pounds—1.6 kg × 2.2 lb/kg = 3.52 lb.

   b. To calculate the number of ounces, Theo knows that there are 16 ounces in 1 lb. He multiplies the fraction of 1 lb (in this case, 0.52) by 16 ounces = 0.52 × 16 = 8.32, or approximately 8 ounces. Thus, Theo is looking to buy a chicken that weighs approximately 3 lb 8 ounces.

2. Converting the weight of the carrots and potatoes from grams into ounces:
   a. To perform this calculation, Theo knows that 1 gram = 0.035 ounce. He multiplies the weight of the carrots or potatoes in grams by 0.035 to get their weight in ounces.
   b. For the carrots—150 grams × 0.035 ounce/gram = 5.25 ounces of carrots
   c. For the potatoes—600 grams × 0.035 = 21 ounces of potatoes

3. To calculate the cooking temperature in Fahrenheit, Theo needs to multiply °C by 9, then divide by 5. Then he needs to add 32 to this value:

   [(°C × 9)/5] + 32 = [(200°C × 9)/5] + 32 = (1,800/5) + 32 = 360 + 32 = 392°F

   The closest setting to this on Theo's oven is 400°F, so he will cook the chicken at this temperature.

4. Now try these steps yourself to calculate the metric equivalents in a recipe from the United States calling for 12 ounces of haddock, 4 ounces of shallots, and a baking temperature of 400°F.

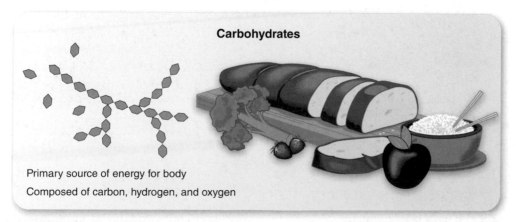

Carbohydrates

Primary source of energy for body

Composed of carbon, hydrogen, and oxygen

FIGURE 1.6 Carbohydrates are a primary source of energy for our body and are found in a wide variety of foods.

What Is a Kilocalorie?

Have you ever wondered what the difference is between the terms *energy*, *kilocalories*, and *calories*? Should these terms be used interchangeably, and what do they really mean? The brief review provided in this Highlight should broaden your understanding. First, here are some precise definitions:

■ *Energy* is defined as the capacity to do work. We derive energy from the energy-containing nutrients in the foods we eat—namely, carbohydrates, lipids, and proteins.

■ A *kilocalorie* (*kcal*) is the amount of heat required to raise the temperature of 1 kilogram (kg) of water by 1 degree Celsius (°C). It is a unit of measurement that nutrition researchers use to quantify the amount of energy in food that can be supplied to the body. For instance, the energy found in 1 gram (g) of carbohydrate is equal to 4 kcal. *Kilo-* is a prefix used in the metric system to indicate 1,000 (think of *kilometer* or *kilobytes*).

Thus, technically speaking, 1 kilocalorie is equal to 1,000 Calories.

■ But what, then, is a *Calorie* (*cal*)? In science, the term *Calorie*, with a capital *C*, is used to indicate a kilocalorie. However, for the sake of simplicity, nutrition labels and publications intended for consumers use the term *calorie* with a lowercase *c* to represent the unit of kilocalories. So if the wrapper on an ice cream bar states that it contains 150 calories, it actually contains 150 kilocalories (150 Calories).

It is most appropriate to use the term *energy* when you are referring to the general concept of energy intake or energy expenditure. If you are discussing the specific *units* related to energy, it is most correct to use either *kilocalories* or *Calories*. In this textbook, we use the term *kilocalorie* (*kcal*) as a unit of energy; we use the term *Calorie* when providing information related to food labels.

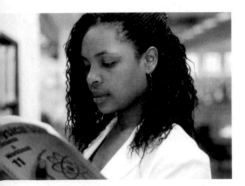

Carbohydrates are the primary source of fuel for the body, particularly for the brain.

to water. You may remember that water is made up of hydrogen and oxygen. Thus, carbohydrates are composed of chains of carbon, hydrogen, and oxygen.

Carbohydrates are found in a wide variety of foods: rice, wheat, and other grains, as well as vegetables and fruits. Carbohydrates are also found in *legumes* (foods that include lentils, beans, and peas), seeds, nuts, and milk and other dairy products. Fiber is also classified as a type of carbohydrate. (Carbohydrates and their role in health are the focus of Chapter 4.)

Lipids Provide Energy and Other Essential Nutrients

Lipids are another important source of energy for the body (**Figure 1.7**). Lipids are a diverse group of organic substances that are largely insoluble in water. Lipids include triglycerides, phospholipids, and sterols. Like carbohydrates, lipids are composed mainly of carbon,

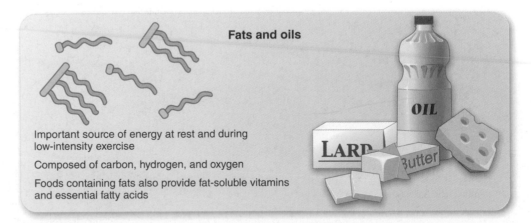

Fats and oils

Important source of energy at rest and during low-intensity exercise

Composed of carbon, hydrogen, and oxygen

Foods containing fats also provide fat-soluble vitamins and essential fatty acids

FIGURE 1.7 Lipids are an important energy source during rest and low-intensity exercise. Foods containing lipids also provide other important nutrients.

hydrogen, and oxygen (and in phospholipids, phosphorus and sometimes nitrogen); however, they contain proportionately much less oxygen and water than do carbohydrates. This quality partly explains why they yield more energy per gram than either carbohydrates or proteins.

Triglycerides (more commonly known as fats) are by far the most common lipid in foods. They are composed of an alcohol molecule called *glycerol* attached to three acid molecules called *fatty acids*. As we'll discuss throughout this book, triglycerides in foods exert different health effects according to the type of fatty acids they contain. Some fatty acids are associated with an increased risk of chronic disease, whereas others—including essential fatty acids—protect our health. Triglycerides are an important energy source when we are at rest and during low- to moderate-intensity exercise. The human body is capable of storing large amounts of triglycerides as adipose tissue, or body fat. These fat stores can be broken down for energy during periods of fasting, such as while we are asleep. Foods that contain lipids are also important in providing fat-soluble vitamins.

Phospholipids are a type of lipid that contains phosphate. The body synthesizes phospholipids, and they are found in a few foods. Cholesterol is a form of lipid that is synthesized in the liver and other body tissues. It is also available in foods of animal origin, such as meat and eggs. (Chapter 5 provides a thorough review of lipids.)

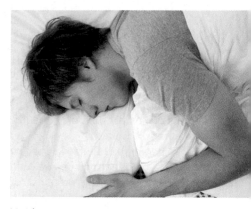

Lipids are an important energy source for our body at rest and can be broken down for energy during periods of fasting, for example, while we are asleep.

Proteins Support Tissue Growth, Repair, and Maintenance

Proteins also contain carbon, hydrogen, and oxygen, but they differ from carbohydrates and lipids in that they contain the element *nitrogen* (**Figure 1.8**). Within proteins, these four elements assemble into small building blocks known as *amino acids*. We break down dietary proteins into amino acids and reassemble them to build our own body proteins—for instance, the proteins in muscles and blood.

Although proteins can provide energy, they are not usually a primary energy source. Proteins play a major role in building new cells and tissues, maintaining the structure and strength of bone, repairing damaged structures, and assisting in regulating metabolism and fluid balance.

Proteins are found in many foods. Meats and dairy products are primary sources, as are seeds, nuts, and legumes. We also obtain small amounts of protein from vegetables and whole grains. (Proteins are explored in detail in Chapter 6.)

Now that you've been introduced to the three energy nutrients, refer to the **You Do the Math** box (page 14) to learn how to calculate the different energy contributions of carbohydrates, lipids, and proteins in 1 day's diet.

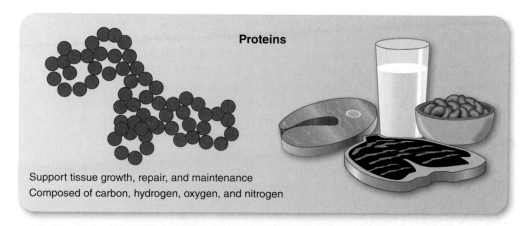

Proteins

Support tissue growth, repair, and maintenance
Composed of carbon, hydrogen, oxygen, and nitrogen

FIGURE 1.8 Proteins contain nitrogen in addition to carbon, hydrogen, and oxygen. Proteins support the growth, repair, and maintenance of body tissues.

Calculating the Energy Contribution of Carbohydrates, Lipids, and Proteins

One of the most useful skills to learn as you study nutrition is determining the percentage of the total energy someone eats that comes from carbohydrates, lipids, or proteins. These data are an important first step in evaluating the quality of an individual's diet. Fortunately, a simple equation is available to help you calculate these values.

To begin, you need to know how much total energy someone consumes each day, as well as how many grams of carbohydrates, lipids, and proteins. You also need to know the kilocalorie (kcal) value of each of these nutrients: the energy value for carbohydrates and proteins is 4 kcal per gram, the energy value for alcohol is 7 kcal per gram, and the energy value for lipids is 9 kcal per gram. Working along with the following example will help you perform the calculations:

1. Let's say you have completed a personal diet analysis for your mother, and she consumes 2,500 kcal per day. From your diet analysis you also find that she consumes 300 g of carbohydrates, 90 g of lipids, and 123 g of proteins.

2. To calculate her percentage of total energy that comes from carbohydrates, you must do two things:

   a. Multiply her total grams of carbohydrate by the energy value for carbohydrate to determine how many kilocalories of carbohydrate she has consumed.

   $$300 \text{ g of carbohydrate} \times 4 \text{ kcal/g} = 1{,}200 \text{ kcal} \\ \text{of carbohydrate}$$

   b. Take the kilocalories of carbohydrate she has consumed, divide this number by the total number of kilocalories she has consumed, and multiply by 100. This will give you the percentage of total energy that comes from carbohydrate.

   $$(1{,}200 \text{ kcal}/2{,}500 \text{ kcal}) \times 100 = 48\% \text{ of total} \\ \text{energy from carbohydrate}$$

3. To calculate her percentage of total energy that comes from lipids, you follow the same steps but incorporate the energy value for lipids:

   a. Multiply her total grams of lipids by the energy value for lipids to find the kilocalories of lipids consumed.

   $$90 \text{ g of fats} \times 9 \text{ kcal/g} = 810 \text{ kcal of lipids}$$

   b. Take the kilocalories of lipids she has consumed, divide this number by the total number of kilocalories she consumed, and multiply by 100 to get the percentage of total energy from lipids.

   $$(810 \text{ kcal}/2{,}500 \text{ kcal}) \times 100 = 32.4\% \text{ of total} \\ \text{energy from lipids}$$

4. Now try these steps to calculate the percentage of the total energy she has consumed that comes from proteins.

These calculations will be useful throughout this course as you learn more about how to design a healthful diet. Later in this book, you will learn how to estimate someone's energy needs and determine the appropriate amount of energy to consume from carbohydrates, fats, and proteins.

Vitamins Assist in the Regulation of Physiologic Processes

Vitamins are organic compounds that assist in the regulation of the body's physiologic processes. Contrary to popular belief, vitamins do not contain energy (or kilocalories); however, they do play an important role in the release and utilization of the energy found in carbohydrates, lipids, and proteins. They are also critical in building and maintaining healthy bone, blood, and muscle; supporting our immune system so we can fight illness and disease; and ensuring healthy vision. Because we need relatively small amounts of these nutrients to support normal health and body functions, the vitamins (in addition to minerals) are referred to as **micronutrients.** Some vitamins can be destroyed by heat, light, excessive cooking, exposure to air, and an alkaline (or basic) environment.

Vitamins are classified according to their solubility in water as either **fat-soluble** or **water-soluble vitamins** (**Table 1.2**). A vitamin's solubility in water affects how it is absorbed, transported, and stored in body tissues. As our body cannot synthesize most vitamins, we must consume them in our diet. Both fat-soluble and water-soluble vitamins are essential for our health and are found in a variety of foods. Learn more about vitamins

micronutrients Nutrients needed in relatively small amounts to support normal health and body functions. Vitamins and minerals are micronutrients.

fat-soluble vitamins Vitamins that are not soluble in water but soluble in fat. These include vitamins A, D, E, and K.

water-soluble vitamins Vitamins that are soluble in water. These include vitamin C and the B-vitamins.

TABLE 1.2 Overview of Vitamins

Type	Names	Distinguishing Features
Fat soluble	A, D, E, K	Soluble in fat Stored in the human body Toxicity can occur from consuming excess amounts, which accumulate in the body
Water soluble	C, B-vitamins (thiamin, riboflavin, niacin, vitamin B_6, vitamin B_{12}, pantothenic acid, biotin, folate)	Soluble in water Not stored to any extent in the human body Excess excreted in urine Toxicity generally only occurs as a result of vitamin supplementation

in Chapter 7, In Depth (pages 300–309). Individual vitamins are discussed in detail later in this text (Chapters 8 through 12).

Minerals Assist in the Regulation of Many Body Functions

Whereas vitamins are organic compounds, *minerals* are inorganic elements. Some important dietary minerals include sodium, potassium, calcium, magnesium, zinc, and iron. Minerals already exist in the simplest possible chemical form; thus, they can't be broken down during digestion or when the body uses them to promote normal function; and unlike certain vitamins, they can't be destroyed by heat or light. Thus, all minerals maintain their structure no matter what environment they are in. This means that the calcium in our bones is the same as the calcium in the milk we drink, and the sodium in our cells is the same as the sodium in our table salt.

Minerals have many important physiologic functions. They assist in fluid regulation and energy production, are essential to the health of our bones and blood, and help rid the body of harmful by-products of metabolism. Minerals are classified according to the amounts we need in our diet and according to how much of the mineral is found in the body. The two categories of minerals in our diet and body are the **major minerals** and the **trace minerals** (**Table 1.3**). Learn more about minerals in the Chapter 7, In Depth (pages 300–309). Individual minerals are discussed in detail later in this text (Chapters 8 through 12).

Water Supports All Body Functions

Water is an inorganic nutrient that is vital for our survival. We consume water in its pure form; in juices, soups, and other liquids; and in solid foods, such as fruits and vegetables. Adequate water intake ensures the proper balance of fluid both inside and outside our cells and assists in the regulation of nerve impulses and body temperature, muscle contractions, nutrient transport, and excretion of waste products. (Chapter 9 focuses on water, its function in the body, and the key role that water plays in our health.)

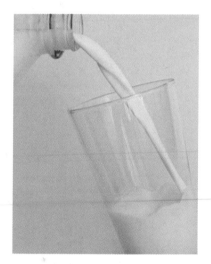

Fat-soluble vitamins are found in a variety of fat-containing foods, including dairy products.

TABLE 1.3 Overview of Minerals

Type	Names	Distinguishing Features
Major minerals	Calcium, phosphorus, sodium, potassium, chloride, magnesium, sulfur	Needed in amounts greater than 100 mg/day in our diet Amount present in the human body is greater than 5 g (5,000 mg)
Trace minerals	Iron, zinc, copper, manganese, fluoride, chromium, molybdenum, selenium, iodine	Needed in amounts less than 100 mg/day in our diet Amount present in the human body is less than 5 g (5,000 mg)

major minerals Minerals we need to consume in amounts of at least 100 mg per day and of which the total amount in our body is at least 5 g (5,000 mg).

trace minerals Minerals we need to consume in amounts less than 100 mg per day and of which the total amount in our body is less than 5 g (5,000 mg).

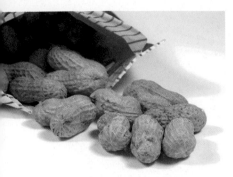

Peanuts are a good source of magnesium and phosphorus, which play an important role in the formation and maintenance of the skeleton.

RECAP

The six essential nutrient groups found in foods are carbohydrates, lipids, proteins, vitamins, minerals, and water. Carbohydrates, lipids, and proteins are energy nutrients. Carbohydrates are the primary energy source; lipids provide fat-soluble vitamins and essential fatty acids and act as energy-storage molecules; and proteins support tissue growth, repair, and maintenance. Vitamins are organic compounds that assist with regulating a multitude of body processes. Minerals are inorganic elements that have critical roles in virtually all aspects of human health and function. Water is essential for survival and is important for regulating nerve impulses and body temperature, muscle contractions, nutrient transport, and excretion of waste products. ■

What Are the Current Dietary Recommendations and How Are They Used?

Now that you know what the six classes of nutrients are, you are probably wondering how much of each a person needs each day. But before you can learn more about specific nutrients and how to plan a healthful diet, you need to become familiar with current dietary standards and how these standards shape nutrition recommendations.

The Dietary Reference Intakes Identify a Healthy Person's Nutrient Needs

In the past, the dietary standards in the United States were referred to as the *Recommended Dietary Allowances (RDAs)*, and the standards in Canada were termed the *Recommended Nutrient Intakes (RNIs)*. These standards defined recommended intake values for various nutrients and were used to plan diets for both individuals and groups. As noted earlier, they were adopted with the goal of preventing nutrient-deficiency diseases; however, in developed countries like the United States and Canada, these diseases are now extremely rare. Thus, nutrition scientists have developed a new set of reference values aimed at preventing and reducing the risk of chronic disease and promoting optimal health. These new reference values in both the United States and Canada are known as the **Dietary Reference Intakes (DRIs) (Figure 1.9)**. These standards include and expand upon the former RDA values, and they set new recommendation standards for nutrients that do not have RDA values.

The DRIs are dietary standards for healthy people only; they do not apply to people with diseases or those who are suffering from nutrient deficiencies. Like the RDAs and RNIs, they identify the amount of a nutrient needed to prevent deficiency diseases in healthy individuals, but they also consider how much of this nutrient may reduce the risk for chronic diseases in healthy people. The DRIs establish an upper level of safety for some nutrients and represent one set of values for both the United States and Canada.

Dietary Reference Intakes (DRIs) A set of nutritional reference values for the United States and Canada that applies to healthy people.

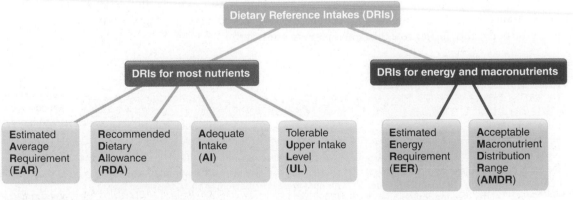

FIGURE 1.9 The Dietary Reference Intakes (DRIs) for all nutrients. Note that the Estimated Energy Requirement (EER) applies only to energy, and the Acceptable Macronutrient Distribution Range (AMDR) applies to the macronutrients.

The DRIs for most nutrients consist of four values:

- Estimated Average Requirement (EAR)
- Recommended Dietary Allowance (RDA)
- Adequate Intake (AI)
- Tolerable Upper Intake Level (UL)

In the case of energy and the macronutrients, different standards are used. The standards for energy and the macronutrients include the Estimated Energy Requirement (EER) and the Acceptable Macronutrient Distribution Range (AMDR). The definitions for each of these DRI values are presented in the following section.

The Estimated Average Requirement Guides the Recommended Dietary Allowance

The first step in determining our nutrient requirements is to calculate the EAR. The **Estimated Average Requirement (EAR)** represents the average daily nutrient intake level estimated to meet the requirement of half of the healthy individuals in a particular life stage or gender group.[4] **Figure 1.10** provides a graph representing this value. As an example, the EAR for iron for women between the ages of 19 and 30 years represents the average daily intake of iron that meets the requirement of half of the women in this age group. Scientists use the EAR to define the Recommended Dietary Allowance (RDA) for a given nutrient. Obviously, if the EAR meets the needs of only half the people in a group, then the recommended intake will be higher.

The Recommended Dietary Allowance Meets the Needs of Nearly All Healthy People

Recommended Dietary Allowance (RDA) was the term previously used to refer to *all* nutrient recommendations in the United States. The RDA is now considered one of many reference standards within the larger umbrella of the DRIs. The RDA represents the average daily nutrient intake level that meets the nutrient requirements of 97% to 98% of healthy individuals in a particular life stage and gender group (**Figure 1.11**).[4] For example, the RDA

Estimated Average Requirement (EAR) The average daily nutrient intake level estimated to meet the requirement of half of the healthy individuals in a particular life stage or gender group.

Recommended Dietary Allowance (RDA) The average daily nutrient intake level that meets the nutrient requirements of 97% to 98% of healthy individuals in a particular life stage and gender group.

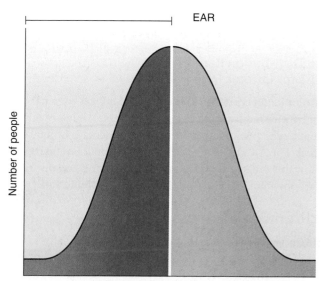

FIGURE 1.10 The Estimated Average Requirement (EAR) represents the average daily nutrient intake level that meets the requirements of half of the healthy individuals in a given group.

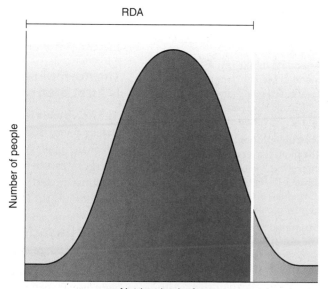

FIGURE 1.11 The Recommended Dietary Allowance (RDA). The RDA represents the average daily nutrient intake level that meets the requirements of almost all (97% to 98%) healthy individuals in a given life stage or gender group.

for iron is 18 mg per day for women between the ages of 19 and 50. This amount of iron will meet the nutrient requirements of almost all women in this age category.

Again, scientists use the EAR to establish the RDA. In fact, if an EAR cannot be determined for a nutrient, then this nutrient cannot have an RDA. When this occurs, an Adequate Intake value is determined for a nutrient.

The Adequate Intake Is Based on Estimates of Nutrient Intakes

The **Adequate Intake (AI)** value is a recommended average daily nutrient intake level based on observed or experimentally determined estimates of nutrient intake by a group of healthy people.[4] These estimates are assumed to be adequate and are used when the evidence necessary to determine an RDA is not available. Many nutrients have an AI value, including vitamin K, chromium, and fluoride. More research needs to be done on human requirements for the nutrients assigned an AI value, so that an EAR, and subsequently an RDA, can be established.

In addition to establishing RDA and AI values for nutrients, an upper level of safety for nutrients, or Tolerable Upper Intake Level, has also been defined.

The Tolerable Upper Intake Level Is the Highest Level That Poses No Health Risk

The **Tolerable Upper Intake Level (UL)** is the highest average daily nutrient intake level likely to pose no risk of adverse health effects to almost all individuals in a particular life stage and gender group.[4] This does not mean that we should consume this intake level or that we will receive more benefits from a nutrient by meeting or exceeding the UL. In fact, as our intake of a nutrient increases in amounts above the UL, the potential for toxic effects and health risks increases. The UL value is a helpful guide to assist you in determining the highest average intake level that is deemed safe for a given nutrient. Note that there is not enough research to define the UL for all nutrients.

The Estimated Energy Requirement Is the Intake Predicted to Maintain a Healthy Weight

The **Estimated Energy Requirement (EER)** is defined as the average dietary energy intake that is predicted to maintain energy balance in a healthy individual. This dietary intake is defined by a person's age, gender, weight, height, and level of physical activity that is consistent with good health.[5] Thus, the EER for an active person is higher than the EER for an inactive person, even if all other factors (age, gender, and so forth) are the same.

The Acceptable Macronutrient Distribution Range Is Associated with Reduced Risk for Chronic Diseases

The **Acceptable Macronutrient Distribution Range (AMDR)** is a range of intakes for a particular energy source that is associated with reduced risk of chronic disease while providing adequate intakes of essential nutrients.[5] The AMDR is expressed as a percentage of total energy or as a percentage of total kcal. The AMDR also has a lower and upper boundary; if we consume nutrients above or below this range, there is a potential for increasing our risk for poor health. The AMDRs for carbohydrate, fat, and protein are listed in **Table 1.4**.

Diets Based on the DRIs Promote Wellness

The primary goal of dietary planning is to develop an eating plan that is nutritionally adequate, meaning that the chances of consuming too little or too much of any nutrient are very low. By eating a diet that provides nutrient intakes that meet the RDA or AI values, a person is more likely to maintain a healthy weight, support his or her daily physical activity, and prevent nutrient deficiencies and toxicities.

The DRI values are listed in several tables at the back of this book; they are also identified with each nutrient as it is introduced throughout this text. Find your own life stage

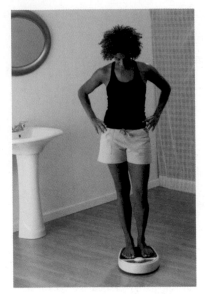

Knowing your daily Estimated Energy Requirement (EER) is a helpful step toward maintaining a healthful body weight. Your EER is defined by your age, gender, weight, height, and physical activity level.

Adequate Intake (AI)   A recommended average daily nutrient intake level based on observed or experimentally determined estimates of nutrient intake by a group of healthy people.

Tolerable Upper Intake Level (UL) The highest average daily nutrient intake level likely to pose no risk of adverse health effects to almost all individuals in a particular life stage and gender group.

Estimated Energy Requirement (EER) The average dietary energy intake that is predicted to maintain energy balance in a healthy individual.

Acceptable Macronutrient Distribution Range (AMDR)   A range of intakes for a particular energy source that is associated with reduced risk of chronic disease while providing adequate intakes of essential nutrients.

TABLE 1.4 Acceptable Macronutrient Distribution Ranges (AMDRs) for Healthful Diets

Nutrient	AMDR*
Carbohydrate	45–65%
Fat	20–35%
Protein	10–35%

*AMDR values expressed as percent of total energy or as percent of total Calories.
Data from: Institute of Medicine, Food and Nutrition Board. © 2005. *Dietary Reference Intakes for Energy, Carbohydrates, Fiber, Fat, Fatty Acids, Cholesterol, Protein, and Amino Acids (Macronutrients).* Washington, DC: National Academies Press. Reprinted by permission.

group and gender in the left-hand column; then simply look across to see each nutrient's value that applies. Using the DRI values in conjunction with diet-planning tools, such as the Dietary Guidelines for Americans or the USDA Food Guide, will ensure a healthful and adequate diet. (Chapter 2 provides details on how you can use these tools to develop a healthful diet.)

RECAP

The Dietary Reference Intakes (DRIs) are dietary standards for nutrients established for healthy people in a particular life stage or gender group. The Estimated Average Requirement (EAR) represents the nutrient intake level that meets the requirement of half of the healthy individuals in a group. The Recommended Dietary Allowance (RDA) represents the level that meets the requirements of 97% to 98% of healthy individuals in a group. The Adequate Intake (AI) is based on estimates of nutrient intake by a group of healthy people when there is not enough information to set an RDA. The Tolerable Upper Intake Level (UL) is the highest daily nutrient intake level that likely poses no health risk. The Estimated Energy Requirement (EER) is the average daily energy intake that is predicted to maintain energy balance in a healthy adult. The Acceptable Macronutrient Distribution Range (AMDR) is a range of intakes associated with reduced risk of chronic disease and adequate intakes of essential nutrients. ∎

How Do Nutrition Professionals Assess the Nutritional Status of Clients?

Before nutrition professionals can make valid recommendations about a client's diet, they need to have a thorough understanding of the client's current nutritional status, including his or her weight, ratio of lean body tissue to body fat, and intake of energy and nutrients. The results of this assessment are extremely important, because they will become the foundation of any dietary or lifestyle changes that are recommended and will provide a baseline against which the success of any recommended changes are evaluated. For instance, if assessments reveal that an adolescent client is 20 lb underweight and consumes less than half the recommended amount of calcium each day, these baseline data are used to support a recommendation of increased energy and calcium intake and to evaluate the success of these recommendations in the future.

A client's nutritional status may fall anywhere along a continuum from healthy to imbalanced. Nutrition professionals use three terms to describe serious nutritional problems:

- **Malnutrition** refers to a situation in which a person's nutritional status is out of balance; the individual is either getting too much or too little of a particular nutrient or energy over a significant period of time.

malnutrition A nutritional status that is out of balance; an individual is either getting too much or not enough of a particular nutrient or energy over a significant period of time.

- **Undernutrition** refers to a situation in which someone consumes too little energy or too few nutrients over time, causing significant weight loss or a nutrient-deficiency disease.
- **Overnutrition** occurs when a person consumes too much energy or too much of a given nutrient over time, causing conditions such as obesity, heart disease, or nutrient toxicity.

Nutrition professionals use a number of tools to determine the nutritional status of a client. As you read about these in the following section, keep in mind that no one method is sufficient to indicate malnutrition. Instead, a combination of tools is used to confirm the presence or absence of nutrient imbalances.

A Physical Examination Is Conducted by a Healthcare Provider

Physical examinations should be conducted by a trained healthcare provider, such as a physician, nurse, nurse practitioner, or physician assistant. The tests conducted during the examination depend on the client's medical history, disease symptoms, and risk factors. Typical tests include checking of vital signs (pulse, blood pressure, body temperature, and respiration rate), auscultation of heart and lung sounds, and laboratory analysis of blood and/or urine samples. Nutritional imbalances may be detected by examining the client's hair, skin, tongue, eyes, and fingernails.

A person's age and health status determine how often he or she needs a physical examination. It is typically recommended that a healthy person younger than 30 years of age have a thorough exam every 2 to 3 years. Adults between the ages of 30 and 50 should have an examination every 1 to 2 years, and people older than 50 years of age should have a yearly exam. However, individuals with established diseases or symptoms of malnutrition may require more frequent examinations.

Questionnaires Elicit Subjective Information

Health-history questionnaires are tools that assist in cataloging a person's history of health, illness, drug use, exercise, and diet. These questionnaires are typically completed just prior to the physical examination by a nurse or other healthcare professional, or the patient may be asked to complete one independently. The questions included in health-history questionnaires usually relate to the following:

- Demographic information, including name, age, contact information, and self-reported height and body weight
- Current medication status, potential drug allergies, and history of drug use
- Family history of disease
- Personal history of illnesses, injuries, and surgeries
- History of menstrual function (for females)
- Exercise history
- Socioeconomic factors, such as education level, access to shopping and cooking facilities, marital status, and racial/ethnic background

In addition, specific questionnaires can be used to assess a person's nutrient and energy intakes. Examples include a diet history, 24-hour dietary recalls, food-frequency questionnaires, and diet records. As you read about each of these tools, bear in mind that they are all subjective; that is, they rely on a person's ability to self-report. The accuracy of the data cannot be empirically verified, as it can, for example, by repeating a measurement of a person's weight. Of these tools, the one or two selected by nutrition professionals will depend on what questions they wish to answer, the population they are working with, and the available resources. Following is a brief description of each.

Diet History

A diet history is typically conducted by a trained nutrition professional. Diet history information is gathered using either an interview process or a questionnaire. Generally included

undernutrition A situation in which too little energy or too few nutrients are consumed over time, causing significant weight loss or a nutrient-deficiency disease.

overnutrition A situation in which too much energy or too much of a given nutrient is consumed over time, causing conditions such as obesity, heart disease, or nutrient-toxicity symptoms.

in the diet history are the patient's current weight, usual weight, and body weight goals; factors affecting appetite and food intake; typical eating patterns (including time, place, dietary restrictions, frequency of eating out, and so forth); disordered eating behaviors (if any); economic status; educational level; living, cooking, and food-purchasing arrangements; medication and/or dietary supplement use; and physical activity patterns. A diet history can help identify any nutrition or eating problems and highlight a person's unique needs.

Twenty-Four-Hour Dietary Recalls

The 24-hour dietary recall is used to assess recent food intake. A trained nutrition professional interviews the person and records his or her responses. The person recalls all of the foods and beverages consumed in the previous 24-hour period. Information that the person needs to know to provide an accurate recall includes serving sizes, food-preparation methods, and brand names of convenience foods or fast foods that were eaten. The 24-hour recall has serious limitations, including the fact that it does not give an indication of a person's typical intake; other limitations include reliance on a person's memory and his or her ability to estimate portion sizes.

Food-Frequency Questionnaires

Food-frequency questionnaires can assist in determining a person's typical dietary pattern over a predefined period of time, such as 1 month, 6 months, or 1 year. These questionnaires include lists of foods with questions regarding the number of times these foods are eaten during the specified time period. Some questionnaires only assess qualitative information, meaning they include only a list of typical foods that are eaten but do not include amounts of foods eaten. Semi-quantitative questionnaires are also available; these assess specific foods eaten and the quantity consumed.

Diet Records

A diet record is a list of all foods and beverages consumed over a specified time period, usually 3 to 7 days. The days selected for recording the person's diet should be representative of typical dietary and activity patterns.

The client is responsible for filling out the record accurately, and both training and take-home instructions are essential. The record is more accurate if all foods consumed are weighed or measured, labels of all convenience foods are saved, and labels of supplements are provided. Providing a food scale and measuring utensils can also assist people in improving the information they provide on diet records.

Although diet records can provide a reasonably good estimate of a person's energy and nutrient intakes, they are challenging to complete accurately and in sufficient detail. Because of this burden, people may change their intake to simplify completing the diet record. They may also change their intake simply because they know it will be analyzed; for example, a client who typically eats ice cream after dinner might forego this indulgence for the duration of the diet record. In addition, analyses are time-consuming and costly.

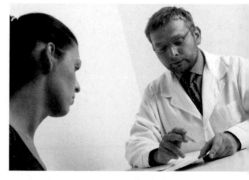

Diet records are a specific type of questionnaire, usually involving some training from a nutrition professional to ensure accuracy.

Anthropometric Assessments Provide Objective Data

Anthropometric assessments are, quite simply, measurements of human beings (*anthropos* is a Greek word meaning "human"). The most common anthropometric measurements are height and body weight. Other measurements that may be taken include head circumference in infants and circumference of limbs. It is critical that the person taking anthropometric measurements is properly trained and uses the correct tools. Measurements are then compared with standards specific for a given age and gender. This allows health practitioners to determine if a person's body size or growth is normal for his or her age and gender. Repeated measurements can also be taken on the same person over time to assess trends in nutritional status and growth.

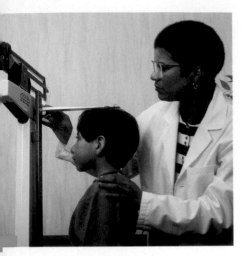

Measuring height is a common anthropometric assessment, and when repeated over time it can help determine a person's nutritional status.

Although not technically considered an anthropometric assessment tool, body composition may also be measured. That is, the health practitioner will use one of several available methods to determine the ratio of fat tissue to nonfat tissue (lean body mass) of which the client's body is composed. (Specific details about body composition assessment are discussed in Chapter 13.)

Think back to the advice that the nutritionist gave to Marilyn in our chapter-opening scenario. Now that you have learned about both subjective and objective methods for assessing a person's nutritional status, you probably recognize that the nutritionist failed to perform even a rudimentary nutritional assessment; instead, she based her weight-loss recommendation solely on a measurement of Marilyn's blood pressure! Later in this chapter, we'll explain what the term *nutritionist* really means and discuss the importance of working within one's scope of practice. But for now, let's look at an example of how healthcare professionals use subjective and objective assessments to determine malnutrition.

A Finding of Malnutrition Requires Further Classification

If the results of nutrition assessment lead to a finding of malnutrition, the nutrition professional classifies the finding further as overnutrition or undernutrition. Overnutrition is further classified as overweight or obesity (see Chapter 13). Nutrient deficiencies are further classified as primary or secondary:

- **Primary deficiency** occurs when a person does not consume enough of a nutrient in the diet; thus, the deficiency occurs as a direct consequence of an inadequate intake.
- **Secondary deficiency** occurs when a person cannot absorb enough of a nutrient in his or her body, when too much of a nutrient is excreted from the body, or when a nutrient is not utilized efficiently by the body. Thus, a secondary deficiency is secondary to, or a consequence of, some other disorder.

Symptoms of a nutrient deficiency are not always obvious. A deficiency in its early stages, when few or no symptoms are observed, is referred to as a **subclinical deficiency.** The symptoms of a subclinical deficiency are typically **covert,** meaning they are hidden and require laboratory tests or other invasive procedures to detect. Once the symptoms of a nutrient deficiency become obvious, they are referred to as **overt.** In the following example, notice that several nutrition assessment tools are used together to determine the presence of a nutrient deficiency.

Bob is a 70-year-old man who has come to his healthcare provider to discuss a number of troubling symptoms. He has been experiencing numbness and tingling in his legs and feet, loses his balance frequently, has memory loss and occasionally feels disoriented, and has intermittent periods of blurred vision. A health history is taken and reveals that Bob has mild hypertension, but he has been regularly physically active and was in good health until the past 6 months. A physical examination shows him to be underweight for his height, with pale skin, and experiencing tremors in his hands. His memory is also poor upon examination. Bob's physician orders some laboratory tests and refers him to the clinic's dietitian, who takes a diet history. During the history, Bob reveals that, a year ago, he began wearing dentures that have made it difficult for him to chew properly. He reports that over time he "gave up on eating anything tough, especially meat." When asked if he eats fish, he says that he has never eaten it, as he does not like the taste. Also, he avoids consuming dairy products because they cause stomach upset, intestinal gas, and diarrhea. When asked if he takes any supplements, Bob explains that he is on a limited income and cannot afford them.

Laboratory test results reveal that Bob is suffering from a deficiency of vitamin B_{12}. This deficiency is primary in nature, as Bob is not consuming meats, fish, or dairy products, which are the primary sources of vitamin B_{12} in our diet. He also does not take a supplement containing vitamin B_{12}. By the time Bob visited his healthcare provider, he was suffering from a clinical deficiency and was showing overt symptoms.

primary deficiency A deficiency that occurs when not enough of a nutrient is consumed in the diet.

secondary deficiency A deficiency that occurs when a person cannot absorb enough of a nutrient, excretes too much of a nutrient from the body, or cannot utilize a nutrient efficiently.

subclinical deficiency A deficiency in its early stages, when few or no symptoms are observed.

covert symptom A symptom that is hidden from a client and requires laboratory tests or other invasive procedures to detect.

overt symptom A symptom that is obvious to a client, such as pain, fatigue, or a bruise.

RECAP

Malnutrition refers to a person's nutritional status being out of balance; undernutrition is a situation in which someone consumes too little energy or too few nutrients over time, and overnutrition occurs when a person consumes too much energy or too much of a nutrient. Assessment tools that can be used to determine if malnutrition exists include a physical examination, a health-history questionnaire, a diet history, a 24-hour dietary recall, a food-frequency questionnaire, a diet record, and anthropometric measures. ■

How Can You Interpret Research Study Results?

"Eat more carbohydrates! Fats cause obesity!"
"Eat more protein and fat! Carbohydrates cause obesity!"

Do you ever feel overwhelmed by the abundant and often conflicting advice in media reports and on the Internet related to nutrition? If so, you are not alone. In addition to the "high-carb, low-carb" controversy, we've been told that calcium supplements are essential to prevent bone loss and that calcium supplements have no effect on bone loss; that high fluid intake prevents constipation and that high fluid intake has no effect on constipation; that coffee and tea can be bad for our health and that both can be beneficial! How can you navigate this sea of changing information? What constitutes valid, reliable evidence, and how can you determine whether or not research findings apply to you?

To become a more informed critic of product claims and nutrition news items, you need to understand the research process and how to interpret the results of different types of studies. Let's now learn more about research.

Research Involves Applying the Scientific Method

When confronted with a claim about any aspect of our world, from "The Earth is flat" to "Carbohydrates cause obesity," scientists, including nutritionists, must first consider whether or not the claim can be tested. In other words, can evidence be presented to substantiate the claim, and if so, what data would qualify as evidence? Scientists worldwide use a standardized method of looking at evidence called the *scientific method.* This method ensures that certain standards and processes are used in evaluating claims. The scientific method usually includes the following steps, which are described in more detail below and summarized in **Figure 1.12**:

- The researcher makes an *observation* and description of a phenomenon.
- The researcher proposes a *hypothesis,* or educated guess, to explain why the phenomenon occurs.
- The researcher develops an *experimental design* that will test the hypothesis.
- The researcher *collects and analyzes data* that will either support or reject the hypothesis.
- If the data do not support the original hypothesis, then an *alternative hypothesis* is proposed and tested.
- If the data support the original hypothesis, then a *conclusion* is drawn.
- The experiment must be *repeatable,* so that other researchers can obtain similar results.
- Finally, a *theory* is proposed offering a conclusion drawn from repeated experiments that have supported the hypothesis time and time again.

Observation of a Phenomenon Initiates the Research Process

The first step in the scientific method is the observation and description of a phenomenon. As an example, let's say you are working in a healthcare office that caters to mostly older adult clients. You have observed that many of these clients have high blood pressure, but

FIGURE 1.12 The scientific method, which forms the framework for scientific research. The researcher makes an observation regarding a phenomenon. This leads the researcher to ask a question. A hypothesis is generated to explain the observations. The researcher conducts an experiment to test the hypothesis. Observations are made during the experiment, and data are generated and documented. The data may either support or refute the hypothesis. If the data support the hypothesis, more experiments are conducted to test and confirm support for the hypothesis. A hypothesis that is supported after repeated testing may be called a theory. If the data do not support the hypothesis, the hypothesis is either rejected or modified and then retested.

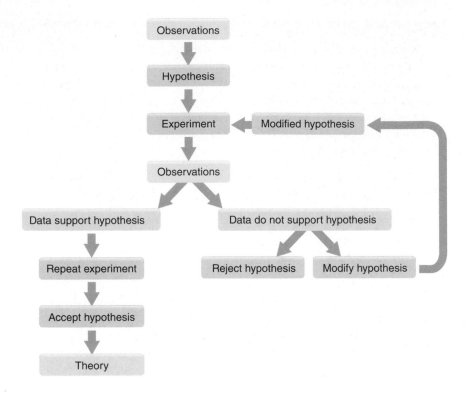

some have normal blood pressure. After talking with a large number of clients, you notice a pattern developing in that the clients who report being more physically active are also those with lower blood pressure readings. This observation leads you to question the relationship that might exist between physical activity and blood pressure. Your next step is to develop a *hypothesis*, or possible explanation for your observation.

A Hypothesis Is a Possible Explanation for an Observation

A **hypothesis** is also sometimes referred to as a research question. In this example, your hypothesis might be "Adults over age 65 with high blood pressure who begin and maintain a program of 45 minutes of aerobic exercise daily will experience a decrease in blood pressure." Your hypothesis must be written in such a way that it can be either supported or rejected. In other words, it must be testable.

An Experiment Is Designed to Test the Hypothesis

An *experiment* is a scientific study that is conducted to test a hypothesis. A well-designed experiment should include several key elements:

- The *sample size*, or the number of people being studied, should be adequate to ensure that the results obtained are not due to chance alone. Would you be more likely to believe a study that tested 5 people or 500?
- Having a *control group* is essential for comparison between treated and untreated individuals. A control group is a group of people who are as much like the treated group as possible except with respect to the *variable* being tested. For instance, in your study, 45 minutes daily of aerobic exercise would be the variable; the experimental group would consist of people over age 65 with high blood pressure who perform the exercise, and the control group would consist of people of the same age with high blood pressure who do not exercise. Using a control group helps a researcher judge if a particular treatment has worked or not.

hypothesis An educated guess as to why a phenomenon occurs.

■ A good experimental design also attempts to control for other variables that may coincidentally influence the results. For example, what if someone in your study is on a diet, smokes, or takes blood pressure–lowering medication? Because any of these factors can affect the results, researchers try to design experiments that have as many constants as possible. In doing so, they increase the chance that their results will be *valid*. To use an old saying, you can think of validity as "comparing apples to apples."

Data Are Collected and Analyzed to Determine Whether They Support or Reject the Hypothesis

As part of the design of the experiment, the researcher must determine the type of data to collect and how to collect them. For example, in your study the data being collected are blood pressure readings. These values could be collected by a person or a machine, but because the data will be closely scrutinized by other scientists, they should be as accurate as technology allows. In this case, an automatic blood pressure gauge would provide more reliable and consistent data than blood pressure measurements taken by research assistants.

Once the data have been collected, they must be interpreted or analyzed. Often, the data will begin to make sense only after being organized and put into different forms, such as tables or graphs, to reveal patterns that at first are not obvious. In your study, you can create a graph comparing blood pressure readings from both your experimental group and your control group to see if there is a significant difference between the blood pressure readings of those who exercised and those who did not.

Most Hypotheses Need to Be Refined

Remember that a hypothesis is basically a guess as to what causes a particular phenomenon. Rarely do scientists get it right the first time. The original hypothesis is often refined after the initial results are obtained, usually because the answer to the question is not clear and leads to more questions. When this happens, an alternative hypothesis is proposed, a new experiment is designed, and the new hypothesis is tested.

An Experiment Must Be Repeatable

One research study does not prove or disprove a hypothesis. Ideally, multiple experiments are conducted over many years to thoroughly test a hypothesis. Indeed, repeatability is a cornerstone of scientific investigation. Supporters and skeptics alike must be able to replicate an experiment and arrive at similar conclusions, or the hypothesis becomes invalid. Have you ever wondered why the measurements used in scientific textbooks are always in the metric system? The answer is repeatability. Scientists use the metric system because it is a universal system and thus allows repeatability in any research facility worldwide.

Unfortunately, media reports on the findings of a research study that has just been published rarely include a thorough review of the other studies conducted on that topic. Thus, you should never accept one report in a newspaper or magazine as absolute fact on any topic.

A Theory May Be Developed Following Extensive Research

If the results of multiple experiments consistently support a hypothesis, then scientists may advance a **theory.** A theory represents a scientific consensus (agreement) as to why a particular phenomenon occurs. Although theories are based on data drawn from repeated experiments, they can still be challenged and changed as the knowledge within a scientific discipline evolves. For example, at the beginning of this chapter, we said that the prevailing theory held that beriberi was an infectious disease. Experiments were conducted over several decades before their consistent results finally confirmed that the disease is due to thiamin deficiency. We continue to apply the scientific method to test hypotheses and challenge theories today.

Nutrition
MILESTONE

In **1782**, the French chemist Antoine Lavoisier invented a device that could measure the heat produced by chemical reactions, including those taking place in an animal. He called his device a *calorimeter*, from the Latin word *calor*, meaning "heat." Using his calorimeter, Lavoisier made the first measurements of the energy (thermal energy, or heat) produced by the consumption of various types of foods. Today, we measure this heat in units called Calories.

theory A scientific consensus, based on data drawn from repeated experiments, as to why a phenomenon occurs.

RECAP

The steps in the scientific method are (1) observing a phenomenon, (2) creating a hypothesis, (3) designing and conducting an experiment, and (4) collecting and analyzing data that support or refute the hypothesis. If the data are rejected, then an alternative hypothesis is proposed and tested. If the data support the original hypothesis, then a conclusion is drawn. A hypothesis that is supported after repeated experiments may be called a theory. ■

Various Types of Research Studies Tell Us Different Stories

You have just learned how the scientific method is applied to test a hypothesis. Establishing nutrition guidelines and understanding the role of nutrition in health involve constant experimentation. Depending on how the research study is designed, we can gather information that tells us different stories. Let's take a look at the various types of research.

Animal Versus Human Studies

In many cases, studies involving animals provide preliminary information that assists scientists in designing human studies. Animal studies also are used to conduct research that cannot be done with humans. For instance, researchers can cause a nutrient deficiency in an animal and study its adverse health effects over the animal's life span, but this type of experiment with humans is not acceptable. Drawbacks of animal studies include ethical concerns and the fact that the results may not apply directly to humans.

Over the past century, animal studies have advanced our understanding of many aspects of nutrition, from micronutrients to obesity. Still, some hypotheses can only be investigated using human subjects. The three primary types of studies conducted with humans are observational studies, case-control studies, and clinical trials.

Observational Studies

Observational studies are used in assessing nutritional habits, disease trends, and other health phenomena of large populations and determining the factors that may influence these phenomena. However, these studies can only indicate *relationships* between factors; they do not prove or suggest that the data are linked by cause and effect. For example, smoking and low vegetable intake appear to be related in some studies, but this does not mean that smoking cigarettes causes people to eat fewer vegetables or that eating fewer vegetables causes people to smoke.

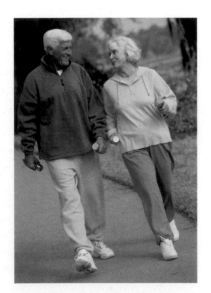

Observational studies indicate relationships between factors, such as between exercise and blood pressure in older adults, but cannot prove cause and effect.

Case-Control Studies

Case-control studies are more complex observational studies with additional design features that allow scientists to gain a better understanding of things that may influence disease. They involve comparing a group of individuals with a particular condition (for instance, 1,000 elderly people with high blood pressure) to a similar group without this condition (for instance, 1,000 elderly people with normal blood pressure). This comparison allows the researcher to identify factors other than the defined condition that differ between the two groups. For example, researchers may find that 75% of the people in their normal blood pressure group are physically active but that only 20% of the people in their high blood pressure group are physically active. Again, this would not prove that physical activity prevents high blood pressure. It would merely suggest a significant relationship between these two factors.

Clinical Trials

Clinical trials are tightly controlled experiments in which an intervention is given to determine its effect on a certain disease or health condition. Interventions include medications, nutritional supplements, controlled diets, and exercise programs. In clinical trials, people in the experimental group are given the intervention, but people in the control group are not. The responses of the two groups are compared. In the case of the blood pressure experiment, researchers could assign one group of elderly people with high blood pressure to an exercise program and assign a second group of elderly people with high blood pressure to a program where no exercise is done. Over the next few weeks, months, or even years, researchers could measure the blood pressure of the people in each group. If the blood pressure of those who exercised decreased and the blood pressure of those who did not exercise rose or remained the same, the influence of exercise on lowering blood pressure would be supported.

Two important questions to consider when evaluating the quality of a clinical trial are whether the subjects were randomly chosen and whether the researchers and subjects were blinded:

■ *Randomized trials.* Ideally, researchers should *randomly* assign research participants to intervention groups (who get the treatment) and control groups (who do not get the treatment). Randomizing participants is like flipping a coin or drawing names from a hat; it reduces the possibility of showing favoritism toward any participants and ensures that the groups are similar on the factors or characteristics being measured in the study. These types of studies are called *randomized clinical (controlled) trials.*

■ *Single- and double-blind experiments.* If possible, it is also important to *blind* both researchers and participants to the treatment being given. A *single-blind experiment* is one in which the participants are unaware of or *blinded* to the treatment they are receiving, but the researchers know which group is getting the treatment and which group is not. A *double-blind experiment* is one in which neither researchers nor participants know which group is really getting the treatment. Double blinding helps prevent the researcher from seeing only the results he or she wants to see, even if these results do not actually occur. In the case of testing medications or nutrition supplements, the blinding process can be assisted by giving the control group a placebo. A *placebo* is an imitation treatment that has no effect on participants; for instance, a sugar pill may be given in place of a vitamin supplement. Studies like this are referred to as *double-blind randomized clinical trials.*

There has been substantial interest in the "placebo effect." This refers to some people experiencing improved health or a reduction in symptoms from a placebo treatment despite the fact that there is no actual treatment given (such as a sham operation) or effective ingredient present in the placebo pill. Although the placebo effect does not occur for all people or across the range of health conditions and diseases affecting the population, it is an intriguing phenomenon that researchers continue to explore to better understand how personal beliefs and attitudes can impact one's response to research and medical treatments.

> **Want to learn more about the placebo effect and how it may lead to improvements in health?** Go to www.cbsnews.com/video/watch/?id=7399364n&tag=segementExtraScroller;housing.

Use Your Knowledge of Research to Help You Evaluate Media Reports

How can all of this research information assist you in becoming a better consumer and critic of media reports and Internet sites? By having a better understanding of the research process and the types of research conducted, you are more capable of discerning the truth or fallacy within media reports. One of the most important points to consider when examining any media report is the issue of conflict of interest.

Conflict of Interest

You probably wouldn't think it strange to see an ad from your favorite brand of ice cream encouraging you to "Go ahead. Indulge." It's just an ad, right? But what if you were to read about a research study in which people who ate your favorite brand of ice cream improved the density of their bones? Could you trust the study results more than you would the ad?

To answer that question, you'd have to ask several more, such as

- Who conducted the research, and who paid for it?
- Was the study funded by a company that stands to profit from certain results?
- Are the researchers receiving goods, personal travel funds, or other perks from the research sponsor, or do they have investments in companies or products related to their study?

If the answer to any of these questions were yes, a *conflict of interest* would exist between the researchers and the funding agency. Whenever a conflict of interest exists, it can seriously compromise the researchers' ability to conduct impartial research and report the results in an accurate and responsible manner. That's why, when researchers submit their results for publication in scientific journals, they are required to reveal any conflicts of interest they may have that could be seen as affecting the integrity of their research. In this way, people who review and eventually read and interpret the study are better able to consider if there are any potential researcher *biases* influencing the results. A bias is any factor—such as investment in the product being studied or gifts from the product manufacturer—that might influence the researcher to favor certain results.

Recent media investigations have reported widespread bias in studies funded by pharmaceutical companies testing the effectiveness of their drugs for medical treatment. In addition, journals in both the United States and Europe have been found less likely to publish negative results (that is, study results suggesting that a therapy is not effective). Also, clinical trials funded by pharmaceutical companies are more likely to report positive results than are trials that were independently financed.[6, 7] This has serious implications: if ineffectiveness and side effects are not fully reported, healthcare providers may be prescribing medications that are ineffective or even harmful.

The seriousness of this issue has inspired researchers around the world to demand a global system whereby all clinical trials are registered and all research results are made accessible to the public. The development of such a system would allow for independent review of research data and work toward ensuring that healthcare decisions were fully informed. As a first step, the US Food and Drug Administration in 2009 launched a Transparency Initiative with the goal of making available to the public useful and understandable information about FDA activities and decision making.

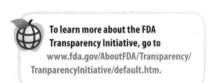

To learn more about the FDA Transparency Initiative, go to www.fda.gov/AboutFDA/Transparency/ TransparencyInitiative/default.htm.

How Can You Determine If a Website Is Reliable?

The Internet provides almost limitless access to a wide variety of health and nutrition information. But how can you determine if the advice given on a website is reliable? Here are some tips to assist you in separating Internet fact from fiction:

- Look at the credentials of the people sponsoring and providing information for the website. Is the individual, group, or company responsible for the website considered a qualified professional in the area of emphasis? Are the names and credentials of those contributing to the website available? Are experts reviewing the content of the website for accuracy and currency?
- Look at the date of the website. Is it fairly recent? As nutrition and medical information are constantly changing, websites should be updated frequently, and the date of the most recent update should be clearly identified on the site.
- Look at the source of the information. The three letters following the "dot" in a World Wide Web address can provide some clues as to the reliability of the information. Government addresses (ending in ".gov"), academic institutions (ending in ".edu"), and professional organizations (ending in ".org") are typically considered to be relatively reliable sources of information. However lecture notes, PowerPoint slides, student assignments, and similar types of documents that can be found on university websites may not be current, accurate, or reliable sources of information. Addresses ending in ".com" designate commercial and business sites. Many of these are reliable

sources, but many are not. It is important to check the qualifications of those contributing to the site and to consider if their primary motivation is to encourage you to buy a product or service.

- Look at the bottom line. What is the message being highlighted on the site? Is it consistent with what is reported by other reliable sources? If the message contradicts what would be considered as common knowledge, then you should question its reliability and intent. An additional clue that a website may be unreliable includes strong and repeated claims of conspiracy theories designed to breed distrust of existing reputable sites.

These suggestions can also be applied to spam. If you have an e-mail account, you're probably familiar with spam ads that make promises such as "Weight-loss miracles for only $19.99!" Do you delete them unread? Or are you tempted to open them to see if you might find something worth exploring? A study from Brooklyn College of the City University of New York found that, in the course of 1 year, 42% of students with weight problems had opened spam e-mails touting weight-loss products, and almost 19% had placed an order! Lead researchers were shocked by the findings and advised physicians to discuss with patients the potential risks of using weight-loss products marketed via spam e-mails.[8]

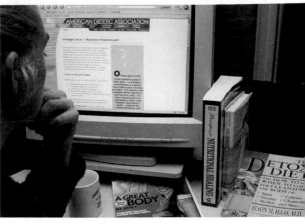

To become a more informed critic of nutrition reports in the media, and a smarter consumer, you need to understand the research process and how to interpret the results of different types of studies.

Other Issues in Evaluating Research

In addition to the considerations mentioned previously, make sure you investigate the following:

- Who is reporting the information? Many people who write for popular magazines, newspapers, and the Internet are not trained in science and are capable of misinter-preting research results. But even trained scientists and physicians can misreport research results for financial gain. For instance, if the report is published on the web-site of a healthcare provider who sells the product or service that was studied, you should be skeptical of the reported results.
- Is the report based on reputable research studies? Did the research follow the scientific method, and were the results reported in a reputable scientific journal? Ideally, the journal is peer-reviewed; that is, the articles are critiqued by other specialists working in the same scientific field. A reputable report should include the reference, or source of the information, and should identify researchers by name. This allows the reader to investigate the original study and determine its merit. Some reputable nutrition journals are identified later in this chapter.
- Is the report based on testimonials about personal experiences? Are sweeping conclusions made from only one study? Be aware of personal testimonials, as they are fraught with bias. In addition, one study cannot answer all of our questions or prove any hypothesis, and the findings from individual studies should be placed in their proper perspective.
- Are the claims in the report too good to be true? Are claims made about curing dis-ease or treating a multitude of conditions? If something sounds too good to be true, it probably is. Claims about curing diseases or treating many conditions with one prod-uct should be a signal to question the validity of the report.

As you may know, **quackery** is the promotion of an unproven remedy, usually by someone unlicensed and untrained, for financial gain. Marilyn, the woman with high blood pressure from our opening story, was a victim of quackery. She probably would not have purchased that weight-loss supplement if she had understood that it was no more effective in promoting weight loss than a generic fiber supplement costing less than half the price. Throughout this text we provide you with information to assist you in becoming a more educated consumer regarding nutrition. You will learn about labeling guidelines, the proper use of supplements, and whether various nutrition topics are myths or facts. Armed with the information in this book, plus plenty of opportunities to test your knowledge, you will become more confident when trying to evaluate nutrition claims.

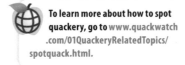

To learn more about how to spot quackery, go to www.quackwatch.com/01QuackeryRelatedTopics/spotquack.html.

quackery The promotion of an un-proven remedy, such as a supplement or other product or service, usually by someone unlicensed and untrained.

RECAP

Studies involving animals provide preliminary information that assists scientists in designing human studies. Human studies include observational studies, case-control studies, and clinical trials. Each type of study can be used to gather a different kind of data. When evaluating media reports, consider whether a conflict of interest exists, who is reporting the information, who conducted and paid for the research, whether or not the research was published in a reputable journal, and whether it involves testimonials or makes claims that sound too good to be true. Quackery is the promotion of an unproven remedy, usually by someone unlicensed and untrained, for financial gain. ■

Nutrition Advice: Whom Can You Trust to Help You Choose Foods Wisely?

After reading this chapter, you can see that nutrition is a relatively new science that plays a critical role in preserving health and preventing and treating disease. As recognition of this vital role has increased over the past few decades, the public has become more and more interested in understanding how nutrition affects their health. One result of this booming interest has been a barrage of nutritional claims on television infomercials; on websites; in magazines; on product packages; and via many other forums. "The noise level is extraordinary," says Marion Nestle, a professor of nutrition at New York University. "I expect health claims from every food in the supermarket."[9] Most individuals do not have the knowledge or training to interpret and evaluate the reliability of this information and thus are vulnerable to misinformation and potentially harmful quackery.

Nutrition professionals are in a perfect position to work in a multitude of settings to counsel and educate their clients and the general public about sound nutrition practices. The following discussion identifies some key characteristics of reliable sources of nutrition information.

Trustworthy Experts Are Educated and Credentialed

It is not possible to list here all of the types of health professionals who provide reliable and accurate nutrition information. The following is a list of the most common groups:

- *Registered dietitian (RD):* To become a **registered dietitian (RD)** requires a minimum of a bachelor's degree, completion of a supervised clinical experience, a passing grade on a national examination, and maintenance of registration with the Academy of Nutrition and Dietetics, formerly the American Dietetic Association (in Canada, the Dietitians of Canada). Individuals who complete the education, experience, exam, and registration are qualified to provide nutrition counseling in a variety of settings. For a reliable list of registered dietitians in your community, you can contact the Academy of Nutrition and Dietetics at www.eatright.org.
- *Licensed dietitian:* A licensed dietitian is a dietitian meeting the credentialing requirement of a given state in the United States to engage in the practice of dietetics.[10] Each state has its own laws regulating dietitians. These laws specify which types of licensure or registration a nutrition professional must obtain in order to provide nutrition services or advice to individuals. Individuals who practice nutrition and dietetics without the required license or registration can be prosecuted for breaking the law.
- *Nutritionist:* This term generally has no definition or laws regulating it. In some cases, it refers to a professional with academic credentials in nutrition who may also be an RD.[10] In other cases, the term may refer to anyone who thinks he or she is knowledgeable about nutrition. There is no guarantee that a person calling himself or herself a nutritionist is necessarily educated, trained, and experienced in the field of nutrition. It is important to research the credentials and experience of any individual calling himself or herself a nutritionist. In the chapter-opening scenario, how might Marilyn have determined whether or not the "nutritionist" was qualified to give her advice?

registered dietitian (RD) A professional designation that requires a minimum of a bachelor's degree in nutrition, completion of a supervised clinical experience, a passing grade on a national examination, and maintenance of registration with the Academy of Nutrition and Dietetics (in Canada, the Dietitians of Canada). RDs are qualified to work in a variety of settings.

- *Professional with an advanced degree* (a master's degree [MA or MS] or doctoral degree [PhD]) *in nutrition:* Many individuals hold an advanced degree in nutrition and have years of experience in a nutrition-related career. For instance, they may teach at community colleges or universities or work in fitness or healthcare settings. Unless these individuals are licensed or registered dietitians, they are not certified to provide clinical dietary counseling or treatment for individuals with disease. However, they are reliable sources of information about nutrition and health.

- *Physician:* The term *physician* encompasses a variety of healthcare professionals. A medical doctor (MD) is educated, trained, and licensed to practice medicine in the United States. However, MDs typically have very limited experience and training in the area of nutrition. Medical students in the United States are not required to take any nutrition courses throughout their academic training, although some may take courses out of personal interest. On the other hand, a number of individuals who started their careers in nutrition go on to become medical doctors and thus have a solid background in nutrition. Nevertheless, if you require a dietary plan to treat an illness or a disease, most medical doctors will refer you to an RD. In contrast, an osteopathic physician, referred to as a doctor of osteopathy (DO), may have studied nutrition extensively, as may a naturopathic physician, a homeopathic physician, or a chiropractor. Thus, it is prudent to determine a physician's level of expertise rather than assuming that he or she has extensive knowledge of nutrition.

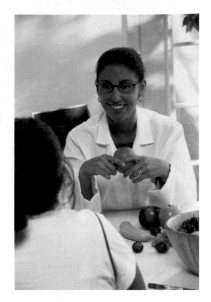

Medical doctors may have limited experience and training in the area of nutrition, but they can refer clients to a registered dietitian (RD) or licensed dietitian to assist them in meeting their dietary needs.

Government Sources of Information Are Usually Trustworthy

Many government health agencies have come together in the past 20 years to address the growing problem of nutrition-related disease in the United States. These organizations are funded with taxpayer dollars, and many of these agencies provide financial support for research in the areas of nutrition and health. Thus, these agencies have the resources to organize and disseminate the most recent and reliable information related to nutrition and other areas of health and wellness. A few of the most recognized and respected of these government agencies are discussed here.

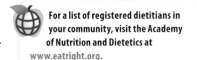

For a list of registered dietitians in your community, visit the Academy of Nutrition and Dietetics at www.eatright.org.

The Centers for Disease Control and Prevention

The **Centers for Disease Control and Prevention (CDC)** is considered the leading federal agency in the United States that protects human health and safety. Located in Atlanta, Georgia, the CDC works in the areas of health promotion, disease prevention and control, and environmental health. The CDC's mission is to promote health and quality of life by preventing and controlling disease, injury, and disability. Among its many activities, the CDC supports two large national surveys that provide important nutrition and health information.

The **National Health and Nutrition Examination Survey (NHANES)** is conducted by the National Center for Health Statistics and the CDC. The NHANES tracks the nutrient consumption of Americans and includes carbohydrates, lipids, proteins, vitamins, minerals, fiber, and other food components. Nutrition and other health information is gathered from interviews and examinations using 24-hour dietary recalls, food-frequency questionnaires, and dietary interviews. The database for the NHANES survey is extremely large, and an abundance of research papers have been generated from it. To learn more about the NHANES, see the Web Links at the end of this chapter.

The **Behavioral Risk Factor Surveillance System (BRFSS)** was established by the CDC to track lifestyle behaviors that increase our risk for chronic disease. The world's largest telephone survey, the BRFSS gathers data at the state level at regular intervals. Although the BRFSS includes questions related to injuries and infectious diseases, it places a particularly

Centers for Disease Control and Prevention (CDC) The leading federal agency in the United States that protects the health and safety of people. Its mission is to promote health and quality of life by preventing and controlling disease, injury, and disability.

National Health and Nutrition Examination Survey (NHANES) A survey conducted by the National Center for Health Statistics and the CDC; this survey tracks the nutrient and food consumption of Americans.

Behavioral Risk Factor Surveillance System (BRFSS) The world's largest telephone survey that tracks lifestyle behaviors that increase our risk for chronic disease.

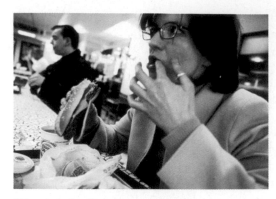

Lifestyle behaviors, such as eating an unhealthful diet, can increase your risk for chronic disease.

strong focus on the health behaviors that increase our risk for the nation's leading killers: heart disease, stroke, cancer, and diabetes. These health behaviors include

- Not engaging in adequate physical activity
- Consuming a diet that is low in fiber and high in saturated fat
- Using tobacco and misusing alcohol
- Not getting medical care that is known to save lives, such as regular Pap smears, mammograms, flu shots, and screening for cancer of the colon and rectum

These behaviors are of particular interest because it is estimated that four out of ten deaths (40%) in the United States can be attributed to smoking, alcohol misuse, lack of physical activity, and an unhealthful diet.[8]

The National Institutes of Health

The **National Institutes of Health (NIH)** is the world's leading medical research center, and it is the focal point for medical research in the United States. The NIH is one of the agencies of the Public Health Service, which is part of the US Department of Health and Human Services. The mission of the NIH is to uncover new knowledge that leads to better health for everyone. This mission is accomplished by supporting medical research throughout the world and by fostering the communication of this information. The NIH has many institutes and centers, which focus on a broad array of nutrition-related health issues. Some of these institutes are

- National Cancer Institute (NCI)
- National Heart, Lung, and Blood Institute (NHLBI)
- National Institute of Diabetes and Digestive and Kidney Diseases (NIDDK)
- National Center for Complementary and Alternative Medicine (NCCAM)

The headquarters of the NIH is located in Bethesda, Maryland. To find out more about the NIH, see the Web Links at the end of this chapter.

Professional Organizations Provide Reliable Nutrition Information

A number of professional organizations represent nutrition professionals, scientists, and educators. These organizations publish cutting-edge nutrition research studies and educational information in journals that are accessible at most university and medical libraries. Some of these organizations are

- *The Academy of Nutrition and Dietetics:* This is the largest organization of food and nutrition professionals in the world. The mission of this organization is to promote nutrition, health, and well-being. The Canadian equivalent is Dietitians of Canada. The Academy of Nutrition and Dietetics publishes a professional journal called the *Journal of the Academy of Nutrition and Dietetics* (formerly the *Journal of the American Dietetic Association*).
- *The American Society for Nutrition (ASN):* The ASN is the premier research society dedicated to improving quality of life through the science of nutrition. The ASN fulfills its mission by fostering, enhancing, and disseminating nutrition-related research and professional education activities. The ASN publishes a professional journal called the *American Journal of Clinical Nutrition.*
- *The Society for Nutrition Education (SNE):* The SNE is dedicated to promoting healthy, sustainable food choices in communities through nutrition research and education. The primary goals of the SNE are to educate individuals, communities, and professionals about nutrition education and to influence policy makers about nutrition, food,

National Institutes of Health (NIH) The world's leading medical research center and the focal point for medical research in the United States.

Liz

*Nutri-*Case

"Am I ever sorry I caught the news last night right before going to bed! They had a report about this study that had just come out saying that ballet dancers are at some super-abnormally high risk for fractures! I couldn't sleep thinking about it, and then today in dance class, every move I made, I was freaking out about breaking my ankle. I can't go on being afraid like this!"

What information should Liz find out about the fracture study to evaluate its merits? Identify at least two factors she should evaluate. Let's say that her investigation of these factors leads her to conclude that the study is trustworthy: what else should she bear in mind about the research process that would help her take a more healthy perspective when thinking about this single study?

and health. The professional journal of the SNE is the *Journal of Nutrition Education and Behavior.*

- *The American College of Sports Medicine (ACSM):* The ACSM is the leading sports medicine and exercise science organization in the world. The mission of the ACSM is to advance and integrate scientific research to provide educational and practical applications of exercise science and sports medicine. Many members are nutrition professionals who combine their nutrition and exercise expertise to promote health and athletic performance. *Medicine and Science in Sports and Exercise* is the professional journal of the ACSM.

- *The North American Association for the Study of Obesity (NAASO):* NAASO is the leading scientific society dedicated to the study of obesity. It is committed to encouraging research on the causes and treatments of obesity and to keeping the medical community and public informed of new advances. The official NAASO journal is *Obesity Research,* which is intended to increase knowledge, stimulate research, and promote better treatment of people with obesity.

For more information on any of these organizations, see the Web Links at the end of this chapter.

RECAP

The Centers for Disease Control and Prevention is the leading federal agency in the United States that protects human health and safety. The CDC supports two large national surveys that provide important nutrition and health information: the National Health and Nutrition Examination Survey (NHANES) and the Behavioral Risk Factor Surveillance System (BRFSS). The National Institutes of Health is the leading medical research agency in the world. The Academy for Nutrition and Dietetics, the American Society for Nutritional Sciences, the Society for Nutrition Education, the American College of Sports Medicine, and the North American Association for the Study of Obesity are examples of professional organizations that provide reliable nutrition information. ■

Chapter Review

TEST YOURSELF | *ANSWERS*

1 **F** A Calorie is a measure of the energy in a food. More precisely, a kilocalorie is the amount of heat required to raise the temperature of 1 kilogram of water by 1 degree Celsius.

2 **T** Carbohydrates and lipids are the primary energy sources for the body.

3 **F** Most water-soluble vitamins need to be consumed daily. However, we can consume foods that contain fat-soluble vitamins less frequently because our body can store these vitamins.

4 **F** The Recommended Dietary Allowance is the average daily nutrient intake level that meets the nutrient requirements of 97% to 98% of healthy individuals in a particular life stage and gender group.

5 **T** Observational studies indicate relationships between nutrition and factors such as disease, but they do not indicate cause and effect.

Summary

- Nutrition is the scientific study of food and how food nourishes the body and influences health.

- Early nutrition research focused on identifying, preventing, and treating nutrient-deficiency diseases. As the Western diet improved, obesity and its associated chronic diseases became an important subject for nutrition research. In the late 20th century, nutrigenomics emerged as a new field of nutrition research.

- Nutrition is an important component of wellness. Healthful nutrition plays a critical role in eliminating deficiency disease and can help reduce our risks for various chronic diseases.

- *Healthy People 2020* is a national health promotion and disease prevention plan that identifies goals we hope to reach as a nation by 2020. Its four overarching goals are to (1) attain high-quality, longer lives free of preventable disease, disability, injury, and premature death; (2) achieve health equity, eliminate disparities, and improve the health of all groups; (3) create social and physical environments that promote good health for all; and (4) promote quality of life, healthy development, and healthy behaviors across all life stages.

- Nutrients are chemicals found in food that are critical to human growth and function.

- The six essential nutrients found in the foods we eat are carbohydrates, lipids, and proteins, which provide energy and are known as the macronutrients; vitamins and minerals, which are micronutrients; and water.

- Carbohydrates are composed of carbon, hydrogen, and oxygen. Carbohydrates are the primary energy source for the human body, particularly for the brain.

- Lipids provide us with fat-soluble vitamins and essential fatty acids in addition to storing large quantities of energy.

- Proteins can provide energy if needed, but they are not a primary fuel source. Proteins support tissue growth, repair, and maintenance.

- Vitamins are organic compounds that assist with the regulation of body processes.

- Minerals are inorganic elements that are not changed by digestion or other metabolic processes.

- Water is critical to support numerous body functions, including fluid balance, the conduction of nervous impulses, and muscle contraction.

- The Dietary Reference Intakes (DRIs) are reference standards for nutrient intakes for healthy people in the United States and Canada.

- The DRIs include the Estimated Average Requirement, the Recommended Dietary Allowance, the Adequate Intake, the Tolerable Upper Intake Level, the Estimated Energy Requirement, and the Acceptable Macronutrient Distribution Range.

- Malnutrition occurs when a person's nutritional status is out of balance. Undernutrition occurs when someone consumes too little energy or nutrients, and overnutrition occurs when too much energy or too much of a given nutrient is consumed over time.

- Nutrition assessment methods include physical examinations, health-history questionnaires, dietary intake tools, and anthropometric assessments. Specific dietary intake tools include diet histories, 24-hour recalls, food-frequency questionnaires, and diet records.

- A primary nutrient deficiency occurs when a person does not consume enough of a given nutrient in the diet. A secondary nutrient deficiency occurs when a person cannot absorb enough of a nutrient, when too much of a nutrient is excreted, or when a nutrient is not efficiently utilized.

- The steps in the scientific method are (1) observing a phenomenon, (2) creating a hypothesis, (3) designing and conducting an experiment, and (4) collecting and analyzing data that support or refute the hypothesis.

- A hypothesis that is supported after repeated experiments may be called a theory.

- Studies involving animals provide preliminary information that assists scientists in designing human studies. Human studies include observational studies, case-control studies, and clinical trials. A double-blind, placebo-controlled study is considered the most trustworthy form of clinical trial.

- When evaluating media reports, consider who is reporting the information, who conducted and paid for the research, whether the research was published in a reputable journal, whether the researchers have a conflict of interest, and whether it involves testimonials or makes claims that sound too good to be true. Quackery is the promotion of an unproven remedy, usually by someone unlicensed and untrained, for financial gain.

- Potentially good sources of reliable nutrition information include registered dietitians, licensed dietitians, and individuals who hold an advanced degree in nutrition. Medical professionals such as physicians, osteopaths, and registered nurses have variable levels of training in nutrition.

- The Centers for Disease Control and Prevention (CDC) is the leading federal agency that protects the health and safety of Americans.

- The National Health and Nutrition Examination Survey (NHANES) is a survey conducted by the CDC and the National Center for Health Statistics that tracks the nutritional status of people in the United States.

- The Behavioral Risk Factor Surveillance System (BRFSS) was established by the CDC and is the world's largest telephone survey; the BRFSS gathers data at the state level on the health behaviors and risks of Americans.

- The National Institutes of Health (NIH) is the leading medical research agency in the world. The mission of the NIH is to uncover new knowledge that leads to better health for everyone.

MasteringNutrition™

To further your understanding, check out www.masteringnutrition.pearson.com (or www.pearsonmylabandmastering.com) and apply what you've learned to real-life case studies that will help you master the content!

Review Questions

1. Vitamins A and C, thiamin, calcium, and magnesium are considered
   a. water-soluble vitamins.
   b. fat-soluble vitamins.
   c. energy nutrients.
   d. micronutrients.

2. Malnutrition plays a role in which of the following?
   a. obesity
   b. iron-deficiency anemia
   c. scurvy
   d. all of the above

3. Ten grams of fat
   a. contain 40 kcal of energy.
   b. contain 90 kcal of energy.
   c. constitute the Dietary Reference Intake for an average adult male.
   d. constitute the Tolerable Upper Intake Level for an average adult male.

4. Which of the following assessment methods provides objective data?
   a. 24-hour dietary recall
   b. history of illnesses, injuries, and surgeries
   c. measurement of height
   d. diet record

5. Which of the following statements about hypotheses is true?
   a. Hypotheses can be proven by clinical trials.
   b. If the results of multiple experiments consistently support a hypothesis, it is confirmed as fact.
   c. "A high-protein diet increases the risk for porous bones" is an example of a valid hypothesis.
   d. "Many inactive people have high blood pressure" is an example of a valid hypothesis.

6. **True or false?** Fat-soluble vitamins provide energy.

7. **True or false?** Carbohydrates, lipids, and proteins all contain carbon, hydrogen, and oxygen.

8. **True or false?** The Recommended Dietary Allowance represents the average daily intake level that meets the requirements of almost all healthy individuals in a given life stage or gender group.

9. **True or false?** An epidemiological study is a clinical trial in which a large population participates as members of the experimental and control groups.

10. **True or false?** Nutrition-related reports in the *Journal of the Academy of Nutrition and Dietetics* are likely to be trustworthy.

11. Explain the role of the control group in a clinical trial.

12. Compare the Estimated Average Requirement with the Recommended Dietary Allowance.

13. Imagine that you are in a gift shop and meet Marilyn, from the chapter-opening scenario. Learning that you are studying nutrition, she tells you of her experience and states that the supplements "didn't seem to do much of anything." She asks you, "How can I find reliable nutrition information?" How would you answer?

14. Your mother, who is a self-described "chocolate addict," phones you. She has read in the newspaper a summary of a research study suggesting that the consumption of a moderate amount of dark chocolate reduces the risk of heart disease in older women. You ask her who funded the research. She says she doesn't know and asks you why it would matter. Explain why such information is important.

15. Intrigued by the idea of a research study on chocolate, you obtain a copy of the full report. In it, you learn the following
   - Twelve women participated in the study.
   - The women's ages ranged from 65 to 78.
   - All the women had been diagnosed with high blood pressure.
   - They all described themselves as sedentary.
   - Six of the twelve smoked at least half a pack of cigarettes a day, but the others did not smoke.

   Your mother is 51 years old, walks daily, and takes a weekly swim class. She does not smoke. Her blood pressure is on the upper end of the normal range. Identify at least three aspects of the study that would cause you to doubt its relevance to your mother.

Math Review

16. You are following a recipe that calls for 200 grams of raisins. How many ounces of raisins is this?

17. Kayla meets with a registered dietitian recommended by her doctor to design a weight-loss diet plan. She is shocked when a dietary analysis reveals that she consumes an average of 2,200 kcal and 60 grams of fat each day. What percentage of Kayla's diet comes from fat, and is this percentage within the AMDR for fat?

Answers to Review Questions and Math Review can be found online in the MasteringNutrition Study Area.

Web Links

www.healthypeople.gov
Healthy People 2020
Search this site for a list of objectives that identify the most significant preventable threats to health in the United States and that establish national goals to reduce these threats.

www.eatright.org
The Academy of Nutrition and Dietetics (formerly the American Dietetic Association)
Obtain a list of registered dietitians in your community from the largest organization of food and nutrition professionals in the United States. Information about careers in dietetics is also available at this site.

www.cdc.gov
Centers for Disease Control and Prevention (CDC)
Visit this site for additional information about the leading federal agency in the United States that protects the health and safety of people.

www.cdc.gov/nchs
National Center for Health Statistics
From the CDC site, click the "National Data" link to learn more about the National Health and Nutrition Examination Survey (NHANES) and other national health surveys.

www.nih.gov
National Institutes of Health (NIH)
Find out more about the National Institutes of Health, an agency under the US Department of Health and Human Services.

www.nutrition.org
American Society for Nutrition (ASN)
Learn more about the American Society for Nutrition and its goal to improve quality of life through the science of nutrition.

www.acsm.org
American College of Sports Medicine (ACSM)
Obtain information about the leading sports medicine and exercise science organization in the world.

www.naaso.org
The North American Association for the Study of Obesity
Learn about this interdisciplinary society and its work to develop, extend, and disseminate knowledge in the field of obesity.

www.iom.edu/Global/Topics/Food-Nutrition
Institute of Medicine of the National Academies
Learn about the Institute of Medicine's history of examining the nation's nutritional well-being and providing sound information about food and nutrition.

www.ncbi.nlm.nih.gov/pubmed
PubMed
Search the more than 21 million citations for biomedical literature, including journals and online books.

References

1. Carpenter, K. J. 2000. *Beriberi, White Rice, and Vitamin B: A Disease, a Cause, and a Cure.* Berkeley: University of California Press.
2. Fung, T. T., R. M. van Dam, S. E. Hankinson, M. Stampfer, W. C. Willett, and F. B. Hu. 2010. Low-carbohydrate diets and all-cause and cause-specific mortality. Two cohort studies. *Ann. Int. Med.* 153(5):289–298.
3. US Department of Health and Human Services. 2012. HealthyPeople.gov. www.healthypeople.gov/2020/default.aspx.
4. Institute of Medicine, Food and Nutrition Board. 2003. *Dietary Reference Intakes: Applications in Dietary Planning.* Washington, DC: National Academies Press.
5. Institute of Medicine, Food and Nutrition Board. 2002. *Dietary Reference Intakes for Energy, Carbohydrates, Fiber, Fat, Protein and Amino Acids (Macronutrients).* Washington, DC: National Academies Press.
6. Rising, K., P. Bacchetti, and L. Bero. 2008. Reporting bias in drug trials submitted to the Food and Drug Administration: review of publication and presentation. *PLos Med.* 5(11):e217. DOI:10.1371/journal.pmed.0050217.
7. Schott, G., H. Pachl, U. Limbach, U. Gundert-Remy, W. Ludwig, and K. Lieb. 2010. The financing of drug trials by pharmaceutical companies and its consequences: part 1. A qualitative systematic review of the literature on possible influences on the findings, protocols, and quality of drug trials. *Deutsch Aerzteblatt International* 107(16):279–285.
8. Fogel, J., and S. B. S. Shlivko. 2010. Weight problems and spam e-mail for weight loss products. *Southern Medical Journal* 103(1):31–36.
9. Elliott, S. 2005. Got bread? A campaign offers an alternative to the low-carb craze. *New York Times,* February 1, p. C9.
10. Winterfeldt, E. A., M. L. Bogle, and L. L. Ebro. 2005. *Dietetics. Practice and Future Trends.* 2nd edn. Sudbury, MA: Jones and Bartlett.

Nutrigenomics: Personalized Nutrition or Pie in the Sky?

Agouti mice are specifically bred for scientific studies. These mice are normally yellow in color, obese, and prone to cancer and diabetes, and they typically have a short life span. When agouti mice breed, these traits are passed on to their offspring. Look at the picture of the agouti mice on this page; do you see a difference? The mouse on the right is obviously brown and of normal weight, but what you can't see is that it did not inherit its parents' susceptibility to disease and therefore will live a longer, healthier life. What caused this dramatic difference between parent and offspring? The answer is diet!

In 2003, researchers at Duke University reported that, when they changed the mother's diet just before conception, they could "turn off" the agouti gene, and any offspring born to that mother would appear normal.[1] As you might know, a *gene* is a segment of DNA, the substance responsible for inheritance, or the passing on of traits from parents to offspring, in both animals and humans. An organism's *genome* is its complete set of DNA, which is found packed into the nucleus of its body cells. Genes are precise regions of DNA that encode instructions for making specific proteins. In other words, genes are *expressed* in proteins; for instance, one way that the agouti gene is expressed is in the pigment proteins that produce yellow fur. (Genes and proteins are discussed in more detail in Chapter 6.)

The Duke University researchers interfered with normal gene expression in their agouti mice by manipulating the mice's diet. Specifically, they fed the mother a diet that was high in methyl donors, compounds that can transfer a methyl group (CH3) to another molecule. Methylation is thought to play a role in genetic expression. Sure enough, the methyl donors attached to the agouti gene and, in essence, turned it off. When the mother conceived, her offspring still carried the agouti gene on their DNA, but their cells no longer used the gene to make proteins. In short, the gene was no longer expressed; thus, the traits, such as obesity, that were linked to the agouti gene did not appear in the offspring. These Duke University studies were some of the first to directly link a dietary intervention to a genetic modification and contributed significantly to the emerging science of *nutrigenomics* (*nutritional genomics*).

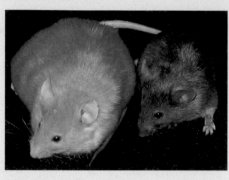

Prompted only by a change in her diet before she conceived, an inbred agouti mouse (left) gave birth to a young mouse (right) that differed not only in appearance but also in its susceptibility to disease.

What Is Nutrigenomics?

Nutrigenomics is a scientific discipline studying the interactions among genes, the environment, and nutrition.[2] Scientists have known for some time that diet and environmental factors can contribute to disease, but what has not been understood before is *how*—namely, by altering how our genes are expressed. Until the late 20th century, scientists believed that the genes a person is born with determined his or her traits rigidly; in other words, that gene expression was not susceptible to outside influences. But the theory behind nutrigenomics is that genetic expression is indeed influenced—perhaps significantly—by the foods we eat and the substances in our environment to which our cells are exposed.

Nutrigenomics proposes that foods and environmental factors can act as a switch in body cells, turning on some genes while turning off others. When a gene is activated, it will instruct the cell to create a protein that will show up as a physical characteristic or functional ability, such as a protein that facilitates the storage of fat. When a gene is switched off, the cell will not create that protein, and the organism's form or function will differ. Some of the factors thought most likely to affect gene activation include tobacco, drugs, alcohol, environmental toxins, radiation, exercise, and the foods most common to an individual's diet.

In addition, nutrigenomics scientists are discovering that what we expose our genes to—such as food and smoke—can affect gene expression not only in the exposed organism but in his or her offspring. In the Duke University study, switching off the agouti gene caused beneficial changes in the offspring mice. But sometimes flipping the switch can be harmful, as when paternal exposure to radiation causes changes in sperm cells that increase the likelihood of birth defects in the offspring.

In short, nutrigenomics proposes that foods and environmental factors can influence the expression of our genes and possibly influence the traits of our children. It's an intriguing theory—but beyond the agouti study, what evidence supports it?

Evidence for Nutrigenomics

Several observations over many decades certainly suggest that the theory has merit. For example, it has long been noted that some people will lose weight on a specific diet and exercise program, whereas others following the same diet and exercise program will experience less weight loss or will even gain weight. The varying results are now thought to depend to a certain extent on how the foods in that diet affect the study participants' genes.

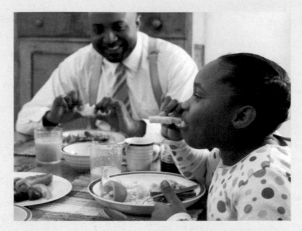

Nutrigenomics suggests that dietary and environmental factors can either activate or turn off some of the genes a person inherits from his or her parents.

Another example is drinking alcohol. Researchers have long understood that consuming too much alcohol is harmful to human health, but they now recognize that people with a particular set of genes may experience considerable reductions in the risk for cardiovascular disease when they consume moderate amounts of alcohol, whereas people who do not have those genes do not gain the same benefits.[2]

Scientists also point to evidence from population studies focusing on fat intake and risk for cardiovascular disease.[2] For example, they observe that, when different ethnic groups are exposed to a high-fat Western diet, the percentage of cardiovascular disease increases in some populations significantly more than in others. There are also genetic differences in how groups respond to types of fat consumed in the diet, which might explain the confusion surrounding whether a low-fat or high-fat diet is beneficial to reducing risks for heart disease.

Evidence of nutrigenomics influencing future generations includes the breakthrough study of agouti mice, as well as recent historical data that suggest a link between the availability of food and type 2 diabetes. Researchers have found that, when one generation experiences a food surplus during critical periods of reproductive development, their offspring are more likely to develop type 2 diabetes.

Promises of Nutrigenomics

Currently, researchers involved in nutrigenomics are making predictions not unlike that of the famous inventor Thomas Edison: "The doctor of the future will give no medicine but will interest his patients in the care of the human frame, in diet, and in the cause and prevention of disease."

One promise of nutrigenomics is that it can assist people in optimizing their health by reducing their risk of developing diet-related diseases and possibly even by treating existing conditions through diet alone. For example, some research is now studying how chemical components of vegetables and certain spices may regulate important genes that suppress cancerous tumors.[3]

Another promise of nutrigenomics is personalized nutrition. Today, dietary advice is based primarily on observations of large populations. Typically, these epidemiological studies do not consider variations within the group. But advice that is generally appropriate for a population might not be appropriate for every individual within that population. For example, most Americans are overweight or obese and need dietary advice that can help them lose weight. But some Americans are chronically underweight and need advice for increasing their energy intake. Advances in nutrigenomics could eliminate this concern by making it possible to provide each individual with a personalized diet. In this future world, you would provide a tissue sample to a healthcare provider, who would send it to a lab for genetic analysis. The results would guide the provider in creating a diet tailored to your genetic makeup. By identifying both foods to eat and foods to avoid, this personalized diet would help you turn on beneficial genes and turn off genes that could be harmful.

Another promise of nutrigenomics is increased understanding of the role of physical activity in human health. Recent research shows that exercise can influence genes involved in certain diseases, such as colon and breast cancer. Researchers have found that regular moderate to vigorous exercise can reduce the risk for cancers of the breast and colon by 20% to 50%.[4, 5] Thus, nutrigenomics is finding that the conventional advice to "eat a balanced diet and exercise" holds true for the majority of people.

A final promise of nutrigenomics is reduction in the global problem of health disparities. Information gained from comparing nutrient/gene interactions as well as environmental factors in different populations may help scientists address the problems of global malnutrition and disease in both developed and developing countries.

Challenges of Nutrigenomics

If the promises of nutrigenomics strike you as pie in the sky, you're not alone. Many researchers caution, for example, that dietary "prescriptions" to prevent or treat chronic diseases would be extremely challenging, because multiple genes may be involved, and environmental, emotional, and even social factors may also play a role.[6] In addition, genetics researchers currently believe that there are about 20,000 to 25,000 genes in human DNA, representing only about 2% of the human genome. [7] The remaining regions of DNA are considered non-coding but are thought to have other functions, many of which may influence nutrition and health. Moreover, the pathways for genetic expression are extremely complex, and turning on a gene may have a beneficial effect on one body function but a harmful effect on another. To complicate the matter further, other factors such as age, gender, and lifestyle will also affect how different foods interact with these different genetic pathways. In short, the number of variables that must be considered in order to develop a "personalized diet" is staggering.

Even by themselves, food interactions are extremely complicated, because when one eats a meal hundreds of nutrient compounds are consumed at one time. Think about all the ingredients found in just one food item, such as pancakes. Each one of these ingredients may interact with a variety of genes directly or indirectly in an uncontrollable and inestimable number of ways. As an example, scientists have determined that at least 150 different genes are linked to type 2 diabetes, and 300 or more have been linked to obesity. Which of the ingredients consumed affect what gene and how? It will be years before researchers are capable of mapping out these complex interactions.

This daunting complexity has not stopped companies from offering naïve consumers nutrigenomics products and services ranging from at-home testing kits to "personalized" diets. A review of the scientific evidence examining online genomic profiling found that there is insufficient evidence that genomic profiles are useful in measuring genetic risk for common diseases or in developing personalized lifestyle recommendations for disease prevention.[8] One study of online sales of nutrigenomics services called such practices premature and concluded that organizations did not provide adequate information about their offerings.[9] Considering these challenges, regulation of the nutrigenomics industry is a growing concern. But what agency should be responsible? Currently the Food and Drug Administration (FDA) monitors and regulates food production and food safety, as well as the safety of medications and many medical devices. In the absence of such oversight, the safety of nutrigenomics services is likely to become a concern as increasing numbers of consumers fall prey to fraudulent or even dangerous dietary advice.

Another potential challenge facing the field of nutrigenomics, discrimination on the basis of an individual's DNA profile, may already have been surmounted. In 2007 the US House of Representatives passed a bill that bans employers and insurance companies from discriminating against people based on their genetic makeup. Under this bill, genetic profiles cannot be used by insurance companies to deny insurance coverage or raise premiums, nor can employers terminate individuals from their jobs for having a genetic mutation.

When Will Nutrigenomics Become a Viable Healthcare Option?

Delivering on the promises of nutrigenomics will require a multidisciplinary approach involving researchers in genetics, nutrition, chemistry, molecular biology, physiology, pathology, sociology, ethics, and many more. The number and complexity of nutritional, environmental, and genetic interactions these scientists will have to contend with are so staggering that decades may pass before nutrigenomics is able to contribute significantly to human health.

Consumers will probably first encounter nutrigenomics in diagnostic testing. In this process, a blood or tissue sample of DNA will be genetically analyzed to determine how food and food supplements interact with that individual's genes and how a change in diet might affect those interactions. Genetic counseling will be required to help consumers understand the meaning and recommendations suggested by their genetic profile.

Second, consumers will probably begin to see more specialized foods promoted for specific conditions. For example, consumers currently have an array of foods they can choose from if they want to lower their cholesterol or enhance their bone health. More such foods will likely be developed, and food packages of the future might even be coded for certain genetic profiles.

We may be decades away from a "personalized diet," but one thing is clear right now: nutrigenomics is showing us the importance of nutrition and environmental factors in preserving our health. In doing so, nutrigenomics is changing not only the way we look at food but also the science of nutrition itself.

CRITICAL THINKING QUESTIONS

■ Are personalized diets and food packages coded for certain genetic profiles part of our future?

■ When you experience poor health, will you consult a nutrigenomics professional instead of a physician and get a prescription for foods instead of medicines?

■ Will nutrigenomics advance preventive medicine and reduce our rate of obesity and other chronic diseases?

■ If so, will it lower healthcare costs?

■ In what other ways could nutrigenomics change the landscape of healthcare in America?

REFERENCES

1. Waterland, R. A., and R. L. Jirtle. 2003. Transposable elements: targets for early nutritional effects on epigenetic gene regulation. *Mol. Cell. Biol.* 23(15):5293–5300.
2. Corella, D., and J. M. Ordovas. 2009. Nutrigenomics in cardiovascular medicine. *Circ. Cardiovasc. Genet.* 2:637–651.
3. Young-Joon, S. 2008. NF-kB and Nrf2 as potential chemopreventive targets of some anti-inflammatory and antioxidative phytonutrients with anti-inflammatory and antioxidative activities. *Asia Pac. J. Clin. Nutr.* 17(S1):269–272.
4. Samad, A. K. A., R. S. Taylor, T. Marshall, and M. A. S. Chapman. 2005. A meta-analysis of the association of physical activity with reduced risk of colorectal cancer. *Colorec. Dis.* 7(3):204–213.
5. McTiernan, A., C. Kooperberg, E. White, S. Wilcox, R. Coates, L. L. Adams-Campbell, N. Woods, and J. Ockene. 2003. Recreational physical activity and the risk of breast cancer in postmenopausal women. The Women's Health Initiative Cohort Study. *JAMA* 290:1331–1336.
6. Kaput, J., and R. Rodriguez. 2004. Nutritional genomics: the next frontier in the post-genomic era. *Physiol. Genomics* 16:166–177.
7. Human Genome Project Information. 2008. How Many Genes Are in the Human Genome? www.ornl.gov/sci/techresources/Human_Genome/faq/genenumber.shtml.
8. Janssens, A. C. J. W., M. Gwinn, L. A. Bradley, B. A. Oostra, C. M. van Duijn, and M. J. Khoury. 2008. A critical appraisal of the scientific basis of commercial genomic profiles used to assess health risks and personalize health interventions. *Am. J. Hum. Genet.* 82(3):593–599.
9. Sterling, R. 2008. The on-line promotion and sale of nutrigenomic services. *Genet. Med.* 10(11):784–796.

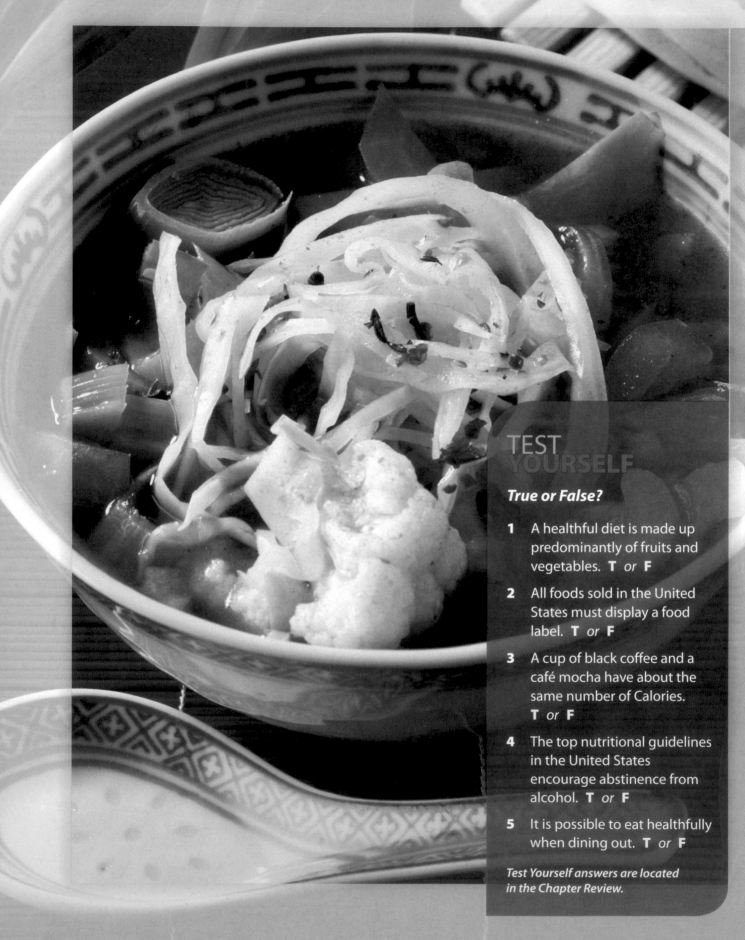

2 Designing a Healthful Diet

Learning Objectives

After studying this chapter, you should be able to:

1. Define the components of a healthful diet, *pp. 44–45*.

2. Read a food label and use the Nutrition Facts Panel to determine the nutritional adequacy of a given food, *pp. 46–49*.

3. Distinguish among label claims related to nutrient content, health, and body structure or function, *pp. 49–50*.

4. Describe the Dietary Guidelines for Americans and discuss how these guidelines can be used to design a healthful diet, *pp. 51–55*.

5. Identify the food groups, number of servings, and serving sizes included in the USDA Food Patterns, *pp. 56–60*.

6. Describe how the USDA Food Patterns can be used to design a healthful diet, *pp. 56–60*.

7. Define *empty Calories* and discuss the role that empty Calories play in designing a healthful diet, *p. 58*.

8. Identify some challenges of using the USDA Food Patterns visual guideline, MyPlate, *pp. 59–60*.

9. List at least four ways to practice moderation and apply healthful dietary guidelines when eating out, *pp. 64–67*.

MasteringNutrition™

Go online for chapter quizzes, pre-tests, Interactive Activities and more!

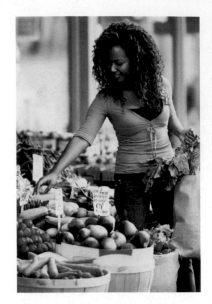

Each person needs to determine his or her own pattern of healthful eating.

Shivani and her parents moved to the United States from India when Shivani was 6 years old. Although delicate in comparison to her American peers, Shivani was healthy and energetic, excelling in school and riding her new bike in her suburban neighborhood. By the time Shivani entered high school, her weight had caught up to that of her American classmates. Now a college freshman, she has joined the almost 17% of US teens who are obese.[1] Shivani explains, "In India, the diet is mostly rice, lentils, and vegetables. Many people are vegetarians, and many others eat meat only once or twice a week, and very small portions. Desserts are only for special occasions. When we moved to America, I wanted to eat like all the other kids: hamburgers, french fries, sodas, and sweets. I gained a lot of weight on that diet, and now my doctor says my cholesterol, my blood pressure, and my blood sugar levels are all too high. I wish I could start eating like my relatives back in India again, but they don't serve rice and lentils at the dorm cafeteria."

What influence does diet have on health? What exactly qualifies as a "poor diet," and what makes a diet healthful? Is it more important to watch how much we eat or what kinds of foods we choose? Is low-carb better, or low-fat? What do the national dietary guidelines advise, and do they apply to "real people" like you?

Many factors contribute to the confusion surrounding healthful eating. First, nutrition is a relatively young science. In contrast with physics, chemistry, and astronomy, which have been studied for thousands of years, the science of nutrition emerged around 1900, with the discovery of the first vitamin in 1897. The initial Recommended Dietary Allowance (RDA) values for the United States were published in 1941. Although we have made substantial discoveries in the area of nutrition during the past century, nutritional research is still considered to be in its infancy. Thus, a growing number of new findings on the benefits of foods and nutrients are discovered almost daily. These new findings contribute to regular changes in how a healthful diet is defined. Second (as stated in Chapter 1), the popular media typically report the results of only selected studies, usually the most recent. This practice does not give a complete picture of all the research conducted in any given area. Indeed, the results of a single study are often misleading. Third, there is no one right way to eat that is healthful and acceptable for everyone. We are individuals with unique needs, food preferences, and cultural influences. For example, a female athlete may need more iron than a sedentary male. One person might prefer to eat three cooked meals a day, whereas another might prefer to eat several smaller snacks, salads, and other quick foods. People following certain religious practices may limit or avoid foods like specific meats and dairy products. Thus, there are literally millions of different ways to design a healthful diet to fit individual needs.

Given all this potential confusion, it's a good thing there are nutritional tools to guide people in designing a healthful diet. In this chapter, we introduce these tools, including food labels, the Dietary Guidelines for Americans, the US Department of Agriculture Food Patterns (and its accompanying graphic, MyPlate), and others. Before exploring the question of how to design a healthful diet, however, it is important to understand what a healthful diet *is*.

What Is a Healthful Diet?

A **healthful diet** provides the proper combination of energy and nutrients. It has four characteristics: it is adequate, moderate, balanced, and varied. No matter if you are young or old, overweight or underweight, healthy or coping with illness, if you keep in mind these characteristics of a healthful diet, you will be able to consciously select foods that provide you with the appropriate combination of nutrients and energy each day.

A Healthful Diet Is Adequate

An **adequate diet** provides enough of the energy, nutrients, and fiber to maintain a person's health. A diet may be inadequate in only one area. For example, as noted, many people in the United States do not eat enough vegetables and therefore are not consuming enough of the fiber and micronutrients found in vegetables. However, their intake of other

healthful diet A diet that provides the proper combination of energy and nutrients and is adequate, moderate, balanced, and varied.

adequate diet A diet that provides enough of the energy, nutrients, and fiber to maintain a person's health.

types of foods may be adequate or even excessive. In fact, some people who eat too few vegetables are overweight or obese, which means that they are eating a diet that exceeds their energy needs.

On the other hand, a generalized state of undernutrition can occur if an individual's diet contains an inadequate level of several nutrients for a long period of time. To maintain a thin figure, some individuals may skip one or more meals each day, avoid foods that contain any fat, and limit their meals to only a few foods, such as a bagel, a banana, or a diet soda. This type of restrictive eating pattern practiced over a prolonged period can cause low energy levels, loss of bone and hair, impaired memory and cognitive function, menstrual dysfunction in women, and even death.

A diet that is adequate for one person may not be adequate for another. For example, the energy needs of a small woman who is lightly active are approximately 1,700 to 2,000 kilocalories (kcal) each day, while a highly active male athlete may require more than 4,000 kcal each day to support his body's demands. These two individuals differ greatly in their activity level and in their quantity of body fat and muscle mass, which means they require very different levels of fat, carbohydrate, protein, and other nutrients to support their daily needs.

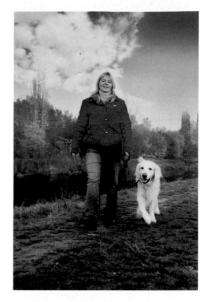

A Healthful Diet Is Moderate

Moderation is one of the keys to a healthful diet. **Moderation** refers to eating any foods in moderate amounts—not too much and not too little. If a person eats too much or too little of certain foods, health goals cannot be reached. For example, some people drink as much as 60 fluid ounces (three 20-oz bottles) of soft drinks on some days. Drinking this much contributes an extra 765 kcal of energy to a person's diet. In order to allow for these extra kilocalories and avoid weight gain, an individual would need to reduce food intake, which could lead to cutting healthful food choices out of his or her diet. In contrast, people who drink mostly water or other beverages containing little or no energy can consume a greater amount of more nourishing foods that will support their wellness.

A Healthful Diet Is Balanced

A **balanced diet** contains the combinations of foods that provide the proper proportions of nutrients. As you will learn in this course, the body needs many types of foods in varying amounts to maintain health. For example, fruits and vegetables are excellent sources of fiber, vitamin C, potassium, and magnesium. Meats are not good sources of fiber and these nutrients, but they are excellent sources of protein, iron, zinc, and copper. By eating the proper balance of all healthful foods, including fruits, vegetables, and meats or meat substitutes, we can be confident that we are consuming the balanced nutrition we need to maintain health.

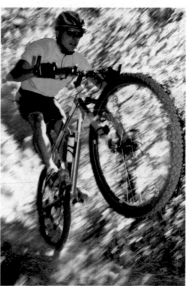

A diet that is adequate for one person may not be adequate for another. A woman who is lightly active will require fewer kilocalories of energy per day than a highly active male.

A Healthful Diet Is Varied

Variety refers to eating many different foods from the different food groups on a regular basis. With thousands of healthful foods to choose from, trying new foods on a regular basis is a fun and easy way to vary your diet. Eat a new vegetable each week or substitute one food for another, such as raw spinach on your turkey sandwich in place of iceberg lettuce. Selecting a wide variety of foods increases the likelihood of consuming the multitude of nutrients the body needs. As an added benefit, eating a varied diet prevents boredom and avoids the potential of getting into a "food rut." Later in this chapter, we provide suggestions for eating a varied diet.

RECAP

A healthful diet provides adequate nutrients and energy, and it includes sweets, fats, and salty foods in moderate amounts only. A healthful diet includes an appropriate balance of nutrients and a wide variety of foods. ■

moderation Eating any foods in moderate amounts—not too much and not too little.

balanced diet A diet that contains the combinations of foods that provide the proper nutrient proportions.

variety Eating a lot of different foods each day.

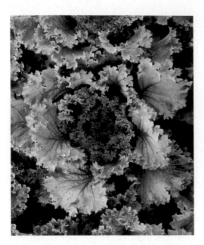

Eating a new vegetable each week is a fun way to vary your diet. Kale is a member of the cabbage family and is an excellent source of calcium, for example.

What Tools Can Help Me Design a Healthful Diet?

Many people feel it is nearly impossible to eat a truly healthful diet. They may mistakenly believe that the foods they would need to eat are too expensive or not available to them, or they may feel too busy to do the necessary planning, shopping, and cooking. Some people rely on dietary supplements to get enough nutrients instead of focusing on eating a variety of foods. But is it really that difficult to eat healthfully?

Although designing and maintaining a healthful diet is not as simple as eating whatever you want, most of us can improve our diets with a just little practice and a little help. Let's look now at some tools for designing a healthful diet.

Reading Food Labels Can Be Easy and Helpful

To design and maintain a healthful diet, it's important to read and understand food labels. It may surprise you to learn that a few decades ago there were no federal regulations for including nutrition information on food labels! The US Food and Drug Administration (FDA) first established such regulations in 1973. These regulations were not as specific as they are today and were not required for many of the foods available to consumers. Throughout the 1970s and 1980s, consumer interest in food quality grew substantially, and many watchdog groups were formed to protect consumers from unclear labeling and false claims made by some manufacturers.

Public interest and concern about how food affects health became so strong that in 1990 the US. Congress passed the Nutrition Labeling and Education Act. This act specifies which foods require a food label, provides detailed descriptions of the information that must be included on the food label, and describes the companies and food products that are exempt from publishing complete nutrition information on food labels. For example, detailed food labels are not required for meat or poultry, as these products are regulated by the US Department of Agriculture, not the FDA. In addition, foods such as coffee, fresh produce, and most spices are not required to follow the FDA labeling guidelines, as they contain insignificant amounts of all the nutrients that must be listed in nutrition labeling.

Five Components Must Be Included on Food Labels

Five primary components of information must be included on food labels (**Figure 2.1**).

1. **A statement of identity:** The common name of the product or an appropriate identification of the food product must be prominently displayed on the label. This information tells us very clearly what the product is.

2. **The net contents of the package:** The quantity of the food product in the entire package must be accurately described. Information may be listed as weight (such as grams), volume (fluid ounces), or numerical count (4 each).

3. **Ingredient list:** The ingredients must be listed by their common names, in descending order by weight. This means that the first product listed in the ingredient list is the predominant ingredient in that food. This information can be useful in many situations, such as when you are looking for foods that are lower in fat or sugar or when you are attempting to identify foods that contain whole-grain flour instead of processed wheat flour.

4. **The name and address of the food manufacturer, packer, or distributor:** This information can be used if you want to find out more detailed

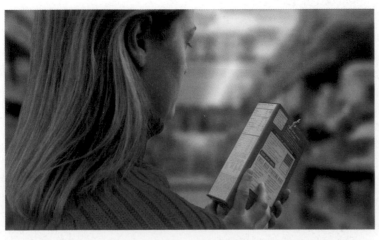

Learning how to read food labels is a skill that can help you meet your nutritional goals.

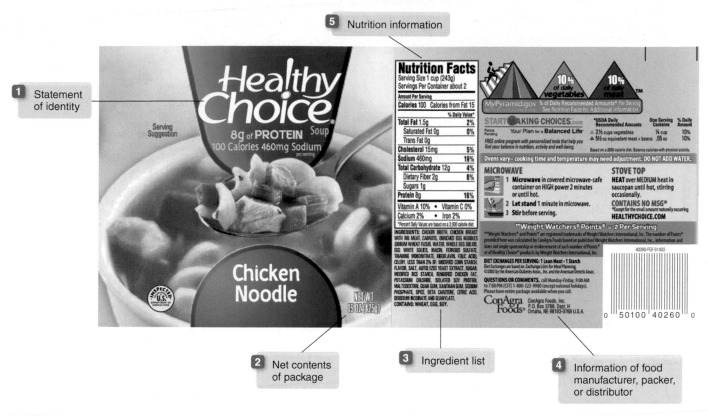

FIGURE 2.1 The five primary components required for food labels. *Source:* (© ConAgra Brands, Inc. Reprinted by permission.)

information about a food product and to contact the company if there is something wrong with the product or you suspect that it caused an illness.

5. **Nutrition information:** The Nutrition Facts Panel contains the nutrition information required by the FDA. This panel is the primary tool to assist you in choosing more healthful foods. An explanation of the components of the Nutrition Facts Panel follows.

How to Read and Use the Nutrition Facts Panel on Foods

Figure 2.2 (page 48) shows an example of a **Nutrition Facts Panel.** You can use the information on this panel to learn more about an individual food, and you can use the panel to compare one food to another. Let's start at the top of the panel and work our way down to better understand how to use this information.

1. **Serving size and servings per container:** describes the serving size in a common household measure (such as cup), a metric measure (grams), and the number of servings contained in the package. The FDA has defined serving sizes based on the amounts people typically eat for each food. However, keep in mind that the serving size listed on the package may not be the same as the amount *you* eat. You must factor in how much of the food you eat when determining the amount of nutrients that this food contributes to your actual diet.

2. **Calories and Calories from fat per serving:** describes the total number of Calories and the total number of Calories that come from fat per one serving of that food. By looking at this section of the label, you can determine if this food is relatively high in fat. For example, one serving of the food on this label (as prepared) contains 320 total Calories, with 90 of those Calories coming from fat. This means that this food contains 28% of its total Calories as fat (90 fat Calories ÷ 320 total Calories).

Think you understand how to read the Nutrition Facts Panel? Take an interactive quiz and find out at www.extension.iastate.edu/healthnutrition/nutrition/diet/nutrition_label.htm.

Nutrition Facts Panel The label on a food package containing the nutrition information required by the FDA.

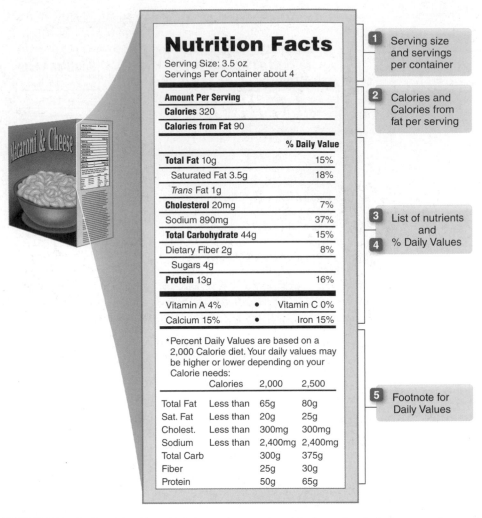

Nutrition Facts

Serving Size: 3.5 oz
Servings Per Container about 4

Amount Per Serving

Calories 320

Calories from Fat 90

	% Daily Value
Total Fat 10g	15%
Saturated Fat 3.5g	18%
Trans Fat 1g	
Cholesterol 20mg	7%
Sodium 890mg	37%
Total Carbohydrate 44g	15%
Dietary Fiber 2g	8%
Sugars 4g	
Protein 13g	16%

Vitamin A 4%	•	Vitamin C 0%
Calcium 15%	•	Iron 15%

*Percent Daily Values are based on a 2,000 Calorie diet. Your daily values may be higher or lower depending on your Calorie needs:

	Calories	2,000	2,500
Total Fat	Less than	65g	80g
Sat. Fat	Less than	20g	25g
Cholest.	Less than	300mg	300mg
Sodium	Less than	2,400mg	2,400mg
Total Carb		300g	375g
Fiber		25g	30g
Protein		50g	65g

1 Serving size and servings per container

2 Calories and Calories from fat per serving

3 List of nutrients and
4 % Daily Values

5 Footnote for Daily Values

FIGURE 2.2 The Nutrition Facts Panel contains a variety of information to help you make more healthful food choices.

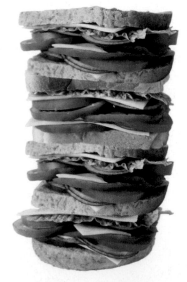

The serving size on a nutrition label may not be the same as the amount you eat.

percent daily values (%DVs)
Information on a Nutrition Facts Panel that identifies how much a serving of food contributes to your overall intake of nutrients listed on the label; based on an energy intake of 2,000 Calories per day.

3. **List of nutrients:** describes various nutrients found in this food. Those nutrients listed toward the top, including total fat, saturated fat, *trans* fat, cholesterol, and sodium, are generally nutrients that we strive to limit in a healthful diet. Some of the nutrients listed toward the bottom are those we try to consume more of, including fiber, vitamins A and C, calcium, and iron.

4. **Percent daily values (%DVs):** tells you how much a serving of food contributes to your overall intake of nutrients listed on the label. For example, 10 grams of fat constitutes 15% of an individual's total daily recommended fat intake. Because we are all individuals with unique nutritional needs, it is impractical to include nutrition information that applies to each person consuming a food. That would require thousands of labels! Thus, when defining the %DV, the FDA based its calculations on a 2,000-Calorie diet. Even if you do not consume 2,000 Calories each day, you can still use the %DV to figure out whether a food is high or low in a given nutrient. For example, foods that contain less than 5% DV of a nutrient are considered low in that nutrient, while foods that contain more than 20% DV are considered high in that nutrient. If you are trying to consume more calcium in your diet, select foods that contain more than 20% DV for calcium. In contrast, if you are trying to consume lower-fat foods, select foods that contain less than 5% or 10% fat. By comparing the %DV between foods for any nutrient, you can quickly decide which food is higher or lower in that nutrient without having to know anything about how many Calories you need.

5. **Footnote (lower part of panel):** tells you that the %DVs are based on a 2,000-Calorie diet and that your needs may be higher or lower. The remainder of the footnote includes a table with values that illustrate the differences in recommendations between a 2,000-Calorie and 2,500-Calorie diet; for instance, someone eating 2,000 Calories should strive to eat less than 65 g of fat per day, whereas a person eating 2,500 Calories should eat less than 80 g of fat per day. The table may not be present on the package if the food label is too small. When present, the footnote and the table are always the same because the information refers to general dietary advice for all Americans rather than to a specific food.

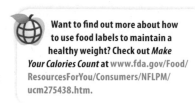

Want to find out more about how to use food labels to maintain a healthy weight? Check out *Make Your Calories Count* at www.fda.gov/Food/ResourcesForYou/Consumers/NFLPM/ucm275438.htm.

Food Labels Can Display a Variety of Claims

Have you ever noticed a food label displaying a claim such as "This food is low in sodium" or "This food is part of a heart-healthy diet"? The claim may have influenced you to buy the food, even if you weren't sure what it meant. So let's take a look.

The FDA regulates two types of claims that food companies put on food labels: nutrient claims and health claims. Food companies are prohibited from using a nutrient or health claim that is not approved by the FDA.

The Daily Values on the food labels serve as a basis for nutrient claims. For instance, if the label states that a food is "low in sodium," that food contains 140 mg or less of sodium per serving. **Table 2.1** (page 50) defines terms approved for use in nutrient claims.

Food labels are also allowed to display certain claims related to health and disease. The health claims that the FDA allows at the present time are listed in **Table 2.2** (page 51). To help consumers gain a better understanding of nutritional information related to health, the FDA has developed a Health Claims Report Card (**Figure 2.3**), which grades the level of confidence in a health claim based on current scientific evidence. For example, if current scientific evidence is not convincing, a particular health claim may have to include a disclaimer, so that consumers are not misled. Complete the **Nutrition Label Activity** (page 52) to determine the strengths of certain health claims made on foods commonly consumed.

In addition to nutrient and health claims, labels may also contain structure–function claims. These are claims that can be made without approval from the FDA. While these claims can be generic statements about a food's impact on the body's structure and function, they cannot refer to a specific disease or symptom. Examples of structure–function claims include "Builds stronger bones," "Improves memory," "Slows signs of aging," and "Boosts your immune system." It is important to remember that these claims can be made with no proof, and thus there are no guarantees that any benefits identified in structure–function claims are true about that particular food.

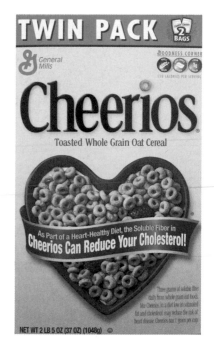

This Cheerios label is an example of an approved health claim.

FDA categories	Health Claims Report Card		Required disclaimers
A	**High confidence** Significant scientific agreement		Applies to claims listed in Table 2.2 No Disclaimer Needed
B	**Moderate confidence** Evidence is not conclusive		..."although there is scientific evidence supporting the claim, the evidence is not conclusive."
C	**Low confidence** Evidence is limited and not conclusive		"Some scientific evidence suggests… however, FDA has determined that this evidence is limited and not conclusive."
D	**Extremely low confidence** Little scientific evidence supporting this claim		"Very limited and preliminary scientific research suggests…FDA concludes that there is little scientific evidence supporting this claim."

FIGURE 2.3 The US Food and Drug Administration's Health Claims Report Card. (*Source:* Data from "Assessing Consumer Perceptions of Health Claims," by Neal Hooker and Ratapol P. Teratanavat, from the Federal Drug Administration website. Updated April 4, 2010.)

TABLE 2.1 US Food and Drug Administration (FDA)–Approved Nutrient-Related Terms and Definitions

Nutrient	Claim	Meaning
Energy	Calorie free	Less than 5 kcal per serving
	Low Calorie	40 kcal or less per serving
	Reduced Calorie	At least 25% fewer kcal than reference (or regular) food
Fat and cholesterol	Fat free	Less than 0.5 g of fat per serving
	Low fat	3 g or less fat per serving
	Reduced fat	At least 25% less fat per serving than reference food
	Saturated fat free	Less than 0.5 g of saturated fat AND less than 0.5 g of *trans* fat per serving
	Low saturated fat	1 g or less saturated fat and less than 0.5 g *trans* fat per serving AND 15% or less of total kcal from saturated fat
	Reduced saturated fat	At least 25% less saturated fat AND reduced by more than 1 g saturated fat per serving as compared to reference food
	Cholesterol free	Less than 2 mg of cholesterol per serving AND 2 g or less saturated fat and *trans* fat combined per serving
	Low cholesterol	20 mg or less cholesterol AND 2 g or less saturated fat per serving
	Reduced cholesterol	At least 25% less cholesterol than reference food AND 2 g or less saturated fat per serving
Fiber and sugar	High fiber	5 g or more fiber per serving*
	Good source of fiber	2.5 g to 4.9 g fiber per serving
	More or added fiber	At least 2.5 g more fiber per serving than reference food
	Sugar free	Less than 0.5 g sugars per serving
	Low sugar	Not defined; no basis for recommended intake
	Reduced/less sugar	At least 25% less sugars per serving than reference food
	No added sugars or without added sugars	No sugar or sugar-containing ingredient added during processing
Sodium	Sodium free	Less than 5 mg sodium per serving
	Very low sodium	35 mg or less sodium per serving
	Low sodium	140 mg or less sodium per serving
	Reduced sodium	At least 25% less sodium per serving than reference food
Relative Claims	Free, without, no, zero	No or a trivial amount of given nutrient
	Light (lite)	This term can have three different meanings: (1) a serving provides one-third fewer kcal than or half the fat of the reference food; (2) a serving of a low-fat, low-Calorie food provides half the sodium normally present; or (3) lighter in color and texture, with the label making this clear (for example, "light molasses")
	Reduced, less, fewer	Contains at least 25% less of a nutrient or kcal than reference food
	More, added, extra, or plus	At least 10% of the Daily Value of nutrient as compared to reference food (may occur naturally or be added); may only be used for vitamins, minerals, protein, dietary fiber, and potassium
	Good source of, contains, or provides	10% to 19% of Daily Value per serving (may not be used for carbohydrate)
	High in, rich in, or excellent source of	20% or more of Daily Value per serving for protein, vitamins, minerals, dietary fiber, or potassium (may not be used for carbohydrate)

*High-fiber claims must also meet the definition of low fat; if not, then the level of total fat must appear next to the high-fiber claim.
Source: "Food Labeling Guide," from FDA.gov.

RECAP

The ability to read and interpret food labels is important for planning and maintaining a healthful diet. Food labels must list the identity of the food, the net contents of the package, the contact information for the food manufacturer or distributor, the ingredients in the food, and a Nutrition Facts Panel. The Nutrition Facts Panel provides specific information about Calories, macronutrients, and selected vitamins and minerals. Food labels may also contain claims related to nutrients, health, and structure–function. ∎

TABLE 2.2 US Food and Drug Administration–Approved Health Claims on Labels

Disease/Health Concern	Nutrient	Example of Approved Claim Statement
Osteoporosis	Calcium	Regular exercise and a healthy diet with enough calcium help teens and young adult white and Asian women maintain good bone health and may reduce their high risk of osteoporosis later in life.
Coronary heart disease	Saturated fat and cholesterol Fruits, vegetables, and grain products that contain fiber, particularly soluble fiber Soluble fiber from whole oats, psyllium seed husk, and beta glucan soluble fiber from oat bran, rolled oats (or oatmeal), and whole-oat flour Soy protein Plant sterol/stanol esters Whole-grain foods	Diets low in saturated fat and cholesterol and rich in fruits, vegetables, and grain products that contain some types of dietary fiber, particularly soluble fiber, may reduce the risk of heart disease, a disease associated with many factors.
Cancer	Dietary fat Fiber-containing grain products, fruits and vegetables Fruits and vegetables Whole-grain foods	Low-fat diets rich in fiber-containing grain products, fruits, and vegetables may reduce the risk of some types of cancer, a disease associated with many factors.
Hypertension and stroke	Sodium Potassium	Diets containing foods that are a good source of potassium and that are low in sodium may reduce the risk of high blood pressure and stroke.*
Neural tube defects	Folate	Healthful diets with adequate folate may reduce a woman's risk of having a child with a brain or spinal cord defect.
Dental caries	Sugar alcohols	Frequent between-meal consumption of foods high in sugars and starches promotes tooth decay. The sugar alcohols in [name of food] do not promote tooth decay.

*Required wording for this claim. Wordings for other claims are recommended model statements but are not required verbatim.
Source: "Food Labeling Guide," from FDA.gov.

Dietary Guidelines for Americans

The **Dietary Guidelines for Americans** are a set of principles developed by the US Department of Agriculture and the US Department of Health and Human Services to promote health, reduce the risk for chronic diseases, and reduce the prevalence of overweight and obesity among Americans through improved nutrition and physical activity.[2] They are updated approximately every 5 years. The 2010 Dietary Guidelines for Americans include twenty-three recommendations for the general population, but you don't have to remember all twenty-three! Instead, they encourage you to focus on the following four main ideas.

Balance Calories to Maintain Weight

Consume adequate nutrients to promote your health while staying within your energy needs. This will help you maintain a healthful weight. You can achieve this by controlling your Calorie intake; if you are overweight or obese, you will need to consume fewer Calories from foods and beverages. At the same time, increase your level of physical activity and reduce the time you spend in sedentary behaviors, such as watching television and sitting at the computer.

An important strategy for balancing your Calories is to consistently choose **nutrient-dense foods** and beverages—that is, foods and beverages that supply the highest level of

Dietary Guidelines for Americans
A set of principles developed by the US Department of Agriculture and the US Department of Health and Human Services to assist Americans in designing a healthful diet and lifestyle.

nutrient-dense foods Foods that provide the highest level of nutrients for the least amount of energy (Calories).

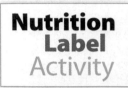

How Do Health Claims on Food Labels Measure Up?

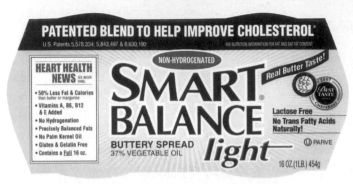

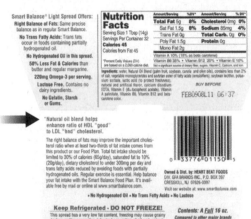

The US Food and Drug Administration has published a Health Claims Report Card to assist consumers in deciphering health claims on food labels (see Figure 2.3, page 49). It is important to note that the claims that are based on a high degree of scientific agreement do not require a label disclaimer. The claims reported in Table 2.2 (page 51) are based on a high degree of scientific agreement. Included here is a food label listing health claims.

Based on the Health Claims Report Card criteria listed in Figure 2.3, what level of confidence do scientists currently have about these health claims? Taking this level of confidence into consideration, would you recommend this product to relatives or friends if they were concerned about their risk for heart disease? Why or why not?

---

nutrients for the least amount of Calories (energy). **Figure 2.4** compares 1 day of meals that are high in **nutrient density** to meals that are low in nutrient density. As you can see in this figure, skim milk is more nutrient dense than whole milk, and a peeled orange is more nutrient dense than an orange-flavored soft drink. This example can help you select the most nutrient-dense foods when planning your meals.

Consume Fewer Foods and Food Components of Concern

The Dietary Guidelines suggest that we reduce our consumption of the following foods and food components. Doing so will help us maintain a healthy weight and lower our risk for chronic diseases.

Sodium   Excessive consumption of sodium, a major mineral found in salt, is linked to high blood pressure in some people. Eating a lot of sodium also can cause some people to lose calcium from their bones, which can increase their risk for bone loss and bone fractures. Although table salt contains sodium and the major mineral chloride, much of the sodium we consume comes from processed and prepared foods. Key recommendations

nutrient density   The relative amount of nutrients per amount of energy (number of Calories).

A Day of Meals: Low vs. High Nutrient Density

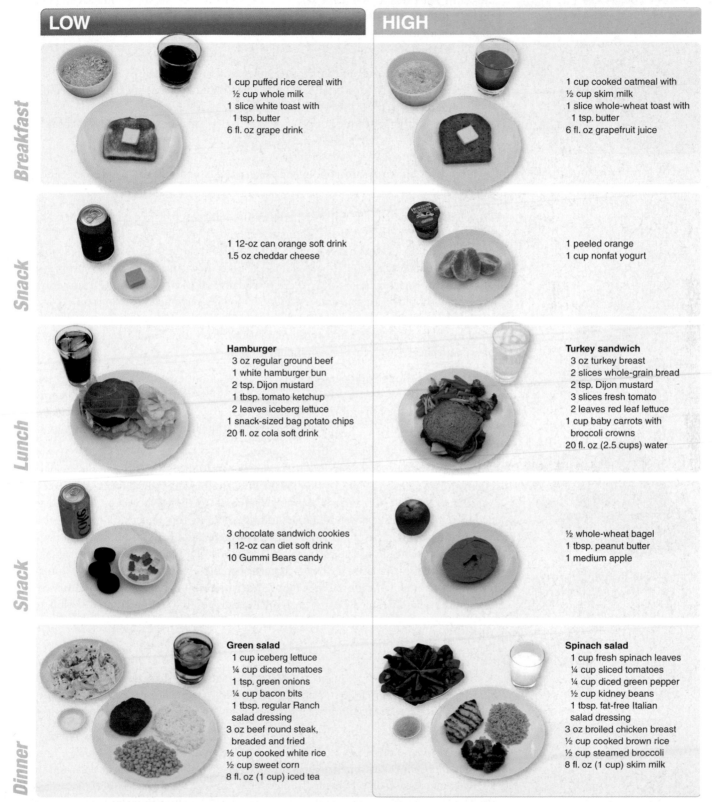

LOW

HIGH

Breakfast

1 cup puffed rice cereal with
½ cup whole milk
1 slice white toast with
1 tsp. butter
6 fl. oz grape drink

1 cup cooked oatmeal with
½ cup skim milk
1 slice whole-wheat toast with
1 tsp. butter
6 fl. oz grapefruit juice

Snack

1 12-oz can orange soft drink
1.5 oz cheddar cheese

1 peeled orange
1 cup nonfat yogurt

Lunch

Hamburger
3 oz regular ground beef
1 white hamburger bun
2 tsp. Dijon mustard
1 tbsp. tomato ketchup
2 leaves iceberg lettuce
1 snack-sized bag potato chips
20 fl. oz cola soft drink

Turkey sandwich
3 oz turkey breast
2 slices whole-grain bread
2 tsp. Dijon mustard
3 slices fresh tomato
2 leaves red leaf lettuce
1 cup baby carrots with
broccoli crowns
20 fl. oz (2.5 cups) water

Snack

3 chocolate sandwich cookies
1 12-oz can diet soft drink
10 Gummi Bears candy

½ whole-wheat bagel
1 tbsp. peanut butter
1 medium apple

Dinner

Green salad
1 cup iceberg lettuce
¼ cup diced tomatoes
1 tsp. green onions
¼ cup bacon bits
1 tbsp. regular Ranch
salad dressing
3 oz beef round steak,
breaded and fried
½ cup cooked white rice
½ cup sweet corn
8 fl. oz (1 cup) iced tea

Spinach salad
1 cup fresh spinach leaves
¼ cup sliced tomatoes
¼ cup diced green pepper
½ cup kidney beans
1 tbsp. fat-free Italian
salad dressing
3 oz broiled chicken breast
½ cup cooked brown rice
½ cup steamed broccoli
8 fl. oz (1 cup) skim milk

FIGURE 2.4 A comparison of 1 day's meals containing foods low in nutrient density to meals with foods high in nutrient density.

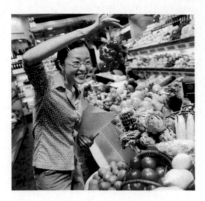

When grocery shopping, try to select foods that are moderate in total fat, sugar, and salt.

include keeping your daily sodium intake below 2,300 milligrams (mg) per day. This is the amount in just 1 teaspoon of table salt! If you are African American; if you have high blood pressure, diabetes, or chronic kidney disease; or if you are over age 50, you should aim for a daily sodium intake below 1,500 mg. Some ways to decrease your sodium intake include the following:

- Eat fresh, plain frozen, or canned vegetables without added salt.
- Limit your intake of processed meats, such as cured ham, sausage, bacon, and most canned meats.
- When shopping for canned or packaged foods, look for those with labels that say "low sodium."
- Add little or no salt to foods at the table.
- Limit your intake of salty condiments, such as ketchup, mustard, pickles, soy sauce, and olives.

Fat Fat is an essential nutrient and therefore an important part of a healthful diet; however, because fats are energy dense, eating a diet high in total fat can lead to overweight and obesity. In addition, eating a diet high in cholesterol and saturated fat (a type of fat abundant in meats and other animal-based foods) is linked to an increased risk for heart disease. For these reasons, less than 7–10% of your total daily Calories should come from saturated fat, and you should try to consume less than 300 mg per day of cholesterol. You can achieve this goal by replacing solid fats, such as butter and lard, with vegetable oils, as well as by eating meat less often and fish or vegetarian meals more often. Finally, replace full-fat milk, yogurt, and cheeses with low-fat or nonfat versions.

Sugars Limit foods and beverages that are high in added sugars, such as sweetened soft drinks and fruit drinks, cookies, and cakes. These foods contribute to overweight and obesity, and they promote tooth decay. Moreover, doughnuts, cookies, cakes, pies, and other pastries are typically made with unhealthful fats and are high in sodium.

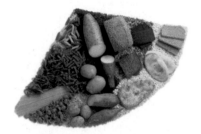

Eating a diet rich in whole-grain foods, such as whole-wheat bread and brown rice, can enhance your overall health.

Alcohol Alcohol provides energy, but not nutrients. In the body, it depresses the nervous system and is toxic to liver and other body cells. Drinking alcoholic beverages in excess can lead to serious health and social problems; therefore, those who choose to drink are encouraged to do so sensibly and in moderation: no more than one drink per day for women and no more than two drinks per day for men, and only by adults of legal drinking age. Adults who should not drink alcohol are those who cannot restrict their intake, women of childbearing age who may become pregnant, pregnant and lactating women, individuals taking medications that can interact with alcohol, people with certain medical conditions, and people who are engaging in activities that require attention, skill, or coordination.

Consume More Healthful Foods and Nutrients

Another goal of the Dietary Guidelines is to encourage people to increase their consumption of healthful foods rich in nutrients, while keeping their Calorie intake within their daily energy needs. Key recommendations for achieving this goal include the following:

- Increase your intake of fruits and vegetables. Each day, try to eat a variety of dark-green, red, and orange vegetables, along with beans and peas.
- Make sure that at least half of all grain foods—such as breads, cereals, pasta, and rice—that you eat each day are made from whole grains.
- Choose fat-free or low-fat milk and milk products, which include milk, yogurt, cheese, and fortified soy beverages.

- When making protein choices, choose protein foods that are lower in solid fat and Calories, such as lean cuts of beef or skinless poultry. Try to eat more fish and shellfish in place of traditional meat and poultry choices. Also choose eggs, beans and peas, soy products, and unsalted nuts and seeds.
- Choose foods that provide an adequate level of dietary fiber as well as nutrients of concern in the American diet, including potassium, calcium, and vitamin D. These nutrients help us maintain healthy blood pressure and reduce our risks for certain diseases. Healthful foods that are good sources of these nutrients include fruits, vegetables, beans and peas, whole grains, and low-fat milk and milk products.

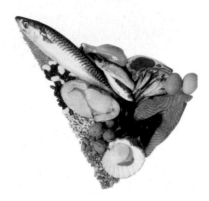

Seafood, meat, poultry, dry beans, eggs, and nuts are examples of foods that are high in protein.

Follow Healthy Eating Patterns

There is no one healthy eating pattern that everyone should follow. Instead, the recommendations made in the Dietary Guidelines are designed to accommodate diverse cultural, ethnic, traditional, and personal preferences and to fit within different individuals' food budgets. Still, the Guidelines offer several flexible templates you can follow to build your healthy eating pattern, including the USDA Food Patterns and the Mediterranean diet (both discussed shortly).

Building a healthy eating pattern also involves following food safety recommendations to reduce your risk for foodborne illnesses, such as those caused by microorganisms and their toxins. The four food-safety principles emphasized in the Dietary Guidelines are

- *Clean* your hands, food contact surfaces, and vegetables and fruits.
- *Separate* raw, cooked, and ready-to-eat foods while shopping, storing, and preparing foods.
- *Cook* foods to a safe temperature.
- *Chill* (refrigerate) perishable foods promptly.

Another important tip is to avoid unpasteurized juices and milk products; raw or undercooked meats, seafood, poultry, and eggs; and raw sprouts.

Table 2.3 provides examples of how you can change your current diet and physical activity habits to meet some of the recommendations in the Dietary Guidelines.

TABLE 2.3 Ways to Incorporate the Dietary Guidelines for Americans into Your Daily Life

If You Normally Do This:	Try Doing This Instead:
Watch television when you get home at night	Do 30 minutes of stretching or lifting of hand weights in front of the television
Drive to the store down the block	Walk to and from the store
Go out to lunch with friends	Take a 15- or 30-minute walk with your friends at lunchtime 3 days each week
Eat white bread with your sandwich	Eat whole-wheat bread or some other bread made from whole grains
Eat white rice or fried rice with your meal	Eat brown rice or try wild rice
Choose cookies or a candy bar for a snack	Choose a fresh nectarine, peach, apple, orange, or banana for a snack
Order french fries with your hamburger	Order a green salad with low-fat salad dressing on the side
Spread butter or margarine on your white toast each morning	Spread fresh fruit compote on whole-grain toast
Order a bacon double cheeseburger at your favorite restaurant	Order a turkey burger or grilled chicken sandwich without the cheese and bacon, and add lettuce and tomato
Drink non-diet soft drinks to quench your thirst	Drink iced tea, ice water with a slice of lemon, seltzer water, or diet soft drinks
Eat salted potato chips and pickles with your favorite sandwich	Eat carrot slices and crowns of fresh broccoli and cauliflower dipped in low-fat or nonfat Ranch dressing

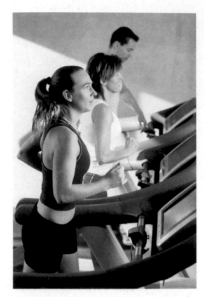

Incorporating daily activity is among the recommendations in the Dietary Guidelines for Americans.

RECAP

The goals of the Dietary Guidelines for Americans are to promote health, reduce the risk for chronic diseases, and reduce the prevalence of overweight and obesity among Americans through improved nutrition and physical activity. This can be achieved by eating whole-grain foods, fruits, and vegetables daily; reducing intake of foods with unhealthful fats and cholesterol, salt, and added sugar; eating more foods rich in potassium, dietary fiber, calcium, and vitamin D; keeping foods safe to eat; and drinking alcohol in moderation, if at all. ■

The USDA Food Patterns

As mentioned, you can use the US Department of Agriculture (USDA) Food Patterns to design healthy eating patterns. The visual representation of the USDA Food Patterns is called **MyPlate** (**Figure 2.5**). MyPlate, which was released in 2011, is an interactive, personalized guide that you can access on the Internet to assess your current diet and physical activity level and to plan appropriate changes. MyPlate replaces the previous MyPyramid graphic (see Appendix A). Although you may continue to see variations of MyPyramid until new MyPlate versions are developed and released, MyPlate is now the primary food icon intended to help Americans make better food choices. In addition, the MyPlate icon and its accompanying website help Americans:

- Eat in moderation to balance Calories
- Eat a variety of foods
- Consume the right proportion of each recommended food group
- Personalize their eating plan
- Increase their physical activity
- Set goals for gradually improving their food choices and lifestyle

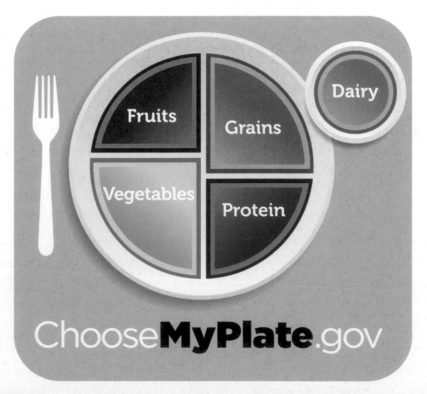

FIGURE 2.5 The USDA MyPlate graphic. MyPlate is an interactive food guidance system based on the 2010 Dietary Guidelines for Americans and the Dietary Reference Intakes from the National Academy of Sciences. Eating more fruits, vegetables, and whole grains and choosing foods low in fat, sugar, and sodium from the five food groups in MyPlate will help you balance your Calories and consume a healthier overall diet. (*Source:* Figure from the United States Department of Agriculture's Choose My Plate website.)

MyPlate The visual representation of the USDA Food Patterns.

Food Groups in the USDA Food Patterns

The food groups emphasized in the USDA Food Patterns are grains, vegetables, fruits, dairy, and protein foods. The food groups are represented in the plate graphic with segments of five different colors. **Figure 2.6** illustrates each of these food groups and provides detailed information on the nutrients they provide and recommended servings each day.

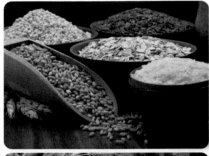

Grains

Make half your grains whole. At least half of the grains you eat each day should come from whole-grain sources.

Eat at least 3 oz of whole-grain bread, cereal, crackers, rice, or pasta every day.

Whole-grain foods provide fiber-rich carbohydrates, riboflavin, thiamin, niacin, iron, folate, zinc, protein, and magnesium.

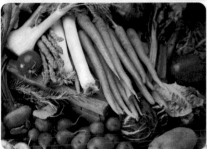

Vegetables

Vary your veggies. Eat a variety of vegetables and increase consumption of dark-green and orange vegetables, as well as dry beans and peas.

Eat at least 2½ cups of vegetables each day.

Vegetables provide fiber and phytochemicals, carbohydrates, vitamins A and C, folate, potassium, and magnesium.

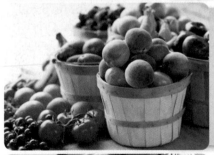

Fruits

Focus on fruits. Eat a greater variety of fruits (fresh, frozen, or dried) and go easy on the fruit juices.

Eat at least 1½ cups of fruit every day.

Fruits provide fiber, phytochemicals, vitamins A and C, folate, potassium, and magnesium.

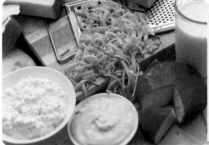

Dairy Foods

Get your calcium-rich foods. Choose low-fat or fat-free dairy products, such as milk, yogurt, and cheese. People who can't consume dairy foods can choose lactose-free dairy products or other sources, such as calcium-fortified juices and soy and rice beverages.

Get 3 cups of low-fat dairy foods, or the equivalent, every day.

Dairy foods provide calcium, phosphorus, riboflavin, protein, and vitamin B_{12} and are often fortified with vitamins D and A.

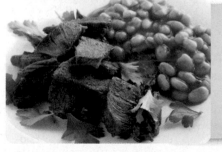

Protein Foods

Go lean with protein. Choose low-fat or lean meats and poultry. Switch to baking, broiling, or grilling more often, and vary your choices to include more fish, processed soy products, beans, nuts, and seeds. Legumes, including beans, peas, and lentils, are included in both the protein and the vegetable groups.

Eat about 5½ oz of lean protein foods each day.

These foods provide protein, phosphorus, vitamin B_6, vitamin B_{12}, magnesium, iron, zinc, niacin, riboflavin, and thiamin.

FIGURE 2.6 Food groups from the USDA Food Patterns.

The Concept of Empty Calories

One concept emphasized in the USDA Food Patterns is that of **empty Calories.** These are Calories from solid fats and/or added sugars that provide few or no nutrients. The USDA recommends that you limit the empty Calories you eat to a small number that fits your Calorie and nutrient needs depending on your age, gender, and level of physical activity. Foods that contain the greatest amount of empty Calories include cakes, cookies, pastries, doughnuts, soft drinks, fruit drinks, cheese, pizza, ice cream, sausages, hot dogs, bacon, and ribs. High-sugar foods, such as candies, desserts, gelatin, soft drinks, and alcoholic beverages, are called *empty Calorie foods*. However, a few foods that contain empty Calories from solid fats and added sugars also provide important nutrients. Examples are sweetened applesauce, sweetened breakfast cereals, regular ground beef, and whole milk. To reduce your intake of empty Calories but ensure you get adequate nutrients, choose the unsweetened, lean, or nonfat versions of these foods.

Number and Size of Servings in the USDA Food Patterns

The USDA Food Patterns also helps you decide *how much* of each food you should eat. The number of servings is based on your age, gender, and activity level. A term used when defining serving sizes that may be new to you is **ounce-equivalent (oz-equivalent)**. It is defined as a serving size that is 1 ounce, or that is equivalent to an ounce, for the grains and meats and beans sections. For instance, both a slice of bread and ½ cup of cooked brown rice qualify as ounce-equivalents.

What is considered a serving size for the foods recommended in the USDA Food Patterns? **Figure 2.7** identifies the number of cups or oz-equivalent servings recommended for a 2,000-Calorie diet and gives examples of amounts equal to 1 cup or 1 oz-equivalent for foods in each group. As you study this figure, notice the variety of examples for each group. For instance, an oz-equivalent serving from the grains group can mean one slice of bread or two small pancakes. Because of their low density, 2 cups of raw, leafy vegetables, such as spinach, actually constitute a 1-cup serving from the vegetables group. Although an oz-equivalent serving of meat is actually 1 oz, ½ oz of nuts also qualifies. One egg, 1 tablespoon of peanut butter, and ¼ cup cooked legumes are also each considered 1 oz-equivalents from the protein group. Although it may seem inconvenient to measure food servings, understanding the size of a serving is crucial to planning a nutritious diet.

> Think you understand the relationship between portion sizes and the physical activity necessary to avoid weight gain? Find out by taking the National Heart, Lung, and Blood Institute's *Portion Distortion Quiz* at www.hp2010.nhlbihin.net/portion.

Nutri-Case

Gustavo

"Until last night, I hadn't stepped inside of a grocery store for 10 years, maybe more. But then my wife fell and broke her hip and had to go to the hospital. On my way home from visiting her, I remembered that we didn't have much food in the house, so I thought I'd do a little shopping. Was I ever in for a shock. I don't know how my wife does it, choosing between all the different brands, reading those long labels. She never went to school past sixth grade, and she doesn't speak English very well, either! I bought a frozen chicken pie for my dinner, but it didn't taste right. So I got the package out of the trash and read the label on the back, and that's when I realized there wasn't any chicken in it at all! It was made out of tofu! This afternoon, my daughter is picking me up, and we're going to do our grocery shopping together!"

Given what you've learned about FDA food labels, what parts of a food package should Gustavo read before he makes a choice? What else can he do to make his grocery shopping easier? Imagine that, like Gustavo's wife, you have only limited skills in mathematics and reading. In that case, what other strategies might you use when shopping for nutritious foods?

empty Calories Calories from solid fats and/or added sugars that provide few or no nutrients.

ounce-equivalent (oz-equivalent) A serving size that is 1 ounce, or equivalent to an ounce, for the grains and the protein foods sections of MyPlate.

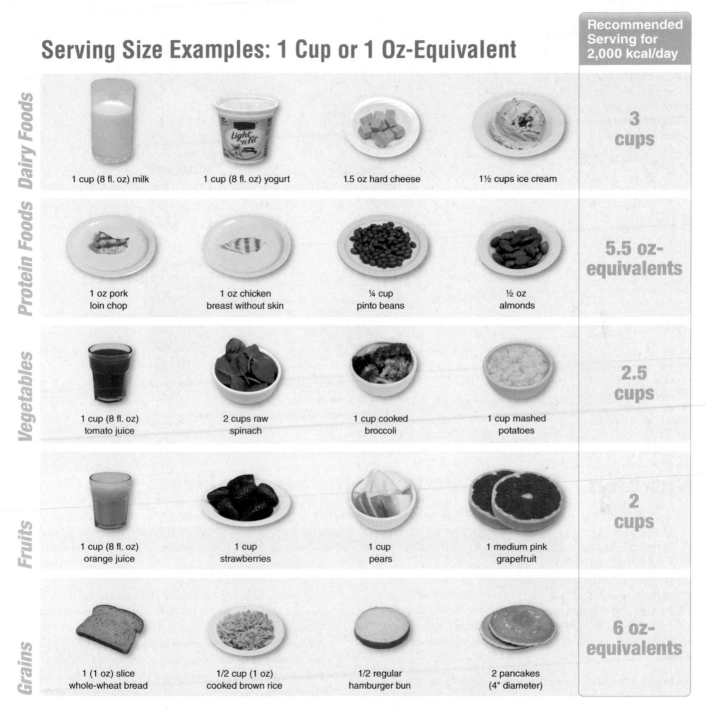

Serving Size Examples: 1 Cup or 1 Oz-Equivalent

				Recommended Serving for 2,000 kcal/day
Dairy Foods	1 cup (8 fl. oz) milk	1 cup (8 fl. oz) yogurt	1.5 oz hard cheese	1½ cups ice cream	**3 cups**
Protein Foods	1 oz pork loin chop	1 oz chicken breast without skin	¼ cup pinto beans	½ oz almonds	**5.5 oz-equivalents**
Vegetables	1 cup (8 fl. oz) tomato juice	2 cups raw spinach	1 cup cooked broccoli	1 cup mashed potatoes	**2.5 cups**
Fruits	1 cup (8 fl. oz) orange juice	1 cup strawberries	1 cup pears	1 medium pink grapefruit	**2 cups**
Grains	1 (1 oz) slice whole-wheat bread	1/2 cup (1 oz) cooked brown rice	1/2 regular hamburger bun	2 pancakes (4" diameter)	**6 oz-equivalents**

FIGURE 2.7 Examples of serving sizes in each food group of MyPlate for a 2,000-Calorie food intake pattern. You can use the following visualizations of common household objects to help you estimate serving sizes: 1.5 oz of hard cheese is equal to four stacked dice, 3 oz of meat is equal in size to a deck of cards, and one-half of a regular hamburger bun is the size of a yo-yo.

Using the USDA Food Patterns (and their visual representation, MyPlate) does have some challenges. For example, no nationally standardized definition for a serving size exists for any food. Thus, a serving size as defined in the USDA Food Patterns may not be equal to a serving size identified on a food label. For instance, the serving size for crackers suggested in the USDA Food Patterns is three to four small crackers, whereas a serving size for crackers on a food label can range from five to eighteen crackers, depending on the size and weight of the cracker.

Also, for food items consumed individually—such as muffins, frozen burgers, and bottled juices—the serving sizes in the USDA Food Patterns are typically much smaller than

FIGURE 2.8 Examples of increases in food portion sizes over the past 30 years. **(a)** A bagel has increased in diameter from 3 inches to 6 inches; **(b)** a cup of coffee has increased from 8 fl. oz to 16 fl. oz and now commonly contains Calorie-dense flavored syrup as well as steamed whole milk.

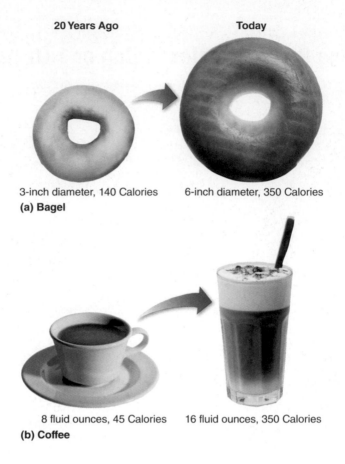

20 Years Ago   Today

3-inch diameter, 140 Calories   6-inch diameter, 350 Calories

(a) Bagel

8 fluid ounces, 45 Calories   16 fluid ounces, 350 Calories

(b) Coffee

Nutrition Label Activity

How Realistic Are the Serving Sizes Listed on Food Labels?

Many people read food labels to determine the energy (Caloric) value of foods, but it is less common to pay close attention to the actual serving size that corresponds to the listed Caloric value. To test how closely your "naturally selected" serving size meets the actual serving size of certain foods, try these label activities:

■ Choose a breakfast cereal that you commonly eat. Pour the amount of cereal that you would normally eat into a bowl. Before adding milk to your cereal, use a measuring cup to measure the amount of cereal you poured. Now read the label of the cereal to determine the serving size (for example, 1/2 cup or 1 cup) and the Caloric value listed on the label. How do your "naturally selected" serving size and the label-defined serving size compare?

■ At your local grocery store, locate various boxes of snack crackers. Look at the number of crackers and total Calories per serving listed on the labels of crackers such as regular Triscuits, reduced-fat Triscuits, Vegetable Thins, and Ritz crackers. How do the number of crackers and total Calories per serving differ for the serving size listed on each box? How do the serving sizes listed in the Nutrition Facts Panel compare to how many crackers you would usually eat?

These activities are just two examples of ways to understand how nutrition labels can assist the consumer with making balanced and healthful food choices. As many people do not know what constitutes a serving size, they are inclined to consume too much of some foods (such as snack foods and meat) and too little of other foods (such as fruits and vegetables).

the items we actually buy and eat. In addition, serving sizes in restaurants, cafés, and movie theaters have grown substantially over the past 30 years (**Figure 2.8**). This "super-sizing" phenomenon, now widespread, indicates a major shift in accepted eating behaviors. It is an important contributor to the rise in obesity rates around the world. For over 10 years it has been recognized[3] that the discrepancy between USDA serving size standards and

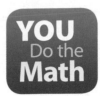

How Much Exercise Is Needed to Combat Increasing Food Portion Sizes?

Although the causes of obesity are complex and multifactorial, it is speculated that one reason obesity rates are rising around the world is a combination of increased energy intake due to expanding food portion sizes and a reduction in overall daily physical activity. This activity should help you better understand how portion sizes have increased over the past 30 years and how much physical activity you would need to do to expend the excess energy resulting from these larger portion sizes.

The two photos in Figure 2.8 give examples of foods whose portion sizes have increased substantially over time. A bagel 30 years ago had a diameter of approximately 3 inches and contained 140 kcal. A bagel today is about 6 inches in diameter and contains 350 kcal. Similarly, a cup of coffee 30 years ago was 8 fl. oz and was typically served with a small amount of whole milk and sugar. It contained about 45 kcal. A standard coffee mocha commonly consumed today is 16 fl. oz and contains 350 kcal; this excess energy comes from the addition of a sweet flavored syrup and whole milk.

On her morning break at work, Judy routinely consumes a bagel and a coffee mocha. Judy has type 2 diabetes, and her doctor has advised her to lose weight. How much physical activity would Judy need to do to "burn" this excess energy? Let's do some simple math to answer this question.

1. Calculate the excess energy Judy consumes from both of these foods:

   a. Bagel: 350 kcal in larger bagel – 140 kcal in smaller bagel = 210 kcal extra

   b. Coffee: 350 kcal in large coffee mocha – 45 kcal in small regular coffee = 305 kcal extra

   Total excess energy for these two larger portions = 515 kcal

2. Judy has started walking each day in an effort to lose weight. Judy currently weighs 200 lb. Based on her relatively low fitness level, Judy walks at a slow pace (approximately 2 miles per hour); it is estimated that walking at this pace expends 1.2 kcal per pound of body weight per hour. How long does Judy need to walk each day to expend 515 kcal?

   a. First, calculate how much energy Judy expends if she walks for a full hour by multiplying her body weight by the energy cost of walking per hour = 1.2 kcal/lb body weight $\times$ 200 lb = 240 kcal.

   b. Next, you need to calculate how much energy she expends each minute she walks by dividing the energy cost of walking per hour by 60 minutes = 240 kcal/hour $\div$ 60 minutes/hour = 4 kcal/minute.

   c. To determine how many minutes she would need to walk to expend 515 kcal, divide the total amount of energy she needs to expend by the energy cost of walking per minute = 515 kcal $\div$ 4 kcal/minute = 103.75 minutes.

Thus, Judy would need to walk for approximately 104 minutes, or about 1 hour and 45 minutes, to expend the excess energy she consumes by eating the larger bagel and coffee. If she wanted to burn off all of the energy in her morning snack, she would have to walk even longer, especially if she enjoyed her bagel with cream cheese!

Now use your own weight in these calculations to determine how much walking you would have to do if you consumed the same foods:

a. 1.2 kcal/lb $\times$ (your weight in pounds) = _____ kcal/hour (If you walk at a brisk pace, use 2.4 kcal/lb.)

b. _____ kcal/hour $\div$ 60 minutes/hour = _____ kcal/minute

c. 515 extra kcal in bagel and coffee $\div$ _____ kcal/minute = _____ minutes

Answers will vary depending on body type and individual nutrient needs.

---

the portion size of many common foods sold outside the home is staggering—chocolate chip cookies have been reported as seven times larger than USDA standards, a serving of cooked pasta in a restaurant can be almost five times larger, and steaks are more than twice as large.[4] Thus, when using diet-planning tools, such as the USDA Food Patterns, learn the definition of a serving size for the tool you're using and *then* measure your food intake to determine whether you are meeting the guidelines. If you don't want to gain weight, it's important to become informed about portion size.

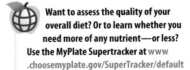

Want to assess the quality of your overall diet? Or to learn whether you need more of any nutrient—or less? Use the MyPlate Supertracker at www .choosemyplate.gov/SuperTracker/default .aspx.

Ethnic Variations of MyPyramid

As you know, the population of the United States is culturally and ethnically diverse, and this diversity influences our food choices. Foods that we may typically consider a part of an Asian, a Latin American, or a Mediterranean diet can also fit into a healthful diet. As previously mentioned, the MyPlate graphic is replacing MyPyramid; however, MyPlate graphics have not yet been developed for various ethnic diets.

FIGURE 2.9 Ethnic variations of healthy eating patterns: the Latin American Diet Pyramid. (*Source:* Latin American Diet Pyramid © 2009 Oldways Preservation and Exchange Trust. www.oldwayspt .org. Reprinted by permission.)

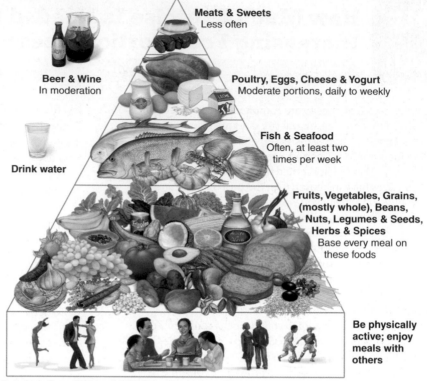

Illustration by Geoge Middleton © 2009 Oldways Preservation and Exchange Trust www.oldwayspt.org

Still, you can easily incorporate foods that match your ethnic, religious, or other life-style preferences into your own personal MyPlate. You can also use one of the many ethnic and cultural variations of the previous USDA Food Guide Pyramid. These include the Latin American Diet Pyramid (**Figure 2.9**) and the Asian Diet Pyramid (**Figure 2.10**). There are also variations for Native Americans, African Americans, and many others.[5] These variations illustrate that anyone can design a healthful diet to accommodate his or her food preferences.

FIGURE 2.10 Ethnic variations of healthy eating patterns: the Asian Diet Pyramid. (*Source:* Asian Diet Pyramid © 2000 Oldways Preservation and Exchange Trust. www .oldwayspt.org. Reprinted by permission.)

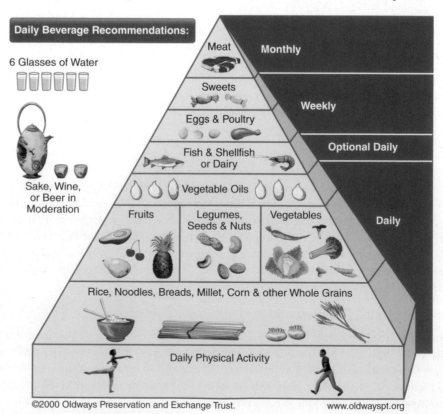

©2000 Oldways Preservation and Exchange Trust.   www.oldwayspt.org

The Mediterranean Diet and Pyramid

A Mediterranean-style diet has received significant attention for many years, largely because the rates of cardiovascular disease in many Mediterranean countries are substantially lower than rates in the United States. There is actually not a single Mediterranean diet, as this region of the world includes Portugal, Spain, Italy, France, Greece, Turkey, and Israel. Each of these countries has different dietary patterns; however, there are similarities that have led to speculation that this type of diet is more healthful than the typical US diet:

- Red meat is eaten only monthly, and eggs, poultry, fish and sweets are eaten weekly, making the diet low in saturated fats and refined sugars.

- The predominant fat used for cooking and flavor is olive oil, making the diet high in monounsaturated fats.

- Foods eaten daily include grains, such as bread, pasta, couscous, and bulgur; fruits; beans and other legumes; nuts; vegetables; and cheese and yogurt. These choices make this diet high in fiber and rich in vitamins and minerals.

- Wine is included, in moderation.

As you can see in **Figure 2.11** (page 64), the base of the Mediterranean Pyramid includes fruits, vegetables, and grains (mostly whole). The Mediterranean Pyramid also highlights daily physical activity.

Whereas MyPlate does not make specific recommendations for protein food choices, the Mediterranean Pyramid recommends beans, other legumes, and nuts as daily sources of protein; fish, poultry, and eggs weekly; and red meat only about once each month. Also, for dairy choices, the Mediterranean Pyramid recommends cheese and yogurt in moderation and suggests drinking water or wine (in moderation) rather than milk.

Interestingly, the Mediterranean diet is not low in fat; in fact, about 40% of the total energy in this diet is derived from fat, which is much higher than the dietary fat recommendations made in the United States. This fact has led some nutritionists to criticize the Mediterranean diet; however, supporters point out that the majority of fats in the Mediterranean diet are plant oils, which are more healthful than the animal fats found in the US diet, and make the Mediterranean diet more protective against cardiovascular disease. (The benefits of plant oils in reducing our risk for heart disease are discussed in Chapter 5.)

Can following a Mediterranean-style diet really improve your health? Evidence has been growing since the mid-1990s indicating that it can lower the risk of recurrent heart attacks,[1] reduce the risks for some forms of cancer,[2] and lower the risk for obesity.[3] A recently published meta-analysis that combined the findings from fifty studies on over 530,000 individuals reported that the Mediterranean diet is consistently associated with a lower waist circumference, lower blood glucose and blood pressure, and a healthier blood lipid profile; taken together, these changes reduce one's risk for cardiovascular disease and type 2 diabetes.[4] These studies indicate that eating a Mediterranean-style diet that includes more fruits and vegetables, less meat, and few high-fat dairy products can reduce the risks for obesity, heart disease and some cancers.

References

1. Renaud, S., M. de Lorgeril, J. Delaye, J. Guidollet, F. Jacquard, N. Mamelle, J.-L. Martin, I. Monjaud, P. Salen, and P. Toubol. 1995. Cretan Mediterranean diet for prevention of coronary heart disease. *Am. J. Clin. Nutr.* 61(suppl.):1360S–1367S.

2. Tavani, A., and C. La Vecchia. 1995. Fruit and vegetable consumption and cancer risk in a Mediterranean population. *Am. J. Clin. Nutr.* 61(suppl):1374S–1377S.

3. Panagiotakos, D. B., C. Chrysohoou, C. Pitsavos, and C. Stefanadis. 2006. Association between the prevalence of obesity and adherence to the Mediterranean diet: the ATTICA study. *Nutrition* 22(5):449–456.

4. Kastorini, C.-M., H. J. Milionis, K. Esposito, D. Giugliano, J. A. Goudevenos, and D. B. Panagiotakos. 2011. The effect of Mediterranean diet on metabolic syndrome and its components. A meta-analysis of 50 studies and 534,906 individuals. *J. Am. Coll. Cardiol.* 57:1299–1313.

Of these variations, the Mediterranean diet has enjoyed considerable popularity. Does it deserve its reputation as a healthful diet? Check out the **Highlight** box (above) to learn more.

RECAP

The USDA Food Patterns can be used to plan a healthful, balanced diet that includes foods from the grains group, vegetables group, fruits group, dairy group, and protein foods group. As defined in the USDA Food Patterns, serving sizes typically are smaller than the amounts we normally eat or are served, so it is important to learn the definitions of serving sizes when using the USDA Food Patterns to design a healthful diet. There are many ethnic and cultural variations of the USDA Food Patterns. This flexibility enables anyone to design a diet that meets the goals of adequacy, moderation, balance, variety, and nutrient density. ■

FIGURE 2.11 The Mediterranean Diet Pyramid. (*Source:* © 2009 Oldways Preservation and Exchange Trust. www.oldwayspt.org. Reprinted by permission).

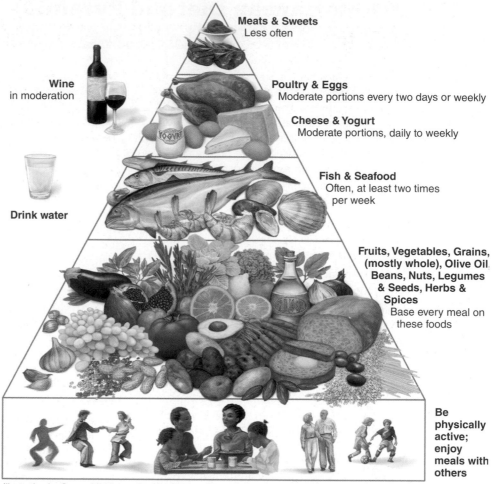

Meats & Sweets
Less often

Wine
in moderation

Poultry & Eggs
Moderate portions every two days or weekly

Cheese & Yogurt
Moderate portions, daily to weekly

Fish & Seafood
Often, at least two times per week

Drink water

Fruits, Vegetables, Grains, (mostly whole), Olive Oil, Beans, Nuts, Legumes & Seeds, Herbs & Spices
Base every meal on these foods

Be physically active; enjoy meals with others

Illustration by Geoge Middleton © 2009 Oldways Preservation and Exchange Trust www.oldwayspt.org

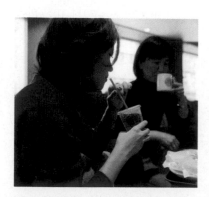

When ordering your favorite coffee drink, avoid those made with flavored syrups, cream, or whipping cream, and request reduced-fat or nonfat milk instead.

Can Eating Out Be Part of a Healthful Diet?

How many times each week do you eat out? A report from the US Department of Agriculture indicates that buying foods away from home now accounts for about half of all food expenditures, and almost 75% of consumers surveyed eat away from home at least once per week.[6] Full-service restaurants and fast-food outlets are the most common sources of foods eaten away from home. Research indicates that, in a given geographic area, there is a positive association between the number of restaurants per person and obesity levels in that area.[7] With so many people eating away from home, combined with recent estimates that more than 35% of all adults in the United States are classified as obese,[1] it is imperative that we learn how to eat more healthfully when eating out.

The Hidden Costs of Eating Out

Table 2.4 shows an example of foods served at McDonald's and Burger King restaurants. As you can see, a regular McDonald's hamburger has only 250 kcal, whereas the Big Mac has 540 kcal. A meal of a Big Mac, large french fries, and a small McCafé Chocolate Shake provides 1,620 kcal. This meal has enough energy to support an entire day's needs for a small, lightly active woman! Similar meals at Burger King and other fast-food chains are also very high in Calories, not to mention total fat and sodium.

TABLE 2.4 Nutritional Value of Selected Fast Foods

Menu Item	Kcal	Fat (g)	Fat (% kcal)	Sodium (mg)
McDonald's				
Hamburger	250	9	32	520
Cheeseburger	300	12	36	750
Quarter Pounder with cheese	510	26	46	1,190
Big Mac	540	29	48	1,040
French fries, small	230	11	43	160
French fries, medium	380	19	45	270
French fries, large	500	25	45	350
Coke, large	310	0	0	0
McCafé Chocolate Shake (small)	580	17	26	240
McCafé Chocolate Shake (large)	880	24	25	370
Burger King				
Hamburger	260	9	31	500
Cheeseburger	300	14	42	710
Whopper	670	40	54	980
Double Whopper	900	57	57	1,050
Bacon Double Cheeseburger	520	31	54	1,180
French fries, small	340	15	40	480
French fries, medium	410	18	40	570
French fries, large	500	22	40	7,100

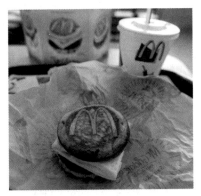

Foods served at fast-food chains are often high in Calories, total fat, and sodium. The popular McDonald's sausage, egg, and cheese McGriddles™ breakfast sandwiches, for example, contain 560 Calories, 32 g of fat, and 1,360 mg of sodium.

Fast-food restaurants are not alone in serving large portions. Most sit-down restaurants also serve large meals, which may include bread with butter, a salad with dressing, sides of vegetables and potatoes, and free refills of sugar-filled drinks. Combined with a high-fat appetizer like potato skins, fried onions, fried mozzarella sticks, or buffalo wings, it is easy to eat more than 2,000 kcal at one meal!

Does this mean that eating out cannot be a part of a healthful diet? Not necessarily. By becoming an educated consumer and making wise meal choices while dining out, you can enjoy both a healthful diet and the social benefits of eating out.

The Healthful Way to Eat Out

Most restaurants, even fast-food restaurants, offer lower-fat menu items that you can choose. For instance, eating a regular McDonald's hamburger, a

Nutrition
MILESTONE

Did you know that in the United States food guides in one form or another have been around for over 125 years? That's right! Back in **1885** a college chemistry professor named Wilber Olin Atwater helped bring the fledging science of nutrition to a broader audience by introducing scientific data boxes that became the basis for the first known US food guide. Those early dietary standards focused on defining the nutrition needs of an "average man" in terms of his daily consumption of proteins and Calories. These became food composition tables defined in three sweeping categories: protein, fats, and carbohydrate; mineral matter; and fuel values. As early as 1902, Atwater advocated for three foundational nutritional principles that we still support today; the concepts of variety, proportionality, and moderation in food choices and eating. (Check out Appendix A for related information on the development of the USDA Food Guide.)

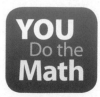

Determining the Healthiest Food Choices When Eating Out

Theo's friend and teammate, Jake, has put on extra weight over the basketball season. He had hoped to start more games this season, but their coach has made it clear that Jake needs to improve his fitness and lose the extra weight to be competitive as a starter.

Jake typically makes healthful food choices when he's on campus or at home, as he has a wide range of meals to choose from in the dining hall, and his family serves healthy foods when he visits them. But Jake really struggles to eat right when the team is on the road, as they typically frequent fast-food outlets or sit-down restaurants that serve meals high in Calories, saturated fat, and salt. Jake knows that Theo is taking a nutrition class and asks him for help in selecting healthier menu items when they are ordering their meals on the road. Theo is happy to help. Fortunately, the fast-food restaurant where they stop for dinner has posted at the counter the nutrition values (Calories, total fat [g and %Daily Value], saturated fat [g and %Daily Value], and sodium [g]) for their menu items. They agree that Jake should order a chicken sandwich, as Theo has learned that chicken has a much lower fat content than beef.

The menu items that Jake selected are

Jake's goal is to select food items that are lower in total Calories, % of Calories from fat, % of Calories from saturated fat, and sodium. As Theo examines these totals, he realizes that the %Daily Values for fat and saturated fat are based on a 2,000-Calorie-per-day intake—as Jake is a highly active male, this value is neither helpful nor appropriate. To determine the % of Calories from fat in the chicken sandwich, Theo does the following calculations:

a. Multiply the total fat (g) in the sandwich by 9 Calories (kcal)/g = 29 g × 9 Calories/g = 261 Calories from fat.

b. Divide the Calories from fat by the total Calories in the sandwich and multiply by 100 = (261 Calories ÷ 620 Calories) × 100 = 42% of total Calories comes from fat in the sandwich.

c. Multiply the saturated fat (g) in the sandwich by 9 Calories/g = 15 g × 9 Calories/g = 135 Calories from saturated fat.

d. Divide the Calories from saturated fat by total Calories in the sandwich = (135 Calories ÷ 620 Calories) = 21.8% of total Calories comes from saturated fat in the sandwich.

After thinking about these figures for % of Calories from fat and saturated fat, Jake decides to select a healthier sandwich that is lower in fat. He selects a grilled chicken club sandwich, at it has only 460 Calories, 16 g of fat, and 6 g of saturated fat.

Now you do the math to calculate the % total Calories from fat and % total Calories from saturated fat in the grilled chicken club sandwich.

What other changes could Jake make to his menu selections to reduce his total intake of Calories, fat, saturated fat, and sodium?

Menu Item	Calories	Total Fat (g)	Total Fat (%Daily Value)	Saturated Fat (g)	Saturated Fat (%Daily Value)	Sodium (g)
Chicken club sandwich	620	29	45%	15	37%	1,200
Large french fries	500	25	38%	3.5	17%	350
Ketchup (4 packets)	60	0	0%	0	0%	440
Side salad	20	0	0%	0	0%	10
Salad dressing (1 packet)	170	15	23%	2.5	12%	530
Total	1,370	69	Not applicable	21	Not applicable	2,530

small order of french fries, and a diet beverage or water provides 480 kcal and 20 g of fat (37.5% of kcal from fat). To provide some vegetables for the day, you could add a side salad with low-fat or nonfat salad dressing. Other fast-food restaurants also offer smaller portions, sandwiches made with whole-grain bread, grilled chicken or other lean meats, and side salads. Many sit-down restaurants offer "lite" menu items, such as grilled chicken and a variety of vegetables, which are usually a much better choice than eating from the regular menu.

Here are some other suggestions on how to eat out in moderation. Practice some of these suggestions every time you eat out:

- Avoid all-you-can-eat buffet-style restaurants.
- Avoid appetizers that are breaded, fried, or filled with cheese or meat, or skip the appetizer altogether.

- Order a healthful appetizer instead of a larger meal as your entrée.
- Order your meal from the children's menu.
- Share an entrée with a friend.
- Order broth-based soups instead of cream-based soups.
- If you order meat, select a lean cut and ask that it be grilled or broiled rather than fried or breaded.
- Instead of a beef burger, order a chicken burger, fish burger, or veggie burger.
- Order a meatless dish filled with vegetables and whole grains. Avoid dishes with cream sauces and a lot of cheese.
- Order a salad with low-fat or nonfat dressing served on the side.
- Order steamed vegetables on the side instead of potatoes or rice. If you order potatoes, make sure you get a baked potato (with very little butter or sour cream on the side).
- Order beverages with few or no Calories, such as water, tea, or diet drinks. Avoid coffee drinks made with syrups, as well as those made with cream, whipping cream, or whole milk.
- Don't feel you have to eat everything you're served. If you feel full, take the rest home for another meal.
- Skip dessert or share one dessert with a lot of friends, or order fresh fruit for dessert.
- Watch out for those "yogurt parfaits" offered at some fast-food restaurants. Many are loaded with sugar, fat, and Calories.

By following the suggestions in this list, you can eat out regularly and still maintain a healthful body weight.

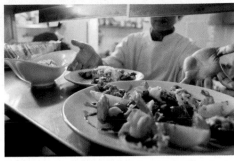

Eating out can be part of a healthful diet if you're careful to choose wisely.

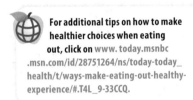 **For additional tips on how to make healthier choices when eating out, click on** www. today.msnbc .msn.com/id/28751264/ns/today-today_ health/t/ways-make-eating-out-healthy- experience/#.T4L_9-33CCQ.

RECAP

Healthful ways to eat out include choosing smaller menu items, ordering meats that are grilled or broiled, avoiding fried foods, choosing items with steamed vegetables, avoiding energy-rich appetizers and desserts, and eating less than half of the food you are served. ■

Chapter Review

TEST YOURSELF | ANSWERS

1. **F** A healthful diet can come in many forms, and particular attention must be paid to adequacy, variety, moderation, and balance. While consuming at least 5 servings of fruits and vegetables each day is important to maintain optimal health, a healthful diet should also include whole grains and cereals, meat or meat substitutes, dairy or dairy substitutes, and small amounts of healthful fats.

2. **F** Detailed food labels are not required for meat or poultry, as these products are regulated by the US Department of Agriculture, and coffee, fresh produce, and most spices are not required to have food labels, as they contain insignificant amounts of all the nutrients that must be listed on food labels.

3. **F** A cup of black coffee has about 5 kcal. Adding 2 teaspoons of sugar and a tablespoon of whole milk would increase that amount to about 45 kcal. In contrast, a café mocha might contain from 350 to 500 kcal, depending on its size and precise contents.

4. **F** The Dietary Guidelines for Americans recommend that people who choose to drink should do so sensibly and in moderation. Moderation is defined as no more than one drink per day for women and no more than two drinks per day for men.

5. **T** Although eating out poses many challenges, it is possible to eat a healthful diet when dining out. Ordering and/or consuming smaller portion sizes, selecting foods that are lower in fat and added sugars, and selecting eating establishments that serve more healthful foods can help.

Summary

- A healthful diet is adequate, moderate, balanced, and varied.

- The US Food and Drug Administration (FDA) regulates the content of food labels; food labels must contain a statement of identity, the net contents of the package, the contact information of the food manufacturer or distributor, an ingredient list, and nutrition information.

- The Nutrition Facts Panel on a food label contains important nutrition information about serving size; servings per package; total Calories and Calories of fat per serving; a list of various macronutrients, vitamins, and minerals; and the %Daily Values for the nutrients listed on the panel.

- The FDA regulates nutrient and health claims found on food labels; however, claims that a food contributes to body structure or function are not regulated.

- The Dietary Guidelines are general directives to promote health, reduce the risk for chronic diseases, and reduce the prevalence of overweight and obesity among Americans through improved nutrition and physical activity. This includes eating whole-grain foods, fruits, and vegetables daily; reducing intake of foods with unhealthful fats and cholesterol, salt, and added sugar; eating more foods rich in potassium, dietary fiber, calcium, and vitamin D; keeping food safe to eat; and drinking alcohol in moderation, if at all.

- The USDA Food Patterns provide a conceptual framework for the types and amounts of foods that make up a healthful diet. MyPlate is the graphic representation of the USDA Food Patterns. The groups in the USDA Food Patterns include grains, fruits, vegetables, dairy foods, and protein foods.

- The concept of empty Calories is emphasized in the USDA Food Patterns. Empty Calories are defined as Calories from solid fats and/or added sugars that provide few or no nutrients. The USDA recommends that you limit your consumption of empty Calories to a small number that fits your Calorie and nutrient needs depending on your age, gender, and level of physical activity.

■ Specific serving sizes are defined for foods in each group of the USDA Food Patterns. However, there is no standard definition for a serving size, and the serving sizes defined in the Food Patterns are generally smaller than those listed on food labels or in the servings generally sold to consumers.

■ There are many ethnic variations of the previous USDA Food Guide Pyramid, including the Mediterranean, Latin American, and Asian diet Pyramids.

■ Eating out can be challenging because of the high fat content and large serving sizes of many fast-food and sit-down restaurant menu items.

■ Behaviors that can improve the quality of your diet when eating out include choosing lower-fat meats that are grilled or broiled, eating vegetables and salads as side or main dishes, asking for low-fat salad dressing on the side, skipping high-fat desserts and appetizers, and drinking low-Calorie or non-Caloric beverages.

MasteringNutrition™

> To further your understanding, go online and apply what you've learned to real-life case studies that will help you master the content!

Review Questions

1. The Nutrition Facts Panel identifies which of the following?
   a. all of the nutrients and Calories in the package of food
   b. the Recommended Dietary Allowance for each nutrient found in the package of food
   c. a footnote identifying the Tolerable Upper Intake Level for each nutrient found in the package of food
   d. the %Daily Values of selected nutrients in a serving of the packaged food

2. An adequate diet is defined as a diet that
   a. provides enough energy to meet minimum daily requirements.
   b. provides enough of the energy, nutrients, and fiber to maintain a person's health.
   c. provides a sufficient variety of nutrients to maintain a healthful weight and to optimize the body's metabolic processes.
   d. contains combinations of foods that provide healthful proportions of nutrients.

3. The USDA Food Patterns recommend eating
   a. at least half your grains as whole grains each day.
   b. 6 to 11 servings of milk, cheese, and yogurt each day.
   c. 200 kcal to 500 kcal of empty Calories each day.
   d. 2 to 3 servings of fruit juice each day.

4. The Dietary Guidelines for Americans recommend which of the following?
   a. choosing and preparing foods without added salt
   b. consuming two alcoholic beverages per day
   c. being physically active each day
   d. following the Mediterranean diet

5. What does it mean to choose foods for their nutrient density?
   a. Dense foods, such as peanut butter or chicken, are more nutritious choices than transparent foods, such as mineral water or gelatin.
   b. Foods with a lot of nutrients per Calorie, such as fish, are more nutritious choices than foods with fewer nutrients per Calorie, such as candy.
   c. Calorie-dense foods, such as cheesecake, should be avoided.
   d. Fat makes foods dense, and thus foods high in fat should be avoided.

6. **True or false?** The USDA has written a standardized definition for a serving size for most foods.

7. **True or false?** Structure–function claims on food labels must be approved by the FDA.

8. **True or false?** Empty Calories are the extra amount of energy a person can consume after meeting all essential needs through eating nutrient-dense foods.

9. **True or false?** The USDA Food Patterns classify beans, peas, and lentils in both the vegetables group and the protein foods group.

10. **True or false?** About half of all Americans eat out at least once a week.

11. Defend the statement that no single diet can be appropriate for every human being.

12. You work for a food company that is introducing a new variety of soup. Design a label for this new soup, including all five label components required by the FDA.

13. Explain why the USDA Food Patterns identify a range in the number of suggested daily servings of each food group instead of telling us exactly how many servings of each food to eat each day.

14. If the label on a box of cereal claims that the cereal is "high in fiber," at least how much fiber does it provide per serving?

15. You are chatting with your nutrition classmate, Sylvia, about her attempts to lose weight. "I tried one of those low-carb diets," Sylvia confesses, "but I couldn't stick with it because bread and pasta are my favorite foods! Now I'm on the Mediterranean diet. I like it because it's a low-fat diet, so I'm sure to lose weight; plus, I can eat all the bread and pasta I want!" Do you think Sylvia's assessment of the Mediterranean diet is accurate? Why or why not?

Math Review

16. Hannah goes to a sandwich shop near the university at least once a week to buy what she considers a healthy lunch, which includes a chicken breast sandwich, garden salad (with Ranch dressing), and a diet cola. Recently, the shop started posting the Calorie and fat content of its menu items. Hannah discovers the following about the Calorie and fat content of the items in her "healthy lunch":
   - Chicken sandwich—317 Calories, 4 g fat
   - Garden salad—49 Calories, 1 g fat

   - Ranch dressing (1 packet)—280 Calories, 28 g fat
   - Diet cola—0 Calories, 0 g fat

   Based on this information, what is the total Calorie and fat content of Hannah's lunch? What is the percentage of Calories from fat for this lunch? Which food item is contributing the highest amount of fat to Hannah's lunch, and what can she do to make a healthier change to this lunch?

Answers to Review Questions and Math Review can be found online in the MasteringNutrition Study Area.

Web Links

www.fda.gov
US Food and Drug Administration (FDA)
Learn more about the government agency that regulates our food and first established regulations for nutrition information on food labels.

www.cnpp.usda.gov/dietaryguidelines
2010 Dietary Guidelines for Americans
Use these guidelines to make changes in your food choices and physical activity habits to help reduce your risk for chronic disease.

www.chooseMyPlate.gov/SuperTracker
The USDA's MyPlate Home Page
Use the SuperTracker on this website to assess the overall quality of your diet and level of physical activity based on the USDA MyPlate.

www.oldwayspt.org
Oldways Preservation and Exchange Trust
Find variations of ethnic and cultural food pyramids and recipes.

www.hp2010.nhlbihin.net/portion
National Institutes of Health (NIH) Portion Distortion Quiz
Take this short quiz to see if you know how today's food portions compare to those of 30 years ago.

www.diabetes.org
American Diabetes Association
Find out more about the nutritional needs of people living with diabetes, as well as meal-planning exchange lists.

www.eatright.org
Academy of Nutrition and Dietetics
Visit the Public Information Center section of this website for additional resources to help you achieve a healthful lifestyle.

www.hsph.harvard.edu/nutritionsource
Harvard School of Public Health
Search this site to learn more about the Healthy Eating Plate, an alternative to the USDA MyPlate.

References

1. Ogden, C. L., M. D. Carroll, B. K. Kit, and K. M. Flegal. 2012. Prevalence of obesity in the United States, 2009–2010. *NCHS Data Brief Number 82*, January. www.cdc.gov/nchs/data/databriefs/db82.htm.

2. US Department of Agriculture and US Department of Health and Human Services. 2010. *Dietary Guidelines for Americans, 2010*, 7th edn. Washington, DC: US Government Printing Office. www.cnpp.usda.gov/dietaryguidelines.htm.

3. Nielsen, S. J., and B. M. Popkin. 2003. Patterns and trends in food portion sizes, 1977–1998. *JAMA* 289(4):450–453.

4. Young, L. R., and M. Nestle. 2002. The contribution of expanding portion sizes to the US obesity epidemic. *Am. J. Pub. Health.* 92(2):246–249.

5. Food and Nutrition Information Center. 2010. Dietary Guidance. Ethnic/Cultural Food Pyramid. http://fnic.nal.usda.gov/nal_display/index.php?info_center=4&tax_level=3&tax_subject=256&topic_id=1348&level3_id=5732.

6. Steward, H., N. Blisard, and D. Joliffe. 2006. Let's Eat Out. Americans Weight Taste, Convenience and Nutrition. *U.S. Department of Agriculture. Economic Research Service. Economic Information Bulletin Number 19.* www.ers.usda.gov/publications/eib19/eib19.pdf.

7. Chou, S.-Y., M. Grossman, and H. Saffer. 2004. An economic analysis of adult obesity: results from the Behavior Risk Factor Surveillance System. *J. Health Econ.* 23:565–587.

Will Revising MyPyramid Promote America's Health?

As you learned in this chapter, the 2005 Dietary Guidelines for Americans (DGAs) were revised in 2010, and the accompanying graphic, MyPlate, and website, www.chooseMyPlate.gov, were released in 2011 to replace the previous MyPyramid versions. The revised DGAs and MyPlate were developed to address the concerns that many public health experts had voiced about the 2005 DGAs and MyPyramid. What were those concerns?

One major criticism was that the serving sizes suggested in MyPyramid were unrealistically small. Critics pointed out that they did not coincide with serving sizes listed on food labels or with servings that people usually eat.

A second criticism was that low-fat and low-Calorie food choices were not clearly defined in each food category. In particular, the 1-oz-equivalent servings of meat, poultry, fish, dry beans, eggs, and nuts suggested in MyPyramid were not differentiated by their fat content or by the type of fat they contain. Fish is low in fat and contains a more healthful type of fat than that found in red meats. In addition, although nuts are relatively high in fat, the type of fat in nuts is more healthful than that found in meats. MyPyramid failed to point out these differences, treating all foods in the protein foods group as equivalent choices.

In addition, MyPyramid recommended that at least half the grains eaten each day should be from whole-grain sources, allowing for eating half of your grain sources from refined foods. In reality, it is more healthful to make all your grain choices whole-grain foods.

Another criticism of MyPyramid was that it had limited value when used as a stand-alone graphic. Without the capacity to access the supplemental text and manipulate the interactive components available on the Internet, individuals could not personalize MyPyramid. Although it may be hard for many people to imagine, a considerable number of Americans still do not have access to the Internet, and many of those who do are not comfortable using interactive programming.

Do the revised DGAs and MyPlate address these criticisms and provide more useful tools to help Americans consume a more healthful diet and reduce their risks for obesity and related chronic diseases? A recent editorial written by experts in public health nutrition highlights some of the progress that has been achieved in the revised DGAs and MyPlate:[1]

- More extensive use of high-quality evidence in developing the guidelines
- Increased emphasis on eating more legumes and other vegetables, fruits, whole grains, and nuts
- Suggestions to replace red meat with fish and chicken
- Greater attention to replacing unhealthy fats with healthy fats

However, concerns about the limitations of these revised guidelines and tools continue. These include the following:

- The new guidelines still recommend that half of the grains we eat should be whole grains, and this continues to support eating half of our grains from refined, low-fiber sources. Some experts feel that the quality of the carbohydrates we consume needs more attention and specific guidance.[1]
- The new guidelines recommend that Americans consume at least 3 servings of dairy foods per day. Some experts feel that this level of dairy consumption is unnecessary, as some evidence suggests that dairy intake may not reduce the risk for bone fractures and could be associated with increased risk for ovarian and prostate cancers.[1,2]
- Although the revised guidelines focus on reducing solid fats and added sugars, more targeted advice specifically advising against the consumption of red meat, butter, cheese, and sugar may be needed to help people improve their dietary patterns.
- Although the DGAs address the benefits of regular physical activity, MyPlate does not illustrate this in any way. Some experts consider this a major oversight, as MyPyramid included a graphic of a person climbing stairs to highlight the importance of daily physical activity.

Given these limitations, it is unclear whether the revised DGAs and MyPlate can halt the current obesity epidemic or promote public health. Although the revisions are grounded in science, more research is needed on the impact of foods, rather than individual nutrients, on health outcomes. Such research should then inform the development of future recommendations. Experts have also called for moving the development of the guidelines to agencies such as the Centers for Disease Control and Prevention to avoid conflicts of interest that may arise within the US Department of Agriculture. They also recommend increased funding to allow for more frequent updates of the DRIs and comprehensive reviews of emerging literature on food patterns and health, as well as more explicit statements about foods that should be avoided or reduced in the diet.[1]

The Harvard School of Public Health has developed a Healthy Eating Plate as an alternative graphic to MyPlate (see Web Links for the URL). Following the design of MyPlate, the Healthy Eating Plate highlights using healthy oils, consuming virtually all grains as whole grains, selecting healthy protein sources, and drinking water, tea, or coffee with little or no added sugar. It also emphasizes daily physical activity. Because the release of MyPlate and the Healthy Eating Plate has been so recent, no studies are yet available comparing the effectiveness of these two graphic tools in reducing risks for obesity and related chronic diseases.

As you can imagine, a great deal of time, effort, and money was invested in the new message, content, and design of MyPlate. In making this investment, nutrition experts at the USDA intend that MyPlate will help reduce the alarmingly high obesity and chronic disease rates in the United States. The primary assumption made by these experts is that people will actually use MyPlate to design their diets. In fact, however, the extent to which people will use MyPlate in their daily lives is debatable.

Think about it; prior to taking this class, did you use the previous MyPyramid or the new MyPlate to help you design a healthful diet? It may be that you had not even seen the various food icons available, or if you did, you had no idea how to use them. This is the case for many Americans. Our work with community members throughout the United States has shown us that some people have no idea what such tools are, and many of those who have seen them do not know how to use them. Others who have tried to use them have found them confusing because of the limitations just discussed. Moreover, as with all government-supported recommendations, consumers

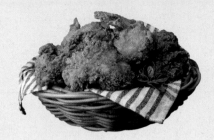

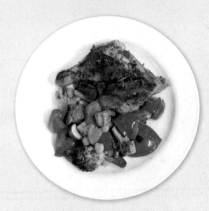

Will MyPlate help you select the most healthful option when you eat?

may not use the revised DGAs and MyPlate because they view them as another confusing mandate from experts who are out of touch with how "real" people eat and how they live their lives.

It is obvious that we need to address the obesity epidemic effectively. In doing so, one of the major challenges we face is to design nutrition recommendations and tools that millions of Americans can, and will, use. Experts in the Department of Health and Human Services intended that the more user-friendly graphic and food group organization of MyPlate would help Americans eat a more healthful diet and maintain a healthier body weight. But until more evidence of their impact on the rates of obesity and chronic disease is assessed, the debate about their value will continue.

CRITICAL THINKING QUESTIONS

- Do you feel that the revised MyPlate has adequately addressed the flaws of the previous USDA MyPyramid?

- Do you think that MyPlate can help people design a more healthful diet?

- Do you think MyPlate can help people lose weight and reduce our nation's rates of obesity and chronic diseases?

REFERENCES

1. Willett, W. C., and D. S. Ludwig. 2011. The 2010 Dietary Guidelines—the best recipe for health? *New Engl. J. Med.* 365(17):1563–1565.
2. World Cancer Research Fund. 2007. *Food, Nutrition, Physical Activity, and the Prevention of Cancer: A Global Perspective.* Washington, DC: American Institute for Cancer Research. www.dietandcancerreport.org/expert_report/.

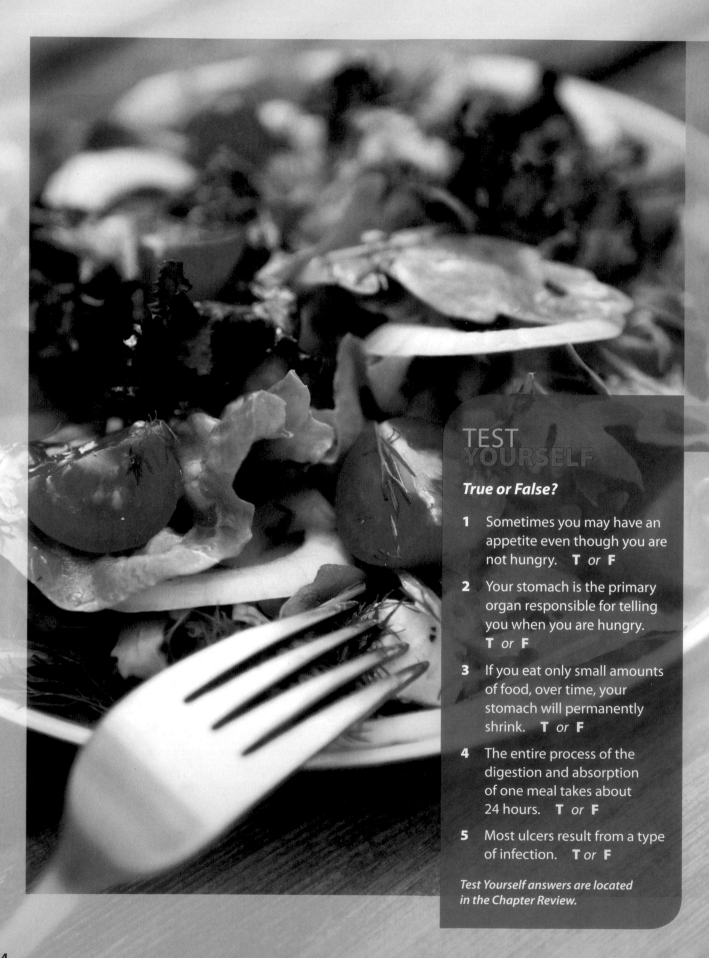

TEST YOURSELF

True or False?

1. Sometimes you may have an appetite even though you are not hungry.   **T** *or* **F**

2. Your stomach is the primary organ responsible for telling you when you are hungry. **T** *or* **F**

3. If you eat only small amounts of food, over time, your stomach will permanently shrink.   **T** *or* **F**

4. The entire process of the digestion and absorption of one meal takes about 24 hours.   **T** *or* **F**

5. Most ulcers result from a type of infection.   **T** *or* **F**

Test Yourself answers are located in the Chapter Review.

74

3 The Human Body: Are We Really What We Eat?

Learning Objectives

After studying this chapter, you should be able to:

1. Distinguish between appetite and hunger, describing the mechanisms, physiology, and other influences behind both conditions, *pp. 76–80.*

2. Draw a picture of the gastrointestinal tract, including all major and accessory organs, *p. 81.*

3. Describe the contribution of each organ of the gastrointestinal tract to the digestion, absorption, and elimination of food, *pp. 82–84, 86–89.*

4. Identify the source and function of the key enzymes involved in digesting foods, *p. 83.*

5. Explain the relationship (or lack of it) between stomach function and the pH scale, *p. 85.*

6. Identify the four major hormones involved in the regulation of the gastrointestinal tract and describe their primary action, *pp. 90–91.*

7. Discuss the roles of the gallbladder, pancreas, and liver in the digestion, absorption, and processing of nutrients, *pp. 92–93.*

8. List and describe the four types of absorption that occur in the small intestine, *pp. 94–96.*

9. Describe the causes, symptoms, and treatments of gastroesophageal reflux disease, ulcers, food allergies, celiac disease, vomiting, inflammatory bowel diseases, and functional gastrointestinal disorders, *pp. 100–109.*

MasteringNutrition™

Go online for chapter quizzes, pre-tests, Interactive Activities and more!

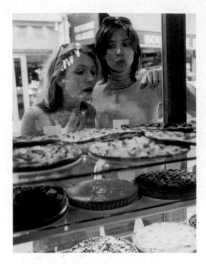

Foods that are artfully prepared, arranged, or ornamented, such as cakes and pies in a bakery display case, appeal to our sense of sight.

Two months ago, Andrea's lifelong dream of becoming a lawyer came one step closer to reality: she moved out of her parents' home in the Midwest to attend law school in Boston. Unfortunately, the adjustment to a new city, new friends, and her intensive course work was more stressful than she'd imagined, and Andrea has been experiencing insomnia and exhaustion. What's more, her always "sensitive stomach" has been getting worse: after every meal, she gets cramps so bad that she can't stand up, and twice she has missed classes because of sudden attacks of pain and diarrhea. She suspects that the problem is related to stress and wonders if she is going to experience it throughout her life. She is even thinking of dropping out of school if that would make her feel well again.

Almost everyone experiences brief episodes of abdominal pain, diarrhea, or other symptoms from time to time. Such episodes are often caused by eating too much or too quickly, food poisoning, or an infection such as influenza. But do you know anyone who experiences these symptoms periodically for days, weeks, or even years? If so, has it made you wonder why? What are the steps in normal digestion and absorption of food, and at what points can the process break down?

We begin this chapter with a look at some of the factors that make us feel as if we want to eat. We then discuss the physiologic processes by which the body digests and absorbs food and eliminates waste products. Finally, we look at some disorders that affect these processes.

Why Do We Want to Eat What We Want to Eat?

You've just finished eating at your favorite Thai restaurant. As you walk back to the block where you parked your car, you pass a bakery window displaying several cakes and pies, each of which looks more enticing than the last, and through the door wafts a complex aroma of coffee, cinnamon, and chocolate. You stop. You know you're not hungry, but you go inside and buy a slice of chocolate torte and an espresso, anyway. Later that night, when the caffeine from the chocolate and espresso keep you awake, you wonder why you succumbed.

Two mechanisms prompt us to seek food: **hunger** is a physiologic drive for food that occurs when the body senses that we need to eat. The drive is *nonspecific;* when you're hungry, a variety of foods could satisfy you. If you've recently finished a nourishing meal, then hunger probably won't compel you toward a slice of chocolate torte. Instead, the culprit is likely to be **appetite,** a psychological desire to consume *specific* foods. It is aroused when environmental cues—such as the sight of chocolate cake or the smell of coffee—stimulate our senses, prompting pleasant emotions and often memories.

People commonly experience appetite in the absence of hunger. That's why you can crave cake and coffee even after eating a full meal. On the other hand, it is possible to have a physiologic need for food yet have no appetite. This state, called *anorexia,* can accompany a variety of illnesses from infectious diseases to mood disorders. It can also occur as a side effect of certain medications, such as the chemotherapy used in treating cancer patients. (Anorexia is covered *In Depth* in Chapter 13.5.) Although in the following sections we describe hunger and appetite as separate entities, ideally the two states coexist: we seek specific, appealing foods to satisfy a physiologic need for nutrients.

The Hypothalamus Prompts Hunger in Response to Various Signals

Because hunger is a physiologic stimulus that drives us to find food and eat, often we experience it as an unpleasant sensation. The primary organ producing that sensation is the brain. That's right—it's not our stomachs, but our brains that tell us when we're hungry. The region of brain tissue that is responsible for prompting us to seek food is called the **hypothalamus** (**Figure 3.1**). It's located just above the pituitary gland and brain stem in a region of the brain

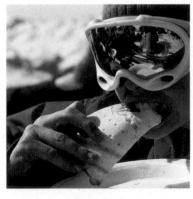

Hunger is a physiologic stimulus that prompts us to find food and eat.

hunger A physiologic sensation that prompts us to eat.

appetite A psychological desire to consume specific foods.

hypothalamus A region of the brain below (*hypo*-) the thalamus and cerebral hemispheres and above the pituitary gland and brain stem where visceral sensations such as hunger and thirst are regulated.

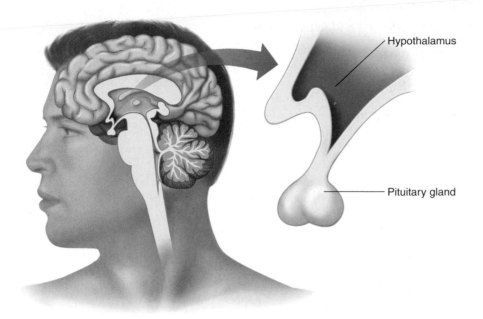

FIGURE 3.1 The hypothalamus triggers hunger by integrating signals from nerve cells throughout the body, as well as from messages carried by hormones.

responsible for regulating many types of involuntary activity. The hypothalamus triggers feelings of hunger or satiation (fullness) by integrating signals from nerve cells in other body regions and from chemical messengers called hormones. Even the amount and type of food we eat influence the hypothalamus to cause us to feel hungry or full. Let's now examine these three types of signals generated from nerve cells, hormones, and the food we eat.

The Role of Nerve Cells

One hunger-regulating signal comes from special cells lining the stomach and small intestine that detect changes in pressure according to whether the organ is empty or distended with food. The cells relay these data to the hypothalamus. For instance, if you have not eaten for many hours and your stomach and small intestine do not contain food, this information is sent to the hypothalamus, which in turn prompts you to experience the sensation of hunger.

The Role of Hormones

Hormones are chemical messengers that are secreted into the bloodstream by one of the many *endocrine glands* of the body. Their presence in the blood helps regulate one or more body functions. Insulin and glucagon are two hormones produced in the pancreas. They are responsible for maintaining blood glucose levels. *Glucose,* a simple sugar, is our bodies' most readily available fuel supply. It's not surprising, then, that its level in our blood is an important signal regulating hunger. When we have not eaten for a while, our blood glucose levels fall, prompting a change in the levels of insulin and glucagon. This chemical message is relayed to the hypothalamus, which then prompts us to eat in order to supply our bodies with more glucose.

After we eat, the hypothalamus picks up the sensation of a distended stomach, other signals from the gut, and a rise in blood glucose levels. When it integrates these signals, we have the experience of feeling full, or *satiated.* However, as noted, even though the brain sends us clear signals about hunger, most of us become adept at ignoring them, and we eat when we are not truly hungry.

In addition to insulin and glucagon, a variety of other hormones and hormone-like substances signal the hypothalamus to cause us to feel hungry or satiated. The various hormones involved in digestion are discussed later in this chapter.

hormone A chemical messenger that is secreted into the bloodstream by one of the many endocrine glands of the body. Hormones act as regulators of physiologic processes at sites remote from the glands that secreted them.

The Role of Amount and Type of Food

Foods containing protein have the highest satiety value.[1] This means that a ham-and-egg breakfast will cause us to feel satiated for a longer period of time than will pancakes with maple syrup, even if both meals have exactly the same number of Calories. High-fat meals have a higher satiety value than high-carbohydrate meals.

Another factor affecting hunger is how bulky the meal is—that is, how much fiber and water are within the food. Bulky meals tend to stretch the stomach and small intestine, which sends signals back to the hypothalamus telling us that we are full, so we stop eating. Beverages tend to be less satisfying than semisolid foods, and semisolid foods have a lower satiety value than solid foods. For example, if you were to eat a bunch of grapes, you would feel a greater sense of fullness than if you drank a glass of grape juice.

Environmental Cues Trigger Appetite

Whereas hunger is prompted by internal signals, appetite is triggered by aspects of our environment. The most significant factors influencing our appetite are sensory data, social and cultural cues, and learning (**Figure 3.2**).

The Role of Sensory Data

Foods stimulate our five senses. Foods that are artfully prepared, arranged, or ornamented appeal to our sense of sight. Food producers know this and spend millions of dollars annually in the United States to promote and package their products in an appealing way.

The aromas of foods can also be powerful stimulants. Much of our ability to taste foods actually comes from our sense of smell. This is why foods are not as appealing when we have a stuffy nose due to a cold. Certain tastes, such as sweetness, are almost universally appealing, whereas others, such as the astringent taste of foods like spinach and kale, are quite individual. Because many natural poisons and spoiled foods are intensely sour or bitter, our distaste for these sensations is thought to be protective.[1]

Texture, or "mouth feel," is also important in food choices, as it stimulates nerve endings sensitive to touch in our mouths and on our tongues. Even our sense of hearing can be stimulated by foods, from the fizz of cola to the crunch of corn chips.

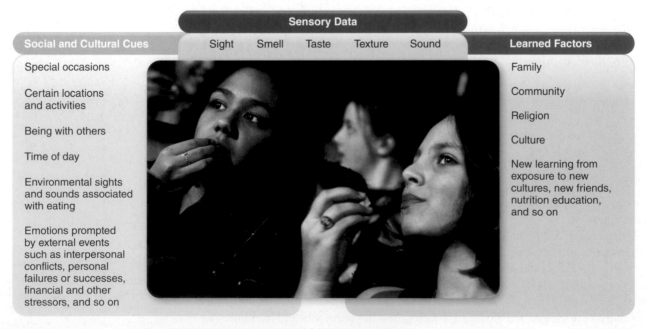

FIGURE 3.2 Appetite is a drive to consume specific foods, such as popcorn at the movies. It is aroused by social and cultural cues and sensory data and is influenced by learning.

The Role of Social and Cultural Cues

In addition to sensory cues, the brain's association with certain social events, such as birthday parties or holiday gatherings, can stimulate our appetite. At these times, our culture gives us permission to eat more than usual or to eat "forbidden" foods.

For some people, being in a certain location, such as at a baseball game or a movie theater, can trigger appetite. Others may get the munchies whenever they watch television or study, or at certain times of day. Many people feel an increase or a decrease in appetite according to whom they are with; for example, they may eat more when at home with family members and less when out on a date. Even visual cues can trigger appetite. Do you start thinking about food every time you pass your refrigerator?

In some cases, appetite masks an emotional response to an external event. For example, after receiving a failing grade or arguing with a close friend, a person might experience a desire for food rather than a desire for emotional comfort. Many people crave food when they're frustrated, worried, or bored or when they are at a party or other gathering where they feel anxious or awkward. Others subconsciously seek food as a "reward." For example, have you ever found yourself heading out for a burger and fries after handing in a term paper?

The Role of Learning

Pigs' feet, anyone? What about blood sausage, stewed octopus, or tripe? These are delicacies in various European cultures. Would you eat grasshoppers? If you'd grown up in certain parts of Africa or Central America, you probably would. That's because your preference for particular foods is largely a learned response. The family, community, religion, and/or culture in which you're raised teach you what plant and animal products are appropriate to eat. If your parents fed you cubes of plain tofu throughout your toddlerhood, then you are probably still eating tofu now.

That said, early introduction to foods is not essential: we can learn to enjoy new foods at any point in our life. Immigrants from developing nations settling in the United States or Canada often adopt a typical Western diet, especially when their traditional foods are not readily available. This happens temporarily when we travel: the last time you were away from home, you probably enjoyed sampling dishes that are not normally part of your diet.

Food preferences also change when people learn what foods are most healthful in terms of nutrient density and the prevention of chronic diseases. Since reading the preceding chapters (Chapters 1 and 2), has your diet changed at all? Chances are, as you learn more about the health benefits of specific types of carbohydrates, fats, and proteins, you'll quite naturally start incorporating more of these foods into your diet.

We can also "learn" to dislike foods we once enjoyed. For example, if we experience an episode of food poisoning after eating undercooked scrambled eggs, we might develop a strong distaste for all types of cooked eggs. Many adults who become vegetarians do so after learning about the treatment of animals in slaughterhouses: they might have eaten meat daily when young but no longer have any appetite for it.

Now that you know the difference between hunger and appetite, you might be wondering which of these states most often motivates you to eat. If so, check out the feature box **Highlight: Do You Eat in Response to External or Internal Cues?** (page 80).

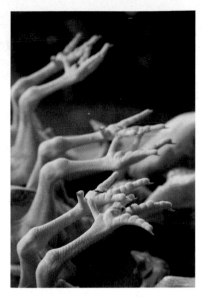

Food preferences are influenced by the family and culture in which you are raised.

RECAP

Hunger is a physiologic sensation triggered by the hypothalamus in response to cues about stomach and intestinal distention and the levels of certain hormones and hormone-like substances. Appetite is a psychological desire to consume specific foods. It is triggered when external stimuli arouse our senses, and it often occurs in combination with social and cultural cues. Our preference for certain foods is largely learned from the culture in which we were raised, but our food choices can change with exposure to new foods or new learning experiences. ■

HIGHLIGHT

Do You Eat in Response to External or Internal Cues?

In this chapter, you learn the differences between appetite and hunger, as well as the influence of learning on food choices. So now you might be curious to investigate your own reasons for eating what and when you do. Whether you're trying to lose weight, gain weight, or maintain your current healthful weight, you'll probably find it intriguing to keep a log of the reasons behind your decisions about what, when, where, and why you eat. Are you eating in response to internal sensations telling you that your body *needs* food, or in response to your emotions, a situation, or a prescribed diet? Keeping a "cues" log for 1 full week would give you the most accurate picture of your eating habits, but even logging 2 days of meals and snacks should increase your cue awareness.

Each day, every time you eat a meal, snack, or beverage other than water, make a quick note of the following:

- **When you eat.** Many people eat at certain times (for example, 6 PM) whether they are hungry or not.

- **What you eat and how much.** A cup of yogurt and a handful of nuts? An apple? A 20-oz cola?

- **Where you eat.** This includes while sitting at the dining room table, watching television, driving in the car, and so on.

- **With whom you eat.** Are you alone or with others? If with others, are they eating as well? Have they offered you food?

- **Your emotions.** Many people overeat when they are happy, especially when celebrating with others. Some people eat excessively when they are anxious, depressed, bored, or frustrated. Still others eat as a way of denying feelings because they don't want to identify and deal with them. For some, food becomes a substitute for emotional fulfillment.

- **Your sensations: what you see, hear, or smell.** Are you eating because you walked past the kitchen and spied a batch of homemade cookies or smelled coffee roasting?

- **Any dietary restrictions.** Are you choosing a particular food because it is allowed on your current diet plan? Or are you hungry but drinking a diet soda to stay within a certain allowance of Calories? Are you restricting yourself because you feel guilty about having eaten too much at another time?

- **Your physiologic hunger.** Rate your hunger on a scale from 1 to 5 as follows:
  1 = you feel full or even stuffed
  2 = you feel satisfied but not uncomfortably full
  3 = neutral; you feel no discernible satiation nor hunger
  4 = you feel hungry and want to eat
  5 = you feel strong physiologic sensations of hunger and need to eat

After keeping a log for 2 or more days, you might become aware of patterns you'd like to change. For example, maybe you notice that you often eat when you are not actually hungry but are worried about homework or personal relationships. Or maybe you notice that you can't walk past the snack bar without going in. This self-awareness may prompt you to take positive steps to change those patterns. For instance, instead of stifling your worries with food, write down exactly what you are worried about, including steps you can take to address your concerns. And the next time you approach the snack bar, before going in, check with your gut: are you truly hungry? If so, then purchase a healthful snack, maybe a yogurt, a piece of fruit, or a bag of peanuts. If you're not really hungry, then take a moment to acknowledge the strength of this visual cue—and then walk on by.

What Happens to the Food We Eat?

digestion The process by which foods are broken down into their component molecules, either mechanically or chemically.

absorption The physiologic process by which molecules of food are taken from the gastrointestinal tract into the circulation.

elimination The process by which the undigested portions of food and waste products are removed from the body.

gastrointestinal (GI) tract A long, muscular tube consisting of several organs: the mouth, esophagus, stomach, small intestine, and large intestine.

When we eat, the food we consume is digested; then the useful nutrients are absorbed; and, finally, the waste products are eliminated. But what does each of these processes really entail? In the simplest terms, **digestion** is the process by which foods are broken down into their component molecules, either mechanically or chemically. **Absorption** is the process of taking these products of digestion through the wall of the intestine. **Elimination** is the process by which the undigested portions of food and waste products are removed from the body.

The processes of digestion, absorption, and elimination occur in the **gastrointestinal (GI) tract,** the organs of which work together to process foods. The GI tract is a long tube: if held out straight, an adult GI tract would be close to 30 feet in length. Food within this tube is digested; in other words, food is broken down into molecules small enough to be absorbed by the cells lining the GI tract and thereby passed into the body.

The GI tract begins at the mouth and ends at the anus (**Figure 3.3**). It is composed of several distinct organs, including the mouth, esophagus, stomach, small intestine, and

The digestive system consists of the organs of the gastrointestinal (GI) tract and associated accessory organs. The processing of food in the GI tract involves ingestion, mechanical digestion, chemical digestion, propulsion, absorption, and elimination.

ORGANS OF THE GI TRACT

MOUTH

Ingestion Food enters the GI tract via the mouth.

Mechanical digestion Mastication tears, shreds, and mixes food with saliva.

Chemical digestion Salivary amylase begins carbohydrate breakdown.

PHARYNX AND ESOPHAGUS

Propulsion Swallowing and peristalsis move food from mouth to stomach.

STOMACH

Mechanical digestion Mixes and churns food with gastric juice into a liquid called chyme.

Chemical digestion Pepsin begins digestion of proteins, and gastric lipase begins to break lipids apart.

Absorption A few fat-soluble substances are absorbed through the stomach wall.

SMALL INTESTINE

Mechanical Digestion and **Propulsion** Segmentation mixes chyme with digestive juices; peristaltic waves move it along tract.

Chemical digestion Digestive enzymes from pancreas and brush border digest most classes of nutrients.

Absorption Nutrients are absorbed into blood and lymph through enterocytes.

LARGE INTESTINE

Chemical digestion Some remaining food residues are digested by bacteria.

Absorption Reabsorbs salts, water, and vitamins.

Propulsion Compacts waste into feces and propels it toward the rectum.

RECTUM

Elimination Temporarily stores feces before voluntary release through the anus.

ACCESSORY ORGANS

SALIVARY GLANDS

Produce saliva, a mixture of water, mucus, enzymes, and other chemicals.

LIVER

Produces bile to digest fats.

GALLBLADDER

Stores bile before release into the small intestine through the bile duct.

PANCREAS

Produces digestive enzymes and bicarbonate, which are released into the small intestine via the pancreatic duct.

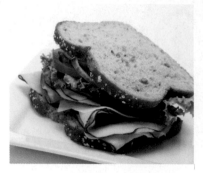

Digestion of a sandwich starts before you even take a bite.

sphincter   A tight ring of muscle separating some of the organs of the GI tract and opening in response to nerve signals indicating that food is ready to pass into the next section.

cephalic phase   The earliest phase of digestion, in which the brain thinks about and prepares the digestive organs for the consumption of food.

saliva   A mixture of water, mucus, enzymes, and other chemicals that moistens the mouth and food, binds food particles together, and begins the digestion of carbohydrates.

salivary glands   A group of glands found under and behind the tongue and beneath the jaw that releases saliva continually as well as in response to the thought, sight, smell, or presence of food.

large intestine. The flow of food between these organs is controlled by muscular **sphincters,** which are tight rings of muscle that open when a nerve signal indicates that food is ready to pass into the next section. The sphincters associated with each region of the GI tract are shown in several figures later in this chapter. Surrounding the GI tract are several accessory organs, including the salivary glands, liver, pancreas, and gallbladder, each of which has a specific role in the digestion and absorption of nutrients.

Now let's take a look at the roles of these organs. Imagine that you ate a turkey sandwich for lunch today. It contained two slices of bread spread with mayonnaise, some turkey, two lettuce leaves, and a slice of tomato. Let's travel along with the sandwich and see what happens as it enters your GI tract and is digested and absorbed into your body.

Digestion Begins in the Mouth

Believe it or not, the first step in the digestive process is not your first bite of that sandwich. It is your first thought about what you wanted for lunch as you stood in line at the deli. In this **cephalic phase** of digestion, hunger and appetite work together to prepare the GI tract to digest food. The nervous system stimulates the release of digestive juices in preparation for food entering the GI tract, and sometimes we experience some involuntary movement commonly called "hunger pangs."

Now, let's stop smelling that sandwich and take a bite and chew! Chewing moistens the food and mechanically breaks it down into pieces small enough to swallow (**Figure 3.4**). The presence of food initiates not only mechanical digestion via chewing but also chemical digestion through the secretion of hormones and other substances throughout the gastrointestinal tract. As the teeth cut and grind the different foods in the sandwich, more surface area of the foods is exposed to the digestive juices in the mouth. Foremost among these is **saliva,** which is secreted from the **salivary glands.**

Without saliva, we could not taste the foods we eat. That's because taste occurs when chemicals dissolved in saliva bind to chemoreceptors called *taste receptors* located in structures called *taste buds* on the surface of the tongue. Taste receptors are able to detect at least five distinct tastes: bitter, sweet, salty, sour, and *umami,* a savory taste due to the presence of glutamic acid, an amino acid that occurs naturally in meats and other protein-rich foods. Flavors, such as turkey or tomato, reflect complex combinations of these five basic tastes. As noted earlier, taste depends significantly on the sense of smell, called *olfaction.* To achieve

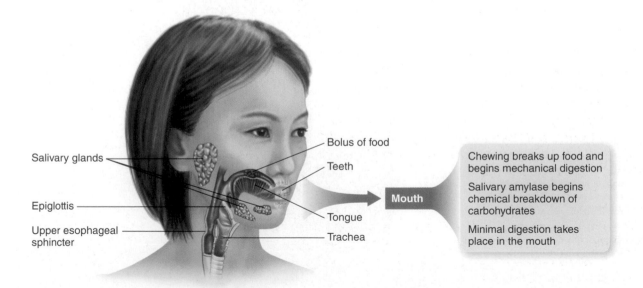

Salivary glands

Epiglottis

Upper esophageal sphincter

Bolus of food

Teeth

Tongue

Trachea

Mouth

Chewing breaks up food and begins mechanical digestion

Salivary amylase begins chemical breakdown of carbohydrates

Minimal digestion takes place in the mouth

FIGURE 3.4 Where your food is now: the mouth. Chewing moistens food and mechanically breaks it down into pieces small enough to swallow, while salivary amylase begins the chemical digestion of carbohydrates.

olfaction, odorants dissolved in mucus bind to chemoreceptors in the nasal cavity called *olfactory receptor cells.* These cells then transmit their data to the olfactory bulb of the brain.

Saliva also initiates the chemical digestion of carbohydrates. It accomplishes this through the actions of salivary amylase, a digestive enzyme. **Enzymes** are compounds, usually proteins, that act as catalysts; that is, they induce chemical changes in other substances to speed up bodily processes. They can be reused because they essentially are unchanged by the chemical reactions they catalyze. Salivary amylase is only one of many enzymes that assist the body in digesting foods. We make hundreds of enzymes in our bodies, and not only digestion but many other biochemical processes as well could not happen without them. By the way, enzyme names usually end in *-ase*, so they are easy to recognize as we go through the digestive process. Various amylases assist in the digestion of carbohydrates, lipases are involved with lipid digestion, and proteases help digest proteins.

Saliva contains many other components, including the following:

- Bicarbonate, which helps neutralize acids
- Mucus, which moistens the food and the oral cavity, ensuring that food easily travels down the esophagus
- Antibodies, proteins that defend against bacteria entering the mouth
- Lysozyme, an enzyme that inhibits bacterial growth in the mouth and may assist in preventing tooth decay

In reality, very little digestion occurs in the mouth. This is because we do not hold food in our mouth for very long and because not all of the enzymes needed to break down foods are present in saliva. Salivary amylase starts the digestion of carbohydrates in the mouth, and this digestion continues until food reaches the stomach. Once in the stomach, salivary amylase is no longer active because it is destroyed by the acidic environment of the stomach.

The Esophagus Propels Food into the Stomach

The mass of food that has been chewed and moistened in the mouth is referred to as a **bolus.** This bolus is swallowed (**Figure 3.5**) and propelled to the stomach through the esophagus. Most of us take swallowing for granted. However, it is a very complex process involving voluntary and involuntary motion. A tiny flap of tissue called the *epiglottis* acts

enzymes Small chemicals, usually proteins, that act on other chemicals to speed up bodily processes but are not changed during those processes.

bolus A mass of food that has been chewed and moistened in the mouth.

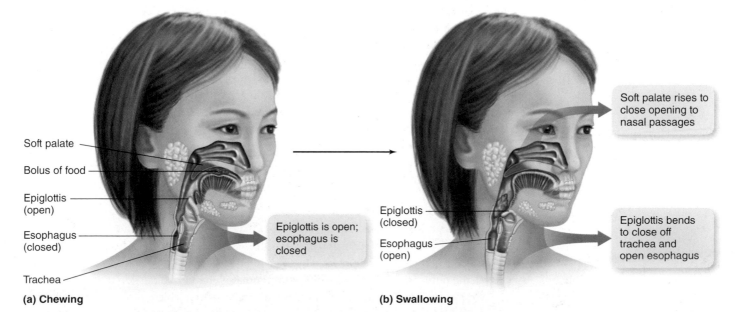

Soft palate rises to close opening to nasal passages

Soft palate

Bolus of food

Epiglottis (open)

Esophagus (closed)

Trachea

Epiglottis is open; esophagus is closed

Epiglottis (closed)

Esophagus (open)

Epiglottis bends to close off trachea and open esophagus

(a) Chewing

(b) Swallowing

FIGURE 3.5 Chewing and swallowing are complex processes. **(a)** During the process of chewing, the epiglottis is open and the esophagus is closed, so that we can continue to breathe as we chew. **(b)** During swallowing, the epiglottis closes, so that food does not enter the trachea and obstruct our breathing. Also, the soft palate rises to seal off the nasal passages to prevent the aspiration of food or liquid into the sinuses.

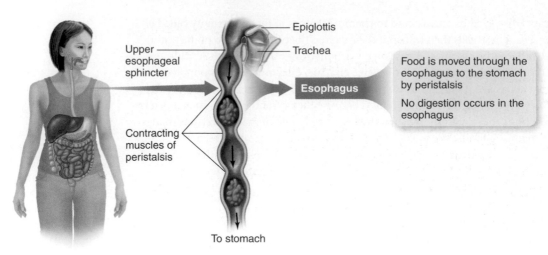

- Epiglottis
- Trachea
- Upper esophageal sphincter
- Contracting muscles of peristalsis
- Esophagus
- To stomach

Food is moved through the esophagus to the stomach by peristalsis

No digestion occurs in the esophagus

FIGURE 3.6 Where your food is now: the esophagus. Peristalsis, the rhythmic contraction and relaxation of both circular and longitudinal muscles in the esophagus, propels food toward the stomach. Peristalsis occurs throughout the GI tract.

as a trapdoor covering the entrance to the trachea (windpipe). The epiglottis is normally open, allowing us to breathe freely even while chewing (Figure 3.5a). As our bite of sandwich moves to the very back of the mouth, the brain is sent a signal to temporarily raise the soft palate and close the openings to the nasal passages, preventing aspiration of food or liquid into the sinuses (Figure 3.5b). The brain also signals the epiglottis to close during swallowing, so that food and liquid cannot enter the trachea. Sometimes this protective mechanism goes awry—for instance, when we try to eat and talk at the same time. When this happens, we experience the sensation of choking and typically cough involuntarily and repeatedly until the offending food or liquid is expelled from the trachea.

As the trachea closes, the sphincter muscle at the top of the esophagus, called the *upper esophageal sphincter*, opens to allow the passage of food. The **esophagus** then transports the food to the stomach (**Figure 3.6**). A muscular tube, the esophagus propels food along its length by contracting two sets of muscles: inner sheets of circular muscle squeeze the food, while outer sheets of longitudinal muscle push food along the length of the tube. Together, these rhythmic waves of squeezing and pushing are called **peristalsis.** We will see later in this chapter that peristalsis occurs throughout the GI tract.

Gravity also helps transport food down the esophagus, which is one reason it is wise to sit or stand upright while eating. Together, peristalsis and gravity can transport a bite of food from the mouth to the opening of the stomach in 5 to 8 seconds. At the end of the esophagus is another sphincter muscle, the *gastroesophageal sphincter* (*gastro-* indicates the stomach), also referred to as the *lower esophageal sphincter,* which is normally tightly closed. When food reaches the end of the esophagus, this sphincter relaxes to allow the passage of food into the stomach. In some people, this sphincter is continually somewhat relaxed. Later in the chapter, we'll discuss this disorder and the unpleasant symptoms it can prompt.

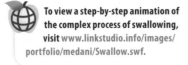

To view a step-by-step animation of the complex process of swallowing, visit www.linkstudio.info/images/portfolio/medani/Swallow.swf.

esophagus A muscular tube of the GI tract connecting the back of the mouth to the stomach.

peristalsis Waves of squeezing and pushing contractions that move food, chyme, and feces in one direction through the length of the GI tract.

RECAP

The cephalic phase of digestion prepares the GI tract for digestion. Chewing initiates the mechanical digestion of food by breaking it into smaller components and mixing all the nutrients together. Chewing also stimulates chemical digestion through the secretion of digestive juices, such as saliva, a component of which is the enzyme salivary amylase. Swallowing causes the nasal passages to close and the epiglottis to cover the trachea to prevent food from entering the sinuses and lungs. The upper esophageal sphincter opens as the trachea closes. The esophagus is a muscular tube that transports food from the mouth to the stomach via peristalsis. Once food reaches the stomach, the gastroesophageal sphincter opens to allow food into the stomach. ■

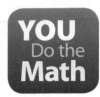

Negative Logarithms and the pH Scale

Have you ever been warned that the black coffee, orange juice, or cola you enjoy is corroding your stomach? If so, relax. It's an urban myth. How can you know for sure? Take a look at the pH scale (**Figure 3.7**). As you can see, the scale shows that hydrochloric acid (HCl) has a pH of 1.0 and gastric juice is 2.0, whereas soft drinks (including cola) are 3.0, orange juice is 4.0, and black coffee is 5.0. Not sure what all of these numbers mean?

An abbreviation for the *potential of hydrogen*, pH is a measure of the hydrogen ion concentration of a solution, or more precisely, the potential of a substance to release or to take up hydrogen ions in solution. Since an acid by definition is a compound that releases hydrogen ions, and a base is a compound that binds them, we can also say that pH is a measure of a compound's acidity or alkalinity. The precise measurements of pH range from 0 to 14, with 7.0 designated as pH neutral. Pure water is exactly neutral, and human blood is close to neutral, normally ranging from about 7.35 to 7.45.

The pH scale is a negative base-10 logarithmic scale. As you may recall from high school math classes, a base-10 logarithm ($\log_{10}$) tells you how many times you multiply by 10 to get the desired number. For example, $\log_{10}(1{,}000) = 3$ because to get 1,000 you have to multiply 10 three times ($10 \times 10 \times 10$). The pH scale is negative because an *increased* number on the scale identifies a corresponding *decrease* in concentration. These facts taken together mean that:

- For every increase of a single digit, the concentration of hydrogen ions decreases by ten-fold.
- For every decrease of a single digit, the concentration of hydrogen ions increases by ten-fold.

For example, milk has a pH of 6, which is one digit lower than 7. Milk is therefore ten times more acidic than pure water. Baking soda, at pH 9, is two digits higher than 7, and thus baking soda is 100 times less acidic than pure water: $2 = \log_{10}(100)$.

Now you do the math:

1. Is the pH of blood normally slightly acidic or slightly alkaline (basic)?

2. Identify the relative acidity of black coffee as compared to pure water and as compared to HCl.

3. Identify the relative acidity of soft drinks as compared to pure water and as compared to HCl.

If you answered correctly, you can appreciate the fact that, since the tissues lining your stomach wall are adequately protected (by mucus and bicarbonate) from the acidity of HCl, they are not likely to be damaged by coffee, cola, or any other standard beverage. On the other hand, if you were to down an entire bottle of pure lemon juice (pH 2.0), the release of all those additional hydrogen ions into the already acidic environment of your stomach would likely make you very sick. Your blood pH would drop, your breathing rate would increase, and you would almost certainly vomit. However, the juice would not corrode your stomach.

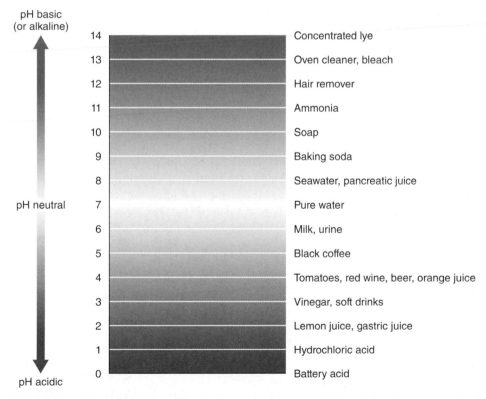

FIGURE 3.7 The pH scale identifies the levels of acidity or alkalinity of various substances. More specifically, pH is defined as the negative logarithm of the hydrogen–ion concentration of any solution. Each one-unit change in pH from high to low represents a tenfold increase in the concentration of hydrogen ions. This means that gastric juice, which has a pH of 2, is 100,000 times more acidic than pure water, which has a pH of 7.

The Stomach Mixes, Digests, and Stores Food

The **stomach** is a J-shaped organ. Its size varies with different individuals; in general, its volume is about 6 fluid ounces (¾ cup) when it is empty. The stomach wall contains four layers, the innermost of which is crinkled into large folds called *rugae,* which flatten progressively to accommodate food. This allows the stomach to expand to hold about 1 gallon of food and liquid.[1] As food is released into the small intestine, the rugae reform, and the stomach gradually returns to its baseline size.

Before any food reaches the stomach, the brain sends signals to the stomach to stimulate and prepare it to receive food. For example, the hormone *gastrin,* secreted by stomach-lining cells called *G cells,* stimulates gastric glands to secrete a digestive fluid referred to as **gastric juice.** Gastric glands are lined with two important types of cells—parietal cells and chief cells—which secrete the various components of gastric juice.

The parietal cells secrete the following:

- *Hydrochloric acid (HCl),* which keeps the stomach interior very acidic. To be precise, the pH of HCl is 1.0, which means that it is ten times more acidic than pure lemon juice and a hundred times more acidic than vinegar! For a review of the negative logarithms behind the pH scale, see the **You Do the Math** box (page 85). The acidic environment of the stomach interior kills any bacteria and/or germs that may have entered the body with the sandwich. HCl is also extremely important for digestion because it starts to denature proteins, which means it breaks the bonds that maintain their structure. This is an essential preliminary step in protein digestion.
- *Intrinsic factor,* a protein critical to the absorption of vitamin B_{12} (discussed in more detail in Chapter 8). Vitamin B_{12} is present in the turkey.

The chief cells secrete the following:

- *Pepsinogen,* an inactive enzyme, which HCl converts into the active enzyme *pepsin.* Recall that salivary amylase begins to digest carbohydrates in the mouth. In contrast, proteins and lipids enter the stomach largely unchanged. Pepsin begins the digestion of protein. It also activates many other GI enzymes that contribute to digesting your sandwich.
- *Gastric lipase,* an enzyme responsible for lipid digestion. Although gastric lipase begins to break apart the lipids in the turkey and mayonnaise in your sandwich, only minimal digestion of lipids occurs in the stomach.

Because gastric juice is normally present in the stomach, the chemical digestion of proteins and lipids begins as soon as food enters (**Figure 3.8**). The stomach also plays a

stomach   A J-shaped organ where food is partially digested, churned, and stored until released into the small intestine.

gastric juice   Acidic liquid secreted within the stomach; it contains hydrochloric acid, pepsin, and other compounds.

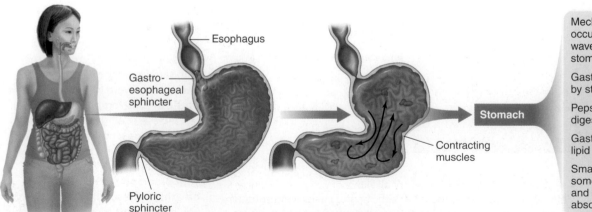

FIGURE 3.8 Where your food is now: the stomach. In the stomach, the protein and lipids in your sandwich begin to be digested. Your meal is churned into chyme and stored until release into the small intestine.

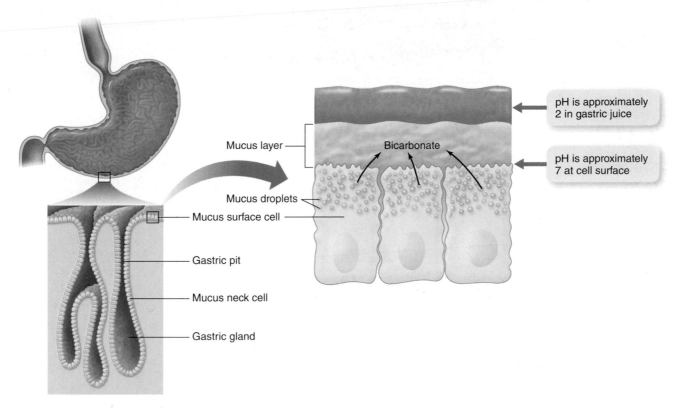

Mucus layer

Bicarbonate

pH is approximately 2 in gastric juice

pH is approximately 7 at cell surface

Mucus droplets

Mucus surface cell

Gastric pit

Mucus neck cell

Gastric gland

FIGURE 3.9 The stomach is protected from the acidity of gastric juice by a layer of mucus.

role in mechanical digestion, by mixing and churning the food with the gastric juice until it becomes a liquid called **chyme.** This mechanical digestion facilitates chemical digestion, because enzymes can access the liquid chyme more easily than solid forms of food.

Despite the acidity of gastric juice, the stomach itself is not eroded because *mucus neck cells* in gastric glands and *mucus surface cells* in the stomach lining secrete a protective layer of mucus (**Figure 3.9**). Any disruption of this mucus barrier can cause gastritis (inflammation of the stomach lining) or an ulcer (a condition that is discussed later in this chapter). Other lining cells secrete bicarbonate, a base, which neutralizes acid near the surface of the stomach's lining.

Although most absorption occurs in the small intestine, some substances are absorbed through the stomach lining and into the blood. These include water, fluoride, some lipids, and some lipid-soluble drugs, including aspirin and alcohol.

Another of the stomach's jobs is to store chyme while the next part of the digestive tract, the small intestine, gets ready for the food. Remember that the capacity of the stomach is about 1 gallon. If this amount of chyme were to move into the small intestine all at once, it would overwhelm it. Chyme stays in the stomach for about 2 hours before it is released periodically in spurts into the duodenum, which is the first part of the small intestine. Regulating this release is the *pyloric sphincter* (see Figure 3.8).

Most Digestion and Absorption Occurs in the Small Intestine

The **small intestine** is the longest portion of the GI tract, accounting for about two-thirds of its length. However, at only an inch in diameter, it is comparatively narrow.

The small intestine is composed of three sections (**Figure 3.10**). The *duodenum* is the section of the small intestine that is connected via the pyloric sphincter to the stomach. The *jejunum* is the middle portion, and the last portion is the *ileum*. It connects to the large intestine at another sphincter, called the *ileocecal valve.*

chyme A semifluid mass consisting of partially digested food, water, and gastric juices.

small intestine The longest portion of the GI tract, where most digestion and absorption takes place.

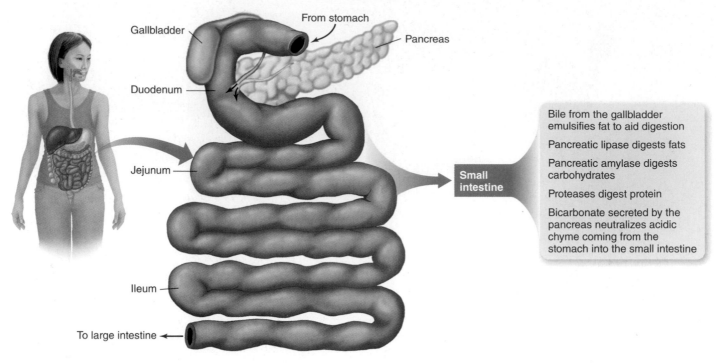

Gallbladder

From stomach

Pancreas

Duodenum

Jejunum

Ileum

To large intestine

Small intestine

Bile from the gallbladder emulsifies fat to aid digestion

Pancreatic lipase digests fats

Pancreatic amylase digests carbohydrates

Proteases digest protein

Bicarbonate secreted by the pancreas neutralizes acidic chyme coming from the stomach into the small intestine

FIGURE 3.10 Where your food is now: the small intestine. Here, most of the digestion and absorption of the nutrients in your sandwich takes place.

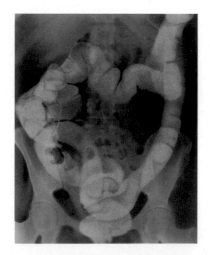

The large intestine is a thick, tubelike structure that stores the undigested mass leaving the small intestine and absorbs any remaining nutrients and water.

large intestine The final organ of the GI tract, consisting of the cecum, colon, rectum, and anal canal and in which most water is absorbed and feces are formed.

Most digestion and absorption take place in the small intestine. Here, the carbohydrates, lipids, and proteins in your turkey sandwich are broken down into their smallest components, molecules that the body can then absorb into the circulation. Digestion and absorption are achieved in the small intestine through the actions of enzymes, accessory organs (the pancreas, gallbladder, and liver), and some unique anatomical features. The details of how these enzymes, organs, and features do their job are described later in this chapter. Once digestion and absorption are completed in the small intestine, the residue is passed into the large intestine.

The Large Intestine Stores Food Waste Until It Is Excreted

The **large intestine** is a thick, tubelike structure that frames the small intestine on three and one-half sides (**Figure 3.11**). It is also referred to as the *colon*. It begins with a tissue sac called the *cecum,* which explains the name of the sphincter—the *ileocecal valve*—which connects it to the ileum of the small intestine. From the cecum, the large intestine continues up along the right side of the small intestine as the *ascending colon.* The *transverse colon* runs across the top of the small intestine, and then the *descending colon* comes down on the left. These regions of the colon are characterized by *haustra,* regular, saclike segmentations that contract to move food toward the *sigmoid colon,* which extends from the bottom left corner to the *rectum.* The last segment of the large intestine is the *anal canal,* which is about 1½ inches long.

What has happened to our turkey sandwich? The residue that finally reaches the large intestine bears little resemblance to the chyme that left the stomach several hours before. This is because a majority of the nutrients have been absorbed, leaving mostly water and non-digestible food material, such as the outer husks of the tomato seeds and the fibers in the lettuce.

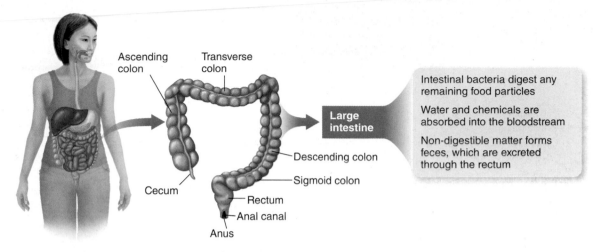

Ascending colon

Transverse colon

Large intestine

Intestinal bacteria digest any remaining food particles

Water and chemicals are absorbed into the bloodstream

Non-digestible matter forms feces, which are excreted through the rectum

Descending colon

Sigmoid colon

Cecum

Rectum

Anal canal

Anus

FIGURE 3.11 Where your food is now: the large intestine. Most water absorption occurs here, as does the formation of food wastes into semisolid feces.

The GI tract hosts a population of trillions of bacterial cells, more than the number of cells making up the human body. Collectively called the *GI flora*, most of these live in the large intestine, where they perform several beneficial functions. First, they finish digesting some of the nutrients remaining in food residues. The by-products of this bacterial digestion are reabsorbed into the body, where they return to the liver and are either stored or used as needed. In addition, the GI flora synthesize certain vitamins, stimulate the immune system, inhibit the growth of harmful bacteria, and reduce the risk for diarrhea.[2] In fact, these bacteria are so helpful that many people consume them deliberately in so-called **probiotic** foods, such as yogurt.

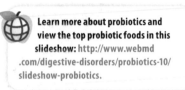

Learn more about probiotics and view the top probiotic foods in this slideshow: http://www.webmd .com/digestive-disorders/probiotics-10/ slideshow-probiotics.

No other digestion occurs in the large intestine. Instead, it stores the digestive mass for 12 to 24 hours, absorbing water, lipid breakdown products, and electrolytes and leaving a semisolid mass called *feces*. Peristalsis occurs weakly to move the feces through the colon, except for one or more stronger waves of peristalsis each day that force the feces more powerfully toward the rectum for elimination.

RECAP

Gastric glands in the stomach secrete gastric juice, which contains hydrochloric acid, the enzymes pepsin and gastric lipase, and intrinsic factor. Bicarbonate and mucus protect the stomach lining from erosion. The stomach mixes food into a substance called chyme, which is released periodically through the pyloric sphincter into the small intestine, where most digestion and absorption occurs. Bicarbonate, bile, and a variety of digestive enzymes play important roles in the process. Small amounts of undigested food, non-digestible food material, and water enter the large intestine. Bacteria in the colon assist with the final digestion of any remaining food particles. The remaining semisolid mass, called feces, is then eliminated from the body. ■

How Does the Body Accomplish Chemical Digestion?

Now that you have learned about the structure and functions of the GI tract, you are ready to delve more deeply into the specific activities of the various enzymes, hormones, and accessory organs involved in digestion.

probiotic Health-promoting; the presence of certain beneficial bacteria in foods that support healthy functioning

TABLE 3.1 Digestive Enzymes Produced in the Gastrointestinal Tract and Their Actions

Organ Where Produced	Enzyme	Site of Action	Primary Action
Mouth	Salivary amylase	Mouth	Digests carbohydrates
Stomach	Pepsin Gastric lipase	Stomach	Digests proteins Digests lipids
Pancreas	Proteases (trypsin, chymotrypsin, carboxypolypeptidase) Elastase Pancreatic lipase Cholesterol esterase Pancreatic amylase (amylase)	Small intestine	Digest proteins Digests fibrous proteins Digests lipids Digests cholesterol Digests carbohydrates
Small intestine	Carboxypeptidase, aminopeptidase, dipeptidase Lipase Sucrase, maltase, and lactase	Small intestine	Digest proteins Digests lipids Digest the simple carbohydrates sucrose, maltose, and lactose

Enzymes Speed Up Digestion via Hydrolysis

Enzymes are released into the gastrointestinal tract as needed, in a process controlled by the nervous system and various hormones. Upon release, they catalyze **hydrolysis** reactions, chemical reactions that break down substances by the addition of water. In this process, which is described in detail in Chapter 7, a reactant, such as a portion of a protein, is broken down into two products.

Although a few digestive enzymes are produced in the mouth and stomach, most are synthesized by the pancreas and small intestine. **Table 3.1** lists many of the enzymes that play a critical role in digestion and specifies where they are produced and their primary actions. Enzymes are usually specific to the substance they act upon, and this is true for the digestive enzymes. As you can see in this table, there are enzymes specific to the digestion of carbohydrates, lipids, and proteins, all of which are too large to be directly absorbed from the gastrointestinal tract. However, water, single-sugar units called monosaccharides, fatty acids, amino acids, vitamins, minerals, and alcohol do not require enzymatic digestion because they are much smaller and therefore can be absorbed in their original form.

Hormones Assist in Regulating Digestion

As introduced earlier in this chapter, hormones are regulatory chemicals produced by endocrine glands. Hormones are released into the bloodstream and travel to target cells that contain the receptor protein specific to that given hormone. Generally, the receptor proteins for hormones are located on the cell membrane. When the hormone arrives at the target cell, it binds to the receptor protein and activates what is referred to as a *second messenger system* within the cell (**Figure 3.12**). This second messenger system achieves the targeted response, such as release of a particular digestive enzyme.

Regulation of the gastrointestinal tract involves the action of more than eighty hormones and hormone-like substances. **Table 3.2** identifies four of the most important of these hormones and the actions they initiate. These are gastrin, secretin, cholecystokinin (CCK), and gastric inhibitory peptide (GIP). Another hormone with an important role in digestion is somatostatin, which is produced by the stomach, small intestine, and pancreas. An inhibitory hormone, it suppresses the release of gastrin and other hormones and enzymes involved in digestion. Finally, ghrelin, a hormone secreted by cells in the stomach as well as the lower gastrointestinal tract, has been identified as playing a role in stimulating

hydrolysis A chemical reaction that breaks down substances by the addition of water.

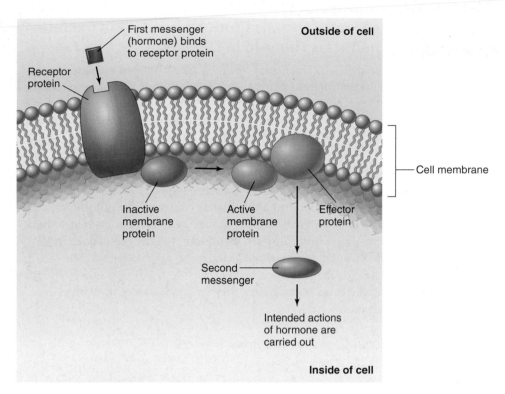

FIGURE 3.12 Hormones travel to target cells to initiate specific actions. When a hormone arrives at its target cell, it binds to the receptor protein on the cell membrane. This binding activates a protein on the interior cell membrane that initiates a second messenger system within the cell. The second messenger system then carries out the action directed by the hormone's "message."

eating, promoting the activity and motility of the GI tract, and regulating carbohydrate metabolism.[3] It has also been shown to have a beneficial effect on the cardiovascular system by improving blood flow and decreasing blood pressure. As ghrelin was just discovered in 1999, the research studying its impact on digestive and cardiovascular health is in its infancy, and there is still much to learn about this hormone.

TABLE 3.2 Hormones Involved in the Regulation of Digestion

Hormone	Production Site	Target Organ	Actions
Gastrin	Stomach	Stomach	Stimulates secretion of HCl and pepsinogen (inactive form of pepsin) Stimulates gastric motility Promotes proliferation of gastric mucosal cells
Secretin	Small intestine (duodenum)	Pancreas	Stimulates secretion of pancreatic bicarbonate (which neutralizes acidic chyme)
		Stomach	Decreases gastric motility
Cholecystokinin (CCK)	Small intestine (duodenum and jejunum)	Pancreas	Stimulates secretion of pancreatic digestive enzymes
		Gallbladder	Stimulates gallbladder contraction
		Stomach	Slows gastric emptying
Gastric inhibitory peptide (GIP)	Small intestine	Stomach	Inhibits gastric acid secretion Slows gastric emptying
		Pancreas	Stimulates insulin release

Nutrition
MILESTONE

Does bile act like soap? As long ago as

1767, a French pharmacist by the name of Cadet presented a chemical analysis of bile to the French Academy, in which he described bile as an "animal soap." Before the close of the century, the French chemist de Fourcroy had repeated Cadet's experiments and confirmed his results: bile caused fatty substances to combine with water in much the same way soap does! Even today, bile from oxen and other animals is mixed with other ingredients to produce bile soap, various preparations of which are marketed for laundry use and even for skin care.

Accessory Organs Produce, Store, and Secrete Chemicals That Aid in Digestion

The gallbladder, pancreas, and liver are considered accessory organs to the gastrointestinal tract. As you will learn in the following sections, these organs are critical to the production, storage, and secretion of enzymes and other substances that are involved in digestion.

The Gallbladder Stores Bile

As noted in Table 3.2, cholecystokinin (CCK) is released in the small intestine in response to the presence of proteins and lipids. This hormone signals the **gallbladder** to contract. The gallbladder is located beneath the liver (see Figure 3.3) and stores a greenish fluid, **bile,** produced by the liver. Contraction of the gallbladder sends bile through the *common bile duct* into the duodenum. Bile then *emulsifies* the lipids; that is, it breaks the lipids into smaller globules and disperses them, so that they are more accessible to digestive enzymes.

The Pancreas Produces Digestive Enzymes and Bicarbonate

The **pancreas** manufactures, holds, and secretes digestive enzymes. It is located behind the stomach (see Figure 3.3). The pancreas stores these enzymes in their inactive forms, and they are activated in the small intestine; this is important because, if the enzymes were active in the pancreas, they would facilitate digestion of the pancreas. Enzymes secreted by the pancreas include *pancreatic amylase, pancreatic lipase,* and *proteases,* which catalyze the digestion of carbohydrates, lipids, and proteins. The pancreas is also responsible for manufacturing hormones that are important in metabolism. Insulin and glucagon, two hormones necessary to regulate the amount of glucose in the blood, are produced by the pancreas.

Another essential role of the pancreas is to secrete bicarbonate into the duodenum. As noted earlier, bicarbonate is a base, whereas chyme leaving the stomach is very acidic. The pancreatic bicarbonate neutralizes this acidic chyme. This allows the pancreatic enzymes to work effectively and ensures that the lining of the duodenum is not eroded. The first portion of the duodenum is also protected by mucus produced by special glands.

The Liver Produces Bile and Regulates Blood Nutrients

The **liver** is a triangular-shaped organ of about 3 lb of tissue that rests almost entirely within the protection of the rib cage on the right side of the body (see Figure 3.3). It is the largest digestive organ; it is also one of the most important organs in the body, performing more than 500 discrete functions. One important job of the liver is to synthesize many of the chemicals the body uses in carrying out metabolic processes. For example, the liver synthesizes bile, which, as we just discussed, is then stored in the gallbladder until needed for the emulsification of lipids.

Another important function of the liver is to receive the products of digestion. Lipids are absorbed from the GI tract into a tissue fluid called lymph, which is drained by lymphatic vessels that eventually drain into the bloodstream. Other types of nutrients are absorbed into capillaries (microscopic blood vessels) that drain into the **portal venous system (Figure 3.13)**. This specialized group of veins drains blood from parts of the stomach, spleen, pancreas, and small and large intestines into a large, central vein, the hepatic portal vein (*hepatic* refers to the liver). This allows the nutrients absorbed by these organs to be transported to the liver for processing before the blood delivers them into the general

gallbladder A pear-shaped organ beneath the liver that stores bile and secretes it into the small intestine.

bile Fluid produced by the liver and stored in the gallbladder; it emulsifies lipids in the small intestine.

pancreas A gland located behind the stomach that secretes digestive enzymes.

liver The largest accessory organ of the GI tract and one of the most important organs of the body. Its functions include the production of bile and processing of nutrient-rich blood from the small intestine.

portal venous system A system of blood vessels that drains blood and various products of digestion from the digestive organs and spleen and delivers them to the liver.

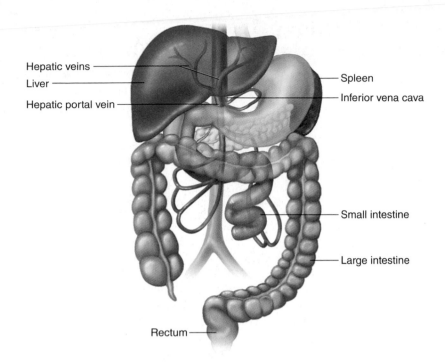

FIGURE 3.13 The portal venous system is a group of veins that drains regions of the digestive system and transports the blood to the liver. There, the blood is filtered through liver cells, which detoxify alcohol and other harmful agents, as well as use or store nutrients or package them before releasing them back into the general circulation for delivery to distant body cells.

circulation. After the liver removes the digestion products from the bloodstream, it can process them for storage or release back into the bloodstream those that are needed elsewhere in the body.

For instance, after we eat a meal, the liver picks up excess glucose from the blood and stores it as glycogen, releasing it into the bloodstream when we need energy later in the day. It stores certain vitamins and manufactures blood proteins. The liver can even make glucose when necessary to ensure that our blood levels stay constant. Thus, the liver plays a major role in regulating the level and type of fuel circulating in our blood.

Have you ever wondered why people who abuse alcohol are at risk for liver damage? That's because another of its functions is to remove from the blood wastes and toxins such as alcohol, medications, and other drugs. When you drink, your liver works hard to replace the cells poisoned with alcohol, but over time scar tissue forms. The scar tissue blocks the free flow of blood through the liver, so any further toxins accumulate in the blood, causing confusion, coma, and, ultimately death. (Alcohol is discussed **In Depth** on pages 160–171.)

RECAP

Enzymes speed up the digestion of food through hydrolysis. Hormones act as chemical messengers to regulate digestion. The digestive accessory organs include the gallbladder, pancreas, and liver. The gallbladder stores bile, which is produced by the liver. Bile emulsifies lipids into pieces that are more easily accessed by digestive enzymes. The pancreas synthesizes and secretes digestive enzymes and bicarbonate. The liver processes nutrients absorbed from the small intestine, regulates blood glucose levels, and stores glucose as glycogen. ■

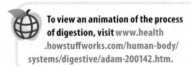

To view an animation of the process of digestion, visit www.health .howstuffworks.com/human-body/ systems/digestive/adam-200142.htm.

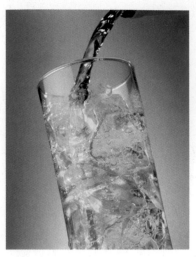

Water is readily absorbed along the entire length of the GI tract.

How Does the Body Absorb and Transport Digested Nutrients?

Although some nutrient absorption occurs in the stomach and large intestine, the majority occurs in the small intestine. With its extensive surface area and specialized absorptive cells, the small intestine is ideally equipped to handle this responsibility. Let's now learn more about how we absorb the nutrients from our food.

A Specialized Lining Enables the Small Intestine to Absorb Food

The lining of the small intestine is especially well suited for absorption. If you looked at the inside of the lining, which is also referred to as the *mucosal membrane,* you would notice that it is heavily folded (**Figure 3.14**). This feature increases the surface area of the small intestine, allowing it to absorb more nutrients than if it were smooth. Within these larger folds, you would notice even smaller, finger-like projections called *villi,* whose constant movement helps them encounter and trap nutrient molecules. The villi are composed of numerous specialized absorptive cells called **enterocytes.** Inside each villus are capillaries and a **lacteal,** which is a small lymphatic vessel. The capillaries and lacteals absorb some of the end products of digestion. Water-soluble nutrients are absorbed directly into the bloodstream, whereas lipids and other fat-soluble nutrients are absorbed into lymph. Each enterocyte of each villus has hairlike projections called *microvilli.* The microvilli look like tiny brushes and are sometimes collectively referred to as the **brush border.** These intricate folds increase the surface area of the small intestine tremendously, increasing its absorptive capacity as well.

Four Types of Absorption Occur in the Small Intestine

Nutrients are absorbed across the mucosal membrane and into the bloodstream or lymph via four mechanisms: passive diffusion, facilitated diffusion, active transport, and endocytosis. These are illustrated in **Figure 3.15** (page 96).

Passive diffusion is a simple process in which nutrients cross into the enterocytes without the use of a carrier protein or the requirement of energy (Figure 3.15a). Passive diffusion can occur when the wall of the intestine is permeable to the nutrient and the concentration of the nutrient in the GI tract is higher than its concentration in the enterocytes. Thus, the nutrient is moving from an area of higher concentration to an area of lower concentration. Lipids, water, vitamin C, and some minerals are absorbed via passive diffusion.

Facilitated diffusion occurs when nutrients are shuttled across the enterocytes with the help of a carrier protein (Figure 3.15b). This process is similar to passive diffusion in that it does not require energy and is driven by a concentration gradient. The monosaccharide fructose is transported via facilitated diffusion.

Active transport requires the use of energy to transport nutrients in combination with a carrier protein (Figure 3.15c). The energy derived from ATP and the assistance of the carrier protein allow for the absorption of nutrients against their concentration gradient, meaning the nutrients can move from areas of low to high concentration. Glucose, galactose, sodium, potassium, magnesium, calcium, iron, and amino acids are some of the nutrients absorbed via active transport. In addition to being absorbed via passive diffusion, vitamin C can be absorbed via active transport.

Endocytosis (also called pinocytosis) is a form of active transport by which a small amount of the intestinal contents is engulfed by the enterocyte's cell membrane and incorporated into the cell (Figure 3.15d). Some proteins and other large particles are absorbed in this way, as are the antibodies contained in breast milk.

---

enterocytes Specialized absorptive cells in the villi of the small intestine.

lacteal A small lymphatic vessel located inside the villi of the small intestine.

brush border The microvilli of the small intestine's lining. These microvilli tremendously increase the small intestine's absorptive capacity.

passive diffusion A transport process in which ions and molecules, following their concentration gradient, cross the cell membrane without the use of a carrier protein or the requirement of energy.

facilitated diffusion A transport process in which ions and molecules are shuttled across the cell membrane with the help of a carrier protein.

active transport A transport process that requires the use of energy to shuttle ions and molecules across the cell membrane in combination with a carrier protein.

endocytosis A transport process in which ions and molecules are engulfed by the cell membrane, which folds inwardly and is released in the cell interior (also called pinocytosis).

Small Intestine Structure/Function

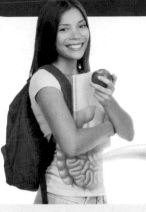

The small intestine is highly adapted for absorbing nutrients. Its length—about 20 feet—provides a huge surface area, and its wall has three structural features—circular folds, villi, and microvilli—that increase its surface area by a factor of more than 600.

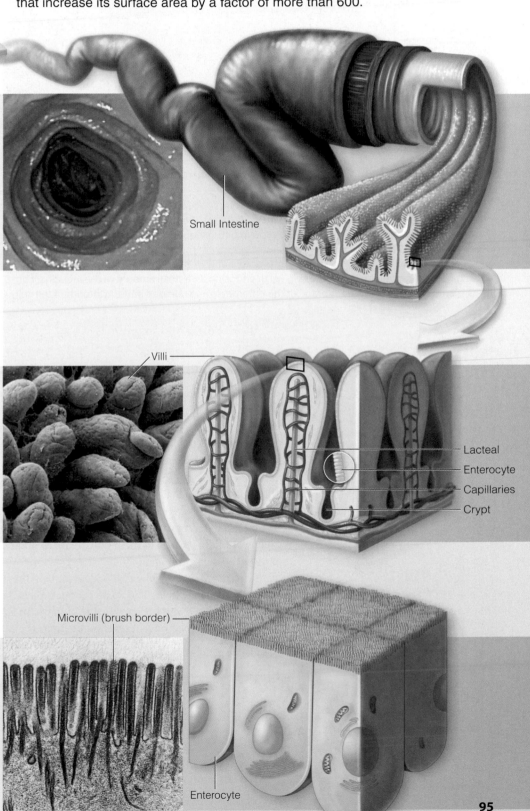

CIRCULAR FOLDS

The lining of the small intestine is heavily folded, resulting in increased surface area for the absorption of nutrients.

Small Intestine

VILLI

The folds are covered with villi, thousands of finger-like projections that increase the surface area even further. Each villus contains capillaries and a lacteal for picking up nutrients absorbed through the enterocytes and transporting them throughout the body.

Villi

Lacteal

Enterocyte

Capillaries

Crypt

MICROVILLI

The cells on the surface of the villi, enterocytes, end in hairlike projections called microvilli that together form the brush border through which nutrients are absorbed.

Microvilli (brush border)

Enterocyte

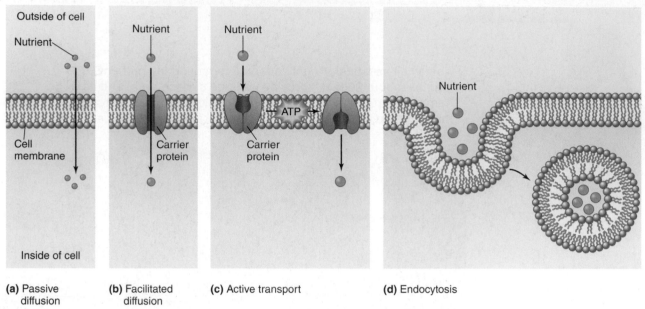

(a) Passive diffusion   **(b)** Facilitated diffusion   **(c)** Active transport   **(d)** Endocytosis

FIGURE 3.15 The four types of absorption that occur in the small intestine. **(a)** In passive diffusion, nutrients at a higher concentration outside the cells diffuse along their concentration gradient into the enterocytes without the use of a carrier protein or the requirement of energy. **(b)** In facilitated diffusion, nutrients are shuttled across the enterocytes with the help of a carrier protein without the use of energy. **(c)** In active transport, energy is used along with a carrier protein to transport nutrients against their concentration gradient. **(d)** In endocytosis, a small amount of the intestinal contents is engulfed by the cell membrane of the enterocyte and released into the interior of the cell.

Blood and Lymph Transport Nutrients and Wastes

Two circulating fluids transport nutrients and waste products throughout the body: blood travels through the cardiovascular system, and lymph travels through the lymphatic system (**Figure 3.16**). The oxygen we inhale into our lungs is carried by our red blood cells. This oxygen-rich blood then travels to the heart, where it is pumped out to the body. Blood travels to all of our tissues to deliver nutrients and other materials and to pick up waste products. In the enterocytes, blood in the capillaries picks up water and water-soluble nutrients, and lymph in the lacteals picks up most lipids and fat-soluble vitamins, as well as any fluids that have escaped from the blood capillaries. Lymph nodes are clusters of immune cells that filter microbes and other harmful agents from the lymph fluid (Figure 3.16). The lymph eventually returns to the bloodstream in an area near the heart where the lymphatic and blood vessels join together.

As discussed earlier, when blood leaves the GI system, it is transported via the portal venous system to the liver. The waste products picked up by the blood as it circulates around the body are filtered and excreted by the kidneys. In addition, much of the carbon dioxide remaining in the blood once it reaches the lungs is exhaled into the outside air, making room for oxygen to attach to the red blood cells and repeat this cycle of circulation again.

RECAP

The mucosal membrane of the small intestine contains multiple villi and microvilli that significantly increase absorptive capacity. Nutrients are absorbed through one of four mechanisms: passive diffusion, facilitated diffusion, active transport, and endocytosis. Most nutrients and waste products are transported throughout the body via the blood, whereas lipids and fat-soluble vitamins are transported through lymph. ■

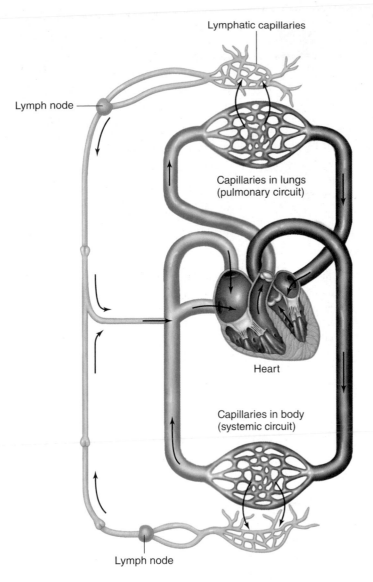

FIGURE 3.16 Blood travels through the cardiovascular system to transport nutrients and fluids and to pick up waste products. Lymph travels through the lymphatic system and transports most lipids and fat-soluble vitamins.

How Does the Body Coordinate and Regulate Digestion?

Now that you can identify the organs involved in digestion and absorption and the complex tasks they each perform, you might be wondering—who's the boss? In other words, what organ or system controls all of these interrelated processes? The answer is the neuromuscular system. Its two components, nerves and muscles, partner to coordinate and regulate the digestion and absorption of food and the elimination of waste.

The Muscles of the Gastrointestinal Tract Mix and Move Food

The purposes of the muscles of the GI tract are to mix food, ensure efficient digestion and optimal absorption of nutrients, and move the intestinal contents from the mouth toward

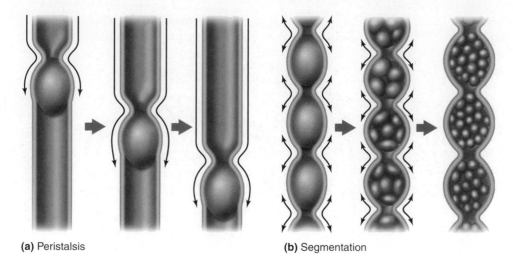

(a) Peristalsis   **(b)** Segmentation

FIGURE 3.17 Peristalsis and segmentation. **(a)** Peristalsis occurs through the actions of circular muscles and longitudinal muscles that run along the entire GI tract. These muscles continuously contract and relax, causing subsequent constriction and bulging of the tract, which pushes the intestinal contents from one area to the next. **(b)** Segmentation occurs through the rhythmic contraction of the circular muscles of the small intestine. This action squeezes the chyme, mixes it, and enhances its contact with digestive enzymes and enterocytes.

the anus. Once we swallow a bolus of food, peristalsis begins in the esophagus and continues throughout the remainder of the gastrointestinal tract. Peristalsis is accomplished through the actions of circular muscles and longitudinal muscles that run along the entire GI tract (**Figure 3.17a**). The circular and longitudinal muscles continuously contract and relax, causing subsequent constriction and bulging of the tract. This action pushes the contents from one area to the next.

The stomach is surrounded by its own set of longitudinal, circular, and diagonal muscles that assist in digestion (**Figure 3.18**). These muscles alternately contract and relax, churning the stomach contents and moving them toward the pyloric sphincter. The pyloric sphincter stays closed while gastric juices are secreted and the chyme is mixed. Once the chyme is completely liquefied, the pyloric sphincter is stimulated to open, and small amounts of chyme are regularly released into the small intestine.

In the small intestine, a unique pattern of motility called **segmentation** occurs (see Figure 3.17b). Segmentation, accomplished by the rhythmic contraction of circular muscles in the intestinal wall, squeezes the chyme, mixes it, and enhances its contact with digestive enzymes and enterocytes.

The colon also exhibits a unique pattern of motility, called **haustration,** in which the haustra contract sluggishly to move wastes toward the sigmoid colon. However, two or more times each day, a much stronger and more sustained **mass movement** of the colon occurs, pushing wastes forcibly toward the rectum.

The muscles of the GI tract contract at varying rates, depending on their location and whether or not food is present. The stomach tends to contract more slowly, about three times per minute, whereas the small intestine may contract up to ten times per minute when chyme is present. The contractions of haustra are very slow, occurring at a rate of about two per hour. As with an assembly line, the entire GI tract functions together, so that materials are moved in one direction, absorption of nutrients is maximized, and wastes are removed as needed.

In order to process the large amount of food we consume daily, we use both voluntary and involuntary muscles. Muscles in the mouth are primarily voluntary; that is, they are

segmentation Rhythmic contraction of the circular muscles of the small intestine, which squeezes chyme, mixes it, and enhances the digestion and absorption of nutrients from the chyme.

haustration Involuntary, sluggish contraction of the haustra of the proximal colon, which moves wastes toward the sigmoid colon.

mass movement Involuntary, sustained, forceful contraction of the colon that occurs two or more times a day to push wastes toward the rectum.

under our conscious control. Once we swallow, the involuntary muscles just described largely take over to propel food through the rest of the GI tract. This enables us to continue digesting and absorbing food while we're working, exercising, and even sleeping. Let's now identify the master controller behind these involuntary muscular actions.

Nerves Control the Contractions and Secretions of the Gastrointestinal Tract

The contractions and secretions of the gastrointestinal tract are controlled by nerves from three divisions of the nervous system:

- The **enteric nervous system (ENS),** which is localized in the wall of the GI tract, and is part of the autonomic nervous system, the division of the peripheral nervous system (PNS) that regulates many internal functions
- The parasympathetic and sympathetic branches of the autonomic nervous system
- The central nervous system (CNS), which includes the brain and spinal cord

Some digestive functions are carried out entirely within the ENS. For instance, the control of peristalsis and segmentation is enteric, occurring without CNS involvement. In addition, enteric nerves regulate the secretions of the various digestive glands whose roles we have discussed in this chapter.

Enteric nerves also work in collaboration with the rest of the PNS and the CNS. For example, we noted earlier in this chapter that, in response to fasting, receptors in the stomach and intestinal walls (ENS receptors) stimulate peripheral nerves to signal the hypothalamus, part of the CNS. We then experience the sensation of hunger.

Finally, some functions, such as the secretion of saliva, are achieved without enteric involvement. A variety of stimuli from the smell, sight, taste, and tactile sensations from food trigger special salivary cells in the CNS; these cells then stimulate increased activity of the salivary glands.

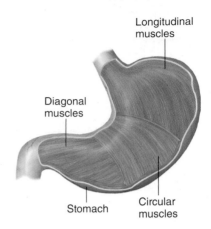

FIGURE 3.18 The stomach has longitudinal, circular, and diagonal muscles. These three sets of muscles aid digestion by alternately contracting and relaxing; these actions churn the stomach contents and move them toward the pyloric sphincter.

RECAP

The coordination and regulation of digestion are directed by the neuromuscular system. Voluntary muscles assist us with chewing and swallowing. Once food is swallowed, involuntary muscles of the GI tract function together, so that materials are processed in a coordinated manner. Involuntary movements include the mixing and churning of chyme by muscles in the stomach wall, as well as peristalsis, segmentation, haustration, and mass movement. The enteric nerves of the GI tract work with the rest of the peripheral nervous system and the central nervous system to achieve the digestion, absorption, and elimination of food. ■

What Disorders Are Related to Digestion, Absorption, and Elimination?

Considering the complexity of digestion, absorption, and elimination, it's no wonder that sometimes things go wrong. Disorders of the neuromuscular system, hormonal imbalances, infections, allergies, and a host of other disorders can disturb gastrointestinal functioning, as can merely consuming the wrong types or amounts of food for our unique needs. Whenever there is a problem with the GI tract, the absorption of nutrients can be affected. If absorption of a nutrient is less than optimal for a long period of time, malnutrition can result. Let's look more closely at some GI tract disorders and what you might be able to do if they affect you.

enteric nervous system (ENS) The autonomic nerves in the walls of the GI tract.

Belching and Flatulence Are Common

Many people complain of problems with belching (eructation) and/or flatulence (passage of intestinal gas). The primary cause of belching is swallowed air. Eating too fast, wearing improperly fitting dentures, chewing gum, sucking on hard candies or a drinking straw, and gulping food or fluid can increase the risk of swallowing air. To prevent or reduce belching, avoid these behaviors.

Although many people find *flatus* (intestinal gas) uncomfortable and embarrassing, its presence in the GI tract is completely normal, as is its expulsion. Flatus is a mixture of many gases, including nitrogen, hydrogen, oxygen, methane, and carbon dioxide. Interestingly, all of these are odorless. It is only when flatus contains sulfur that it causes the embarrassing odor associated with flatulence.

Foods most commonly reported to cause flatus include those rich in fibers, starches, and sugars, such as beans, dairy products, and some vegetables. The partially digested carbohydrates from these foods pass into the large intestine, where they are fermented by bacteria, producing gas. Other food products that may cause flatus, intestinal cramps, and diarrhea include products made with the fat substitute olestra, sugar alcohols, and quorn (a meat substitute made from fungus).

Because many of the foods that can cause flatus are healthful, it is important not to avoid them. Eating smaller portions can help reduce the amount of flatus produced and passed. In addition, products such as Beano can offer some relief. Beano is an over-the-counter supplement that contains alpha-galactosidase, an enzyme that digests the complex sugars in gas-producing foods. Although flatus is generally normal, some people have malabsorption diseases that cause painful bloating and require medical treatment. Some of these disorders are described later in this section.

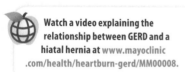

Although the exact causes of gastroesophageal reflux disease (GERD) are unknown, smoking and being overweight may be contributing factors.

Heartburn and Gastroesophageal Reflux Disease (GERD) Are Caused by Reflux of Stomach Acid

As explained earlier, when you eat food, your stomach secretes gastric juice to start the digestive process. Sometimes, the amount of HCl in the gastric juice is excessive, or the gastroesophageal sphincter opens too soon or does not fully close. As a result, gastric juice seeps back up into the esophagus (**Figure 3.19**). Although the stomach lining is protected by bicarbonate and a thick coat of mucus, the esophagus does not have these defenses. Thus, the gastric juice burns it. When this happens, a person experiences a painful sensation in the chest region above the sternum (breastbone). This condition is commonly called **heartburn.** People often take over-the-counter antacids to neutralize the pH of the gastric juice in their stomach, thereby relieving the heartburn. A non-drug approach is to repeatedly swallow: this action causes any acid within the esophagus to be swept down into the stomach, eventually relieving the symptoms.

Gastroesophageal reflux disease (GERD) is a more painful type of heartburn that occurs more than twice per week, sometimes daily. GERD affects about 15 million Americans; like heartburn, it occurs when gastric juice flows back into the esophagus. Although people who experience occasional heartburn usually have no structural abnormalities, many people with GERD have a permanently relaxed or damaged esophageal sphincter or damage to the esophagus itself. Some people have a *hiatal hernia,* which occurs when the upper part of the stomach protrudes through the opening in the diaphragm muscle through which the esophagus normally passes as it nears the top of stomach. As shown in Figure 3.19, the diaphragm muscle normally separates the stomach and other abdominal organs from the chest cavity. It also exerts pressure on the lower esophagus, which helps keep gastric juice out. Stomach acid can more easily enter the esophagus in people with a hiatal hernia.

Symptoms of GERD include persistent heartburn and acid regurgitation. Some people have GERD without heartburn and instead experience chest pain, asthma, trouble

Watch a video explaining the relationship between GERD and a hiatal hernia at www.mayoclinic .com/health/heartburn-gerd/MM00008.

heartburn   The painful sensation that occurs over the sternum when hydrochloric acid backs up into the lower esophagus.

gastroesophageal reflux disease (GERD)   A painful type of heartburn that occurs more than twice per week.

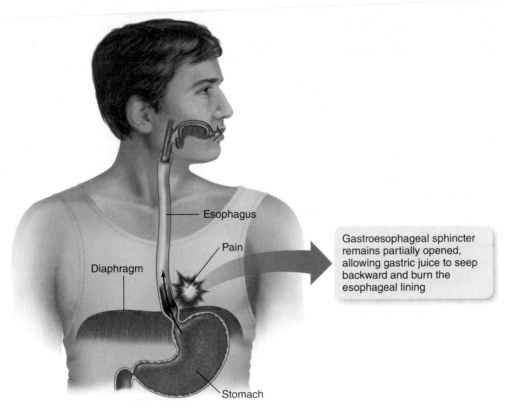

Esophagus

Pain

Diaphragm

Gastroesophageal sphincter remains partially opened, allowing gastric juice to seep backward and burn the esophageal lining

Stomach

FIGURE 3.19 The mechanism of heartburn and gastroesophageal reflux disease is the same: acidic gastric juices seep backward through an open, or relaxed, sphincter into the lower portion of the esophagus, burning its lining. The pain is felt above the sternum, over the heart.

swallowing, burning in the mouth, the feeling that food is stuck in the throat, or hoarseness in the morning.[4]

A number of factors may contribute to GERD, including the following:[4]

- Cigarette smoking
- Alcohol use
- Overweight
- Pregnancy
- Foods such as citrus fruits, chocolate, caffeinated drinks, fried foods, garlic and onions, spicy foods, and tomato-based foods such as chili, pizza, and spaghetti sauce
- Large, high-fat meals; these meals stay in the stomach longer and increase stomach pressure, making it more likely that acid will be pushed up into the esophagus
- Lying down within 1 to 2 hours after a meal; this is almost certain to bring on symptoms in susceptible people because it positions the body so that it is easier for the stomach acid to back up into the esophagus

There are ways to reduce the symptoms of GERD. One way is to identify the types of foods or situations that trigger episodes and then avoid them. Eating smaller meals also helps. After a meal, waiting at least 3 hours before lying down is recommended. Some people relieve their nighttime symptoms by elevating the head of the bed 4 to 6 inches—for instance, by placing a wedge between the mattress and the box spring. This keeps the chest area elevated and minimizes the amount of acid that can back up into the esophagus. It is also suggested that, if people smoke, they should stop and, if they are overweight, they should lose weight. Taking an antacid before a meal can help, and many prescription medications are available to treat GERD. The most effective medications currently available are called *proton pump inhibitors*; these drugs reduce the secretion of HCl from the stomach's parietal cells.

Left untreated, GERD can cause serious health problems, including bleeding and ulceration of the esophagus. Scar tissue can develop in the esophagus, making swallowing very difficult. Some people can also develop a condition called Barrett esophagus, which can lead to cancer.

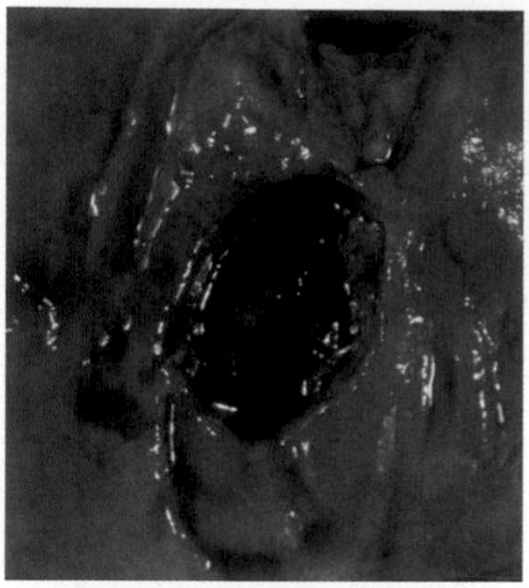

An Ulcer Is an Area of Erosion in the GI Tract

A **peptic ulcer** is an area of the GI tract that has been eroded away by a combination of hydrochloric acid and the enzyme pepsin (**Figure 3.20**). In almost all cases, it is located in the stomach area (*gastric ulcer*) or the part of the duodenum closest to the stomach (*duodenal ulcer*). It causes a burning pain in the abdominal area, typically 1 to 3 hours after eating a meal. In serious cases, eroded blood vessels bleed into the GI tract, causing vomiting of blood and/or blood in the stools, as well as anemia. If the ulcer entirely perforates the tract wall, stomach contents can leak into the abdominal cavity, causing a life-threatening infection. Peptic ulcers are common, affecting about 500,000 Americans annually.[5]

The bacterium *Helicobacter pylori* (*H. pylori*) plays a key role in the development of most peptic ulcers, which include both gastric and duodenal ulcers.[5] *H. pylori* infection is common; however, most people with *H. pylori* infection do not develop ulcers, and the reason for this is not known.[5]

Because of the role of *H. pylori* in ulcer development, treatment usually involves antibiotics and other types of medications to reduce gastric secretions. Antacids are used to weaken the gastric acid, and the same medications used to treat GERD can be used to treat peptic ulcers. Special diets are not recommended as often as they once were because they do not reduce acid secretion. In fact, we now know that ulcers are not caused by stress or spicy foods.

Although most peptic ulcers are caused by *H. pylori* infection, some are caused by a prolonged use of nonsteroidal anti-inflammatory drugs (NSAIDs), including the pain relievers aspirin, ibuprofen, and naproxen sodium. Acetaminophen use does not cause ulcers. The NSAIDs appear to cause ulcers by preventing the stomach from protecting itself from acidic gastric juices. Ulcers caused by NSAID use generally heal once a person stops taking the medication.[6]

FIGURE 3.20 A peptic ulcer.

RECAP

Belching is commonly caused by behaviors that cause us to swallow air. Foods that may cause flatulence include those rich in fibers, starches, and sugars. Heartburn is caused by the seepage of gastric juices into the esophagus. Gastroesophageal reflux disease (GERD) is a painful type of heartburn that occurs more than twice per week. Peptic ulcers are caused by erosion of the GI tract by hydrochloric acid and pepsin. The two major causes of peptic ulcers are *Helicobacter pylori* infection and the use of nonsteroidal anti-inflammatory drugs. ■

Some People Experience Disorders Related to Specific Foods

You check out the ingredients list on your energy bar, and you notice that it says "Produced in a facility that processes peanuts." The carton of soy milk you're drinking from proclaims "Gluten free!" What's all the fuss about? To some people, consuming certain food ingredients can be dangerous, even life-threatening. To learn more about product labeling for potential food offenders, see the **Nutrition Label Activity** box.

Disorders related to specific foods can be clustered into three main groupings: food intolerances, food allergies, and a genetic disorder called celiac disease. We discuss these separately.

peptic ulcer An area of the GI tract that has been eroded away by the acidic gastric juice of the stomach. The two main causes of peptic ulcers are *Helicobacter pylori* infection and the use of nonsteroidal anti-inflammatory drugs.

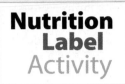

Recognizing Common Allergens in Foods

The US Food and Drug Administration (FDA) requires food labels to clearly identify any ingredients containing protein derived from the eight major allergenic foods.[1] Manufacturers must identify "in plain English" the presence of ingredients that contain protein derived from the following:

- Milk
- Eggs
- Fish
- Crustacean shellfish (crab, lobster, shrimp, and so on)
- Tree nuts (almonds, pecans, walnuts, and so on)
- Peanuts
- Wheat
- Soybeans

Although more than 160 foods have been identified as causing food allergies in sensitive individuals, the FDA requires labeling for only these eight foods because together they account for over 90% of all documented food allergies in the United States and represent the foods most likely to result in severe or life-threatening reactions.[1]

These eight allergenic foods must be indicated in the list of ingredients; alternatively, adjacent to the ingredients list, the label must say "Contains" followed by the name of the food. For example, the label of a product containing the milk-derived protein casein would have to use the term *milk* in addition to the term *casein*, so that those who have milk allergies would clearly understand the presence of an allergen they need to avoid.[1] Any food product found to contain an undeclared allergen is subject to recall by the FDA.

Look at the ingredients list from an energy bar, shown below, and answer the following questions:

- Which of the FDA's eight allergenic foods does this bar definitely contain?
- If you were allergic to peanuts, would eating this bar pose any risk to you?

  Yes or No
- If you were allergic to almonds, would eating this bar pose any risk to you?

  Yes or No

(Answers are located online in the MasteringNutrition Study Area.)

Ingredients: Soy protein isolate, rice flour, oats, milled flax-seed, brown rice syrup, evaporated cane juice, sunflower oil, soy lecithin, cocoa, nonfat milk solids, salt.
   Contains soy and dairy. May contain traces of peanuts and other nuts.

Reference

1. US Food and Drug Administration. 2012. Food Allergies: What You Need to Know. www.fda.gov/food/resourcesforyou/consumers/ucm079311.htm.

Food Intolerance

A **food intolerance** is a cluster of GI symptoms (often gas, abdominal pain, and diarrhea) that occurs following consumption of a particular food. The immune system plays no role in intolerance, and although episodes are unpleasant, they are usually transient, resolving after the offending food has been eliminated from the body. An example is lactose intolerance. It occurs in people whose bodies do not produce sufficient quantities of the enzyme lactase, which facilitates the breakdown of the milk sugar lactose. (Lactose intolerance is discussed in more detail in Chapter 4.) People can also have an intolerance to wheat, soy, and other foods, but as with lactose intolerance, the symptoms pass once the offending food is out of the person's system.

Food Allergy

A **food allergy** is a hypersensitivity reaction of the immune system to a particular component (usually a protein) in a food. This reaction causes the immune cells to release chemicals that cause either limited or systemic (whole-body) inflammation. Although much less common than food intolerances, food allergies can be far more serious. Approximately 30,000 consumers require emergency room treatment and 150 Americans die each year because of allergic reactions to foods.[7]

food intolerance Gastrointestinal discomfort caused by certain foods that is not a result of an immune system reaction.

food allergy An allergic reaction to food, caused by a reaction of the immune system.

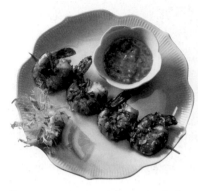

For some people, eating a meal of grilled shrimp with peanut sauce would cause a severe allergic reaction.

You may have heard stories of people being allergic to foods as common as peanuts. This is the case for Liz (see the **Nutri-Case** at the end of this discussion). She was out to dinner with her parents, celebrating her birthday, when the dessert cart came around. The caramel custard looked heavenly and was probably a safe choice, but she asked the waiter, just to be sure that it contained no peanuts. He checked with the chef, then returned and assured her that, no, the custard was peanut-free—but within minutes of consuming it, Liz's skin became flushed, and she struggled to breathe. As her parents were dialing 911, she lost consciousness. Fortunately, the paramedics arrived within minutes and were able to resuscitate her. It was subsequently determined that, unknown to the chef, the spoon that his prep cook had used to scoop the baked custard into serving bowls had been resting on a cutting board where he had chopped peanuts for a different dessert. Just this small exposure to peanuts was enough to cause a severe allergic reaction in Liz.

How can a food that most people consume regularly, such as peanuts, shellfish, eggs, or milk, cause another person's immune system to react so violently? In Liz's case, a trace amount of peanut stimulated immune cells throughout her body to release their inflammatory chemicals. In many people, the inflammation is localized, so the damage is limited; for instance, a person's mouth and throat might itch whenever he or she eats cantaloupe. Other localized reactions include swelling of the mouth or face, a skin rash, vomiting, and wheezing.[7] What made Liz's experience so terrifyingly different was that the inflammation was widespread. Thus, her airways became constricted and clogged with mucus, leading to respiratory collapse. At the same time, her blood vessels dilated and became so permeable that her blood pressure plummeted, leading to circulatory collapse. This state, called *anaphylactic shock*, is nearly always fatal if not treated immediately. For this reason, many people with known food allergies carry with them a kit containing an injection of a powerful stimulant called epinephrine. This drug can reduce symptoms long enough to buy the victim time to get emergency medical care.

Celiac Disease

Celiac disease, also known as *celiac sprue*, is a digestive disease that severely damages the lining of the small intestine and interferes with the absorption of nutrients.[8] As in food allergy, the body's immune system causes the disorder. There is a strong genetic predisposition to celiac disease, with the risk now linked to specific gene markers. Approximately 1 in every 133 Americans is thought to have celiac disease, but among those with a close family member with the disease, the rate is 1 in 22.[8]

celiac disease A disorder characterized by an immune reaction that damages the lining of the small intestine when the individual is exposed to a component of a protein called gluten.

*Nutri-*Case

Liz

"I used to think my peanut allergy was no big deal, but ever since my experience at that restaurant last year, I've been pretty obsessive about it. For months afterward, I refused to eat anything that I hadn't prepared myself. I do eat out now, but I always insist that the chef prepare my food personally, with clean utensils, and I avoid most desserts. They're just too risky. Shopping is a lot harder, too, because I have to check every label. The worst, though, is eating at my friends' houses. I have to ask them "Do you keep peanuts or peanut butter in your house?" Some of them are really sympathetic, but others look at me as if I'm a hypochondriac! I wish I could think of something to say to them to make them understand that this isn't something I have any control over."

What could Liz say in response to friends who don't understand the cause and seriousness of her food allergy? Do you think it would help Liz to share her fears with her doctor and discuss possible strategies? If so, why? In addition to shopping, dining out, and eating at friends' houses, what other situations might require Liz to be cautious about her food choices?

Whereas many foods prompt food allergies, in celiac disease the offending food component is always *gliadin*, a fraction of a protein called *gluten* that is found in wheat, rye, and barley. When people with celiac disease eat a food made with one of these grains, their immune system triggers an inflammatory response that erodes the villi of the small intestine. If the person is unaware of the disorder and continues to eat gluten, repeated immune reactions cause the villi to become greatly decreased, so that there is less absorptive surface area. In addition, the enzymes secreted at the brush border of the small intestine become reduced. As a result, the person becomes unable to absorb certain nutrients properly—a condition known as *malabsorption*. Over time, malabsorption can lead to malnutrition (poor nutrient status). Deficiencies of fat-soluble vitamins A, D, E, and K, as well as iron, folic acid, and calcium, are common in those suffering from celiac disease, as are inadequate intakes of protein and total energy.[8]

Symptoms of celiac disease often mimic those of other intestinal disturbances, such as irritable bowel syndrome (discussed shortly), so the condition is often misdiagnosed. Some of the symptoms of celiac disease include fatty stools (due to poor fat absorption) with an odd odor; abdominal bloating and cramping; diarrhea, constipation, or vomiting; and weight loss. However, other puzzling symptoms do not appear to involve the GI tract. These include an intensely itchy rash called *dermatitis herpetiformis*, unexplained anemia, fatigue, osteoporosis (poor bone density), arthritis, infertility, seizures, anxiety, irritability, and depression, among others.[8]

Diagnostic tests for celiac disease include a variety of blood tests that screen for the presence of immune proteins called antibodies or for the genetic markers of the disease. However, these are considered first steps in diagnosis. Positive findings should be followed by a biopsy of the small intestine, in which a small portion of tissue is removed and analyzed for atrophy of the villi. Because long-term complications of undiagnosed celiac disease include an increased risk for intestinal cancer, early diagnosis can be life-saving. Unfortunately, celiac disease is currently thought to be widely underdiagnosed in the United States.[9] We'll explore some reasons for this in the **Nutrition Debate** box (pages 114–115).

Currently, there is no cure for celiac disease. Treatment is with a special diet that excludes all forms of wheat, rye, and barley. Oats are allowed, but they are often contaminated with wheat flour from processing, and even a microscopic amount of wheat can cause an immune response. The diet is especially challenging because many binding agents and other unfamiliar ingredients in processed foods are derived from gluten. Thus, nutritional counseling is essential. Although many gluten-free foods are now available, they are typically more expensive and less palatable than traditional wheat-based foods. Someday, however, gluten-free foods may be unnecessary. Earlier, we discussed the beneficial functions of certain types of bacteria in the GI tract. Now, researchers have discovered that beneficial mouth bacteria are able to degrade gluten.[10] Thus, researchers are looking into the potential of developing probiotic breads and other gluten-containing foods that would be safe for people with celiac disease to consume. Another line of research is exploring the use of certain combinations of enzymes that could detoxify gluten before it entered the small intestine.[8]

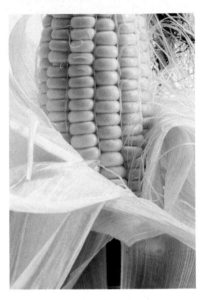

For people with celiac disease, corn is a gluten-free source of carbohydrates.

Vomiting Can Be Acute or Chronic

Vomiting is the involuntary expulsion of the contents of the stomach and duodenum from the mouth. The reflex is triggered when substances or sensations stimulate a cluster of cells in the brain stem to signal a strong wave of "backwards" peristalsis that begins in the small intestine and surges upward. The sphincter muscles of the GI tract relax, allowing the chyme to pass.

One or two episodes of vomiting often accompany a gastrointestinal infection, typically with the norovirus, which is often spread via contaminated water or food. Vomiting triggered by infection is classified as one of the body's innate defenses, as it removes harmful agents before they are absorbed. Certain medical procedures, medications, illicit drugs, motion sickness, and even severe pain can also trigger acute vomiting.

vomiting The involuntary expulsion of the contents of the stomach and duodenum from the mouth.

In contrast, *cyclic vomiting syndrome (CVS)* is a chronic condition characterized by recurring cycles of severe nausea and vomiting that can last for hours or days, alternating with symptom-free periods.[11] The number of people affected is unknown, but the condition is thought to be somewhat common, and people of all ages can be affected.

In CVS, the person typically experiences an initial period of a few minutes or hours of nausea before suddenly beginning to vomit, commonly several times in a single hour. The vomiting may be severe enough to cause dehydration, and the person may need to be hospitalized.

Anxiety, excitement, allergies, infections, and a variety of other disturbances may trigger CVS. These triggers are similar to those involved in migraine headaches, and the same medications used for migraines are often prescribed for CVS, along with anti-nausea and anti-emesis drugs.[11]

Crohn's Disease and Colitis Are Inflammatory Bowel Diseases

Two inflammatory bowel diseases are Crohn's disease and ulcerative colitis. The precise causes of these disorders are unknown, but both have been linked to an immune response to a virus or bacterium. Both also are associated with similar symptoms.

Crohn's Disease

Crohn's disease causes inflammation in the small intestine, usually the ileum, and affects the entire thickness of the wall. Experts speculate that the inflammation is caused by an accumulation of white blood cells as a result of an inappropriate immune reaction to an otherwise harmless bacterium or even a food.[12]

The symptoms of Crohn's disease include diarrhea, abdominal pain, rectal bleeding, weight loss, and fever. People with this disease may also suffer from anemia due to the persistent bleeding that occurs, and children with Crohn's disease can experience delayed physical and mental development. If allowed to progress, Crohn's disease can cause blockage of the intestine and the development of ulcers that tunnel through the areas surrounding the inflammation, such as the bladder, vagina, skin, anus, or rectum. These tunnels are referred to as *fistulas,* and they become infected and commonly require surgical treatment. Crohn's disease also results in deficiencies in protein, energy, and vitamins and is associated with arthritis, kidney stones, gallstones, and diseases of the liver.

Because it shares many symptoms with other intestinal disorders, Crohn's disease can be difficult to diagnose. Treatment may involve a combination of prescription anti-inflammatory drugs and medications that suppress the immune response, as well as nutritional supplements. About two-thirds of patients eventually require surgery to remove an intestinal blockage or abscess or to relieve bleeding, diarrhea, or other problems.[12]

Ulcerative Colitis

Ulcerative colitis (UC) is a chronic disease characterized by inflammation and ulceration of the mucosa, or innermost lining, of the colon. Ulcers form on the surface of the mucosa, where they bleed and produce pus and mucus. The disease affects men and women equally and typically develops between ages 15 and 30.[13]

The causes of UC are unknown. Researchers believe it results from an interaction between bacteria residing in the colon and the immune system. This interaction might either trigger the disease or directly cause the damage to the intestinal wall. This abnormal interaction may be due to certain genetic abnormalities that are found more often in people with UC.

The resulting signs and symptoms are similar to those of Crohn's disease and include diarrhea (which may be bloody), abdominal discomfort, weight loss, anemia, nausea, fever, and fatigue. Complications of ulcerative colitis include profuse bleeding, rupture of the GI tract wall, severe abdominal distention, dehydration, and nutritional deficiencies.

Treatment usually involves taking anti-inflammatory medications. Surgery to remove the affected portion of the colon may be needed for patients who do not respond adequately to medications.[13] No particular foods cause ulcerative colitis, but it may be necessary for people with this disease to avoid large meals, high-fiber foods, and carbonated beverages, as these can cause intestinal discomfort.

Crohn's disease A chronic disease that causes inflammation in the small intestine, leading to diarrhea, abdominal pain, rectal bleeding, weight loss, and fever.

ulcerative colitis A chronic disease of the large intestine, or colon, indicated by inflammation and ulceration of the mucosa, or innermost lining of the colon.

RECAP

Food intolerances are digestive problems caused by the consumption of certain foods, but not due to an immune reaction. Food allergies are hypersensitivities to food ingredients caused by an immune reaction. Food allergies can cause localized symptoms, such as itching and swelling, or life-threatening inflammation and anaphylactic shock. In people with celiac disease, the consumption of gluten, a protein found in wheat, rye, and barley, causes an immune reaction that erodes the lining of the small intestine. Crohn's disease and ulcerative colitis are inflammatory bowel diseases. Crohn's disease usually affects the entire thickness of the ileum of the small intestine, whereas colitis is inflammation and ulceration of the innermost lining of the colon. Vomiting is a defensive response to the presence of harmful agents in the GI tract. Cyclic vomiting syndrome is a pattern of recurring episodes of severe vomiting that can last hours or days. ■

Diarrhea, Constipation, and Irritable Bowel Syndrome Are Functional Disorders

As their name implies, functional disorders affect the regular function of the gastrointestinal tract. Food may move through the small or large intestine too quickly or too slowly, prompting discomfort, bloating, or other symptoms.

Diarrhea

Diarrhea is the frequent (more than three times in one day) passage of loose, watery stools. Other symptoms may include cramping, abdominal pain, bloating, nausea, fever, and blood in the stools. Diarrhea is usually caused by an infection of the gastrointestinal tract, stress, food intolerances, reactions to medications, or an underlying inflammatory bowel disorder or other chronic disease.[14]

Acute diarrhea lasts less than 4 weeks and is usually caused by an infection from bacteria, a virus, or a parasite. Chronic diarrhea, which lasts 4 weeks or longer, is usually caused by allergies to cow's milk, irritable bowel syndrome (discussed shortly), lactose intolerance, celiac disease, or conditions such as Crohn's disease or ulcerative colitis.

Whatever the cause, diarrhea can be harmful if it persists for a long period of time because the person can lose large quantities of water and electrolytes and become severely dehydrated. **Table 3.3** reviews the signs and symptoms of dehydration, which is particularly dangerous in infants and young children. In fact, a child can die from dehydration in just a few days. Adults, particularly the elderly, can also become dangerously ill if severely dehydrated.

A condition referred to as *traveler's diarrhea* has become a common health concern due to the expansion in global travel. Traveler's diarrhea is discussed in the **Highlight** box (page 108).

TABLE 3.3 Signs and Symptoms of Dehydration in Adults and Children

Signs and Symptoms in Adults	Signs and Symptoms in Children
Thirst	Dry mouth and tongue
Light-headedness	No tears when crying
Less frequent urination	No wet diapers for 3 hours or more
Dark-colored urine	High fever
Fatigue	Sunken abdomen, eyes, or cheeks
Dry skin	Irritable or listless
	Skin that does not flatten when pinched and released

Source: Data from National Digestive Diseases Information Clearinghouse (NDDIC). 2001. Diarrhea. NIH Publication No. 01–2749.

diarrhea A condition characterized by the frequent passage of loose, watery stools.

HIGHLIGHT

Traveler's Diarrhea—What Is It and How Can You Prevent It?

Diarrhea is the rapid movement of fecal matter through the large intestine, often accompanied by large volumes of water. *Traveler's diarrhea* (also called *dysentery*) is experienced by people traveling to countries outside of their own and is usually caused by a viral or bacterial infection. Diarrhea is the body's way of ridding itself of the invasive agent. The large intestine and even some of the small intestine become irritated by the microbes and the resulting immune response. This irritation leads to increased secretion of fluid and increased peristalsis of the large intestine, causing watery stools and a higher-than-normal frequency of bowel movements.

Travelers generally get diarrhea from consuming water or food that is contaminated with fecal matter. High-risk destinations include developing countries in Africa, Asia, Latin America, and the Caribbean.[1]

Symptoms include fatigue, lack of appetite, abdominal cramps, and watery diarrhea. In some cases, you may also experience nausea, vomiting, and low-grade fever. Usually, this diarrhea passes within 4 to 6 days, and people recover completely.

What can you do to prevent traveler's diarrhea? The National Digestive Diseases Clearinghouse advises that travelers to high-risk areas avoid the following:[1]

- Drinking tap water, using tap water to brush their teeth, and using ice made from tap water

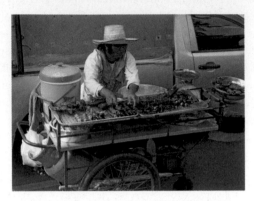

When traveling in developing countries, it is wise to avoid food from street vendors.

- Drinking unpasteurized milk or milk products
- Eating raw fruits and vegetables, including lettuce and fruit salads, unless they peel the fruits or vegetables themselves
- Eating raw or rare meat and fish
- Eating meat or shellfish that is not hot when served
- Eating food from street vendors

Travelers can drink bottled water, soft drinks, and hot drinks, such as coffee or tea.

If you do suffer from traveler's diarrhea, it is important to replace the fluid and nutrients lost as a result of the illness. Specially formulated oral rehydration solutions are usually available in most countries at local pharmacies or stores. Antibiotics may also be prescribed to kill the bacteria. Once treatment is initiated, the diarrhea should cease within 2 to 3 days. If the diarrhea persists for more than 10 days after the initiation of treatment, or if there is blood in your stools, you should return to a physician immediately to avoid serious medical consequences.

Reference

1. National Digestive Diseases Information Clearinghouse (NDDIC). 2011. Diarrhea. NIH Publication No. 11–2749. http://digestive.niddk.nih.gov/ddiseases/pubs/diarrhea/index.htm.

Constipation

At the opposite end of the spectrum is **constipation,** which is typically defined as a condition in which no stools are passed for 2 or more days; however, it is important to recognize that some people normally experience bowel movements only every second or third day. Thus, the definition of constipation varies from one person to another. In addition to being infrequent, the stools are usually hard, small, and difficult to pass.

Constipation is frequent in people who have disorders affecting the nervous system, which in turn affect the muscles of the large intestine, as they do not receive the appropriate neurologic signals needed for involuntary muscle movement to occur. For these individuals, drug therapy is often needed to maintain bowel functioning.

Many people experience temporary constipation at some point in their lives in response to a variety of factors. Often people have trouble with it when they travel, when

constipation A condition characterized by the absence of bowel movements for a period of time that is significantly longer than normal for the individual.

their schedule is disrupted, if they change their diet, or if they are on certain medications. Increasing fiber and fluid in the diet is one of the mainstays of preventing constipation. Five servings of fruits and vegetables each day and six or more servings of whole grains is helpful to most people. If you eat breakfast cereal, make sure you buy one containing at least 2 to 3 g of fiber per serving. (The dietary recommendation for fiber and the role it plays in maintaining healthy elimination is discussed in detail in Chapter 4.) Staying well hydrated by drinking lots of water is especially important when increasing fiber intake. Exercising also helps reduce the risk for constipation.

Irritable Bowel Syndrome

Irritable bowel syndrome (IBS) is a disorder that interferes with normal functions of the colon. Symptoms include abdominal cramps, bloating, and either constipation or diarrhea. It is one of the most common disorders, affecting as many as 20% of Americans. More women than men are diagnosed with IBS, which typically first appears before age 35.[15]

IBS causes no digestive damage that can be observed or measured, nor does it lead to a serious disease, such as cancer.[15] However, it appears that the colon is more sensitive to physiologic or emotional stress in people with IBS than in healthy people. Some researchers believe that the problem stems from conflicting messages between the central nervous system and the enteric nervous system. The immune system may also trigger symptoms of IBS. Whatever the cause, the normal movement of the colon appears to be disrupted. In some people with IBS, food moves too quickly through the colon and fluid cannot be absorbed fast enough, which causes diarrhea. In others, the movement of the colon is too slow and too much fluid is absorbed, leading to constipation. The following are some of the foods thought to cause physiologic stress linked to IBS:

- Caffeinated drinks, such as tea, coffee, and colas
- Chocolate, alcohol, dairy products, and wheat
- Large meals

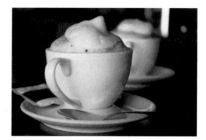

Consuming caffeinated drinks is one of several factors that have been linked with irritable bowel syndrome (IBS), a disorder that interferes with normal functioning of the colon.

Some women with IBS find that their symptoms worsen during their menstrual period, indicating a possible link between reproductive hormones and IBS. Certain medications may also increase the risk.

The high prevalence of the diagnosis in the United States, along with the lack of any sign of physical disease, has led to charges that IBS is overdiagnosed or misdiagnosed. Some physicians do not agree that IBS qualifies as a disease, pointing out that stress has always affected the enteric nervous system. Others argue that US physicians too often apply the diagnosis of IBS before screening for more serious disorders. For example, it is not uncommon for patients who have been diagnosed with IBS to test positive for celiac disease.[15] If you think you have IBS, it is important to have a complete physical examination to rule out any other disorders.

Treatment options include certain medications to treat diarrhea or constipation, stress management, and regular physical activity. Dietary modifications can also help. These include eating smaller meals, avoiding foods that exacerbate symptoms, eating a higher-fiber diet, and drinking at least six to eight glasses of water each day.[15]

RECAP

Diarrhea is the frequent passage of loose or watery stools, whereas constipation is the failure to have a bowel movement for 2 or more days or within a time period that is normal for the individual. Diarrhea should be treated quickly to avoid dehydration. Constipation often can be corrected by increasing your intake of fiber and water. Irritable bowel syndrome (IBS) causes abdominal cramps, pain, bloating, and constipation or diarrhea. Factors linked by some studies to the exacerbation of IBS include stress, the consumption of certain foods and fluids, large meals, and certain medications. ■

irritable bowel syndrome (IBS)   A stress-related disorder that interferes with normal functions of the colon. Symptoms are abdominal cramps, bloating, and constipation or diarrhea.

Chapter Review

1 **T** Sometimes you may have an appetite even though you are not hungry. These feelings are referred to as "cravings" and are associated with physical or emotional cues.

2 **F** Your brain, not your stomach, is the primary organ responsible for telling you when you are hungry.

3 **F** Even extreme food restriction, such as near-starvation, does not cause the stomach to shrink permanently. Likewise, the stomach doesn't stretch permanently. The folds in the wall of the stomach flatten as it expands to accommodate a large meal, but they re-form over the next few hours as the food empties into the small intestine. Only after gastric surgery, when a very small stomach "pouch" remains, can stomach tissue stretch permanently.

4 **T** Although there are individual variations in how we respond to food, the entire process of digestion and absorption of one meal usually takes about 24 hours.

5 **T** Most ulcers result from an infection by the bacterium *Helicobacter pylori* (*H. pylori*). Contrary to popular belief, ulcers are not caused by stress or spicy food.

Summary

- Hunger is a physiologic drive that prompts us to eat. It is regulated by the hypothalamus.

- Foods that contain fiber, water, and large amounts of protein have the highest satiety value.

- Appetite is a psychological desire to consume specific foods; this desire is influenced by sensory data, social and cultural cues, and learning.

- Digestion is the process of breaking down foods into molecules small enough to be transported into enterocytes. Absorption is the process of taking molecules of food out of the gastrointestinal tract and into the circulation. Elimination is the process of removing undigested food and waste products from the body.

- In the mouth, chewing starts the mechanical digestion of food. Saliva contains salivary amylase, an enzyme that initiates the chemical digestion of carbohydrates.

- Food moves down to the stomach through the esophagus via a process called peristalsis. Peristalsis involves rhythmic waves of squeezing and pushing food through the gastrointestinal tract.

- The stomach mixes and churns food together with gastric juices. Hydrochloric acid and the enzyme pepsin initiate protein digestion, and a minimal amount of fat digestion begins through the action of gastric lipase.

- The stomach periodically releases the partially digested food, referred to as chyme, into the small intestine.

- Most of the digestion and absorption of nutrients occurs in the small intestine.

- The large intestine digests any remaining food particles, absorbs water and chemicals, and moves feces to the rectum for elimination.

- Enzymes guide the digestion of food via the process of hydrolysis. Most digestive enzymes are synthesized by the pancreas and small intestine.

- The four primary hormones that regulate digestion are gastrin, secretin, cholecystokinin, and gastric inhibitory peptide.

- The gallbladder stores bile and secretes it into the small intestine to assist with the digestion of lipids.

- The pancreas manufactures and secretes digestive enzymes into the small intestine. Pancreatic amylase digests carbohydrates, pancreatic lipase digests lipids, and proteases digest proteins. The pancreas also synthesizes two hormones that play a critical role in carbohydrate metabolism, insulin and glucagon.

- The liver processes, packages, and stores nutrients, detoxifies the blood, synthesizes bile, and regulates the metabolism of monosaccharides, fatty acids, and amino acids.

- The lining of the small intestine has folds, villi, and microvilli that increase its surface area and absorptive capacity.

- The four types of absorption that occur in the small intestine are passive diffusion, facilitated diffusion, active transport, and endocytosis.

- The neuromuscular system involves coordination of the muscles as well as the enteric, peripheral, and central nervous systems to move food along the gastrointestinal tract and to control digestion, absorption, and elimination.

- Belching results from swallowed air, and flatulence can be caused by the consumption of foods rich in fibers, starches, and sugars, such as beans, dairy products, and some vegetables.

- Heartburn occurs when hydrochloric acid seeps into the esophagus and burns its lining. Gastroesophageal reflux disease (GERD) is a more painful type of heartburn that occurs more than twice per week.

- A peptic ulcer is an area in the stomach or duodenum that has been eroded away by hydrochloric acid and pepsin.

- Food allergies can cause either localized reactions, such as a minor skin rash, or systemic inflammation resulting in respiratory and circulatory collapse.

- People with celiac disease cannot eat gluten, a protein found in wheat, rye, and barley, as it causes an immune reaction that damages intestinal villi, leading to malabsorption of nutrients and malnutrition.

- Acute vomiting is usually a protective response, whereas cyclic vomiting syndrome is a chronic disorder that can lead to severe dehydration.

- Crohn's disease is a chronic disease that causes inflammation in the small intestine, whereas ulcerative colitis damages the mucosal lining of the colon. The causes of these diseases are unknown.

- Diarrhea is the frequent (more than three times per day) elimination of loose, watery stools. Constipation is a condition in which no stools are passed for 2 or more days or for a length of time considered abnormally long for the individual. Irritable bowel syndrome is a stress-related disorder that interferes with normal functions of the colon, causing pain, diarrhea, and/or constipation.

MasteringNutrition™

To further your understanding, go online and apply what you've learned to real-life case studies that will help you master the content!

Review Questions

1. Which of the following processes moves food along the entire GI tract?
   a. mass movement
   b. peristalsis
   c. haustration
   d. segmentation

2. Bile is a greenish fluid that
   a. is produced by the gallbladder.
   b. is stored by the pancreas.
   c. denatures proteins.
   d. emulsifies lipids.

3. The region of brain tissue that is responsible for prompting us to seek food is the
   a. pituitary gland.
   b. brain.
   c. hypothalamus.
   d. thalamus.

4. Heartburn is caused by
   a. seepage of gastric acid into the esophagus.
   b. seepage of gastric acid into the cardiac muscle.
   c. seepage of bile into the stomach.
   d. seepage of salivary amylase into the trachea.

5. Which of the following foods is likely to keep a person satiated for the longest period of time?
   a. a bean and cheese burrito
   b. a serving of full-fat ice cream
   c. a bowl of rice cereal in whole milk
   d. a tossed salad with oil and vinegar dressing

6. **True or false?** Hunger is more physiological, and appetite is more psychological.

7. **True or false?** The autonomic nerves in the walls of the GI tract are collectively known as the enteric nervous system.

8. **True or false?** Vitamins and minerals are digested in the small intestine.

9. **True or false?** Vomiting is regulated by a cluster of cells in the brain stem.

10. **True or false?** The specialized absorptive cells of the small intestine are called enterocytes.

11. Explain why it can be said that you are what you eat.

12. Imagine that the lining of your small intestine were smooth, like the inside of a rubber tube. Would this design be efficient in performing the main function of this organ? Why or why not?

13. Why doesn't the acidic environment of the stomach cause it to digest itself?

14. Create a table comparing the area of inflammation, symptoms, and treatment options for celiac disease, Crohn's disease, and ulcerative colitis.

15. After dinner, your roommate lies down to rest for a few minutes before studying. When he gets up, he complains of a sharp, burning pain in his chest. Offer a possible explanation for his pain.

Math Review

16. Some people use baking soda as an antacid. The pH of baking soda is 9.0. The pH of gastric juice is 2.0. Express the alkalinity of baking soda in relation to gastric juice using a logarithmic equation.

Answers to Review Questions and Math Review are located on the MasteringNutrition Study Area.

Web Links

www.digestive.niddk.nih.gov
National Digestive Diseases Information Clearinghouse (NDDIC)
Explore this site to learn more about the disorders covered in this chapter.

www.healthfinder.gov
Health Finder
This site has further information on the disorders related to digestion, absorption, and elimination.

www.foodallergy.org
Food Allergy & Anaphylaxis Network (FAN)
Visit this site to learn more about common food allergies.

www.csaceliacs.org
Celiac Sprue Association—National Celiac Disease Support Group
The website for this national educational organization provides information and referral services for individuals with celiac disease.

www.celiaccenter.org
University of Maryland Center for Celiac Research
This university-based research website has useful information and resources on celiac disease.

www.ccfa.org
Crohn's & Colitis Foundation of America
Search this site to learn more about the most current research, news and advocacy information on ulcerative colitis and Crohn's disease.

References

1. Marieb, E., and K. Hoehn. 2013. *Human Anatomy and Physiology*. 9th edn. San Francisco: Benjamin Cummings, p. 569.
2. Saulnier, D. M., S. Kolida, and G. R. Gibson. 2009. Microbiology of the human intestinal tract and approaches for its dietary modulation. *Curr. Pharm. Des*. 15(13):1403–1414.
3. Fetissov, S. O., A. Laviano, S. Kalra, and A. Inui. 2010. Update on ghrelin. *Int. J. Pept. 963501*.
4. National Institute of Diabetes and Digestive and Kidney Diseases (NIDDK). 2012. Heartburn, Gastroesophageal Reflux (GER), and Gastroesophageal Reflux Disease (GERD). NIH Publication No. 07–0882. http://digestive.niddk.nih.gov/ddiseases/pubs/gerd/index.htm.
5. National Digestive Diseases Information Clearinghouse (NDDIC). 2012. *H. pylori* and Peptic Ulcer. NIH Publication No. 10–4225. http://digestive.niddk.nih.gov/ddiseases/pubs/hpylori/index.htm.
6. National Digestive Diseases Information Clearinghouse (NDDIC). 2012. NSAIDs and Peptic Ulcers. NIH Publication No. 10–4644. http://digestive.niddk.nih.gov/ddiseases/pubs/nsaids/index.htm.
7. US Food and Drug Administration (FDA). 2012. Food Allergies: What You Need to Know. www.fda.gov/food/resourcesforyou/consumers/ucm079311.htm.
8. National Digestive Diseases Information Clearinghouse (NDDIC). 2012. Celiac Disease. NIH Publication No. 12-4269. http://digestive.niddk.nih.gov/ddiseases/pubs/celiac/.
9. National Institutes of Health (NIH). 2012. Celiac Disease Awareness Campaign: Frequently Asked Questions about the Campaign. http://celiac.nih.gov/FAQ.aspx.
10. National Institutes of Health (NIH). 2011. NIH-funded scientists discover gluten-degrading enzymes in the mouth. *Celiac Disease News*. www.celiac.nih.gov/NewsletterSummer11.aspx.
11. National Digestive Diseases Information Clearinghouse (NDDIC). 2012. Cyclic Vomiting Syndrome. NIH Publication No. 09-4548. http://digestive.niddk.nih.gov/ddiseases/pubs/cvs/index.aspx.
12. National Digestive Diseases Information Clearinghouse (NDDIC). 2011. Crohn's Disease. NIH Publication No. 12–3410. http://digestive.niddk.nih.gov/ddiseases/pubs/crohns/index.htm.
13. National Digestive Diseases Information Clearinghouse (NDDIC). 2011. Ulcerative Colitis. NIH Publication No. 12-1597. http://digestive.niddk.nih.gov/ddiseases/pubs/colitis/index.aspx.
14. National Digestive Diseases Information Clearinghouse (NDDIC). 2011. Diarrhea. NIH Publication No. 11–2749. http://digestive.niddk.nih.gov/ddiseases/pubs/diarrhea/index.htm.
15. National Digestive Diseases Information Clearinghouse (NDDIC). 2012. Irritable Bowel Syndrome. NIH Publication No. 07–693. http://digestive.niddk.nih.gov/ddiseases/pubs/ibs/.

Should All School-Age Children Be Screened for Celiac Disease?

A *screening test* is a diagnostic procedure that elicits data about the presence or absence of characteristic signs of a disorder. Every baby born in a U.S. hospital undergoes at least two screening tests within the first 48 hours of life.[1] These are for a metabolic disorder called phenylketonuria and for hypothyroidism, a disorder affecting the thyroid gland. In addition, it is recommended that states require their hospitals to test newborns for more than fifty other conditions that may affect childhood health. Once they get to school, most children in the United States are also screened for vision and hearing impairment, learning disorders, excessive sleepiness, head lice, and other problems. With all this screening going on, should school-age children also be screened for celiac disease?

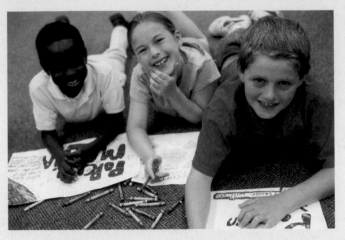

School-age children may have celiac disease and not know it. Undiagnosed celiac disease can lead to a variety of serious health problems as children grow.

Researchers and healthcare professionals in favor of screening children for celiac disease point to several factors in support of their position. First, the prevalence in the United States is high enough to be of general concern: about 1 in every 133 Americans is believed to have celiac disease.[2] This is in line with prevalence rates in Europe, where many countries do have screening programs.

In addition, celiac disease is thought to be greatly underdiagnosed. This is in part because many healthcare providers in the United States are not knowledgeable about the disease or familiar with its manifestations, especially those that don't involve the digestive system, and therefore attribute their patients' symptoms to other causes. In fact, the National Institutes of Health (NIH) in 2006 launched the Celiac Disease Awareness Campaign to raise awareness of the disease among healthcare providers and share information about appropriate diagnostic tests and treatment. In a 2009 study, researchers found that among children age 3 and up with positive results on a screening test for celiac disease, the majority had an "atypical gastrointestinal presentation" or no symptoms at all.[3] Many other studies, in both Europe and the United States, also reveal a significant prevalence of "silent celiac disease"; that is, the individual

is not aware of having any illness symptoms, but a screening test comes back positive, and a follow-up biopsy reveals atrophy of the intestinal villi. The intestinal damage in these people puts them at risk for all of the complications of untreated celiac disease. In one study of Swedish families who had a teen diagnosed with celiac after a routine screening, 92% said they were grateful for the screening, even when the diagnosis "came out of the blue."[4]

In children, one of the potentially serious consequences of a missed diagnosis is short stature, which results when childhood celiac disease prevents nutrient absorption during the years when nutrition is critical to normal growth and development.[2] Children who are diagnosed and treated before their growth period ends may be able to catch up to the growth of their peers, but after that time, the short stature is irreversible. Other possible consequences of a missed diagnosis include an increased risk for depression, anxiety, learning disorders, seizures, autoimmune disorders, type 1 diabetes, thyroid disease, liver disease, poor bone density, and GI cancers.[2]

Arguments against routine testing center on the invasiveness of current screening techniques, questions of reliability of the available tests, and uncertainty about when to recommend a gluten-free diet.[5] Let's look at these one at a time:

- *Invasiveness:* Unlike the screening tests for vision, hearing, or head lice, the antibody test for celiac disease is invasive, requiring that the healthcare provider draw a small amount of blood. Some families object to invasive medical tests for religious or other reasons.
- *Reliability:* Although the antibody test is considered generally reliable for diagnosing celiac disease, false negatives are not uncommon, even among adults. However, because a child's immune system is still developing, the reliability of the test for children is even lower. The only definitive proof of celiac disease is a biopsy of the small intestine that shows atrophy of the villi. But

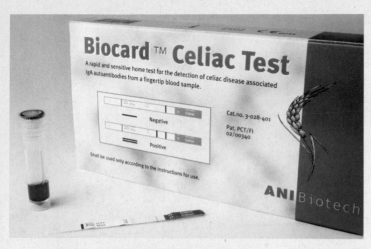

A simple blood test can identify celiac disease.

few people would argue that all children should undergo a biopsy.

- *Uncertainty about need for gluten-free diet:* Many children who test positive with the antibody screen do not have symptoms or any damage to the intestinal villi. Do these children need to go on the highly restrictive gluten-free diet? And when? Because current research data do not indicate a clear benefit of a gluten-free diet in people with latent disease, this question is the subject of debate.[5]

Finally, the concept of routine screening itself is a matter of some controversy. While few would argue against simple, low-cost screening tests such as those for vision or hearing problems, some people hesitate when tests become more costly. The United States does not currently require screening of all children for type 1 or type 2 diabetes, obesity, or many other serious health problems, so why should the public be burdened with screening for celiac disease?

At this time, national healthcare agencies do not support routine screening for celiac disease. Instead, the NIH Celiac Disease Awareness Campaign recommends more research into the benefits and cost-effectiveness of screening in the general population. Ongoing with this research, the campaign recommends increased education of physicians, registered dietitians, and other healthcare providers.[6]

CRITICAL THINKING QUESTIONS

- Now that you've read the arguments for and against routine screening of American children for celiac disease, do you think that all children should have the test? Why or why not?
- If you said yes to the first question, who should pay for it? Parents? School districts? The public health department?
- Given the number of children who are home-schooled or in private schools, how could we ensure that all families were offered screening?
- Would you be in favor of routine screening of children for type 2 diabetes, hypertension, obesity, and other disorders?
- What factors seem most important to consider when deciding which diseases we screen for in American children?

REFERENCES

1. Davidson, M., M. London, and P. Ladewig. 2012. *Maternal–Newborn Nursing & Women's Health.* 9th edn. Upper Saddle River, NJ: Pearson Prentice Hall, p. 843.
2. National Digestive Diseases Information Clearinghouse (NDDIC). 2012. Celiac Disease. NIH Publication No. 12-4269. http://digestive.niddk.nih.gov/ddiseases/pubs/celiac/.
3. McGowan, K. E., D. A. Castiglione, and J. D. Butzner. (2009). The changing face of childhood celiac disease in North America: impact of serological testing. *Pediatrics* 124(6):1572–1578.
4. Rosen, A., M. Emmelin, A. Carlsson, S. Hammarroth, E. Karlsson, and A. Ivarsson. 2011. Mass screening for celiac disease from the perspective of newly diagnosed adolescents and their parents: a mixed-method study. *BMC Public Health* 11:822.
5. Hoffenberg, E. J. 2005. Should all children be screened for celiac disease? *Gastroenterology* 128(suppl.):S98–S103.
6. National Institutes of Health (NIH). 2012. Celiac Disease Awareness Campaign. http://celiac.nih.gov/.

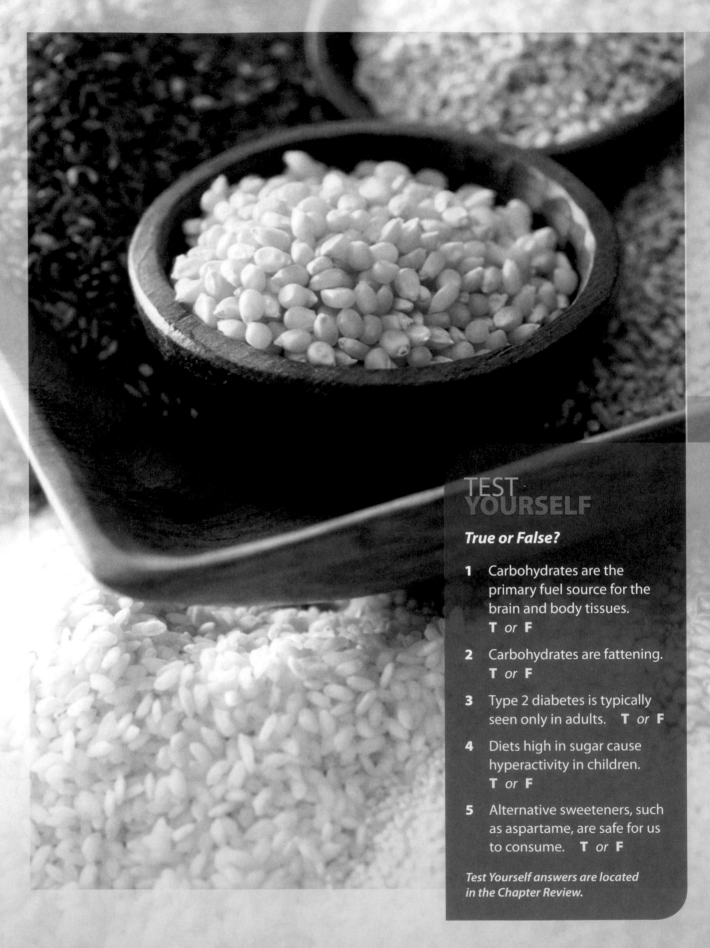

TEST YOURSELF

True or False?

1 Carbohydrates are the primary fuel source for the brain and body tissues. **T** *or* **F**

2 Carbohydrates are fattening. **T** *or* **F**

3 Type 2 diabetes is typically seen only in adults. **T** *or* **F**

4 Diets high in sugar cause hyperactivity in children. **T** *or* **F**

5 Alternative sweeteners, such as aspartame, are safe for us to consume. **T** *or* **F**

Test Yourself answers are located in the Chapter Review.

4 Carbohydrates: Plant-Derived Energy Nutrients

Learning Objectives

After studying this chapter, you should be able to:

1. Describe the difference between simple and complex carbohydrates, *pp. 119–122*.

2. Describe the difference between alpha and beta bonds, and discuss how these bonds are related to the digestion of fiber and lactose intolerance, *pp. 121–122*.

3. Compare and contrast soluble and insoluble fibers, *pp. 123–124*.

4. Discuss how carbohydrates are digested and absorbed by the body, *pp. 125–128*.

5. List four functions of carbohydrates in the body, *pp. 131–132*.

6. Define the Acceptable Macronutrient Distribution Range for carbohydrates and the Adequate Intake for fiber, *pp. 134, 139*.

7. Identify the potential health risks associated with diets high in added sugars, *pp. 135–136*.

8. List five foods that are good sources of carbohydrates, *pp. 138–139*.

9. Identify three alternative sweeteners, *pp. 142, 144–145*.

10. Describe type 1 and type 2 diabetes, and discuss how diabetes differs from hypoglycemia, *pp. 145–150*.

MasteringNutrition™

Go online for chapter quizzes, pre-tests, Interactive Activities, and more!

It's common for college seniors to stress out about their future: Will I get into grad school? Find a good job? Be able to make new friends? But Sara, a 21-year-old college senior, has a more critical concern. She wonders when her legs will be amputated, and whether or not she'll go blind. Sara was diagnosed with type 2 diabetes when she was 16 years old. Her doctor prescribed weight loss and oral medication, but she's been unable to keep the weight off and recently her blood glucose soared out of control despite the drugs. As a result, she was started on insulin injections. Sara is not alone: A 2012 study found that a combination of oral medication and an intensive weight-loss program failed to control blood glucose in 47% of young participants, including those who adhered strictly to the treatment protocol.[1]

Thirty years ago, type 2 diabetes was so rare in anyone younger than middle age it was known as *adult-onset diabetes.* Now it is diagnosed in thousands of children and teens each year. A similar escalation has been seen among adult Americans: The US Centers for Disease Control and Prevention report that, if current trends continue, the prevalence of diabetes may skyrocket from 1 in 10 to 1 in 3 by 2050. Diabetes is the leading cause of surgical leg and foot amputations, blindness, and kidney failure among U.S. adults. It is also the seventh leading cause of death.[2]

What is diabetes, and why are we discussing it in a chapter on carbohydrates? Does carbohydrate consumption somehow lead to diabetes—or, for that matter, to obesity or any other disorder? Several popular diets—including the Zone Diet,[3] Sugar Busters,[4] and Dr. Atkins' New Diet Revolution[5]—claim that carbohydrates are bad for your health and waistline. Are carbohydrates a health menace, and should we reduce our intake?

In this chapter, we explore the differences between simple and complex carbohydrates and learn why some carbohydrates are better than others. We also learn how the human body breaks down carbohydrates and uses them to maintain our health and to fuel our activity and exercise. Because carbohydrate metabolism sometimes goes wrong, we also discuss its relationship to some common health disorders, including diabetes.

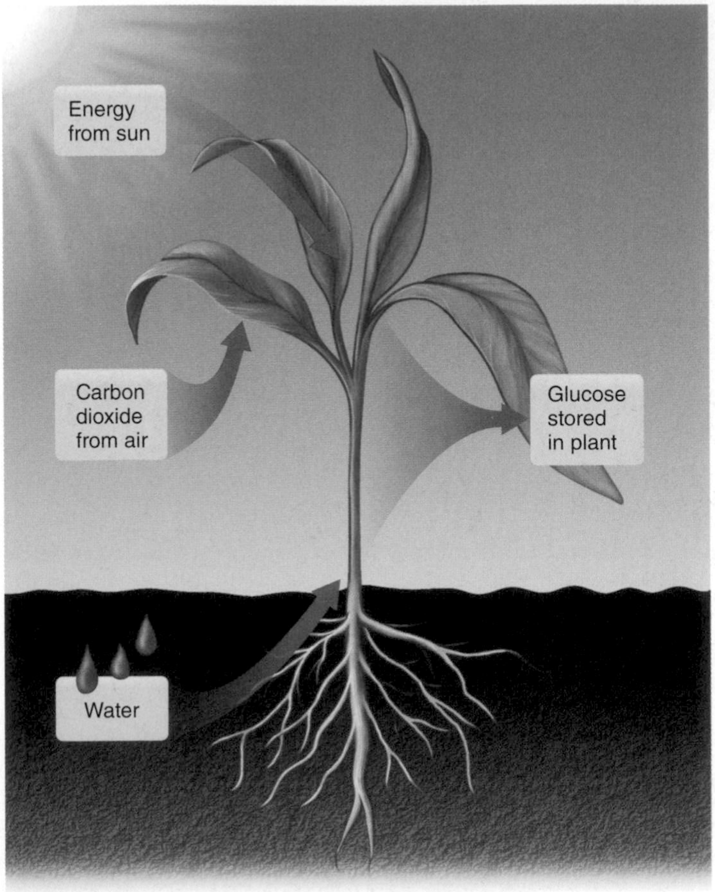

FIGURE 4.1 Plants make carbohydrates through the process of photosynthesis. Water, carbon dioxide, and energy from the sun are combined to produce glucose.

carbohydrates One of the three macronutrients, a compound made up of carbon, hydrogen, and oxygen that is derived from plants and provides energy.

glucose The most abundant sugar molecule, a monosaccharide generally found in combination with other sugars; the preferred source of energy for the brain and an important source of energy for all cells.

photosynthesis A process by which plants use sunlight to fuel a chemical reaction that combines carbon and water into glucose, which is then stored in their cells.

What Are Carbohydrates?

As mentioned previously (in Chapter 1), **carbohydrates** are one of the three macronutrients. As such, they are an important energy source for the entire body and are the preferred energy source for nerve cells, including those of the brain. We will say more about their functions later in this chapter.

The term *carbohydrate* literally means "hydrated carbon." When something is said to be *hydrated,* it contains water, which is made up of hydrogen and oxygen (H_2O). The chemical abbreviation for carbohydrate (CHO) indicates the atoms it contains: carbon, hydrogen, and oxygen.

We obtain carbohydrates predominantly from plant foods, such as fruits, vegetables, and grains. Plants make the most abundant form of carbohydrate, called **glucose,** through a process called **photosynthesis.** During photosynthesis, the green pigment of plants, called *chlorophyll,* absorbs sunlight, which provides the energy needed to fuel the manufacture of glucose. As shown in **Figure 4.1**, water absorbed from the earth by the roots of plants combines with carbon dioxide present in the leaves to produce the carbohydrate glucose. Plants continually store glucose and use it to support their own growth. Then, when we eat plant foods, our bodies digests, absorbs, and uses the stored glucose.

Carbohydrates can be classified as *simple* or *complex*. Simple carbohydrates contain either one or two molecules, whereas complex carbohydrates contain hundreds to thousands of molecules.

Simple Carbohydrates Include Monosaccharides and Disaccharides

Simple carbohydrates are commonly referred to as *sugars*. Four of these sugars are called **monosaccharides** because they consist of a single sugar molecule (*mono*, meaning "one," and *saccharide*, meaning "sugar"). The other three sugars are **disaccharides**, which consist of two molecules of sugar joined together (*di*, meaning "two").

Glucose, Fructose, Galactose, and Ribose Are Monosaccharides

Glucose, fructose, and *galactose* are the three most common monosaccharides in our diet. Each of these monosaccharides contains 6 carbon atoms, 12 hydrogen atoms, and 6 oxygen atoms (**Figure 4.2**). Very slight differences in the structure of these three monosaccharides cause major differences in their level of sweetness.

Given what you've just learned about how plants manufacture glucose, it probably won't surprise you to discover that glucose is the most abundant monosaccharide found in our diet and in our bodies. Glucose does not generally occur by itself in foods but attaches to other sugars to form disaccharides and complex carbohydrates. In our bodies, glucose is the preferred source of energy for the brain, and it is a very important source of energy for all cells.

Fructose, the sweetest natural sugar, occurs in fruits and vegetables. Fructose is also called *levulose,* or *fruit sugar.* In many processed foods, it is a component of *high-fructose corn syrup.* This syrup is made from corn and is used to sweeten soft drinks, desserts, candies, and jellies.

Galactose does not occur alone in foods. It joins with glucose to create lactose, one of the three most common disaccharides.

Ribose is a five-carbon monosaccharide. Very little ribose is found in our diet; our bodies produce ribose from the foods we eat, and ribose is contained in the genetic material of our cells: deoxyribonucleic acid (DNA) and ribonucleic acid (RNA).

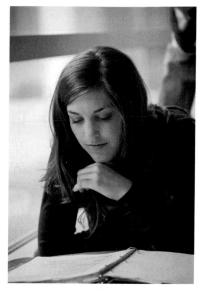

Glucose is the preferred source of energy for the brain.

simple carbohydrate   A monosaccharide or disaccharide, such as glucose; commonly called *sugar.*

monosaccharide   The simplest of carbohydrates; consists of one sugar molecule, the most common form of which is glucose.

disaccharide   A carbohydrate compound consisting of two monosaccharide molecules joined together.

fructose   The sweetest natural sugar; a monosaccharide that occurs in fruits and vegetables; also called *levulose,* or *fruit sugar.*

galactose   A monosaccharide that joins with glucose to create lactose, one of the three most common disaccharides.

ribose   A five-carbon monosaccharide that is located in the genetic material of cells.

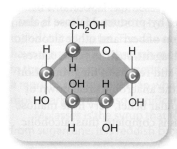

Glucose
Most abundant sugar molecule in our diet; good energy source

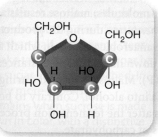

Fructose
Sweetest natural sugar; found in fruit, high-fructose corn syrup

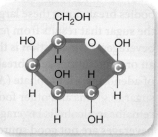

Galactose
Does not occur alone in foods; binds with glucose to form lactose

FIGURE 4.2 The three most common monosaccharides. Notice that all three monosaccharides contain identical atoms: 6 carbon, 12 hydrogen, and 6 oxygen. It is only the arrangement of these atoms that differs.

Carbohydrate Digestion Overview

The primary goal of carbohydrate digestion is to break down polysaccharides and disaccharides into monosaccharides that can then be converted to glucose.

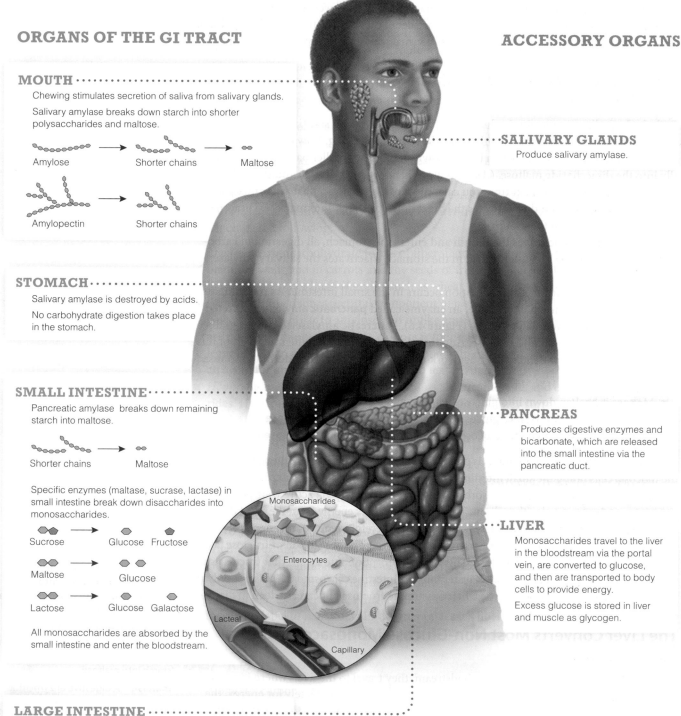

ORGANS OF THE GI TRACT

MOUTH
Chewing stimulates secretion of saliva from salivary glands.

Salivary amylase breaks down starch into shorter polysaccharides and maltose.

Amylose → Shorter chains → Maltose

Amylopectin → Shorter chains

STOMACH
Salivary amylase is destroyed by acids.

No carbohydrate digestion takes place in the stomach.

SMALL INTESTINE
Pancreatic amylase breaks down remaining starch into maltose.

Shorter chains → Maltose

Specific enzymes (maltase, sucrase, lactase) in small intestine break down disaccharides into monosaccharides.

Sucrose → Glucose Fructose

Maltose → Glucose

Lactose → Glucose Galactose

All monosaccharides are absorbed by the small intestine and enter the bloodstream.

LARGE INTESTINE
Some carbohydrates pass into the large intestine undigested.

Bacteria ferment some undigested carbohydrate.

Remaining fiber is excreted in feces.

ACCESSORY ORGANS

SALIVARY GLANDS
Produce salivary amylase.

PANCREAS
Produces digestive enzymes and bicarbonate, which are released into the small intestine via the pancreatic duct.

LIVER
Monosaccharides travel to the liver in the bloodstream via the portal vein, are converted to glucose, and then are transported to body cells to provide energy.

Excess glucose is stored in liver and muscle as glycogen.

Monosaccharides

Enterocytes

Lacteal

Capillary

combines with carbon dioxide present in the leaves to produce the carbohydrate glucose. Plants continually store glucose and use it to support their own growth. Then, when we eat plant foods, our bodies digests, absorbs, and uses the stored glucose.

Carbohydrates can be classified as *simple* or *complex*. Simple carbohydrates contain either one or two molecules, whereas complex carbohydrates contain hundreds to thousands of molecules.

Simple Carbohydrates Include Monosaccharides and Disaccharides

Simple carbohydrates are commonly referred to as *sugars*. Four of these sugars are called **monosaccharides** because they consist of a single sugar molecule (*mono*, meaning "one," and *saccharide*, meaning "sugar"). The other three sugars are **disaccharides,** which consist of two molecules of sugar joined together (*di*, meaning "two").

Glucose, Fructose, Galactose, and Ribose Are Monosaccharides

Glucose, fructose, and *galactose* are the three most common monosaccharides in our diet. Each of these monosaccharides contains 6 carbon atoms, 12 hydrogen atoms, and 6 oxygen atoms (**Figure 4.2**). Very slight differences in the structure of these three monosaccharides cause major differences in their level of sweetness.

Given what you've just learned about how plants manufacture glucose, it probably won't surprise you to discover that glucose is the most abundant monosaccharide found in our diet and in our bodies. Glucose does not generally occur by itself in foods but attaches to other sugars to form disaccharides and complex carbohydrates. In our bodies, glucose is the preferred source of energy for the brain, and it is a very important source of energy for all cells.

Fructose, the sweetest natural sugar, occurs in fruits and vegetables. Fructose is also called *levulose,* or *fruit sugar.* In many processed foods, it is a component of *high-fructose corn syrup.* This syrup is made from corn and is used to sweeten soft drinks, desserts, candies, and jellies.

Galactose does not occur alone in foods. It joins with glucose to create lactose, one of the three most common disaccharides.

Ribose is a five-carbon monosaccharide. Very little ribose is found in our diet; our bodies produce ribose from the foods we eat, and ribose is contained in the genetic material of our cells: deoxyribonucleic acid (DNA) and ribonucleic acid (RNA).

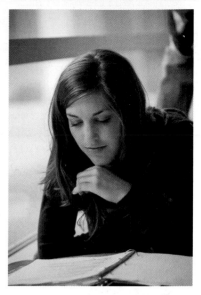

Glucose is the preferred source of energy for the brain.

simple carbohydrate A monosaccharide or disaccharide, such as glucose; commonly called *sugar*.

monosaccharide The simplest of carbohydrates; consists of one sugar molecule, the most common form of which is glucose.

disaccharide A carbohydrate compound consisting of two monosaccharide molecules joined together.

fructose The sweetest natural sugar; a monosaccharide that occurs in fruits and vegetables; also called *levulose,* or *fruit sugar.*

galactose A monosaccharide that joins with glucose to create lactose, one of the three most common disaccharides.

ribose A five-carbon monosaccharide that is located in the genetic material of cells.

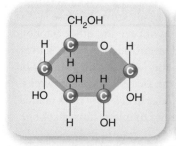

Glucose
Most abundant sugar molecule in our diet; good energy source

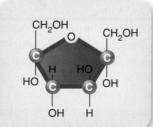

Fructose
Sweetest natural sugar; found in fruit, high-fructose corn syrup

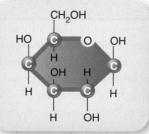

Galactose
Does not occur alone in foods; binds with glucose to form lactose

FIGURE 4.2 The three most common monosaccharides. Notice that all three monosaccharides contain identical atoms: 6 carbon, 12 hydrogen, and 6 oxygen. It is only the arrangement of these atoms that differs.

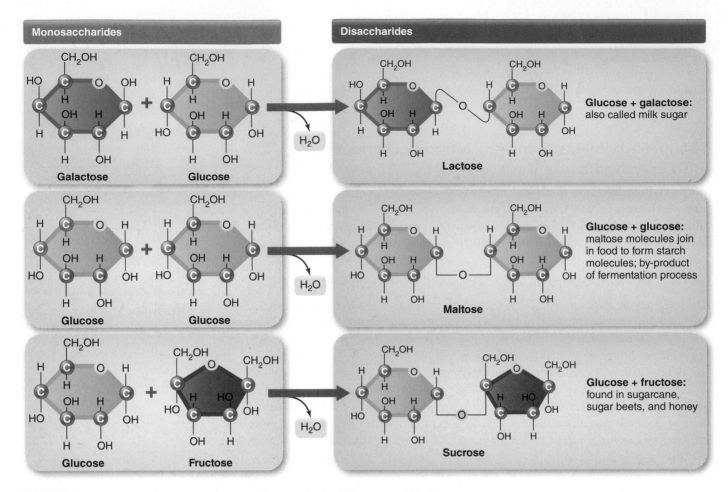

FIGURE 4.3 Galactose, glucose, and fructose join together in different combinations to make the disaccharides lactose, maltose, and sucrose.

Lactose, Maltose, and Sucrose Are Disaccharides

The three most common disaccharides found in foods are *lactose, maltose,* and *sucrose* (**Figure 4.3**). **Lactose** (also called *milk sugar*) consists of one glucose molecule and one galactose molecule. Interestingly, human breast milk has a higher amount of lactose than cow's milk, which makes human breast milk taste sweeter.

Maltose (also called *malt sugar*) consists of two molecules of glucose. It does not generally occur by itself in foods but rather is bound together with other molecules. As our bodies break down these larger molecules, maltose results as a by-product. Maltose is also the sugar that results from *fermentation* during the production of beer and other alcoholic beverages. **Fermentation** is the anaerobic process in which an agent, such as yeast, causes an organic substance to break down into simpler substances and results in the production of adenosine triphosphate (ATP). Maltose is formed during the anaerobic breakdown of sugar in grains and other foods into alcohol. Contrary to popular belief, very little maltose remains in alcoholic beverages after the fermentation process is complete; thus, alcoholic beverages are not good sources of carbohydrate.

Sucrose is composed of one glucose molecule and one fructose molecule. Because sucrose contains fructose, it is sweeter than lactose or maltose. Sucrose provides much of the sweet taste found in honey, maple syrup, fruits, and vegetables. Table sugar, brown sugar, powdered sugar, and many other products are made by refining the sucrose found in sugarcane and sugar beets. Are honey and other naturally occurring forms of sucrose more healthful than manufactured forms? The feature box **Nutrition Myth or Fact? Is Honey More Nutritious Than Table Sugar?** investigates this question.

lactose Also called *milk sugar,* a disaccharide consisting of one glucose molecule and one galactose molecule; found in milk, including human breast milk.

maltose A disaccharide consisting of two molecules of glucose; does not generally occur independently in foods but results as a by-product of digestion; also called *malt sugar.*

fermentation The anaerobic process in which an agent causes an organic substance to break down into simpler substances and results in the production of ATP.

sucrose A disaccharide composed of one glucose molecule and one fructose molecule; sweeter than lactose or maltose.

Is Honey More Nutritious Than Table Sugar?

Liz's friend Tiffany is dedicated to eating healthful foods. She advises Liz to avoid sucrose and to eat foods that contain honey, molasses, or raw sugar. Like many people, Tiffany believes these sweeteners are more natural and nutritious than refined table sugar. How can Liz sort sugar fact from fiction?

Remember that sucrose consists of one glucose molecule and one fructose molecule joined together. From a chemical perspective, honey is almost identical to sucrose, because honey also contains glucose and fructose molecules in almost equal amounts. However, enzymes in bees' "honey stomachs" separate some of the glucose and fructose molecules; as a result, honey looks and tastes slightly different from sucrose. As you know, bees store honey in combs, and they fan it with their wings to reduce its moisture content. This also alters the appearance and texture of honey.

Honey does not contain any more nutrients than sucrose, so it is not a more healthful choice than sucrose. In fact, per tablespoon, honey has more Calories (energy) than table sugar. This is because the crystals in table sugar take up more space on a spoon than the liquid form of honey, so a tablespoon contains less sugar. However, some people argue that honey is sweeter, so you use less.

It is important to note that honey commonly contains bacteria that can cause fatal food poisoning in infants. The more mature digestive system of older children and adults is immune to the effects of these bacteria, but babies younger than 12 months should never be given honey.

Are raw sugar and molasses more healthful than table sugar? Actually, the "raw sugar" available in the United States is not really raw. Truly raw sugar is made up of the first crystals obtained when sugar is processed. Sugar in this form contains dirt, parts of insects, and other by-products that make it illegal to sell in the United States. The raw sugar products in American stores have actually gone through more than half of the same steps in the refining process used to make table sugar. Raw sugar has a more coarse texture than white sugar and is unbleached; in most markets, it is also significantly more expensive.

Molasses is the syrup that remains when sucrose is made from sugarcane. It is reddish brown in color, with a distinctive taste that is less sweet than table sugar. It does contain some iron, but this iron does not occur naturally. It is a contaminant from the machines that process the sugarcane! Incidentally, blackstrap molasses is the residue of a third boiling of the syrup. It contains less sugar than light or dark molasses but more minerals.

Table 4.1 compares the nutrient content of white sugar, honey, blackstrap molasses, and raw sugar. As you can see, none of them contain many nutrients that are important for health. This is why highly sweetened products are referred to as "empty Calories."

TABLE 4.1 Nutrient Comparison of Four Different Sugars

	Table Sugar	Raw Sugar	Honey	Molasses
Energy (kcal)	49	55	64	58
Carbohydrate (g)	12.6	13.8	17.3	14.95
Fat (g)	0	0	0	0
Protein (g)	0	0	0.06	0
Fiber (g)	0	0	0	0
Vitamin C (mg)	0	0	0.1	0
Vitamin A (IU)	0	0	0	0
Thiamin (mg)	0	0	0	0.008
Riboflavin (mg)	0.002	0.003	0.008	0
Folate (µg)	0	0	0	0
Calcium (mg)	0	2	1	41
Iron (mg)	0.01	0.05	0.09	0.94
Sodium (mg)	0	0	1	7
Potassium (mg)	0	4	11	293

Note: Nutrient values are identified for 1 tablespoon of each product.

Source: US Department of Agriculture, Agricultural Research Service. 2011. USDA National Nutrient Database for Standard Reference, Release 24.

The two monosaccharides that compose a disaccharide are attached by a bond between oxygen and one carbon on each of the monosaccharides (**Figure 4.4**, page 122). Two forms of this bond occur in nature: an **alpha bond** and a **beta bond**. As you can see in Figure 4.4a, sucrose is produced by an alpha bond joining a glucose molecule and a fructose molecule. The disaccharide maltose is also produced by an alpha bond. In contrast,

alpha bond   A type of chemical bond that can be digested by enzymes found in the human intestine.

beta bond   A type of chemical bond that cannot be easily digested by enzymes found in the human intestine.

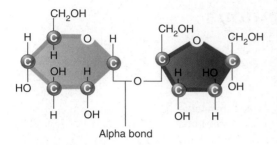

(a) Sucrose

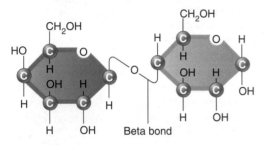

(b) Lactose

FIGURE 4.4 The two monosaccharides that compose a disaccharide are attached by either (a) an alpha bond or (b) a beta bond between oxygen and one carbon of each monosaccharide.

lactose is produced by a beta bond joining a glucose molecule and a galactose molecule (Figure 4.4b). Alpha bonds are easily digestible by humans, whereas beta bonds are very difficult to digest and may even be nondigestible. As you will learn later in this chapter, many people do not possess enough of the enzyme lactase, needed to break the beta bond present in lactose, which causes the condition referred to as *lactose intolerance.* Beta bonds are also present in high-fiber foods, leading to our inability to digest most forms of fiber.

RECAP

Carbohydrates contain carbon, hydrogen, and oxygen. Simple carbohydrates include monosaccharides and disaccharides. Glucose, fructose, galactose, and ribose are monosaccharides; lactose, maltose, and sucrose are disaccharides. In disaccharides, two monosaccharides are linked together with either an alpha bond or a beta bond. Alpha bonds are easily digestible by humans, whereas beta bonds are not easily digestible. ■

Oligosaccharides and Polysaccharides Are Complex Carbohydrates

Complex carbohydrates, the second major classification of carbohydrate, generally consist of long chains of glucose molecules. Technically, any carbohydrates with three or more monosaccharides are considered complex carbohydrates.

Oligosaccharides are carbohydrates that contain 3 to 10 monosaccharides (*oligo,* meaning "few"). Two of the most common oligosaccharides found in our diet are **raffinose** and **stachyose.** Raffinose is composed of galactose, glucose, and fructose. It is commonly found in beans, cabbage, brussels sprouts, broccoli, and whole grains. Stachyose is composed of two galactose molecules, a glucose molecule, and a fructose molecule. It is found in many beans and other legumes.

Raffinose and stachyose are part of the raffinose family of oligosaccharides (RFOs).[6] Because humans do not possess the enzyme needed to break down these RFOs, they pass into the large intestine undigested. Once they reach the large intestine, they are fermented by bacteria that produce gases such as carbon dioxide, methane, and hydrogen. The product Beano® contains the enzyme alpha-galactosidase; this is the enzyme needed to break down the RFOs in the intestinal tract. Thus, this product can help to reduce the intestinal gas caused by eating beans and various vegetables.

Most **polysaccharides** consist of hundreds to thousands of glucose molecules (*poly,* meaning "many").[6] The polysaccharides include starch, glycogen, and most fibers (**Figure 4.5**).

complex carbohydrate A nutrient compound consisting of long chains of glucose molecules, such as starch, glycogen, and fiber.

oligosaccharides Complex carbohydrates that contain 3 to 10 monosaccharides.

raffinose An oligosaccharide composed of galactose, glucose, and fructose. Also called melitose, it is found in beans, cabbage, broccoli, and other vegetables.

stachyose An oligosaccharide composed of two galactose molecules, a glucose molecule, and a fructose molecule; found in the Chinese artichoke and various beans and legumes.

polysaccharide A complex carbohydrate consisting of long chains of glucose.

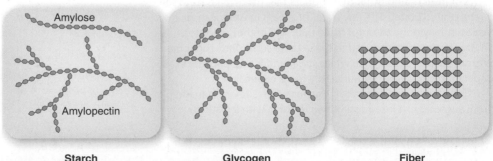

Starch	Glycogen	Fiber
Storage form of glucose in plants; found in grains, legumes, and tubers	Storage form of glucose in animals; stored in liver and muscles	Forms the support structures of leaves, stems, and plants

FIGURE 4.5 Polysaccharides, also referred to as complex carbohydrates, include starch, glycogen, and fiber.

Starch Is a Polysaccharide Stored in Plants

Plants store glucose not as single molecules but as polysaccharides in the form of **starch.** The two forms of starch are *amylose* and *amylopectin* (see Figure 4.5). Amylose is a straight chain of glucose molecules, whereas amylopectin is highly branched. Both forms of starch are found in starch-containing foods. The more open-branched structure of amylopectin increases its surface area and thus its exposure to digestive enzymes; as a result, it is more rapidly digested than amylose. In turn, amylopectin raises blood glucose more quickly than amylose.

Excellent food sources of starch include grains (wheat, rice, corn, oats, and barley), legumes (peas, beans, and lentils), and tubers (potatoes and yams). Our cells cannot use the complex starch molecules exactly as they occur in plants. Instead, the body must break them down into the monosaccharide glucose, from which we can then fuel our energy needs.

Our bodies easily digest most starches, in which alpha bonds link the numerous glucose units; however, starches linked by beta bonds are largely indigestible and are called *resistant.* Technically, resistant starch is classified as a type of fiber. When our intestinal bacteria ferment resistant starch, a short-chain fatty acid called *butyrate* is produced. Consuming resistant starch may be beneficial: some research suggests that butyrate reduces the risk for cancer.[7] Legumes contain more resistant starch than do grains, fruits, or vegetables. This quality, plus their high protein and fiber content, makes legumes a healthful food.

Glycogen Is a Polysaccharide Stored by Animals

Glycogen is the storage form of glucose for animals, including humans. After an animal is slaughtered, most of the glycogen is broken down by enzymes found in animal tissues. Thus, very little glycogen exists in meat. As plants contain no glycogen, it is not a dietary source of carbohydrate. We can very quickly break down the glycogen stored in the body into glucose when we need it for energy. We store glycogen in our muscles and liver; the storage and use of glycogen are discussed in more detail on pages 125–127.

Fiber Is a Polysaccharide That Gives Plants Their Structure

Like starch, fiber is composed of long polysaccharide chains; however, the body does not easily break down the bonds that connect fiber molecules. This means that most fibers pass through the digestive system without being digested and absorbed, so they contribute no energy to our diet. However, fiber offers many other health benefits (see pages 132–133).

There are currently a number of definitions of fiber. The Food and Nutrition Board of the Institute of Medicine uses three distinctions: *dietary fiber, functional fiber,* and *total fiber.*[6]

- **Dietary fiber** is the non-digestible parts of plants that form the support structures of leaves, stems, and seeds (see Figure 4.5). In a sense, you can think of dietary fiber as the plant's "skeleton."
- **Functional fiber** consists of nondigestible forms of carbohydrates that are extracted from plants or manufactured in a laboratory and have known health benefits. Functional fiber is added to foods and is the form found in fiber supplements. Examples of functional fiber sources you might see on nutrition labels include cellulose, guar gum, pectin, and psyllium.
- **Total fiber** is the sum of dietary fiber and functional fiber.

Fiber can also be classified according to its chemical and physical properties as soluble or insoluble.

Soluble Fibers **Soluble fibers** dissolve in water. They are also **viscous,** forming a gel when wet, and they are fermentable; that is, they are easily digested by bacteria in the colon. Soluble fibers are typically found in citrus fruits, berries, oat products, and beans.

Research suggests that regular consumption of soluble fibers reduces the risks for cardiovascular disease and type 2 diabetes by lowering blood cholesterol and blood glucose levels. The possible mechanisms by which fiber reduces the risk for various diseases are discussed in more detail on pages 132–133.

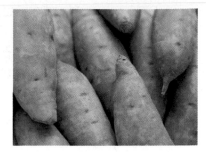

Tubers, such as these sweet potatoes, are excellent food sources of starch.

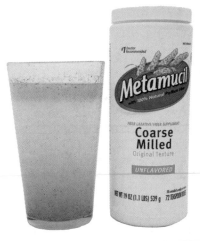

Dissolvable laxatives are examples of soluble fiber.

starch The storage form of glucose (as a polysaccharide) in plants.

glycogen The storage form of glucose (as a polysaccharide) in animals.

dietary fiber The nondigestible carbohydrate parts of plants that form the support structures of leaves, stems, and seeds.

functional fiber The nondigestible forms of carbohydrate that are extracted from plants or manufactured in the laboratory and have known health benefits.

total fiber The sum of dietary fiber and functional fiber.

soluble fibers Fibers that dissolve in water.

viscous Having a gel-like consistency; viscous fibers form a gel when dissolved in water.

Soluble fibers include the following:

- *Pectins,* which contain chains of galacturonic acid and other monosaccharides. Pectins are found in the cell walls and intracellular tissues of many fruits and berries. They can be isolated and used to thicken foods, such as jams and yogurts.
- *Gums* contain galactose, glucuronic acid, and other monosaccharides. Gums are a diverse group of polysaccharides that are viscous. They are typically isolated from seeds and are used as thickening, gelling, and stabilizing agents. Guar gum and gum arabic are common gums used as food additives.
- *Mucilages* are similar to gums and contain galactose, mannose, and other monosaccharides. Two examples include psyllium and carrageenan. Psyllium is the husk of psyllium seeds, which are also known as plantago or flea seeds. Carrageenan comes from seaweed. Mucilages are used as food stabilizers.

Insoluble Fibers **Insoluble fibers** are those that do not typically dissolve in water. These fibers are usually nonviscous and cannot be fermented by bacteria in the colon. They are generally found in whole grains, such as wheat, rye, and brown rice, as well as in many vegetables. These fibers are not associated with reducing cholesterol levels but are known for promoting regular bowel movements, alleviating constipation, and reducing the risk for a bowel disorder called diverticulosis (discussed later in this chapter). Examples of insoluble fibers include the following:

- *Lignins* are noncarbohydrate forms of fiber. Lignins are found in the woody parts of plant cell walls and in carrots and the seeds of fruits and berries. Lignins are also found in brans (the outer husk of grains such as wheat, oats, and rye) and other whole grains.
- *Cellulose* is the main structural component of plant cell walls. Cellulose is a chain of glucose units similar to amylose, but unlike amylose, cellulose contains beta bonds that are nondigestible by humans. Cellulose is found in whole grains, fruits, vegetables, and legumes. It can also be extracted from wood pulp or cotton, and it is added to foods as an agent for anti-caking, thickening, and texturizing.
- *Hemicelluloses* contain glucose, mannose, galacturonic acid, and other monosaccharides. Hemicelluloses are found in plant cell walls and they surround cellulose. They are the primary component of cereal fibers and are found in whole grains and vegetables. Although many hemicelluloses are insoluble, some are also classified as soluble.

Fiber-Rich Carbohydrates Materials written for the general public usually don't refer to the carbohydrates found in foods as complex or simple; instead, resources such as the Dietary Guidelines for Americans 2010 emphasize eating **fiber-rich carbohydrates,** such as fruits, vegetables, and whole grains.[8] This term is important, because fiber-rich carbohydrates are known to contribute to good health, but not all complex carbohydrate foods are fiber-rich. For example, potatoes that have been processed into frozen hash browns retain very little of their original fiber. On the other hand, some foods rich in simple carbohydrates (such as fruits) are also rich in fiber. So when you're reading labels, it pays to check the grams of dietary fiber per serving. And if the food you're considering is fresh produce and there's no label to read, that almost guarantees it's fiber-rich.

insoluble fibers Fibers that do not dissolve in water.

fiber-rich carbohydrates A group of foods containing either simple or complex carbohydrates that are rich in dietary fiber. These foods, which include most fruits, vegetables, and whole grains, are typically fresh or moderately processed.

RECAP

Complex carbohydrates include oligosaccharides and polysaccharides. The three types of polysaccharides are starch, glycogen, and fiber. Starch is the storage form of glucose in plants, whereas glycogen is the storage form of glucose in animals. Fiber forms the support structures of plants. Soluble fibers dissolve in water, are viscous, and can be digested by bacteria in the colon, whereas insoluble fibers do not dissolve in water, are not viscous, and cannot be digested. Fiber-rich carbohydrates are known to contribute to good health. ■

How Do Our Bodies Break Down Carbohydrates?

Glucose is the form of sugar that our bodies use for energy, and the primary goal of carbohydrate digestion is to break down polysaccharides and disaccharides into monosaccharides, which can then be converted to glucose. The previous chapter (Chapter 3) provided an overview of digestion of the three types of macronutrients, as well as vitamins and minerals. Here, we focus specifically and in more detail on the digestion and absorption of carbohydrates. **Figure 4.6** (page 126) provides a visual tour of carbohydrate digestion.

Digestion Breaks Down Most Carbohydrates into Monosaccharides

Carbohydrate digestion begins in the mouth (Figure 4.6). As you saw (in Chapter 3), the starch in the foods you eat mixes with your saliva during chewing. Saliva contains an enzyme called **salivary amylase,** which breaks down starch into smaller particles and eventually into the disaccharide maltose. (*Amyl-* is a prefix referring to starch, and the suffix *–ase* indicates an enzyme.) The next time you eat a piece of bread, notice that you can actually taste it becoming sweeter; this indicates the breakdown of starch into maltose. Disaccharides are not digested in the mouth.

As the bolus of food leaves the mouth and enters the stomach, all digestion of carbohydrates ceases. This is because the acid in the stomach inactivates the salivary amylase enzyme (Figure 4.6).

The majority of carbohydrate digestion occurs in the small intestine. As the contents of the stomach enter the small intestine, an enzyme called **pancreatic amylase** is secreted by the pancreas into the small intestine (Figure 4.6). Pancreatic amylase continues to digest any remaining starch into maltose. Additional enzymes found in the microvilli of the mucosal cells that line the intestinal tract work to break down disaccharides into monosaccharides (Figure 4.6):

- Maltose is broken down into glucose by the enzyme **maltase.**
- Sucrose is broken down into glucose and fructose by the enzyme **sucrase.**
- Lactose is broken down into glucose and galactose by the enzyme **lactase.**

Once digestion of carbohydrates is complete, all monosaccharides are then absorbed into the mucosal cells lining the small intestine, where they pass through and enter into the bloodstream. Glucose and galactose are absorbed across the enterocytes via active transport using a carrier protein saturated with sodium. This process requires energy from the breakdown of ATP. Fructose is absorbed via facilitated diffusion and therefore requires no energy. (Refer to Chapter 3 for a description of these transport processes.) The absorption of fructose takes longer than that of glucose or galactose. This slower absorption rate means that fructose stays in the small intestine longer and draws water into the intestines via osmosis. This not only results in a smaller rise in blood glucose when consuming fructose but can also lead to diarrhea.

The Liver Converts Most Non-Glucose Monosaccharides into Glucose

Once the monosaccharides enter the bloodstream, they travel to the liver, where fructose and galactose are converted to glucose (Figure 4.6). If needed immediately for energy, the glucose is released into the bloodstream, where it can travel to the cells to provide energy. If glucose is not needed immediately for energy, it is stored as glycogen in the liver and muscles. Enzymes in liver and muscle cells combine glucose molecules to form glycogen (an anabolic, or building, process) and break glycogen into glucose (a catabolic, or destructive, process), depending on the body's energy needs. On average, the liver can store 70 g (280 kcal) and the muscles can store about 120 g (480 kcal) of glycogen. Between meals, our

salivary amylase An enzyme in saliva that breaks starch into smaller particles and eventually into the disaccharide maltose.

pancreatic amylase An enzyme secreted by the pancreas into the small intestine that digests any remaining starch into maltose.

maltase A digestive enzyme that breaks maltose into glucose.

sucrase A digestive enzyme that breaks sucrose into glucose and fructose.

lactase A digestive enzyme that breaks lactose into glucose and galactose.

The primary goal of carbohydrate digestion is to break down polysaccharides and disaccharides into monosaccharides that can then be converted to glucose.

ORGANS OF THE GI TRACT

ACCESSORY ORGANS

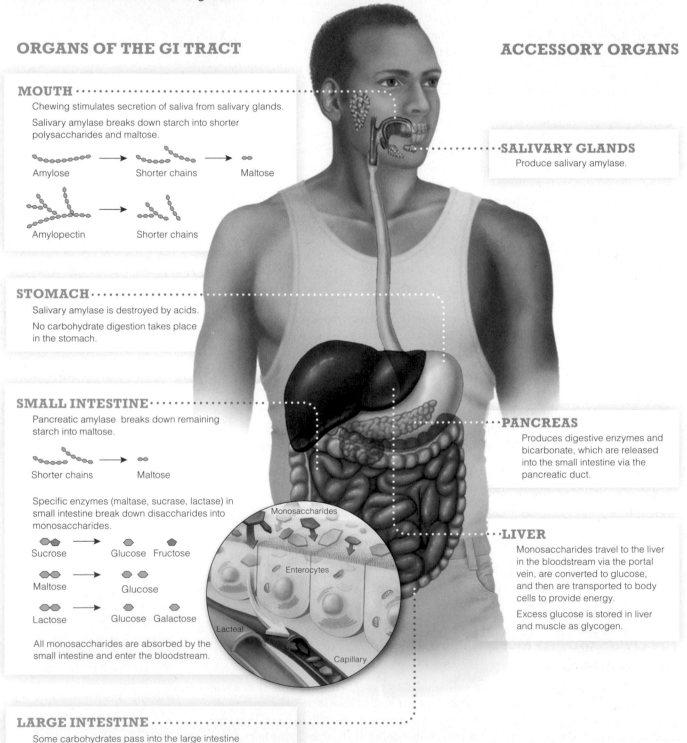

MOUTH

Chewing stimulates secretion of saliva from salivary glands.

Salivary amylase breaks down starch into shorter polysaccharides and maltose.

Amylose → Shorter chains → Maltose

Amylopectin → Shorter chains

STOMACH

Salivary amylase is destroyed by acids.

No carbohydrate digestion takes place in the stomach.

SMALL INTESTINE

Pancreatic amylase breaks down remaining starch into maltose.

Shorter chains → Maltose

Specific enzymes (maltase, sucrase, lactase) in small intestine break down disaccharides into monosaccharides.

Sucrose → Glucose Fructose

Maltose → Glucose

Lactose → Glucose Galactose

All monosaccharides are absorbed by the small intestine and enter the bloodstream.

Monosaccharides

Enterocytes

Lacteal

Capillary

LARGE INTESTINE

Some carbohydrates pass into the large intestine undigested.

Bacteria ferment some undigested carbohydrate.

Remaining fiber is excreted in feces.

SALIVARY GLANDS

Produce salivary amylase.

PANCREAS

Produces digestive enzymes and bicarbonate, which are released into the small intestine via the pancreatic duct.

LIVER

Monosaccharides travel to the liver in the bloodstream via the portal vein, are converted to glucose, and then are transported to body cells to provide energy.

Excess glucose is stored in liver and muscle as glycogen.

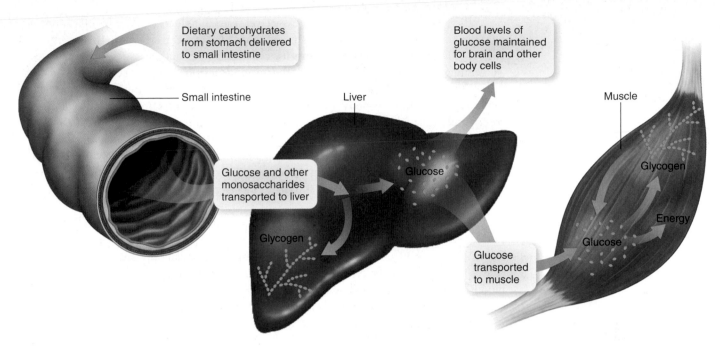

FIGURE 4.7 Glucose is stored as glycogen in both the liver and muscle. The glycogen stored in the liver maintains blood glucose between meals; muscle glycogen provides immediate energy to the muscle during exercise.

bodies draw on liver glycogen reserves to maintain blood glucose levels and support the needs of our cells, including those of our brain, spinal cord, and red blood cells (**Figure 4.7**).

The glycogen stored in our muscles continually provides energy to the muscles, particularly during intense exercise. Endurance athletes can increase their storage of muscle glycogen from two to four times the normal amount through a process called *glycogen,* or *carbohydrate, loading* (see Chapter 14). Any excess glucose is stored as glycogen in the liver and muscles and saved for such future energy needs as exercise. Once the carbohydrate storage capacity of the liver and muscles is reached, any excess glucose can be stored as fat in adipose tissue.

Fiber Is Excreted from the Large Intestine

As previously mentioned, humans do not possess enzymes in the small intestine that can break down fiber. Thus, fiber passes through the small intestine undigested and enters the large intestine, or colon. There, bacteria ferment some previously undigested carbohydrates, causing the production of gases such as hydrogen, methane, and sulfur and a few short-chain fatty acids such as acetic acid, butyric acid, and propionic acid. The cells of the large intestine use these short-chain fatty acids for energy. It is estimated that fermented fibers yield about 1.5 to 2.5 kcal/g.[5,6] This is less than the 4 kcal/g provided by carbohydrates that are digested and absorbed in the small intestine; the discrepancy is due to the fact that fermentation of the fibers in the colon is an anaerobic process, which yields less energy than the aerobic digestive process of other carbohydrates. Obviously, the fibers that remain totally undigested contribute no energy to our bodies. Fiber remaining in the colon adds bulk to our stools and is excreted in feces (Figure 4.6). In this way, fiber assists in maintaining bowel regularity. The health benefits of fiber are discussed later in this chapter.

A Variety of Hormones Regulate Blood Glucose Levels

Our bodies regulate blood glucose levels within a fairly narrow range to provide adequate glucose to the brain and other cells. A number of hormones, including insulin, glucagon, epinephrine, norepinephrine, cortisol, and growth hormone, assist the body with maintaining blood glucose.

When we eat a meal, our blood glucose level rises. But glucose in our blood cannot help the nerves, muscles, and other tissues function unless it can cross into their cells. Glucose molecules are too large to cross the cell membranes of our tissues independently. To get in, glucose needs assistance from the hormone **insulin,** which is secreted by the beta cells of the pancreas (**Figure 4.8** top panel). Insulin is transported in the blood to the cells of tissues throughout the body, where it stimulates special carrier proteins, called *glucose transporters,* located in cells. The arrival of insulin at the cell membrane stimulates glucose transporters to travel to the surface of the cell, where they assist in transporting glucose across the cell membrane and into the cell. Insulin can be thought of as a key that opens the gates of the cell membrane, enabling the transport of glucose into the cell interior, where it can be used for energy. Insulin also stimulates the liver and muscles to take up glucose and store it as glycogen.

When you have not eaten for a period of time, your blood glucose level declines. This decrease in blood glucose stimulates the alpha cells of the pancreas to secrete another hormone, **glucagon** (Figure 4.8 bottom panel). Glucagon acts in an opposite way to insulin: it causes the liver to convert its stored glycogen into glucose, which is then secreted into the bloodstream and transported to the cells for energy. Glucagon also assists in the breakdown of body proteins to amino acids, so that the liver can stimulate *gluconeogenesis* ("generating new glucose"), the production of glucose from amino acids.

Epinephrine, norepinephrine, cortisol, and growth hormone are additional hormones that work to increase blood glucose. Epinephrine and norepinephrine are secreted by the adrenal glands and nerve endings when blood glucose levels are low. They act to increase glycogen breakdown in the liver, resulting in a subsequent increase in the release of glucose into the bloodstream. They also increase gluconeogenesis. These two hormones are also responsible for our "fight-or-flight" reaction to danger; they are released when we need a burst of energy to respond quickly. Cortisol and growth hormone are secreted by the adrenal glands to act on liver, muscle, and adipose tissue. Cortisol increases gluconeogenesis and decreases the use of glucose by muscles and other body organs. Growth hormone decreases glucose uptake by the muscles, increases our mobilization and use of the fatty acids stored in our adipose tissue, and increases the liver's output of glucose.

Normally, the effects of these hormones balance each other to maintain blood glucose within a healthy range. If this balance is altered, it can lead to health conditions such as diabetes (pages 146–149) or hypoglycemia (page 150).

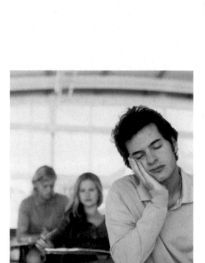

Our red blood cells, brain, and nerve cells primarily rely on glucose. This is why we get tired, irritable, and shaky when we have not eaten for a prolonged period of time.

insulin A hormone secreted by the beta cells of the pancreas in response to increased blood levels of glucose that facilitates uptake of glucose by body cells.

glucagon A hormone secreted by the alpha cells of the pancreas in response to decreased blood levels of glucose; it stimulates the liver to convert stored glycogen into glucose, which is released into the bloodstream and transported to cells for energy.

glycemic index A rating of the potential of foods to raise blood glucose and insulin levels.

RECAP

Carbohydrate digestion starts in the mouth and continues in the small intestine. Glucose and other monosaccharides are absorbed into the bloodstream and travel to the liver, where non-glucose monosaccharides are converted to glucose. Glucose is used by the cells for energy, converted to glycogen and stored in the liver and muscles for later use, or converted to fat and stored in adipose tissue. Various hormones are involved in regulating blood glucose. Insulin lowers blood glucose levels by facilitating the entry of glucose into cells. Glucagon, epinephrine, norepinephrine, cortisol, and growth hormone raise blood glucose levels by a variety of mechanisms. ■

The Glycemic Index Shows How Foods Affect Our Blood Glucose Levels

The term **glycemic index** refers to the potential of foods to raise blood glucose levels. Foods with a high glycemic index cause a sudden surge in blood glucose. This in turn triggers a large increase in insulin, which may be followed by a dramatic drop in blood glucose. Foods with a low glycemic index cause low to moderate fluctuations in blood glucose. When foods are assigned a glycemic index value, they are often compared to the glycemic effect of pure glucose.

Regulation of Blood Glucose

Our bodies regulate blood glucose levels within a fairly narrow range to provide adequate glucose to the brain and other cells. Insulin and glucagon are two hormones that play a key role in regulating blood glucose.

HIGH BLOOD GLUCOSE

1 **Insulin secretion:** When blood glucose levels increase after a meal, the pancreas secretes the hormone insulin from the beta cells into the bloodstream.

2 **Cellular uptake:** Insulin travels to the tissues. There, it stimulates glucose transporters within cells to travel to the cell membrane, where they facilitate glucose transport into the cell to be used for energy.

3 **Glucose storage:** Insulin also stimulates the storage of glucose in body tissues. Glucose is stored as glycogen in the liver and muscles (glycogenesis), and is stored as triglycerides in adipose tissue (lipogenesis).

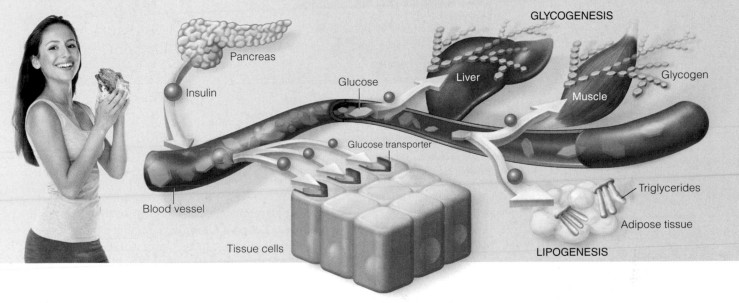

Pancreas

Insulin

Blood vessel

Glucose

Glucose transporter

Tissue cells

GLYCOGENESIS

Liver

Muscle

Glycogen

Triglycerides

Adipose tissue

LIPOGENESIS

LOW BLOOD GLUCOSE

1 **Glucagon secretion:** When blood glucose levels are low, the pancreas secretes the hormone glucagon from the alpha cells into the bloodstream.

2 **Glycogenolysis:** Glucagon stimulates the liver to convert stored glycogen into glucose, which is released into the blood and transported to the cells for energy.

3 **Gluconeogenesis:** Glucagon also assists in the breakdown of proteins and the uptake of amino acids by the liver, which creates glucose from amino acids.

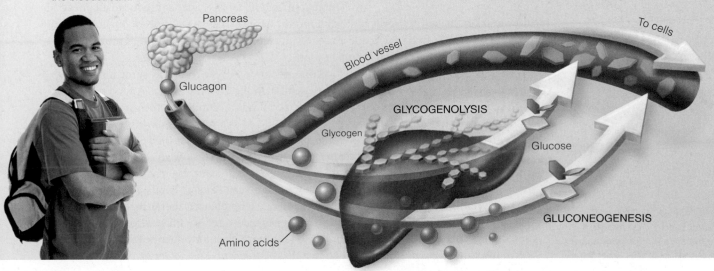

Pancreas

Glucagon

Blood vessel

To cells

GLYCOGENOLYSIS

Glycogen

Glucose

Amino acids

GLUCONEOGENESIS

129

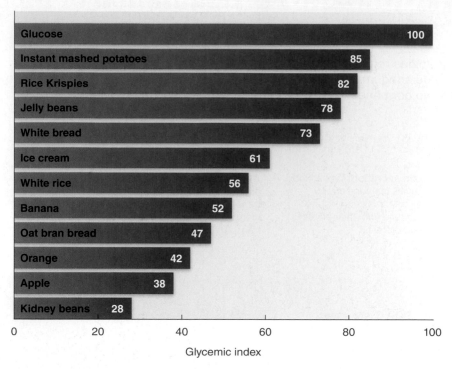

FIGURE 4.9 Glycemic index values for various foods as compared to pure glucose. (*Source:* Data adapted from International Table of Glycemic Index and Glycemic Load Values," by Foster-Powell, K.,S. H. A. Holt, and J. C. Brand-Miller, from *American Journal of Clinical Nutrition*, 2002.)

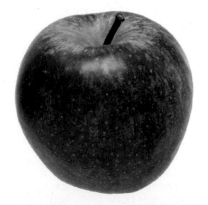

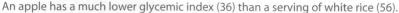

An apple has a much lower glycemic index (36) than a serving of white rice (56).

The glycemic index of a food is not always easy to predict. **Figure 4.9** ranks certain foods according to their glycemic index. Do any of these rankings surprise you? Most people assume that foods containing simple sugars have a higher glycemic index than starches, but this is not always the case. For instance, compare the glycemic index for apples and instant potatoes. Although instant potatoes are a starchy food, they have a glycemic index value of 85, while the value for an apple is only 38!

The type of carbohydrate, the way the food is prepared, and its fat and fiber content can all affect how quickly the body absorbs it. It is important to note that we eat most of our foods combined into a meal. In this case, the glycemic index of the total meal becomes more important than the ranking of each food.

For determining the effect of a food on a person's glucose response, some nutrition experts believe the **glycemic load** is more useful than the glycemic index. A food's glycemic load is the number of grams of carbohydrate it contains multiplied by the glycemic index of that carbohydrate. For instance, carrots are recognized as a vegetable having a relatively high glycemic index of about 68; however, the glycemic load of carrots is only 3.[9] This is because there is very little total carbohydrate in a serving of carrots. The low glycemic load of carrots means that carrot consumption is unlikely to cause a significant rise in glucose and insulin.

Why do we care about the glycemic index and glycemic load? Foods or meals with a lower glycemic load are a better choice for someone with diabetes, because they will not trigger dramatic fluctuations in blood glucose. They may also reduce the risk for heart disease and colon cancer, because they generally contain more fiber, and fiber helps decrease fat levels in the blood. Recent studies have shown that people who eat a lower glycemic index diet

glycemic load The amount of carbohydrate in a food multiplied by the glycemic index of the carbohydrate.

have higher levels of high-density lipoprotein, or HDL (a healthful blood lipid), and lower levels of low-density lipoprotein, or LDL (a blood lipid associated with increased risk for heart disease), and their blood glucose values are more likely to be normal.[10, 11] Diets with a low glycemic index and load are also associated with a reduced risk for prostate cancer.[12]

Despite some encouraging research findings, the glycemic index and glycemic load remain controversial. Many nutrition researchers feel that the evidence supporting their health benefits is weak. In addition, many believe the concepts of the glycemic index/load are too complex for people to apply to their daily lives. Other researchers insist that helping people choose foods with a lower glycemic index/load is critical to the prevention and treatment of many chronic diseases. Until this controversy is resolved, people are encouraged to eat a variety of fiber-rich and less processed carbohydrates, such as beans and lentils, fresh vegetables, and whole-wheat bread, because these forms of carbohydrates have a lower glycemic load and they contain a multitude of important nutrients.

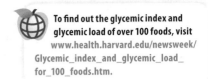

To find out the glycemic index and glycemic load of over 100 foods, visit **www.health.harvard.edu/newsweek/ Glycemic_index_and_glycemic_load_ for_100_foods.htm.**

RECAP

The glycemic index is a value that indicates the potential of foods to raise blood glucose and insulin levels. The glycemic load is the amount of carbohydrate in a food multiplied by the glycemic index of the carbohydrate in that food. Foods with a high glycemic index/load cause sudden surges in blood glucose and insulin, whereas foods with a low glycemic index/load cause low to moderate fluctuations in blood glucose. Diets with a low glycemic index/load are associated with a reduced risk for chronic diseases such as cardiovascular disease, type 2 diabetes, and prostate cancer. ■

Why Do We Need Carbohydrates?

We have seen that carbohydrates are an important energy source for our bodies. Let's learn more about this and discuss other functions of carbohydrates.

Carbohydrates Provide Energy

Carbohydrates, an excellent source of energy for all of our cells, provide 4 kcal of energy per gram. Some of our cells can also use lipids and even protein for energy if necessary. However, our red blood cells can use only glucose, and the brain and other nervous tissues rely primarily on glucose. This is why you get tired, irritable, and shaky when you have not eaten carbohydrates for a prolonged period of time.

Carbohydrates Fuel Daily Activity

Many popular diets—such as Dr. Atkins' New Diet Revolution and the Sugar Busters plan—are based on the idea that our bodies actually "prefer" to use dietary fats and/or protein for energy. They claim that current carbohydrate recommendations are much higher than we really need.

In reality, the body relies mostly on both carbohydrates and fats for energy. In fact, as shown in **Figure 4.10** (page 132), our bodies always use some combination of carbohydrates and fats to fuel daily activities. Fat is the predominant energy source used by our bodies at rest and during low-intensity activities, such as sitting, standing, and walking. Even during rest, however, our brain cells and red blood cells still rely on glucose.

Carbohydrates Fuel Exercise

When we exercise, whether running, briskly walking, bicycling, or performing any other activity that causes us to breathe harder and sweat, we begin to use more glucose than fat. Whereas fat breakdown is a slow process and requires oxygen, we can break down glucose very quickly either with or without oxygen. Even during very intense exercise, when less

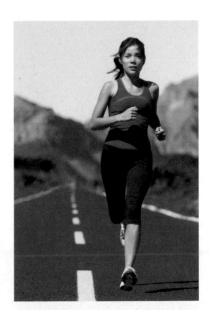

When we exercise or perform any other activity that causes us to breathe harder and sweat, we begin to use more glucose than fat.

Carbohydrate Use by Exercise Intensity

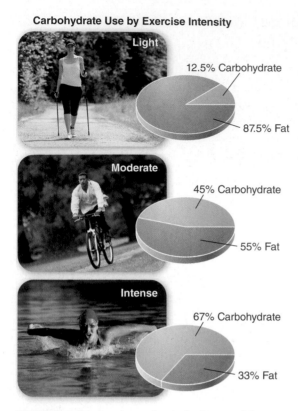

FIGURE 4.10 Amounts of carbohydrate and fat used during light, moderate, and intense exercise. (*Source:* Figure data adapted from the "Regulation of endogenous fat and carbohydrate metabolism in relation to exercise intensity and duration" by Romijn et al., from *American Journal of Physiology*, September 1, 1993. Copyright © 1993 by The American Physiological Society. Reprinted with permission.)

oxygen is available, we can still break down glucose very quickly for energy. That's why when you are exercising at maximal effort carbohydrates are providing almost 100% of the energy your body requires.

If you are physically active, it is important to eat enough carbohydrates to provide energy for your brain, red blood cells, and muscles. Later in this text (in Chapter 14) we discuss in more detail the carbohydrate recommendations for active people. In general, if you do not eat enough carbohydrate to support regular exercise, your body will have to rely on fat and protein as alternative energy sources. One advantage of becoming highly trained for endurance-type events, such as marathons and triathlons, is that our muscles are able to store more glycogen, which provides us with additional glucose we can use during exercise. (See Chapter 14 for more information on how exercise improves our use and storage of carbohydrates.)

Low Carbohydrate Intake Can Lead to Ketoacidosis

When we do not eat enough carbohydrates, the body seeks an alternative source of fuel for the brain and begins to break down stored fat. This process, called **ketosis,** produces an alternative fuel called **ketones.** (The metabolic process of ketosis is discussed in more detail in Chapter 7.)

Ketosis is an important mechanism for providing energy to the brain during situations of fasting, low carbohydrate intake, or vigorous exercise. However, ketones also suppress appetite and cause dehydration and acetone breath (the breath smells like nail polish remover). If inadequate carbohydrate intake continues for an extended period of time, the body will produce excessive amounts of ketones. Because many ketones are acids, high ketone levels cause the blood to become very acidic, leading to a condition called **ketoacidosis.** The high acidity of the blood interferes with basic body functions, causes the loss of lean body mass, and damages many body tissues. People with untreated diabetes are at high risk for ketoacidosis, which can lead to coma and even death. (See pages 146–149 for further details about diabetes.)

Carbohydrates Spare Protein

If the diet does not provide enough carbohydrate, the body will make its own glucose from protein. As noted earlier, this process, called gluconeogenesis, involves breaking down the proteins in blood and tissues into amino acids, then converting them to glucose.

When our bodies use proteins for energy, the amino acids from these proteins cannot be used to make new cells, repair tissue damage, support the immune system, or perform any other function. During periods of starvation or when eating a diet that is very low in carbohydrate, our bodies will take amino acids from the blood first, and then from other tissues, such as muscles and the heart, liver, and kidneys. Using amino acids in this manner over a prolonged period of time can cause serious, possibly irreversible, damage to these organs. (See Chapter 6 for more details on using protein for energy.)

Fiber Helps Us Stay Healthy

The terms *simple* and *complex* can cause confusion when discussing the health effects of carbohydrates. As we explained earlier, these terms are used to designate the number of sugar molecules present in the carbohydrate. However, when distinguishing carbohydrates in terms of their effect on our health, it is more appropriate to talk about them in terms of their nutrient density and their fiber content. Although we cannot digest fiber, research

ketosis The process by which the breakdown of fat during fasting states results in the production of ketones.

ketones Substances produced during the breakdown of fat when carbohydrate intake is insufficient to meet energy needs. They provide an alternative energy source for the brain when glucose levels are low.

ketoacidosis A condition in which excessive ketones are present in the blood, causing the blood to become very acidic, which alters basic body functions and damages tissues. Untreated ketoacidosis can be fatal. This condition is often found in individuals with untreated diabetes mellitus.

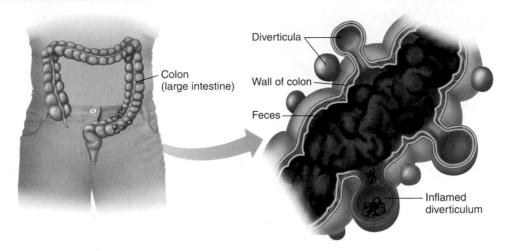

FIGURE 4.11 Diverticulosis occurs when bulging pockets form in the wall of the colon. These pockets become infected and inflamed, demanding proper treatment.

indicates that it helps us stay healthy and may prevent many digestive and chronic diseases. The following are potential benefits of fiber consumption:

- May reduce the risk of colon cancer. Although there is some controversy surrounding this claim, many researchers believe that fiber binds cancer-causing substances and speeds their elimination from the colon. However, recent studies of colon cancer and fiber have shown that their relationship is not as strong as previously thought.
- Helps prevent hemorrhoids, constipation, and other intestinal problems by keeping our stools moist and soft. Fiber gives gut muscles "something to push on" and makes it easier to eliminate stools.
- Reduces the risk for *diverticulosis,* a condition that is caused in part by trying to eliminate small, hard stools. A great deal of pressure must be generated in the large intestine to pass hard stools. This increased pressure weakens intestinal walls, causing them to bulge outward and form pockets (**Figure 4.11**). Feces and fibrous materials can get trapped in these pockets, which become infected and inflamed. This painful condition is typically treated with antibiotics or surgery.
- May reduce the risk of heart disease by delaying or blocking the absorption of dietary cholesterol into the bloodstream (**Figure 4.12**, page 134). In addition, when soluble fibers are digested, bacteria in the colon produce short-chain fatty acids that may reduce the production of low-density lipoprotein (LDL) to healthful levels.
- May enhance weight loss, as eating a high-fiber diet causes a person to feel more full. Fiber absorbs water, expands in our large intestine, and slows the movement of food through the upper part of the digestive tract. Also, people who eat a fiber-rich diet tend to eat fewer fatty and sugary foods.
- May lower the risk for type 2 diabetes. In slowing digestion and absorption, fiber also slows the release of glucose into the blood. It thereby improves the body's regulation of insulin production and blood glucose levels.

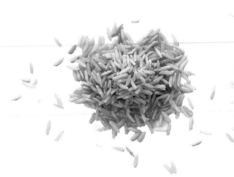

Brown rice is a good food source of dietary fiber.

RECAP

Carbohydrates are an important energy source at rest and during exercise, and they provide 4 kcal of energy per gram. Carbohydrates are necessary in the diet to spare body protein and prevent ketosis. Complex carbohydrates contain fiber and other nutrients that can reduce the risk for obesity, heart disease, and type 2 diabetes. Fiber helps prevent hemorrhoids, constipation, and diverticulosis; may reduce the risk for colon cancer and heart disease; and may assist with weight loss. ■

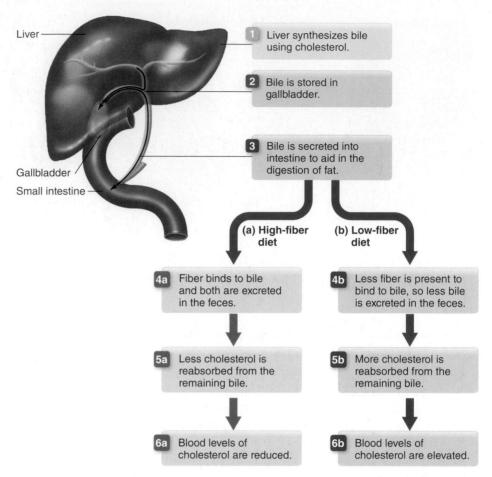

FIGURE 4.12 How fiber might help decrease blood cholesterol levels. **(a)** When we eat a high-fiber diet, fiber binds to the bile that is produced from cholesterol, resulting in relatively more cholesterol being excreted in the feces. **(b)** When a lower-fiber diet is consumed, less fiber (and thus cholesterol) is bound to bile and excreted in the feces.

How Much Carbohydrate Should We Eat?

Proponents of low-carbohydrate diets claim that eating carbohydrates makes you gain weight. However, anyone who consumes more Calories than he or she expends will gain weight, whether those Calories are in the form of simple or complex carbohydrates, protein, or fat. Moreover, fat is twice as "fattening" as carbohydrate: it contains 9 kcal per gram, whereas carbohydrate contains only 4 kcal per gram. In fact, eating carbohydrate sources that are high in fiber and micronutrients has been shown to reduce the overall risk for obesity, heart disease, and diabetes. Thus, not all carbohydrates are bad, and even foods with added sugars—in limited amounts—can be included in a healthful diet.

The Recommended Dietary Allowance (RDA) for carbohydrate is based on the amount of glucose the brain uses.[6] The current RDA for adults 19 years of age and older is 130 g of carbohydrate per day. It is important to emphasize that this RDA does not cover the amount of carbohydrate needed to support daily activities; it covers only the amount of carbohydrate needed to supply adequate glucose to the brain.

As discussed (in Chapter 1), carbohydrates have been assigned an Acceptable Macronutrient Distribution Range (AMDR). This is the range of intake associated with a decreased risk for chronic diseases. The AMDR for carbohydrates is 45% to 65% of total energy intake.

Table 4.2 compares the carbohydrate recommendations from the Institute of Medicine with the Dietary Guidelines for Americans related to carbohydrate-containing foods.[6, 8]

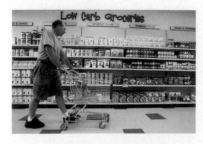

Many popular diets claim that current carbohydrate recommendations are much higher than we really need.

TABLE 4.2 Dietary Recommendations for Carbohydrates

Institute of Medicine Recommendations*	Dietary Guidelines for Americans†
Recommended Dietary Allowance (RDA) for adults 19 years of age and older is 130 g of carbohydrate per day.	Limit the consumption of foods that contain refined grains, especially refined grain foods that contain solid fats, added sugars, and sodium.
The Acceptable Macronutrient Distribution Range (AMDR) for carbohydrate is 45–65% of total daily energy intake.	Reduce the intake of Calories from solid fats and added sugars.
Added sugar intake should be 25% or less of total energy intake each day.	Increase vegetable and fruit intake. Eat a variety of vegetables, especially dark-green and red and orange vegetables and beans and peas. Consume at least half of all grains as whole grains. Increase whole-grain intake by replacing refined grains with whole grains. Choose foods that provide more potassium, dietary fiber, calcium, and vitamin D, which are nutrients of concern in American diets. These foods include vegetables, fruits, whole grains, and milk and milk products.

Source: *Institute of Medicine, Food and Nutrition Board. 2005. Dietary Reference Intakes for Energy, Carbohydrates, Fiber, Fat, Fatty Acids, Cholesterol, Protein, and Amino Acids (Macronutrients). Washington, DC: The National Academy of Sciences. Reprinted by permission.
Source: †US Department of Health and Human Services and US Department of Agriculture. 2010. Dietary Guidelines for Americans.

As you can see, the Institute of Medicine provides specific numeric recommendations, whereas the Dietary Guidelines for Americans are general suggestions about eating foods high in fiber and low in added sugars. Most health agencies agree that most of the carbohydrates you eat each day should be high in fiber, whole-grain, and unprocessed. As recommended in the USDA Food Guide, eating at least half your grains as whole grains and eating the suggested amounts of fruits and vegetables each day will ensure that you get enough fiber-rich carbohydrates in your diet. Although fruits are predominantly composed of simple sugars, they are good sources of vitamins, some minerals, and fiber.

Most Americans Eat Too Much Added Sugar

The average carbohydrate intake per person in the United States is approximately 50% of total energy intake. For some people, almost half of this amount consists of sugars. Where does all this sugar come from? Some sugar comes from healthful food sources, such as fruit and milk. Some comes from foods made with refined grains, such as soft white breads, saltine crackers, and pastries. Much of the rest comes from **added sugars**—that is, sugars and syrups that are added to foods during processing or preparation.[6] For example, many processed foods include high-fructose corn syrup (HFCS), an added sugar.

The most common source of added sugars in the U.S. diet is sweetened soft drinks; we drink an average of 40 gallons per person each year. Consider that one 12-oz sugared cola contains 38.5 g of sugar, or almost 10 teaspoons. If you drink the average amount, you are consuming more than 16,420 g of sugar (about 267 cups) each year! Other common sources of added sugars include cookies, cakes, pies, fruit drinks, fruit punches, and candy. Even many nondessert items, such as peanut butter, yogurt, flavored rice mixes, and even salad dressing, contain added sugars.

If you want a quick way to figure out the amount of sugar in a processed food, check the Nutrition Facts Panel on the box for the line that identifies "Sugars." You'll notice that the amount of sugar in a serving is identified in grams. Divide the total grams by 4 to get teaspoons. For instance, one national brand of yogurt contains 21 grams of sugar in a half-cup serving. That's more than 5 teaspoons of sugar! Doing this simple math before you buy may help you choose among different, more healthful versions of the same food.

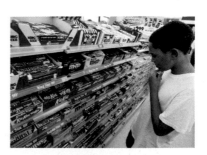

Foods with added sugars, such as candy, have lower levels of vitamins, minerals, and fiber than foods that naturally contain simple sugars.

added sugars Sugars and syrups that are added to food during processing or preparation.

HIGHLIGHT

Forms of Sugars Commonly Added to Foods

Brown sugar A highly refined sweetener made up of approximately 99% sucrose and produced by adding to white table sugar either molasses or burnt table sugar for coloring and flavor

Concentrated fruit juice sweetener A form of sweetener made with concentrated fruit juice, commonly pear juice

Confectioner's sugar A highly refined, finely ground white sugar; also referred to as powdered sugar

Corn sweeteners A general term for any sweetener made with corn starch

Corn syrup A syrup produced by the partial hydrolysis of corn starch

Dextrose An alternative term for glucose

Fructose A monosaccharide that occurs in fruits and vegetables; also called levulose, or fruit sugar

Galactose A monosaccharide that joins with glucose to create lactose

Granulated sugar Another term for white sugar, or table sugar

High-fructose corn syrup A type of corn syrup in which part of the sucrose is converted to fructose, making it sweeter than sucrose or regular corn syrup; most high-fructose corn syrup contains 42% to 55% fructose

Honey A sweet, sticky liquid sweetener made by bees from the nectar of flowers; contains glucose and fructose

Invert sugar A sugar created by heating a sucrose syrup with a small amount of acid; inverting sucrose results in its breakdown into glucose and fructose, which reduces the size of the sugar crystals; due to its smooth texture, it is used in making candies, such as fondant and some syrups.

Levulose Another term for fructose, or fruit sugar

Mannitol A type of sugar alcohol

Maple sugar A sugar made by boiling maple syrup

Molasses A thick, brown syrup that is separated from raw sugar during manufacturing; it is considered the least refined form of sucrose

Natural sweeteners A general term for any naturally occurring sweeteners, such as fructose, honey, and raw sugar

Raw sugar The sugar that results from the processing of sugar beets or sugarcane; it is approximately 96% to 98% sucrose; true raw sugar contains impurities and is not stable in storage; the raw sugar available to consumers has been purified to yield an edible sugar

Sorbitol A type of sugar alcohol

Turbinado sugar The form of raw sugar that is purified and safe for human consumption; it is sold as "Sugar in the Raw" in the United States.

White sugar Another name for sucrose, or table sugar

Xylitol A type of sugar alcohol

Added sugars are not chemically different from naturally occurring sugars. However, foods and beverages with added sugars have lower levels of vitamins, minerals, and fiber than fruits and other foods that naturally contain simple sugars. That's why most healthcare organizations recommend that we limit our consumption of added sugars. The Nutrition Facts Panel includes a list of total sugars, but a distinction is not generally made between added sugars and naturally occurring sugars. Thus, you need to check the ingredients label. (Refer to the feature box **Highlight: Forms of Sugars Commonly Added to Foods** for a list of terms indicating added sugars.) To maintain a diet low in added sugars, limit foods in which a form of added sugar is listed as one of the first few ingredients on the label.

Sugars Are Blamed for Many Health Problems

Why do sugars have such a bad reputation? First, they are known to contribute to tooth decay. Second, many people believe they cause hyperactivity in children. Third, eating a lot of sugar could increase the levels of unhealthful lipids in our blood, increasing our risk for heart disease. High intakes of sugar have also been blamed for causing diabetes and obesity. Let's learn the truth about these accusations.

Sugar Causes Tooth Decay

Sugars do play a role in dental problems, because the bacteria that cause tooth decay thrive on sugar. These bacteria produce acids, which eat away at tooth enamel and can eventually cause cavities and gum disease (**Figure 4.13**). Eating sticky foods that adhere to teeth—such as caramels, crackers, sugary cereals, and licorice—and sipping sweetened beverages over a period of time are two behaviors that increase the risk for tooth decay. This means that people shouldn't suck on hard candies or caramels, slowly sip soda or juice, or put babies to bed with a bottle unless it contains water. As we have seen, even breast milk contains sugar, which can slowly drip onto the baby's gums. As a result, infants should not routinely be allowed to fall asleep at the breast.

To reduce your risk for tooth decay, brush your teeth after each meal, after drinking sugary drinks, and after snacking on sweets. Drinking fluoridated water and using a fluoride toothpaste will also help protect your teeth.

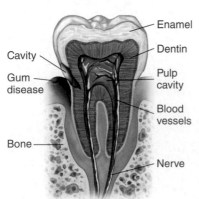

FIGURE 4.13 Eating sugar can cause an increase in cavities and gum disease. This is because bacteria in the mouth consume sugars present on the teeth and gums and produce acids, which eat away at these tissues.

Labels on figure: Cavity, Gum disease, Bone, Enamel, Dentin, Pulp cavity, Blood vessels, Nerve

There Is No Link Between Sugar and Hyperactivity in Children

Although many people believe that eating sugar causes hyperactivity and other behavioral problems in children, there is little scientific evidence to support this claim. Some children actually become less active shortly after a high-sugar meal! However, it is important to emphasize that most studies of sugar and children's behavior have only looked at the effects of sugar a few hours after ingestion. We know very little about the long-term effects of sugar intake on the behavior of children. Behavioral and learning problems are complex issues, most likely caused by a multitude of factors. Because of this complexity, the Institute of Medicine has stated that, overall, there does not appear to be enough evidence that eating too much sugar causes hyperactivity or other behavioral problems in children.[6] Thus, there is no Tolerable Upper Intake Level for sugar.

High Sugar Intake Can Lead to Unhealthful Levels of Blood Lipids

Research evidence does suggest that consuming a diet high in sugars, particularly fructose, can lead to unhealthful changes in blood lipids. You will learn more about blood lipids (including cholesterol and lipoproteins) in Chapter 5. Briefly, higher intakes of sugars are associated with increases in our blood of both low-density lipoproteins (LDL, commonly referred to as "bad cholesterol") and triglycerides. At the same time, high sugar intake appears to *decrease* our high-density lipoproteins (HDL), which are protective and are often referred to as "good cholesterol."[6, 13] These changes are of concern, as increased levels of triglycerides and LDL and decreased levels of HDL are risk factors for heart disease. Although there is not enough scientific evidence at the present time to state with confidence that eating a diet high in sugar causes heart disease, it is prudent for those at risk for heart disease to eat a diet low in sugars. Because fructose, especially in the form of high-fructose corn syrup, is a component of many processed foods and beverages, careful label reading is advised.

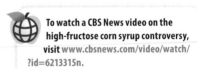

To watch a CBS News video on the high-fructose corn syrup controversy, visit www.cbsnews.com/video/watch/?id=6213315n.

High Sugar Intake Does Not Cause Diabetes But May Contribute to Obesity

There is no scientific evidence that eating a diet high in sugar causes diabetes. In fact, studies examining the relationship between sugar intake and type 2 diabetes report no association.[14] However, people who already have diabetes do need to moderate their intake of sugar and closely monitor their blood glucose levels.

We have somewhat more evidence linking sugar intake with obesity. For example, a recent study found that overweight children consumed more sugared soft drinks than did children of normal weight.[15] Another study found that for every extra sugared soft drink consumed by a child per day, the risk of obesity increases by 60%.[16] We also know that if you consume more energy than you expend, you will gain weight. It makes intuitive sense that people who consume extra energy from high-sugar foods are at risk for obesity, just as people who consume extra energy from fat or protein gain weight. In addition to the increased potential for obesity, another major concern about high-sugar diets is that they tend to be low in nutrient density because the intake of high-sugar foods tends to replace that of more nutritious foods. The relationship between sugared soft drinks and obesity is highly controversial and discussed in more detail in the **Nutrition Debate** at the end of this chapter.

RECAP

The RDA for carbohydrate is 130 g per day; this amount is sufficient only to supply adequate glucose to the brain. The AMDR for carbohydrate is 45% to 65% of total energy intake. Added sugars are sugars and syrups added to foods during processing or preparation. Sugar causes tooth decay but does not appear to cause hyperactivity in children. High intakes of sugars are associated with increases in unhealthful blood lipids. Diets high in sugar are not confirmed to cause diabetes but may contribute to obesity. ■

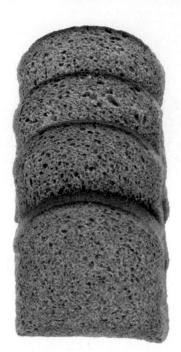

Whole-grain foods provide more nutrients and fiber than foods made with enriched flour.

Most Americans Eat Too Little Fiber-Rich Carbohydrate

Do you get enough fiber-rich carbohydrate each day? Most people in the United States eat only about two servings of fruits or vegetables each day, and most don't consistently choose whole-grain breads, pastas, and cereals. As explained earlier, fruits, vegetables, and whole-grain foods are rich in micronutrients and fiber. Whole grains also have a lower glycemic index than refined carbohydrates; thus, they prompt a more gradual release of insulin and result in less severe fluctuations in both insulin and glucose.

Table 4.3 defines the terms commonly used on nutrition labels for breads and cereals. Read the label for the bread you eat—does it list *whole-wheat* flour or just *wheat* flour? Although most labels for breads and cereals list wheat flour as the first ingredient, this term actually refers to enriched white flour, which is made when flour is processed. To gain a better understanding of the difference between whole-grain and processed grain products, it's important to learn about what makes a whole grain whole, and how whole grains are processed to reduce their fiber content.

What Makes a Whole Grain Whole?

Grains are grasses that produce edible kernels. A kernel of grain is the seed of the grass. If you were to plant a kernel of barley, a blade of grass would soon shoot up. Kernels of different grains all share a similar design. As shown in **Figure 4.14**, they consist of three parts:

- The outermost covering, called the *bran*, is very high in fiber and contains most of the grain's vitamins and minerals.
- The *endosperm* is the grain's midsection and contains most of the grain's carbohydrates and protein.
- The *germ* sits deep in the base of the kernel, surrounded by the endosperm, and is rich in healthful fats and some vitamins.

Whole grains are kernels that retain all three of these parts.

TABLE 4.3 Terms Used to Describe Grains and Cereals on Nutrition Labels

Term	Definition
Brown bread	Brown bread may or may not be made using whole-grain flour. Many brown breads are made with white flour with brown (caramel) coloring added.
Enriched (or fortified) flour or grain	Enriching or fortifying grains involves adding nutrients to refined foods. In order to use this term in the United States, a minimum amount of iron, folate, niacin, thiamin, and riboflavin must be added. Other nutrients can also be added.
Refined flour or grain	Refining involves removing the coarse parts of food products; refined wheat flour is flour in which all but the internal part of the kernel has been removed.
Stone ground	This term refers to a milling process in which limestone is used to grind any grain. Stone ground does not mean that bread is made with whole grain, as refined flour can be stone ground.
Unbleached flour	Unbleached flour has been refined but not bleached; it is very similar to refined white flour in texture and nutritional value.
Wheat flour	This term means any flour made from wheat; it includes white flour, unbleached flour, and whole-wheat flour.
White flour	White flour has been bleached and refined. All-purpose flour, cake flour, and enriched baking flour are all types of white flour.
Whole-grain flour	This is flour made from grain that is not refined; whole grains are milled in their complete form, with only the husk removed.
Whole-wheat flour	Whole-wheat flour is an unrefined, whole-grain flour made from whole wheat kernels.

The kernels of some grains also have a *husk* (hull): a thin, dry coat that is inedible. Removing the husk is always the first step in milling (grinding) these grains for human consumption.

People worldwide have milled grains for centuries, usually using heavy stones. A little milling removes only a small amount of the bran, leaving a crunchy grain suitable for cooked cereals. For example, cracked wheat and hulled barley retain much of the kernel's bran. Whole-grain flours are produced when whole grains are ground and then recombined. Because these hearty flours retain a portion of the bran, endosperm, and germ, foods such as breads made with them are rich in fiber and a wide array of vitamins and minerals.

With the advent of modern technology, processes for milling grains became more sophisticated, with seeds being repeatedly ground and sifted into increasingly finer flours, retaining little or no bran and therefore little fiber and few vitamins and minerals. For instance, white wheat flour, which consists almost entirely of endosperm, is high in carbohydrate but retains only about 25% of the wheat's fiber, vitamins, and minerals. In the United States, manufacturers of breads and other baked goods made with white flour are required by law to enrich their products with vitamins and minerals to replace some of those lost in processing. **Enriched foods** are foods in which nutrients that were lost during processing have been added back, so the food meets a specified standard. However, enrichment replaces only a handful of nutrients and leaves the product low in fiber. Notice that the terms *enriched* and *fortified* are not synonymous: **fortified foods** have nutrients added that did not originally exist in the food (or existed in insignificant amounts). For example, some breakfast cereals have been fortified with iron, a mineral that is not present in cereals naturally.

When choosing breads, crackers, and other baked goods, look for whole wheat, whole oats, or similar whole grains on the ingredient list. This ensures that the product contains the fiber and micronutrients that nature packed into the plant's seed.

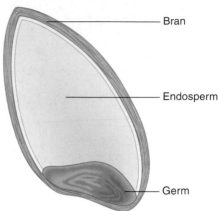

FIGURE 4.14 A whole grain includes the bran, endosperm, and germ.

We Need at Least 25 Grams of Fiber Daily

How much fiber do we need? The Adequate Intake for fiber is 25 g per day for women and 38 g per day for men, or 14 g of fiber for every 1,000 kcal per day that a person eats.[6] Most people in the United States eat only 12 to 18 g of fiber each day, getting only half of the fiber they need. Although fiber supplements are available, it is best to get fiber from food, because foods contain additional nutrients, such as vitamins and minerals.

It's important to drink plenty of fluid as you increase your fiber intake, as fiber binds with water to soften stools. Inadequate fluid intake with a high-fiber diet can actually result in hard, dry stools that are difficult to pass through the colon. At least eight 8-oz glasses of fluid each day are commonly recommended.

Can you eat too much fiber? Excessive fiber consumption can lead to problems such as intestinal gas, bloating, and constipation. Also, because fiber causes the body to eliminate more water in the feces, a very-high-fiber diet could result in dehydration. Fiber also binds certain vitamins and minerals: a diet with too much fiber can reduce our absorption of iron, zinc, calcium, and vitamin D. In children, some elderly, the chronically ill, and other at-risk populations, extreme fiber intake can even lead to malnutrition—they feel full before they have eaten enough to provide adequate energy and nutrients. Although some societies are accustomed to a very-high-fiber diet, most people in the United States find it difficult to tolerate more than 50 g of fiber per day.

Hunting for Fiber

Eating the amounts of whole grains, vegetables, fruits, nuts, and legumes recommended in the USDA Food Guide will ensure that you get adequate fiber. **Figure 4.15** (page 140) lists some common foods and their fiber content. You can use this information to design a diet that includes adequate fiber.

enriched foods Foods in which nutrients that were lost during processing have been added back, so that the food meets a specified standard.

fortified foods Foods in which nutrients are added that did not originally exist in the food or existed in insignificant amounts.

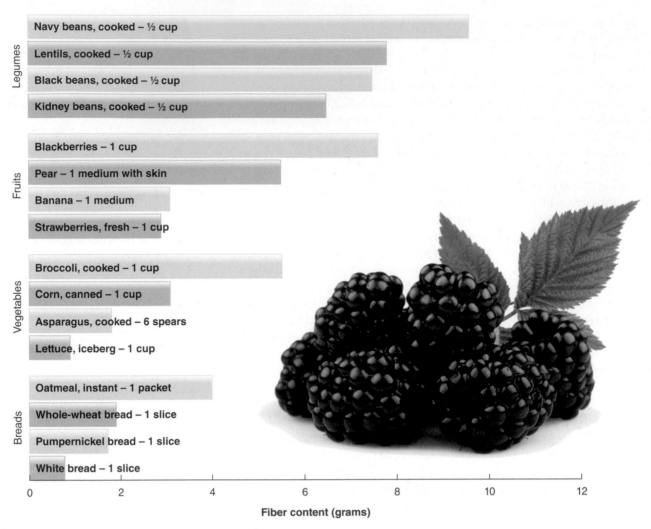

FIGURE 4.15 Fiber content of common foods. *Note*: The Adequate Intake for fiber is 25 g per day for women and 38 g per day for men. (*Source:* Data from US Department of Agriculture, Agricultural Research Service. 2011. USDA National Nutrient Database for Standard Reference, Release 24. Nutrient Data Laboratory home page. www.ars.usda.gov/ba/bhnrc/ndl.)

Figure 4.16 compares the food and fiber content of two diets, one high in fiber-rich carbohydrates and one high in refined carbohydrates. Here are some hints for selecting healthful carbohydrate sources:

■ Select breads and cereals that are made with *whole* grains, such as wheat, oats, barley, and rye (make sure the label says "whole" before the word *grain*). Two slices of whole-grain bread provide 4–6 grams of fiber.

■ Switch from a low-fiber breakfast cereal to one that has at least 4 grams of fiber per serving.

■ For a mid-morning snack, stir 1–2 tablespoons of whole ground flaxseed meal (4 grams of fiber) into a cup of low-fat or nonfat yogurt. Or choose an apple or a pear, with the skin left on (approximately 5 grams of fiber).

■ Instead of potato chips with your lunchtime sandwich, have a side of carrot sticks or celery sticks (approximately 2 grams of fiber per serving).

■ Eat legumes frequently, every day if possible (approximately 6–8 grams of fiber per serving). Canned or fresh beans, peas, and lentils are excellent sources of fiber-rich carbohydrates, vitamins, and minerals. Have them as your main dish, as a side, or in soups, chili, and other dishes.

To see a vast menu of high-fiber choices for each meal of the day, and find out how much fiber the foods you eat provide, visit the Fiber-o-Meter at www.webmd.com/diet/healthtool-fiber-meter.

A Day of Meals: Two High-Carb Diets

High in Refined Carbs

Breakfast

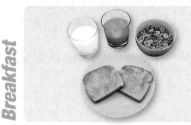

1½ cups Fruit Loops cereal
1 cup skim milk
2 slices white bread toasted,
  with 1 tbsp. light margarine
8 fl. oz fresh orange juice

Lunch

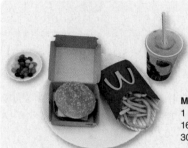

McDonald's Quarter Pounder
1 large order french fries
16 fl. oz cola beverage
30 jelly beans

Snack

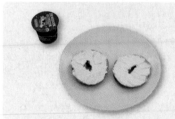

1 cinnamon raisin bagel
(3½ -inch diameter)
2 tbsp. cream cheese
8 fl. oz low-fat strawberry yogurt

Dinner

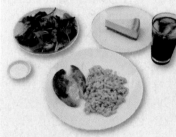

1 whole roasted chicken breast
2 cups mixed green salad
2 tbsp. ranch salad dressing
1 serving macaroni and cheese
12 fl. oz cola beverage
Cheesecake (1/8 of cake)

Snack

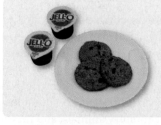

2 cups gelatin dessert
(cherry flavored)
3 raspberry oatmeal no-fat
cookies

Nutrient Analysis
4,012 kcal
60% of energy from carbohydrates
25% of energy from fat
15% of energy from protein
18.5 grams of dietary fiber

High in Fiber-Rich Carbs

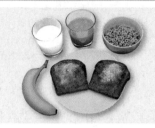

1½ cups Cheerios
1 cup skim milk
2 slices whole-wheat toast
  with 1 tbsp. light margarine
1 medium banana
8 fl. oz fresh orange juice

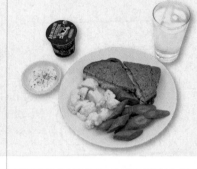

Tuna sandwich
  2 slices whole-wheat bread;
  1/4 cup tuna packed in water,
  drained; 1 tsp. Dijon mustard;
  2 tsp. low-calorie mayonnaise
2 carrots, raw, with peel
1 cup raw cauliflower
1 tbsp. peppercorn ranch
  salad dressing
8 fl. oz low-fat blueberry yogurt

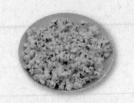

3 cups nonfat popcorn

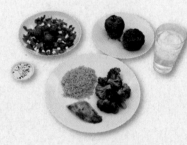

1/2 chicken breast roasted
1 cup brown rice, cooked
1 cup cooked broccoli
Spinach salad
  (1 cup chopped spinach,
  1 whole egg white, 2 slices
  turkey bacon, 3 cherry
  tomatoes, and 2 tbsp. creamy
  bacon salad dressing)
2 baked apples (no added sugar)

(No Snack)

Nutrient Analysis
2,150 kcal
60% of energy from carbohydrates
22% of energy from fat
18% of energy from protein
38 grams of dietary fiber

FIGURE 4.16 Comparison of two high-carbohydrate diets. (Diets were analyzed using Food Processor Version 7.21. Data from ESHA Research, Salem, OR.)

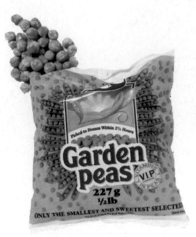

Frozen vegetables and fruits can be a healthful alternative when fresh produce is not available.

- Don't forget the vegetables! A cup of cooked leafy greens provides about 4 grams of fiber, and a salad is rich in fiber.
- For dessert, try fresh, frozen, or dried fruit or a high-fiber granola with sweetened soy milk.
- When shopping, choose fresh fruits and vegetables whenever possible. Buy frozen vegetables and fruits when fresh produce is not available. Check frozen selections to make sure there is no sugar or salt added.
- Be careful when buying canned fruits, vegetables, and legumes, as they may be high in added sugar or sodium. Select versions without added sugar or salt, or rinse before serving.

Try the **Nutrition Label Activity** to learn how to recognize various carbohydrates on food labels. Armed with this knowledge, you'll be ready to make more healthful food choices.

RECAP

The Adequate Intake for fiber is 25 g per day for women and 38 g per day for men. Most Americans eat only half of the fiber they need each day. Foods high in fiber include whole grains and cereals, fruits, and vegetables. The more processed the food, the less fiber it is likely to contain. ■

What's the Story on Alternative Sweeteners?

Most of us love sweets but want to avoid the extra Calories and tooth decay that go along with them. Remember that all carbohydrates, whether simple or complex, contain 4 kcal of energy per gram. Because sweeteners such as sucrose, fructose, honey, and brown sugar contribute energy, they are called **nutritive sweeteners.**

Other nutritive sweeteners include the *sugar alcohols,* such as mannitol, sorbitol, isomalt, and xylitol. Popular in sugar-free gums, mints, and diabetic candies, sugar alcohols are less sweet than sucrose. Foods with sugar alcohols have health benefits that foods made with sugars do not have, such as a reduced glycemic response and decreased risk for dental caries. Also, because sugar alcohols are absorbed slowly and incompletely from the intestine, they provide less energy than sugar, usually 2 to 3 kcal of energy per gram. However, because they are not completely absorbed from the intestine, they can attract water into the large intestine and cause diarrhea. A number of other products have been developed to sweeten foods without promoting tooth decay and weight gain. Because these products provide little or no energy, they are called **non-nutritive,** or *alternative*, **sweeteners.**

Limited Use of Alternative Sweeteners Is Not Harmful

Research has shown alternative sweeteners to be safe for adults, children, and individuals with diabetes. Women who are pregnant should discuss the use of alternative sweeteners with their healthcare provider. In general, it appears safe for pregnant women to consume alternative sweeteners in amounts within the Food and Drug Administration (FDA) guidelines.[17] These amounts, known as the **Acceptable Daily Intake (ADI),** are estimates of the amount of a sweetener that someone can consume each day over a lifetime without adverse effects. The estimates are based on studies conducted on laboratory animals, and they include a 100-fold safety factor. It is important to emphasize that actual intake by humans is typically well below the ADI.

Saccharin

Discovered in the late 1800s, *saccharin* is about 300 times sweeter than sucrose. Concerns arose in the 1970s that saccharin could cause cancer; however, more than 20 years of

nutritive sweeteners Sweeteners, such as sucrose, fructose, honey, and brown sugar, that contribute Calories (energy).

non-nutritive sweeteners Also called *alternative sweeteners;* manufactured sweeteners that provide little or no energy.

Acceptable Daily Intake (ADI) An estimate made by the Food and Drug Administration of the amount of a non-nutritive sweetener that someone can consume each day over a lifetime without adverse effects.

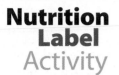
Recognizing Carbohydrates on the Label

Figure 4.17 shows labels for two breakfast cereals. The cereal on the left (a) is processed and sweetened, whereas the one on the right (b) is a whole-grain product with no added sugar. Which is the better breakfast choice? Fill in the label data below to find out!

■ Check the center of each label to locate the amount of total carbohydrate.

   1. For the sweetened cereal, the total carbohydrate is _____ g.

   2. For the whole-grain cereal, the total carbohydrate is _____ g for a smaller serving size.

■ Look at the information listed as subgroups under Total Carbohydrate. The label for the sweetened cereal lists all types of carbohydrates in the cereal: dietary fiber, sugars, and other carbohydrate (which refers to starches). Notice that this cereal contains 13 g of sugar—half of its total carbohydrates.

   3. How many grams of dietary fiber does the sweetened cereal contain? _____

■ The label for the whole-grain cereal lists only 1 g of sugar, which is 4% of its total carbohydrates.

   4. How many grams of dietary fiber does the whole-grain cereal contain? _____

■ To calculate the percentage of Calories that comes from carbohydrate, do the following:

   a. Calculate the *Calories* in the cereal that come from carbohydrate. Multiply the total grams of carbohydrate per serving by the energy value of carbohydrate:

$$26 \text{ g of carbohydrate} \times 4 \text{ kcal/g} = 104 \text{ kcal from carbohydrate}$$

   b. Calculate the *percentage of Calories* in the cereal that comes from carbohydrate. Divide the kcal from carbohydrate by the total Calories for each serving:

$$(104 \text{ kcal/120 kcal}) \times 100 = 87\% \text{ Calories from carbohydrate}$$

Which cereal should you choose to increase your fiber intake? Check the ingredients for the sweetened cereal. Remember that they're listed in order from highest to lowest amount. The second and third ingredients listed are sugar and brown sugar, and the corn and oat flours are not whole-grain. Now look at the ingredients for the other cereal—it contains whole-grain oats. Although the sweetened product is enriched with more B vitamins, iron, and zinc, the whole-grain cereal packs 4 g of fiber per serving, not to mention 5 g of protein, and it contains no added sugars. Overall, it is a more healthful choice.

(a)

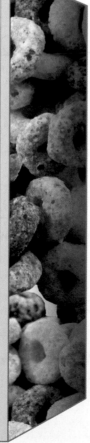

Nutrition Facts

Serving Size: 3/4 cup (30g)
Servings Per Package: About 14

Amount Per Serving		Cereal With 1/2 Cup Cereal Skim Milk
Calories	120	160
Calories from Fat	15	15
	% Daily Value**	
Total Fat 1.5g*	2%	2%
Saturated Fat 0g	0%	0%
Trans Fat 0g		
Polyunsaturated Fat 0g		
Monounsaturated Fat 0.5g		
Cholesterol 0mg	0%	1%
Sodium 220mg	9%	12%
Potassium 40mg	1%	7%
Total Carbohydrate 26g	9%	11%
Dietary Fiber 1g	3%	3%
Sugars 13g		
Other Carbohydrate 12g		
Protein 1g		

INGREDIENTS: Corn Flour, Sugar, Brown Sugar, Partially Hydrogenated Vegetable Oil (Soybean and Cottonseed), Oat Flour, Salt, Sodium Citrate (a flavoring agent), Flavor added [Natural & Artificial Flavor, Strawberry Juice Concentrate, Malic Acid (a flavoring agent)], Niacinamide (Niacin), Zinc Oxide, Reduced Iron, Red 40, Yellow 5, Red 3, Yellow 6, Pyridoxine Hydrochloride (Vitamin B6), Riboflavin (Vitamin B2), Thiamin Mononitrate (Vitamin B1), Folic Acid (Folate) and Blue 1.

(b)

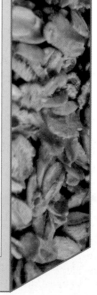

Nutrition Facts

Serving Size: 1/2 cup dry (40g)
Servings Per Container: 13

Amount Per Serving	
Calories	150
Calories from Fat	25
	% Daily Value*
Total Fat 3g	5%
Saturated Fat 0.5g	2%
Trans Fat 0g	
Polyunsaturated Fat 1g	
Monounsaturated Fat 1g	
Cholesterol 0mg	0%
Sodium 0mg	0%
Total Carbohydrate 27g	9%
Dietary Fiber 4g	15%
Soluble Fiber 2g	
Insoluble Fiber 2g	
Sugars 1g	
Protein 5g	

INGREDIENTS: 100% Natural Whole Grain Rolled Oats.

FIGURE 4.17 Labels for two breakfast cereals: **(a)** processed and sweetened cereal; **(b)** whole-grain cereal with no sugar added.

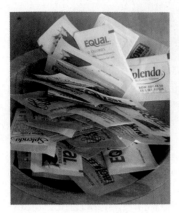

Contrary to recent media reports claiming severe health consequences related to the consumption of alternative sweeteners, major health agencies have determined that these products are safe for us to consume.

subsequent research failed to link saccharin to cancer in humans. Based on this evidence, in May 2000 the National Toxicology Program of the US government removed saccharin from its list of products that may cause cancer. No ADI has been set for saccharin, and it is used in foods and beverages and as a tabletop sweetener. It is sold as Sweet 'n Low (also known as "the pink packet") in the United States.

Acesulfame-K

Acesulfame-K (acesulfame potassium) is marketed under the names Sunette and Sweet One. It is a calorie-free sweetener that is 200 times sweeter than sugar. It is used to sweeten gums, candies, beverages, instant tea, coffee, gelatins, and puddings. The taste of acesulfame-K does not change when it is heated, so it can be used in cooking. The body does not metabolize acesulfame-K, so it is excreted unchanged by the kidneys. The ADI for acesulfame-K is 15 mg per kg body weight per day. For example, the ADI in an adult weighing 150 pounds (68 kg) would be 1,020 mg.

Aspartame

Aspartame, also called Equal ("the blue packet") and NutraSweet, is one of the most popular alternative sweeteners currently in use. Aspartame is composed of two amino acids: phenylalanine and aspartic acid. When these amino acids are separate, one is bitter and the other has no flavor—but joined together, they make a substance that is 180 times sweeter than sucrose. Although aspartame contains 4 kcal of energy per gram, it is so sweet that only small amounts are used; thus, it ends up contributing little or no energy. Heat destroys the dipeptide bonds that bind the two amino acids in aspartame (see Chapter 6), so it cannot be used in cooking because it loses its sweetness.

Although there are numerous claims that aspartame causes headaches and dizziness and can increase a person's risk for cancer and nerve disorders, studies do not support these claims.[18] A significant amount of research has been done to test the safety of aspartame.

The ADI for aspartame is 50 mg per kg body weight per day. For an adult weighing 150 pounds (68 kg), the ADI would be 3,400 mg. **Table 4.4** shows how many servings of aspartame-sweetened foods would have to be consumed to exceed the ADI. Because the ADI is a very conservative estimate, it would be difficult for adults or children to exceed this amount of aspartame intake. However, drinks sweetened with aspartame, which are extremely popular among children and teenagers, are very low in nutritional value. They should not replace more healthful beverages, such as milk, water, and 100% fruit juice.

Some people should not consume aspartame at all: those with the disease *phenylketonuria (PKU).* This is a genetic disorder that prevents the breakdown of the amino acid phenylalanine. Because a person with PKU cannot metabolize phenylalanine, it builds up to toxic levels in the tissues of the body and causes irreversible brain damage. In the United States, all newborn babies are tested for PKU; those who have it are placed on a phenylalanine-limited diet. Some foods that are common sources of protein and other nutrients for many growing children, such as meats and milk, contain phenylalanine. Thus, it

TABLE 4.4 Foods and Beverages That a Child and an Adult Would Have to Consume Daily to Exceed the ADI for Aspartame

Foods and Beverages	50-lb Child	150-lb Adult
12 fl. oz carbonated soft drink OR	7	20
8 fl. oz powdered soft drink OR	11	34
4 fl. oz gelatin dessert OR	14	42
Packets of tabletop sweetener	32	97

Source: "Information About Aspartame" from Aspartame Resource website, September 4, 2012. Copyright © 2005 by Calorie Control Council. Reprinted with permission.

is critical that children with PKU not waste what little phenylalanine they can consume on nutrient-poor products sweetened with aspartame.

Sucralose

Sucralose is marketed under the brand name Splenda and is known as "the yellow packet." It is made from sucrose, but chlorine atoms are substituted for the hydrogen and oxygen normally found in sucrose, and it passes through the digestive tract unchanged, without contributing any energy. It is 600 times sweeter than sucrose and is stable when heated, so it can be used in cooking. It has been approved for use in many foods, including chewing gum, salad dressings, beverages, gelatin and pudding products, canned fruits, frozen dairy desserts, and baked goods. Studies have shown sucralose to be safe. The ADI for sucralose is 5 mg per kg body weight per day. For example, the ADI of sucralose in an adult weighing 150 pounds (68 kg) would be 340 mg.

Neotame and Stevia

Neotame is an alternative sweetener that is 7,000 times sweeter than sugar. Manufacturers use it to sweeten a variety of products, such as beverages, dairy products, frozen desserts, and chewing gums.

Stevia was approved as an alternative sweetener by the FDA in 2008. It is produced from a purified extract of the stevia plant, native to South America. Stevia is 200 times sweeter than sugar. It is currently used commercially to sweeten beverages and is available in powder and liquid forms for tabletop use. Stevia is also called Rebiana, Reb-A, Truvia, and Purevia.

Using Artificial Sweeteners Does Not Necessarily Prevent Weight Gain

Remember that, to prevent weight gain, you need to balance the total number of kcal you consume against the number you expend. If you're expending an average of 2,000 kcal a day and you consume about 2,000 kcal per day, then you'll neither gain nor lose weight. But if, in addition to your normal diet, you regularly indulge in "treats," you're bound to gain weight, whether they are sugar free or not. Consider the Calorie count of these artificially sweetened foods:

- One cup of nonfat chocolate frozen yogurt with artificial sweetener = 199 Calories
- One sugar-free chocolate cookie = 100 Calories
- One serving of no-sugar-added hot cocoa = 55 Calories

Does the number of Calories in these foods surprise you? *Remember, sugar free doesn't mean Calorie free.* Make it a habit to check the Nutrition Facts Panel to find out how much energy is really in your food!

RECAP

Alternative sweeteners can be used in place of sugar to sweeten foods. Most of these products do not promote tooth decay and contribute little or no energy. The alternative sweeteners approved for use in the United States are considered safe when consumed in amounts less than the acceptable daily intake. ■

What Disorders Are Related to Carbohydrate Metabolism?

Health conditions that affect the body's ability to absorb and/or use carbohydrates include diabetes, hypoglycemia, and lactose intolerance.

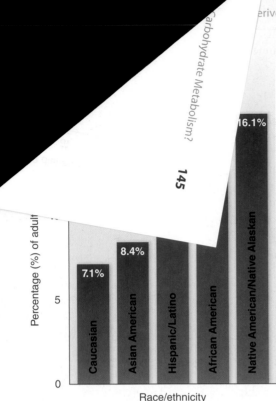

FIGURE 4.18 The percentage of adults from various ethnic and racial groups in the United States with type 2 diabetes. (*Source:* The National Diabetes Information Clearinghouse [NDIC]. 2011. National diabetes statistics. National Institutes of Health [NIH] publication no. 11–3892.)

To calculate your current level of risk for type 2 diabetes, go to www .facebook.com/AmericanDiabetes Association/app_283844141683657?loc= hpfeature2_alertday-test_apr2012.

hyperglycemia A condition in which blood glucose levels are higher than normal.

diabetes A chronic disease in which the body can no longer regulate glucose.

type 1 diabetes A disorder in which the pancreas cannot produce enough insulin.

Diabetes: Impaired Regulation of Glucose

Hyperglycemia is the term referring to higher-than-normal levels of blood glucose. **Diabetes** is a chronic disease in which the body can no longer regulate glucose within normal limits, and blood glucose levels become dangerously high. It is imperative to detect and treat the disease as soon as possible, because excessive fluctuations in glucose injure tissues throughout the body. As we noted at the beginning of this chapter, if not controlled, diabetes can lead to blindness, seizures, stroke, kidney failure, nerve disease, and cardiovascular disease.

Diabetes causes disease when chronic exposure to elevated blood glucose levels damages the body's blood vessels and nerves. Damage to large blood vessels results in problems referred to as *macrovascular complications,* including cardiovascular disease. Damage to small blood vessels results in problems referred to as *microvascular complications*. For example, damage to the kidneys' microscopic blood vessels, which filter blood and produce urine, impairs kidney function and can result in kidney failure. Damage to blood vessels that serve the eyes can lead to blindness. Damage to the nerves can also occur, particularly in the limbs. This condition leads to a loss of sensation in the hands and feet and is referred to as *neuropathy*. At the same time, microvascular damage reduces circulation to the limbs. Together, these changes increase the risk for injury, infection, and tissue death (necrosis), leading to a greatly increased number of toe, foot, and lower leg amputations in people with diabetes. Uncontrolled diabetes can also lead to ketoacidosis, which may result in coma and death.

As noted previously (in Chapter 1), diabetes is the seventh leading cause of death in the United States.[19] Approximately 18.8 million people in the United States—7% of the total population, including adults and children—are currently diagnosed with diabetes. It is speculated that another 7 million people have diabetes but do not know it.[20] **Figure 4.18** shows the percentage of adults with diabetes from various ethnic groups in the United States.[21] As you can see, diabetes is more common in African Americans, Hispanic or Latino Americans, and American Indians and Alaska Natives than in Caucasians.

The two main forms of diabetes are type 1 and type 2. Some women develop a third form, *gestational diabetes*, during pregnancy (we will review this in more detail in Chapter 16).

In Type 1 Diabetes, the Body Does Not Produce Enough Insulin

Approximately 5% to 10% of people with diabetes have **type 1 diabetes,** in which the body cannot produce enough insulin. When people with type 1 diabetes eat a meal and their blood glucose rises, the pancreas is unable to secrete insulin in response. Glucose therefore cannot move into body cells and remains in the bloodstream. The kidneys try to expel the excess blood glucose by excreting it in the urine. In fact, the medical term for the disease is *diabetes mellitus* (from the Greek *diabainein,* "to pass through," and Latin *mellitus,* "sweetened with honey"), and frequent urination is one of its warning signs (see **Table 4.5** for other symptoms). If blood glucose levels are not controlled, a person with type 1 diabetes will become confused and lethargic and have trouble breathing. This is because the brain cells are not getting enough glucose to function properly. As discussed earlier, uncontrolled diabetes can lead to ketoacidosis; left untreated, the ultimate result is coma and death.

Type 1 diabetes is classified as an *autoimmune disease.* This means that the body's immune system attacks and destroys its own tissues—in this case, the beta cells of the pancreas.[20]

Most cases of type 1 diabetes are diagnosed in adolescents around 10 to 14 years of age, although the disease can appear in infants, young children, and adults. It has a genetic link, so siblings and children of those with type 1 diabetes are at greater risk.[22]

is critical that children with PKU not waste what little phenylalanine they can consume on nutrient-poor products sweetened with aspartame.

Sucralose

Sucralose is marketed under the brand name Splenda and is known as "the yellow packet." It is made from sucrose, but chlorine atoms are substituted for the hydrogen and oxygen normally found in sucrose, and it passes through the digestive tract unchanged, without contributing any energy. It is 600 times sweeter than sucrose and is stable when heated, so it can be used in cooking. It has been approved for use in many foods, including chewing gum, salad dressings, beverages, gelatin and pudding products, canned fruits, frozen dairy desserts, and baked goods. Studies have shown sucralose to be safe. The ADI for sucralose is 5 mg per kg body weight per day. For example, the ADI of sucralose in an adult weighing 150 pounds (68 kg) would be 340 mg.

Neotame and Stevia

Neotame is an alternative sweetener that is 7,000 times sweeter than sugar. Manufacturers use it to sweeten a variety of products, such as beverages, dairy products, frozen desserts, and chewing gums.

Stevia was approved as an alternative sweetener by the FDA in 2008. It is produced from a purified extract of the stevia plant, native to South America. Stevia is 200 times sweeter than sugar. It is currently used commercially to sweeten beverages and is available in powder and liquid forms for tabletop use. Stevia is also called Rebiana, Reb-A, Truvia, and Purevia.

Using Artificial Sweeteners Does Not Necessarily Prevent Weight Gain

Remember that, to prevent weight gain, you need to balance the total number of kcal you consume against the number you expend. If you're expending an average of 2,000 kcal a day and you consume about 2,000 kcal per day, then you'll neither gain nor lose weight. But if, in addition to your normal diet, you regularly indulge in "treats," you're bound to gain weight, whether they are sugar free or not. Consider the Calorie count of these artificially sweetened foods:

- One cup of nonfat chocolate frozen yogurt with artificial sweetener = 199 Calories
- One sugar-free chocolate cookie = 100 Calories
- One serving of no-sugar-added hot cocoa = 55 Calories

Does the number of Calories in these foods surprise you? *Remember, sugar free doesn't mean Calorie free.* Make it a habit to check the Nutrition Facts Panel to find out how much energy is really in your food!

RECAP

Alternative sweeteners can be used in place of sugar to sweeten foods. Most of these products do not promote tooth decay and contribute little or no energy. The alternative sweeteners approved for use in the United States are considered safe when consumed in amounts less than the acceptable daily intake. ■

What Disorders Are Related to Carbohydrate Metabolism?

Health conditions that affect the body's ability to absorb and/or use carbohydrates include diabetes, hypoglycemia, and lactose intolerance.

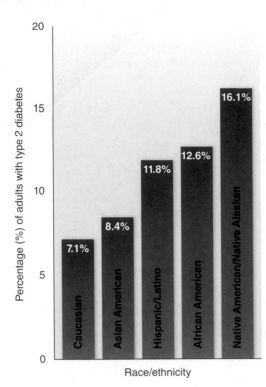

FIGURE 4.18 The percentage of adults from various ethnic and racial groups in the United States with type 2 diabetes. (*Source:* The National Diabetes Information Clearinghouse [NDIC]. 2011. National diabetes statistics. National Institutes of Health [NIH] publication no. 11–3892.)

To calculate your current level of risk for type 2 diabetes, go to www.facebook.com/AmericanDiabetes Association/app_283844141683657?loc=hpfeature2_alertday-test_apr2012.

hyperglycemia A condition in which blood glucose levels are higher than normal.

diabetes A chronic disease in which the body can no longer regulate glucose.

type 1 diabetes A disorder in which the pancreas cannot produce enough insulin.

Diabetes: Impaired Regulation of Glucose

Hyperglycemia is the term referring to higher-than-normal levels of blood glucose. **Diabetes** is a chronic disease in which the body can no longer regulate glucose within normal limits, and blood glucose levels become dangerously high. It is imperative to detect and treat the disease as soon as possible, because excessive fluctuations in glucose injure tissues throughout the body. As we noted at the beginning of this chapter, if not controlled, diabetes can lead to blindness, seizures, stroke, kidney failure, nerve disease, and cardiovascular disease.

Diabetes causes disease when chronic exposure to elevated blood glucose levels damages the body's blood vessels and nerves. Damage to large blood vessels results in problems referred to as *macrovascular complications,* including cardiovascular disease. Damage to small blood vessels results in problems referred to as *microvascular complications.* For example, damage to the kidneys' microscopic blood vessels, which filter blood and produce urine, impairs kidney function and can result in kidney failure. Damage to blood vessels that serve the eyes can lead to blindness. Damage to the nerves can also occur, particularly in the limbs. This condition leads to a loss of sensation in the hands and feet and is referred to as *neuropathy.* At the same time, microvascular damage reduces circulation to the limbs. Together, these changes increase the risk for injury, infection, and tissue death (necrosis), leading to a greatly increased number of toe, foot, and lower leg amputations in people with diabetes. Uncontrolled diabetes can also lead to ketoacidosis, which may result in coma and death.

As noted previously (in Chapter 1), diabetes is the seventh leading cause of death in the United States.[19] Approximately 18.8 million people in the United States—7% of the total population, including adults and children—are currently diagnosed with diabetes. It is speculated that another 7 million people have diabetes but do not know it.[20] **Figure 4.18** shows the percentage of adults with diabetes from various ethnic groups in the United States.[21] As you can see, diabetes is more common in African Americans, Hispanic or Latino Americans, and American Indians and Alaska Natives than in Caucasians.

The two main forms of diabetes are type 1 and type 2. Some women develop a third form, *gestational diabetes,* during pregnancy (we will review this in more detail in Chapter 16).

In Type 1 Diabetes, the Body Does Not Produce Enough Insulin

Approximately 5% to 10% of people with diabetes have **type 1 diabetes,** in which the body cannot produce enough insulin. When people with type 1 diabetes eat a meal and their blood glucose rises, the pancreas is unable to secrete insulin in response. Glucose therefore cannot move into body cells and remains in the bloodstream. The kidneys try to expel the excess blood glucose by excreting it in the urine. In fact, the medical term for the disease is *diabetes mellitus* (from the Greek *diabainein,* "to pass through," and Latin *mellitus,* "sweetened with honey"), and frequent urination is one of its warning signs (see **Table 4.5** for other symptoms). If blood glucose levels are not controlled, a person with type 1 diabetes will become confused and lethargic and have trouble breathing. This is because the brain cells are not getting enough glucose to function properly. As discussed earlier, uncontrolled diabetes can lead to ketoacidosis; left untreated, the ultimate result is coma and death.

Type 1 diabetes is classified as an *autoimmune disease.* This means that the body's immune system attacks and destroys its own tissues—in this case, the beta cells of the pancreas.[20]

Most cases of type 1 diabetes are diagnosed in adolescents around 10 to 14 years of age, although the disease can appear in infants, young children, and adults. It has a genetic link, so siblings and children of those with type 1 diabetes are at greater risk.[22]

TABLE 4.5 Signs and Symptoms of Type 1 and Type 2 Diabetes

Type 1 Diabetes	Type 2 Diabetes*
Increased or frequent urination	Any of the type 1 signs and symptoms
Excessive thirst	Greater frequency of infections
Constant hunger	Sudden vision changes
Unexplained weight loss	Slow healing of wounds or sores
Extreme fatigue	Tingling or numbness in the hands or feet
Blurred vision	Very dry skin

Source: Data adapted from U.S. Dept. of Health and Human Services, National Diabetes Information Clearinghouse (NDIC). Available online at http://diabetes.niddk.nih.gov/dm/pubs/overview/index.aspx#types and from Centers for Disease Control and Infection, Basics about Diabetes, available at http://www.cdc.gov/diabetes/consumer/learn.htm.

*Some people with type 2 diabetes experience no symptoms.

The only treatment for type 1 diabetes is the administration of insulin by injection or pump several times daily. Insulin is a hormone composed of protein, so it would be digested in the intestine if taken as a pill. Individuals with type 1 diabetes must also monitor their blood glucose levels closely to ensure that they remain within a healthful range (**Figure 4.19**). The feature box **Highlight: Living with Diabetes** (page 148) describes how one young man with type 1 diabetes stays healthy.

In Type 2 Diabetes, Cells Become Less Responsive to Insulin

In **type 2 diabetes,** body cells become resistant (less responsive) to insulin. This type of diabetes develops progressively, meaning that the biological changes resulting in the disease occur over a long period of time. Approximately 90% to 95% of all cases of diabetes are classified as type 2.

Obesity is the most common trigger for a cascade of changes that eventually results in the disorder. It is estimated that 80% to 90% of the people with type 2 diabetes are overweight or obese. One factor linking obesity to diabetes is the inappropriate accumulation of lipids in muscle, the liver, and beta cells, which reduces the ability of body cells to respond to insulin.[23] As a result, the cells of many obese people begin to exhibit a condition called *insulin insensitivity* (insulin resistance). The pancreas attempts to compensate for this insensitivity by secreting more insulin. At first, the increased secretion of insulin is sufficient to maintain normal blood glucose levels. However, over time, a person who is insulin insensitive will have to circulate very high levels of insulin to use glucose for energy. Eventually, this excessive production becomes insufficient for preventing a rise in fasting blood glucose. The resulting condition is referred to as **impaired fasting glucose,** meaning glucose levels are higher than normal but not high enough to indicate a diagnosis of type 2 diabetes. Some health professionals refer to this condition as *pre-diabetes*, as people with impaired fasting glucose are more likely to get type 2 diabetes than are people with normal fasting glucose levels. Ultimately, the pancreas becomes incapable of secreting these excessive amounts of insulin and stops producing the hormone altogether. Thus, blood glucose levels may be elevated in a person with type 2 diabetes because (1) the person has developed insulin insensitivity, (2) the pancreas can no longer secrete enough insulin, or (3) the pancreas has entirely stopped insulin production.

Who Is at Risk for Type 2 Diabetes?

As noted, obesity is the most common trigger for type 2 diabetes. But many other factors also play a role. For instance, relatives of people with type 2 diabetes are at increased risk, as are people with a sedentary lifestyle. A cluster of risk factors referred to as *metabolic syndrome* is also known to increase the risk for type 2 diabetes. The criteria for metabolic syndrome include a waist circumference ≥88 cm (35 in.) for women and ≥102 cm (40 in.)

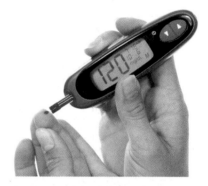

FIGURE 4.19 Monitoring blood glucose requires pricking the fingers several times each day and measuring the blood glucose level using a glucometer.

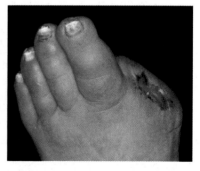

Amputations are a common complication of uncontrolled diabetes.

type 2 diabetes A progressive disorder in which body cells become less responsive to insulin.

impaired fasting glucose Fasting blood glucose levels that are higher than normal but not high enough to lead to a diagnosis of type 2 diabetes.

HIGHLIGHT

Living with Diabetes

Vincent is a young man who was diagnosed with type 1 diabetes when he was 10 years old. At first, Vincent and his family were frightened by the disease and found it difficult to adapt their lifestyle to provide a safe and health-promoting environment for Vincent. For example, Vincent's mother felt frustrated because her son could no longer eat the cakes, pies, and other sweets she had always enjoyed baking for her family, and his sister found herself watching over her brother's meals and snacks, running to her parents whenever she feared that he was about to eat something that would harm him. Within a few months, though, Vincent's mother learned to adapt her recipes and cooking techniques to produce a variety of foods that Vincent could enjoy, and the entire family learned to allow Vincent the responsibility for his food choices and his health.

Vincent is now a college sophomore and has been living with diabetes for 9 years. Although diabetes has its challenges, he lives an active and fulfilling life. He plays baseball for his college team and ice hockey with friends on weekends. He has learned to maintain healthy control of his blood glucose by taking his insulin regularly, monitoring his blood glucose, drinking plenty of water, and eating a wide variety of foods. For inspiration, he enjoys reading about the many professional and Olympic athletes and other famous people who have diabetes, showing that the disease shouldn't prevent people from realizing their dreams.

Vincent is smart and a good student, and he has learned the importance of balancing his meals and insulin therapy; if his blood glucose declines, he has trouble concentrating. He eats three nutritious meals a day on a regular schedule and snacks as needed to keep his blood glucose from dropping too low. He can also enjoy occasional treats, such as cake, cookies, and candy, and he eats fast-food meals from time to time with his friends and family. He is aware of his increased risk for various

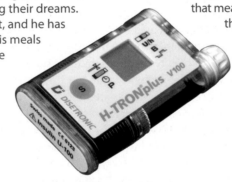

Insulin pumps can help those with diabetes eat a wider range of foods.

diseases and tries to make dietary choices that support his active lifestyle and help him maintain a healthful body weight.

To maintain his blood glucose level in a healthy range, Vincent checks it several times a day. He has to prick his fingers to do this, and they get tender and develop calluses. During his first few years with diabetes, he had to give himself two to four shots of insulin each day. He learned to measure the insulin into a syringe, and he monitored where the shots were injected, because each insulin shot had to be given in a different place on his body to avoid damaging the skin and underlying tissue. Technological advances now offer easier and less painful alternatives than a needle and syringe. Vincent wears an insulin infusion pump, which looks like a small pager and delivers insulin into the body through a long, thin tube in very small amounts throughout the day. Because insulin delivery via his pump is continuous throughout the day, he can eat more of his favorite foods with less concern for their effect on his blood glucose. One of Vincent's friends also has diabetes but can't use a pump; instead, he uses an insulin pen, which includes a needle and a cartridge of insulin.

Currently, there is no cure for type 1 diabetes. However, many new treatments and potential cures are being researched. The FDA has approved several devices that measure blood glucose without pricking the finger. Some of them can read glucose levels through the skin, and others insert a small needle into the body to monitor glucose continually. Tests are also being conducted on insulin nasal sprays and inhalers. Advances in genetic engineering may soon make it possible to transplant healthy beta cells into the pancreas of virtually anyone with type 1 diabetes, so that the normal cells will secrete insulin. Vincent looks forward to seeing major changes in the treatment of diabetes in the next few years.

---

for men, elevated blood pressure, and unhealthful levels of certain blood lipids and blood glucose.

Increased age is another risk factor for type 2 diabetes. Most cases develop after age 45, and almost 27% of Americans 65 years of age and older have diabetes.

As mentioned in the chapter-opening story, type 2 diabetes in children and adolescents was virtually unheard of until about 20 years ago. Unfortunately, the prevalence of the disease has been increasing dramatically in this age group. In a 2004 study, more than 6% of college students were found to have pre-diabetes.[24] And each year, about 3,600 people under age 20 are newly diagnosed with full-blown type 2 diabetes.[21]

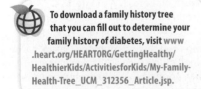

To download a family history tree that you can fill out to determine your family history of diabetes, visit www.heart.org/HEARTORG/GettingHealthy/HealthierKids/ActivitiesforKids/My-Family-Health-Tree_UCM_312356_Article.jsp.

Lifestyle Choices Can Help Prevent or Control Diabetes

Type 2 diabetes is thought to have become an epidemic in the United States because of a combination of our poor eating habits, sedentary lifestyles, increased obesity, and an aging population. We can't control our age, but we can and do control how much and what types of foods we eat and how much physical activity we engage in—and that, in turn, influences our risk for obesity. Currently, over 34% of American college students are either overweight or obese.[25] Although adopting a healthful diet is important, moderate daily exercise may prevent the onset of type 2 diabetes more effectively than dietary changes alone. (See Chapter 14 for examples of moderate exercise programs.) Exercise will also assist in weight loss, and studies show that losing only 10 to 30 pounds can reduce or eliminate the symptoms of type 2 diabetes.[26] In summary, by eating a healthy diet, staying active, and maintaining a healthful body weight, you should be able to keep your risk for type 2 diabetes low.

What if you've already been diagnosed with type 2 diabetes? In general, you should follow many of the same dietary guidelines recommended for people without diabetes (see Chapter 2). One difference is that you may need to eat less carbohydrate and slightly more fat or protein to help regulate your blood glucose levels. Carbohydrates are still an important part of the diet, so, if you're eating less, make sure your choices are rich in nutrients and fiber. Precise nutritional recommendations vary according to each individual's responses to foods, so consulting with a registered dietitian is essential.

In addition, people with diabetes should avoid alcoholic beverages, which can cause a drop in blood glucose that can cause confusion, clumsiness, and fainting. If left untreated, this can lead to seizures, coma, and death. The symptoms of alcohol intoxication and hypoglycemia are very similar. People with diabetes, their companions, and even healthcare providers may confuse these conditions; this can result in a potentially life-threatening situation.

When blood glucose levels can't be adequately controlled with lifestyle changes, oral medications may be required. These drugs work in either of two ways: they improve body cells' sensitivity to insulin or reduce the amount of glucose the liver produces. As noted earlier, a 2012 study found that oral medications are not as effective in children and teens with type 2 diabetes as compared to adults.[1] Finally, if the pancreas can no longer secrete enough insulin, then people with type 2 diabetes must have daily insulin injections, just like people with type 1 diabetes.

RECAP

Diabetes is a disease that results in dangerously high levels of blood glucose. Type 1 diabetes typically appears at a young age; the pancreas cannot secrete sufficient insulin, so insulin injections are required. Type 2 diabetes develops over time and may be triggered by obesity: body cells become insensitive to the effects of insulin or the pancreas no longer secretes sufficient insulin for bodily needs. Supplemental insulin may or may not be needed to treat type 2 diabetes. Diabetes increases the risk for dangerous complications, such as heart disease, blindness, kidney disease, and amputations. Many cases of type 2 diabetes could be prevented or delayed with eating a balanced diet, getting regular exercise, and achieving and/or maintaining a healthful body weight. ■

Nutrition
MILESTONE

By the late 19th century, scientists had discovered a link between the pancreas and diabetes. Experiments had shown that, without a pancreas, an otherwise healthy animal would develop the disease quickly. Still, no one knew how to treat diabetes: nutritional therapies ranged from low-carbohydrate diets to starvation. For children, a diagnosis of diabetes was essentially a death sentence.

Then, in **1921**, Canadian surgeon Frederick Banting had an idea. He and his medical assistant removed the pancreas from a dog, thereby inducing diabetes. They then injected the diabetic dog with secretions extracted from a cluster of cells in the pancreas called the islets of Langerhans. They called this extraction *isletin*. A few injections of isletin a day cured the dog of diabetes. They then purified the substance—which we now call insulin—and repeated their experiment several times before trying it on a 14-year-old boy dying of diabetes. The injection reversed all signs of the disease in the boy. Banting published a paper on his research in 1922 and received a Nobel Prize the following year.

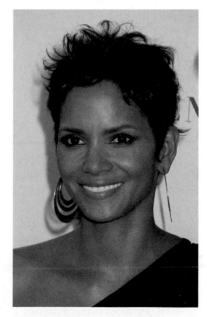

Actress Halle Berry has type 2 diabetes.

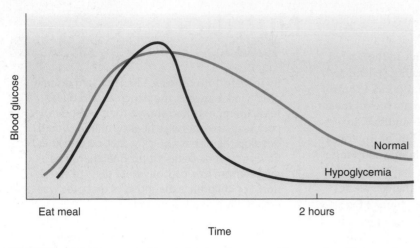

FIGURE 4.20 Changes in blood glucose after a meal for people with hypoglycemia (lower than normal) and without hypoglycemia (normal).

Hypoglycemia: Low Blood Glucose

In **hypoglycemia,** fasting blood sugar falls to lower-than-normal levels (**Figure 4.20**). One cause of hypoglycemia is excessive production of insulin, which lowers blood glucose too far. People with diabetes can develop hypoglycemia if they inject too much insulin or if they exercise and fail to eat enough carbohydrates. Two types of hypoglycemia can develop in people who do not have diabetes: reactive and fasting.

Reactive hypoglycemia occurs when the pancreas secretes too much insulin after a high-carbohydrate meal. The symptoms of reactive hypoglycemia usually appear about 1 to 4 hours after the meal and include nervousness, shakiness, anxiety, sweating, irritability, headache, weakness, and rapid or irregular heartbeat. Although many people experience these symptoms from time to time, they are rarely caused by true hypoglycemia. A person diagnosed with reactive hypoglycemia must eat smaller meals more frequently to level out blood insulin and glucose levels.

Fasting hypoglycemia occurs when the body continues to produce too much insulin, even when someone has not eaten. This condition is usually secondary to another disorder, such as cancer; liver infection; alcohol-induced liver disease; or a tumor in the pancreas. Its symptoms are similar to those of reactive hypoglycemia but occur more than 4 hours after a meal.

Lactose Intolerance: Inability to Digest Lactose

Sometimes our bodies do not produce enough of the enzymes necessary to break down certain carbohydrates before they reach the colon. A common example is **lactose intolerance,** in which the body does not produce sufficient amounts of the enzyme lactase in the small intestine and therefore cannot digest foods containing lactose.

Lactose intolerance should not be confused with a milk allergy. People who are allergic to milk experience an immune reaction to the proteins found in cow's milk. Symptoms of milk allergy include skin reactions, such as hives and rashes; intestinal distress, such as nausea, vomiting, cramping, and diarrhea; and respiratory symptoms, such as wheezing, runny nose, and itchy and watery eyes. In severe cases, anaphylactic shock can occur. In contrast, symptoms of lactose intolerance are limited to the GI tract and include intestinal gas, bloating, cramping, nausea, diarrhea, and discomfort. These symptoms resolve spontaneously within a few hours.

Although some infants are born with lactose intolerance, it is more common to see lactase enzyme activity decrease after 2 years of age. In fact, it is estimated that up to 70% of the world's adult population will lose some ability to digest lactose as they age. In the United States, lactose intolerance is more common in Native American, Asian, Hispanic, and African American adults than in Caucasians.

Not everyone experiences lactose intolerance to the same extent. Some people cannot tolerate any dairy products. However, many people who are lactose intolerant can consume multiple small servings of dairy products without symptoms. This will enable them to meet their calcium requirements.[27] People with more severe lactose intolerance need to find foods that can supply enough calcium for normal growth, development, and maintenance of bones. Many can tolerate specially formulated milk products that are low in lactose, whereas others take pills or use drops that contain the lactase enzyme when they eat dairy products. Calcium-fortified soy milk and orange juice are excellent substitutes for cow's

hypoglycemia A condition marked by blood glucose levels that are below normal fasting levels.

lactose intolerance A disorder in which the body does not produce sufficient lactase enzyme and therefore cannot digest foods that contain lactose, such as cow's milk.

milk. Many lactose-intolerant people can also digest yogurt and aged cheese, as the bacteria or molds used to ferment these products break down the lactose during processing.

How can you tell if you are lactose intolerant? Many people discover that they have problems digesting dairy products by trial and error. But because intestinal gas, bloating, and diarrhea may indicate other health problems, you should consult a physician to determine the cause.

Tests for lactose intolerance include drinking a lactose-rich beverage and testing blood glucose levels over a 2-hour period. If you do not produce the normal amount of glucose, this means that your body is unable to digest the lactose in the beverage. A similar test involves measuring hydrogen levels in the breath, as lactose-intolerant people breathe out more hydrogen when they drink a beverage that contains lactose.

Milk products, such as ice cream, are hard to digest for people who are lactose intolerant.

RECAP

Hypoglycemia refers to lower-than-normal blood glucose levels. It results from overproduction of insulin. Lactose intolerance is an inability to digest lactose because of insufficient production of the enzyme lactase. ■

*Nutri-*Case — Hannah

"Last night, my mom called and said she'd be late getting home from work, so I made dinner. I was tired after my classes and I had a lot of homework to get to, so I kept it simple. I made us each a cheeseburger—no bun!—served with frozen french fries and some carrot sticks with guacamole on the side. We both had a cola, too. Later that night, though, when I was studying, I got a snack attack and raided a package of sugar-free cookies. I ate maybe three or four, but I didn't think it was a big deal because they're sugar-free. Then when I checked the package label this morning, I found out that each cookie has 90 Calories! It bummed me out—until those cookies, I'd been doing pretty well on my new low-carb diet!"

Hannah takes public transportation to the community college she attends and does not engage in regular physical activity. Without analyzing the precise grams of carbohydrate or number of Calories in Hannah's meal, would you agree that before the cookies she'd been "doing pretty well" on her low-carb diet? In other words, would you describe her meal as low carb? Would you characterize her meal as low in energy? About how many grams of dietary fiber do you think were in the meal?

Chapter Review

TEST YOURSELF | *ANSWERS*

1 **T** Our brains rely almost exclusively on glucose for energy, and our bodies tissue utilizes glucose for energy both at rest and during exercise.

2 **F** At 4 kcal/g, carbohydrates have less than half the energy of a gram of fat. Eating a high-carbohydrate diet will not cause people to gain body fat unless their total diet contains more energy (kcal) than they expend. In fact, eating a diet high in complex, fiber-rich carbohydrates is associated with a lower risk for obesity.

3 **F** Although specific estimates are not yet available, significantly higher rates of type 2 diabetes are now being reported in children and adolescents; these higher rates are attributed to increasing obesity rates in young people.

4 **F** There is no evidence that diets high in sugar cause hyperactivity in children.

5 **T** Contrary to recent reports claiming harmful consequences related to the consumption of alternative sweeteners, major health agencies have determined that these products are safe for most of us to consume in limited quantities.

Summary

- Carbohydrates contain carbon, hydrogen, and oxygen. Plants make the carbohydrate glucose during photosynthesis.

- Simple sugars include mono- and disaccharides. The three primary monosaccharides are glucose, fructose, and galactose.

- Two monosaccharides joined together are called disaccharides. Glucose and fructose join to make sucrose; glucose and glucose join to make maltose; and glucose and galactose join to make lactose.

- The two monosaccharides that compose a disaccharide are attached by a bond between oxygen and one carbon on each of the monosaccharides. There are two forms of this bond: alpha bonds are easily digestible by humans, whereas beta bonds are very difficult to digest.

- Oligosaccharides are complex carbohydrates that contain 3 to 10 monosaccharides.

- Polysaccharides are complex carbohydrates that typically contain hundreds to thousands of monosaccharides. The three types of polysaccharides are starches, glycogen, and fiber.

- Starches are the storage form of glucose in plants.

- Glycogen is the storage form of glucose in humans. Glycogen is stored in the liver and in muscles.

- Dietary fiber is the nondigestible parts of plants, whereas functional fiber is a nondigestible form of carbohydrate extracted from plants or manufactured in the laboratory. Fiber may reduce the risk for certain diseases.

- Carbohydrate digestion starts in the mouth, where chewing and an enzyme called salivary amylase start breaking down the carbohydrates in food.

- Digestion continues in the small intestine. Specific enzymes are secreted to break starches into smaller mono- and disaccharides. As disaccharides pass through the intestinal cells, they are digested into monosaccharides.

- Glucose and other monosaccharides are absorbed into the bloodstream and travel to the liver, where all non-glucose molecules are converted to glucose.

- Glucose is transported in the bloodstream to the cells, where it is used for energy, stored in the liver or muscle as glycogen, or converted to fat and stored in adipose tissue.

- Insulin is secreted when blood glucose increases sufficiently, and it assists with the transport of glucose into cells.

- Glucagon, epinephrine, norepinephrine, cortisol, and growth hormone are secreted when blood glucose levels are low, and they assist with the conversion of glycogen to glucose, with gluconeogenesis, and with reducing the use of glucose by muscles and other organs.

- The glycemic index and the glycemic load are values that indicate how much a food increases glucose levels. High-glycemic foods can trigger detrimental increases in blood glucose for people with diabetes.

- All cells can use glucose for energy. The red blood cells, brain, and central nervous system prefer to use glucose exclusively.

- Using glucose for energy helps spare body proteins, and glucose is an important fuel for the body during exercise.

- Fiber helps us maintain the healthy elimination of waste products. Eating adequate fiber may reduce the risk for colon cancer, type 2 diabetes, obesity, heart disease, hemorrhoids, and diverticulosis.

- The Acceptable Macronutrient Distribution Range for carbohydrate is 45% to 65% of total energy intake.

- High sugar intake can cause tooth decay, elevate triglyceride and low-density lipoprotein levels in the blood, and contribute to obesity. It does not appear to cause hyperactivity in children.

- The Adequate Intake for fiber is 25 g per day for women and 38 g per day for men, or 14 g of fiber for every 1,000 kcal of energy consumed.

- Foods high in fiber include whole grains and cereals, fruits, and vegetables. Eating 6 to 11 servings of breads/grains and 5 to 9 servings of fruits and vegetables helps ensure that you meet your fiber-rich carbohydrate goals.

- Alternative sweeteners are added to some foods because they sweeten foods without promoting tooth decay and add little or no Calories to foods.

- All alternative sweeteners approved for use in the United States are believed to be safe when consumed at levels at or below the Acceptable Daily Intake levels defined by the FDA.

- Diabetes is caused by insufficient insulin or by the cells becoming resistant or insensitive to insulin. It causes dangerously high blood glucose levels. The two primary types of diabetes are type 1 and type 2.

- A lower-than-normal blood glucose level is defined as hypoglycemia. There are two types: reactive and fasting. Reactive hypoglycemia occurs when too much insulin is secreted after a high-carbohydrate meal; fasting hypoglycemia occurs when blood glucose drops even though no food has been eaten.

- Lactose intolerance results from an insufficient amount of the enzyme lactase. Symptoms include intestinal gas, bloating, cramping, diarrhea, and discomfort following consumption of dairy products.

MasteringNutrition™

To further your understanding, go online and apply what you've learned to real-life case studies that will help you master the content!

Review Questions

1. The glycemic index rates
   a. the acceptable amount of alternative sweeteners to consume in 1 day.
   b. the potential of foods to raise blood glucose and insulin levels.
   c. the risk of a given food for causing diabetes.
   d. the ratio of soluble to insoluble fiber in a complex carbohydrate.

2. Carbohydrates contain
   a. carbon, nitrogen, and water.
   b. carbonic acid and a sugar alcohol.
   c. hydrated sugar.
   d. carbon, hydrogen, and oxygen.

3. The most common source of added sugar in the American diet is
   a. table sugar.
   b. white flour.
   c. alcohol.
   d. sweetened soft drinks.

4. Glucose, fructose, and galactose are
   a. monosaccharides.
   b. disaccharides.
   c. oligosaccharides.
   d. polysaccharides.

5. Aspartame should not be consumed by people who have
   a. phenylketonuria.
   b. type 1 diabetes.
   c. lactose intolerance.
   d. diverticulosis.

6. **True or false?** Sugar alcohols are non-nutritive sweeteners.

7. **True or false?** Insulin and glucagon are both pancreatic hormones.

8. **True or false?** A person with lactose intolerance is allergic to milk.

9. **True or false?** Plants store glucose as fiber.

10. **True or false?** Salivary amylase breaks down starches into galactose.

11. Describe the role of insulin in regulating blood glucose levels.

12. Identify at least four ways in which fiber helps us maintain a healthy digestive system.

13. Your niece, Lilly, is 6 years old and is learning about MyPlate in her first-grade class. She points out the "grains" group and proudly lists her favorite food choices from this group: "saltine crackers, pancakes, and spaghetti." Explain to Lilly, in words she could understand, the difference between fiber-rich carbohydrates and refined carbohydrates and why fiber-rich carbohydrates are more healthful food choices.

14. Explain how obesity can trigger type 2 diabetes.

15. Create a table listing the molecular composition and food sources of each of the following carbohydrates: glucose, fructose, lactose, and sucrose.

Math Review

16. Simon is trying to determine how much carbohydrate he should consume in his diet to meet the AMDR for health. His total energy intake needed to maintain his current weight is 3,500 kcal per day. Simon has learned that the AMDR for carbohydrate is 45% to 65% of total energy intake. How many (a) kcal and (b) grams of carbohydrate should Simon consume each day?

Answers to Review Questions and Math Review can be found online in the MasteringNutrition Study Area.

Web Links

www.eatright.org
Academy of Nutrition and Dietetics
Visit this website to learn more about diabetes, low- and high-carbohydrate diets, and general healthful eating habits.

www.foodinsight.org
Food Insight—International Food Information Council Foundation (IFIC)
Search this site to find out more about sugars and low-calorie sweeteners.

www.ada.org
American Dental Association
Go to this site to learn more about tooth decay, as well as other oral health topics.

www.nidcr.nih.gov
National Institute of Dental and Craniofacial Research (NIDCR)
Find out more about recent oral and dental health discoveries, and obtain statistics and data on the status of dental health in the United States.

www.diabetes.org
American Diabetes Association
Find out more about the nutritional needs of people living with diabetes.

www2.niddk.nih.gov
National Institute of Diabetes and Digestive and Kidney Diseases (NIDDK)
Learn more about diabetes, including treatment, complications, U.S. statistics, clinical trials, and recent research.

www.caloriecontrol.org
Calorie Control Council
This site provides information about reducing energy and fat in the diet, achieving and maintaining a healthy weight, and eating various low-calorie, reduced-fat foods and beverages.

References

1. TODAY Study Group. 2012. A clinical trial to maintain glycemic control in youth with type 2 diabetes. *N. Engl. J. Med*. Epub ahead of print. April 29, 2012. 10.1056/NEJMoa1109333.

2. US Centers for Disease Control and Prevention. 2010. Number of Americans with diabetes projected to double or triple by 2050. Press Release, October 22, 2010. www.cdc.gov/media/pressrel/2010/r101022.html.

3. Sears, B. 1995. *The Zone. A Dietary Road Map*. New York: HarperCollins.

4. Steward, H. L., M. C. Bethea, S. S. Andrews, and L. A. Balart. 1995. *Sugar Busters! Cut Sugar to Trim Fat*. New York: Ballantine Books.

5. Atkins, R. C. 1992. *Dr. Atkins' New Diet Revolution*. New York: M. Evans & Company.

6. Institute of Medicine, Food and Nutrition Board. 2002. *Dietary Reference Intakes for Energy, Carbohydrates, Fiber, Fat, Protein and Amino Acids (Macronutrients)*. Washington, DC: National Academy of Sciences.

7. Scharlau, D., A. Borowicki, N. Habermann, T. Hofmann, S. Klenow, C. Miene, U. Munjal, K. Stein, and M. Glei. 2009. Mechanisms of primary prevention by butyrate and other products formed during gut flora-mediated fermentation of dietary fibre. *Mutat. Res*. 682(1):39–53.

8. US Department of Agriculture and US Department of Health and Human Services. 2010. *Dietary Guidelines for Americans, 2010*. 7th ed. Washington, DC: US Government Printing Office. www.cnpp.usda.gov/dietaryguidelines.htm.

9. Foster-Powell K., S. H. A. Holt, and J. C. Brand-Miller. 2002. International table of glycemic index and glycemic load values: 2002. *Am. J. Clin. Nutr*. 76:5–56.

10. Levitan, E. B., N. R. Cook, M. J. Stampfer, P. M. Ridker, K. M. Rexrode, J. E. Buring, J. E. Manson, and S. Liu. 2008. Dietary glycemic index, dietary glycemic load, blood lipids, and C-reactive protein. *Metab*. 57(3):437–443.

11. Denova-Gutiérrez, E., G. Huitrón-Bravo, J. O. Talavera, S. Castañon, K. Gallegos-Carrillo, Y. Flores, and J. Salmerón. 2010. Dietary glycemic index, dietary glycemic load, blood lipids, and coronary heart disease. *J. Nutr. Metab*. DOI:10.1155/2010/170680.

12. Augustin, L., S. A., C. Galeone, L. Dal Maso, C. Pelucchi, V. Ramazzotti, D. J. A. Jenkins, M. Montella, R. Talamini, E. Negri, S. Franceschi, and C. La Vecchia. 2004. Glycemic index, glycemic load and risk of prostate cancer. *Int. J. Cancer*. 112:446–450.

13. Howard, B. V., and J. Wylie-Rosett. 2002. Sugar and cardiovascular disease. A statement for healthcare professionals from the Committee on Nutrition of the Council on Nutrition, Physical Activity, and Metabolism of the American Heart Association. *Circulation* 106:523–527.

14. Janket, S.-J., J. E. Manson, H. Sesso, J. E. Burring, and S. Liu. 2003. A prospective study of sugar intake and risk of type 2 diabetes in women. *Diab. Care*. 26(4):1008–1015.

15. Gillis, L. J., and O. Bar-Or. 2003. Food away from home, sugar-sweetened drink consumption and juvenile obesity. *J. Am. Coll. Nutr*. 22(6):539–545.

16. Ludwig, D. S., K. E. Peterson, and S. L. Gortmaker. 2001. Relation between consumption of sugar-sweetened drinks and childhood obesity: a prospective, observational analysis. *Lancet* 357:505–508.

17. International Food Information Council Foundation. 2009. Facts About Low-Calorie Sweeteners. www.foodinsight.org/Content/6/LCS%20Fact%20Sheet_11-09.pdf.

18. International Food Information Council Foundation. 2012. Everything You Need to Know About Aspartame. www.foodinsight.org/Resources/Detail.aspx?topic=Everything_You_Need_to_Know_About_Aspartame.

19. Centers for Disease Control and Prevention (CDC). National Center for Health Statistics. 2009. FastStats. Leading Causes of Death. www.cdc.gov/nchs/fastats/lcod.htm.

20. American Diabetes Association. 2010. Position statement. Diagnosis and classification of diabetes mellitus. *Diab. Care*. 33(suppl 1):562–569.

21. National Diabetes Information Clearinghouse (NDIC). 2011. National Diabetes Statistics, 2011. http://diabetes.niddk.nih.gov/dm/pubs/statistics/#fast.

22. American Diabetes Association. 2010. Genetics of Diabetes. www.diabetes.org/diabetes-basics/genetics-of-diabetes.html.

23. Savage, D. B., K. F. Petersen, and G. I. Shulman. 2005. Mechanisms of insulin resistance in humans and possible links with inflammation. *Hypertension* 45:828–833.

24. Huang, T. T.-K., A. M. Kempf, M. L. Strother, C. Li, R. E. Lee, K. J. Harris, and H. Kaur. 2004. Overweight and components of the metabolic syndrome in college students. *Diab. Care*. 27(12):3000–3001.

25. American College Health Association (ACHA). National College Health Assessment (NCHA). 2011. ACHA NCHA II. Reference Group Executive Summary Fall 2011. www.achancha.org/reports_ACHA-NCHAII.html.

26. American College of Sports Medicine and the American Diabetes Association. 2010. Exercise and type 2 diabetes: American College of Sports Medicine and American Diabetes Association joint position statement. *Med. Sci. Sports Exerc*. 42(12):2282–2303.

27. National Digestive Diseases Information Clearinghouse. 2010. What I Need to Know About Lactose Intolerance. NIH Publication No. 10-2751. http://digestive.niddk.nih.gov/ddiseases/pubs/lactoseintolerance_ez/#top.

Is High-Fructose Corn Syrup the Cause of the Obesity Epidemic?

Almost every day in the news we see headlines about obesity: "More Americans Overweight!" "The Fattening of America," "Obesity Is a National Epidemic!" These headlines accurately reflect the state of weight in the United States. Over the past 30 years, obesity rates have increased dramatically for both adults and children. Obesity has become public health enemy number one, as many chronic diseases, such as type 2 diabetes, heart disease, high blood pressure, and arthritis, go hand in hand with obesity.

Of particular concern are the rising obesity rates in children. Recent evidence from the Centers for Disease Control and Prevention indicates that the prevalence of obesity is 10.4% in young children aged 2 to 5 years, 19.6% in children aged 6 to 11 years, and 18.1% in adolescents aged 12 to 19 years.[1]

Why should we concern ourselves with fighting obesity in children? First, it is well established that the treatment of existing obesity is extremely challenging, and our greatest hope of combating this disease is through prevention. Most agree that prevention should start with children at a very early age. Second, approximately 30% of children who are obese will remain obese as adults, suffering all of the health problems that accompany this disease. Young children are now experiencing type 2 diabetes, high blood pressure, and high cholesterol at increasingly younger ages,

only compounding the devastating effects of these illnesses as they get older. We have reached the point at which serious action must be taken immediately to curb this growing crisis.

How can we prevent obesity? This is a difficult question to answer. One way is to better understand the factors that contribute to obesity, and then take actions to alter these factors. We know of many factors that contribute to overweight and obesity. These include genetic influences, lack of adequate physical activity, and consumption of foods that are high in fat, added sugar, and energy. Although it is easy to blame our genetics, they cannot be held entirely responsible for the rapid rise in obesity that has occurred over the past 30 years. Our genetic makeup takes thousands of years to change; thus, humans who lived 100 years ago have essentially the same genetic makeup as humans who live now. The fact that obesity rates have risen so dramatically in recent years illustrates that we need to look more closely at how our lifestyle changes over the same period have contributed to obesity.

One factor that has recently come to the forefront of nutrition research and policy making is the contribution of added sugars, particularly in the form of high-fructose corn syrup (HFCS), to overweight and obesity. As discussed earlier in this chapter, there is disagreement about whether added sugar does cause, and how much it might contribute to, obesity. Many nutrition researchers are beginning to draw attention to the potential role of HFCS in rising obesity rates. Before we discuss why these researchers are pointing to HFCS as a major cause of the obesity epidemic, it is important to understand what HFCS is and how it is metabolized in our bodies.

What Is HFCS?

HFCS is made by first converting the starch in corn to glucose, and then converting some of the glucose to fructose through a process referred to as *enzymatic isomerization*. The result is an inexpensive, corn-based syrup that has been used to replace sucrose and other simple sugars as a sweetener in foods and beverages. Fructose is sweeter than glucose. It is also metabolized differently than glucose, as it is absorbed farther down in the small intestine and, unlike glucose, it does not stimulate insulin release

It is estimated that the rate of overweight in children in the United States has increased 100% since the mid-1970s.

from the pancreas. It also enters the cell by a transport protein that does not require the presence of insulin. Interestingly, brain cells do not have this transport protein; thus, unlike glucose, fructose cannot enter brain cells and stimulate satiety signals. In addition, consumption of fructose increases the production of triglycerides in the blood significantly more than consumption of glucose and in animals can lead to excessive insulin production, resistance to insulin, and impaired glucose regulation—all factors that can lead to type 2 diabetes.

Arguments Linking HFCS to Obesity

How might the consumption of HFCS contribute to obesity? Bray et al.[2] speculate that HFCS could lead to increased obesity because of its effect on appetite regulation and its contribution to excessive energy intake. Both insulin and the hormone leptin inhibit food intake in humans, and as previously stated, fructose does not stimulate insulin release. As insulin increases the release of leptin, it is possible that consuming fructose results in lower circulating levels of both insulin and leptin, which results in an increase in appetite and food intake.

At the same time, HFCS could contribute to obesity because people consume significant amounts of excess energy in the form of HFCS-sweetened soft drinks and foods.

Bray et al.[2] emphasize that HFCS is the sole caloric sweetener in sugared soft drinks and represents more than 40% of caloric sweeteners added to other foods and beverages in the United States. These researchers have linked the increased use and consumption of HFCS in beverages and foods with the rising rates of obesity since the 1970s, when HFCS was first developed and marketed (see the accompanying graph).

Consumption of sweetened soft drinks is thought to play a much greater role in obesity than consumption of sugary foods. Why? Evidence indicates that the body does not recognize the energy in sweetened beverages in the same way as it recognizes the energy in solid food. Studies suggest that, when we snack on cookies, we unconsciously compensate for these Calories by reducing our intake of other foods in the next several hours. But when we consume energy in the form of soft drinks and other sweetened beverages, we do not adjust our intake of foods accordingly.[3]

How significant a problem is soft drink consumption in children? Data from the National Health and Examination Survey indicate that boys aged 12 to 19 years consume 273 kcal per day of sugar-sweetened beverages, which is the highest average intake of any age group in the United States.[4] Children aged 6 to 11 years consume 112 to 141 kcal per day of sugar-sweetened beverages, and even young children aged 2 to 5 years consume 70 kcal per day! High consumption of sweetened beverages has been associated with significantly higher energy intakes and a lower intake of fruit in 4th to 6th graders.[5] A recent pilot intervention study found that replacing sweetened soft drinks with noncaloric beverages in the diets of 13- to 18-year-old adolescents resulted in a significant decrease in body mass index in the adolescents who were the most overweight when starting the study.[6]

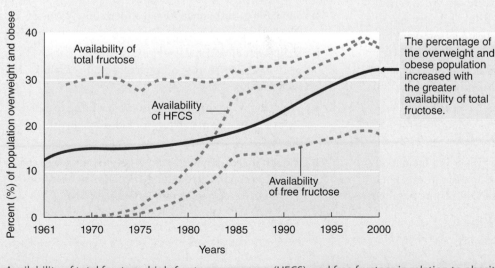

Availability of total fructose, high-fructose corn syrup (HFCS), and free fructose in relation to obesity prevalence in the United States. *Source:* (Data adapted from Bray, G. A., S. J. Nielsen, and B. M. Popkin. 2004. Consumption of high-fructose corn syrup in beverages may play a role in the epidemic of obesity. *Am. J. Clin. Nutr.* 79:537–543. Used with permission.)

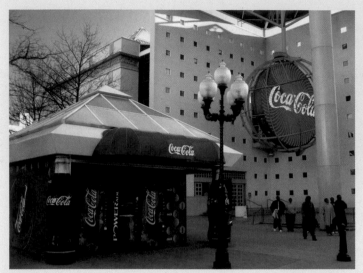

Aggressive marketing and easy availability of soft drinks make them a tempting choice for children and adults, adding HFCS and Calories to their diet.

In addition to providing significant quantities of nutritionally empty Calories, soft drinks may also have a detrimental effect on bone density: soft drinks typically displace milk in the diet, and the phosphorus available in some sodas, whether sugared or diet, binds with calcium, causing it to be drawn out of the bones. This is especially harmful during childhood and adolescence, when bones are still growing.[7]

All of this alarming information has led to dramatic changes in soft drink availability in schools and at school-sponsored events. In 2006, the soft drink industry agreed to a voluntary ban on sales of all sweetened soft drinks in elementary and high schools, to take effect by the start of the 2009–2010 school year. Despite these positive changes in schools, foods and beverages containing HFCS are still widely available in the marketplace.

Arguments Defending HFCS

Although the evidence pinpointing HFCS as a major contributor to the obesity epidemic may appear strong, not all nutrition professionals find them valid. Some point out that HFCS is not meaningfully different from any other sweeteners, and that soft drinks would have contributed to the obesity epidemic no matter whether the sweetener was sucrose or fructose and that their contribution to obesity is due to increased consumption resulting from massive increases in advertising, substantial increases in serving sizes of soft drinks, and virtually unlimited access to soft drinks throughout our everyday lives.[8,9] A recent study has also indicated that, although 4 weeks of increased fructose consumption in humans does cause an increased production of triglycerides, as previously stated, it does not cause weight gain or increased resistance to insulin.[10] Thus, it may be that animals respond differently than humans to diets high in fructose.

It is entirely possible that the obesity epidemic has resulted from increased consumption of energy not only in the form of sweetened soft drinks but also in other high-energy foods, along with a reduction in physical activity levels. If that's the case, HFCS plays only a minor role in the obesity epidemic. Evidence to support this supposition stems from the fact that obesity rates are rising around the world, and many of the countries experiencing this epidemic do not use HFCS as a sweetener.

This issue is extremely complex, and more research needs to be done in humans before we can fully understand how HFCS contributes to our diet and our health.

CRITICAL THINKING QUESTIONS

- After reading this, do you think HFCS is unhealthful and a major contributor to the obesity epidemic?
- Should HFCS be banned from our food supply? Why or why not?
- Should soft drink companies be encouraged to replace HFCS with sucrose or some other form of caloric sweetener?
- Should reducing soft drink consumption be up to individuals, or should it be mandatory for those at high risk for obesity?
- Should families, schools, and our government play a central role in controlling the types of foods and beverages offered to young people throughout their day?

REFERENCES

1. Ogden, C., and M. Carroll. 2010. NCHS Public Health E-Stat Prevalence of Obesity Among Children and Adolescents: United States, Trends 1962–1965 Through 2007–2008. www.cdc.gov/nchs/data/hestat/obesity_child_07_08/obesity_child_07_08.htm#table1.

2. Bray G. A., S. J. Nielsen, and B. M. Popkin. 2004. Consumption of high-fructose corn syrup in beverages may play a role in the epidemic of obesity. *Am. J. Clin. Nutr.* 79:537–543.

3. Flood, J. E., L. S. Roe, and B. J. Rolls. 2006. The effect of increased beverage portion size on energy intake at a meal. *J. Am. Diet. Assoc.* 106:1984–1990.

4. Ogden, C. L., B. K. Kit, M. D. Carroll, and S. Park. 2011. Consumption of Sugar Drinks in the United States, 2005–2008. NCHF Data Brief Number 71. www.cdc.gov/nchs/data/databriefs/db71.htm.

5. Cullen, K. W., D. M. Ahs, C. Warneke, and C. de Moor. 2002. Intake of soft drinks, fruit-flavored beverages, and fruits and vegetables by children in grades 4 through 6. *Am. J. Public Health.* 92(9):1475–1478.

6. Ebbeling, C. B., H. A. Feldman, S. K. Osganian, V. R. Chomitz, S. H. Ellenbogen, and D. S. Ludwig. 2006. Effects of decreasing sugar-sweetened beverage consumption on body weight in adolescents: a randomized, controlled pilot study. *Pediatrics* 117:673–680.

7. Wolf, A., G. A. Bray, and B. M. Popkin. 2008. A short history of beverages and how our body treats them. *Obesity Rev.* 9:151–164.

8. Jacobson, M. F. 2004. Letter to the editor. High-fructose corn syrup and the obesity epidemic. *Am. J. Clin. Nutr.* 80:1081–1090.

9. White, J. S. 2008. Straight talk about high-fructose corn syrup: what it is and what it ain't. *Am. J Clin. Nutr.* 88(6 supplement):1716S–1721S.

10. Lê, K.-A., D. Faeh, R. Stettler, M. Ith, R. Kreis, P. Vermathen, C. Boesch, E. Ravussin, and L. Tappy. 2006. A 4-wk high-fructose diet alters lipid metabolism without affecting insulin sensitivity or ectopic lipids in healthy humans. *Am. J. Clin. Nutr.* 84:1374–1379.

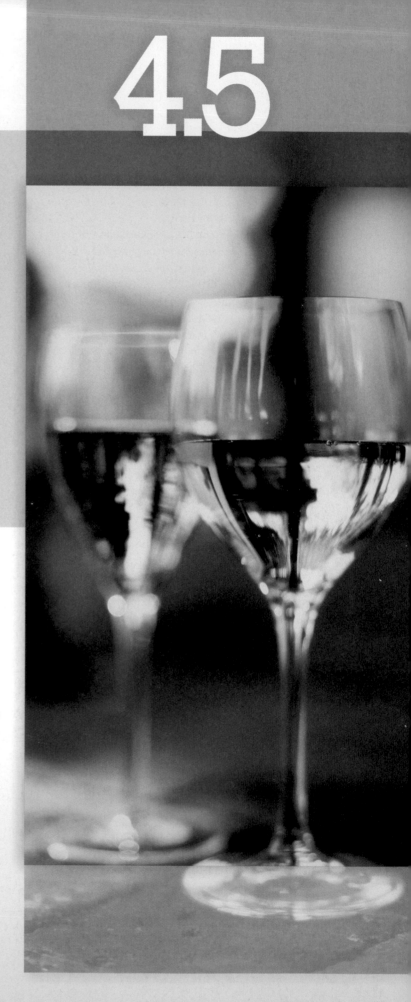

Alcohol

Want to find out . . .

- what "moderate drinking" really means?
- how many Americans die in alcohol-related incidents each year?
- if you should be concerned about your alcohol intake?
- how to talk to someone who might have a drinking problem?

READ ON.

No one should have to spend his 21st birthday in an emergency room, but that's what happened to Todd the night he turned 21. His friends took him off campus to celebrate, and, with their encouragement, he attempted to drink 21 shots before the bar closed at 2:00 AM. Fortunately for Todd, when he passed out and couldn't be roused, his best friend noticed his cold, clammy skin and erratic breathing and drove him to the local emergency room. There, his stomach was pumped and he was treated for alcohol poisoning. He regained consciousness but felt sick and shaky for several more hours. Not everyone is so lucky. Some people with alcohol poisoning never wake up.

What makes excessive alcohol intake so dangerous, and why is moderate alcohol consumption often considered healthful? How can you tell if someone is struggling with alcohol addiction, and what can you do to help? What if that someone is you? We explore these questions *In Depth* here.

Alcohols are chemical compounds structurally similar to carbohydrates, with one or more hydroxyl (OH) groups. **Ethanol,** the specific type of alcohol found in beer, wine, and distilled spirits such as whiskey and vodka, has one hydroxyl group. Throughout this discussion, the common term *alcohol* will be used to represent the specific compound *ethanol.*

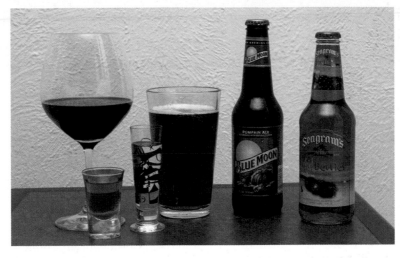

FIGURE 1 What does one drink look like? A drink is equivalent to 1½ oz of distilled spirits, 4 to 5 oz of wine, 10 oz of wine cooler, or 12 oz of beer.

What Do We Know About Moderate Alcohol Intake?

Alcohol intake is usually described as "drinks per day." A **drink** is defined as the amount of a beverage that provides ½ fluid ounce of pure alcohol. For example, 12 oz of beer, 10 oz of a wine cooler, 4–5 oz of wine, and 1½ oz of 80-**proof** whiskey, scotch, gin, or vodka are each equivalent to one drink (**Figure 1**).

The 2010 Dietary Guidelines for Americans advise "If alcohol is consumed, it should be consumed in moderation—up to one drink per day for women and two drinks per day for men—and only by adults of legal drinking age." Notice that this definition of **moderate drinking** is based on a maximal daily intake; a person who does not drink any alcohol on weekdays but downs a six-pack of beer most Saturday nights would *not* be classified as a "moderate drinker"! The 2010 Dietary Guidelines for Americans also identify groups of individuals who should not consume alcohol at all, including women who are or may become pregnant and women who are breastfeeding. In addition, people who cannot restrict their drinking to moderate levels and those taking medications that interact with alcohol should not drink at all, nor should individuals driving, operating machinery, or engaging in other tasks that require attention and coordination. Finally, anyone younger than the legal drinking age should not consume alcohol.

As we discuss here, both health benefits and concerns are associated with moderate alcohol intake. When deciding whether or how much alcohol to drink, you need to weigh the pros and cons of alcohol consumption against your own personal health history.

Benefits of Moderate Alcohol Intake

In most people, moderate alcohol intake offers some psychological benefits; it can reduce stress and anxiety while improving self-confidence. It can also have nutritional benefits. Moderate use of alcohol can improve appetite and dietary intake, which can be of great value to the elderly and people with a chronic disease that suppresses appetite.[1]

In addition, moderate alcohol consumption has been linked to lower rates of heart disease, especially in older adults and those already at risk for heart disease, such as people with type 2 diabetes.[2] Alcohol increases levels of the "good" type of cholesterol (HDL) while lowering the concentration of "bad" cholesterol (LDL); it also reduces the risk of abnormal clot formation in the blood vessels.

Recently, there has been a great deal of interest in **resveratrol,** a chemical found in red wines, grapes, and other plant foods. Some researchers, based on experiments with mice, are proposing that resveratrol may be able to lower our risk for certain chronic diseases, such as diabetes, heart disease, and liver disease.[3] However, the amount in red wine is too minimal to provide a health benefit. Instead, if resveratrol were found to be effective in promoting human health, it would have to be given as a purified supplement.

---

alcohol　Chemically, a compound characterized by the presence of a hydroxyl group; in common usage, a beverage made from fermented fruits, vegetables, or grains and containing ethanol.

ethanol　A specific alcohol compound (C_2H_5OH) formed from the fermentation of dietary carbohydrates and used in a variety of alcoholic beverages.

drink　The amount of an alcoholic beverage that provides approximately 0.5 fl. oz of pure ethanol.

proof　A measure of the alcohol content of a liquid; 100-proof liquor is 50% alcohol by volume, 80-proof liquor is 40% alcohol by volume, and so on.

moderate drinking　Alcohol consumption of up to one drink per day for women and up to two drinks per day for men.

resveratrol　A chemical known to play a role in limiting cell damage from the by-products of metabolic reactions. It is found in red wine and certain other plant-based foods.

Concerns of Moderate Alcohol Intake

Not everyone responds to alcohol in the same manner. A person's age, genetic makeup, state of health, and use of medications can influence both immediate and long-term responses to alcohol intake, even at moderate levels. For example, some women appear to be at increased risk for breast cancer when consuming low to moderate amounts of alcohol. Consumption of less than 30 g of alcohol per day (roughly equivalent to two drinks) has been shown to increase blood pressure in men over the age of 40 years.[4] In some studies, moderate use of alcohol has been linked to a higher rate of bleeding in the brain, resulting in what is termed *hemorrhagic stroke;* however, other research has found that light to moderate alcohol consumption does not increase the risk for stroke.[5]

Another concern is the effect of alcohol on our waistlines! As noted earlier (in Chapter 1), alcohol is not classified as a nutrient because it does not serve any unique metabolic role in humans. Although it provides virtually no nutritional value, alcohol does provide energy: at 7 kcal/g, alcohol has a relatively high Calorie content. Only fat (9 kcal/g) has more Calories per gram. If you are watching your weight, it makes sense to strictly limit your consumption of alcohol to stay within your daily energy needs. Alcohol intake may also increase your *total* energy intake, increasing your risk for overweight or obesity. That's because alcoholic beverages enhance appetite, particularly during social events, leading some people to overeat. Both current and lifelong intakes of alcohol increase the risk for obesity in both males and females.[6]

The potential for drug–alcohol interactions is well known; many medications carry a warning label advising consumers to avoid alcohol while taking the drug. Alcohol magnifies the effect of certain painkillers, sleeping pills, antidepressants, and anti-anxiety medications and can lead to loss of consciousness.

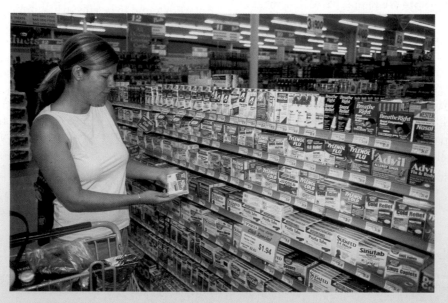

Alcohol can interfere with and increase the risks of using some over-the-counter and prescription medications.

It also increases the risk for gastrointestinal bleeding in people taking aspirin or ibuprofen, as well as the risk for stomach bleeding and liver damage in people taking acetaminophen (Tylenol). In diabetics using insulin or oral medications to lower blood glucose, alcohol can exaggerate the drug's effect, leading to an inappropriately low level of blood glucose.

As you can see, there are both benefits and risks to moderate alcohol consumption. Experts agree that people who are currently consuming alcohol in moderation and who have low or no risk for alcohol addiction or medication interaction can safely continue their current level of use. Adults who abstain from alcohol, however, should not start drinking just for the possible health benefits. Individuals who have a personal or family history of alcoholism or fall into any other risk category should consider abstaining from alcohol use, even at a moderate level.

How Is Alcohol Metabolized?

Alcohol is absorbed directly from both the stomach and the small intestine; it does not require digestion prior to absorption. Consuming foods with some fat, protein, and fiber slows the absorption of alcohol and can reduce *blood alcohol concentration (BAC)* by as much as 50% compared to peak BAC when drinking on an empty stomach. Carbonated alcoholic beverages are absorbed very rapidly, which explains why champagne and sparkling wines are so quick to generate an alcoholic "buzz."

The process of alcohol metabolism is discussed in detail later in this text (in Chapter 7), but a brief overview will introduce you to the basics. Although most alcohol is oxidized, or broken down, in the liver, a small amount is metabolized in the stomach before it has even been absorbed. Cells in both the stomach and the liver secrete the enzyme *alcohol dehydrogenase (ADH),* which triggers the first step in alcohol degradation, while *aldehyde dehydrogenase (ALDH)* takes the breakdown process one step further (**Figure 2**). In women, ADH in the stomach is less active than in men; thus, women do not oxidize as much alcohol in their

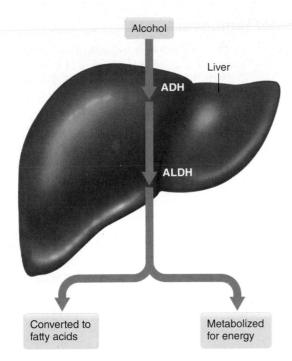

Alcohol

Liver

ADH

ALDH

Converted to fatty acids

Metabolized for energy

FIGURE 2 Metabolism of alcohol.

TABLE 1 Myths About Alcohol Metabolism

The Claim	The Reality
Physical activity, such as walking around, will speed up the breakdown of alcohol.	Muscles don't metabolize alcohol; the liver does.
Drinking a lot of coffee will keep you from getting drunk.	Coffee does not cause alcohol to be excreted in the urine.
Using a sauna or steam room will force the alcohol out of your body.	Very little alcohol is lost in sweat; the alcohol will remain in your bloodstream.
Herbal and nutritional products are available that speed up the breakdown of alcohol.	There is no scientific evidence that commercial supplements will increase the rate of alcohol metabolism; they will not lower blood alcohol levels.

stomach, leaving up to 30% to 35% more intact alcohol to be absorbed.

Once absorbed, the alcohol moves through the bloodstream to the liver, where it is broken down at a fairly steady rate. On average, a healthy adult metabolizes the equivalent of one drink per hour. If someone drinks more than that, such as two or three alcoholic drinks in an hour, the excess alcohol is released back into the bloodstream, where it elevates BAC and triggers a variety of behavioral and metabolic reactions. Through the blood, alcohol is readily distributed throughout all body fluids and tissues, including the brain. Anytime you consume more than one alcoholic beverage per hour, you are exposing every tissue in your body to the toxic effects of alcohol.

Despite what you may have heard, there is no effective intervention to speed up the breakdown of alcohol (**Table 1**). The key to keeping your BAC below the legal limit is to drink alcoholic beverages while eating a meal or large snack, to drink very slowly, to have no more than one drink per hour, and to limit your total consumption of alcohol on any one occasion.

A person who steadily increases his or her alcohol consumption over time becomes more tolerant of a given intake of alcohol. Chronic drinkers experience *metabolic tolerance*, a condition in which the liver becomes more efficient in its breakdown of alcohol. This means that the person's BAC rises more slowly after consuming a certain number of drinks. In addition, chronic drinkers develop what is called *functional tolerance*, meaning they show few, if any, signs of

impairment or intoxication, even at high BACs. As a result, these individuals may consume twice as much alcohol as when they first started drinking before they reach the same state of euphoria.

What Is Alcohol Abuse?

The National Institute on Alcohol Abuse and Alcoholism (NIAAA) recognizes two general types of *alcohol use disorders*: alcohol abuse and alcohol dependence, commonly known as alcoholism. In the United States, about 18 million people have an alcohol use disorder.[7]

Alcohol abuse is a pattern of alcohol consumption, whether chronic or occasional, that results in distress, danger, or harm to one's health, functioning, or interpersonal relationships. Both chronic and occasional alcohol abuse can eventually lead to alcoholism.

Binge drinking, the consumption of five or more alcoholic drinks on one occasion by a man or four or more drinks for a woman, is a form of alcohol abuse that occurs in about 15% of US adults and in youth as young as 12 years of age.[8] Males between the ages of 18 and 25 have the highest rate of binge drinking.[9] Binge drinking by college students and other young adults (or even underage adolescents) increases the risk for potentially fatal falls, drownings, and automobile accidents. Acts of physical violence, including vandalism and physical and sexual assault, are also associated with binge drinking. The consequences also carry over beyond a particular episode: binge drinking impairs cognition, planning, problem solving, memory, and inhibition, leading to significant social, educational, and employment

---

alcohol abuse A pattern of alcohol consumption, whether chronic or occasional, that results in harm to one's health, functioning, or interpersonal relationships.

binge drinking The consumption of five or more alcoholic drinks on one occasion for a man, or four or more drinks for a woman.

problems. Finally, hangovers, which are discussed shortly, are practically inevitable, given the amount of alcohol consumed during a binge.

Alcoholism is a disease characterized by chronic dependence on alcohol, notably the following:

- *Craving:* a strong need or urge to drink alcoholic beverages
- *Loss of control:* the inability to stop once drinking has begun
- *Physical dependence:* the presence of nausea, sweating, shakiness, and other signs of withdrawal after stopping alcohol intake
- *Tolerance:* the need to drink larger and larger amounts of alcohol to get the same "high," or pleasurable sensations, associated with alcohol intake

What Are the Effects of Alcohol Abuse?

Alcohol is a drug. It exerts a narcotic effect on virtually every part of the brain, acting as a sedative and depressant. Alcohol also has the potential to act as a direct toxin; in high concentrations, it can damage or destroy cell membranes and internal cell structures. As shown in **Figure 3**, an alcohol intake between ½ and 1 drink per day is associated with the lowest risk of mortality for both men and women. The risk of death increases sharply as alcohol intake increases above 2 drinks per day for women, and 3½ drinks per day for men. These increased mortality risks are related to alcohol's damaging effects on the brain, the liver, and other organs, as well as its role in motor vehicle accidents and other traumatic injuries.

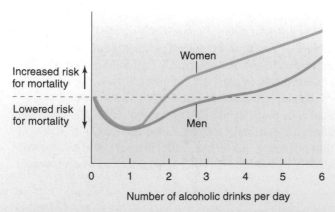

FIGURE 3 The effect of alcohol consumption on mortality risk. Consuming ½ to 1 drink per day is associated with the lowest mortality risk for all adults. The risk of death increases sharply at levels of alcohol intake above 2 drinks per day for women and about 3½ drinks per day for men.

Alcohol Hangovers

Alcohol hangover is an extremely unpleasant consequence of drinking too much alcohol. It lasts up to 24 hours, and its symptoms include headache, fatigue, dizziness, muscle aches, nausea and vomiting, sensitivity to light and sound, and extreme thirst. Some people also experience depression, anxiety, irritability, and other mood disturbances. While some of the aftereffects of a binge may be due to nonalcoholic compounds known as *congeners* (found in red wines, brandy, and whiskey, for example), most of the consequences are directly related to the alcohol itself. These include the following:

- *Fluid and electrolyte imbalance:* Some of the symptoms occur because of alcohol's effect as a *diuretic,* a compound that increases urine output. Alcohol inhibits the release of the hormones that normally regulate urine production, prompting an excessive loss of fluid and electrolytes and contributing to dizziness and lightheadedness.
- *Irritation and inflammation:* Alcohol irritates the lining of the stomach, causing inflammation (gastritis) and increasing gastric acid production. This may account for the abdominal pain, nausea, and vomiting seen in most hangovers.
- *Metabolic disturbances:* Alcohol disrupts normal body metabolism, leading to low levels of blood glucose and elevated levels of lactic acid. These disturbances contribute to the characteristic fatigue, weakness, and mood changes seen after excessive alcohol intake.
- *Biological disturbances:* Alcohol disrupts various biological rhythms, such as sleep patterns and cycles of hormone secretion, leading to an effect similar to that of jet lag.

While many folk remedies, including various herbal products, claim to prevent or reduce hangover effects, few have proven effective. Drinking water or other nonalcoholic beverages will minimize the risk for dehydration, and toast or dry cereal is effective in bringing blood glucose levels back to normal. Getting adequate sleep can counteract the fatigue, and the use of antacids can help reduce nausea and abdominal pain. Whereas aspirin, acetaminophen, and ibuprofen might be useful for headaches, they may, in fact, worsen stomach pain, increase the risk for GI bleeding, and, if taken regularly over an extended period of time, increase the risk for liver damage.

alcoholism A disease state characterized by chronic dependence on alcohol.

alcohol hangover A consequence of drinking too much alcohol; symptoms include headache, fatigue, dizziness, muscle aches, nausea and vomiting, sensitivity to light and sound, extreme thirst, and mood disturbances.

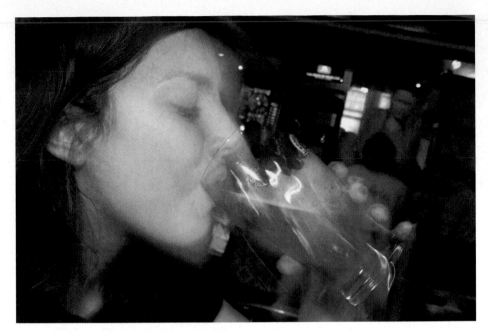

Alcohol abuse can lead to a number of negative consequences.

Reduced Brain Function

Alcohol is known for its ability to alter behavior, mainly through its effects on the brain. Even at low intakes, alcohol impairs reasoning and judgment (**Table 2**). Alcohol also interferes with normal sleep patterns, alters sight and speech, and leads to loss of both fine and gross motor skills such as handwriting, hand–eye coordination, and balance. Many people who drink experience unexpected mood swings, intense anger, or unreasonable irritation. Others react in the opposite direction, becoming sad, withdrawn, and lethargic. When teens or young adults chronically consume excessive amounts of alcohol, they may permanently damage brain structure and function.[10] Intellectual functioning and memory can be lost or compromised. In addition, early exposure to alcohol increases the risk for future alcohol addiction and may contribute to lifelong deficits in memory, motor skills, and muscle coordination.[11]

Alcohol Poisoning

At very high intakes of alcohol, a person is at risk for **alcohol poisoning,** a metabolic state that occurs in response to binge drinking. At high BACs, the respiratory center of the brain is depressed. This reduces the level of oxygen reaching the brain and increases the individual's risk for death by respiratory or cardiac failure. Like Todd in our opening story, many binge drinkers lose consciousness before alcohol poisoning becomes fatal, but emergency care is often essential.

If someone passes out after a night of hard drinking, he or she should never be left alone to "sleep it off." Instead, the person should be placed on his or her side to prevent aspiration if vomiting occurs. The person should also be watched carefully for cold and clammy skin, a bluish tint to the skin, or slow, irregular breathing. If any of these signs become evident, if the person cannot be awakened, or there is any other reason to believe he or she has alcohol poisoning, emergency healthcare should be sought immediately.

Reduced Liver Function

The liver performs an astonishing number and variety of body functions, including nutrient metabolism, glycogen storage, the synthesis of many essential compounds, and the detoxification of medications and other potential poisons. As noted earlier, it is the main site of alcohol metabolism. When an individual's rate of alcohol intake exceeds the rate at which the liver can break down the alcohol, liver cells are damaged or destroyed. The longer the alcohol abuse continues, the greater the damage to the liver.

Fatty liver (also called *alcoholic steatosis*), is a condition in which abnormal amounts of fat build up in the liver, is an early yet reversible sign of liver damage commonly linked to alcohol abuse. Once alcohol intake stops and a healthful diet is maintained, the liver is able to heal and resume normal function.

TABLE 2 Effects of Blood Alcohol Concentration (BAC) on Brain Activity

Blood Alcohol Concentration	Typical Response
0.02–0.05%	Feelings of relaxation, euphoria, relief
0.06–0.10%	Impaired judgment, fine motor control, and coordination; loss of normal emotional control; legally drunk in many states (at the upper end of the range)
0.11–0.15%	Impaired reflexes and gross motor control; staggered gait; legally drunk in all states; slurred speech
0.16–0.20%	Impaired vision; unpredictable behavior; further loss of muscle control
0.21–0.35%	Total loss of coordination; stupor
0.40% and above	Loss of consciousness; coma; suppression of respiratory response; death

alcohol poisoning   A potentially fatal condition in which an overdose of alcohol results in cardiac and/or respiratory failure.

fatty liver   An early and reversible stage of liver disease often found in people who abuse alcohol, characterized by the abnormal accumulation of fat within liver, and cells; also called alcoholic steatosis.

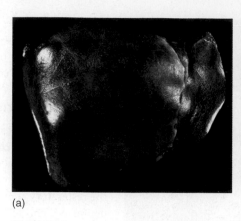 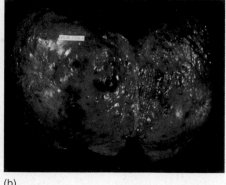

(a)   (b)

FIGURE 4 Cirrhosis of the liver is often caused by chronic alcohol abuse. **(a)** A healthy liver; **(b)** a liver damaged by cirrhosis.

Alcoholic hepatitis is a more severe condition of liver inflammation, resulting in loss of appetite, nausea and vomiting, abdominal pain, and jaundice (a yellowing of the skin and eyes, reflecting reduced liver function). Mental confusion and impaired immune response often occur with alcoholic hepatitis. Whereas avoidance of alcohol and a healthful diet often result in full recovery, many people experience lifelong complications from alcoholic hepatitis.

Cirrhosis of the liver is often the result of long-term alcohol abuse; liver cells are scarred, blood flow through the liver is impaired, and liver function declines (**Figure 4**). This condition almost always results in irreversible damage to the liver and can be life-threatening. Blood pressure increases dramatically, large amounts of fluid are retained in the abdominal cavity, and metabolic wastes accumulate. In some cases, liver function fails completely, resulting in the need for a liver transplant or the likelihood of death.

Increased Risk for Chronic Disease

While moderate drinking may provide some health benefits, it is clear that chronically high intakes of alcohol damage a number of body organs and systems, increasing a person's risk for chronic disease and death:

- *Bone health:* Men and women who are alcohol dependent experience an increased loss of calcium in the urine, impaired vitamin D activation, and decreased production of certain hormones that enhance bone formation.[12]
- *Pancreatic injury and diabetes:* Alcohol damages the pancreas, which produces insulin, and decreases the body's ability to properly respond to insulin. The result is chronically elevated blood glucose levels and an increased risk for diabetes.
- *Cancer:* Research has most strongly linked alcohol consumption, particularly at high intakes, to increased risk for

cancer of the mouth and throat, esophagus, stomach, liver, colon, and female breast.[13,14]

Malnutrition

As alcohol intake increases to 30% or more of total energy intake, appetite is lost and intake of healthful foods declines. Over time, the diet becomes deficient in protein, fats, carbohydrates, vitamins A and C, and minerals such as iron, zinc, and calcium (**Figure 5**). End-stage alcoholics may consume as much as 90% of their daily energy intake from alcohol, displacing virtually all foods. Even if food intake is maintained, the toxic effects of alcohol lead to impaired food digestion, nutrient absorption, and nutrient metabolism.

Long-term exposure to alcohol damages not only the liver but also the stomach, small intestine, and pancreas. Alcohol increases gastric acid production, leading to stomach ulcers, gastric bleeding, and damage to the cells that produce gastric enzymes, mucus, and other proteins. The lining of the small intestine is also damaged by chronic alcohol abuse, reducing nutrient absorption, whereas damage to the pancreas reduces the production of pancreatic digestive enzymes. As a result, the digestion of foods and absorption of nutrients, such as the fat-soluble vitamins (A, D, E, and K), vitamin B_6, folate, and zinc, become inadequate, leading to malnutrition and inappropriate weight loss.

Not only are dietary intake, food digestion, and nutrient absorption negatively impacted by alcohol abuse but so, too, is the ability of body cells to utilize nutrients. For example, even if an alcoholic were to take vitamin D

---

alcoholic hepatitis A serious condition of inflammation of the liver caused by alcohol.

cirrhosis of the liver End-stage liver disease characterized by significant abnormalities in liver structure and function; may lead to complete liver failure.

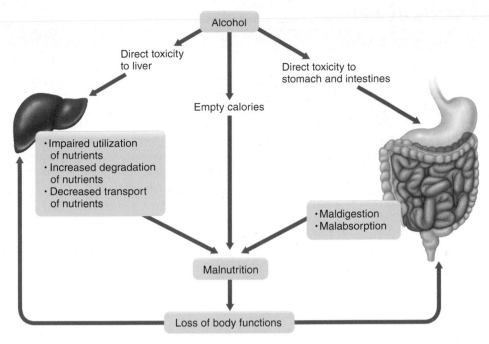

FIGURE 5 Alcohol-related malnutrition. Excess alcohol consumption contributes directly and indirectly to widespread nutrient deficiencies.

supplements, his or her liver would be so damaged that its cells could not activate the vitamin D. Many chronic alcoholics are unable to synthesize the liver proteins that carry vitamins and minerals to target tissues. Other vitamins and minerals are negatively affected because the liver is too damaged to maintain normal nutrient storage capacity. Across the whole spectrum, from food intake to cell nutrient metabolism, alcohol abuse increases the risk for malnutrition.

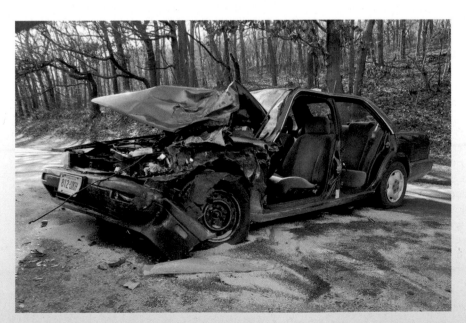

Excessive alcohol intake greatly increases the risks for car accidents and other traumatic injuries.

Increased Risk for Traumatic Injury

Excessive alcohol intake is the third leading cause of preventable death for Americans, contributing to nearly 80,000 deaths per year.[15] It has been estimated that as many as 6,000 young Americans die each year from alcohol-related motor vehicle accidents, suicides, and homicides. As previously noted, rates of physical and sexual assaults, vandalism, accidental falls, and drownings also increase when people are under the influence of alcohol.

Fetal and Infant Health Problems

No level of alcohol consumption is considered safe for pregnant women. Women who are or think they may be pregnant should abstain from all alcoholic beverages. As discussed in the **Highlight** box (page 168), fetal alcohol syndrome, which is caused by alcohol intake in a childbearing woman, is a critical problem in the United States.

Women who are breastfeeding should also abstain from alcohol because it easily passes into the breast milk at levels equal to blood alcohol concentrations. If consumed by the infant, the alcohol in breast milk can slow motor development, depress the central nervous system, and increase sleepiness in the child. Alcohol also reduces the mother's ability to produce milk, putting the infant at risk for malnutrition.

Taking Control of Your Alcohol Intake

Knowing that a moderate intake of alcohol may provide some health benefits and that excessive intake results in a wide range of problems, what can you do to control your drinking? The following are practical strategies that can help you avoid the negative consequences of excessive alcohol consumption:

■ Think about *why* you are planning to drink. Is it to relax and socialize, or are you using alcohol to release stress? If the latter, try some stress-reduction

Fetal Alcohol Syndrome

Alcohol is a known **teratogen** (a substance that causes fetal harm) that readily crosses the placenta into the fetal bloodstream. Because the immature fetal liver cannot effectively break down the alcohol, it accumulates in the fetal blood and tissues, increasing the risk for various birth defects. The effects of maternal alcohol intake are dose-related: the more the mother drinks, the greater the potential harm to the fetus. In addition to the amount of alcohol consumed during pregnancy, the timing of the mother's alcohol intake influences the risk for fetal complications. Binge or frequent drinking during the first trimester of pregnancy is more likely to result in birth defects and other permanent abnormalities, whereas alcohol consumption in the third trimester typically results in low birth weight and growth retardation.

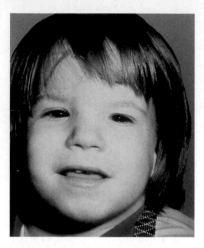

FIGURE 6 A child with fetal alcohol syndrome (FAS). The facial features typical of children with FAS include a short nose with a low, wide bridge; drooping eyes with an extra skinfold; and a flat, thin upper lip. These external traits are typically accompanied by behavioral problems and learning disorders. The effects of FAS are irreversible.

Fetal alcohol syndrome (FAS) is the most severe consequence of maternal alcohol consumption. The Centers for Disease Control and Prevention, using data from the Fetal Alcohol Syndrome Surveillance Network (FASSNet), found prevalence estimates of 0.3 to 1.5 cases of FAS per 1,000 live births in certain areas in the United States.[1] FAS is a condition characterized by malformations of the face, limbs, heart, and nervous system. The characteristic facial features of FAS persist throughout the child's life (**Figure 6**). Exposure to alcohol while in the womb impairs fetal growth; FAS babies are often underweight at birth and rarely normalize their growth after birth. Newborn and infant death rates are abnormally high, and those who do survive suffer from emotional, behavioral, social, learning, and developmental problems throughout life. FAS is one of the most common causes of mental retardation in the United States and the only one that is completely preventable.

Conditions associated with maternal alcohol consumption are collectively known as **fetal alcohol spectrum disorders (FASD).** In addition to FAS, they include the following:

- *Alcohol-related birth defects (ARBD):* Children with ARBD are born with heart, skeletal, kidney, ear, and eye malformations.

- *Alcohol-related neurodevelopmental disorder (ARND):* Children with ARND demonstrate a range of life-long developmental, behavioral, and mental problems, including hyperactivity and attention deficit disorder.

- *Fetal alcohol effects (FAE):* A more subtle set of consequences related to maternal alcohol intake, FAE is usually not identified at birth but becomes evident when the child enters preschool or kindergarten, where the child may exhibit impaired learning abilities. It is estimated that the incidence of FAE is ten times greater than that of FAS.

Can a pregnant woman safely consume any amount of alcohol? Although some pregnant women do have an occasional alcoholic drink with no apparent ill effects, there is no amount of alcohol known to be safe. In one study, researchers identified a number of subtle but long-term negative consequences of light to moderate alcohol consumption during pregnancy: girls born to women who had as little as one alcoholic drink a week during their pregnancy were more likely to experience mental health problems through the age of 7 years compared to children who had no fetal exposure to alcohol.[2] The best advice regarding alcohol intake during pregnancy is to abstain if there is any chance of becoming pregnant, as well as throughout the pregnancy.

References:

1. Centers for Disease Control and Prevention. 2010. Tracking Fetal Alcohol Syndrome. www.cdc.gov/ncbddd/fasd/research-tracking.html. (Accessed May 2012.)
2. Sayal, K., J. Heron, J. Golding, and A. Emond. 2007. Prenatal alcohol exposure and gender differences in childhood mental health problems: a longitudinal population-based study. *Pediatrics* 119:e426–e434.

techniques that don't involve alcohol, such as exercise, yoga, meditation, or simply talking with a friend.[16]

- Make sure you have a protein-containing meal or snack before your first alcoholic drink; having food in the stomach delays gastric emptying, which means more of the alcohol can be broken down in the stomach before it even gets the chance to be absorbed into the bloodstream.
- Rotate between alcoholic and nonalcoholic drinks. Start with a large glass of water, iced tea, or soda. Once your thirst has been satisfied, your rate of fluid intake will drop. Remember, a glass of pure orange juice doesn't look any different from one laced with vodka, so no one will even know what it is you are or are not drinking! Dilute hard liquor with large amounts of soda, water, juice, or iced tea. These diluted beverages are cheaper and lower in Calories, too!
- Whether or not your drink is diluted, sip slowly to allow your liver time to keep up with your alcohol intake.
- If your friends pressure you to drink, volunteer to be the designated driver. You'll have a "free pass" for the night in terms of saying no to alcoholic drinks.
- Decide in advance what your alcohol intake will be, and plan some strategies for sticking to your limit. If you are going to a bar, for example, take only enough money to buy two beers and two sodas. If you are at a party, stay occupied dancing, sampling the food, or talking with friends, and stay as far away from the bar area as you can.

Should You Be Concerned About Your Alcohol Intake?

Even if you are not dependent on alcohol, you should be concerned about your alcohol intake if you engage in binge drinking or drink at inappropriate times (while pregnant, before or while driving a car, to deal with negative emotions, or while at work/school). If you answer "yes" to one or more of the following questions, provided by the National Institute on Alcohol Abuse and Alcoholism, you may have a problem with alcohol abuse:

- Have you ever felt you should cut down on your drinking?
- Have people annoyed you by criticizing your drinking?
- Have you ever felt bad or guilty about your drinking?
- Do you drink alone when you feel angry or sad?
- Has your drinking ever made you late for school or work?
- Have you ever had a drink first thing in the morning to steady your nerves or get rid of a hangover?
- Do you ever drink after promising yourself you won't?

If you think you have an alcohol problem, it is important for you to speak with a trusted friend, coach, teacher, counselor, or healthcare provider. In addition, many campuses have support groups that can help. Taking control of your alcohol intake will allow you to take control of your life.

Talking to Someone About Alcohol Addiction

You may suspect that a close friend or relative might be one of the nearly 18 million Americans with an alcohol use disorder. If your friend or relative uses alcohol to calm down, cheer up, or relax, that may be a sign of alcohol dependency. The appearance of tremors or other signs of withdrawal as well as the initiation of secretive behaviors when consuming alcohol are other indications that alcohol has become a serious problem.

Many people become defensive or hostile when asked about their use of alcohol; denial is very common. The single

---

teratogen A substance or compound known to cause fetal harm or birth defects.

fetal alcohol syndrome (FAS) A set of serious, irreversible alcohol-related birth defects characterized by certain physical and mental abnormalities, including malformations of the face, limbs, heart, and nervous system; impaired growth; and a spectrum of mild to severe cognitive, emotional, and physical problems.

fetal alcohol spectrum disorders (FASD) An umbrella designation for a wide range of clinical outcomes that can result from prenatal exposure to alcohol. Fetal alcohol syndrome (FAS), alcohol-related neurodevelopmental disorder (ARND), and alcohol-related birth defects (ARBD) are components of FASD.

*Nutri-*Case

Theo

"I was driving home from a post-game party last night when I was pulled over by the police. The officer said I seemed to be driving 'erratically' and asked me how many drinks I'd had. I told him I'd only had three beers and explained that I was pretty tired from the game. Then, just to prove I was fine, I offered to count backward from a hundred, but I must have sounded sober, because he didn't make me do it. I can't believe he thought I was driving drunk! Still, maybe three beers after a game really is too much."

Do you think it is physiologically possible that Theo's driving had been impaired after consuming three beers? To answer, you'll need to consider both Theo's body weight and the effect of playing a long basketball game. What other factors that influence the rate of alcohol absorption or breakdown could have affected Theo's BAC? How could all of these factors influence a decision about whether "three beers after a game really is too much"?

hardest step toward sobriety is often the first: accepting the fact that help is needed. Some people respond well when confronted by a single person, while others benefit more from a group intervention. There should be no blaming or shaming; alcohol use disorders are medical conditions with a genetic component. The National Institute on Alcoholism and Alcohol Abuse suggests the following approaches when trying to get a friend or relative into treatment:

- *Stop "covering" and making excuses*: Often, family and friends will make excuses to others to protect the person from the results of his or her drinking. It is important, however, to stop covering for that person so he or she can experience the full consequences of inappropriate alcohol consumption.
- *Intervene at a vulnerable time*: The best time to talk to someone about problem drinking is shortly after an alcohol-related incident, such as a DUI arrest, an alcohol-related traffic accident, or a public scene. Wait until the person is sober and everyone is relatively calm.
- *Be specific*: Tell the person exactly why you are concerned; use examples of specific problems associated with his or her drinking habits (e.g., poor school or work performance; legal problems; inappropriate behaviors). Explain what will happen if the person chooses not to get help—for example, no longer going out with the person if alcohol will be available, no longer riding with him or her in motor vehicles, moving out of a shared home, and so on.
- *Get help*: Professional help is available from community agencies, healthcare providers, online sites, school or work-site wellness centers, and some religious organizations. Several contacts and websites are listed at the end of this *In Depth*. If the person indicates a willingness to get help, call immediately for an appointment and/or immediately take him or her to a treatment center. The longer the delay, the more likely it is that the person will experience a change of heart.
- Enlist the support of others. Whether or not the person agrees to get help, calling upon other friends and relatives can often be effective, especially if one of these people has battled alcohol abuse. Formal support groups, such as Al-Anon and Alateen, can provide additional information and guidance.

Treatment for alcohol use disorders works for many, but not all, individuals. Success is measured in small steps, and relapses are common. Most scientists agree that people who abuse alcohol cannot just "cut down." Complete avoidance of all alcoholic beverages is the only way for most people who abuse alcohol to achieve full and ongoing recovery.

Web Links

www.aa.org
Alcoholics Anonymous, Inc.
This site provides both links to local AA groups and information on the AA program.

www.al-anon.alateen.org
Al-Anon Family Group Headquarters, Inc.
This site provides links to local Al-Anon and Alateen groups, which offer support to spouses, children, and other loved ones of people addicted to alcohol.

www.niaaa.nih.gov
National Institute on Alcohol Abuse and Alcoholism
Visit this website for information on the prevalence, consequences, and treatments of alcohol-related disorders. Information for healthcare providers, people struggling with alcohol abuse, and family members is available free of charge.

www.collegedrinkingprevention.gov
College Drinking: Changing the Culture
The NIAAA developed this website for college students seeking information and advice on the subject of college drinking. Services include self-assessment questionnaires, answers to frequently asked questions, news articles, research, and links to support groups.

References

1. Yeomans, M. R. 2010. Alcohol, appetite and energy balance: is alcohol intake a risk factor for obesity? *Physio. Behav.* 100:82–89.
2. Rajpathak, S. N., M. S. Freiber, C. Wang, J. Wylie-Rosett, R. P. Wildman, T. E. Rohan, J. G. Robinson, S. Liu, and S. Wassertheil-Smoller. 2010. Alcohol consumption and the risk of coronary heart disease in postmenopausal women with diabetes: Women's Health Initiative Observational Study. *Eur. J. Nutr.* 49:211–218.
3. National Institutes of Health. 2012. NIH study uncovers probable mechanism underlying resveratrol activity. *NIH News.* www.nih.gov/news/health/feb2012/nhlbi-02.htm.
4. Wakabayaski, I., and Y. Araki. 2010. Influences of gender and age on relationships between alcohol drinking and atherosclerotic risk factors. *Alcohol. Clin. Exp. Res.* 34(suppl1):S54–60.
5. Jimenez, M., S. E. Chiuve, R. J. Glynn, M. J. Stampfer, C. A. Camargo, W. C. Willett, J. E. Manson, and K. M. Rexrode. 2012. Alcohol consumption and risk of stroke in women. *Stroke* 43:939–945.
6. Lourenço, S., A. Oliveira, and C. Lopes. 2012. The effect of current and lifetime alcohol consumption on overall and central obesity. *Europ. J. Clinic. Nutr.* 1–6.
7. NIAAA. 2012. Alcohol Use Disorders. www.niaaa.nih .gov/alcohol-health/overview-alcohol-consumption/ alcohol-use-disorders.
8. Xiao-Jun, W., D. Kanny, W. W. Thompson, C. A. Okoro, M. Town, and L. S. Balluz. 2012. Binge drinking intensity and health-related quality of life among US adult binge drinkers. *Prev. Chronic Dis* 9:110204.

9. Centers for Disease Control and Prevention. 2010. Vital signs: binge drinking among high school students and adults—United States, 2009. *MMWR Morb. Mortal Wkly. Rep.* 59:1274–1279.

10. Parada, M., M. Corral, N. Mota, A. Crego, S. Rodríguez Holguín, and F. Cadaveira. 2012. Executive functioning and alcohol binge drinking in university students. *Addictive Behaviors* 37:167–172.

11. Guerri, C., and M. Pascual. 2010. Mechanisms involved in the neurotoxic, cognitive, and neurobehavioral effects of alcohol consumption during adolescence. *Alcohol* 44:15–26.

12. Maurel, D. B., N. Boisseau, C. L. Benhamou, and C. Jaffre. 2012. Alcohol and bone: review of dose effects and mechanisms. *Osteoporosis* 23:1–16.

13. Chen, W. Y., B. Rosner, S. E. Hankinson, et al. 2011. Moderate alcohol consumption during adult life, drinking pattern, and breast cancer risk. *JAMA* 306:1884–1890.

14. Tramacere, I., E. Negri, C. Pelucchi, V. Bagnardi, M. Rota, L. Scotti, F. Islami, G. Corrao, C. La Vecchia, and P. Boffetta. 2012. A meta-analysis on alcohol drinking and gastric cancer risk. *Annals of Oncology* 23:28–36.

15. Dalye, J. I., M. A. Stahre, F. J. Chaloupka, and T. S. Naimi. 2012. The impact of a 25-cent-per-drink alcohol tax increase. *Am. J. Prev. Med.* 42:382–389.

16. National Institute on Alcohol Abuse and Alcoholism (NIAAA). 2007. Alcohol: How to Cut Down on Your Drinking. www.collegedrinkingprevention.gov/otheralcoholinformation/cutdownondrinking.aspx. (Accessed May 2012.)

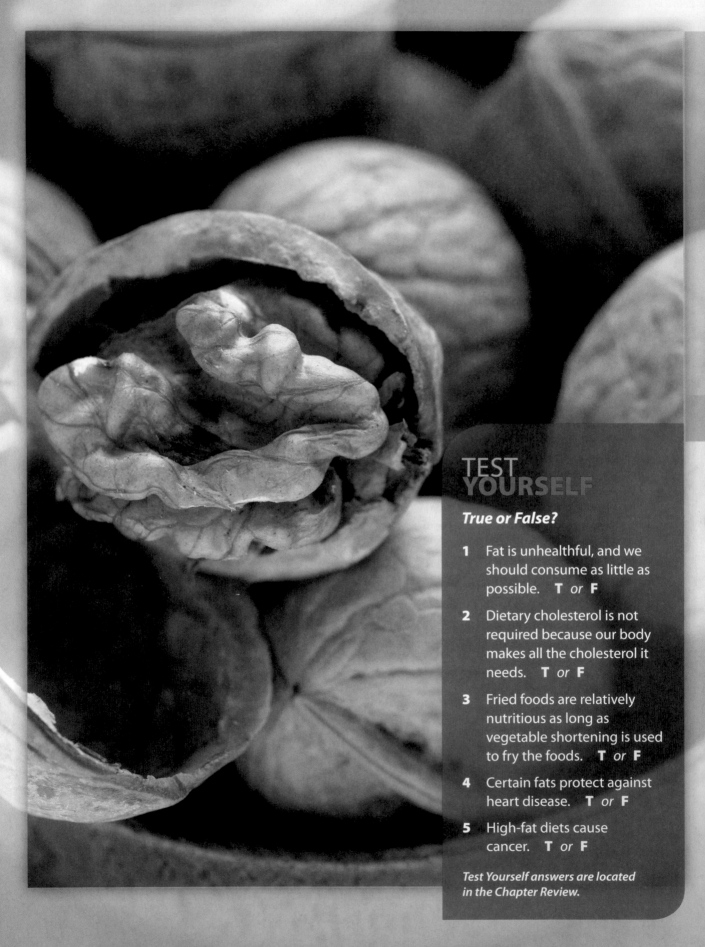

TEST YOURSELF

True or False?

1 Fat is unhealthful, and we should consume as little as possible. **T** *or* **F**

2 Dietary cholesterol is not required because our body makes all the cholesterol it needs. **T** *or* **F**

3 Fried foods are relatively nutritious as long as vegetable shortening is used to fry the foods. **T** *or* **F**

4 Certain fats protect against heart disease. **T** *or* **F**

5 High-fat diets cause cancer. **T** *or* **F**

Test Yourself answers are located in the Chapter Review.

5

Lipids: Essential Energy-Supplying Nutrients

Learning Objectives

After studying this chapter, you should be able to:

1. List and describe the three types of lipids found in foods, *pp. 174–183*.

2. Discuss how the level of saturation of a fatty acid affects its shape and the form it takes, *pp. 176–179*.

3. Explain the derivation of the term *trans* fatty acid and how *trans* fatty acids can negatively affect health, *pp. 178–179*.

4. Identify the beneficial functions of the two essential fatty acids, *pp. 179–181*.

5. Describe the steps involved in fat digestion, absorption, and transport, *pp. 183–188*.

6. List three physiologic functions of fat in the body, *pp. 189–191*.

7. Define the recommended dietary intakes for total fat, saturated fat, and the two essential fatty acids, *pp. 192–193*.

8. Identify at least three common food sources of unhealthful fats and three common sources of beneficial fats, *pp. 193–197*.

9. Describe the role of blood lipids and dietary fats in the development of cardiovascular disease, *p. 206*.

10. Identify lifestyle recommendations for the prevention or treatment of cardiovascular disease, *pp. 206–207*.

MasteringNutrition™

Go online for chapter quizzes, pre-tests, Interactive Activities and more!

H ow would you feel if you purchased a bag of potato chips and were charged an extra 5% "fat tax"? What if you ordered fish and chips in your favorite restaurant only to be told that, in an effort to avoid lawsuits, fried foods were no longer being served? Sound surreal? Believe it or not, these and dozens of similar scenarios are being proposed, threatened, and defended in the current "obesity wars" raging around the globe. From Maine to California, from Iceland to New Zealand, local and national governments and healthcare policy advisors are scrambling to find effective methods for combating their rising rates of obesity. For reasons we explore in this chapter, many of their proposals focus on limiting consumption of foods high in saturated fats—for instance, requiring food vendors and manufacturers to reduce the portion size of these foods; taxing them, or increasing their purchase price; levying fines on manufacturers who produce them; removing these foods from vending machines; banning advertisements of these foods to children; and using food labels and public service announcements to warn consumers away from these foods. At the same time, "food litigation" lawsuits have been increasing, including allegations against restaurant chains and food companies for failing to warn consumers of the health dangers of eating their energy-dense, high-saturated-fat foods.

Is saturated fat really such a menace? Does a diet high in saturated fat cause obesity, heart disease, or diabetes? What exactly *is* saturated fat, anyway? And are other types of fat just as bad?

Although some people think that all dietary fat should be avoided, a certain amount of fat is absolutely essential for life and health. In this chapter, we'll discuss the function of fat in the human body; explain how dietary fat is digested, absorbed, transported, and stored; and help you distinguish between beneficial and harmful types of dietary fat. You'll also assess how much fat you need in your diet and learn about the role of dietary fat in the development of heart disease and other disorders.

What Are Lipids?

Lipids are a large and diverse group of substances that are distinguished by the fact that they are insoluble in water. Think of a salad dressing made with vinegar (which is mostly water) and olive oil—a lipid. Shaking the bottle *disperses* the oil but doesn't *dissolve* it; that's why it separates back out again so quickly. Lipids are found in all sorts of living things, from bacteria to plants to human beings. In fact, their presence on your skin explains why you can't clean your face with water alone—you need some type of soap to break down the insoluble lipids before you can wash them away. In this chapter, we focus on lipids that are found in foods and some of the lipids synthesized within the body.

Many different forms of lipids occur in the body and in foods. In the body, lipids are stored in adipose tissues that protect and insulate organs, are combined with phosphorus in cell membranes, and occur as steroids in bile salts, sex hormones, and other substances.[1] In foods, lipids occur as both fats and oils. These two forms are distinguished by the fact that fats, such as butter and lard, are solid at room temperature, whereas oils, such as olive oil, are liquid at room temperature. Dietary guidelines, food labels, and other nutrition information intended for the general public use the term *fats* when referring to the lipid content of diets and foods. We adopt this practice throughout this textbook, reserving the term *lipids* for discussions of chemistry and metabolism.

Three types of lipids are commonly found in foods and in the cells and tissues of the human body. These are triglycerides, phospholipids, and sterols. Let's take a look at each.

Triglycerides Are the Most Common Food-Based Lipid

Most of the fat we eat (95%) is in the form of triglycerides (also called triacylglycerols), which is the same form in which most body fat is stored. As reflected in the prefix *tri-*,

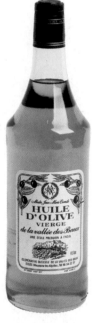

Some lipids, such as olive oil, are liquid at room temperature.

lipids A diverse group of organic substances that are insoluble in water; lipids include triglycerides, phospholipids, and sterols.

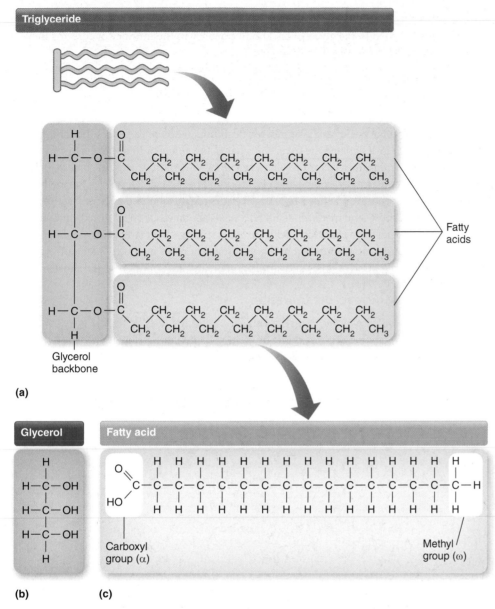

FIGURE 5.1 **(a)** A triglyceride consists of three fatty acids attached to a three-carbon glycerol backbone. **(b)** Structure of glycerol. **(c)** Structure of a fatty acid showing the carboxyl carbon (α) and the methyl carbon (ω) ends.

a **triglyceride** is a molecule consisting of *three* fatty acids attached to a *three*-carbon glycerol backbone (**Figure 5.1a**). **Fatty acids** are long chains of carbon atoms bound to each other as well as to hydrogen atoms. They are acids because they contain an acid group (carboxyl group) at one end of their chain. **Glycerol**, the backbone of a triglyceride molecule, is an alcohol composed of three carbon atoms (Figure 5.1b). One fatty acid attaches to each of these three carbons to make the triglyceride.

Triglycerides can be classified by their chain length (number of carbons in each fatty acid), by their level of saturation (how much hydrogen is attached to each carbon atom in the fatty acid chain), and by their shape, which is determined in some cases by how they are commercially processed. All of these factors influence how the triglyceride is used within the body and how it affects our health.

triglyceride A molecule consisting of three fatty acids attached to a three-carbon glycerol backbone.

fatty acids Long chains of carbon atoms bound to each other as well as to hydrogen atoms.

glycerol An alcohol composed of three carbon atoms; it is the backbone of a triglyceride molecule.

Triglycerides Vary in Chain Length

The fatty acids attached to the glycerol backbone can vary in the number of carbons they contain, a quality referred to as their *chain length*.

- **Short-chain fatty acids** are usually fewer than six carbon atoms in length.
- **Medium-chain fatty acids** are six to twelve carbons in length.
- **Long-chain fatty acids** are fourteen or more carbons in length.

The carbons of a fatty acid can be numbered beginning with the carbon of the carboxyl end (COOH), which is designated the α-carbon (that is, the *alpha*, or first, carbon), or from the carbon of the terminal methyl group (CH_3), called the ω-carbon (that is, the *omega*, or last, carbon) (Figure 5.1c). Fatty acid chain length is important because it determines the method of digestion and absorption and affects how triglycerides are metabolized and used within the body. For example, short- and medium-chain fatty acids are digested, transported, and metabolized more quickly than long-chain fatty acids. In general, long-chain fatty acids are more abundant in nature, and thus more abundant in our diet, than short- or medium-chain fatty acids. We will discuss the digestion of lipids and absorption of fatty acids in more detail shortly.

Triglycerides Vary in Level of Saturation

Triglycerides can also vary by the types of bonds found in the fatty acids. If a fatty acid has no carbons bonded together with a double bond anywhere along its length, it is referred to as a **saturated fatty acid (SFA)** (**Figure 5.2a**). This is because every carbon atom in the chain

short-chain fatty acids Fatty acids fewer than six carbon atoms in length.

medium-chain fatty acids Fatty acids that are six to twelve carbon atoms in length.

long-chain fatty acids Fatty acids that are fourteen or more carbon atoms in length.

saturated fatty acid (SFAs) Fatty acids that have no carbons joined together with a double bond; these types of fatty acids are generally solid at room temperature.

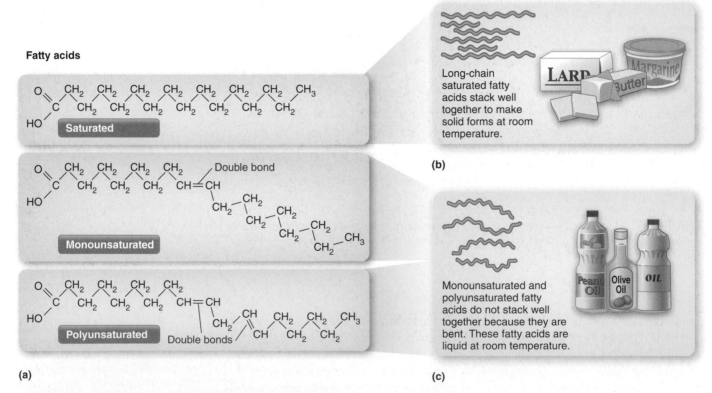

FIGURE 5.2 Examples of levels of saturation among fatty acids and how these levels of saturation affect the shape of fatty acids. **(a)** Saturated fatty acids are saturated with hydrogen, meaning they have no carbons bonded together with a double bond. Monounsaturated fatty acids contain two carbons bound by one double bond. Polyunsaturated fatty acids have more than one double bond linking carbon atoms. **(b)** Saturated fats have straight fatty acids packed tightly together and are solid at room temperature. **(c)** Unsaturated fats have "kinked" fatty acids at the area of the double bond, preventing them from packing tightly together; they are liquid at room temperature.

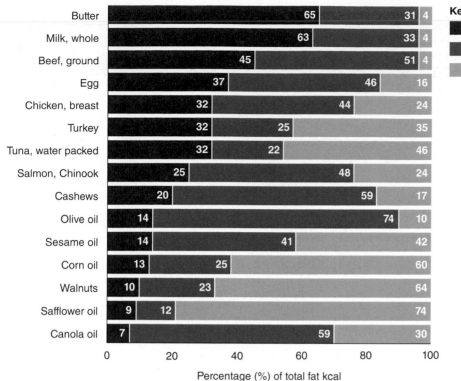

Key:
- ■ Saturated fatty acids
- ■ Monounsaturated fatty acids
- ■ Polyunsaturated fatty acids

Food	Saturated	Monounsaturated	Polyunsaturated
Butter	65	31	4
Milk, whole	63	33	4
Beef, ground	45	51	4
Egg	37	46	16
Chicken, breast	32	44	24
Turkey	32	25	35
Tuna, water packed	32	22	46
Salmon, Chinook	25	48	24
Cashews	20	59	17
Olive oil	14	74	10
Sesame oil	14	41	42
Corn oil	13	25	60
Walnuts	10	23	64
Safflower oil	9	12	74
Canola oil	7	59	30

Percentage (%) of total fat kcal

FIGURE 5.3 Major sources of dietary fat.

is *saturated* with hydrogen: each has the maximum amount of hydrogen bound to it. Some foods that are high in saturated fatty acids are coconut oil, palm kernel oil, butter, cheese, whole milk, cream, lard, and beef fat.

If, within the chain of carbon atoms, two are bound to each other with a double bond, then this double carbon bond excludes hydrogen. This lack of hydrogen at *one* part of the molecule results in a fat that is referred to as *monounsaturated* (recall from Chapter 4 that the prefix *mono-* means "one"). A monounsaturated molecule is shown in Figure 5.2a. **Monounsaturated fatty acids (MUFAs)** are usually liquid at room temperature. Foods that are high in monounsaturated fatty acids are olive oil, canola oil, peanut oil, and cashew nuts.

If the fat molecules have *more than one* double bond, they contain even less hydrogen and are referred to as **polyunsaturated fatty acids (PUFAs)** (see Figure 5.2a). Polyunsaturated fatty acids are also liquid at room temperature and include cottonseed, canola, corn, and safflower oils.

Foods vary in the types of fatty acids they contain. For example, animal fats provide approximately 40% to 60% of their energy from saturated fats, whereas plant fats provide 80% to 90% of their energy from monounsaturated and polyunsaturated fats (**Figure 5.3**). Notice that most oils are a good source of both MUFAs and PUFAs. Diets higher in plant foods are usually lower in saturated fats than diets high in animal products.

Carbon Bonding Affects Shape

Have you ever noticed how many toothpicks are packed into a small box? Two hundred or more! But if you were to break a bunch of toothpicks into V shapes anywhere along their length, how many could you then fit into the same box? It would be very few because the bent toothpicks would jumble together, taking up much more space. Molecules of saturated fat are like straight toothpicks: they have no double carbon bonds and always form straight, rigid chains. As they have no kinks, these chains can pack together tightly (see Figure 5.2b). That is why saturated fats, such as the fat in meats, are solid at room temperature.

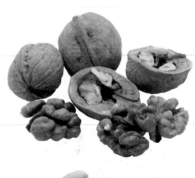

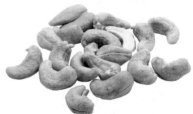

Walnuts and cashews are high in monounsaturated fatty acids.

monounsaturated fatty acids (MUFAs) Fatty acids that have two carbons in the chain bound to each other with one double bond; these types of fatty acids are generally liquid at room temperature.

polyunsaturated fatty acids (PUFAs) Fatty acids that have more than one double bond in the chain; these types of fatty acids are generally liquid at room temperature.

FIGURE 5.4 Structure of **(a)** a *cis* and **(b)** a *trans* polyunsaturated fatty acid. Notice that *cis* fatty acids have both hydrogen atoms located on the same side of the double bond. This positioning makes the molecule kinked. In *trans* fatty acids, the hydrogen atoms are attached on diagonally opposite sides of the double carbon bond. This positioning makes them straighter and more rigid.

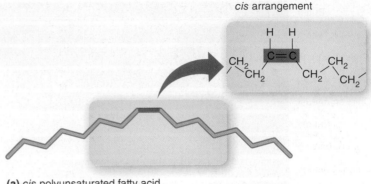

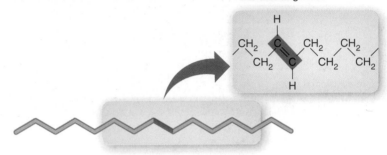

(a) *cis* polyunsaturated fatty acid

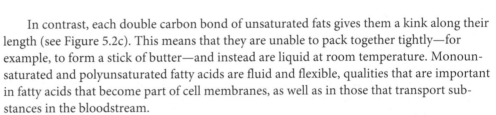

(b) *trans* polyunsaturated fatty acid

In contrast, each double carbon bond of unsaturated fats gives them a kink along their length (see Figure 5.2c). This means that they are unable to pack together tightly—for example, to form a stick of butter—and instead are liquid at room temperature. Monounsaturated and polyunsaturated fatty acids are fluid and flexible, qualities that are important in fatty acids that become part of cell membranes, as well as in those that transport substances in the bloodstream.

Unsaturated fatty acids can occur in either a *cis* or a *trans* shape. The prefix *cis-* indicates a location on the same side, whereas *trans-* is a prefix that denotes across or opposite. In lipid chemistry, these terms describe the positioning of the hydrogen atoms around the double carbon bond.

A *cis fatty acid* has both hydrogen atoms located on the same side of the double bond (**Figure 5.4a**). This positioning gives the *cis* molecule a pronounced kink at the double carbon bond. We typically find the *cis* fatty acids in nature and thus in foods such as olive oil.

In contrast, in a *trans fatty acid*, the hydrogen atoms are attached on diagonally opposite sides of the double carbon bond (Figure 5.4b). This positioning makes *trans* fatty acid fats straighter and more rigid, just like saturated fats. Although a limited amount of *trans* fatty acids is found in full-fat cow's milk, the majority of *trans* fatty acids are commercially produced by manipulating the fatty acid during food processing. For example, in the **hydrogenation** of oils, such as corn or safflower oil, hydrogen is added to the fatty acids. In this process, the double bonds found in the monounsaturated and polyunsaturated fatty acids in the oil are broken, and additional hydrogen is inserted at diagonally opposite sides of the double bonds. This process straightens out the molecules, making the oil more solid at room temperature—as well as more saturated. The hydrogenation of fats helps foods containing these fats, such as cakes, cookies, and crackers, resist rancidity, because the additional hydrogen reduces the tendency of the carbon atoms in the fatty acid chains to undergo oxidation.

The hydrogenation process can be controlled to make the oil more or less saturated: if only some of the double bonds are broken, the fat produced is called *partially hydrogenated*, a term you will see frequently on food labels. For example, corn oil margarine is a

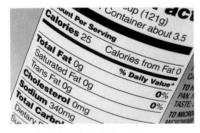

The U.S. Food and Drug Administration (FDA) requires that both saturated and *trans* fats be listed as separate line items on Nutrition Facts Panels for conventional foods and some dietary supplements. Research studies show that diets high in these fatty acids can increase the risk of cardiovascular disease.

hydrogenation The process of adding hydrogen to unsaturated fatty acids, making them more saturated and thereby more solid at room temperature.

partially hydrogenated fat made from corn oil. Margarines that are even partially hydrogenated have more *trans* fatty acids than butter, unless the label indicates otherwise.

Does the straight, rigid shape of the saturated and *trans* fats we eat have any effect on our health? Absolutely! Research during the past two decades has shown that both saturated and *trans* fatty acids raise blood cholesterol levels and appear to change cell membrane function and the way cholesterol is removed from the blood. For these reasons, diets high in saturated or *trans* fatty acids are associated with an increased risk for cardiovascular disease.

Because of these health concerns, food manufacturers are required to list the amount of saturated and *trans* fatty acids per serving on the Nutrition Facts Panel of food labels. However, the U.S. Food and Drug Administration (FDA) allows products that have less than 1 g of *trans* fat per serving to claim that they are *trans* fat free. So even if the Nutrition Facts panel states 0 g *trans* fats, the product can still have ½ g of *trans* fat per serving. If the ingredients list states that the product contains partially hydrogenated oils, it contains *trans* fats.

Given the fact that most margarines have more *trans* fatty acids than butter does, which is the more healthful choice for your morning toast? Check out the feature box **Nutrition Myth or Fact? Is Margarine More Healthful Than Butter?** to find out.

Some Triglycerides Contain Essential Fatty Acids

The length of the fatty acid chain and the placement of the double bonds determine the function of the fatty acid within the body. As noted earlier, the carbons of a fatty acid can be numbered beginning with the carbon of the terminal methyl group, called the ω-carbon (ω [omega] is the last letter in the Greek alphabet), or from the α-carbon of the beginning carboxyl group (α [alpha] is the first letter in the Greek alphabet). In **Figure 5.5**, we have illustrated this numbering system and have numbered the carbons from the ω-carbon.[2] When synthesizing fatty acids, the body cannot insert double bonds before the ninth carbon from the ω-carbon.[2] For this reason, fatty acids with double bonds closer to the methyl end (at ω-3 and at ω-6) are considered **essential fatty acids (EFAs)**—because the body cannot synthesize them, they must be obtained from food.

EFAs are precursors to important biological compounds called *eicosanoids* and are therefore essential to growth and health. Eicosanoids get their name from the Greek word *eicosa,* which means "twenty," as they are synthesized from fatty acids with twenty carbon atoms. They include prostaglandins, thromboxanes, and leukotrienes. Among the most potent regulators of cellular function in nature, eicosanoids are produced in nearly every cell within the body.[3] They help regulate gastrointestinal tract motility, secretory activity, blood clotting, vasodilatation and vasoconstriction, vascular permeability, and inflammation. There must be a balance between the various eicosanoids to assure that the appropriate amount of blood clotting or dilation/constriction of the blood vessels occurs.

The body's synthesis of various eicosanoids depends on the abundance of the EFAs available as precursors and the enzymes within each pathway. The two essential fatty acids in our diet are linoleic acid and alpha-linolenic acid.

Linoleic Acid   Also known as an *omega-6 fatty acid,* **linoleic acid** is found in vegetable and nut oils, such as sunflower, safflower, corn, soy, and peanut oils. If you eat lots of vegetables or use vegetable-oil-based margarines or vegetable oils, you are probably getting adequate amounts of this essential fatty acid in your diet. Linoleic acid is metabolized in the body to arachidonic acid, which is a precursor to a number of eicosanoids.

Alpha-Linolenic Acid   Also known as an *omega-3 fatty acid,* **alpha-linolenic acid** was only recognized to be essential in the mid-1980s. It is found primarily in dark green, leafy vegetables, flaxseeds and flaxseed oil, soybeans and soybean oil, walnuts and walnut oil, and canola oil. Alpha-linolenic acid is also a precursor of two omega-3 fatty acids now recognized for their role in protecting against cardiovascular disease: **eicosapentaenoic acid (EPA)** and **docosahexaenoic acid (DHA).** Unfortunately, only a limited amount of

essential fatty acids (EFAs)   Fatty acids that must be consumed in the diet because they cannot be made by the body. The two essential fatty acids are linoleic acid and alpha-linolenic acid.

linoleic acid   An essential fatty acid found in vegetable and nut oils; also known as omega-6 fatty acid.

alpha-linolenic acid   An essential fatty acid found in leafy green vegetables, flaxseed oil, soy oil, fish oil, and fish products; an omega-3 fatty acid.

eicosapentaenoic acid (EPA)   A metabolic derivative of alpha-linolenic acid.

docosahexaenoic acid (DHA)   A metabolic derivative of alpha-linolenic acid; together with EPA, it appears to reduce the risk of heart disease.

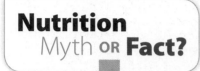

Is Margarine More Healthful Than Butter?

Your toast just popped up! Which will it be: butter or margarine? As you've seen in Figure 5.3, butter is 65% saturated fat. Moreover, 1 tablespoon provides 30 grams of cholesterol! In contrast, corn oil margarine is just 2% saturated fat, with no cholesterol. But how much *trans* fat does that margarine contain? And which is better—the more natural and more saturated butter or the more processed and less saturated margarine?

You're not the only one asking this question. Until recently, vegetable-based oils were hydrogenated to make margarines. These products were filled with *trans* fats, which can increase the consumer's risk of heart disease, as well as harm cell membranes, weaken immune function, and inhibit the body's natural anti-inflammatory hormones. Some margarines also contained harmful amounts of toxic metals, such as nickel and aluminum, as by-products of the hydrogenation process. These are among some of the reasons researchers began warning consumers against these margarines several years ago.

So does that mean that the saturated-fat, cholesterol-rich butter is the better choice? A decade ago, that may have been the case, but food manufacturers now offer "*trans*-fat-free margarines and spreads" that contain no *trans* fats, no cholesterol, and low amounts of saturated fats. The American Heart Association[1] advises consumers to choose these *trans*-fat-free margarines over butter. However, some whole-food advocates point out that such manufactured products are still "non-foods" and recommend that consumers choose unprocessed nut butters (peanut, walnut, cashew, and almond butters). These natural alternatives are rich in essential fatty acids and other heart-healthy unsaturated fats.

Remember, a label claiming that a margarine has zero *trans* fatty acids doesn't guarantee that the product is *trans* fatty acid free (see the accompanying table). You have to look for margarines with no "partially hydrogenated" oil in them. That is the only way you will know your spread is entirely free of *trans* fatty acids. Check out the table to help you decide which spreads you're going to include in your diet.

Spreads for Your Bread*

Brand Name	Energy (kcal)	Sat Fat (g)	*Trans* fat (g)	Sodium (mg)
Tubs and Squeezes Made Without Partially Hydrogenated Oil				
Promise Fat Free; I Can't Believe It's Not Butter (fat free)	5	0	0	90
Country Crock Omega Plus Light	50	1	0	80
Smart Balance Omega Light	50	1.5	0	80
Parkay Squeeze	70	1.5	0	110
Canola Harvest Original	100	1.5	0	100
Tubs and Sticks Made with Partially Hydrogenated Oil				
Blue Bonnet Light	50	1	1	80
Blue Bonnet	60	1	0.4	130
I Can't Believe It's Not Butter! Original	80	2	0.3	90
Fleischmann's Original	100	2	2.5	120
Butter				
Butter, any brand, stick	100	7.5	0.4	80
Land O'Lakes Light with Canola Oil	50	2	0	90
Shortening				
Crisco, stick or tub	100	3	0.5	0
Nut Butters				
Peanut butter	95	1.5	0	78
Almond butter	99	1	0	70

*All portion sizes are 1 tablespoon.

Source: Hurley, J., and B. Liebman. 2009. Covering the Spreads. Tracking down the butters and margarines. *Nutrition Action Health Letter*, September, 13–15. Food Processor-SQL, Version 10.3, ESHA Research, Salem, OR.

Reference

1. Lichtenstein, A. H., L. J. Appel, M. Brands, M. Carnethon, S. Daniels, H. A. Franch, B. Franklin, P. Kris-Etherton, W. S. Harris, B. Howard, N. Karanja, M. Lefevre, L. Rudel, F. Sacks, L. Van Horn, M. Winston, and J. Wylie-Rosett. 2006. Diet and lifestyle recommendations revision 2006: scientific statement from the American Heart Association Nutrition Committee. *Circulation* 114:82–96.

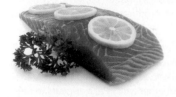

Salmon is high in omega-3 fatty acid content.

dietary alpha-linolenic acid is converted to EPA and DHA within the body; therefore, it is important to get these key fatty acids from marine sources.[4] They are found in fish, shellfish, and fish oils. Fish that naturally contain more oil, such as salmon and tuna, are higher in EPA and DHA than lean fish, such as cod and flounder. Research indicates that diets high in EPA and DHA stimulate the production of prostaglandins and thromboxanes that reduce inflammatory responses in the body, reduce blood clotting and plasma triglycerides, and thereby reduce an individual's risk for heart disease.

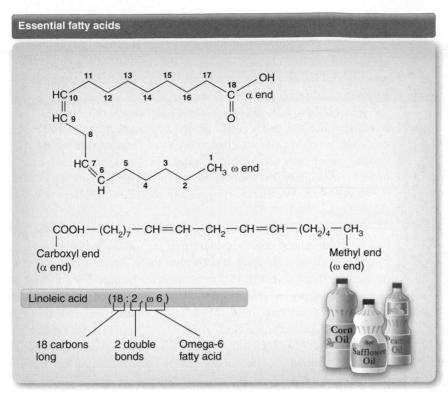

Essential fatty acids

(a)

(b)

FIGURE 5.5 The two essential fatty acids. **(a)** In linoleic acid (omega-6 fatty acid), counting from the terminal methyl group (the ω-carbon), the first double bond occurs at the sixth carbon. **(b)** In alpha-linolenic acid (omega-3 fatty acid), counting from the terminal methyl group (the ω-carbon), the first double bond occurs at the third carbon.

RECAP

Fat is essential for health. Triglycerides are the most common fat found in food. A triglyceride is made up of glycerol and three fatty acids. These fatty acids can be classified based on chain length, level of saturation, and shape. The essential fatty acids, linoleic acid and alpha-linolenic acid, cannot be synthesized by the body and must be consumed in the diet. ■

Nutrition
MILESTONE

In **1935**, J. A. Urquhart, a physician working among the Inuit people of the Arctic Circle in Canada, reported that in 7 years of serving this population he had encountered no cases of heart disease, diabetes, or cancer. Over the next 50 years, studies from other researchers working among Inuit groups in Canada and Greenland continued to report similar surprising findings. How could the Inuit—whose diets were made up of as much as 75% fat—have had such extremely low rates of heart disease? The key, the researchers soon discovered, was in the *type* of fat the Inuit consumed. Cold-water fish and sea mammals, such as seal, walrus, and whales, which were staples of the Inuit diet, are very low in saturated fats, high in monounsaturated fats, and particularly rich in polyunsaturated omega-3 fatty acids—particularly EPA and DHA.

Phospholipids Combine Lipids with Phosphate

Along with the triglycerides just discussed, we also find **phospholipids** in the foods we eat. They are abundant, for example, in egg yolks, peanuts, and soybeans and are present in processed foods containing emulsifiers, additives that help foods stay blended.

Phospholipids consist of a glycerol backbone with fatty acids attached at the first and second carbons and another compound that contains phosphate attached at the third carbon (**Figure 5.6a**). Because phosphates are soluble in water, phospholipids are soluble in water, a property that enables them to assist in transporting fats in the bloodstream. We discuss this concept in more detail later in this chapter (page 184).

The phospholipids are unique in that they have a hydrophobic (water-avoiding) end, which is their lipid "tail," and a hydrophilic (water-attracting) end, which is their phosphate "head." In the cell membrane, this quality helps them regulate the transport of substances into and out of the cell (Figure 5.6b). Phospholipids also help with digestion of dietary fats. In the liver, phospholipids called *lecithins* combine with bile salts and electrolytes to make bile. As you recall (from Chapter 3), bile emulsifies lipids. Note that the body manufactures phospholipids, so it is not essential to include them in the diet.

Sterols Have a Ring Structure

Sterols are a type of lipid with a multiple-ring structure quite different from that of triglycerides or phospholipids (**Figure 5.7a**). Plant foods contain some sterols, but they are not very well absorbed. However, plant sterols have a healthful function: they appear to block

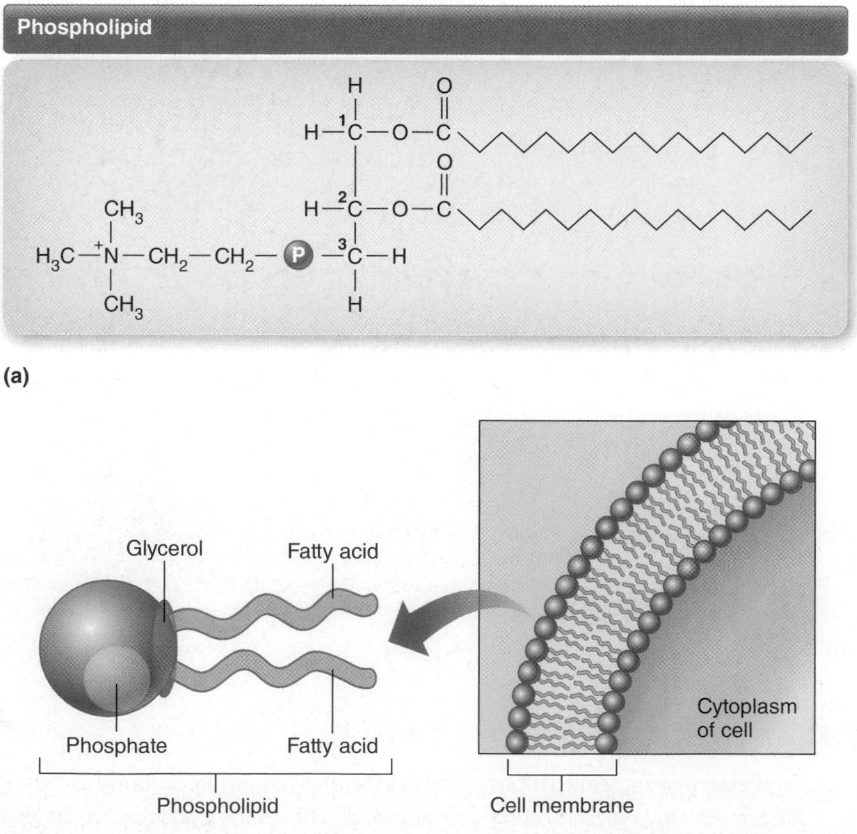

FIGURE 5.6 The structure of a phospholipid. **(a)** Detailed biochemical drawing of the phospholipid phosphatidylcholine, in which the phosphate is bound to choline and attached to the glycerol backbone at the third carbon. This phospholipid is commonly called lecithin and is found in foods such as egg yolks, as well as in the body. **(b)** Phospholipids consist of a glycerol backbone with two fatty acids and a compound that contains phosphate. This diagram illustrates the placement of the phospholipids in the cell membrane structure.

Phospholipid

(a)

(b)

phospholipids A type of lipid in which a fatty acid is combined with another compound that contains phosphate; unlike other lipids, phospholipids are soluble in water.

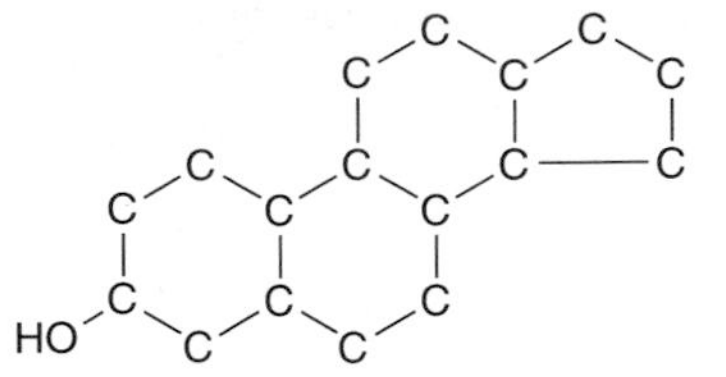

FIGURE 5.7 Sterol structure. **(a)** Sterols are lipids that contain multiple ring structures. **(b)** Cholesterol is the most commonly occurring sterol in the diet. **(c)** When a fatty acid is attached to the cholesterol molecule, it is called a cholesterol ester. Cholesterol esters are a common form of cholesterol in our diet.

(a) Sterol ring structure

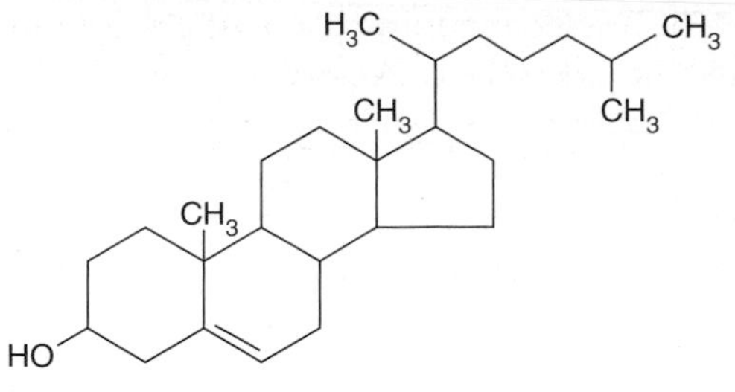

(b) Cholesterol

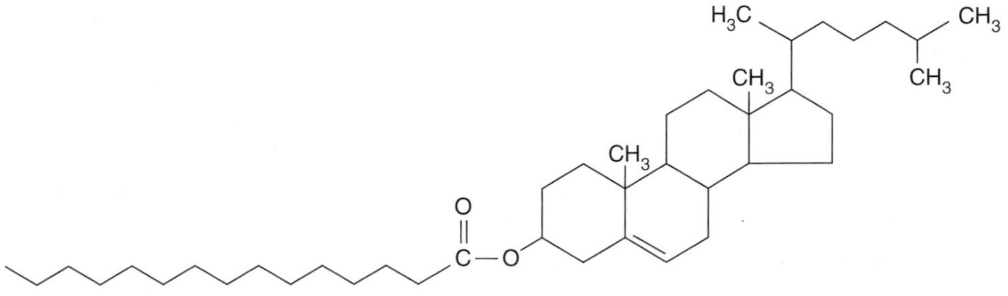

(c) Cholesterol ester

the absorption of dietary cholesterol, the most commonly occurring sterol in the diet and the sterol associated with an increased risk for cardiovascular disease (Figure 5.7b). We'll discuss plant sterols and their ability to lower blood cholesterol in more depth later in this chapter. Cholesterol is found in animal-based foods primarily as cholesterol esters, in which a fatty acid is attached to the cholesterol ring structure (Figure 5.7c). It is abundant in the fatty part of animal products, such as butter, egg yolks, whole milk, meats, and poultry. Lean meats and low- or reduced-fat milk, yogurt, and cheeses have little cholesterol.

It is not necessary to consume exogenous (dietary) cholesterol because nearly every cell in the body continually synthesizes all the cholesterol it needs. Most of the body's endogenous cholesterol production occurs in the liver, which releases the cholesterol into the blood to supply other tissues. Whether exogenous or endogenous, cholesterol is used in the structure of every cell membrane, where it works in conjunction with fatty acids and phospholipids to help maintain cell membrane integrity and modulate fluidity. It is particularly plentiful in the neural cells that make up the brain, spinal cord, and nerves. The body also uses cholesterol to make several important sterol compounds, including sex hormones (estrogen, androgens such as testosterone, and progesterone), adrenal hormones, and vitamin D. In addition, cholesterol is the precursor for the bile salts that are a primary component of bile, which helps emulsify lipids in the gut prior to digestion. Thus, despite cholesterol's bad reputation, it is absolutely essential to human health.

Concerned about the saturated fat and cholesterol in the meat you eat? Use this guide to choosing the leanest cuts of beef at www.mayoclinic.com/health/cuts-of-beef/MY01387.

RECAP

Phospholipids combine two fatty acids and a glycerol backbone with a phosphate-containing compound, making them soluble in water. Sterols have a multiple-ring structure; cholesterol is the most commonly occurring sterol in our diet. ■

How Does the Body Break Down Lipids?

Because lipids are not soluble in water, they cannot enter the bloodstream easily from the digestive tract. Thus, their digestion, absorption, and transport within the body differ from those of carbohydrates and proteins, which are water-soluble substances.

sterols A type of lipid found in foods and the body that has a ring structure; cholesterol is the most common sterol that occurs in our diets.

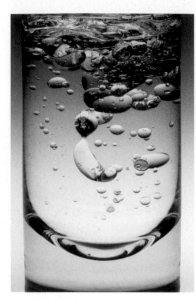

Fats and oils do not dissolve readily in water.

The digestion and absorption of lipids were discussed in detail in Chapter 3, but we briefly review the process here (**Figure 5.8**). Dietary fats are usually mixed with other foods. Lingual lipase, a salivary enzyme released during chewing, plays a minor role in the breakdown of lipids in food, so most lipids reach the stomach intact. The primary role of the stomach in lipid digestion is to mix and break up the lipid into smaller droplets. Because lipids are not soluble in water, these droplets typically float on top of the watery digestive juices in the stomach until they are passed into the small intestine.

The Gallbladder, Liver, and Pancreas Assist in Fat Digestion

Because lipids are not soluble in water, their digestion requires the help of bile from the gallbladder and digestive enzymes from the pancreas. Recall (from Chapter 3) that the gallbladder is a sac attached to the underside of the liver and the pancreas is an oblong-shaped organ sitting below the stomach. Both have a duct connecting them to the small intestine. As lipids enter the small intestine from the stomach, the gallbladder contracts and releases bile. The contraction of the gallbladder is primarily caused by the release of cholecystokinin (CCK) (also called pancreozymin) from the duodenal mucosal cells into the circulation. Secretin, another hormone released from the duodenal mucosa, also plays a role in gallbladder contraction. The same gut hormones also cause the release of the pancreatic aqueous phase (bicarbonate and water) and the pancreatic digestive enzymes into the gut.

Although bile is stored in the gallbladder, it is actually produced in the liver. It is composed primarily of bile salts made from cholesterol, lecithins and other phospholipids, and electrolytes (for example, sodium, potassium, chloride, and calcium). *Lecithins* (also called phosphatidylcholine; see Figure 5.6a) are phospholipids in which a phosphate-containing compound and choline are combined and attached at the third carbon on the glycerol backbone. They are the primary emulsifiers in bile: the hydrophobic tails of lecithin molecules attract lipid droplets, clustering them together in tiny spheres, while the hydrophilic heads form a water-attracting shell. Lecithins enable bile to act much as soap, breaking up lipids into smaller and smaller droplets with a greater surface area. The more droplets there are, the greater the chance that digestive enzymes will be able to reach their target. Interestingly, lecithins are abundant in egg yolk, which is frequently used as an emulsifier in cooking—for instance, when oil and vinegar are combined to make mayonnaise.

At the same time the bile is mixing with the lipids to emulsify them, lipid-digesting enzymes produced in the pancreas travel through the pancreatic duct into the small intestine. Each lipid product requires a specific digestive enzyme or enzymes. For example, triglycerides require both pancreatic lipase and co-lipase for digestion. The co-lipase anchors the pancreatic lipase to the lipid droplet, so that it can break the fatty acids away from their glycerol backbones. Each triglyceride molecule is broken down into two free fatty acids, which are removed from the first and third carbons on the glycerol backbone, and one *monoacylglyceride*, a glycerol molecule with one fatty acid still attached at the second carbon on the glycerol backbone (**Figure 5.9a**).

Specific enzymes also assist in the digestion of cholesterol esters and phospholipids. As noted in Figure 5.7c, when a fatty acid is attached to cholesterol it is called a cholesterol ester. Some of the cholesterol in our diet is in this form; thus, we need *cholesterol esterase*, an enzyme released from the pancreas, to break the ester bond between cholesterol and its attached fatty acid and release a free cholesterol molecule and a free fatty acid. Phospholipase enzymes are responsible for breaking phospholipids into smaller parts. Thus, the end products of digestion are much smaller molecules, which can be more easily captured and transported to the enterocytes for absorption.

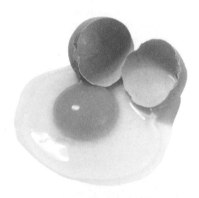

Lecithins are abundant in egg yolk, which is used as an emulsifier in products such as mayonnaise.

Absorption of Lipids Occurs Primarily in the Small Intestine

The majority of lipid absorption occurs in the mucosal lining of the small intestine with the help of micelles (see Figure 5.8). A **micelle** is a spherical compound made up of bile salts and biliary phospholipids that can capture the lipid digestion products, such as free fatty acids, free cholesterol, and the monoglycerides, and transport them to the enterocytes for

micelle A spherical compound made up of bile salts and biliary phospholipids that transports lipid digestion products to the intestinal mucosal cell.

The majority of lipid digestion takes place in the small intestine, with the help of bile from the liver and digestive enzymes from the pancreas. Micelles transport the end products of lipid digestion to the enterocytes for absorption and eventual transport via the blood or lymph.

ORGANS OF THE GI TRACT

MOUTH

Lingual lipase secreted by tongue cells and mixed with saliva digests some triglycerides.

Little lipid digestion occurs here.

STOMACH

Most fat arrives intact at the stomach, where it is mixed and broken into droplets.

Gastric lipase digests some triglycerides.

SMALL INTESTINE

Bile from the gallbladder breaks fat into smaller droplets.

Lipid-digesting enzymes from the pancreas break triglycerides into monoacylglycerides and fatty acids.

Lipid-digesting enzymes from the pancreas break dietary cholesterol esters and phospholipids into their components.

Products of fat digestion combine with bile salts to form micelles.

Micelles transport lipid digestion products to the enterocytes.

Within enterocytes, components from micelles reform triglycerides and are repackaged as chylomicrons for transport into the lymphatic system.

Shorter fatty acids can be absorbed directly into the bloodstream.

ACCESSORY ORGANS

SALIVARY GLANDS

Produce saliva.

LIVER

Produces bile, which is stored in the gallbladder.

GALLBLADDER

Contracts and releases bile into the small intestine.

PANCREAS

Produces lipid-digesting enzymes, which are released into the small intestine.

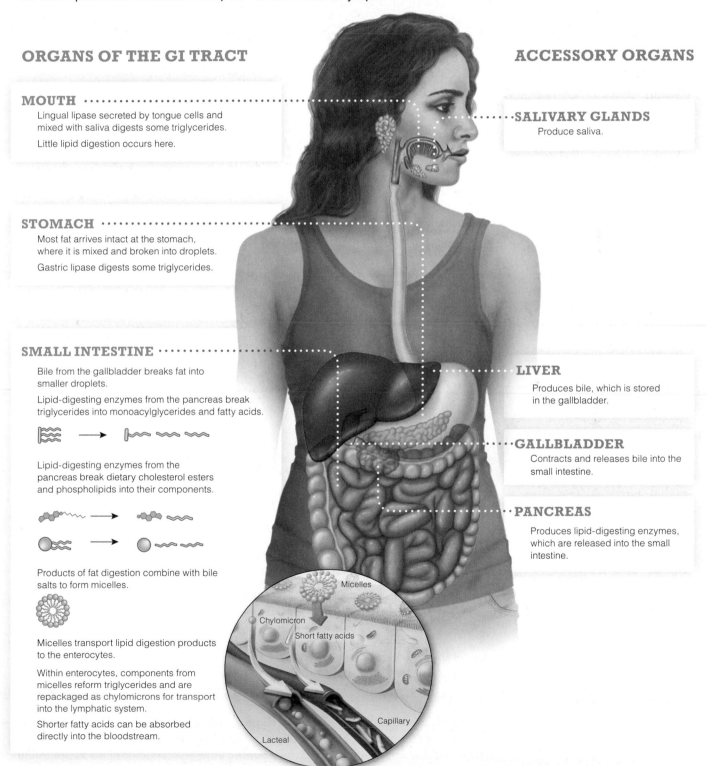

Micelles

Chylomicron

Short fatty acids

Capillary

Lacteal

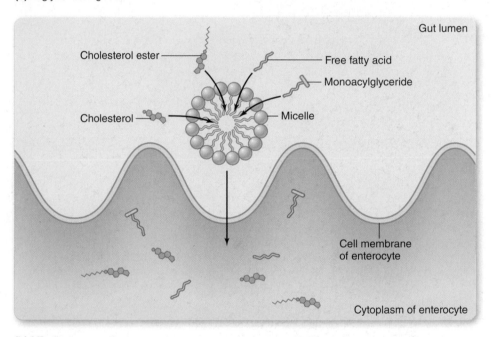

(a) Triglyceride digestion

(b) Micelle transport into enterocyte

FIGURE 5.9 Lipid digestion and absorption. **(a)** In the presence of enzymes, triglycerides are broken down into fatty acids and monoacylglycerides. **(b)** These products, along with cholesterol and cholesterol esters, are trapped in the micelle, a spherical compound made up of bile salts and biliary phospholipids. The micelle then transports these lipid digestion products to the intestinal mucosal cell, and these products are then absorbed into the cell.

lipoprotein A spherical compound in which fat clusters in the center and phospholipids and proteins form the outside of the sphere.

chylomicron A lipoprotein produced in the mucosal cell of the intestine; transports dietary fat out of the intestinal tract.

absorption (Figure 5.9b). The micelle has a hydrophobic core and a hydrophilic surface, which is excellent for transporting lipids in the watery environment of the gut.

How do the absorbed lipids—which do not mix with water—get into the bloodstream? Within the enterocytes, the fatty acids and monoglycerides are reformulated back into triglycerides and then packaged into lipoproteins before they're released into the bloodstream. A **lipoprotein** is a spherical compound with triglycerides clustered in the center along with cholesterol esters, free cholesterol, and other hydrophobic lipids and phospholipids and proteins forming the outside of the sphere (**Figure 5.10**). The specific lipoprotein produced in the enterocytes to transport lipids from a meal is called a **chylomicron.**

The process of forming a chylomicron begins with the re-creation of the triglycerides and the cholesterol esters in the enterocytes (**Figure 5.11**, page 188). These products are then loosely enclosed within an outer shell made of phospholipids and proteins. The chylomicron is now soluble in water because phospholipids and proteins are water soluble. Once chylomicrons are formed, they are transported out of the enterocytes to the lymphatic system, which empties into the bloodstream through the thoracic duct at the left subclavian vein in the neck. In this way, the dietary fat consumed in a meal is transported into the blood. This is why, soon after a meal containing fat, there is an increase of chylomicrons in the blood.

The triglycerides within chylomicrons are used by cells throughout the body. They are released with the help of an enzyme called **lipoprotein lipase,** or LPL, which is found on the outside of body cells. When chylomicrons touch the surface of a cell, they come into contact with LPL, which breaks apart the triglycerides in their core. This process frees individual fatty acids to move into the cell.

As body cells take up these fatty acids, the chylomicrons decrease in size and become more dense. These smaller chylomicrons, called *chylomicron remnants,* are now filled with cholesterol, phospholipid, and protein. The remnants are removed from the blood by the liver, which recycles their contents. Liver cells also synthesize two additional types of lipoprotein that play important roles in cardiovascular disease. We discuss these later in the chapter. For most individuals, chylomicrons are cleared rapidly from the blood, usually within 6 to 8 hours after a moderate-fat meal, which is why patients are instructed to fast overnight before having blood drawn for a laboratory analysis of blood lipid levels.

As mentioned earlier, short- and medium-chain fatty acids (those less than fourteen carbons in length) can be transported in the body more readily than long-chain fatty acids. This is because short- and medium-chain fatty acids transported to the mucosal cells do not have to be re-formed into triglycerides and incorporated into chylomicrons (see Figure 5.11). Instead, they can travel in the portal bloodstream bound to either the transport protein albumin or a phospholipid. In general, our diet is low in short- and medium-chain fatty acids; however, they can be extracted from certain oils for clinical use in feeding patients who cannot digest long-chain fatty acids.

Fat Is Stored in Adipose Tissues for Later Use

We've said that, after a meal, the chylomicrons begin to circulate through the blood. There are three primary fates of the fatty acids in their core:

1. They can be taken up and used as a source of energy for body cells, especially muscle cells.
2. They can be used to make lipid-containing compounds in the body.
3. They can be stored in the muscle or adipose tissue for later use. (See **Figure 5.12**, page 188, for an illustration of an adipose cell.)

If body cells don't need the fatty acids for immediate energy, they will have to be stored. However, cells cannot store individual fatty acids; instead, cells convert these fatty acids back into a triglyceride for storage. Because adipose cells are the only body cells that have significant storage capacity for triglycerides, most fat not needed for energy is stored in adipose tissues for later use.

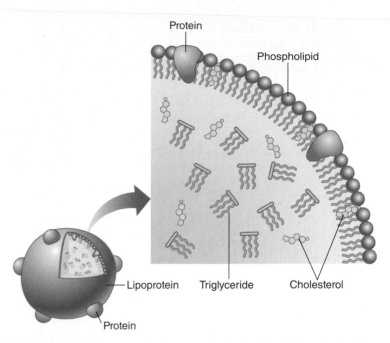

FIGURE 5.10 Structure of a lipoprotein. Notice that the fat clusters in the center of the molecule and the phospholipids and proteins, which are water soluble, form the outside of the sphere. This enables lipoproteins to transport fats in the bloodstream.

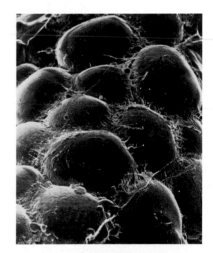

Adipose tissue. During times of weight gain, excess fat consumed in the diet is stored in the adipose tissue.

lipoprotein lipase   An enzyme that sits on the outside of cells and breaks apart triglycerides, so that their fatty acids can be removed and taken up by the cell.

FIGURE 5.11 The reassembly of the lipid components (for example, triglycerides) into a chylomicron, which is then released into the lymphatic circulation and then into the bloodstream at the thoracic duct. Short- and medium-chain fatty acids are transported directly into the portal circulation (for example, the blood going to the liver).

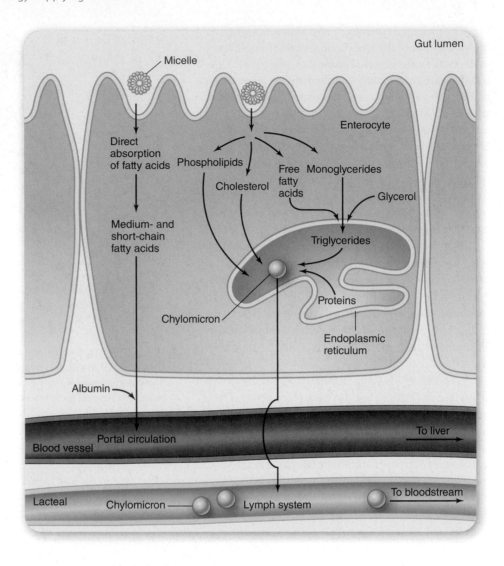

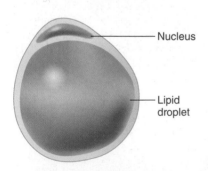

FIGURE 5.12 Diagram of an adipose cell.

Although the primary storage site for triglycerides is the body's adipose tissues, if you are physically active, your body will preferentially store this extra fat in your muscle tissues. This ensures that, the next time you go out for a run, the fat will be readily available for energy. Thus, people who engage in physical activity are more likely to have extra triglyceride stored in the muscle tissue and to have less body fat—something many of us would prefer. Of course, fat stored in your adipose tissues can also be used for energy during exercise, but it must be broken down first and then transported to your muscle cells.

RECAP

Fat digestion begins when fats are emulsified by bile. Lipid-digesting enzymes from the pancreas subsequently digest the triglycerides into two free fatty acids and one monoglyceride. These are transported into the intestinal mucosal cells with the help of micelles. Once inside the mucosal cells, triglycerides are re-formed and packaged into lipoproteins called chylomicrons. Dietary fat, in the form of triglycerides, is transported by the chylomicrons to cells within the body that need energy. Triglycerides stored in the muscle tissue are used as a source of energy during physical activity. Excess triglycerides are stored in the adipose tissue and can be used whenever the body needs energy. ■

Why Do We Need Lipids?

Lipids, in the form of dietary fat, provide energy and help our body perform essential physiologic functions.

Lipids Provide Energy

Dietary fat is a primary source of energy because fat has more than twice the energy per gram as carbohydrate or protein. Fat provides 9 kilocalories (kcal) per gram, whereas carbohydrate and protein provide only 4 kcal per gram. This means that fat is much more energy dense. For example, 1 tablespoon of butter or oil contains approximately 100 kcal, whereas it takes 2.5 cups of steamed broccoli or 1 slice of whole-wheat bread to provide 100 kcal.

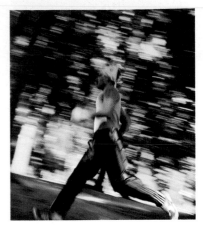

Dietary fat provides energy.

Lipids Are a Major Fuel Source When We Are at Rest

At rest, we are able to deliver plenty of oxygen to our cells, so that metabolic functions can occur. Just as a candle needs oxygen for the flame to continue burning, our cells need oxygen to use fat for energy. Thus, approximately 30% to 70% of the energy used at rest by the muscles and organs comes from lipids.[5] The exact amount of energy coming from lipids at rest will depend on how much fat you are eating in your diet, how physically active you are, and whether you are gaining or losing weight. If you are dieting, more lipid will be used for energy than if you are gaining weight. During times of weight gain, more of the fat consumed in the diet is stored in the adipose tissue, and the body uses more dietary protein and carbohydrate as fuel sources at rest.

Lipids Fuel Physical Activity

Lipids are the major energy source during physical activity, and one of the best ways to lose body fat is to exercise and reduce energy intake. During aerobic exercise, such as running or cycling, lipids can be mobilized from any of the following sources of body fat: muscle tissue, adipose tissue, and blood lipoproteins. A number of hormonal changes signal the body to break down stored energy to fuel the working muscles. The hormonal responses, and the amount and source of the lipids used, depend on your level of fitness; the type, intensity, and duration of the exercise; and how well fed you are before you exercise.

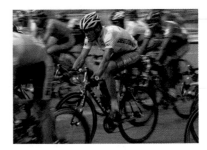

The longer you exercise, the more fat you use for energy. Cyclists in a long-distance race make greater use of fat stores as the race progresses.

For example, adrenaline (that is, epinephrine) strongly stimulates the breakdown of stored fat. Within minutes of beginning exercise, blood levels of epinephrine rise dramatically. Through a cascade of events, this surge of epinephrine activates an enzyme within adipose cells called *hormone-sensitive lipase*. This enzyme works to remove single fatty acids from the stored triglycerides. When all three free fatty acids on the glycerol backbone have been removed, the free fatty acids and the glycerol are released into the blood.

Epinephrine also signals the pancreas to *decrease* insulin production. This is important, because insulin inhibits fat breakdown. Thus, when the need for fat as an energy source is high, blood insulin levels are typically low. As you might guess, blood insulin levels are high when we are eating, because during this time our need for energy from stored fat is low and the need for fat storage is high.

Once fatty acids are released from the adipose cells, they travel in the blood attached to the transport protein albumin, to the muscle cells. There, they enter the mitochondria, the cell's energy-generating structures, and use oxygen to produce ATP, which is the cell's energy source. Becoming more physically fit means you can deliver more oxygen to the muscle cells to use the fatty acids delivered there. In addition, you can exercise longer when you are fit. Because the body has only a limited supply of stored carbohydrate as glycogen in muscle tissue, the longer you exercise, the more fatty acids you use for energy. This point is illustrated in **Figure 5.13**. In this example, an individual is running for 4 hours at a moderate intensity. As the muscle glycogen levels become depleted, the body relies on fatty acids from the adipose tissue as a fuel source.

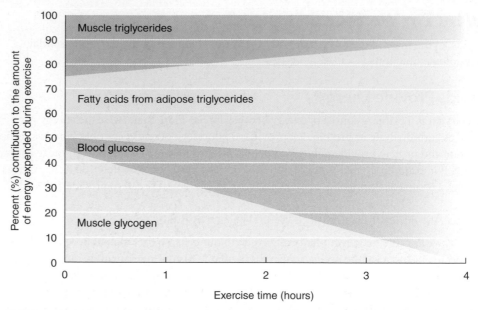

FIGURE 5.13 Various sources of energy used during exercise. As a person exercises for a prolonged period of time, fatty acids from adipose cells contribute relatively more energy than do carbohydrates stored in the muscle or circulating in the blood. (*Source:* Data from Coyle, E. F. 1995. Substrate utilization during exercise in active people. *Am. J. Clin. Nutr.* 61[Suppl.]:968S–979S. Used with permission.)

Under normal circumstances, fatty acids cannot be used to produce glucose[6]; however, recall that the breakdown of triglycerides also frees molecules of glycerol into the bloodstream. Some of this free glycerol travels to the liver, where it can be used for the production of modest amounts of glucose (in the process of gluconeogenesis).

Body Fat Stores Energy for Later Use

The body stores extra energy in the form of body fat, which then can be used for energy at rest, during exercise, or during periods of low energy intake. Having a readily available energy source in the form of fat allows the body to always have access to energy even when we choose not to eat (or are unable to eat), when we are exercising, and while we are sleeping. The body has small amounts of stored carbohydrate in the form of glycogen—only enough to last about 1 to 2 days—and there is no place that the body can store extra protein. We cannot consider our muscles and organs as a place where "extra" protein is stored! For these reasons, the fat stored in adipose and muscle tissues is necessary to fuel the body between meals. Although too much stored adipose tissue can harm our health, some fat storage is essential to protect our health.

Essential Fatty Acids Are Components of Important Biological Compounds

As discussed earlier, EFAs are needed to make a number of important biological compounds. They also are important constituents of cell membranes, help prevent DNA damage, help fight infection, and are essential for fetal growth and development. In the growing fetus, EFAs are necessary for normal growth, especially for the development of the brain and visual centers.

Dietary Fat Enables the Transport of Fat-Soluble Vitamins

Dietary fat enables the absorption and transport of the fat-soluble vitamins (A, D, E, and K) needed by the body for many essential metabolic functions. The fat-soluble vitamins are transported in the gut to the intestinal cells for absorption as part of micelles, and they are transported in the blood to the body cells as part of chylomicrons.[7] Vitamin A is important for normal vision and night vision. Vitamin D helps regulate blood calcium and phosphorus concentrations within normal ranges, which indirectly helps maintain bone health. Vitamin E keeps cell membranes healthy throughout the body, and vitamin K is important for the proteins involved in blood clotting and bone health. We discuss these vitamins in detail in later chapters.

Lipids Help Maintain Cell Function and Provide Protection to the Body

Lipids, especially PUFAs, phospholipids, and cholesterol, are a critical part of every cell membrane, where they help maintain membrane integrity, determine what substances are transported into and out of the cell, and regulate what substances can bind to the cell. Thus, lipids strongly influence the function of cells.

In addition, lipids help maintain cell fluidity. For example, wild salmon live in very cold water and have high levels of omega-3 fatty acids in their cell membranes. These fatty acids stay fluid and flexible even at very low temperatures, thereby enabling the fish to swim in extremely cold water. In the same way, lipids help our cell membranes stay fluid and flexible. This quality enables red blood cells, for example, to bend and move through the smallest capillaries in the body, delivering oxygen to all body cells.

Lipids are also primary components of the tissues of the nervous system. The body uses lipids for the development, growth, and maintenance of these tissues and for the transmission of impulses from one nerve cell to another.

Although we often think of body fat as "bad," it plays an important role in keeping the body healthy and functioning properly. Besides being the primary site of stored energy, adipose tissue pads the body and protects the organs, such as the kidneys and liver, when we fall or are bruised. Fat under the skin also acts as insulation to help retain body heat.

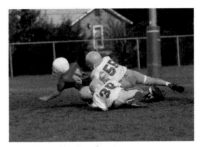

Adipose tissue pads the body and protects the organs when we fall or are bruised.

Fats Contribute to the Flavor and Texture of Foods

Dietary fat adds texture and flavor to foods. Fat makes salad dressings smooth and ice cream "creamy," and it gives cakes and cookies their moist, tender texture. Frying foods in melted fat or oil, as with doughnuts or french fries, gives them a crisp, flavorful coating; however, eating such foods regularly can be unhealthful because they are high in saturated and/or *trans* fatty acids.

Fats Help Us Feel Satiated

We often hear that fats contribute to satiation and satiety. First, what does this mean? A food or nutrient is said to contribute to *satiation* if that food makes you feel full and causes you to stop eating. A food or nutrient is said to contribute to *satiety* if it contributes to a feeling of fullness that subsequently reduces the amount of food you eat at the next meal or lengthens the time between meals.

A number of research studies have compared the effects of fat and carbohydrate on both satiation and satiety. In general, this research has found little difference between these two macronutrients when energy intake has been controlled.[8, 9] However, research also indicates that the energy density of a food contributes significantly to both satiety and satiation. Fat is more energy dense (kcal/g) than carbohydrate and protein; that is, for every gram of fat you consume, you get more than twice the energy. Thus, foods that contain a high proportion of fat are higher in energy density. Foods high in fat also stimulate the release of satiety factors in the small intestine, but our response to these satiety factors becomes blunted with chronic fat ingestion. This may explain why it is so easy to overeat high-fat, palatable foods and end up consuming more Calories than we would if we selected foods with lower energy densities. Satiety is also affected by the level of gastric distention produced by the food consumed, and by how quickly food empties from the stomach, which can also be affected by the energy density of food.[10]

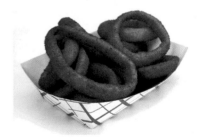

Fat adds texture and flavor to foods.

RECAP

Dietary fats provide the majority of energy required at rest and are a major fuel source during exercise, especially endurance exercise. They also provide essential fatty acids (linoleic and alpha-linolenic acid). Dietary fats help transport the fat-soluble vitamins into the body, help regulate cell function, and maintain cell membrane integrity. Stored body fat in the adipose tissue helps protect vital organs and pads the body. Fats contribute to the flavor and texture of foods, and because fats are energy dense, they are one factor that contributes to the satiety we feel after a meal. ■

How Much Dietary Fat Should We Eat?

The latest research comparing low-carbohydrate to low-fat diets has made Americans wonder what, exactly, is a healthful level of dietary fat and what foods contain the most beneficial fats. We'll explore these issues here.

Dietary Reference Intake for Total Fat

The Acceptable Macronutrient Distribution Range (AMDR) for fat is 20% to 35% of total energy.[11] This recommendation is based on evidence indicating that higher intakes of fat increase the risk for obesity and its complications, especially heart disease and diabetes, but that diets too low in fat and too high in carbohydrate can also increase the risk for heart disease if they cause an unhealthful shift in blood lipids.[11] Within this range of fat intake, we're also advised to minimize our intake of saturated and *trans* fatty acids as much as possible; these changes will lower our risk for heart disease.

Because carbohydrate is essential in replenishing glycogen, athletes and other physically active people are advised to consume less fat and more carbohydrate, especially if they participate in endurance activities. Specifically, it is recommended that athletes consume 20% to 25% of their total energy from fat, 55% to 60% of energy from carbohydrate, and 12% to 15% of energy from protein.[12] This percentage of fat intake is still within the AMDR and represents approximately 45 to 55 g of fat per day for an athlete consuming 2,000 kcal per day, and 78 to 97 g of fat per day for an athlete consuming 3,500 kcal per day.

Although many people trying to lose weight consume less than 20% of their energy from fat, this practice may do more harm than good, especially if they are also limiting their energy intake (eating fewer than 1,500 kcal per day). Research suggests that very-low-fat diets, or those with less than 15% of energy from fat, do not provide additional health or performance benefits over moderate-fat diets and are usually very difficult to follow.[13] In fact, most people find that they feel better, are more successful in weight maintenance, and are less preoccupied with food if they keep their fat intakes at 20–25% of energy intake. Additionally, people attempting to reduce their dietary fat frequently eliminate protein-rich foods, such as meat, dairy, eggs, and nuts. These foods are also potential sources of many essential vitamins and minerals important for good health and for maintaining an active lifestyle. Diets extremely low in fat may also be deficient in essential fatty acids.

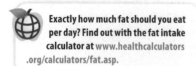

Exactly how much fat should you eat per day? Find out with the fat intake calculator at www.healthcalculators.org/calculators/fat.asp.

Dietary Reference Intakes for Essential Fatty Acids

Dietary Reference Intakes (DRIs) for the two essential fatty acids are[11]

- *Linoleic acid.* The Adequate Intake (AI) for linoleic acid is 14 to 17 g per day for men and 11 to 12 g per day for women 19 years and older. Using the typical energy intakes for adult men and women, this translates into an AMDR of 5% to 10% of energy.
- *Alpha-linolenic acid.* The AI for alpha-linolenic acid is 1.6 g per day for adult men and 1.1 g per day for adult women. This translates into an AMDR of 0.6% to 1.2% of energy.

For example, an individual consuming 2,000 kcal per day should consume about 11–22 g per day of linoleic acid and about 1.3–2.6 g per day of alpha-linolenic acid. This level of intake would keep one within the 5:1 to 10:1 ratio of linoleic:alpha-linolenic acid recommended by the World Health Organization and supported by the Institute of Medicine.[11] Because these fatty acids compete for the same enzymes to produce various eicosanoids that regulate body functions, this ratio helps keep the eicosanoids produced in balance; that is, one isn't overproduced at the expense of another.

Americans appear to get adequate amounts of linoleic acid, probably because of the high amount of salad dressings, vegetable oils, margarine, and mayonnaise we eat. In contrast, our consumption of alpha-linolenic acid is more variable and can be low in the diet of people who do not eat dark green, leafy vegetables; fish or fish oil; walnuts; soy products; canola oil; or flaxseeds or their oil.

Most Americans Eat Too Much Saturated and *Trans* Fat

Many nutrition experts have been recommending the reduction of dietary fat for more than 20 years. According to recent data, relative fat intake decreased from 36.6% of total energy intake in 1971 to 33.7% of energy intake in 2006 for both men and women.[14, 15] However, this reduction in the percentage of fat consumed is misleading, because Americans are consuming 9–16% more energy overall. This additional energy comes mostly in the form of carbohydrates, and less in fats, but the end result is that daily fat consumption in absolute levels has not decreased.

Of the dietary fat we eat, saturated and *trans* fats are most highly correlated with an increased risk for heart disease because they increase blood cholesterol levels by altering the way cholesterol is removed from the blood. Thus, the recommended intake of saturated fat is less than 7–10% of our total energy; unfortunately, our average intake of saturated fats is between 11% and 12% of energy.[16] According to data from the National Health and Nutrition Examination Survey, about 64% of adults in the United States exceed the dietary recommendation for saturated fats.[17] The Institute of Medicine also recommends that we keep our intake of *trans* fatty acids to an absolute minimum.[11] Currently, the average consumption of industrially produced *trans* fatty acids is about 2–3% of total energy intake, with the majority coming from deep-fried fast or frozen foods, some tub margarines, and bakery products.[11, 18, 19]

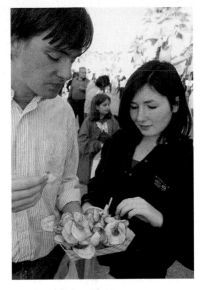

Americans consume more saturated and *trans* fats than is recommended.

Watch Out for Invisible Fats

Americans not only eat lots of high-fat foods but also commonly add fat to foods to improve their taste. Added fats, such as oils, butter, cream, shortening, margarine, mayonnaise, and salad dressings, are called **visible fats** because we can easily see that we are adding them to our food.

When we add cream to coffee or butter to pancakes, we know how much fat we are adding and what kind. In contrast, when fat is added in the preparation of a frozen entrée or a fast-food burger and fries, we are less aware of how much or what type of fat is actually there. In fact, we might not realize that a food contains any fat at all. We call fats in prepared and processed foods **invisible fats** because they are hidden within the food. In fact, their invisibility often tricks us into choosing them over more healthful foods. For example, a slice of yellow cake is much higher in fat (40% of total energy) than a slice of angel food cake (1% of total energy), yet many consumers assume that the fat content of these foods is the same, because they are both cake.

The majority of the fat in the average American diet is invisible. Foods that can be high in invisible fats are baked goods, regular-fat dairy products, processed meats or meats that are highly marbled or not trimmed, and most convenience and fast foods, such as hamburgers, hot dogs, chips, ice cream, french fries, and other fried foods.

Because high-fat diets have been associated with obesity, many Americans have tried to reduce their total fat intake. Food manufacturers have been more than happy to provide consumers with low-fat alternatives to their favorite foods. However, these lower-fat foods may not always have fewer Calories. See the box **Highlight: Low-Fat, Reduced-Fat, Nonfat . . . What's the Difference?** and **Table 5.1**.

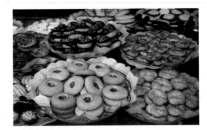

Baked goods are often high in invisible fats.

visible fats Fats we can see in our foods or see added to foods, such as butter, margarine, cream, shortening, salad dressings, chicken skin, and untrimmed fat on meat.

invisible fats Fats that are hidden in foods, such as the fats found in baked goods, regular-fat dairy products, marbling in meat, and fried foods.

Select Beneficial Fats

We know that high-fat diets, especially those high in saturated and *trans* fatty acids, can contribute to chronic diseases, including heart disease and cancer. However, as we have

Low-Fat, Reduced-Fat, Nonfat . . . What's the Difference?

Although most people love high-fat foods, we also know that eating too much fat isn't good for our health or our waistline. Because of this concern, food manufacturers have produced a host of modified-fat foods—so you can have your cake and eat it too! Today there are thousands of low- or reduced-fat modified foods in the market. This means that similar foods may come in a wide range of fat contents. For example, you can purchase full-fat, low-fat, or fat-free milk, ice cream, sour cream, cheese, and yogurt.

In Table 5.1, we list a number of full-fat foods with their lower-fat alternatives. These products, if incorporated into the diet on a regular basis, can significantly reduce the amount of fat consumed but may or may not reduce the amount of energy consumed. For example, drinking nonfat milk (86 kcal and 0.5 g of fat per serving) instead of whole milk (150 kcal and 8.2 g of fat per serving)

will dramatically reduce both fat and energy intake. However, eating fat-free Fig Newton cookies (three cookies have 204 kcal and 0 g of fat) instead of regular Fig Newton cookies (three cookies have 210 kcal and 4.5 g of fat) does not significantly reduce your energy intake, even though it reduces your fat intake by 4.5 g per serving. Thus, those who think that they can eat all the low-fat foods they want without gaining weight are mistaken. The reduced fat is often replaced with added carbohydrate, resulting in a very similar total energy intake. Thus, if you want to reduce both the amount of fat and the number of Calories you consume, you must read the labels of modified-fat foods carefully before you buy.

TABLE 5.1 Comparison of Full-Fat, Reduced-Fat, and Low-Fat Foods

Product and Serving Size	Version	Energy (kcal)	Protein (g)	Carbohydrate (g)	Fat (g)
Milk, 8 oz	Whole, 3.3% fat	150	8.0	11.4	8.2
	2% fat	121	8.1	11.7	4.7
	Skim (nonfat)	86	8.4	11.9	0.5
Mayonnaise, 1 tbsp.	Regular	100	0.0	0.0	11.0
	Light	50	0.0	1.0	5.0
Margarine, corn oil, 1 tbsp.	Regular	100	0.0	0.0	11.0
	Reduced-fat	60	0.0	0.0	7.0
Peanut butter, 1 tbsp.	Regular	95	4.1	3.1	8.2
	Reduced-fat	81	4.4	5.2	5.4
Wheat Thins, 18 crackers	Regular	158	2.3	21.4	6.8
	Reduced-fat	120	2.0	21.0	4.0
Cookies, Oreo, 3 cookies	Regular	160	2.0	23.0	7.0
	Reduced-fat	130	2.0	25.0	3.5
Cookies, Fig Newton, 3 cookies	Regular	210	3.0	30.0	4.5
	Fat-free	204	2.4	26.8	0.0

Source: Data from Food Processor-SQL, Version 9.9, ESHA Research, Salem, OR.

explored in this chapter, unsaturated fatty acids do not have this negative effect and are absolutely essential to good health. Thus, a sensible health goal would be to eat the appropriate amounts and types of fat.

In general, it is prudent to switch to more healthful sources of fats without increasing your total fat intake. For example, use olive oil and canola oil for cooking and a nut butter on your toast. Dairy products, including cheeses, can be high in saturated fats, so select low- and reduced-fat versions when possible. What about processed foods? Review the box **Nutrition Label Activity: How Much Fat Is in This Food?** (on page 196) to learn how to calculate the Calories from fat in the foods you buy.

Eat More Fish

Table 5.2 identifies the omega-3 fatty acid content of various foods. As you can see, the best source of DHA and EPA is fish. Moreover, fish is low in saturated fats. So select fish at least twice a week instead of meat sources of protein.

It is important to recognize that there can be some risk associated with eating large amounts of fish on a regular basis. Depending on the species of fish and the level of pollution in the water in which it is caught, the fish may contain high levels of toxins, such as mercury, polychlorinated biphenyls (PCBs), and other environmental contaminants. Types of fish that are currently considered safe to consume include salmon (except from the Great Lakes region), farmed trout, flounder, sole, mahi mahi, and cooked shellfish. Line-caught tuna, either fresh or canned, is low in mercury. These tuna are smaller, usually less

TABLE 5.2 Omega-3 Fatty Acid Content of Selected Foods

Food Item	Total Omega-3	DHA	EPA
	g/Serving		
Flaxseed oil, 1 tbsp.	7.25	0.00	0.00
Salmon oil (fish oil), 1 tbsp.	4.39	2.48	1.77
Sardine oil, 1 tbsp.	3.01	1.45	1.38
Flaxseed, whole, 1 tbsp.	2.50	0.00	0.00
Herring, Atlantic, broiled, 3 oz	1.83	0.94	0.77
Salmon, Coho, steamed, 3 oz	1.34	0.71	0.46
Canola oil, 1 tbsp.	1.28	0.00	0.00
Sardines, Atlantic, w/ bones, oil, 3 oz	1.26	0.43	0.40
Trout, rainbow fillet, baked, 3 oz	1.05	0.70	0.28
Walnuts, English, 1 tbsp.	0.66	0.00	0.00
Halibut, fillet, baked, 3 oz	0.53	0.31	0.21
Shrimp, canned, 3 oz	0.47	0.21	0.25
Tuna, white, in oil, 3 oz	0.38	0.19	0.04
Crab, Alaska King, steamed, 3 oz	0.36	0.10	0.25
Scallops, broiled, 3 oz	0.31	0.14	0.17
Smart Balance Omega-3 Buttery Spread (1 tbsp.)	0.32	0.01	0.01
Tuna, light, in water, 3 oz	0.23	0.19	0.04
Avocado, California, fresh, whole	0.22	0.00	0.00
Spinach, cooked, 1 cup	0.17	0.00	0.00
Eggland's Best, 1 large egg, with omega-3	0.12	0.06	0.03

EPA = eicosapentaenoic acid; DHA = docosahexaenoic acid

Source: Data from Food Processor SQL, Version 10.3, ESHA Research, Salem, OR, and manufacturer labels.

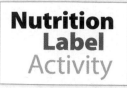

How Much Fat Is in This Food?

One simple way to determine the amount of fat in the foods you buy is to read the Nutrition Facts Panel on the label. Two cracker labels are shown in **Figure 5.14**; one cracker is higher in fat than the other. Let's review how you can determine the percentage of energy coming from fat in each product. These calculations are relatively simple.

1. Divide the total kcal from fat by the total kcal per serving, and multiply the answer by 100.
- For the regular wheat crackers: 50 kcal/150 kcal = 0.33 × 100 = 33%.
  Thus, for the regular crackers, the total energy coming from fat is 33%.
- For the reduced-fat wheat crackers: 35 kcal/130 kcal = 0.269 × 100 = 27%.
  Thus, for the reduced-fat crackers, the total energy coming from fat is 27%.

You can see that, although the total amounts of energy per serving are not very different between these two crackers, the levels of fat are quite different.

2. If the total kcal per serving from fat is not indicated on the label, you can quickly calculate this value by multiplying the grams of total fat per serving by 9 (as there are 9 kcal per gram of fat).
- For the regular wheat crackers: 6 g fat × 9 kcal g = 54 kcal of fat.
- To calculate percentage of kcal from fat: 54 kcal/150 kcal = 0.36 × 100 = 36%.

You can see that this value is not exactly the same as the 50 kcal reported on the label or the 33% of kcal from fat calculated in example 1. The values on food labels are rounded off, so your estimations may not be identical when you do this second calculation.

Refer to Table 5.1, which lists regular, reduced-fat, and fat-free foods. You can quickly calculate the percentage of fat per serving for these foods by following the same series of steps:

1. Multiply the grams of fat per serving by 9 kcal per gram.

2. Divide this number by the total kcal per serving.

3. Multiply by 100.

Using the previous calculations and Table 5.1, compare regular cheddar cheese to low-fat cheddar cheese; then answer the following questions:

1. What is the percentage of energy from fat in the regular-fat cheddar cheese vs. the low-fat cheese?

2. How much does the percentage of fat decrease by selecting the low-fat cheese?

3. If you select the low-fat cheese, how many kcal do you save? How many grams of fat do you save?

---

than 20 pounds, and have had less exposure to mercury in their lifetime. Fish more likely to be contaminated are shark, swordfish, golden bass, golden snapper, marlin, bluefish, and largemouth and smallmouth bass. (For more information on food safety, see Chapter 15.)

Pick Plants

Of course, healthful fats include not only the essential fatty acids but also polyunsaturated and monounsaturated fats in general. An easy way to shift your diet toward these healthful fats—without increasing your total fat intake—is to replace animal-based foods with versions derived from plants. For example, drink soy milk or almond milk instead of cow's milk. Order your Chinese take-out with tofu instead of beef. Plant oils are excellent sources of unsaturated fats, so cook with olive, canola, soybean, or walnut oil in place of butter. Use thin slices of avocado in a sandwich in place of cheese, or serve tortilla chips with guacamole instead of nachos.

Nuts and seeds provide another way to increase the healthful fats in your diet. They are rich in unsaturated fats and provide protein, minerals, vitamins, and fiber. They are high in energy: a 1 oz serving of nuts (about 4 tablespoons) contains 160–180 kcal. So eat them in moderation, for instance by sprinkling a few on your salad, yogurt, or breakfast cereal. Spread a nut butter on your morning toast, or pack a peanut butter and jelly sandwich instead of a meat sandwich for lunch. Or add some pumpkin seeds, flaxseeds, or sunflower seeds to raisins and pretzel sticks for a quick trail mix.

One particular seed that is growing in popularity is flaxseed. Flax is a flowering plant grown in many parts of the world for centuries. Its fibers are used in making fabrics,

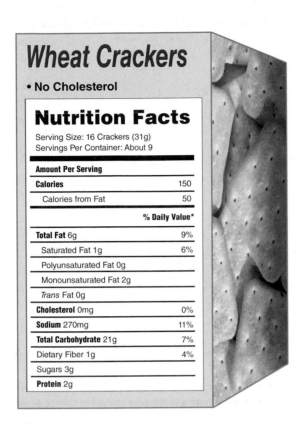

(a)

(b)

FIGURE 5.14 Labels for two types of wheat crackers. **(a)** Regular wheat crackers. **(b)** Reduced-fat wheat crackers.

paper, and other products, and its seeds are crushed for their oil. Flaxseed oil provides both omega-6 and omega-3 fatty acids. It is available in many markets today and can be consumed directly by teaspoon; mixed into yogurt, puddings, or applesauce; or taken as a capsule. Flaxseeds themselves are largely undigestible, but when ground they provide EFAs as well as fiber and phytochemicals called *lignans*. Ground flaxseeds, like their oil, can be mixed into yogurt and other creamy foods. You can also sprinkle them on breakfast cereal or mix them into the batter of pancakes, breads, and other baked goods.

Look for Low-Fat

When shopping, look for lower-fat versions of all processed foods you buy. Read food labels and do the math! Most importantly, look for foods with no hydrogenated oils and low amounts of saturated fat per serving.

Here are a few more tips to help you choose and cook foods low in saturated and *trans* fats:

- Select liquid or tub margarines/butters over hard stick forms. Fats that are solid at room temperature are usually high in *trans* or saturated fats. Also, select margarines made from healthful fats, such as canola oil.
- Buy naturally occurring plant oils, such as olive and canola oil. These types of oils have not been hydrogenated and contain healthful unsaturated fatty acids and no *trans* fatty acids. Make sure to cook with these oils instead of butter. Use cooking spray instead of oil or butter when possible.
- Buy reduced-fat salad dressings and mayonnaise or those made with healthful fats, such as olive oil and vinegar blends. Remember, a tablespoon of full-fat salad dressing or mayonnaise contains 100 kcal.

- Select low-fat or nonfat milk, yogurt, cheese, and cheese spreads. If you can't imagine life without "real" cheese, then buy sharp cheddar and hard, drier cheeses, such as Parmesan. These have less fat than mild cheeses, and they provide more flavor.
- When purchasing meat and poultry, choose cuts lower in fat. When preparing these foods at home, trim any visible fat before cooking, and remove the skin from poultry. Bake or broil instead of frying.
- Buy fish more often, especially those high in omega-3 fatty acids, such as salmon, line-caught tuna, herring, and sardines.
- Use beans, peas, and lentils more frequently as the main source of protein in your meal, or add them to your meat-based dish, so that you use less meat overall.

Putting these tips into practice can make a big reduction in your intake of saturated and *trans* fats as well as total energy. Need more convincing? Compare the two sets of meals in **Figure 5.15**.

Watch Out When You're Eating Out!

Many college students eat most of their meals in dining halls, fast-food restaurants, and other food establishments. If that describes you, watch out! The menu items you choose each day may be increasing the amount of fat in your diet, including your intake of saturated and *trans* fats. A high fat intake is especially difficult to avoid if you regularly eat fast food. According to national data, fast-food consumers have higher total energy, total fat, and saturated fat intakes than those who eat fast food infrequently.[20] And although many fast food restaurants have eliminated *trans* fatty acids from their menus, McDonald's still has a few items, such as desserts and shakes, that contain *trans* fatty acids. The following are a few tips and strategies you can use to improve the amount and type of fat in your menu choices.

- When dining out, select a fish high in omega-3 fatty acid, such as salmon, or try a vegetarian entrée made with tofu or tempeh. If you do choose meat, ask that it be trimmed of fat and broiled rather than fried.
- Cut back on packaged or bakery pastries, such as Danish, croissants, doughnuts, cakes, tarts, pies, and brownies. These baked goods are typically high in saturated and *trans* fatty acids.
- Consider splitting an entrée with your dinner companion and have a dinner salad or broth-based soup as a first course.
- On your salad, choose olive oil and vinegar instead of a high-fat dressing. Always order the dressing on the side, so that you can monitor the amount you use. Use olive oil instead of butter for your bread.
- Order a baked potato or rice instead of french fries or potatoes au gratin. At fast-food restaurants, either skip the french fries or order the smallest serving for portion control. Some fast-food restaurants allow you to replace the french fries in a meal order with fruit.
- Order pizza with vegetable toppings instead of pepperoni or sausage.
- Share or skip dessert or choose fat-free sorbet, fruit, or angel-food cake.
- Order coffee drinks with skim milk instead of cream or whole milk, and accompany them with a biscotti instead of a brownie.

Be Aware of Fat Replacers

The rising rates of obesity and its associated health concerns have increased the demand for low-fat versions of our favorite foods, which in turn has created a booming industry for *fat replacers*, substances that mimic the palate-pleasing and flavor-enhancing properties of fats with fewer Calories. Snack foods and desserts have been the primary target for fat replacers because it is difficult to simply eliminate all or most of the fat in these products without dramatically changing their taste. In the mid-1990s, both food industry executives and nutritionists thought that fat replacers would be the answer to our growing obesity problem. They reasoned that, if we replace some of the fats in snack and fast foods with these products, we might be able to reduce both energy and fat intake and help Americans manage their weight better.

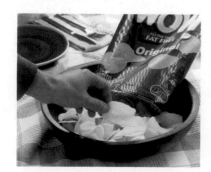

Snack foods have been the primary target for fat replacers, such as Olean, because it is more difficult to significantly reduce the fat in these types of foods without dramatically changing the taste.

A Day of Meals: High vs. Low in Saturated Fat

High		Low	

Breakfast

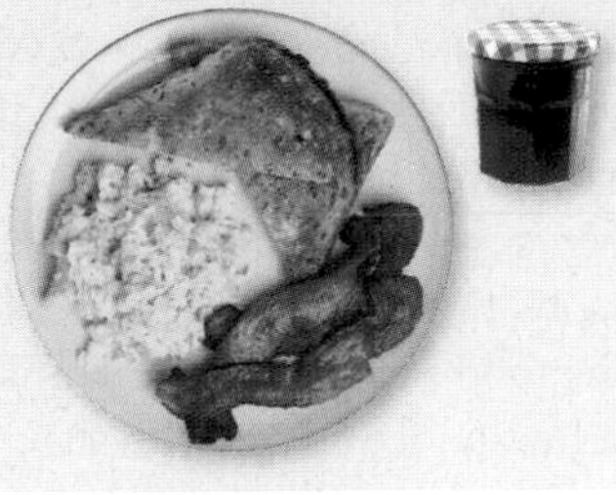

2 slices pan-fried bacon
2 eggs, scrambled
2 slices toast
1 TB butter
1 TB jam

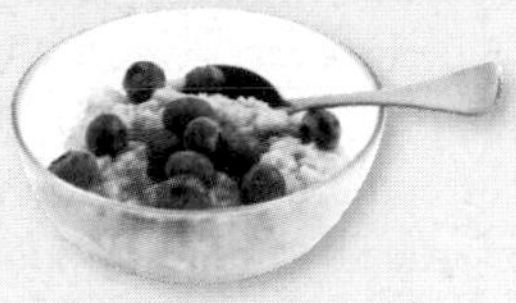

1 cup cooked oatmeal
¾ cup skim milk
½ cup fresh/frozen blueberries
2 TB almonds
1 TB brown sugar
1 tsp cinnamon

Snack

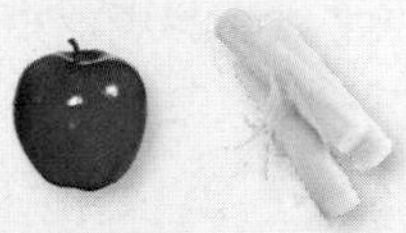

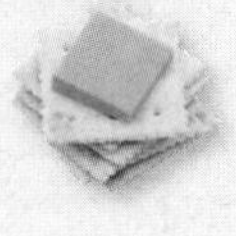

7 saltine crackers
2 slices cheddar cheese

1 medium apple
1 piece low-fat string cheese

Lunch

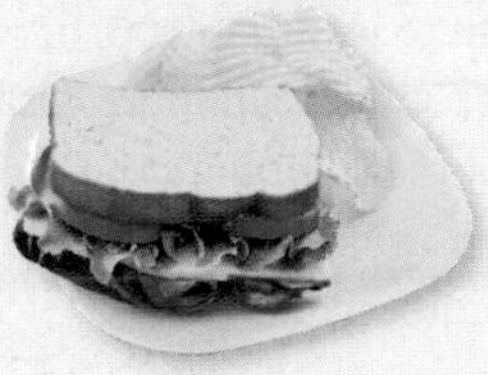

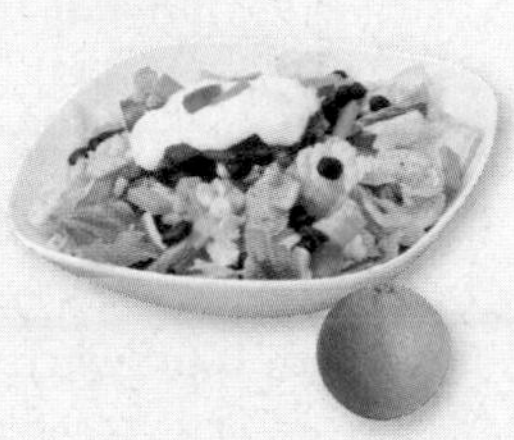

Roast beef sandwich
2 oz roast beef
2 slices white bread
1 slice cheddar cheese
2 lettuce leaves
3 slices tomato
1 TB mayonnaise
1 oz potato chips

Taco salad
2 cups lettuce
¼ cup chopped carrots
¼ cup chopped cabbage
½ cup chopped tomato
2 oz shredded skinless
chicken breast
1 oz shredded cheddar cheese
1 oz tortilla chips
⅓ cup low-fat sour cream
1 medium orange

Snack

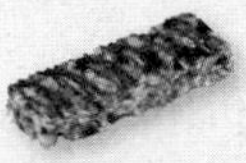

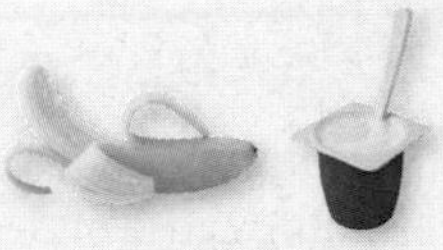

1 chocolate chip granola bar

¾ cup plain, low-fat yogurt
½ banana

Dinner

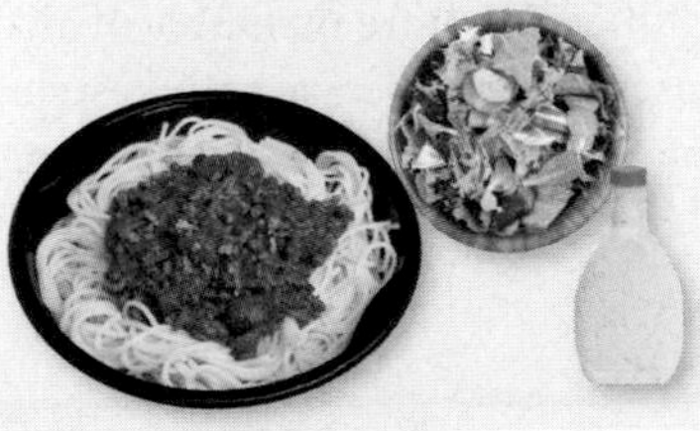

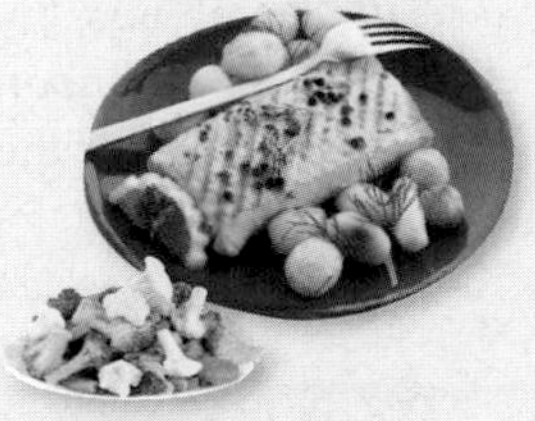

Spaghetti
1 cup spaghetti noodles
½ cup ground beef
½ pasta sauce
½ cup green beans
1 cup green salad
1 TB ranch dressing

3 oz salmon
½ cup roasted small potatoes
with rosemary
1 cup roasted broccoli, cauliflower,
onions
1 TB olive oil

Snack

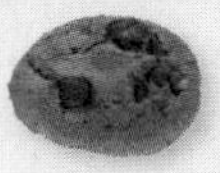

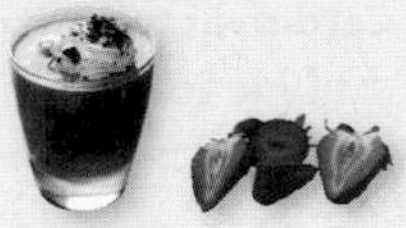

1 med. chocolate chip cookie

½ cup chocolate pudding (made
with 2% milk)
1 cup sliced strawberries
2 TB non-fat whipped topping

Nutrient Analysis
2125 kcals
44% of energy from fat
 18% of energy from
 saturated fat
 13.8% of energy from
 MUFA
 6.5% of energy from PUFA
 3.3 g of trans fat (1.4% of
 energy)

1.5 g of omega 3 FA
10.8 g of omega 6 FA
38% of energy from
carbohydrates
18% of energy from protein
653 g of cholesterol
3977 mg of sodium
15 g of dietary fiber
1087 g total weight
Energy density 2.0 kcal/g

Nutrient Analysis
2030 kcals
23% of energy from fat
 4% of energy from
 saturated fat
 12% of energy from MUFA
 6% of energy from PUFA
 0.01 g of trans fat (0% of
 energy)

2.7 g of omega 3 FA
8.9 g of omega 6 FA
57% of energy from
carbohydrates
20% of energy from protein
138 g of cholesterol
972 mg of sodium
41 g of dietary fiber
2250 g total weight
Energy Density 0.94 kcal/g

FIGURE 5.15 Comparison of a day of meals high in saturated fat and a day of meals low in saturated fat with appropriate unsaturated fats and essential fatty acids. Diets were analyzed using Food Processor Version 7.21 (*Source:* ESHA Research, Salem, OR).

Products such as olestra (brand name Olean) hit the market in 1996 with a lot of fanfare, but the hype was short-lived. Initially, foods containing olestra had to bear a label warning of potential gastrointestinal side effects. In 2003, the U.S. Food and Drug Administration (FDA) announced that this warning was no longer necessary, as more recent research indicated that olestra caused only mild, infrequent discomfort. However, even with the new labeling, only limited foods in the marketplace now contain olestra. It is also evident from our growing obesity problem that fat replacers, such as olestra, did not help Americans lose weight or even maintain their current weight.

More recently, a new group of fat replacers has been developed using proteins, such as the whey protein found in milk. Like their predecessors, these new fat replacers lower the fat content of food, but in addition they improve the food's total nutrient profile and decrease its Calorie content. This means we can have a low-fat ice cream with the mouth-feel, finish, and texture of a full-fat ice cream that is also higher in protein and lower in Calories than traditional ice cream. So don't be surprised if you see more products containing protein-based fat replacers on your supermarket shelves in the next few years.

RECAP

The AMDR for total fat is 20–35% of total energy. The AI for linoleic acid is 14–17 g per day for adult men and 11–12 g per day for adult women. The AI for alpha-linolenic acid is 1.6 g per day for adult men and 1.1 g per day for adult women. Health professionals recommend that we reduce our intake of saturated fat to less than 10% of our total energy intake and our intake of *trans* fatty acids to the absolute minimum. Visible fats can be easily recognized, but invisible fats are added to our food during manufacturing or cooking, so we are not aware of how much we are consuming. A healthful dietary strategy is to switch from saturated and *trans* fats to unsaturated fats. ■

What Role Do Lipids Play in Cardiovascular Disease and Cancer?

According to the Centers for Disease Control and Prevention, diseases of the heart are the leading cause of death in the United States, accounting for nearly 600,000 deaths in 2010. Cancer is a close second, with over 567,000 deaths, and stroke is the fourth leading cause of death. Combined, these three disease categories accounted for more than 31% of all deaths in 2010. So it's important to take a look at these diseases and the dietary and lifestyle factors that can influence their development. Let's start with a look at cardiovascular disease, since it is projected that, by the year 2030, 40% of the United States population will have some form of cardiovascular disease.[21]

What Is Cardiovascular Disease?

Cardiovascular disease is a general term used to refer to any abnormal condition involving dysfunction of the heart (*cardio-* means "heart") and blood vessels (*vasculature*). There are many forms of this disease, but the three most common are the following:

- *Coronary heart disease* occurs when blood vessels supplying the heart (the *coronary arteries*) become blocked or constricted; such blockage reduces the flow of blood—and the oxygen and nutrients it carries—to the heart. This can result in chest pain, called *angina pectoris*, and lead to a heart attack.
- *Stroke* is caused by blockage or rupture of one of the blood vessels supplying the brain (the *cerebral arteries*). When this occurs, the region of the brain depending on that artery for oxygen and nutrients cannot function. As a result, the movement, speech, or other body functions controlled by that part of the brain suddenly stop.

cardiovascular disease A general term that refers to abnormal conditions involving dysfunction of the heart and blood vessels; cardiovascular disease can result in heart attack or stroke.

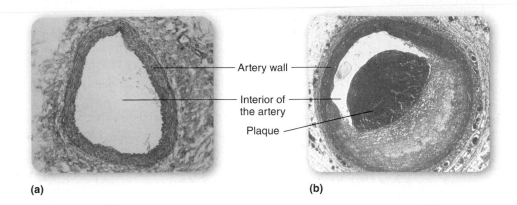

Artery wall

Interior of
the artery

Plaque

(a)

(b)

FIGURE 5.
These light mic
cross section of **(a)**
containing little chole
plaque and allowing ade
blood flow through the hea
(b) an artery that is partially bl
with cholesterol-rich plaque, whic
can lead to a heart attack.

- *Hypertension,* also called *high blood pressure*, is a condition that may not cause any symptoms, but it increases your risk for a heart attack or stroke. If your blood pressure is high, that means that the force of the blood flowing through your arteries is above normal. (We discuss hypertension and the dietary and lifestyle factors that affect it in Chapter 9.)

To understand cardiovascular disease, we need to look at a condition called *atherosclerosis*, which is responsible for the blockage of arteries that leads to heart attacks and strokes.

Atherosclerosis Is Narrowing of Arteries

Atherosclerosis is a disease in which arterial walls accumulate deposits of lipids and scar tissue, which build up to such a degree that they impair blood flow. It's a complex process that begins with injury to the cells that line the insides of all arteries. Factors that commonly promote such injury are the forceful pounding of blood under high pressure and blood-vessel damage from irritants, such as the nicotine in tobacco or the excessive blood glucose in people with poorly controlled diabetes. Whatever the cause, the injury leads to vessel inflammation, which is increasingly being recognized as an important marker of cardiovascular disease.[22] Inflamed vessels become weakened, allowing lipids, mainly cholesterol, to seep through the layers of the vessel wall and eventually become trapped in thick, grainy deposits called *plaque*. The term *atherosclerosis* reflects the presence of these deposits: *athere* is a Greek word meaning "a thick porridge."

As plaque forms, the interior of the blood vessel narrows and slowly diminishes the blood supply to any tissues "downstream," including the heart muscle or the brain (**Figure 5.16**). As a result, these tissues—including heart muscle—wither and gradually lose their ability to function. Alternatively, the blockage may occur suddenly because a plaque ruptures and *platelets*, substances in blood that promote clotting, stick to the damaged area. This quickly obstructs the artery, causing the death of the tissue it supplies. As a result, the person experiences a heart attack or stroke.

Risk Factors for Cardiovascular Disease

During the past two decades, researchers have identified a number of factors that contribute to an increased risk for cardiovascular disease. Some of these risk factors are nonmodifiable, meaning they are beyond your control. These include age (the older you are, the higher your risk), male gender, and family history. For example, you have an increased risk for cardiovascular disease if one of your parents has suffered a heart attack, especially at a young age.

Other risk factors are modifiable, meaning they are at least partly within your control. Following is a brief description of each of these modifiable risk factors. Notice that many of them have a dietary component.[23, 24, 25]

- *Overweight.* Being overweight is associated with higher rates of cardiovascular disease and higher rates of death from cardiovascular disease. The risk is due primarily

Atherosclerosis A disease in which arterial walls accumulate deposits of lipids and scar tissue, which build up to a point at which they impair blood flow.

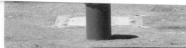

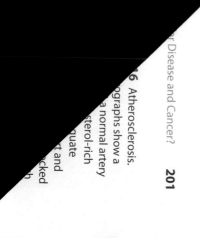

Being overweight is associated with higher rates of death from cardiovascular disease.

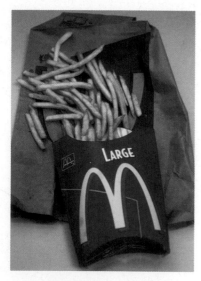

Lowering your intake of saturated and *trans* fats—such as those found in french fries—can help improve your blood lipid profile, especially when accompanied by increasing your physical activity and soluble fiber intake.

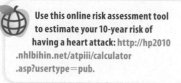

Use this online risk assessment tool to estimate your 10-year risk of having a heart attack: http://hp2010 .nhlbihin.net/atpiii/calculator .asp?usertype=pub.

to a greater occurrence of hypertension, inflammation, abnormal blood lipids (discussed in more detail shortly), and type 2 diabetes in individuals who are overweight. In general, an overweight condition develops from an energy imbalance from eating too much and getting too little physical activity. (Chapter 13 explores energy balance and discusses the role of obesity in increasing an individual's overall cardiometabolic risk.)

- *Physical inactivity.* Numerous research studies have shown that physical activity can reduce your risk for cardiovascular disease by improving several risk factors associated with the disease. Regular physical activity can reduce body fat and weight, improve blood lipids, lower resting blood pressure, and reduce blood glucose levels both at rest and after eating. Physical activity can also significantly reduce the risk for type 2 diabetes, a major cardiovascular disease risk factor.[25] According to the 2008 US Physical Activity Guidelines,[26] physical activity can reduce your risk for heart disease by 20–30%, stroke by 25–30%, and type 2 diabetes by 25–35%.

- *Smoking.* There is strong evidence that smoking increases your risk for blood-vessel injury and cardiovascular disease. Research indicates that smokers have a two- to six-fold greater chance of developing cardiovascular disease than nonsmokers, depending on age and gender.[27] If you smoke, quitting is one of the best ways to reduce your risk for cardiovascular disease. People who stop smoking live longer than those who continue to smoke, and smokers who quit by age 30 reduce their chances of dying from a smoking-related disease by more than 90%.[28]

- *Hypertension.* High blood pressure stresses the heart and blood vessels, increasing the chance that blockage or rupture of a blood vessel will occur. Hypertension is associated with a number of modifiable factors, including obesity, diet (for example, high sodium intake, low calcium intake, or high caffeine intake), smoking, and physical inactivity.

- *Type 2 diabetes.* As discussed (in Chapter 4), many individuals with type 2 diabetes, the condition is directly related to being overweight or obese. The risk for cardiovascular disease is three times higher in women with diabetes and two times higher in men with diabetes compared to individuals without diabetes.

- *Inflammation.* Earlier, we explained the role of blood-vessel inflammation in the development of atherosclerosis. C-reactive protein (CRP) is a nonspecific marker of inflammation that is associated with cardiovascular disease. Risk for cardiovascular disease appears to be higher in individuals who have high blood inflammatory markers, such as CRP, in addition to other risk factors, such as abnormal blood lipids.[29] Thus, reducing the factors that promote inflammation, such as obesity and a diet low in omega-3 fatty acids and high in saturated fats, can reduce the risk for cardiovascular disease.

- *Abnormal blood lipids.* As we explain next, levels of certain blood lipids are associated with an increased or decreased risk for cardiovascular disease. Making lifestyle changes, such as lowering your intake of saturated and *trans* fat, increasing your physical activity and soluble fiber intake, and achieving a healthful body weight, can help improve your blood lipid profile. These lipoproteins are discussed in more detail in the following section.

The Role of Blood Lipids in Cardiovascular Disease

Recall that lipids are transported in the blood by lipoproteins made up of a lipid center and a protein outer coat. Because lipoproteins are soluble in blood, they are commonly called *blood lipids.*

The names of lipoproteins reflect their proportion of lipid, which is less dense, to protein, which is very dense. For example, very-low-density lipoproteins (VLDLs) have a high ratio of lipid to protein (**Figure 5.17**). Let's look at each of these blood lipids in more detail to determine how they are linked to heart disease risk.

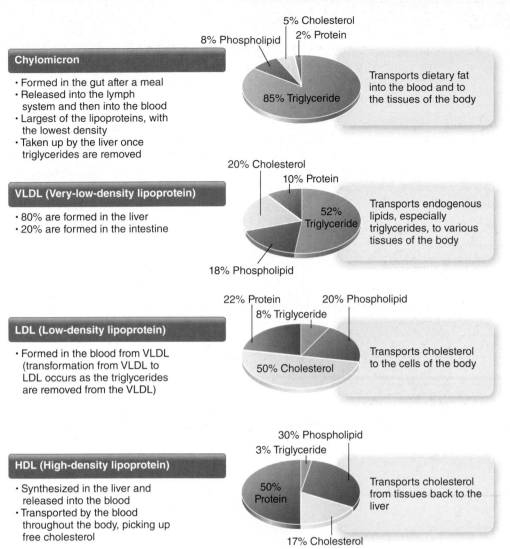

FIGURE 5.17 The chemical components of various lipoproteins. Notice that chylomicrons contain the highest proportion of triglycerides, making them the least dense, and high-density lipoproteins (HDLs) have the highest proportion of protein, making them the most dense.

Chylomicrons Only after a meal does the blood contain chylomicrons, which we learned earlier are produced in the enterocytes to transport dietary fat into the lymph system and from there into the bloodstream. At 85% triglyceride, chylomicrons have the lowest density.

Very-Low-Density Lipoproteins More than half of the substance of **very-low-density lipoproteins (VLDLs)** is triglyceride. The liver is the primary source of VLDLs, but they are also produced in the intestines. VLDLs are primarily transport vehicles ferrying triglycerides from their source to the body's cells, including to adipose tissues for storage (**Figure 5.18**). The enzyme lipoprotein lipase (LPL) frees most of the triglyceride from the VLDL molecules, resulting in its uptake by the body's cells.

Diets high in fat, simple sugars, and extra Calories can increase the production of endogenous VLDLs, whereas diets high in omega-3 fatty acids can help reduce their production. In addition, exercise can reduce VLDLs, because the fat produced in the body is quickly used for energy instead of remaining to circulate in the blood.

Low-Density Lipoproteins The molecules resulting when VLDLs release their triglyceride load are much higher in cholesterol, phospholipids, and protein and therefore somewhat more dense. These **low-density lipoproteins (LDLs)** circulate in the blood, delivering their cholesterol to cells with specialized LDL receptors. Diets high in saturated fat *decrease* the removal of LDLs by body cells, apparently by blocking these receptor sites.

very-low-density lipoprotein (VLDL) A lipoprotein made in the liver and intestine that functions to transport endogenous lipids, especially triglycerides, to the tissues of the body.

low-density lipoprotein (LDL) A lipoprotein formed in the blood from VLDLs that transports cholesterol to the cells of the body; often called "bad cholesterol."

Lipoprotein Transport/ Distribution

Dietary and endogenous lipids are transported in the body via several different lipoprotein compounds, such as chylomicrons, VLDLs, LDLs, and HDLs.

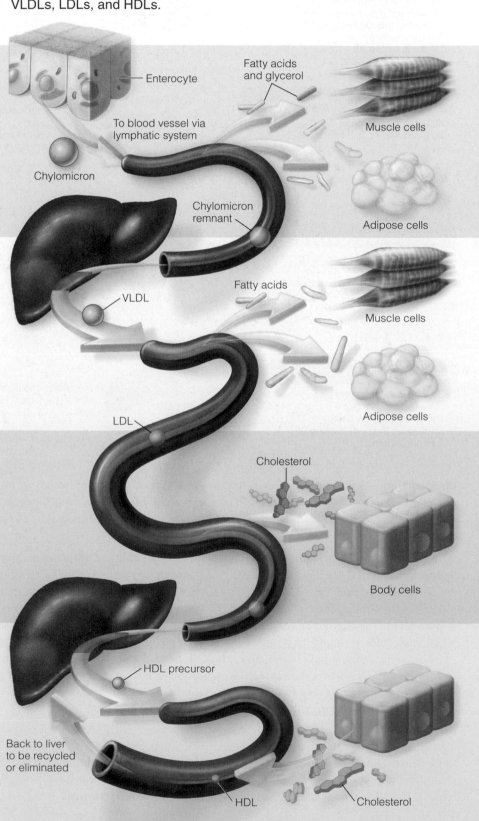

CHYLOMICRONS

Chylomicrons are produced in the enterocytes to transport dietary lipids. The enzyme lipoprotein lipase (LPL), found on the endothelial cells in the capillaries, hydrolyzes the triglycerides in the chylomicrons into fatty acids and glycerol, which enter body cells (such as muscle and adipose cells), leaving a chylomicron remnant. Chylomicron remnants are dismantled in the liver.

VLDLs

VLDLs (very-low-density lipoproteins) are produced primarily in the liver to transport endogenous fat in the form of triglycerides into the bloodstream. Lipoprotein lipase hydrolyzes the triglycerides in the VLDLs, allowing the fatty acids to enter body cells, especially muscle and adipose cells. Glycerol is also released and is transported back to the liver.

LDLs

LDLs (low-density lipoproteins) are created with the removal of most of the VLDLs' triglyceride load. LDLs are rich in cholesterol, which they deliver to body cells with LDL receptors. LDLs not taken up by the cells are primarily taken up by the liver for degradation.

HDLs

HDLs (high-density lipoproteins) are produced in the liver and circulate in the blood, picking up cholesterol from dying cells, other lipoproteins, and arterial plaques. They return this cholesterol to the liver, where it can be recycled or eliminated from the body through bile.

Enterocyte

Fatty acids and glycerol

To blood vessel via lymphatic system

Muscle cells

Chylomicron

Chylomicron remnant

Adipose cells

VLDL

Fatty acids

Muscle cells

Adipose cells

LDL

Cholesterol

Body cells

HDL precursor

Back to liver to be recycled or eliminated

HDL

Cholesterol

What happens to LDLs not taken up by body cells? As shown in Figure 5.18, such LDLs are primarily taken up by the liver for degradation. As they degrade over time, they release their cholesterol; thus, failure to remove LDLs from the bloodstream results in an increased load of cholesterol in the blood. The more cholesterol circulating in the blood, the greater the risk that some of it will adhere to the walls of the blood vessels. The presence of such adhesions signals "scavenger" white blood cells to rush to the site and bind cholesterol to their receptors. As more and more cholesterol binds to these cells, they form the plaque that characterizes atherosclerosis. This plaque becomes hard and calcified and blocks arterial blood flow (see Figure 5.16). Because high blood levels of LDL-cholesterol increase the risk for heart disease, it is commonly called "bad cholesterol."

High-Density Lipoproteins   As their name indicates, **high-density lipoproteins (HDLs)** are small, dense lipoproteins with a very low cholesterol content and a high protein content. They are released from the liver and intestines to circulate in the blood, picking up cholesterol from dying cells and arterial plaques and transferring it to other lipoproteins, which return it to the liver. The liver takes up the cholesterol and uses it to synthesize bile, thereby removing it from the circulatory system. High blood levels of HDL-cholesterol are therefore associated with a low risk for coronary artery disease. That's why HDL-cholesterol is often referred to as "good cholesterol." There is some evidence that diets high in omega-3 fatty acids and participation in regular physical exercise can modestly increase HDL-cholesterol levels. Refer to the box **Highlight: Blood Lipid Levels: Know Your Numbers!** to gain more insight into your own blood lipid levels.

Total Serum Cholesterol   Normally, as the dietary level of cholesterol increases, the body decreases the amount of cholesterol it makes, which keeps the body's level of cholesterol constant. Unfortunately, this feedback mechanism does not work well in everyone. For some individuals, eating dietary cholesterol doesn't decrease the amount of cholesterol produced in the body, and their total body cholesterol level rises. This also increases the level

high-density lipoprotein (HDL) A lipoprotein made in the liver and released into the blood. HDLs function to transport cholesterol from the tissues back to the liver; often called "good cholesterol."

HIGHLIGHT

Blood Lipid Levels: Know Your Numbers!

One of the most important steps you can take to reduce your own risk for heart disease is to know your "numbers"—that is, your blood lipid values. In addition, if you are considering a career in nutrition or healthcare, you'll need to be able to work with your clients to track their blood lipid levels as they change their diet and lifestyle to decrease their risk for cardiovascular disease. So it's important to keep a record of blood lipid values and have them checked every 1 to 2 years.

How are blood lipids, such as LDL-cholesterol or HDL-cholesterol, actually measured? First, a blood sample is taken and the lipoproteins in the blood are extracted. Total cholesterol is determined by breaking apart all the lipoproteins and measuring their combined cholesterol content. You can see from Figure 5.17 that each of the lipoproteins contains some cholesterol and some triglycerides. The same process is used to determine total blood triglyceride level. The next step is to measure the amount of cholesterol in the LDLs and HDLs, because these two lipoproteins can either raise or lower an individual's risk for heart disease. These lipoproteins are separated and the amount of cholesterol in each one is determined to give an LDL-cholesterol and an HDL-cholesterol value. Once these values are determined, you can compare them to the following "target" levels, which identify healthful ranges for each blood lipid, and see how you measure up.

The target lipid values are as follows:[1]

Total cholesterol (mg/dl): <200 mg/dl
LDL-cholesterol (mg/dl): <130 mg/dl
HDL-cholesterol (mg/dl): >40 mg/dl
Triglycerides (mg/dl): <150 mg/dl

Reference

1. National Institutes of Health. 2002. *Third Report of the National Cholesterol Education Program: Detection, Evaluation and Treatment of High Blood Cholesterol in Adults (ATP III)*. Bethesda, MD: National Cholesterol Education Program, National Heart, Lung, and Blood Institute, NIH. Available at www.nhlbi.nih.gov/guidelines/cholesterol/atp3xsum.pdf.

of cholesterol in the blood. These individuals benefit from reducing their intake of dietary cholesterol.

Both dietary cholesterol and saturated fats are found in animal foods; thus, by limiting their intake of animal products or selecting low-fat animal products, people reduce their intake of both saturated fat and cholesterol. According to the 2010 Dietary Guidelines, Americans get the majority of their dietary cholesterol from eggs and egg mixed dishes (25%), chicken and chicken mixed dishes (12%), beef and beef mixed dishes (6%), and all types of beef burgers (5%). Selecting fish, poultry without the skin, lean cuts of meat, plant sources of protein, and low-fat dairy products, as well as consuming egg whites without yolks, can dramatically reduce the amount of cholesterol in the diet.

The Role of Dietary Fats in Cardiovascular Disease

Research indicates that high intakes of saturated and *trans* fatty acids increase the blood's level of the lipids associated with cardiovascular disease—namely, total blood cholesterol and the cholesterol found in VLDLs and LDLs. It has also been shown that *trans* fatty acids can raise blood LDL-cholesterol, and lower HDL-cholesterol levels, more than saturated fatty acids.[16] Moreover, in vegetable oils converted to solids (for example, corn oil to corn oil margarine), the level of saturated fat dramatically increases, along with the level of *trans* fatty acids. Hence, to reduce the risk for heart disease, we must reduce our intake of high-fat animal products, hydrogenated vegetable products, and commercially prepared foods high in *trans* fatty acids.

The FDA requires that both saturated fat and *trans* fatty acid content be listed on labels for conventional foods and some dietary supplements. Unfortunately, no federal regulations require restaurants to provide nutrition facts for any of their foods at the present time, although some local ordinances do require restaurants to post this information. Until all restaurants are required to identify the nutrient composition of their foods, use healthy eating practices (see Chapter 2, pages 64–67, for some tips) whenever you're eating out.

Conversely, omega-3 fatty acids decrease our risk for heart disease by reducing inflammation and blood triglycerides and increasing HDLs.[30] Moreover, replacing saturated fats with monounsaturated and polyunsaturated fatty acids lowers both total and LDL-cholesterol levels.[23, 31]

Lifestyle Changes Can Prevent or Reduce Cardiovascular Disease

Diet and exercise interventions aimed at reducing the risk for cardiovascular disease center on reducing high levels of triglycerides and LDL-cholesterol while raising HDL-cholesterol. The Centers for Disease Control and Prevention (CDC); the NIH Expert Panel on Detection, Evaluation, and Treatment of High Blood Cholesterol in Adults (ATP III), and the American Heart Association have made the following dietary and lifestyle recommendations to improve blood lipid levels and reduce the risk for cardiovascular disease:[16, 22, 30, 32, 33, 34]

- Maintain total fat intake to within 20% to 35% of energy.[11] Polyunsaturated fats (for example, soy and canola oil) can comprise up to 10% of total energy intake, and monounsaturated fats (for example, olive oil) can comprise up to 20% of total energy intake. For some people, a lower fat intake may help them maintain a healthful body weight.
- Decrease dietary saturated fat to less than 7% of total energy intake. Decrease cholesterol intake to less than 300 mg per day, and keep *trans* fatty acid intake to an absolute minimum (<1% of energy). Lowering the intakes of these fats will lower your LDL-cholesterol level. Replace saturated and *trans* fats (for example, butter, margarine, vegetable shortening, or lard) with more healthful fats, such as olive oil or canola oil. Select fish, lean meats, and vegetable alternatives and use nonfat or low-fat dairy products.
- Increase intake of dietary omega-3 fatty acids from dark green, leafy vegetables; fatty fish; soybeans or soybean oil; walnuts or walnut oil; flaxseed meal or oil; or canola oil. Consuming fish, especially oily fish, at least twice a week will increase omega-3 fatty acid intake.

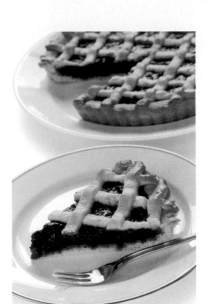

Invisible and *trans* fats are hidden in processed and prepared foods, such as pies. Without a label, it is impossible to know the amount of fat in each serving of these types of foods, so their intake should be limited.

- Increase dietary intakes of whole grains, fruits, and vegetables, so that total dietary fiber is 20–30 g per day, with 10–25 g per day coming from fiber sources such as oat bran, beans, and fruits. Approximately 5–10 g/day of this type of fiber will reduce LDL-cholesterol by approximately 5%.[16]
- Consume 400 μg/day of folate from dietary or supplemental sources to help maintain low blood levels of the amino acid homocysteine. High homocysteine levels in the blood are associated with increased risk for cardiovascular disease. (Folate is discussed in Chapter 12.)
- Maintain blood glucose and insulin concentrations within normal ranges. High blood glucose levels are associated with high blood triglycerides. Consume whole foods (such as whole-wheat breads and cereals, whole fruits and vegetables, and beans and legumes), and select low-saturated-fat meats and dairy products, while limiting your intake of foods high in refined carbohydrates and saturated and *trans* fats.
- Eat throughout the day (for example, smaller meals and snacks) instead of eating most of your Calories in the evening before bed.
- Consume no more than two alcoholic drinks per day for men and one drink per day for women. Alcohol consumption is discussed in detail in the In Depth (Chapter 4.5, pages 160–171).
- If you smoke, stop. As noted earlier, smoking significantly increases the risk for cardiovascular disease.
- Maintain an active lifestyle. Exercise most days of the week for 30–60 minutes whenever possible. Exercise increases HDL-cholesterol while lowering blood triglyceride levels. Exercise also helps maintain a healthful body weight and a lower blood pressure and reduces your risk for diabetes.
- Maintain a healthy body weight by balancing your energy intake and physical activity level. Blood lipids and glucose levels typically improve when obese individuals lose weight and engage in regular physical activity. Obesity promotes inflammation; thus, keeping body weight within a healthy range helps keep inflammation low.[35] In addition, blood pressure values have been shown to decrease three to four points in people who have lost 10 pounds of body weight.[36]
- Select and prepare foods with little or no salt to help keep your blood pressure normal (<120/80 mm Hg). Sodium intake can increase blood pressure in sodium-sensitive individuals. Hypertension is an independent risk factor for cardiovascular disease.
- Add plant sterols to your diet. There is now strong clinical research evidence that the consumption of 2–3 g/day of plant sterols can reduce blood LDL-cholesterol concentrations by 6–15%.[16] The U.S. Food and Drug Administration has approved a health claim for plant-sterol-fortified foods in the reduction of cardiovascular disease. Plant sterols are isolated from plant oils and then mixed into commercial margarines, salad dressings, milk, yogurt, or pills and chews. Researchers do not know exactly how plant sterols reduce cholesterol absorption, but one suggested mechanism is that they compete with dietary cholesterol for incorporation into the micelle, which reduces dietary cholesterol absorption. However, very little of the plant sterols are absorbed (<1%) from the micelle;[37] that is, they block the absorption of dietary cholesterol but are not absorbed themselves. Thus, total blood cholesterol is significantly reduced in the presence of plant sterols.[38]

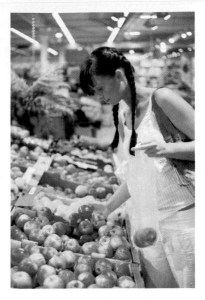

Consuming whole fruits and vegetables can reduce your risk for cardiovascular disease.

The impact of diet on reducing the risk for cardiovascular disease was clearly demonstrated in the Dietary Approaches to Stop Hypertension (DASH) study, which is discussed in detail later in this text (Chapter 9). Although this study focused on dietary interventions to reduce hypertension, the results showed that eating the DASH way can also dramatically improve blood lipids. The DASH diet includes high intakes of fruits, vegetables, whole grains, low-fat dairy products, poultry, fish, and nuts and low intakes of fats, red meat, sweets, and sugar-containing beverages. Combining the DASH dietary approach with an active lifestyle significantly reduces the risk for cardiovascular disease.

*Nutri-*Case

Gustavo

"Sometimes I wonder where doctors get their funny ideas. Yesterday I had my annual checkup and my doctor says, 'You're doing great! Your weight is fine, your blood sugar's good. . . . The only thing that concerns me is that your blood pressure is a little high. So I want you to watch your diet. Don't sprinkle salt on your food. Eat fish more often. When you eat meat, trim off all the fat. Use one of the new heart-healthy margarines instead of butter, and olive oil instead of lard. And when you have eggs, don't eat the yolks.'

I know he means well, but my wife's just starting to get around again after breaking her hip. How am I supposed to go home and tell her that now she has to learn a whole new way to cook too?"

Do you think Gustavo's objection to his physician's advice is valid? Why or why not? Identify at least two interventions or resources that might help Gustavo and his wife.

Prescription Medications Can Reduce Cardiovascular Disease Risk

Sometimes medications are needed in addition to lifestyle changes to reduce cardiovascular risk. A number of medications on the market help lower LDL-cholesterol. The following are some of the most common:

- *Endogenous cholesterol synthesis inhibitors.* These types of drugs, typically called *statins,* block an enzyme in the cholesterol synthesis pathway. Thus, these drugs lower blood levels of LDL-cholesterol and VLDL-cholesterol. Statins also have an important anti-inflammatory effect that contributes to the reduction in cardiovascular disease risk independent of their effect on blood lipids.[39]
- *Bile acid sequestrants.* These types of drugs bind the bile acids, preventing them from being reabsorbed by the intestinal tract. Because bile acids are made from cholesterol, blocking their reabsorption means the liver must use cholesterol already in the body to make new bile acids. Continually eliminating bile acids from the body reduces the total cholesterol pool.
- *Nicotinic acid.* Therapeutic doses of nicotinic acid, a form of niacin, favorably affect all blood lipids when given pharmacologically. (The form of niacin found in multivitamin supplements does not affect lipids.) Unfortunately, this drug has a number of side effects, such as flushing of the skin, gastrointestinal distress, and liver problems.[16] Because of this, it is used less frequently than the other two drugs.

Does a High-Fat Diet Cause Cancer?

Cancer develops as a result of a poorly understood interaction between the environment and genetic factors. In addition, most cancers take years to develop, so examining the impact of diet on cancer development can be a long and difficult process. Diet and lifestyle are two of the most important factors that have been identified in the development of cancer.[40, 41] Currently, research shows that obesity, poor nutrition, and physical inactivity may account for 25% to 30% of several major cancers, including colon cancer and postmenopausal breast cancer.[42] Of course, a diet high in fat can contribute to obesity, but there is no strong evidence that a certain type or amount of fat causes cancer. Three types of cancer that have been studied extensively for their possible relationship to dietary fat intake are breast cancer, colon cancer, and prostate cancer:

- *Breast cancer.* Currently, no clinical trials show a link between the amount or type of fat consumed and increased risk for breast cancer.[43, 44, 45]
- *Colon cancer.* Recent research shows that a Western diet high in red meat, fat, refined grains, and desserts is associated with a greater occurrence of colon cancer compared

to a diet high in fruits, vegetables, poultry, and fish.[46] Because we now know that physical activity can reduce the risk for colon cancer, earlier diet and colon cancer studies that did not control for this factor are now being questioned.

- *Prostate cancer.* As with other cancers, the exact link between dietary fat intake and prostate cancer is not clear.[47, 48] Research shows that there is a consistent link between prostate cancer risk and consumption of animal fats, but not other types of fats. The exact mechanism by which animal fats may contribute to prostate cancer has not yet been identified. Men who consume diets high in animal fat also have lower intakes of fruits and vegetables.

Until we know more about the link between diet, especially fat, and cancer, the American Institute for Cancer Research[40] recommends the following diet and lifestyle changes to reduce your risk:

- Maintain a healthy body weight. Avoid weight gain and increases in waist circumference throughout adulthood.
- Engage in moderate physical activity, the equivalent of brisk walking, for at least 30 minutes a day. For improved fitness, aim for 60 minutes or more of moderate activity, or 30 minutes of vigorous activity every day. Limit nonessential sedentary behaviors, such as watching television and playing video games.
- Limit consumption of sugary drinks and other sources of empty Calories.
- Eat a variety of fruits, legumes and other vegetables, and whole unprocessed grains.
- Limit consumption of red meats, such as beef, pork, and lamb, and avoid processed meats.
- If you drink alcohol, limit intake to two drinks/day for men and one drink/day for women.
- Limit consumption of salty foods and foods processed with salt.
- Don't use supplements to protect against cancer.

RECAP

The types of fats we eat can significantly influence our health and risk for disease. Saturated and *trans* fatty acids increase our risk for heart disease, whereas omega-3 fatty acids can reduce our risk. Other risk factors for heart disease include being overweight, being physically inactive, smoking, having high blood pressure, and having diabetes. High levels of LDL-cholesterol and low levels of HDL-cholesterol increase your risk for heart disease. Making appropriate changes in diet and lifestyle behaviors may reduce your risk for some types of cancer. ■

Chapter Review

1. **F** Eating too much fat, or too much of unhealthful fats such as saturated and trans fatty acids, can increase our risk for diseases such as cardiovascular disease and obesity. However, fat is an important part of a nutritious diet, and we need to consume a certain minimum amount to provide adequate levels of essential fatty acids and fat-soluble vitamins.

2. **T** Cholesterol is required for good health; however; our body can make all the cholesterol we need, so we do not need to consume cholesterol in our diet.

3. **F** Even foods fried in vegetable shortening can be unhealthful, because they are higher in *trans* fatty acids. In addition, fried foods are high in total fat and energy and can contribute to overweight and obesity.

4. **T** Certain essential fatty acids, including EPA and DHA, reduce inflammation, blood clotting, and plasma triglycerides and thereby reduce an individual's risk for heart disease.

5. **F** Cancer develops as a result of a poorly understood interaction between environmental and genetic factors. Some research indicates an association between high dietary fat consumption and certain cancers, but this research is inconclusive.

Summary

- Fats and oils are forms of a larger and more diverse group of substances called lipids; most lipids are insoluble in water.

- The three types of lipids commonly found in foods are triglycerides, phospholipids, and sterols.

- Most of the fat we eat is in the form of triglycerides; a triglyceride is a molecule that contains three fatty acids attached to a glycerol backbone.

- Short-chain fatty acids are usually less than six carbon atoms in length; medium-chain fatty acids are six to twelve carbons in length; and long-chain fatty acids are fourteen or more carbons in length.

- Saturated fatty acids have no carbons attached together with a double bond, which means that every carbon atom in the fatty acid chain is saturated with hydrogen. They are straight in shape and solid at room temperature.

- Monounsaturated fatty acids contain one double bond between two carbon atoms. Polyunsaturated fatty acids contain more than one double bond between carbon atoms. Unsaturated fatty acids are usually liquid at room temperature.

- A *cis* fatty acid has hydrogen atoms located on the same side of the double bond in an unsaturated fatty acid. This *cis* positioning produces a kink in the unsaturated fatty acid and is the shape found in naturally occurring fatty acids.

- A *trans* fatty acid has hydrogen atoms located on opposite sides of the double carbon bond. This positioning causes *trans* fatty acids to be straighter and more rigid, like saturated fats. This *trans* positioning results when oils are hydrogenated during food processing.

- The essential fatty acids (linoleic acid and alpha-linolenic acid) must be obtained from food. These fatty acids are precursors to important biological compounds called eicosanoids, which are essential for growth and health.

- Linoleic acid is found primarily in vegetable and nut oils, whereas alpha-linolenic acid is found in dark green, leafy vegetables; flaxseeds and oil; walnuts and walnut oil; soybean oil and soy foods; canola oil; and fish products and fish oil.

- Phospholipids consist of a glycerol backbone and two fatty acids with a phosphate group; phospholipids are soluble in water and assist with transporting fats in the bloodstream.

- Sterols have a ring structure; cholesterol is the most common sterol in our diet.

- The majority of fat digestion and absorption occurs in the small intestine. Fat is broken into smaller components by bile, which is produced by the liver and stored in the gallbladder.

- Lipid digestion products are transported to enterocytes by micelles.

- Because fats are not soluble in water, triglycerides are packaged into lipoproteins before being released into the bloodstream for transport to the cells.

- Dietary fat is primarily used either as an energy source for the cells or to make lipid-containing compounds in the body, or it is stored in the muscle and adipose tissue as triglyceride for later use.

- Fats are a primary energy source during rest and exercise, are our major source of stored energy, provide essential fatty acids, enable the transport of fat-soluble vitamins, help maintain cell function, provide protection for body organs, contribute to the texture and flavor of foods, and help us feel satiated after a meal.

- The AMDR for fat is 20–35% of total energy intake. Our intake of saturated fats and *trans* fatty acids should be kept to a minimum. Individuals who limit fat intake to less than 15%

of energy intake need to make sure that essential fatty acid needs are met, as well as protein and energy needs.

■ For the essential fatty acids, 5–10% of energy intake should be in the form of linoleic acid and 0.6–1.2% as alpha-linolenic acid.

■ Watch for invisible fats found in cakes, cookies, marbling in meat, regular-fat dairy products, and fried foods. Select beneficial unsaturated fats.

■ Diets high in saturated fat and *trans* fatty acids can increase our risk for cardiovascular disease. Other risk factors for cardiovascular disease are overweight or obesity, physical inactivity, smoking, high blood pressure, and diabetes.

■ High levels of circulating low-density lipoproteins, or LDLs, increase total blood cholesterol concentrations and the formation of plaque on arterial walls, leading to an increased risk for cardiovascular disease. This is why LDL-cholesterol is sometimes called the "bad cholesterol."

■ High levels of circulating high-density lipoproteins, or HDLs, reduce our blood cholesterol levels and our risk for cardiovascular disease. This is why HDL-cholesterol is sometimes called the "good cholesterol."

■ Research shows that dietary behaviors can increase or decrease the risk for certain cancers. Key modifiable behaviors that reduce the risk for cancer are maintaining normal body weight, being physically active, limiting intake of empty Calories, eating mostly plant-based foods, and limiting intake of red meat.

Mastering Nutrition™

To further your understanding, go online and apply what you've learned to real-life case studies that will help you master the content!

Review Questions

1. Omega-3 fatty acids are
   a. a form of *trans* fatty acid.
   b. metabolized in the body to arachidonic acid.
   c. synthesized in the liver and small intestine.
   d. found in flaxseeds, walnuts, and fish.

2. One of the most sensible ways to reduce body fat is to
   a. limit intake of dietary fat to less than 15% of total energy consumed.
   b. exercise regularly.
   c. avoid all consumption of *trans* fatty acids.
   d. restrict total energy to 1,200 kcal per day.

3. Lipids in chylomicrons are taken up by cells with the help of
   a. lipoprotein lipase.
   b. micelles.
   c. sterols.
   d. pancreatic enzymes.

4. The risk for heart disease is reduced in people who have high blood levels of
   a. triglycerides.
   b. very-low-density lipoproteins.
   c. low-density lipoproteins.
   d. high-density lipoproteins.

5. Fatty acids with a double bond at one part of the molecule are referred to as
   a. monounsaturated.
   b. hydrogenated.
   c. saturated.
   d. essential.

6. **True or false?** Lecithin is a protein found in egg whites that assists in the transport of lipids.

7. **True or false?** During exercise, lipids cannot be mobilized from adipose tissue for use as energy.

8. **True or false?** Triglycerides are the same as fatty acids.

9. **True or false?** *Trans* fatty acids are produced by food manufacturers; they do not occur in nature.

10. **True or false?** A serving of food labeled *reduced fat* has at least 25% less fat and 25% fewer Calories than a full-fat version of the same food.

11. Explain how the straight, rigid shape of the saturated and *trans* fatty acids we eat affects our health.

12. Explain the contribution of dietary fat to bone health.

13. You have volunteered to participate in a 20-mile walk-a-thon to raise money for a local charity. You have been training for several weeks, and the event is now 2 days away. An athlete friend of yours advises you to "load up on carbohydrates" today and tomorrow and says you should avoid eating any foods that contain fat during the day of the walk-a-thon. Do you take this advice? Why or why not?

14. Caleb's father is feeling down after an appointment with his doctor. He tells Caleb that his "blood test didn't turn out so good." He then adds, "My doctor told me I can't eat any of my favorite foods anymore. He says red meat and butter have too much fat. I guess I'll have to switch to cottage cheese and margarine!" What type of blood test do you think Caleb's father had? How should Caleb respond to his father's intention to switch to cottage cheese and margarine? Finally, suggest a nondietary lifestyle choice that might improve his health.

Math Review

15. Your friend Maria has determined that she needs to consume about 2,000 kcal per day to maintain her healthful weight. Create a chart for Maria showing the recommended maximum number of Calories she should consume in each of the following forms: unsaturated fat, saturated fat, linoleic acid, alpha-linolenic acid, and *trans* fatty acids.

16. Hannah believes that, if she limits her fat intake, she will lose weight. After classes, she treats herself to a cup (8 ounces) of nonfat frozen yogurt topped with 4 tablespoons of fat-free chocolate syrup. The yogurt contains 35 grams of carbohydrate, 0.5 gram of fat, and 6 grams of protein. The chocolate syrup contains 48 grams of carbohydrate and 2 grams of protein. First, what do you think of Hannah's approach to weight loss? Second, approximately how many kcal are in her after-class snack? Third, propose a nutrient-dense snack with approximately the same number of kcal and a healthful level of unsaturated fat.

Answers to Review Questions and Math Review can be found online in the MasteringNutrition Study Area.

Web Links

www.heart.org/HEARTORG
American Heart Association
Learn the best way to lower, and manage, your blood cholesterol levels.

www.nhlbi.nih.gov/chd
National Cholesterol Education Program
Check out this site for information on how a healthful diet can lower your cholesterol levels.

www.nhlbi.nih.gov
National Heart, Lung, and Blood Institute
Use the online risk assessment tool to estimate your personal risks for having a heart attack.

www.nlm.nih.gov/medlineplus
MEDLINE Plus Health Information
Search for "fats" or "lipids" to locate resources and learn the latest news on dietary lipids, heart disease, and cholesterol.

www.nih.gov
National Institutes of Health
Go to this clearinghouse site for a wide range of resources, reports, and other useful tools on the subjects we cover in this chapter.

References

1. Marieb, E. N., and K. Hoehn. 2013. *Human Anatomy and Physiology.* 9th edn. San Francisco: Benjamin Cummings, p. 46.

2. Champe, P. C., R. A. Harvey, and D. R. Ferrier. 2008. *Lippincott's Illustrated Reviews: Biochemistry.* 4th edn. Philadelphia: Lippincott Williams & Wilkins.

3. Gropper, S. S., J. L. Smith, and J. L. Groff. 2009. *Advanced Nutrition and Human Development.* 5th edn. Belmont, CA: Thompson Wadsworth.

4. Whelan, J., and C. Rust. 2006. Innovative dietary sources of n-3 fatty acids. *Annu. Rev. Nutr.* 26:75–103.

5. Manore, M. M., N. L. Meyer, and J. Thompson. 2009. *Sport Nutrition for Health and Performance.* 2nd edn. Champaign, IL: Human Kinetics.

6. Kaleta, C., L. F. de Figueiredo, S. Werner, R. Guthke, M. Ristow, and S. Schuster. 2011. In silico evidence for gluconeogenesis from fatty acids in humans. *PLoS Computational Biology* 7(7):e1002116.

7. Institute of Medicine, Food and Nutrition Board. 2000. *Dietary Reference Intakes for Vitamin C, Vitamin E, Selenium and Carotenoids.* Washington, DC: National Academies Press.

8. Rolls, B. J. 2000. The role of energy density in the overconsumption of fat. *J. Nutr.* 130:268S–271S.

9. Gerstein, D. E., G. Woodward-Lopez, A. E. Evans, K. Kelsey, and A. Drewnowski. 2004. Clarifying concepts about macronutrients' effects on satiation and satiety. *J. Am. Diet. Assoc.* 104:1151–1153.

10. Rolls, B. J. 2009. The relationship between dietary energy density and energy intake. *Physiol. Behav.* 97(5):609–615.

11. Institute of Medicine, Food and Nutrition Board. 2005. *Dietary Reference Intakes for Energy, Carbohydrate, Fiber, Fat, Fatty Acids, Cholesterol, Protein, and Amino Acids (Macronutrients).* Washington, DC: National Academies Press.

12. Rodriguez, N. R., N. M. DiMarco, and S. Langley. 2009. Position of the American Dietetic Association, Dietitians of Canada, and the American College of Sports Medicine: nutrition and athletic performance. *J. Am. Diet. Assoc.* 109(3):509–527.

13. Lichtenstein, A. H., and L. Van Horn. 1998. Very low fat diets. *Circulation* 98:935–939.

14. Briefel, R. R., and C. L. Johnson. 2004. Secular trend in dietary intake in the United States. *Ann. Rev. Nutr.* 24:401–431.

15. Austin, G. L., L. G. Ogden, and J. O. Hill. 2011. Trends in carbohydrate, fat, and protein intakes and association with energy intake in normal-weight, overweight, and obese individuals: 1971–2006. *Am. J. Clin. Nutr.* 93(4):836–843.

16. National Institutes of Health, Expert Panel on Detection, Evaluation, and Treatment of High Blood Cholesterol in Adults, 2002. Third report of the National Cholesterol Education Program (NCEP) Expert Panel on Detection, Evaluation, and Treatment of High Blood Cholesterol in Adults (Adult Treatment Panel III) final report. *Circulation* 106:3143–3421. www.nhlbi.nih.gov/guidelines/cholesterol/atp3xsum.pdf.

17. United States Department of Agriculture, Agriculture Research Service. 2008. Weighing in on Fats. www.ars.usda.gov/is/AR/archive/mar08/fats308.htm.

18. Ratnayake, W., M. R. L'Abbe, S. Farnworth, et al. 2009. Trans fatty acids: current contents in Canadian foods and estimated intake levels for the Canadian opulation. *Journal of AOAC International* 92(5):1258–1276.

19. Teegala, S. M., W. C. Willett, and D. Mozaffarian. 2009. Consumption and health effects of trans fatty acids: a review. *Journal of AOAC International* 92(5):1250–1257.

20. Sabastian R., C. Enns, J. Goldman, and A. Moshfegh. 2008. Effect of fast food consumption on dietary intake and likehood of meeting MyPyramid recommendations in adults: results from What We Eat in America, NHANES 2003–2004. *FASEB Journal* 22:868.7.

21. Heidenreich, P. A., J. G. Trogdon, O. A. Khavjou, J. Butler, K. Dracup, M. D. Ezekowitz, E. A. Finkelstein, Y. Hong, S. C. Johnson, A. Khera, D. M. Lloyd-Jones, S. A. Nelson, G. Nichol, D. Orenstein, P. W. F. Wilson, and J. Y. Woo. 2011. Forecasting the future of cardiovascular disease in the United States: a policy statement from the American Heart Association. *Circulation* 123. DOI: 10.1161/CIR.0b013e31820a55f5.

22. Wilson, P. W. F. 2004. CDC/AHA workshop on markers of inflammation and cardiovascular disease. Application to clinical and public health practice. Ability of inflammatory markers to predict disease in asymptomatic patients. A background paper. *Circulation* 110:e568–e571.

23. United States Department of Agriculture and Department of Health and Human Services. 2010. *Dietary Guidelines for Americans 2010.* 7th edn. Washington, DC: US Government Printing Office.

24. Rippe, J. M., T. J. Angelopoulos, and L. Zukley. 2007. The rationale for intervention to reduce the risk of coronary heart disease. *Am. J. Lifestyle Med.* 1(1):10–19.

25. Marwick, T. H., M. D. Hordern, T. Miller, D. A. Chyun, A. G. Bertoni, R. S. Blumenthal, G. Philippides, and A. Rocchini. 2009. Exercise training for type 2 diabetes mellitus: impact on cardiovascular risk: a scientific statement from the American Heart Association. *Circulation* 119:3244–3262.

26. Department of Health and Human Services. 2008. *Physical Activity Guidelines Advisory Committee Report.* Washington, DC:.US Government Printing Office.

27. Department of Health and Human Services. 2010. *How Tabacco Smoke Causes Disease: The Biology and Behavioral Basis for Smoking-Attributable Disease: A Report of the Surgeon General.* Atlanta, GA: US Department of Health and Human Services, Centers for Disease Control and Prevention, National Center for Chronic Disease Prevention and Health Promotion, Office on Smoking and Health.

28. National Cancer Institute. 2011. Harms of Smoking and Health Benefits of Quitting. www.cancer.gov/cancertopics/factsheet/Tobacco/cessation. (Accessed February 2012.)

29. Hohensinner, P. J., A. Niessner, K. Huber, C. M. Weyand, and J. Wojta. 2011. Inflammation and cardiac outcome. *Current Opinion in Infectious Diseases* 24(3):259–264.

30. Kris-Etherton, P. M., W. S. Harris, L. J. Appel, and the Nutrition Committee of the American Heart Association. 2002. Fish consumption, fish oil, omega-3 fatty acids and cardiovascular disease. *Circulation* 106:2747–2757.

31. Harris, W. S., D. Mozffarian, E. Rimm, P. Kris-Etherton, L. L. Rudel, L. J. Appel, M. M. Engler, M. B. Engler, and F. Sacks. 2009. Omega-6 fatty acids and risk for cardiovascular disease. *Circulation* 119. DOI: 10.1161/CIRCULATIONAHA.108.19167.

32. National Center for Chronic Disease Prevention and Health Promotion. 2008. Division for Heart Disease and Stroke Prevention addressing the nation's leading killers. At a glance 2008. www.cdc.gov/print.do?url= http://www.cdc.gov/nccdphp/publications/AAG/dhdsp.htm.

33. Lichtenstein, A. H., L. J. Appel, M. Brands, M. Carnethon, S. Daniels, H. A. Franch, B. Franklin, P. Kris-Etherton, W. S. Harris, B. Howard, N. Karanja, M. Lefevre, L. Rudel, F. Sacks, L. Van Horn, M. Winston, and J. Wylie-Rosett. 2006. Diet and lifestyle recommendations revision 2006: scientific statement from the American Heart Association Nutrition Committee. *Circulation* 114:82–96.

34. Gidding, S. S., A. H. Lichtenstein, M. S. Faith, A. Karpyn, J. A. Mennella, B. Popkin, J. Rowe, L. Van Horn, and L. Whitsel. 2009. Implementing American Heart Association Pediatric and Adult Nutrition Guidelines. *Circulation* 119:1161–1175.

35. Despres, J. P., and I. Lemieux. 2006. Abdominal obesity and metabolic syndrome. *Nature* 444(14):881–887.

36. Appel, L. J., M. W. Brands, S. R. Daniels, N. Karaja, P. J. Elmer, and F. M. Sacks. 2006. Dietary approaches to prevent and treat hypertenesion: a scientific statement from the American Heart Association. *Hypertension* 47:296–308.

37. Tso, P. P., K. Crissinger, and F. J. Jandacek. 2006. Digestion and absorption of lipids. In: Stipanuk, M. H., ed. *Biochemical, Physiological, and Molecular Aspects of Human Nutrition.* Philadelphia: Saunders/Elsevier, pp. 219–239.

38. Rideout, T. C., and P. J. H. Jones. 2010. Plant sterols: an essential component of preventive cardiovascular medicine. *SCAN Pulse* 29(1):1–6.

39. Mizuno, Y., F. R. Jacob, and R. P. Mason. 2011. Inflammation and the development of atherosclerosis. *Journal of Atherosclerosis and Thrombosis* 28(5):351–358.

40. American Institute for Cancer Research (AICR) World Cancer Research Fund. 2007. *Food, Nutrition, Physical Activity, and the Prevention of Cancer: A Global Perspective.* Washington, DC: AICR.

41. Liebman B. 2012. Cancer. How to lower your risk. *Nutrition Action.* January/February, 1–7.

42. American Cancer Society. January 2012. Body Weight and Cancer Risk. www.cancer.org/Cancer/CancerCauses/. (Accessed February 2012.)

43. Prentice, R. L., C. Bette, R. Chlebowski, et al. 2006. Low-fat dietary patterns and risk of invasive breast cancer. The Women's Health Initiative Randomized Controlled Dietary Modification Trial. *JAMA.* 295:629–642.

44. Willette, W. C., and M. J. Stamper. 2006. Foundations of a healthy diet. In: Shils, M. E., M. Shike, A. C. Ross, B. Caballero, and R. J. Cousins, eds., *Modern Nutrition in Health and Disease.* 10th edn. Baltimore: Williams & Wilkins, pp. 1625–1637.

45. Alexander, D. D., L. M. Morimoto, P. J. Mink, and K. A. Lowe. 2010. Summary and meta-analysis of prospective studies of animal fat intake and breast cancer. *Nutrition Research Reviews* 23(1):169–179.

46. Meyerhardt, J. A., D. Niedzwiecki, D. Hollis, L. B. Saltz, F. B. Hu, R. J. Mayer, H. Nelson, R. Whittom, A. Hantel, J. Thomas, and C. S. Fuchs. 2007. Association of dietary patterns with cancer recurrence and survival in patients with stage III colon cancer. *JAMA* 298(7):754–764.

47. American Cancer Society. October 2011. What Are the Risk Factors for Prostate Cancer? www.cancer.org/Cancer/ProstateCancer/. (Accessed February 2012.)

48. Ma, R. W., and K. Chapman. 2009. A systemic review of the effect of diet in prostate cancer prevention and treatment. *Journal of Human Nutrition and Dietetics* 22(3):187–199.

Should Nutrition Professionals Speak Out Against "Bad" Foods?

Look around you. How many fast-food restaurants are within walking distance of your home, place of work, or campus? These restaurants are notorious for the high-fat, high-Calorie meals and high-sugar beverages they serve. So why do consumers choose them? Fast food has three major advantages over traditional restaurant meals and home-cooked meals: it is quick to obtain, tastes good to a majority of consumers, and is relatively cheap for the number of Calories it provides.[1] Many Americans view the large portions served in fast-food restaurants as evidence that they are getting good "value" for their money. It took the documentary film *Super Size Me* to make many Americans realize just how quickly eating these large portions of high-fat, high-sugar foods can pack on the pounds and significantly harm their health.

Several questions are raised by the high-fat, high-sugar, low-cost, fast-food environment in which we live. First, can all foods fit into a healthful diet, or are there certain high-fat, high-sugar foods, like many of those offered at fast-food outlets, that we should avoid entirely? As a nation, how are we going to curb our growing obesity problem? Do populations respond better to guidelines or proscriptions? What type of food recommendations should nutrition professionals make to government agencies, media, clients, and friends and family members? Fundamentally, these questions all contribute to the same debate—that is, whether nutrition professionals should advise their clients to avoid specific foods.

This debate touches on the interaction between science and politics in the matter of nutrition advice and interventions. On one side of the debate, we have a growing body of scientific evidence that identifies specific foods that promote health and specific foods that detract from health. Many dietitians and healthcare professionals say that they have an obligation to share this information with their clients.[2] They argue that consumers have a right to know which foods protect against disease and which increase the risk for disease. Some support proposed FDA regulations requiring eating establishments to publish the nutrient composition of their meals alongside the price in their menu. Some within this group also argue that we should tax unhealthful foods in the

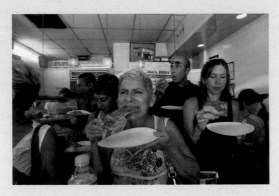

Fast food can be convenient for students and others with busy lifestyles. Should nutrition professionals tell people not to eat it at all?

same way that we tax alcohol and cigarettes. Such a tax might reduce purchases of these foods and promote better health.[3]

On the other side of the debate are the politics of food and food preferences. Every nutrition professional knows that quick, good-tasting, and low-cost food sells extremely well, even among consumers who know it does not promote their health.[2] Thus, many nutrition professionals attempt to work with clients' food preferences to the extent possible. Many dietitians and professional groups, including the Academy of Nutrition and Dietetics, share the philosophy that all foods can fit into a healthful diet.[4] They believe that it is important to look at an individual's total diet and dietary patterns, including portion sizes, and not focus just on "bad" foods. They also argue that you cannot assign "moral" qualities to foods. They believe their responsibility is to communicate positive nutrition messages that inspire people to make better food choices.

Dietitians on this side of the debate believe it is unrealistic to tell people to stop eating their favorite foods and that change will be achieved by encouraging clients to eat these foods in moderation. They point out that a significant percentage of people advised to make dramatic dietary changes get discouraged and give up. They also point to studies showing that, in restaurants that post Calorie and nutrient data for their meals, patrons' choices are not affected.[5] Thus,

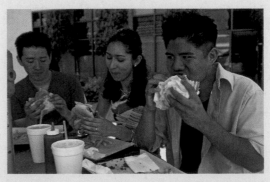

What kind of information will help you make the best dietary choices?

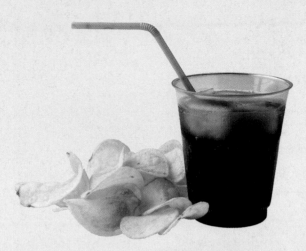

Should some foods be avoided entirely?

in working with a client who eats fast food daily, they would not tell the client to stop eating it altogether but rather would suggest the client eat it less often and make better food choices at fast-food restaurants. Their goal is to help individuals set achievable goals and make small steps toward changing their diet.

In controlled environments, when health-promoting food messages are reinforced by increased availability of healthful foods, it appears that study participants improve their diet. But the real world is not a lab. Certainly, more research is needed to determine what kinds of advice and messages are most helpful in producing health-promoting dietary changes in large populations.

CRITICAL THINKING QUESTIONS

- Prior to taking this class, how often did you think about the fat and energy content of the foods you ordered when eating out? Did you frequently order high-fat, large-portion meals at fast-food restaurants? Did you "super-size" your serving?

- Now that you know more about nutrition, do you think that all foods can fit into a healthful diet, or should some foods just be avoided completely?

- Should professional nutrition organizations warn people against "bad" foods? Why or why not?

- Do you feel a tax should be imposed on certain foods with empty Calories? What are the pros and cons to this proposition?

- What approach do you think would be the most effective for encouraging Americans to make positive dietary changes?

REFERENCES

1. Variyam, J. N. 2004. The price is right. Economics and the rise of obesity. *Amber Waves. USDA Economic Research Service* 3(1):20–27.

2. Nestle, M., and L. B. Dixon. 2004. *Taking Sides: Clashing Views on Controversial Issues in Food and Nutrition.* New York: McGraw-Hill/Dushkin, pp. 24–39.

3. Colson, J. M. 2012. *Taking Sides: Clashing Views on Controversial Issues in Food and Nutrition.* 2nd edn. New York: McGraw-Hill/Dushkin, pp. 231–243.

4. American Dietetic Association. 2002. Position of the American Dietetic Association: Total diet approaches to communicating food and nutrition information. *J. Am. Diet. Assoc.* 102(1):100–108.

5. Elbel, B., J. Gyamfi, and R. Kersh. 2011. Child and adolescent fast-food choice and the influence of calorie labeling: a natural experiment. *International Journal of Obesity* 35(4):493–500.

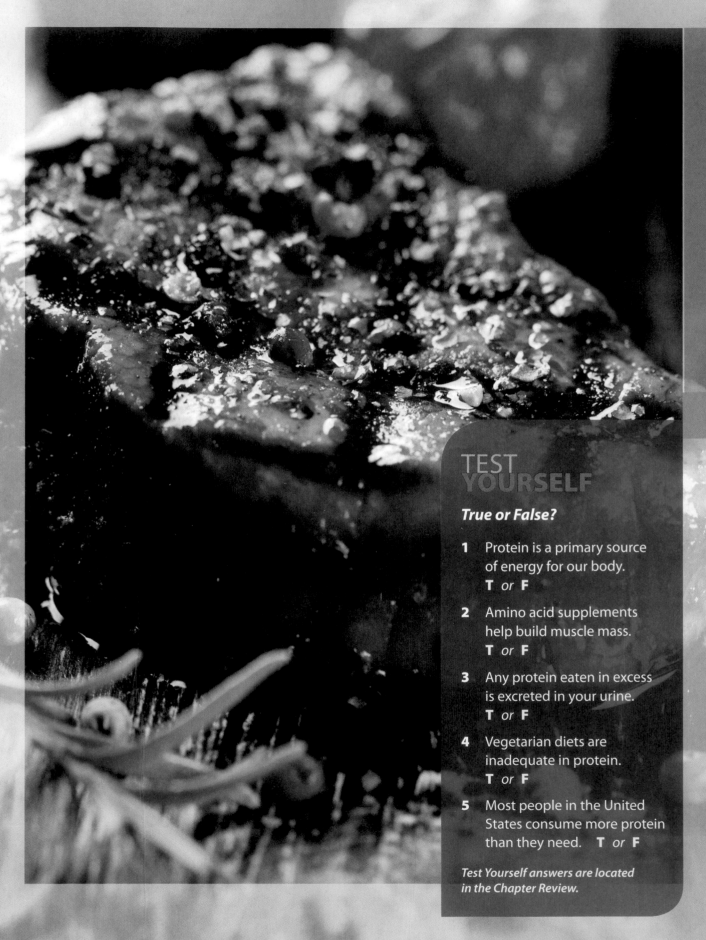

TEST YOURSELF

True or False?

1 Protein is a primary source of energy for our body. **T** *or* **F**

2 Amino acid supplements help build muscle mass. **T** *or* **F**

3 Any protein eaten in excess is excreted in your urine. **T** *or* **F**

4 Vegetarian diets are inadequate in protein. **T** *or* **F**

5 Most people in the United States consume more protein than they need. **T** *or* **F**

Test Yourself answers are located in the Chapter Review.

6 Proteins: Crucial Components of All Body Tissues

Learning Objectives

After studying this chapter, you should be able to:

1. Describe how proteins differ from carbohydrates and lipids, *p. 218.*

2. Identify the structure of an amino acid molecule including its five essential components, *p. 218.*

3. Differentiate among essential amino acids, nonessential amino acids, and conditionally essential amino acids, *pp. 219–221.*

4. Explain how proteins are made and the relationship between protein shape and function, *pp. 221–226.*

5. Discuss how proteins are digested and absorbed by the body, *pp. 228–230.*

6. Describe at least four functions of proteins in the body, *pp. 230–235.*

7. Calculate your Recommended Dietary Allowance for protein, *p. 238.*

8. Identify the potential health risks associated with high-protein diets, *pp. 239–240.*

9. List six foods that are good sources of protein, including at least three non-meat sources, *pp. 240–245.*

10. Describe two disorders related to inadequate protein intake or genetic abnormalities, *pp. 249–251.*

MasteringNutrition™

Go online for chapter quizzes, pre-tests, Interactive Activities and more!

What do professional skateboarder Forrest Kirby, tennis pro Venus Williams, fitness guru Bob Harper, and hundreds of other athletes have in common? They're all vegetarians! Boxing champ Mike Tyson says that his vegetarian diet "feels awesome . . . I wish I was born this way!"[1] Although statistics on the number of vegetarian athletes aren't available, in a 2011 poll nationwide, 5% of all U.S. adults reported that they never eat meat, poultry, or fish, and 17% said they eat meat, poultry, or fish at fewer than half their weekly meals.[2]

What is a protein, and what makes it so different from carbohydrates and fats? How much protein do people really need, and do most people get enough in their daily diet? What exactly is a vegetarian, anyway? Do you qualify? If so, how do you plan your diet to include sufficient protein, especially if you play competitive sports? Are there real advantages to eating meat, or is plant protein just as good?

It seems as if everybody has an opinion about protein, both how much you should consume and from what sources. In this chapter, we address these and other questions to clarify the importance of protein in the diet and dispel common myths about this crucial nutrient.

What Are Proteins?

Proteins are large, complex molecules found in the cells of all living things. Although proteins are best known as a part of our muscle mass, they are, in fact, critical components of all tissues of the human body, including bones, blood, and skin. Proteins also function in metabolism, immunity, fluid balance, and nutrient transport, and they can provide energy in certain circumstances. The functions of proteins will be discussed in detail later in this chapter.

How Do Proteins Differ from Carbohydrates and Lipids?

As we have seen (in Chapter 1), proteins are one of the three macronutrients. Like carbohydrates and lipids, proteins are found in a wide variety of foods; plus, the human body is able to synthesize them. But unlike carbohydrates and lipids, proteins are made according to instructions provided by our genetic material, or DNA. We'll explore how DNA dictates the structure of proteins shortly.

Another key difference between proteins and the other macronutrients lies in their chemical makeup. In addition to the carbon, hydrogen, and oxygen also found in carbohydrates and lipids, proteins contain a special form of nitrogen that the body can readily use. Our bodies are able to break down the proteins in foods and utilize the nitrogen for many important processes. Carbohydrates and lipids do not provide nitrogen.

The Building Blocks of Proteins Are Amino Acids

The proteins in our body are made from a combination of building blocks called **amino acids,** molecules composed of a central carbon atom connected to four other groups: an amine group, an acid group, a hydrogen atom, and a side chain (**Figure 6.1a**). The word *amine* means "nitrogen-containing," and nitrogen is indeed the essential component of the amine portion of the molecule.

As shown in Figure 6.1b, the portion of the amino acid that makes each unique is its side chain. The amine group, acid group, and carbon and hydrogen atoms do not vary. Variations in the structure of the side chain give each amino acid its distinct properties.

The singular term *protein* is misleading, as there are potentially an infinite number of unique types of proteins in living organisms. Most of the body's proteins are made from combinations of just 20 amino acids, identified in **Table 6.1** (page 219). Two of the twenty amino acids listed in Table 6.1, cysteine and methionine, are unique in that their side chains contain sulfur. This property affects the types of chemical bonds they form. By combining a few

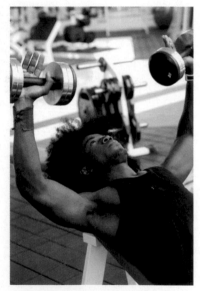

Proteins are an integral part of our body tissues, including our muscle tissue.

proteins Large, complex molecules made up of amino acids and found as essential components of all living cells.

amino acids Nitrogen-containing molecules that combine to form proteins.

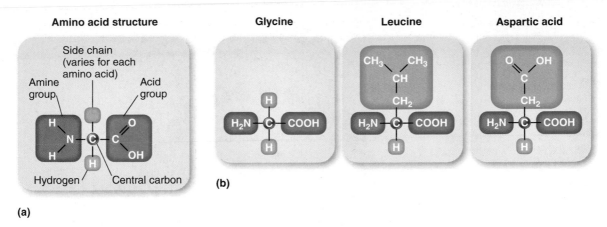

FIGURE 6.1 Structure of an amino acid. **(a)** All amino acids contain five parts: a central carbon atom, an amine group that contains nitrogen, an acid group, a hydrogen atom, and a side chain. **(b)** Only the side chain differs for each of the twenty amino acids, giving each its unique properties.

dozen to more than 300 of these 20 amino acids in various sequences, our body synthesizes an estimated 10,000 to 50,000 unique proteins. **Figure 6.2** (page 220) illustrates how the components of a protein differ from that of a carbohydrate, such as starch. As you can see, starch is composed of a chain of glucose molecules. In contrast, the protein insulin is composed of 51 amino acids connected in a specific order, or sequence. Notice that different regions of the molecule are connected by unique disulfide bridges linking the sulfur-containing cysteine amino acids. We'll discuss the structure of proteins in more detail shortly.

We Must Obtain Essential Amino Acids from Food

Of the twenty amino acids in the body, nine are classified as essential. This does not mean that they are more important than the others. Instead, an **essential amino acid** is one that the body cannot produce at all or cannot produce in sufficient quantities to meet its physiologic needs. Thus, essential amino acids must be obtained from food. Without the proper amount of essential amino acids in our bodies, we lose our ability to make the proteins and other nitrogen-containing compounds we need.

TABLE 6.1 Amino Acids of the Human Body

Essential Amino Acids	Nonessential Amino Acids
These amino acids must be consumed in the diet.	*These amino acids can be manufactured by the body.*
Histidine	Alanine
Isoleucine	Arginine
Leucine	Asparagine
Lysine	Aspartic acid
Methionine	Cysteine
Phenylalanine	Glutamic acid
Threonine	Glutamine
Tryptophan	Glycine
Valine	Proline
	Serine
	Tyrosine

essential amino acids Amino acids not produced by the body, or not produced in sufficient amounts, so they must be obtained from food.

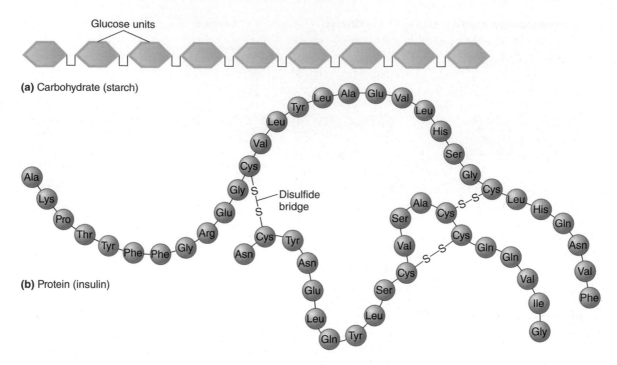

FIGURE 6.2 How proteins differ from starch. **(a)** Starch is composed of a chain of glucose molecules, whereas proteins are composed of multiple amino acids connected together. **(b)** Insulin is a protein that contains fifty-one amino acids in two chains that are connected by three disulfide bridges—two that connect the two amino acid chains and a third that connects a section of the shortest amino acid chain.

The Body Can Make Nonessential Amino Acids

Nonessential amino acids are just as important to the body as essential amino acids, but the body can synthesize them in sufficient quantities, so we do not need to consume them in our diet. We make nonessential amino acids by transferring the amine group from other amino acids to a different acid group and side chain. This process is called **transamination** and it is shown in **Figure 6.3**. The acid groups and side chains can be donated by amino acids, or they can be made from the breakdown products of carbohydrates and fats. Thus, by combining parts of different amino acids, the necessary nonessential amino acid can be made.

nonessential amino acids Amino acids that can be manufactured by the body in sufficient quantities and therefore do not need to be consumed regularly in our diet.

transamination The process of transferring the amine group from one amino acid to another in order to manufacture a new amino acid.

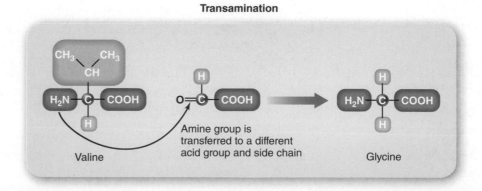

FIGURE 6.3 Transamination. Our bodies can make nonessential amino acids by transferring the amine group from an essential amino acid to a different acid group and side chain.

Under some conditions, a nonessential amino acid can become an essential amino acid. In this case, the amino acid is called a **conditionally essential amino acid.** Consider what occurs in the disease known as phenylketonuria (PKU). As previously discussed (in Chapter 4), someone with PKU cannot metabolize phenylalanine (an essential amino acid). Normally, the body uses phenylalanine to produce the nonessential amino acid tyrosine, so the inability to metabolize phenylalanine results in failure to make tyrosine. If PKU is not diagnosed immediately after birth, it results in irreversible brain damage. In this situation, tyrosine becomes a conditionally essential amino acid that must be provided by the diet. Other conditionally essential amino acids include arginine, cysteine, and glutamine.

RECAP

Proteins are critical components of all the tissues of the human body. Like carbohydrates and lipids, they contain carbon, hydrogen, and oxygen. Unlike the other macronutrients, they also contain nitrogen and some contain sulfur, and their structure is dictated by DNA. The building blocks of proteins are amino acids. The amine group of the amino acid contains nitrogen. The portion of the amino acid that changes, giving each amino acid its distinct identity, is the side chain. The body cannot make essential amino acids, so we must obtain them from our diet. The body can make nonessential amino acids from parts of other amino acids, carbohydrates, and fats. ■

Nutrition MILESTONE

In **1934**, Dr. Asbjøn Følling, a Norwegian physician and biochemist, examined children with mental retardation who were excreting urine that smelled unusually strong. He found that the urine contained a substance called phenylpyruvic acid, which is a by-product of the breakdown of the amino acid phenylalanine. Although a small amount of this by-product in the urine is normal, a large amount indicates an inability to completely break down phenylalanine. Initially named Følling's disease, this condition is now known as phenylketonuria, or PKU. It is a genetic disorder that causes a deficiency in the enzyme that breaks down phenylalanine.

In people with PKU, phenylalanine can build up in the body, causing brain damage, seizures, and psychiatric disorders. As a result of Følling's discovery, United States healthcare providers now screen the blood of all newborns for PKU. Those newborns found to have PKU are prescribed a diet low in phenylalanine, and they can develop into healthy children and adults.

How Are Proteins Made?

As stated, our bodies can synthesize proteins by selecting the needed amino acids from the pool of all amino acids available at any given time. Let's look more closely at how this occurs.

Amino Acids Bond to Form a Variety of Peptides

Figure 6.4 shows that, when two amino acids join together, the amine group of one binds to the acid group of another in a unique type of chemical bond called a **peptide bond.** In this dehydration synthesis reaction, a molecule of water is released as a by-product.

Two amino acids joined together form a *dipeptide*, and three amino acids joined together are called a *tripeptide*. The term *oligopeptide* is used to identify a string of four to

conditionally essential amino acids   Amino acids that are normally considered nonessential but become essential under certain circumstances when the body's need for them exceeds the ability to produce them.

peptide bonds   Unique types of chemical bonds in which the amine group of one amino acid binds to the acid group of another in order to manufacture dipeptides and all larger peptide molecules.

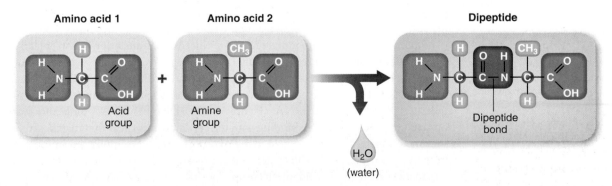

FIGURE 6.4 Amino acid bonding. Two amino acids join together to form a dipeptide. By combining multiple amino acids, proteins are made.

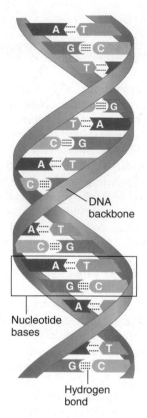

FIGURE 6.5 The double helix of DNA. DNA is a complex compound made up of molecules called nucleotides, each of which consists of a deoxyribose sugar and phosphate backbone and a nitrogenous base. Hydrogen bonding of complementary bases holds the two strands of DNA together.

gene expression The process of using a gene to make a protein.

nucleotide A molecule composed of a phosphate group, a pentose sugar called deoxyribose, and one of four nitrogenous bases: adenine (A), guanine (G), cytosine (C), or thymine (T).

transcription The process through which messenger RNA copies genetic information from DNA in the nucleus.

translation The process that occurs when the genetic information carried by messenger RNA is translated into a chain of amino acids at the ribosome.

nine amino acids, and a *polypeptide* is ten or more amino acids bonded together. As a polypeptide chain grows longer, it begins to fold into any of a variety of complex shapes that give proteins their sophisticated structure.

Genes Regulate Amino Acid Binding

Each of us is unique because we inherited a specific "code" that integrates the code from each of our parents. Each person's genetic code dictates minor differences in amino acid sequences, which in turn lead to differences in our bodies' individual proteins. These differences in proteins result in the unique physical and physiologic characteristics each one of us possesses. **Gene expression** is the process by which cells use genes to make proteins.

The Structure of Genes

A *gene* is a segment of deoxyribonucleic acid (DNA) that serves as a template for the synthesis—or expression—of a particular protein.

The building blocks of DNA are **nucleotides,** molecules composed of a "backbone" made up of a phosphate group and a pentose sugar called deoxyribose, to which is attached one of four nitrogenous bases: adenine (A), guanine (G), cytosine (C), or thymine (T). Within DNA molecules, these nucleotides occur in two long, parallel chains coiled into the shape of a double helix (**Figure 6.5**). Because nucleotides vary only in their nitrogenous bases, the astonishing variability of DNA arises from the precise sequencing of nucleotides along these chains.

Chains of nucleotides are held together by hydrogen bonds that link their nitrogenous bases. Each base can bond only to its *complementary base:* A always bonds to T, and G always bonds to C. The complementary nature of bases guides the transfer of genetic instructions from DNA into the resulting protein.

Transcription and Translation

Proteins are actually manufactured at the site of ribosomes in the cell's cytoplasm. But DNA never leaves the nucleus. So for gene expression to occur, a gene's DNA has to replicate itself—that is, it must make an exact copy of itself, which can then be carried out to the cytoplasm. DNA replication ensures that the genetic information in the original gene is identical to the genetic information used to build the protein. Through the process of replication, DNA provides the instructions for building every protein in the body.

Cells use a special molecule to copy, or transcribe, the information from DNA and carry it to the ribosomes. This molecule is *messenger RNA (messenger ribonucleic acid, or mRNA).* In contrast with DNA, RNA is a single strand of nucleotides, and its four nitrogenous bases are A, G, C, and U ("U" stands for uracil, which takes the place of the thymine found in DNA). Also, as its name suggests, it contains the pentose sugar ribose instead of deoxyribose. During **transcription,** mRNA copies to its own base sequence the genetic information from DNA's base sequence (**Figure 6.6**, no. 1). The mRNA then detaches from the DNA and leaves the nucleus, carrying its genetic "message" to the ribosomes in the cytoplasm (Figure 6.6, no. 2).

Once the genetic information reaches the ribosomes, **translation** occurs; that is, the language of the mRNA nucleotide sequences is translated into the language of amino acid sequences, or proteins. At the ribosomes, mRNA binds with ribosomal RNA (rRNA) and its nucleotide sequences are distributed, somewhat like orders for parts in an assembly plant, to molecules of transfer RNA (tRNA) (Figure 6.6, no. 3). Now the tRNA molecules roam the cytoplasm until they succeed in binding with the specific amino acid that matches their "order." They then transfer their amino acid to the ribosome, which assembles the amino acids into proteins (Figure 6.6, no. 4). Once the amino acids are loaded onto the ribosome, tRNA works to maneuver each amino acid into its proper position (Figure 6.6, no. 5). When synthesis of the new protein is completed, it is released from the ribosome and can either go through further modification in the cell or can be functional in its current state (Figure 6.6, no. 6).

Protein Synthesis

Cell ——

Nucleus ——

In the nucleus, genetic information from DNA is transcribed by messenger RNA (mRNA), which then carries it to ribosomes in the cytoplasm, where this genetic information is translated into a chain of amino acids that eventually make a protein.

1 Part of the DNA unwinds, and a section of its genetic code is transcribed to the mRNA inside the nucleus.

2 The mRNA leaves the nucleus via a nuclear pore and travels to the cytoplasm.

3 Once the mRNA reaches the cytoplasm, it binds to a ribosome via ribosomal RNA (rRNA). The code on the mRNA is translated into the instructions for a specific order of amino acids.

4 The transfer RNA (tRNA) binds with specific amino acids in the cytoplasm and transfers the amino acids to the ribosome as dictated by the mRNA code.

5 The amino acid is added to the growing amino acid chain, and the tRNA returns to the cytoplasm.

6 Once the synthesis of the new protein is complete, the protein is released from the ribosome. The protein may go through further modifications in the cell or can be functional in its current state.

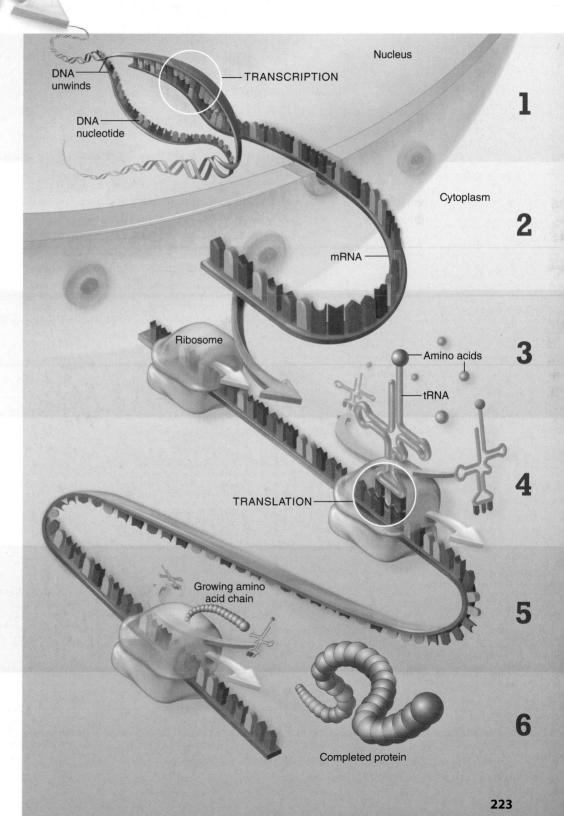

DNA unwinds

DNA nucleotide

TRANSCRIPTION

Nucleus

Cytoplasm

mRNA

Ribosome

Amino acids

tRNA

TRANSLATION

Growing amino acid chain

Completed protein

1

2

3

4

5

6

The proper sequencing of amino acids determines both the shape and function of a particular protein. Genetic abnormalities can occur when the DNA contains errors in proper nucleotide sequencing or when mistakes occur in the translation of this sequencing. Two examples of the consequences of these types of genetic abnormalities, sickle cell anemia and cystic fibrosis, are discussed later in this chapter.

Although the DNA for making every protein in our bodies is contained within each cell nucleus, not all genes are expressed and each cell does not make every type of protein. For example, each cell contains the DNA to manufacture the hormone insulin. However, only the beta cells of the pancreas *express* the insulin gene to produce insulin. As we explored (in the **Nutrition Debate** in Chapter 1), our physiologic needs alter gene expression, as do various nutrients. For instance, a cut in the skin that causes bleeding will prompt the production of various proteins that clot the blood. Or if we consume more dietary iron than we need, the gene for ferritin (a protein that stores iron) will be expressed, so that we can store this excess iron. Our genetic makeup and how appropriately we express our genes are important factors in our health.

Protein Turnover Involves Synthesis and Degradation

Our bodies constantly require new proteins to function properly. *Protein turnover* involves both the synthesis of new proteins and the degradation of existing proteins to provide the building blocks for those new proteins (**Figure 6.7**). This process allows the cells to respond to the constantly changing demands of physiologic functions. For instance, skin cells live only for about 30 days and must continually be replaced. The amino acids needed to produce these new skin cells can be obtained from the body's *amino acid pool*, which includes those amino acids we consume in our diet as well as those that are released from the breakdown of other cells in our bodies. The body's pool of amino acids is used to produce not only new amino acids but also other products, including glucose, fat, and urea.

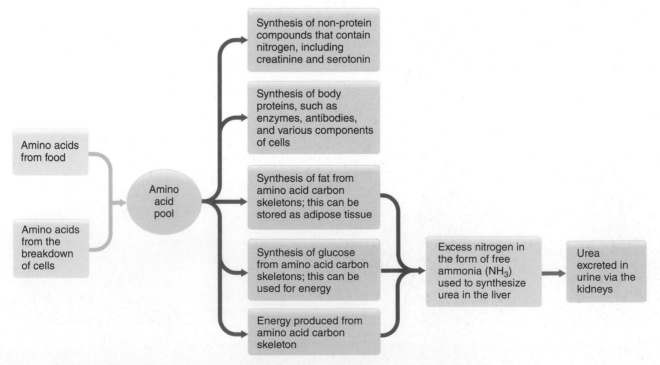

FIGURE 6.7 Protein turnover involves the synthesis of new proteins and the breakdown of existing proteins to provide building blocks for new proteins. Amino acids are drawn from the body's amino acid pool and can be used to build proteins, fat, glucose, and non-protein nitrogen-containing compounds. Urea is produced as a waste product from any excess nitrogen, which is then excreted by the kidneys.

Protein Organization Determines Function

Four levels of protein structure have been identified (**Figure 6.8**). The sequential order of the amino acids in a protein is called the *primary structure* of the protein. The different amino acids in a polypeptide chain possess unique chemical attributes that cause the chain to twist and turn into a characteristic spiral shape, or to fold into a so-called pleated sheet. These shapes are also referred to as the protein's *secondary structure*. The stability of the secondary structure is achieved by hydrogen bonds that create a bridge between two protein strands or two parts of the same strand of protein (see Figure 6.2). The spiral or pleated sheet of the secondary structure further folds into a unique three-dimensional shape, referred to as the protein's *tertiary structure*. Both hydrogen bonds and disulfide bridges between sulfur atoms maintain the tertiary shape, which is critically important because it determines each protein's function in the body. Often, two or more identical or different polypeptides bond to form an even larger protein with a *quaternary structure*, which may be *globular* or *fibrous*.

The importance of the shape of a protein to its function cannot be overemphasized. For example, the protein strands in muscle fibers are much longer than they are wide (Figure 6.8d). This structure plays an essential role in enabling muscle contraction and relaxation. In contrast, the proteins that form red blood cells are globular in shape, and they result in the red blood cells being shaped like flattened discs with depressed centers, similar to a miniature doughnut (**Figure 6.9**, page 226). This structure and the flexibility of the proteins in the red blood cells permit them to change shape and flow freely through even the tiniest capillaries to deliver oxygen and still return to their original shape.

Protein Denaturation Affects Shape and Function

Proteins can uncoil and lose their shape when they are exposed to heat, acids, bases, heavy metals, alcohol, and other damaging substances. The term used to describe this change in

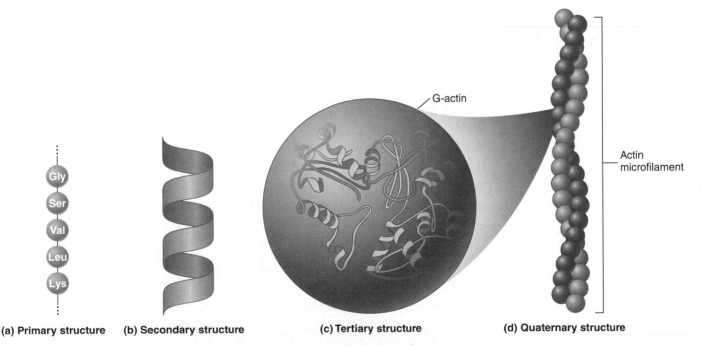

(a) Primary structure   **(b) Secondary structure**   **(c) Tertiary structure**   **(d) Quaternary structure**

FIGURE 6.8 Levels of protein structure. **(a)** The primary structure of a protein is the sequential order of amino acids. **(b)** The secondary structure of a protein is the twisting or folding of the amino acid chain. **(c)** The tertiary structure is a further folding that results in the three-dimensional shape of the protein. **(d)** In proteins with a quaternary structure, two or more polypeptides interact, forming a larger protein, such as the actin molecule illustrated here. In this figure, strands of actin molecules intertwine to form contractile elements involved in generating muscle contractions.

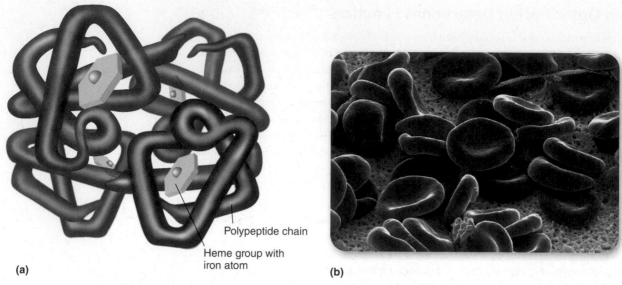

(a)

Polypeptide chain

Heme group with
iron atom

(b)

FIGURE 6.9 Protein shape determines function. **(a)** Hemoglobin, the protein that forms red blood cells, is globular in shape. **(b)** The globular shape of hemoglobin results in red blood cells being shaped like flattened discs.

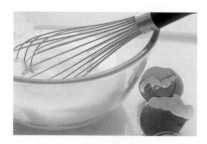

Stiffening egg whites adds air through the beating action, which denatures some of the proteins within them.

denaturation The process by which proteins uncoil and lose their shape and function when they are exposed to heat, acids, bases, heavy metals, alcohol, and other damaging substances.

limiting amino acid The essential amino acid that is missing or in the smallest supply in the amino acid pool and is thus responsible for slowing or halting protein synthesis.

incomplete proteins Foods that do not contain all of the essential amino acids in sufficient amounts to support growth and health.

complete proteins Foods that contain sufficient amounts of all nine essential amino acids.

the shape of proteins is **denaturation.** Everyday examples of protein denaturation that we can see are the stiffening of egg whites when they are whipped, the curdling of milk when lemon juice or another acid is added, and the solidifying of eggs as they cook.

Denaturation does not affect the primary structure of proteins. However, when a protein is denatured, its function is also lost. For instance, denaturation of critical body proteins on exposure to heat or acidity is harmful, because it prevents them from performing their functions. This type of denaturation can occur during times of high fever or when blood pH is out of the normal range. In some cases, however, denaturation is helpful. For instance, denaturation of proteins during the digestive process allows for their breakdown into amino acids and the absorption of these amino acids from the digestive tract into the bloodstream.

Protein Synthesis Can Be Limited by Missing Amino Acids

For protein synthesis to occur, all essential amino acids must be available to the cell. If this is not the case, the amino acid that is missing or in the smallest supply is called the **limiting amino acid.** Without the proper combination and quantity of essential amino acids, protein synthesis slows to the point at which proteins cannot be generated. For instance, the protein hemoglobin contains the essential amino acid histidine. If we do not consume enough histidine, it becomes the limiting amino acid in hemoglobin production. As no other amino acid can be substituted, our bodies become unable to produce adequate hemoglobin, and we lose the ability to transport oxygen to our cells.

Inadequate energy consumption also limits protein synthesis. If there is not enough energy available from our diets, our bodies will use any accessible amino acids for energy, thus preventing them from being used to build new proteins.

Protein that do not contain all of the essential amino acids in sufficient quantities to support growth and health are called **incomplete** (*low-quality*) **proteins.** Proteins that have all nine of the essential amino acids in sufficient quantities are considered **complete** (*high-quality*) **proteins.** The most complete protein sources are foods derived from animals and include egg whites, meat, poultry, fish, and milk. Soybeans are the most complete source of plant protein. In general, the typical American diet is very high in complete proteins, as we eat proteins from a variety of food sources.

Protein Synthesis Can Be Enhanced by Mutual Supplementation

Many people believe that we must consume meat or dairy products to obtain complete proteins. Not true! Consider a meal of beans and rice. Beans are low in the amino acids methionine and cysteine but have adequate amounts of isoleucine and lysine. Rice is low in isoleucine and lysine but contains sufficient methionine and cysteine. By combining beans and rice, a complete protein source is created.

Mutual supplementation is the process of combining two or more incomplete protein sources to make a complete protein. The two foods involved are called complementary foods; these foods provide **complementary proteins (Figure 6.10)** which, when combined, provide all nine essential amino acids.

It is not necessary to eat complementary proteins at the same meal. Recall that we maintain a free pool of amino acids in the blood; these amino acids come from food and sloughed-off cells. When we eat one complementary protein, its amino acids join those in the free amino acid pool. These free amino acids can then combine to synthesize complete proteins. However, it is wise to eat complementary-protein foods during the same day, as partially completed proteins cannot be stored and saved for a later time. Mutual supplementation is important for people eating a vegetarian diet, particularly if they consume no animal products whatsoever.

mutual supplementation The process of combining two or more incomplete protein sources to make a complete protein.

complementary proteins Proteins contained in two or more foods that together contain all nine essential amino acids necessary for a complete protein. It is not necessary to eat complementary proteins at the same meal.

Combining Complementary Foods

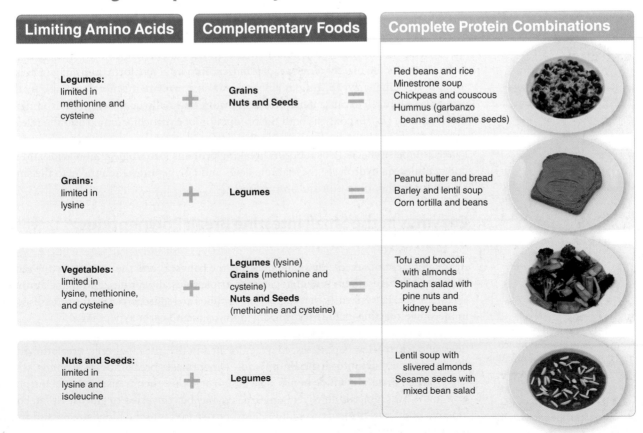

Limiting Amino Acids	Complementary Foods	Complete Protein Combinations
Legumes: limited in methionine and cysteine	**+** **Grains** **Nuts and Seeds** **=**	Red beans and rice Minestrone soup Chickpeas and couscous Hummus (garbanzo beans and sesame seeds)
Grains: limited in lysine	**+** **Legumes** **=**	Peanut butter and bread Barley and lentil soup Corn tortilla and beans
Vegetables: limited in lysine, methionine, and cysteine	**+** **Legumes** (lysine) **Grains** (methionine and cysteine) **Nuts and Seeds** (methionine and cysteine) **=**	Tofu and broccoli with almonds Spinach salad with pine nuts and kidney beans
Nuts and Seeds: limited in lysine and isoleucine	**+** **Legumes** **=**	Lentil soup with slivered almonds Sesame seeds with mixed bean salad

FIGURE 6.10 Complementary food combinations.

Amino acids bind together to form proteins. Genes regulate the amino acid sequence, and thus the structure, of all proteins. During transcription, mRNA copies to its own base sequence the genetic information from DNA. mRNA carries this information from the cell nucleus to the ribosomes in the cytoplasm, where translation into proteins occurs. Protein turnover involves the synthesis and degradation of proteins, so that the body can constantly adapt to a changing environment. The shape of a protein determines its function. When a protein is denatured by heat or damaging substances, such as acids, it loses its shape and its function. When a particular amino acid is limiting, protein synthesis cannot occur. A complete protein provides all nine essential amino acids. Mutual supplementation combines two or more complementary-protein sources to make a complete protein. ■

How Does the Body Break Down Proteins?

The body does not directly use proteins from the diet to make the proteins it needs. Dietary proteins are first digested and broken into amino acids, so that they can be absorbed and transported to the cells. In this section, we will review how proteins are digested and absorbed. As you review each step in this process, refer to **Figure 6.11** for a visual overview of the process of protein digestion.

Stomach Acids and Enzymes Break Proteins into Short Polypeptides

Virtually no enzymatic digestion of proteins occurs in the mouth. As shown in Figure 6.11, proteins in food are chewed, crushed, and moistened with saliva to ease swallowing and to increase the surface area of the protein for more efficient digestion. There is no further digestive action on proteins in the mouth.

When proteins reach the stomach, hydrochloric acid denatures the protein strands. It also converts the inactive enzyme, *pepsinogen,* into its active form, **pepsin,** which is a protein-digesting enzyme. Although pepsin is itself a protein, it is not denatured by the acid in the stomach because it has evolved to work optimally in an acidic environment. The hormone *gastrin* controls both the production of hydrochloric acid and the release of pepsin; thinking about food or actually chewing food stimulates the gastrin-producing cells located in the stomach. Pepsin begins breaking proteins into single amino acids and shorter polypeptides via hydrolysis; these amino acids and polypeptides then travel to the small intestine for further digestion and absorption.

Enzymes in the Small Intestine Break Polypeptides into Single Amino Acids

As the polypeptides reach the small intestine, the pancreas and the small intestine secrete enzymes that digest them into oligopeptides, tripeptides, dipeptides, and single amino acids (Figure 6.11). The enzymes that digest polypeptides are called **proteases;** proteases found in the small intestine include trypsin, chymotrypsin, and carboxypeptidase.

The cells in the wall of the small intestine then absorb the single amino acids, dipeptides, and tripeptides. Peptidases, enzymes located in the intestinal cells, break the dipeptides and tripeptides into single amino acids. Dipeptidases break dipeptide bonds, whereas tripeptidases break tripeptide bonds. The amino acids are then transported via the portal vein to the liver. Once in the liver, amino acids may be converted to glucose or fat, combined to build new proteins, used for energy, or released into the bloodstream and transported to other cells as needed (Figure 6.11).

pepsin   An enzyme in the stomach that begins the breakdown of proteins into shorter polypeptide chains and single amino acids.

proteases   Enzymes that continue the breakdown of polypeptides in the small intestine.

Protein Digestion Overview

Digestion of dietary proteins into single amino acids occurs primarily in the stomach and small intestine. The single amino acids are then transported to the liver, where they may be converted to glucose or fat, used for energy or to build new proteins, or transported to cells as needed.

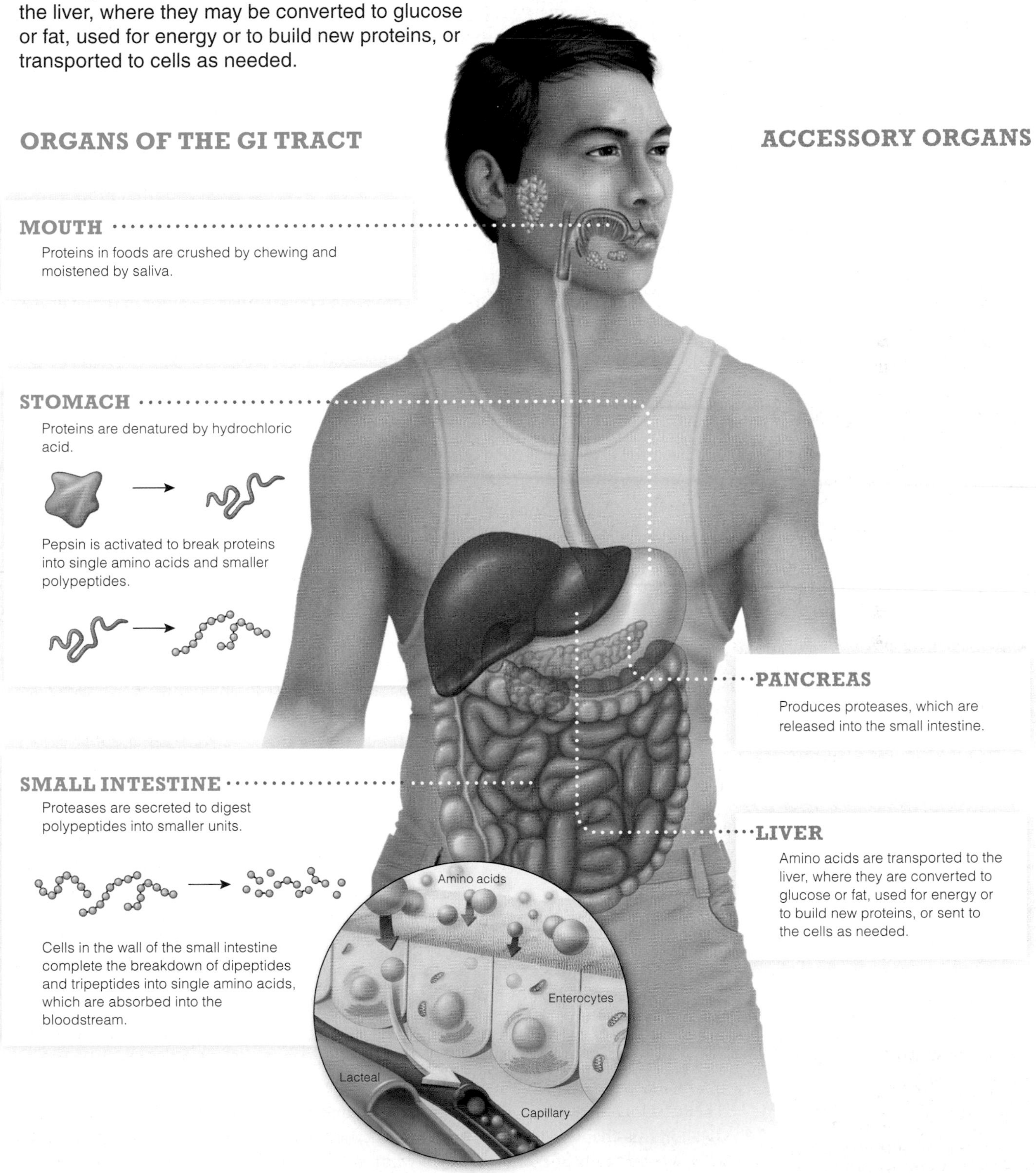

ORGANS OF THE GI TRACT

ACCESSORY ORGANS

MOUTH

Proteins in foods are crushed by chewing and moistened by saliva.

STOMACH

Proteins are denatured by hydrochloric acid.

Pepsin is activated to break proteins into single amino acids and smaller polypeptides.

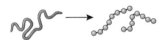

SMALL INTESTINE

Proteases are secreted to digest polypeptides into smaller units.

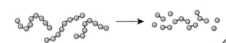

Cells in the wall of the small intestine complete the breakdown of dipeptides and tripeptides into single amino acids, which are absorbed into the bloodstream.

PANCREAS

Produces proteases, which are released into the small intestine.

LIVER

Amino acids are transported to the liver, where they are converted to glucose or fat, used for energy or to build new proteins, or sent to the cells as needed.

Amino acids

Enterocytes

Lacteal

Capillary

The cells of the small intestine have different sites that specialize in transporting certain types of amino acids, dipeptides, and tripeptides. This fact has implications for users of amino acid supplements. When very large doses of supplements containing single amino acids are taken on an empty stomach, they typically compete for the same absorption sites. This competition can block the absorption of other amino acids and could in theory lead to deficiencies. In reality, people rarely take very large doses of single amino acids on an empty stomach. We discuss the use of amino acid supplements in more detail later in this chapter.

Protein Digestibility Affects Protein Quality

Earlier in this chapter, we discussed how various protein sources differ in quality of protein. The quantity of essential amino acids in a protein determines its quality: higher-protein-quality foods are those that contain more of the essential amino acids in sufficient quantities needed to build proteins, and lower-protein-quality foods contain fewer essential amino acids.

A number of methods are used to estimate a food's protein quality. One method is to calculate a *chemical score*. A **chemical score** is a comparison of the amount of the limiting amino acid in a food to the amount of the same amino acid in a reference food. The amino acid that is found to have the lowest proportion in the test food as compared to the reference food is defined as the limiting amino acid. Thus, the chemical score of a protein gives an indication of the lowest amino acid ratio calculated for any amino acid in a particular food.

Another factor in protein quality is *digestibility*, or how well our bodies can digest a protein. The **protein digestibility corrected amino acid score (PDCAAS)** uses the chemical score and a correction factor for digestibility to calculate a value for protein quality. Proteins with higher digestibility are more complete. Animal protein sources, such as meat and dairy products, are highly digestible, as are many soy products; we can absorb more than 90% of these protein sources. Legumes are also highly digestible (about 70% to 80%). Grains and many vegetable proteins are less digestible, with PDCAAS values ranging from 60% to 90%.

These measures of protein quality are useful when determining the quality of protein available to populations of people. However, these measures are impractical and are not used for individual diet planning.

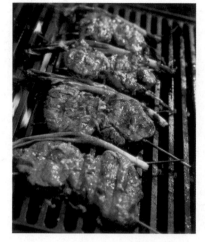

Meats are highly digestible sources of dietary protein.

RECAP

In the stomach, hydrochloric acid denatures proteins and converts pepsinogen to pepsin; pepsin breaks proteins into smaller polypeptides and individual amino acids. In the small intestine, proteases break polypeptides into smaller fragments and single amino acids. Enzymes in the cells in the wall of the small intestine break the smaller peptide fragments into single amino acids, which are then transported to the liver for distribution to our cells. Taking high doses of individual amino acid supplements can lead to deficiencies of other amino acids. Protein digestibility and the provision of essential amino acids influence protein quality. ■

chemical score A method used to estimate a food's protein quality; it is a comparison of the amount of the limiting amino acid in a food to the amount of the same amino acid in a reference food.

protein digestibility corrected amino acid score (PDCAAS) A measurement of protein quality that considers the balance of amino acids as well as the digestibility of the protein in the food.

Why Do We Need Proteins?

The functions of proteins in the body are so numerous that only a few can be described in detail in this chapter. Note that proteins function most effectively when we also consume adequate amounts of energy as carbohydrates and fat. When there is not enough energy available, the body uses proteins as an energy source, limiting their availability for the functions described in this section.

Proteins Contribute to Cell Growth, Repair, and Maintenance

The proteins in the body are dynamic, meaning that they are constantly being broken down, repaired, and replaced. When proteins are broken down, many amino acids are recycled into new proteins. Think about all of the new proteins that are needed to allow an embryo to develop and grow. In this case, an entirely new human body is being made! In fact, a newborn baby has more than 10 trillion body cells.

Even in adulthood, all cells are constantly turning over, as damaged or worn-out cells are broken down and their components are used to create new cells. Red blood cells live for only 3 to 4 months and then are replaced by new cells that are produced in bone marrow. The cells lining the intestinal tract are replaced every 3 to 6 days. The "old" intestinal cells are treated just like the proteins in food; they are digested and the amino acids absorbed back into the body. The constant turnover of proteins from our diet is essential for such cell growth, repair, and maintenance.

Proteins Act as Enzymes and Hormones

Recall that enzymes are compounds—usually proteins—that speed up chemical reactions, without being changed by the chemical reaction themselves. Enzymes can increase the rate at which reactants bond, break apart, or exchange components. **Figure 6.12** shows how an enzyme can facilitate bonding between two compounds.

Each cell contains thousands of enzymes that facilitate specific cellular reactions. For example, the enzyme phosphofructokinase (PFK) is critical to driving the rate at which we break down glucose and use it for energy during exercise. Without PFK, we would be unable to generate energy at a fast enough rate to allow us to be physically active.

Hormones are substances that act as chemical messengers in the body. Some hormones are made from amino acids, whereas others are made from lipids (refer to Chapter 5). Hormones are stored in various glands in the body, which release them in response to changes in the body's environment. They then act on the body's organs and tissues to restore the body to normal conditions. For example, recall that insulin, a hormone made from amino acids, acts on cell membranes to facilitate the transport of glucose into cells. Other examples of amino-acid-containing hormones are glucagon, which responds to conditions of low blood glucose, and thyroid hormone, which helps control our resting metabolic rate.

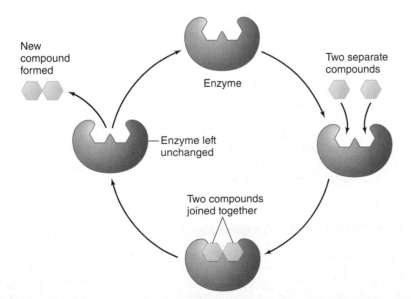

FIGURE 6.12 Proteins act as enzymes. Enzymes facilitate chemical reactions, such as joining two compounds together.

Proteins Help Maintain Fluid and Electrolyte Balance

Electrolytes are electrically charged atoms (ions) that assist in maintaining fluid balance. For our bodies to function properly, fluids and electrolytes must be maintained at healthy levels inside and outside cells and within blood vessels. Proteins attract fluids, and the proteins that are in the bloodstream, in the cells, and in the spaces surrounding the cells work together to keep fluids moving across these spaces in the proper quantities to maintain fluid balance and blood pressure. When protein intake is deficient, the concentration of proteins in the bloodstream is insufficient to draw fluid from the tissues and across the blood vessel walls; fluid then collects in the tissues, causing **edema** (**Figure 6.13**). In addition to being uncomfortable, edema can lead to serious medical problems.

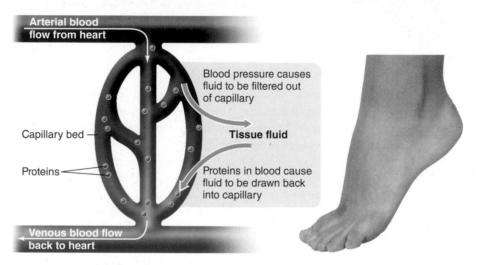

(a) Normal fluid balance

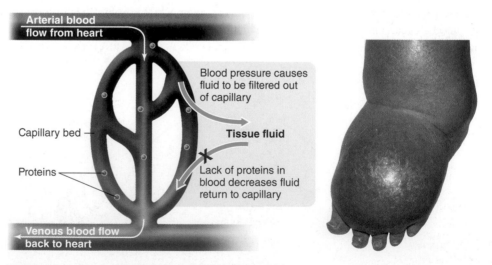

(b) Edema caused by insufficient protein in bloodstream

FIGURE 6.13 The role of proteins in maintaining fluid balance. The heartbeat exerts pressure that continually pushes fluids in the bloodstream through the arterial walls and out into the tissue spaces. By the time blood reaches the veins, the pressure of the heartbeat has greatly decreased. In this environment, proteins in the blood are able to draw fluids out of the tissues and back into the bloodstream. **(a)** This healthy (non-swollen) tissue suggests that body fluids in the bloodstream and in the tissue spaces are in balance. **(b)** When the level of proteins in the blood is insufficient to draw fluids out of the tissues, edema can result. This foot with edema is swollen due to fluid imbalance.

edema A potentially serious disorder in which fluids build up in the tissue spaces of the body, causing fluid imbalances and a swollen appearance.

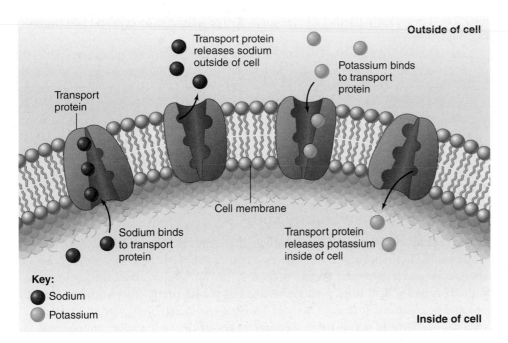

FIGURE 6.14 Transport proteins help maintain electrolyte balance. Transport proteins in the cell membrane pick up potassium and sodium and transport them across the cell membrane.

Sodium (Na^+) and potassium (K^+) are examples of common electrolytes. Under normal conditions, Na^+ is more concentrated outside the cell, and K^+ is more concentrated inside the cell. This proper balance of Na^+ and K^+ is accomplished by the action of **transport proteins** located within the cell membrane. **Figure 6.14** shows how these transport proteins work to pump Na^+ outside and K^+ inside of the cell. The conduction of nerve signals and contraction of muscles depend on a proper balance of electrolytes. If protein intake is deficient, we lose our ability to maintain these functions, resulting in potentially fatal changes in the rhythm of the heart. Other consequences of chronically low protein intakes include muscle weakness and spasms, kidney failure, and, if conditions are severe enough, death.

Proteins Help Maintain Acid–Base Balance

The body's cellular processes result in the constant production of acids and bases. These substances are transported in the blood to be excreted through the kidneys and the lungs. The human body maintains very tight control over the **pH,** or the acid–base balance, of the blood. The body goes into a state called **acidosis** when the blood becomes too acidic. **Alkalosis** results if the blood becomes too basic. Both acidosis and alkalosis can be caused by respiratory or metabolic problems. Acidosis and alkalosis can cause coma and death by denaturing body proteins.

Proteins are excellent **buffers,** meaning they help maintain proper acid–base balance. Acids contain hydrogen ions, which are positively charged. The side chains of proteins have negative charges that attract the hydrogen ions and neutralize their detrimental effects on the body. Proteins can release the hydrogen ions when the blood becomes too basic. By buffering acids and bases, proteins maintain acid–base balance and blood pH.

Proteins Help Maintain a Strong Immune System

Antibodies are special proteins that are critical components of the immune system. When a foreign substance attacks the body, the immune system produces antibodies to defend against it. Bacteria, viruses, toxins, and allergens (substances that cause allergic reactions) are examples of antigens that can trigger antibody production. (An *antigen* is any

transport proteins Protein molecules that help transport substances throughout the body and across cell membranes.

pH An abbreviation for percentage of hydrogen. It is a measure of the acidity—or level of hydrogen—of any solution, including human blood.

acidosis A disorder in which the blood becomes acidic; that is, the level of hydrogen in the blood is excessive. It can be caused by respiratory or metabolic problems.

alkalosis A disorder in which the blood becomes basic; that is, the level of hydrogen in the blood is deficient. It can be caused by respiratory or metabolic problems.

buffers Proteins that help maintain proper acid–base balance by attaching to, or releasing, hydrogen ions as conditions change in the body.

antibodies Defensive proteins of the immune system. Their production is prompted by the presence of bacteria, viruses, toxins, and allergens.

To learn more about how blood clots and wounds heal, go to www.nlm.nih.gov/medlineplus/ency/anatomyvideos/000011.htm.

substance—but typically a protein—that our bodies recognize as foreign and that triggers an immune response.)

Each antibody is designed to target one specific invader. When that substance invades the body, antibodies are produced to neutralize or target the specific antigen so that it can be subsequently destroyed. Once antibodies have been made, the body "remembers" this process and can respond more quickly the next time that invader appears. *Immunity* refers to the development of the molecular memory to produce antibodies quickly upon subsequent invasions.

Adequate protein is necessary to support the increased production of antibodies that occurs in response to a cold, flu, or an allergic reaction. If we do not consume enough protein, our resistance to illnesses and disease is weakened. On the other hand, eating more protein than we need does not improve immune function.

Proteins Serve as an Energy Source

The body's primary energy sources are carbohydrate and fat. Remember that both carbohydrate and fat have specialized storage forms that can be used for energy—glycogen for carbohydrate and triglycerides for fat. Proteins do not have a specialized storage form for energy. This means that, when proteins need to be used for energy, they are taken from the blood and body tissues, such as the liver and skeletal muscle. In healthy people, proteins contribute very little to energy needs. Because we are efficient at recycling amino acids, protein needs are relatively low compared to needs for carbohydrate and fat.

To use proteins for energy, the liver removes the amine group from the amino acids in a process called **deamination.** The nitrogen bonds with hydrogen, creating ammonia, which is a toxic compound that can upset acid–base balance. To avoid this, the liver quickly combines ammonia with carbon dioxide to make *urea*, which is much less toxic. The urea is then transported via the bloodstream to the kidneys, where the urea is filtered out of the blood and is subsequently excreted in the urine (**Figure 6.15**). The remaining fragments of the amino acid contain carbon, hydrogen, and oxygen. The body can use these fragments to generate energy or to build carbohydrates. Certain amino acids can be converted into glucose via gluconeogenesis. This is a critical process during times of low carbohydrate intake or starvation. Fat cannot be converted into glucose, but body proteins can be broken down and converted into glucose to provide needed energy to the brain.

To protect the proteins in our body tissues, it is important that we regularly eat an adequate amount of carbohydrate and fat to provide energy. We also need to consume enough dietary protein to perform the required work without using up the proteins that already are playing an active role in our bodies. Unfortunately, the body cannot store excess dietary protein. As a consequence, eating too much protein results in the removal and excretion of the nitrogen in the urine and the use of the remaining components for energy. Any remaining components not used for energy can be converted and stored as body fat.

Proteins Assist in the Transport and Storage of Nutrients

Proteins act as carriers for many important nutrients in the body. As previously discussed (in Chapter 5), lipoproteins contain lipids bound to proteins, which allows the transport of hydrophobic lipids through the watery medium of blood. Another example of a transport protein is transferrin, which carries iron in the blood. Ferritin, in contrast, is an example of a storage protein: it is the compound in which iron is stored in the liver.

As discussed on page 233, transport proteins are located in cell membranes and allow for the proper transport of many nutrients across the cell membrane. These transport proteins also help in the maintenance of fluid and electrolyte balance and conduction of nerve impulses.

Other Roles of Proteins

The amino acids from proteins can also be used to make compounds such as **neurotransmitters,** which are chemical messengers that transmit messages from one nerve cell to another. Examples of neurotransmitters include epinephrine and norepinephrine, both of

deamination The process by which an amine group is removed from an amino acid. The nitrogen is then transported to the kidneys for excretion in the urine, and the carbon and other components are metabolized for energy or used to make other compounds.

neurotransmitters Chemical messengers that transmit messages from one nerve cell to another.

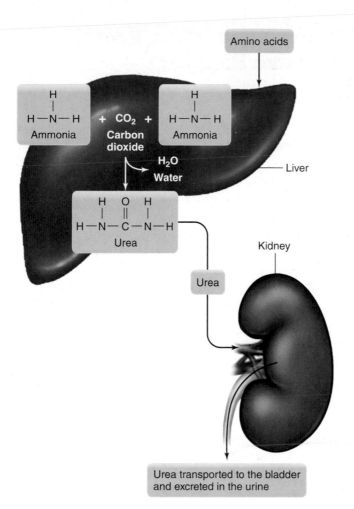

FIGURE 6.15 Urea excretion. The process of deamination leads to the creation of ammonia, which the liver quickly combines with carbon dioxide to make urea. The urea is then transported via the bloodstream to the kidneys, where the urea is filtered out of the blood and is subsequently excreted in the urine.

which stimulate the sympathetic nervous system, and *melatonin*, which plays a critical role in the regulation of sleep. Proteins also assist in blood clotting via a mass of protein fibers called *fibrin*; fibrin is developed from the protein *fibrinogen*. The scar tissue that is formed to heal wounds is comprised of another protein, *collagen*.

RECAP

Proteins serve many important functions: (1) enabling growth, repair, and maintenance of body tissues; (2) acting as enzymes and hormones; (3) maintaining fluid and electrolyte balance; (4) maintaining acid–base balance; (5) making antibodies, which strengthen the immune system; (6) providing energy when carbohydrate and fat intake are inadequate; (7) transporting and storing nutrients; and (8) producing compounds such as neurotransmitters, fibrin, and collagen. Proteins function best when adequate amounts of energy, carbohydrate, and fat are consumed. ◼

How Much Protein Should We Eat?

Consuming adequate protein is a major concern of many people. In fact, one of the most common issues among active people and athletes is that their diets are deficient in protein (see the **Nutrition Myth or Fact?** box (page 236) for a discussion of this topic). This concern about dietary protein is generally unnecessary, as we can easily consume the protein our bodies need by eating an adequate and varied diet.

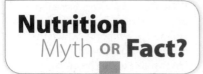

Nutrition
Myth OR **Fact?**

Do Athletes Need More Protein Than Inactive People?

At one time, it was believed that the Recommended Dietary Allowance (RDA) for protein, which is 0.8 g/kg body weight, was sufficient for both inactive people and athletes. Recent studies, however, show that athletes' protein needs are higher.

Why do athletes need more protein? Regular exercise increases the transport of oxygen to body tissues, requiring changes in the oxygen-carrying capacity of the blood. To carry more oxygen, we need to produce more of the protein that carries oxygen in the blood (hemoglobin). During intense exercise, we use a small amount of protein directly for energy. We also use protein to make glucose to maintain adequate blood glucose levels and to prevent hypoglycemia (low blood sugar) during exercise. Regular exercise stimulates tissue and causes tissue damage, which must be repaired by additional proteins. Current consensus from the American College of Sports Medicine, American Dietetic Association, and Dietitians of Canada is that strength athletes (such as bodybuilders and weightlifters) need 1.8 to 2 times more protein than the current RDA, and endurance athletes (such as distance runners and triathletes) need 1.5 to 1.75 times more protein than the current RDA.[1] More recent evidence suggests that the optimal protein needs for both types of athletes may be 1.6 to 2.25 times higher than the current RDA.[2]

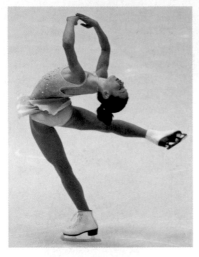

Some athletes who diet persistently are at risk for low protein intake.

Later in this chapter, we will calculate the protein needs for inactive and active people.

If you're active, does this mean you should add more protein to your diet? Not necessarily. Contrary to popular belief, most Americans, including inactive people *and athletes*, already consume more than twice the RDA for protein. For healthy individuals, evidence does not support eating more than two times the RDA for protein to increase strength, build muscle, or improve athletic performance. In fact, eating more protein as food or supplements or taking individual amino acid supplements does not cause muscles to become bigger or stronger. Only regular strength training can achieve these goals. By eating a balanced diet and consuming a variety of foods, both inactive and active people can easily meet their protein requirements.

References

1. American College of Sports Medicine, American Dietetic Association, and Dietitians of Canada. 2009. Joint position statement. Nutrition and athletic performance. *Med. Sci. Sports Exerc.* 41(3):709–731.
2. Phillips, S. M., and L. J. C. van Loon. 2011. Dietary protein for athletes: from requirements to optimum adaptation. *J. Sports Sci.* 29(suppl. 1):S29–S38.

Nitrogen Balance Is a Method Used to Determine Protein Needs

A highly specialized procedure referred to as *nitrogen balance* is used to determine a person's protein needs. Nitrogen is excreted through the body's processes of recycling or using proteins; thus, the balance can be used to estimate if protein intake is adequate to meet protein needs.

Typically performed only in experimental laboratories, the nitrogen-balance procedure involves measuring both nitrogen intake and nitrogen excretion over a 2-week period. A standardized diet, the nitrogen content of which has been measured and recorded, is fed to the study participant. The person is required to consume all of the foods provided. Because the majority of nitrogen is excreted in the urine and feces, laboratory technicians directly measure the nitrogen content of the subject's urine and fecal samples. Small amounts of nitrogen are excreted in the skin, hair, and body fluids such as mucus and semen, but because of the complexity of collecting nitrogen excreted via these routes, the measurements are estimated. Then, technicians add the estimated nitrogen losses to the nitrogen measured in the subject's urine and feces. Nitrogen balance is then calculated as the difference between nitrogen intake and nitrogen excretion.

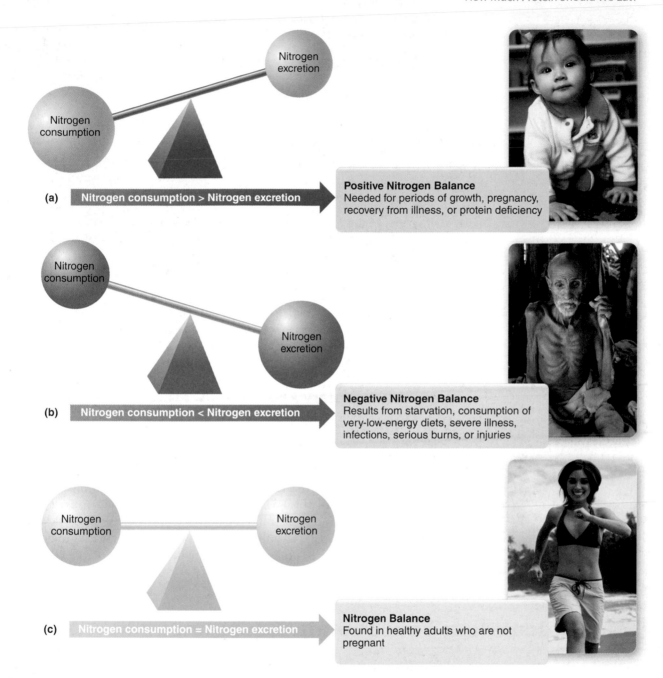

FIGURE 6.16 *Nitrogen balance* describes the relationship between how much nitrogen (protein) we consume and how much we excrete each day. **(a)** Positive nitrogen balance occurs when nitrogen consumption is greater than excretion. **(b)** Negative nitrogen balance occurs when nitrogen consumption is less than excretion. **(c)** Nitrogen balance is maintained when nitrogen consumption equals excretion.

People who consume more nitrogen than is excreted are considered to be in positive nitrogen balance (**Figure 6.16**). This state indicates that the body is retaining or adding protein, and it occurs during periods of growth, pregnancy, or recovery from illness or a protein deficiency. People who excrete more nitrogen than is consumed are in negative nitrogen balance. This situation indicates that the body is losing protein, and it occurs during starvation or when people are consuming very-low-energy diets. This is because, when energy intake is too low to meet energy demands over a prolonged period of time, the body metabolizes body proteins for energy. The nitrogen from these proteins is excreted in the urine and feces. Negative nitrogen balance also occurs during severe illness, infections,

TABLE 6.2 Recommended Protein Intakes

Group	Protein Intake (grams per kilogram* body weight)
Sedentary adults[1]	0.8
Nonvegetarian endurance athletes[2]	1.2 to 1.4
Nonvegetarian strength athletes[2]	1.2 to 1.7
Vegetarian endurance athletes[2]	1.3 to 1.5
Vegetarian strength athletes[2]	1.3 to 1.8

*To convert body weight to kilograms, divide weight in pounds by 2.2.
Weight (lb)/2.2 Weight (kg)
Weight (kg) × protein recommendation (g/kg body weight per day) = protein intake (g/day)

[1]Data from Food and Nutrition Board, Institute of Medicine. 2005. Dietary Reference Intakes for Energy, Carbohydrate, Fiber, Fat, Fatty Acids, Cholesterol, Protein, and Amino Acids (Macronutrients). Washington, DC: National Academies Press. Available at http://www.nap.edu/openbook.php?isbn=0309085373.
[2]Data American College of Sports Medicine, American Dietetic Association, and Dietitians of Canada. 2009. Joint position statement. Nutrition and athletic performance. Med. Sci. Sports Exerc. 41(3): 709–731.

high fever, serious burns, or injuries that cause significant blood loss. People in these situations require increased dietary protein. A person is in nitrogen balance when nitrogen intake equals nitrogen excretion. This indicates that protein intake is sufficient to cover protein needs. Healthy adults who are not pregnant are in nitrogen balance.

Recommended Dietary Allowance for Protein

How much protein should we eat? The RDA for sedentary people is 0.8 g per kilogram of body weight per day. The recommended percentage of energy that should come from protein is 10% to 35% of total energy intake. Protein needs are higher for children, adolescents, and pregnant/lactating women because more protein is needed during times of growth and development (refer to Chapters 16 and 17 for details on protein needs during these phases of the life cycle). Protein needs can also be higher for active people and for vegetarians.

Table 6.2 lists the daily recommendations for protein for a variety of lifestyles. How can we convert this recommendation into total grams of protein for the day? In the **You Do the Math** box, let's calculate Theo's protein requirements.

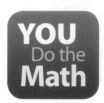

Calculating Your Protein Needs

Theo wants to know how much protein he needs each day. During the off-season, he works out three times a week at a gym and practices basketball with friends every Friday night. He is not a vegetarian. Although Theo exercises regularly, he would not be considered an endurance athlete or as a strength athlete during the off-season. At this level of physical activity, Theo's requirement for protein probably ranges from the RDA of 0.8 up to 1.0 g per kg body weight per day. To calculate the total number of grams of protein Theo should eat each day,

1. Convert Theo's weight from pounds to kilograms. Theo presently weighs 200 lb. To convert this value to kilograms, divide by 2.2:

    (200 lb)/(2.2 lb/kg) = 91 kg

2. Multiply Theo's weight in kilograms by his RDA for protein, like so:

    (91 kg) × (0.8 g/kg) = 72.8 g of protein per day
    (91 kg) × (1.0 g/kg) = 91 g of protein per day

What happens during basketball season, when Theo practices, lifts weight, and has games 5 or 6 days a week? This will probably raise his protein needs to approximately 1.2 to 1.7 g per kg body weight per day. How much more protein should he eat? See below:

91 kg × 1.2 g/kg = 109.2 g of protein per day
91 kg × 1.7 g/kg = 154.7 g of protein per day

Now calculate your own recommended protein intake based on your activity level.

Answers will vary depending on body weight and individual activity levels.

Most Americans Meet or Exceed the RDA for Protein

Surveys indicate that Americans eat 14% to 16% of their total daily energy intake as protein.[3] Men report eating about 73 to 104 g of protein each day, and women consume 59 to 72 g per day. Putting these values into perspective, let's assume that the average man weighs 75 kg (165 lb) and the average woman weighs 65 kg (143 lb). Their protein requirements (assuming they are not athletes or vegetarians) are 60 g and 52 g per day for men and women at this average weight, respectively. As you can see, many adults in the United States eat more than the RDA for protein.

Research indicates that the protein intake of athletes participating in a variety of sports can also well exceed current recommendations.[4] For instance, the protein intake for some female distance runners is 1.2 g per kg body weight per day, accounting for 15% of their total daily energy intake. In addition, some male bodybuilders consume 3 g per kg body weight per day, accounting for almost 38% of their total daily energy intake! However, certain groups of athletes are at risk for low protein intakes. Athletes who consume inadequate energy and limit food choices, such as some distance runners, figure skaters, female gymnasts, and wrestlers who are dieting, are all at risk for low protein intakes. Unlike people who consume adequate energy, individuals who are restricting their total energy intake (kilocalories) need to pay close attention to their protein intake.

Can Too Much Dietary Protein Be Harmful?

High protein intakes have been identified with increased health risks. Three health conditions that have received particular attention are heart disease, bone loss, and kidney disease.

High Protein Intake and High Blood Cholesterol

High-protein diets composed of predominantly animal sources have been associated with higher blood cholesterol levels. This is probably due to the saturated fat in animal products, which is known to increase both blood cholesterol levels and the risk for heart disease. However, a review of studies examining this issue indicates that moderately high-protein diets, particularly those including protein sources low in saturated fat, are associated with a significantly healthier blood lipid profile, reduced blood pressure, and reduced risk for cardiovascular disease.[5] These experts state than the optimal amount and sources of protein to reduce the risk for cardiovascular disease are not yet known, and they encourage partially replacing refined carbohydrate foods in the diet with protein sources that are low in saturated fat. These sources do not necessarily have to come from animals, as vegetarians have been shown to have a greatly reduced risk for heart disease.[6, 7]

High Protein Intake and Bone Loss

How might a high-protein diet lead to bone loss? Until recently, nutritionists have been concerned about high-protein diets because they increase calcium excretion. This may be because animal products contain more of the sulfur amino acids (methionine and cysteine). Metabolizing these amino acids makes the blood more acidic, and calcium is pulled from the bone to buffer these acids. Although eating more protein can cause an increased excretion of calcium, it is very controversial whether high protein intakes actually cause bone loss. In fact, we do know that eating too little protein causes bone loss, which increases the risk for fractures and osteoporosis. Higher intakes of animal and soy protein have been shown to protect bone in middle-aged and older women. A recent systematic review of the literature has concluded that there is no evidence to support the contention that high-protein diets lead to bone loss, except in people consuming inadequate calcium.[8]

High Protein Intake and Kidney Disease

A third risk associated with high protein intakes is kidney disease. A high-protein diet can increase the risk of acquiring kidney disease in people who are susceptible. People with diabetes have higher rates of kidney disease and may benefit from a lower-protein diet.

The American Diabetes Association states that people with diabetes have a higher protein need than people without diabetes, but a protein intake of 15% to 20% of total energy is adequate to meet these increased needs.[9] This level of protein intake is deemed safe for people with diabetes who have normal renal function. There is no evidence, however, that eating more protein causes kidney disease in healthy people who are not susceptible to this condition.[10] In fact, a review of studies assessing the effect of high protein intakes on renal function in athletes has found that regularly consuming over 2 g of protein per kg body weight per day does not appear to cause unhealthy changes in kidney function.[10] Thus, experts agree that eating no more than 2 g of protein per kg body weight each day is safe for healthy people.

It is important for people who consume a lot of protein to drink more water. This is because eating more protein increases protein metabolism and urea production. As mentioned earlier, urea is a waste product that forms when nitrogen is removed during amino acid metabolism. Adequate fluid is needed to flush excess urea from the kidneys. This is particularly important for athletes, who need more fluid due to higher sweat losses.

Protein: Much More Than Meat!

Table 6.3 compares the protein content of a variety of foods. Although some people think that the only good sources of protein are meats (beef, pork, poultry, seafood), many other foods are rich in proteins. These include dairy products (milk, cheese, yogurt, and so on), eggs, legumes (including soy products), whole grains, and nuts. Fruits and many vegetables are not particularly high in protein; however, these foods provide fiber and many vitamins and minerals and are excellent sources of carbohydrates. Thus, eating them can help provide the carbohydrates and energy you need, so that your body can use proteins for building and maintaining tissues.

After reviewing Table 6.3, you might be wondering how much protein you typically eat. See the **Nutrition Label Activity** box (page 242) to find out.

Legumes

Legumes include soybeans, kidney beans, pinto beans, black beans, garbanzo beans (chickpeas), lima beans, green peas, black-eyed peas, and lentils. Would you be surprised to learn that the quality of the protein in some of these legumes is almost equal to that of meat? It's true! The quality of soybean protein is almost identical to that of meat and is available as soy milk, tofu, textured vegetable protein, and tempeh, a firm cake made by cooking and fermenting whole soybeans. For more information about the nutrients in soy, claims regarding its health benefits, and ways to enjoy soy, check out the **Highlight** box (page 244).

The protein quality of other legumes is also relatively high. In addition to being excellent sources of protein, legumes are high in fiber, iron, calcium, and many of the B-vitamins. They are also low in saturated fat and cholesterol. Eating legumes regularly, including foods made from soybeans, may help reduce the risk for heart disease by lowering blood cholesterol levels. Diets high in legumes and soy products are also associated with lower rates of some cancers. Legumes are not nutritionally complete, however, as they do not contain vitamins B_{12}, C, or A. They're also deficient in methionine, an essential amino acid; however, combining them with grains, nuts, or seeds gives you a complete protein.

How can you add more legumes to your daily diet? Try these suggestions:

- Instead of cereal, eggs, or a doughnut, microwave a frozen bean burrito for a quick, portable breakfast.
- If you normally have a side of bacon, ham, or sausage with your eggs for breakfast, have a side of black beans instead.
- For lunch, try a sandwich made with hummus (a garbanzo bean spread), cucumbers, tomato, avocado, and/or lettuce on whole-wheat bread or in a whole-wheat pocket.

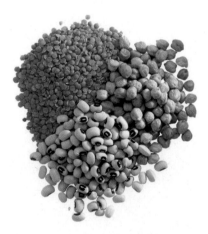

The quality of the protein in some legumes, such as these black-eyed peas, lentils, and garbanzo beans, is almost equal to that of meat.

TABLE 6.3 Protein Content of Commonly Consumed Foods

Food	Serving Size	Protein (g)
Beef		
Ground, lean, baked (15% fat)	3 oz	22
Beef tenderloin steak, broiled (1/8-in. fat)	3 oz	21.5
Top sirloin, broiled (1/8-in. fat)	3 oz	23
Poultry		
Chicken breast, broiled, no skin (bone removed)	½ breast	27
Chicken thigh, bone and skin removed	1 thigh	20
Turkey breast, roasted, Louis Rich	3 oz	15
Seafood		
Cod, cooked	3 oz	19
Salmon, Chinook, baked	3 oz	22
Shrimp, steamed	3 oz	19
Tuna, light, in water, drained	3 oz	22
Pork		
Pork loin chop, broiled	3 oz	21
Ham, roasted, extra lean (5% fat)	3 oz	18
Dairy		
Whole milk (3.3% fat)	8 fl. oz	7.7
1% milk	8 fl. oz	8.2
Skim milk	8 fl. oz	8.3
Low-fat, plain yogurt	8 fl. oz	12
American cheese, processed	1 oz	5
Cottage cheese, low-fat (2%)	1 cup	27
Soy Products		
Tofu	½ cup	10
Tempeh, cooked	3 oz	15.5
Soy milk beverage	1 cup	8
Beans		
Refried	½ cup	6
Kidney, red	½ cup	8
Black	½ cup	7.6
Nuts		
Peanuts, dry roasted	1 oz	6.7
Peanut butter, creamy	2 tbsp.	8
Almonds, blanched	1 oz	6
Cereals, Grains, and Breads		
Oatmeal, quick instant	1 packet	6.6
Cheerios	1 cup	3
Grape Nuts	1/2 cup	7.2
Raisin Bran	1 cup	4.7
Brown rice, cooked	1 cup	5
Whole-wheat bread	1 slice	3.6
Bagel, 3½-in. diameter	1 each	10.5
Vegetables		
Carrots, raw (7.5 × 1 1/8 in.)	1 each	0.7
Broccoli, raw, chopped	1 cup	2.6
Collards, cooked from frozen	1 cup	5
Spinach, raw	1 cup	0.9

Source: Values obtained from U.S. Department of Agriculture, Agricultural Research Service. 2011. USDA National Nutrient Database for Standard Reference, Release 24. Available online at http://ndb.nal.usda.gov/.

- Add garbanzo beans, kidney beans, or fresh peas to tossed salads, or make a three-bean salad with kidney beans, green beans, and garbanzo beans.
- Make a side dish using legumes, such as peas with pearl onions; succotash (lima beans, corn, and tomatoes); or homemade chili with kidney beans and tofu instead of meat.
- Make black bean soup, lentil soup, pea soup, minestrone soup, or a batch of dal (a type of yellow lentil used in Indian cuisine) and serve over brown rice. Top with plain yogurt, a traditional accompaniment in many Asian cuisines.

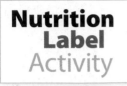

How Much Protein Do You Eat?

Theo wants to know if his diet contains enough protein. To calculate his protein intake, he records all the foods he eats for 3 days in a food diary. The foods Theo consumed for 1 of his 3 days are listed on the left in the following table, and the protein content of those foods is listed on the right. Theo recorded the protein content listed on the Nutrition Facts Panel for those foods with labels. For products without labels, he used the nutrient analysis program that came with this book. There is also a US Department of Agriculture website that lists the energy and nutrient content of thousands of foods (http://ndb.nal .usda.gov/).

Foods Consumed	Protein Content (g)
Breakfast	
Brewed coffee (2 cups) with 2 tbsp. half and half	1.4
1 large bagel (5-in. diameter)	13
Low-fat cream cheese (2 tbsp.)	1.6
Mid-Morning Snack	
Cola beverage (32 fl. oz)	0
Low-fat strawberry yogurt (1 cup)	10
Fruit and nut granola bar (2; 37 g each)	5.7
Lunch	
Ham and cheese sandwich:	
Whole-wheat bread (2 slices)	4
Mayonnaise (1.5 tbsp.)	0.2
Extra-lean ham (4 oz)	24
Swiss cheese (2 oz)	15
Iceberg lettuce (2 leaves)	0.3
Sliced tomato (3 slices)	0.5
Banana (1 large)	1.5
Wheat Thin crackers (20)	3.6
Bottled water (20 fl. oz)	0.0

Foods Consumed	Protein Content (g)
Dinner	
Cheeseburger:	
Broiled ground beef (1/2 lb, cooked)	52
American cheese (1 oz)	5
Seeded bun (1 large)	8
Ketchup (2 tbsp.)	0.5
Mustard (1 tbsp.)	0.7
Shredded lettuce (1/2 cup)	0.3
Sliced tomato (3 slices)	0.5
French fries (30; 2- to 3-in. strips)	5
Baked beans (2 cups)	24
2% low-fat milk (2 cups)	16
Evening Snack	
Chocolate chip cookies (4; 3-in.-diameter)	3
2% low-fat milk (1 cup)	8
Total protein intake for the day:	**203.8 g**

As calculated in the **You Do the Math** box (page 238), Theo's RDA during the off-season is 72.8 to 91 g of protein. He is consuming 2.3 to 2.8 times that amount! You can see that he does not need to use amino acid or protein supplements, because he has more than adequate amounts of protein to build lean tissue. Now calculate your own protein intake using food labels and a diet analysis program. Do you obtain more protein from animal or non-animal sources? If you consume mostly non-animal sources, are you eating soy products and complementary foods throughout the day? If you eat animal-based products on a regular basis, notice how much protein you consume from even small servings of meat and dairy products.

- Make burritos with black or pinto beans instead of shredded meat.
- Make a "meatloaf" using cooked, mashed lentils instead of ground beef.
- For fast food at home, keep canned beans on hand. Serve over rice with a salad for a complete and hearty meal.
- Instead of potato chips or pretzels for snacks, try one of the new bean chips.
- Dip fresh vegetables in bean dip.
- Serve hummus on wedge of pita bread.

Nuts

Nuts are another healthful high-protein food. In the past, the high fat and energy content of nuts was assumed to be harmful, and people were advised to eat nuts only occasionally and in very small amounts. The results from recent epidemiological studies have helped to substantially change the way nutrition experts view nuts. These studies show that consuming about 2 to 5 oz of nuts per week significantly reduced people's risk for cardiovascular disease.[11, 12] Although the exact mechanism for the reduction in cardiovascular disease risk with increased nut intake is not known, nuts contain many nutrients and other substances that are associated with health benefits, including fiber, unsaturated fats, potassium, folate, and plant sterols that inhibit cholesterol absorption.

"New" Foods

A new source of non-meat protein that is available on the market is *quorn,* a protein product derived from fermented fungus. It is mixed with a variety of other foods to produce various types of meat substitutes. Other "new" foods high in protein include some very ancient grains! For instance, you may have heard of pastas and other products made with quinoa (pronounced keen-wah), a plant so essential to the diet of the ancient Incas that they considered it sacred. No wonder: quinoa, which is cooked much like rice, provides 8 g of protein in a 1-cup serving. It's highly digestible and, unlike many more familiar grains, provides all nine essential amino acids. A similar grain, called amaranth, also provides complete protein. Teff, millet, and sorghum are grains long cultivated in Africa as rich sources of protein. They are now widely available in the United States. Although these three grains are low in the essential amino acid lysine, combining them with legumes produces a complete-protein meal.

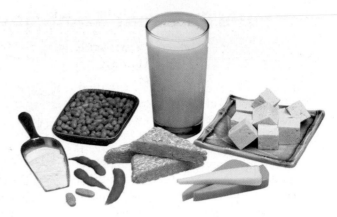

Soy products are also a good source of dietary protein.

Amino Acid Supplements—Are They Necessary?

"Amino acid supplements—you can't gain without them!" This is just one of the headlines found in bodybuilding magazines and Internet sites touting amino acid supplements as the key to achieving increased power, strength, and performance "perfection." Many athletes who read these claims believe that taking amino acid supplements will boost their energy during performance, replace proteins metabolized for energy during exercise, enhance muscle growth and strength, and hasten recovery from intense training or injury. Should you believe the hype?

As noted earlier in this chapter, we use very little protein for energy during exercise, and many Americans already consume nearly twice the RDA for protein. Consuming adequate energy and following the recommended intakes for protein listed in Table 6.2 will more than support either strength or endurance exercising training and performance. What about the claims related to muscle-building? Although some research has shown that intravenous infusions of various amino acids in the laboratory can stimulate certain hormones that enhance the building of muscle, there is little evidence that taking individual amino acids or protein supplements orally can build muscle or improve strength.[4] Since many of these supplements can be expensive, ensuring that you get enough protein solely from your diet will put a lot less strain on your wallet!

RECAP

The RDA for protein for most nonpregnant, nonlactating, nonvegetarian sedentary adults is 0.8 g per kg body weight. Children, pregnant women, nursing mothers, vegetarians, and active people need slightly more. Most people who eat enough kilocalories and carbohydrates have no problem meeting their RDA for protein. Eating too much protein may increase a susceptible person's risk for kidney disease. Good sources of protein include meats, eggs, dairy products, soy products, legumes, quorn, whole grains, and nuts. Amino acid supplements are not necessary to support muscle growth or exercise performance, assuming energy and protein intakes are adequate. ■

HIGHLIGHT

What's So Great About Soy?

Twenty years ago, if you were able to find a soy-based food in a traditional grocery store in the United States or Canada, it was probably soy milk. Now, it seems there are soy products in almost every aisle, from marinated tofu and tempeh to miso soup to soy-based cheeses, cereals, hot dogs, burgers, frozen dinners, and even tofu ice cream. Why the explosion? What's so great about soy, and should you give it a try?

What Is Soy?

Before we explore the many health claims tied to soy-based foods, let's define some terms. First, all soy-based foods start with soybeans, a staple in many Asian countries. Soybeans provide all essential amino acids and have almost twice as much protein as any other legume (7–10 grams of protein in 1 cup of soy milk). Although they also pack three to ten times as much fat as other beans, almost all of it is unsaturated, and soy has no cholesterol. Soy is also rich in a group of phytochemicals called *isoflavones*. These plant chemicals mimic the effect of the hormone estrogen in the human body. Here are some common varieties of soy-based foods you might find in your local supermarket:

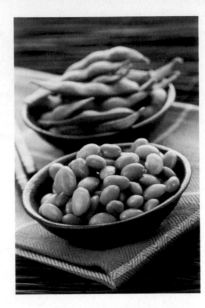

- *Soy milk* is a beverage produced when soybeans are ground with water. Flavorings are added to make the drink palatable, and many brands of soy milk are fortified with calcium and vitamin D.

- *Tofu* is made from soy milk coagulated to form curds. If the coagulant used is calcium sulfate, the resulting product is high in calcium. Tofu is usually sold in blocks, like cheese, and is used as a meat substitute. Although many people object to its bland taste and mushy texture, tofu adapts well to many seasonings, and when drained and frozen before cooking it develops a chewy texture similar to meat. Tofu is also the basis of many processed foods, such as meatless hot dogs and burgers.

- *Tempeh* is a more flavorful and firmer-textured meat substitute made from soybeans fermented with grains. It is often used in stir-fried dishes.

- *Miso* is a paste made from fermented soybeans and grains. It is used sparingly as a base for soups and sauces, as it is very high in sodium.

- *Edamame* are precooked, frozen soybeans eaten as a snack or in salads and other dishes.

Soy May Reduce Your Risk for Chronic Disease

Now let's look at the health claims. Proponents say that a diet high in soy protein can reduce your risk for heart disease, certain types of cancer, and osteoporosis (loss of bone density). Let's review the research behind each of these claims.

Heart Disease

In 1999, the US Food and Drug Administration (FDA) gave food manufacturers permission to put labels on products high in soy protein stating that a daily diet containing 25 grams of soy protein and low in saturated fat and cholesterol may reduce the risk for heart disease.[1] Until recently, there was general agreement that soy consumption resulted in a modest reduction in LDL-cholesterol, with this cholesterol-reducing benefit of soy being linked only to soy-based foods, not supplements. In 2006, the American Heart Association (AHA) issued a science advisory stating that the reductions in LDL-cholesterol observed with soy-based foods is relatively small and that these foods do not improve lipid profiles overall or reduce blood pressure.[2] Despite these findings, the AHA recommends consuming soy-based foods (such as soy milk, tofu, and tempeh) as part of a heart-healthy diet because of their high content of polyunsaturated fats, fiber, and vitamins and minerals and their low saturated fat content.[2]

Cancer

Many studies suggest that soy protects against prostate cancer, which is the most common cancer in men.[3] Although it is theorized that the isoflavones in soy foods may be responsible for this protective effect, researchers recommend eating soy-based foods, not isoflavone supplements.

Whereas the risk-reducing benefits of soy seem clear in the case of prostate cancer, the claims for soy's effect on breast cancer risk are controversial. Some studies have suggested that the isoflavones in soy may reduce a woman's risk for breast cancer; however, their findings conflict with those of other studies indicating a possible increased risk. The American Cancer Society (ACS) explains that the plant estrogens in soy "may have both a protective role and a stimulatory role in breast cancer cell growth depending on several factors, including at what age they're consumed and whether they're consumed as food or as supplement."[4] Several federally funded studies are currently being conducted to further our understanding of the effect of soy on breast cancer risk, but for now, the ACS recommends consuming naturally occurring soy foods as part of a balanced, plant-based diet.[4]

Bone Loss

Published studies of the effect of soy on bone density, a particular concern for older women, have also been inconclusive. Whereas some suggest that soy can help keep bones strong, others suggest little benefit. A recent review combining the results of ten randomized, controlled trials found that consuming soy helped prevent bone loss in the spine in white, postmenopausal women.[5] Several new studies investigating the potential link between soy and bone health are underway.

Adding Soy to Your Diet

If you decide that you want to try soy, how do you go about it? A first step for many people is to substitute soy milk for cow's milk on its own, on cereal, in smoothies, or in recipes for baked goods. Different brands of soy milk can have very different flavors, so try a few before you decide you don't like the taste.

Here are some other possibilities for adding soy to your diet:[5]

- Try one of the breakfast cereals made with soy.
- Use soy nut butter (similar to peanut butter), soy deli meats, or soy cheese in sandwiches.
- Try soy sausages, bacon, hot dogs, burgers, ground "beef," and "chicken" patties.
- Use soy "crumbles" in any recipe calling for ground beef.
- Toss cubes of prepackaged, flavored, baked tofu or tempeh or a handful of edamame into stir-fried vegetables and serve over Chinese noodles or rice.
- Order soy-based dishes, such as spicy bean curd and miso soup, at Asian restaurants.
- Eat roasted soy nuts, edamame, or a soy protein bar for a snack.
- Try soy yogurt and ice cream.

References

1. Henkel, J. 2000. Soy: health claims for soy protein, questions about other components. *FDA Consumer Magazine*, May–June. www.fda.gov/fdac/features/2000/300_soy.html.
2. Sacks, F. M., A. Lichtenstein, L. Van Horn, W. Harris, P. Kris-Etherton, and M. Winston for the American Heart Association Nutrition Committee. 2006. Soy protein, isoflavones, and cardiovascular health. An American Heart Association Science Advisory for Professionals from the Nutrition Committee. *Circulation* 113:1034–1044.
3. Centers for Disease Control and Prevention. 2011. Cancer and Men. www.cdc.gov/Features/CancerandMen/.
4. American Cancer Society. 2010. Find Support and Treatment. Soybean. www.cancer.org/Treatment/TreatmentsandSideEffects/ComplementaryandAlternativeMedicine/DietandNutrition/soybean.
5. Ma, D.-F., L.-Q. Qin, P.-Y. Wang, and R. Katoh. 2008. Soy isoflavone intake increases bone mineral density in the spine of menopausal women: meta-analysis of randomized-controlled trials. *Clin. Nutr.* 27(1):57–64.

Can a Vegetarian Diet Provide Adequate Protein?

Vegetarianism is the practice of restricting the diet to food substances of plant origin, including vegetables, fruits, grains, and nuts. As many as 15 million Americans are vegetarians; about half of these are vegans, people who do not eat any kind of animal product, including dairy foods and eggs.[2] Many vegetarians are college students; moving away from home and taking responsibility for one's eating habits appears to influence some young adults to try vegetarianism as a lifestyle choice.

Types of Vegetarian Diets

There are almost as many types of vegetarian diets as there are vegetarians. Some people who consider themselves vegetarians regularly eat poultry and fish. Others avoid the flesh of animals but consume eggs, milk, and cheese liberally. Still others strictly avoid

> Maybe you're not considering adopting a vegetarian diet but would like to explore your options for eating less meat. For help doing just that, watch this video from ABC News at http://abcnews.go.com/Health/video/vegetarian-diet-10450710.

vegetarianism The practice of restricting the diet to food substances of plant origin, including vegetables, fruits, grains, and nuts.

TABLE 6.4 Terms and Definitions of a Vegetarian Diet

Type of Diet	Foods Consumed	Comments
Semivegetarian (also called partial vegetarian or flexitarian)	Vegetables, grains, nuts, fruits, legumes; sometimes seafood, poultry, eggs, dairy products	Typically exclude or limit red meat; may also avoid other meats
Pescovegetarian	Similar to semivegetarian but excludes poultry	*Pesco* means "fish," the only animal source of protein in this diet
Lacto-ovo-vegetarian	Vegetables, grains, nuts, fruits, legumes, dairy products (*lacto*), eggs (*ovo*)	Excludes animal flesh and seafood
Lactovegetarian	Similar to lacto-ovo-vegetarian but excludes eggs	Relies on milk and cheese for animal sources of protein
Ovovegetarian	Vegetables, grains, nuts, fruits, legumes, eggs	Excludes dairy, flesh, seafood products
Vegan (also called strict vegetarian)	Only plant-based foods (vegetables, grains, nuts, seeds, fruits, legumes)	May not provide adequate vitamin B_{12}, zinc, iron, or calcium
Macrobiotic diet	Vegan type of diet; becomes progressively more strict until almost all foods are eliminated; at the extreme, only brown rice and small amounts of water or herbal tea	Taken to the extreme, can cause malnutrition and death
Fruitarian	Only raw or dried fruit, seeds, nuts, honey, vegetable oil	Very restrictive diet; deficient in protein, calcium, zinc, iron, vitamin B_{12}, riboflavin, other nutrients

all products of animal origin, including milk and eggs, and even by-products such as candies and puddings made with gelatin. A type of "vegetarian" diet receiving significant media attention recently is the *flexitarian* diet: flexitarians are considered semivegetarians who eat mostly plant foods, eggs, and dairy but occasionally eat red meat, poultry, and/or fish.

Table 6.4 identifies the various types of vegetarian diets, ranging from the most inclusive to the most restrictive. Notice that the more restrictive the diet, the more challenging it becomes to achieve an adequate protein intake.

Why Do People Become Vegetarians?

When discussing vegetarianism, one of the most often-asked questions is why people would make this food choice. The most common responses are included here.

Religious, Ethical, and Food-Safety Reasons

Some make the choice for religious or spiritual reasons. Several religions prohibit or restrict the consumption of animal flesh; however, generalizations can be misleading. For example, whereas certain sects within Hinduism forbid the consumption of meat, perusing the menu at any Indian restaurant will reveal that many other Hindus regularly consume small quantities of meat, poultry, and fish. Many Buddhists are vegetarians, as are some Christians, including Seventh Day Adventists.

Many vegetarians are guided by their personal philosophy to choose vegetarianism. These people feel that it is morally and ethically wrong to consume animals and any products from animals (such as dairy or egg products) because they view the practices in the modern animal industries as inhumane. They may consume milk and eggs but choose to purchase them only from family farms where they feel animals are treated humanely.

There is also a great deal of concern about meat-handling practices, because contaminated meat has occasionally made its way into our food supply. For example, several outbreaks of severe illness, sometimes resulting in permanent disability and even death, have been traced to hamburgers served at fast-food restaurants, as well as ground

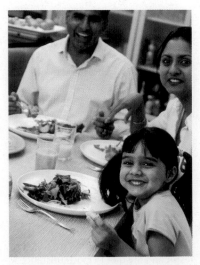

People who follow certain sects of Hinduism refrain from eating meat.

beef sold in markets and consumed at home. A concern surrounding beef is the potential for contracting the human variant of *mad cow disease*. (See the **Nutrition Myth or Fact** box in Chapter 15 [page 605] for a look at mad cow disease and its impact in the United States and other countries.)

Ecological Benefits

Many people choose vegetarianism because of their concerns about the effect of meat production on the global environment. Due to the high demand for meat in developed nations, meat production has evolved from small family farming operations into the larger system of agribusiness. Critics point to the environmental costs of agribusiness, including massive uses of water and grain to feed animals, methane gases and other wastes produced by animals themselves, and increased land use to support livestock. For an in-depth discussion of this complex and emotionally charged topic, refer to the **Nutrition Debate** at the end of this chapter.

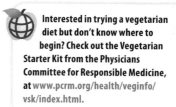

Interested in trying a vegetarian diet but don't know where to begin? Check out the Vegetarian Starter Kit from the Physicians Committee for Responsible Medicine, at www.pcrm.org/health/veginfo/vsk/index.html.

Health Benefits

Still others practice vegetarianism because of its health benefits. Research over several years has consistently shown that a varied and balanced vegetarian diet can reduce the risk for many chronic diseases. Its health benefits include the following:[13]

- Reduced intake of fat and total energy, which reduces the risk for obesity. This may in turn lower a person's risk for type 2 diabetes.
- Lower blood pressure, which may be due to a higher intake of fruits and vegetables. People who eat vegetarian diets tend to be nonsmokers, to drink little or no alcohol, and to exercise more regularly, which are also factors known to reduce blood pressure and help maintain a healthy body weight.
- Reduced risk for heart disease, which may be due to lower saturated fat intake and a higher consumption of *antioxidants,* which are found in plant-based foods. Antioxidants (discussed in detail in Chapter 10) are substances that can protect our cells from damage. They are abundant in fruits and vegetables.
- Fewer digestive problems, such as constipation and diverticular disease, perhaps due to the higher fiber content of vegetarian diets. Diverticular disease (discussed in Chapters 3 and 4) occurs when the wall of the bowel (large intestine) pouches and becomes inflamed.
- Reduced risk for some cancers. Research shows that vegetarians may have lower rates of cancer, particularly colorectal cancer. Many components of a vegetarian diet could contribute to reducing cancer risks, including higher fiber, no intake of red meats and processed meats (which increase the risk for colorectal cancer), and lower consumption of *carcinogens* (cancer-causing agents) that are formed when cooking meat.[14]
- Reduced risk for kidney disease, kidney stones, and gallstones. The lower protein contents of vegetarian diets, plus the higher intake of legumes and vegetable proteins such as soy, may be protective against these conditions.

A well-balanced vegetarian diet can provide adequate protein.

What Are the Challenges of a Vegetarian Diet?

Although a vegetarian diet can be healthful, it also presents some challenges. Limiting the consumption of flesh and dairy products introduces the potential for inadequate intakes of certain nutrients, especially for people consuming a vegan, macrobiotic, or fruitarian diet. **Table 6.5** (page 248) lists the nutrients that can be deficient in a vegan type of diet plan and describes good non-animal sources that can provide these nutrients. Vegetarians who consume dairy and/or egg products obtain these nutrients more easily.

Research indicates that some female athletes at risk for disordered eating will switch to a vegetarian diet.[15] Instead of eating a healthful variety of non-animal foods, people with disordered eating problems may use vegetarianism as an excuse to restrict

TABLE 6.5 Nutrients of Concern in a Vegan Diet

Nutrient	Functions	Non-Meat/Nondairy Food Sources
Vitamin B_{12}	Assists with DNA synthesis; protection and growth of nerve fibers	Vitamin B_{12}–fortified cereals, yeast, soy products, and other meat analogues; vitamin B_{12} supplements
Vitamin D	Promotes bone growth	Vitamin D–fortified cereals, margarines, and soy products; adequate exposure to sunlight; supplementation may be necessary for those who do not get adequate exposure to sunlight
Riboflavin (vitamin B_2)	Promotes release of energy; supports normal vision and skin health	Whole and enriched grains, green leafy vegetables, mushrooms, beans, nuts, seeds
Iron	Assists with oxygen transport; involved in making amino acids and hormones	Whole-grain products, prune juice, dried fruits, beans, nuts, seeds, leafy vegetables such as spinach
Calcium	Maintains bone health; assists with muscle contraction, blood pressure, and nerve transmission	Fortified soy milk and tofu, almonds, dry beans, leafy vegetables, calcium-fortified juices, fortified breakfast cereals
Zinc	Assists with DNA and RNA synthesis, immune function, and growth	Whole-grain products, wheat germ, beans, nuts, seeds

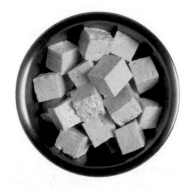

Vegetarians should eat two to three servings of beans, nuts, seeds, eggs, or meat substitutes (such as tofu) daily.

many foods from their diet. Experts suggest that the possibility of disordered eating should be considered if the switch to a vegetarian diet is accompanied by unnecessary weight loss.[15]

Can a vegetarian diet provide enough protein? Because high-quality non-meat protein sources are quite easy to obtain in developed countries, a well-balanced vegetarian diet can provide adequate protein. In fact, the American Dietetic Association endorses an appropriately planned vegetarian diet as healthful, nutritionally adequate, and beneficial in reducing and preventing various diseases.[13] As you can see, the emphasis is on a *balanced* and *adequate* vegetarian diet; thus, it is important for vegetarians to consume soy products, eat complementary proteins, and obtain enough energy from other macronutrients to spare protein from being used as an energy source. Although the digestibility of a vegetarian diet is potentially lower than that of an animal-based diet, there is no separate protein recommendation for vegetarians who consume complementary plant proteins.[16]

Using MyPlate

Although the USDA has not designed a version of MyPlate specifically for people following a vegetarian diet, healthy eating tips for vegetarians are available at MyPlate online (see the Web Links section at the end of this chapter). For example, to meet their needs for protein and calcium, lacto-vegetarians can consume low-fat or nonfat dairy products. Vegans and ovovegetarians can consume calcium-fortified soy milk or one of the many protein bars fortified with calcium.

In addition to protein and calcium, vegans need to pay special attention to consuming foods high in vitamins D, B_{12}, and riboflavin (B_2) and the minerals zinc and iron. Supplementation of these micronutrients may be necessary for certain individuals if they cannot consume adequate amounts in their diet.

RECAP

A balanced vegetarian diet may reduce the risk for obesity, type 2 diabetes, heart disease, digestive problems, some cancers, kidney disease, kidney stones, and gallstones. Whereas varied vegetarian diets can provide enough protein, vegetarians who consume no animal products need to make sure they consume adequate plant sources of protein and supplement their diet with good sources of vitamin B_{12}, vitamin D, riboflavin, iron, calcium, and zinc. ■

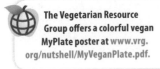

The Vegetarian Resource Group offers a colorful vegan MyPlate poster at www.vrg.org/nutshell/MyVeganPlate.pdf.

What Disorders Are Related to Protein Intake or Metabolism?

Consuming inadequate protein can result in severe illness and death. Typically, this occurs when people do not consume enough total energy, but a diet deficient specifically in protein can have similar effects.

Protein–Energy Malnutrition Can Lead to Debility and Death

When a person consumes too little protein and energy, the result is **protein–energy malnutrition** (also called *protein–Calorie malnutrition*). Two diseases that can follow are marasmus and kwashiorkor (**Figure 6.17**).

Marasmus Results from Grossly Inadequate Energy Intakes

Marasmus is a disease that results from grossly inadequate intakes of protein, energy, and other nutrients. Essentially, people with marasmus slowly starve to death. It is most common in young children (6 to 18 months of age) living in impoverished conditions who are severely undernourished. For example, the children may be fed diluted cereal drinks that are inadequate in energy, protein, and most nutrients. People suffering from marasmus have the look of "skin and bones," as their body fat and tissues are wasting. The consequences of marasmus include the following:

- Wasting and weakening of muscles, including the heart muscle
- Stunted brain development and learning impairment
- Depressed metabolism and little insulation from body fat, causing a dangerously low body temperature
- Stunted physical growth and development
- Deterioration of the intestinal lining, which further inhibits absorption of nutrients
- *Anemia* (abnormally low levels of hemoglobin in the blood)
- Severely weakened immune system
- Fluid and electrolyte imbalances

If marasmus is left untreated, death from dehydration, heart failure, or infection will result. Treating marasmus involves carefully correcting fluid and electrolyte imbalances. Protein and carbohydrates are provided once the body's condition has stabilized. Fat is

protein–energy malnutrition A disorder caused by inadequate consumption of protein. It is characterized by severe wasting.

marasmus A form of protein-energy malnutrition that results from grossly inadequate intakes of protein, energy, and other nutrients.

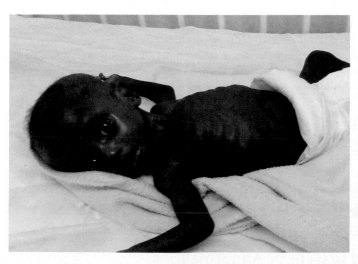
(a)

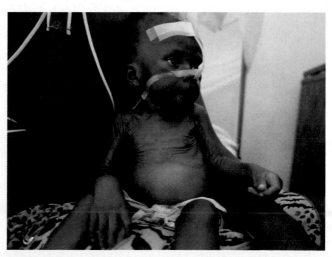
(b)

FIGURE 6.17 Two forms of protein-energy malnutrition: **(a)** marasmus and **(b)** kwashiorkor.

*Nutri-*Case

Theo

"No way would I ever become a vegetarian! The only way to build up your muscles is to eat meat. I was reading in a bodybuilding magazine last week about a new diet called the *Protein Path to Power* that says if you eat a diet really high in lean meats and cut out the junk foods, you'll gain muscle but not fat because 'protein makes protein, but fat and sugar make fat.' That makes sense to me. Besides, after a game I just crave meat. If I don't have it, I feel sort of like my batteries don't get recharged. Competitive athletes just can't perform without meat."

What specific claims does Theo make here about the role of meat in the diet? Do you think these claims are valid? Why or why not?

introduced much later, as the protein levels in the blood must improve to the point at which the body can use them to carry fat, so that it can be safely metabolized by the body.

Kwashiorkor Results from a Low-Protein Diet

Kwashiorkor often occurs in developing countries when infants are weaned early due to the arrival of a subsequent baby. This deficiency disease is typically seen in young children (1 to 3 years of age) who no longer drink breast milk. Instead, they often are fed a low-protein, starchy cereal. Unlike marasmus, kwashiorkor often develops quickly and causes the person to look swollen, particularly in the belly. This is because the low protein content of the blood is inadequate to keep fluids from seeping into the tissue spaces. These are other symptoms of kwashiorkor:

- Some weight loss and muscle wasting, with some retention of body fat
- Retarded growth and development but less severe than that seen with marasmus
- Edema, which results over time in extreme distension of the belly and is caused by fluid and electrolyte imbalances
- Fatty degeneration of the liver
- Loss of appetite, sadness, irritability, and apathy
- Development of sores and other skin problems; skin pigmentation changes
- Dry, brittle hair that changes color, straightens, and falls out easily

Kwashiorkor can be reversed if adequate protein and energy are given in time. Because of their severely weakened immune systems, many individuals with kwashiorkor die from infectious diseases they contract in their weakened state. Of those who are treated, many return home to the same impoverished conditions, only to develop this deficiency once again.

Many people think that only children in developing countries suffer from these diseases. However, protein–energy malnutrition occurs in all countries and affects both children and adults. In the United States, poor people living in inner cities and isolated rural areas are especially affected. Others at risk include the elderly, the homeless, people with eating disorders, those addicted to alcohol and other drugs, and individuals with wasting diseases, such as AIDS or cancer. (Chapter 19 provides more information on malnutrition and hunger.)

kwashiorkor A form of protein–energy malnutrition that is typically seen in developing countries in infants and toddlers who are weaned early. Denied breast milk, they are fed a cereal diet that provides adequate energy but inadequate protein.

Disorders Related to Genetic Abnormalities

Numerous disorders are caused by defective DNA. These genetic disorders include phenylketonuria (PKU), sickle cell anemia, and cystic fibrosis.

As previously discussed (in Chapter 4), *phenylketonuria* is an inherited disease in which a person does not have the ability to break down the amino acid phenylalanine. As a result, phenylalanine and its metabolic by-products build up in tissues and can cause brain damage. Individuals with PKU must eat a diet that is severely limited in phenylalanine.

Sickle cell anemia is an inherited disorder of the red blood cells in which a single amino acid present in hemoglobin is changed. As shown in Figure 6.9, normal hemoglobin is globular, giving red blood cells a round, doughnut-like shape. The genetic alteration that occurs with sickle cell anemia causes the red blood cells to be shaped like a sickle or a crescent (**Figure 6.18**). Because sickled red blood cells are stiff and sticky, they cannot flow smoothly through the smallest blood vessels. Instead, they block the vessels, depriving nearby tissues of their oxygen supply and eventually damaging vulnerable organs, particularly the spleen. Sickled cells also have a life span of only about 10 to 20 days, as opposed to the 120-day average for globular red blood cells. The body's greatly increased demand for new red blood cells leads to severe anemia. Other signs and symptoms of sickle cell anemia include impaired vision, headaches, convulsions, bone degeneration, and decreased function of various organs. This disease occurs in any person who inherits the sickle cell gene from both parents.

Cystic fibrosis is an inherited disease that primarily affects the respiratory system and digestive tract. It is caused by a defective gene that causes cells to build and then reject an abnormal version of a protein that normally allows the passage of chloride into and out of certain cells. This alteration in chloride transport causes cells to secrete thick, sticky mucus. The linings of the lungs and pancreas are particularly affected, causing breathing difficulties, lung infections, and digestion problems that lead to nutrient deficiencies. Symptoms include wheezing, coughing, and stunted growth. The severity of this disease varies greatly; some individuals with cystic fibrosis live relatively normal lives, whereas others are seriously debilitated and die in childhood.

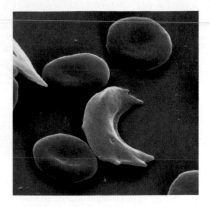

FIGURE 6.18 A sickled red blood cell.

RECAP

Protein–energy malnutrition can lead to marasmus and kwashiorkor. These diseases primarily affect impoverished children in developing nations. However, residents of developed countries are also at risk, especially the elderly, the homeless, people who abuse alcohol or other drugs, and people with AIDS, cancer, and other wasting diseases. Genetic disorders involving abnormal proteins include phenylketonuria, sickle cell anemia, and cystic fibrosis. ■

sickle cell anemia A genetic disorder that causes red blood cells to be shaped like a sickle or crescent. These cells cannot travel smoothly through blood vessels, causing cell breakage and anemia.

cystic fibrosis A genetic disorder that causes an alteration in chloride transport, leading to the production of thick, sticky mucus that causes life-threatening respiratory and digestive problems.

Chapter Review

TEST YOURSELF | ANSWERS

1 F Although protein can be used for energy in certain circumstances, fats and carbohydrates are the primary sources of energy for our bodies.

2 F There is no evidence that consuming amino acid supplements assists in building muscle tissue. Consuming adequate energy and exercising muscles, specifically using weight training, build muscle tissue.

3 F Excess protein is broken down and its component parts are either stored as fat or used for energy or tissue building and repair. Only the nitrogen component of protein is excreted in the urine.

4 F Vegetarian diets can meet and even exceed an individual's protein needs, assuming that adequate energy-yielding macronutrients, a variety of protein sources, and complementary protein sources are consumed.

5 T Most people in the United States consume 1.5 to 2 times more protein than they need.

Summary

- Unlike carbohydrates and fat, the structure of proteins is dictated by DNA, and proteins contain nitrogen.

- Amino acids are the building blocks of proteins; they are composed of an amine group, an acid group, a hydrogen atom, and a unique side chain.

- There are twenty different amino acids in our bodies: nine are essential amino acids, meaning that our bodies cannot produce them, and we must obtain them from food; eleven are nonessential, meaning our bodies can make them, so they do not need to be consumed in the diet.

- Our genetic makeup determines the sequence of amino acids in our proteins. *Gene expression* refers to using a gene in a cell to make a protein.

- Deoxyribonucleic acid (DNA) is the genetic template for gene expression and protein synthesis. The building blocks of DNA are nucleotides, molecules composed of a phosphate group, a pentose sugar called deoxyribose, and one of four nitrogenous bases.

- Protein turnover involves the synthesis of new proteins and the degradation of existing proteins.

- The three-dimensional shape of proteins determines their function in the body.

- When proteins are exposed to damaging substances, such as heat, acids, bases, and alcohol, they are denatured, meaning they lose their shape and function.

- A limiting amino acid is one that is missing or in limited supply, preventing the synthesis of adequate proteins.

- Mutual supplementation is the process of combining two incomplete protein sources to make a complete protein. The two foods involved in this process are called complementary proteins.

- Most of the digestion of proteins occurs in the small intestine.

- Protein quality is determined by its amino acid content and digestibility. Higher-quality proteins contain more essential amino acids and are more digestible. Animal sources, soy protein, and legumes are highly digestible forms of protein.

- Proteins are needed to promote cell growth, repair, and maintenance. They act as enzymes and hormones; help maintain the balance of fluids, electrolytes, acids, and bases; and support healthy immune function. They are also critical for nutrient transport and storage.

- The RDA for protein for sedentary adults is 0.8 g of protein per kilogram of body weight per day; protein should comprise 10% to 35% of total energy intake. Most people in the United States routinely eat much more than the RDA for protein.

■ High protein intakes are claimed to be harmful. Recent evidence suggests that high-protein diets do not lead to increased blood cholesterol levels if protein sources low in saturated fat are consumed, and bone health should not be compromised with high protein intakes if adequate calcium is consumed. High-protein diets can increase the risk for kidney disease in susceptible people.

■ There are many forms of vegetarianism: lacto-ovo-vegetarians eat plant foods plus eggs and dairy products; pescovegetarians consume plant foods and rely on fish as the only meat source; vegans consume only plant foods.

■ Consuming a well-planned vegetarian diet may reduce the risk for obesity, heart disease, type 2 diabetes, and some forms of cancer.

■ Vegans may need to supplement their diet with vitamins B_{12} and D, riboflavin, iron, calcium, and zinc.

■ Marasmus and kwashiorkor are two forms of protein–energy malnutrition that results from grossly inadequate energy and protein intake.

■ Phenylketonuria is a genetic disease in which the person cannot break down the amino acid phenylalanine. The buildup of phenylalanine and its by-products leads to brain damage.

■ Sickle cell anemia is a genetic disorder of the red blood cells. Because of an alteration of one amino acid in hemoglobin, the red blood cells become sickle-shaped and cannot travel smoothly through blood vessels. This blocks the vessels, causing inadequate oxygenation of nearby tissues, organ damage, and anemia.

■ Cystic fibrosis is a genetic disease that causes an alteration in chloride transport, leading to the production of thick, sticky mucus. This mucus causes serious respiratory and digestive problems, which lead to variable levels of debilitation and, in some cases, premature death.

MasteringNutrition™

To further your understanding, go online and apply what you've learned to real-life case studies that will help you master the content!

Review Questions

1. The process of combining peanut butter and whole-wheat bread to make a complete protein is called
   a. deamination.
   b. vegetarianism.
   c. transamination.
   d. mutual supplementation.

2. Which of the following meals would be appropriate in a well-planned vegan diet?
   a. rice, pinto beans, acorn squash, soy butter, and almond milk
   b. veggie dog, bun, and a banana–yogurt milkshake
   c. brown rice and green tea
   d. egg salad on whole-wheat toast, broccoli, carrot sticks, and soy milk

3. The substance that breaks down polypeptides in the small intestine is called
   a. hydrochloric acid.
   b. pepsin.
   c. protease.
   d. ketones.

4. The portion of an amino acid that contains nitrogen is called the
   a. R group.
   b. amine group.
   c. acid group.
   d. nitrate cluster.

5. All proteins contain
   a. carbon, oxygen, iron, and nitrogen.
   b. iron, oxygen, and hydrogen.
   c. carbon, hydrogen, oxygen, and nitrogen.
   d. carbon, hydrogen, oxygen, and sulfur.

6. **True or false?** After leaving the small intestine, amino acids are transported to the liver for distribution throughout the body.

7. **True or false?** When a protein is denatured, its shape is lost but its function is retained.

8. **True or false?** All hormones are proteins.

9. **True or false?** Buffers help the body maintain acid–base balance.

10. **True or false?** Athletes typically require about three times as much protein as nonactive people.

11. Explain the relationship between inadequate protein intake and the swollen bellies of children with kwashiorkor.

12. Explain the relationship between excessive protein intake and an increased risk for kidney disease.

13. Differentiate between the roles of mRNA and tRNA in DNA replication.

14. You've always thought of your dad as a bit of a "health nut," so you're not surprised when you come home on spring break and he offers you a dinner of stir-fried vegetables and something called *quorn*. Over dinner, he announces that he has joined an online vegetarian chat group. "But, Dad," you protest, "you still eat meat, don't you?" "Sure I do," he answers, "but only once or twice a week. Lots of the other people in my chat group occasionally eat meat, too!" In your opinion, is vegetarianism an identity, a lifestyle choice, or a fad? Defend your position.

15. Draw a sketch showing how amino acids bond to form proteins.

Math Review

16. Barry is concerned he is not eating enough protein. After reading this chapter, he recorded his diet each day for 1 week to calculate how much protein he is eating. Barry's average protein intake for the week is equal to 190 g, and his daily energy intake averages 3,000 kcal. Barry weighs 182 lb. Based on your calculations, is Barry (a) meeting or exceeding the AMDR for protein and (b) meeting or exceeding the RDA for protein?

Answers to Review Questions and Math Review can be found online in the MasteringNutrition Study Area.

Web Links

www.eatright.org
Academy of Nutrition and Dietetics
Search for "vegetarian diets" to learn how to plan healthful meat-free meals.

www.fnic.nal.usda.gov
USDA Food and Nutrition Information Center
Click on "food consumption" in the left navigation bar to find a searchable database of the nutrient values of foods.

www.cdc.gov
Centers for Disease Control and Prevention
Click on "Health Topics A-Z" to learn more about E. coli and mad cow disease.

www.who.int/nutrition/en/
World Health Organization Nutrition Site
Visit this site to learn more about the worldwide scope of protein-deficiency diseases and related topics.

www.nlm.nih.gov/medlineplus
MEDLINE Plus Health Information
Search for "sickle cell anemia" and "cystic fibrosis" to obtain additional information and resources, and the latest developments for these diseases.

www.vrg.org
Vegetarian Resource Group
Visit this site for additional information on how to build a balanced vegetarian diet.

www.choosemyplate.gov/healthy-eating-tips/tips-for-vegetarian.html
MyPlate.gov
This section of the MyPlate website contains useful, healthy eating tips for vegetarians.

www.meatlessmonday.com
Meatless Monday Campaign
Find out how to start going meatless one day a week with this innovative campaign's website.

References

1. Huffington Post. 2011. Vegetarian Celebrities Highlighted on World Vegetarian Day. www.huffingtonpost.com/2011/10/01/world-vegetarian-day-2011_n_989218.html#s381790&title=Mike_Tyson_.

2. Vegetarian Resource Group. 2011. How Many Vegetarians Are There? *Vegetarian Journal*, www.vrg.org/press/2009poll.htm.

3. Fulgoni, V. L. 2008. Current protein intake in America: analysis of the National Health and Nutrition Examination Survey, 2003–2004. *Am. J. Clin. Nutr.* 87(suppl):1554S–1557S.

4. Manore, M. M., N. L. Meyer, and J. Thompson. 2009. *Sport Nutrition for Health and Performance.* 2nd edn. Champaign, IL: Human Kinetics.

5. Halton, T. L., and F. B. Hu. 2004. The effects of high protein diets on thermogenesis, satiety and weight loss: a critical review. *J. Am. Coll. Nutr.* 23(5):373–385.

6. Leitzmann, C. 2005. Vegetarian diets: what are the advantages? *Forum Nutr.* 57:147–156.

7. Szeto, Y. T., T. C. Y. Kwok, and I. F. F. Benzie. 2004. Effects of a long-term vegetarian diet on biomarkers of antioxidant status and cardiovascular disease risk. *Nutrition* 20:863–866.

8. Calvez, J., N. Poupin, C. Chesneau, C. Lassale, and D. Tomé. 2012. Protein intake, calcium balance and health consequences. *Eur. J. Clin. Nutr.* 66:281–295.

9. American Diabetes Association (ADA). 2003. Evidence-based nutrition principles and recommendations for the treatment and prevention of diabetes and related complications. *Diabetes Care* 26:S51–S61.

10. Martin, W. F., L. E. Armstrong, and N. R. Rodriguez. 2005. Dietary protein intake and renal function. *Nutr. Metabol.* 2:25. www.nutritionandmetabolism.com/content/2/1/25.

11. Sabaté, J.m and Y. Ang. 2009. Nuts and health outcomes: new epidemiological evidence. *Am. J. Clin. Nutr.* 89(suppl):1643S–1648S.

12. Li, T. Y., A. M. Brennan, N. M. Wedick, C. Mantzoros, N. Rifai, and F. B. Hu. 2009. Regular consumption of nuts is associated with a lower risk of cardiovascular disease in women with type 2 diabetes. *J. Nutr.* 139(7):1333–1338.

13. American Dietetic Association. 2009. Position of the American Dietetic Association: vegetarian diets. *J. Am. Diet. Assoc.* 109:1266–1282.

14. World Cancer Research Fund and the American Institute for Cancer Research. 2012. Continuous Update Project. Colorectal Cancer. Latest Evidence. www.dietandcancerreport.org/cup/current_progress/colorectal_cancer.php.

15. Barr, S. I., and C. A. Rideout. 2004. Nutrition considerations for vegetarian athletes. *Nutrition* 20:696–703.

16. Institute of Medicine, Food and Nutrition Board. 2005. *Dietary Reference Intakes for Energy, Carbohydrate, Fiber, Fat, Fatty Acids, Cholesterol, Protein, and Amino Acids (Macronutrients).* Washington, DC: National Academies Press.

Meat Consumption and Global Warming: Tofu to the Rescue?

Which causes more greenhouse gas emissions: livestock production or traffic? The answer may surprise you: according to the Food and Agriculture Organization of the United Nations (FAO), livestock production generates more of the gases responsible for global warming—18%—than does transportation.[1] In a landmark 2006 report called *Livestock's Long Shadow*, the FAO estimated that livestock production accounts for

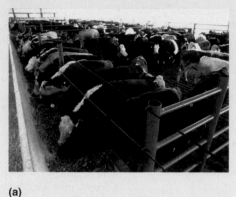
(a)

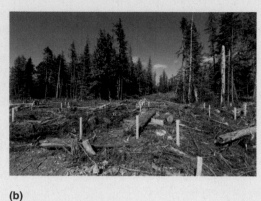
(b)

(a) Livestock production and **(b)** aggressive deforestation contribute to increased greenhouse gas emissions.

- 9% of all carbon dioxide (CO_2) production derived from human activity,
- 37% of all human-induced methane,
- 64% of ammonia, and
- 65% of human-related production of nitrous oxide.

The report generated considerable concern internationally. For example, in 2008, Dr. Rajendra Pachauri, chair of the United Nations Intergovernmental Panel on Climate Change, released a statement calling upon individuals to have one meat-free day a week and to progressively reduce their meat consumption even further.[2] Pachauri noted that reducing meat consumption is an action that anyone can take immediately, and one that can have a significant impact on global warming in a short period of time.

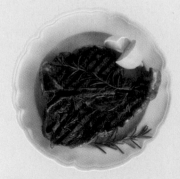
(a)

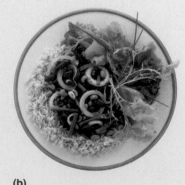
(b)

The difference in greenhouse gas emissions associated with **(a)** meat-based versus **(b)** vegetarian meals is similar to the difference between driving an SUV and driving an average sedan.

But in 2009, two environmental researchers from the World Bank published a report with far more disturbing conclusions.[3] Their data included factors that had been overlooked in the FAO report, leading the researchers to conclude that the actual contribution of livestock production to greenhouse gas emissions is 51%! Although some researchers immediately insisted that this percentage was inflated, the authors of the report have stood by it, insisting that their analysis is accurate.

Although the precise percentage is open to debate, no one disputes that livestock production does emit greenhouse gases, and thereby promotes global warming. In contrast, plants absorb carbon dioxide from the atmosphere (as you learned in Chapter 4, plants use carbon dioxide to synthesize glucose).

Livestock production is also a major source of land degradation, using 30% of the earth's land surface for pasture or feed production. Aggressive deforestation has cleared about 70% of former forests in the Amazon region for grazing.[1] Again, this loss of plant mass reduces the capture of greenhouse gases. In addition, the production of feed crops for livestock uses 33% of global arable land. Livestock's presence in vast tracts of land and its demand for feed crops also have contributed significantly to a reduction in biodiversity and a decline in ecosystems.[1]

Another environmental concern is the effect of livestock production on the global water supply. The Water Footprint Network, a project founded by the United Nations Educational, Scientific, and

Cultural Organization (UNESCO), explains that, whereas the production of a soy burger requires an investment of about 150 liters of water, the production of a beef burger of the same size requires 1,000 liters. [4] Moreover, animal waste, antibiotics, hormones, and fertilizers and pesticides used on feed crops can run off into neighboring streams, rivers, and lakes and into nearby irrigation fields used to produce crops for human consumption.

In response to many of these claims of environmental degradation due to livestock production, meat industry organizations have published information in defense of their practices. The Cattlemen's Beef Board and National Cattlemen's Beef Association website disputes many of the claims made by environmental impact scientific experts and critics. They state the following:[5]

- The waste produced by cattle is very minor, accounting for only 2.6% of the country's greenhouse gas emissions, compared to 25% for transportation.
- Approximately 85% of all land is not suitable for growing vegetable or grain crops. Double the land area can be used to produce food by grazing animals on this land.
- Beef production is significantly more environmentally sustainable than 30 years ago. As compared to 1977, each pound of beef today produces 18% less carbon emissions, takes 30% less land, and requires 14% less water.

Although some individuals choose vegetarianism to protect the environment, it is not practical or realistic to expect every human around the world to adopt this lifestyle. Animal products provide important nutrients for our bodies, and many people on the brink of starvation cannot survive without small amounts of milk and meat.

Still, if people were to reduce their consumption of meat even modestly, the change would have a powerful collective impact. A 2011 report from the Environmental Working Group found that, if every American ate only plant foods just 1 day a week, the reduction in greenhouse gas emissions would be the equivalent of taking 7.6 million cars off the road.[6] If Americans were to reduce their intake more significantly, it could be possible to return to the system of small family farming, which is more environmentally friendly. When animals are raised on smaller farms and/or allowed

to range freely, they consume grass, crop wastes, and scraps recycled from the kitchen, which is an efficient means of utilizing food sources that humans do not consume. What's more, the waste produced by these animals can be used for fertilizer and fuel.

CRITICAL THINKING QUESTIONS

- Are the data convincing that meat consumption increases global warming?
- Given the accelerated pace of climate change, as well as land and water degradation, is it our ethical responsibility as citizens of the earth to reduce our consumption of meat?
- What adverse impact might reducing meat consumption have on farmers and ranchers? Would this be greater or worse than the impact of climate change?
- Would eating less meat be practical for you?
- Whether or not you decide to eat less meat, what other actions can you take to reduce the "carbon footprint" of your diet?

REFERENCES

1. Food and Agriculture Organization of the United Nations. 2006. Livestock's Long Shadow: Environmental Issues and Options. www.fao.org/docrep/010/a0701e/a0701e00.HTM.
2. Jowit, J. 2008. UN says eat less meat to curb global warming. *The Observer.* www.guardian.co.uk/environment/2008/sep/07/food.foodanddrink.
3. Goodland, R., and J. Anhang. 2009. Livestock and Climate Change. *World Watch.* www.worldwatch.org/files/pdf/Livestock%20and%20Climate%20Change.pdf.
4. Water Footprint Network. 2012. Direct and Indirect Water Use. www.waterfootprint.org/?page=files/home.
5. Cattlemen's Beef Board and National Cattlemen's Beef Association. 2010. Explore Beef. http://www.explorebeef.org/environment.aspx.
6. Hamerschlag, K. (2011, July). Meat-Eater's Guide to Climate Change and Health. Environmental Working Group. http://static.ewg.org/reports/2011/meateaters/pdf/report_ewg_meat_eaters_guide_to_health_and_climate_2011.pdf.

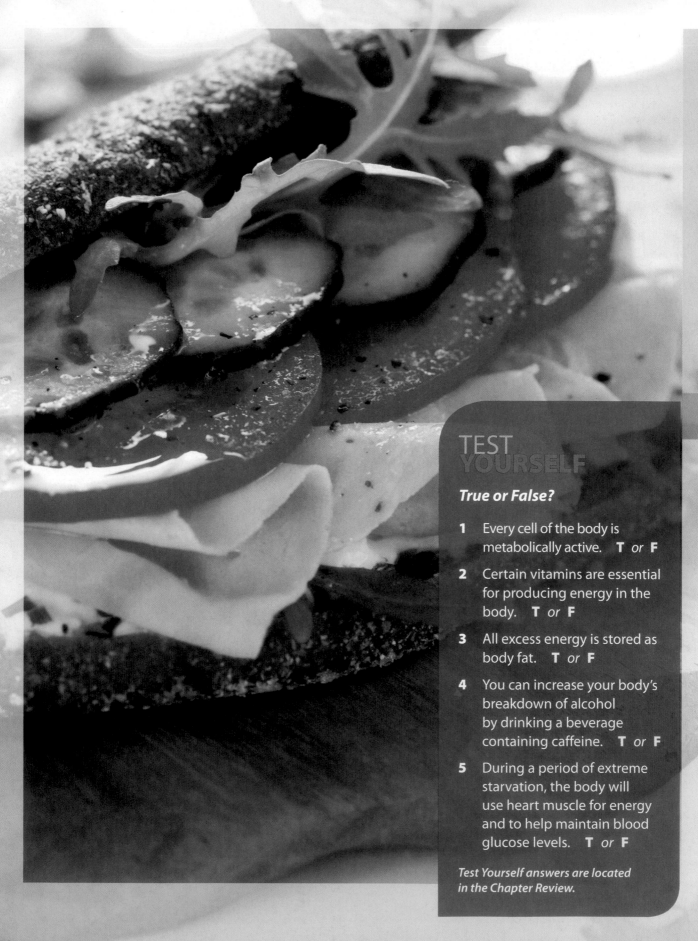

7

Metabolism: From Food to Life

Learning Objectives

After studying this chapter, you should be able to:

1. Describe the properties of metabolism, catabolism, and anabolism, including the roles of ATP, ADP, and AMP, *pp. 260–262.*

2. Illustrate the following types of metabolic reactions: hydrolysis, dehydration synthesis, oxidation–reduction, and phosphorylation, *pp. 264–265.*

3. Explain the role of enzymes, cofactors, and coenzymes during chemical reactions, *pp. 265–266.*

4. Identify the metabolic processes and stages involved in extracting energy from carbohydrates, *pp. 266–272.*

5. Identify the metabolic processes and stages involved in extracting energy from fats, *pp. 272–277.*

6. Explain how the catabolism of proteins differs from the catabolism of carbohydrates and lipids, *pp. 277–280.*

7. Delineate the process by which alcohol is metabolized, *pp. 280–282.*

8. Identify the body's mechanisms for storing excess glucose, triglycerides, and proteins, *pp. 283–284.*

9. Describe the processes by which macronutrients are synthesized, and the role of hormones in regulating metabolism, *pp. 284–287.*

10. Explain how the states of feasting and fasting affect metabolism, *pp. 288–291.*

MasteringNutrition™

Go online for chapter quizzes, pre-tests, Interactive Activities and more!

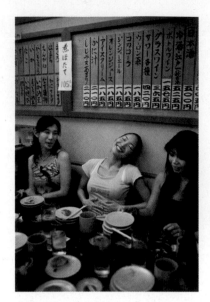

The food we eat is converted to fuel and other necessary substances through metabolism.

Malia, just 12 hours old, was fussing in her father's arms when the hospital pediatrician and a neonatal nurse entered the room. While the nurse soothed Malia, the pediatrician broke the news: the results of a routine screening test indicated that Malia had been born with maple syrup urine disease (MSUD), a metabolic disorder, and further tests confirmed the diagnosis. He explained that MSUD occurs when a baby lacks an enzyme necessary to break down certain amino acids. If the disorder is not treated, the unmetabolized amino acids quickly build up in the body's tissues, especially the brain, resulting in severe and sometimes fatal neurologic damage. Malia's parents had never heard of MSUD and immediately asked if their daughter would be all right. The pediatrician assured them that, when the disease is detected and dietary treatment initiated in the first days of life, children with MSUD develop normally. He explained that Malia would not be able to breastfeed but would have to be fed a special formula low in the amino acids leucine, isoleucine, and valine. "Are you saying that the only thing we have to do to keep Malia healthy is switch her from breast milk to a special formula?" Malia's father asked. "For now, yes," the pediatrician replied. "But as she grows, you'll have to pay careful and consistent attention to her diet." He scheduled them to meet with the hospital's registered dietitian that afternoon to discuss Malia's dietary needs.

Metabolic disorders such as MSUD, phenylketonuria (see Chapter 4), galactosemia (an error of carbohydrate metabolism), and others are rare, but because they interrupt the normal processes of metabolism, their consequences can be severe or fatal. Why is metabolism so critical to our health and life, and how does it occur? We explore these and other questions in this chapter.

Why Is Metabolism Essential for Life?

Although some people say they live to eat, we all have to eat to live. The food we eat each day provides the energy and nutrients the body needs to sustain life. **Metabolism** is the sum of all the chemical and physical processes by which the body breaks down and builds up molecules. When nutrition researchers burn food in a **calorimeter** to determine how much energy the food contains, carbon dioxide, water, and thermal energy (heat) are released. In a similar way, when the body uses food for fuel, carbon dioxide, water, and energy, both chemical and thermal energy are released. Cells throughout the body require chemical energy to grow, reproduce, repair themselves, and maintain their functions. Indeed, every chemical reaction in the body either requires or releases energy. In addition, energy released as heat helps keep us warm. When cell metabolism functions properly, so, too, does the body.

Anabolism and Catabolism Require or Release Energy

As you learned in previous chapters, the end products of digestion are absorbed into the small intestine and then circulated to the body's cells. There, they may be broken down even further for energy. Alternatively, the cells may use these small, basic molecules as building blocks to synthesize compounds, such as glycogen, cholesterol, hormones, enzymes, or cell membranes, according to the body's needs. The process of making larger, chemically complex molecules from smaller, more basic ones is called **anabolism** (**Figure 7.1**). Because the process of anabolism supports the building of compounds, it is critical for growth, repair and maintenance of the body's tissues, and synthesis of the chemical products essential for human functioning. From a small subset of metabolic "building blocks," including glucose, amino acids, and fatty acids, the body is able to use anabolism to synthesize thousands of chemically complex substances.

Anabolic reactions require energy. If you've studied physics, you know that *energy* can be broadly defined as the capacity to perform work. Mechanical energy is necessary for movement, electrical energy sparks nerve impulses, and thermal energy maintains body temperature. The energy that fuels anabolic reactions is chemical energy. How exactly does the body generate this chemical energy?

metabolism The sum of all the chemical and physical changes that occur in body tissues.

calorimeter A special instrument in which food can be burned and the amount of heat that is released can be measured; this process demonstrates the energy (caloric) content of the food.

anabolism The process of making new molecules from smaller ones.

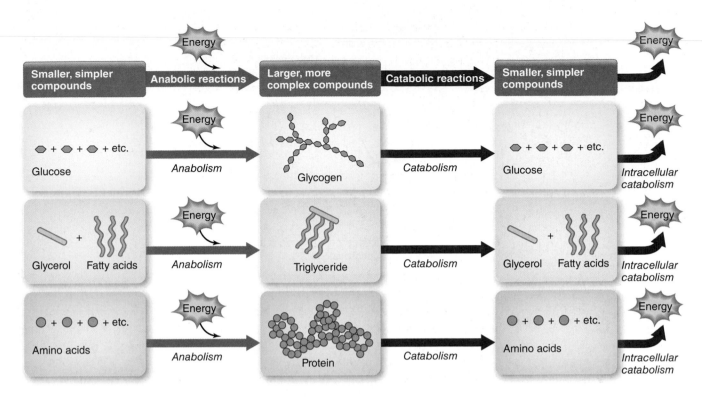

FIGURE 7.1 Anabolic reactions use energy to convert simple chemical compounds into larger, more complex structures. Catabolic reactions degrade complex compounds and produce energy.

Catabolism is the breakdown, or degradation, of larger, more complex molecules to smaller, more basic molecules (see Figure 7.1). The opposite of anabolism, it releases chemical energy. Catabolism of food begins with digestion, when chemical reactions break down the macronutrients we consume. The thousands of different proteins, lipids, and carbohydrates in the human diet are all broken down into the same small group of end products: amino acids, fatty acids, glycerol, and monosaccharides (usually glucose). After absorption, these basic components are transported to body cells. When a cell needs energy, it can catabolize these components into even smaller molecules. Energy is released as a by-product of this intracellular catabolism. Catabolism is also used to break down old cells or tissues that need to be repaired or replaced. The energy gained via catabolic reactions is used not only to fuel the body's work but also to build new compounds, cells, and tissues via anabolism. Thus, in response to our earlier question, the energy to fuel anabolic reactions comes from the body's catabolic reactions.

Overall, a balance between anabolism and catabolism maintains health and function. However, there are times when one of these two processes dominates. For example, fetal and childhood growth represents a net anabolic state, because more tissue is formed than broken down. However, disease is often dominated by catabolism, with more tissue being broken down than repaired. Of course, one goal of treatment is to stop or minimize these catabolic processes and allow the anabolic phase of recovery to begin.

Energy Stored in Adenosine Triphosphate Fuels the Work of All Body Cells

When cells catabolize nutrients such as glucose, they package the energy that is released during the reaction in a compound called **adenosine triphosphate (ATP)**. As you might guess from its name, a molecule of ATP includes an organic compound called adenosine and three phosphate groups (**Figure 7.2a**). The bonds between the phosphate groups store a significant amount of potential energy and are sometimes termed *high-energy phosphate bonds*.[1] When these bonds are broken, their energy is released and can be used to do the work

catabolism   The breakdown, or degradation, of larger molecules to smaller molecules.

adenosine triphosphate (ATP)   A high-energy compound made up of the purine adenine, the simple sugar ribose, and three phosphate units; it is used by cells as a source of metabolic energy.

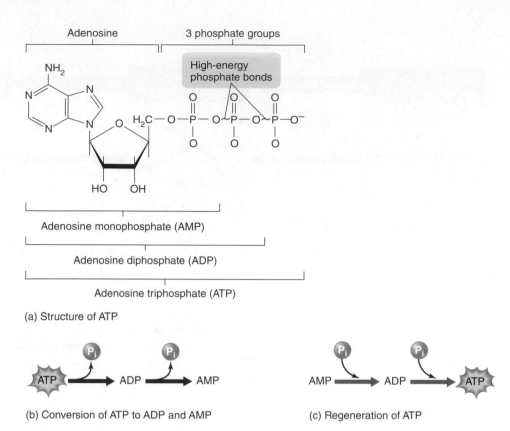

(a) Structure of ATP

(b) Conversion of ATP to ADP and AMP

(c) Regeneration of ATP

FIGURE 7.2 (a) Structure of adenosine triphosphate (ATP). (b) When one high-energy phosphate group is removed, adenosine diphosphate (ADP) is formed. When two high-energy phosphate groups are removed, adenosine monophosphate (AMP) is formed. (c) ATP can be regenerated by adding phosphate groups back to AMP and ADP through the process of phosphorylation.

of the cell. This explains why ATP is often called the molecular "currency" of the cell: its phosphate bonds store energy to build new molecules, break down old molecules, and keep the cell functioning optimally.

When one high-energy phosphate bond is broken and a single phosphate group released, **adenosine diphosphate (ADP)** is produced (Figure 7.2b). When two phosphates are removed, **adenosine monophosphate (AMP)** is produced. ATP can be regenerated by adding phosphate groups back to these molecules (Figure 7.2c).

A small amount of ATP is stored in every cell for immediate use. When cells need more ATP, they can generate it via the catabolism of glucose, glycerol, fatty acids, and amino acids. Thus, the food we eat each day continues to help the body regenerate the ATP required by the cells.

RECAP

All forms of life are dependent upon metabolic pathways for survival. A balance between anabolic and catabolic reactions helps the body achieve growth and repair and maintain health and functioning. The body uses and produces energy in the form of ATP. ■

adenosine diphosphate (ADP) A metabolic intermediate that results from the removal of one phosphate group from ATP.

adenosine monophosphate (AMP) A low-energy compound that results from the removal of two phosphate groups from ATP.

What Chemical Reactions Are Fundamental to Metabolism?

Metabolic pathways are clusters of chemical reactions that occur sequentially and achieve a particular goal, such as the breakdown of glucose for energy. Cells use different, yet related, metabolic pathways to release the energy in each of the major energy-containing

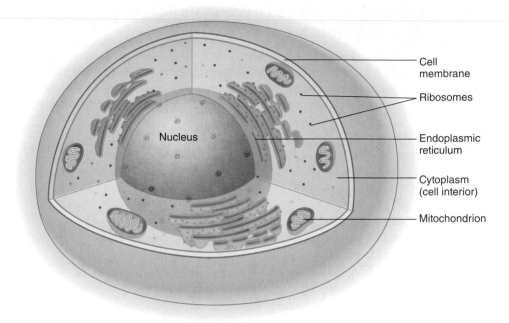

FIGURE 7.3 Structure of a typical cell. The cell membrane separates the cell from the extracellular fluid. The nucleus contains the genetic information. The cytoplasm contains the organelles, surrounded by a fluid called cytosol. Organelles include mitochondria, endoplasmic reticulum, and ribosomes.

nutrients—glucose, fatty acids, and amino acids. These pathways typically occur within a specific part of a cell. This is because many metabolic enzymes are restricted to one or a few locations within the cell. As an example, the process of glycolysis, to be discussed shortly, occurs in the cytosol, the liquid portion of the cytoplasm, because all of the enzymes needed for that process can be found in the cytosol. **Figure 7.3** shows the general structure of a cell and its components.

The cell's mitochondria, which might be compared to the furnace in your house, are the location of many other metabolic reactions. The mitochondria contain large numbers of metabolic enzymes and are the primary sites where chemical energy, in the form of ATP, is produced. Cells that lack mitochondria, such as red blood cells, are limited in their ability to produce energy. These cells must rely on less efficient energy-producing processes that can occur in their cytoplasm.

Metabolic pathways are limited not only to certain types of cells and certain cell structures, but they may also be limited to specific body organs or tissues. Glycogen stored in the liver can be catabolized and the resulting glucose released into the bloodstream, yet the catabolism of muscle glycogen does not allow for the release of glucose into the blood. Why the difference? Muscle lacks one enzyme that catalyzes one simple step in the metabolic pathway that is found in the liver; thus, the glucose released from the catabolism of muscle glycogen is not able to pass through the muscle cell membrane into the blood.

Although all cells are metabolically active, many nutritionists view liver, muscle, and adipose cells as key locations for the integration of metabolic pathways. As this chapter unfolds, it will be possible to visualize the "networking" of metabolic pathways that occurs between these and other body cells.

Before describing each of the unique metabolic pathways involving carbohydrates, fats, and proteins, we will review a few simple chemical reactions common to all of them.

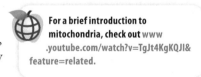

For a brief introduction to mitochondria, check out www .youtube.com/watch?v=TgJt4KgKQJI& feature=related.

In Dehydration Synthesis and Hydrolysis Reactions, Water Reacts with Molecules

Dehydration synthesis and **hydrolysis** are chemical reactions involving water. Dehydration synthesis, also called *condensation*, is an anabolic process. It occurs when small, chemically simple units combine to produce a larger, more complex molecule. In the process, water is released as a by-product. The general formula for these reactions is written as follows:

$$A{-}OH + H{-}B \rightarrow A{-}B + H_2O$$

One example is the synthesis of disaccharides from individual monosaccharides. As previously discussed (in Chapter 4), the formation of a chemical bond between two simple sugars occurs when one monosaccharide donates a hydroxyl (OH) group and the other donates a hydrogen (H) atom. The dehydration synthesis of glucose and fructose to yield sucrose is shown in **Figure 7.4a**.

Again, dehydration synthesis is typically an anabolic process. Its opposite, termed *hydrolysis,* is usually catabolic. Recall that *hydro-* refers to water, whereas *lysis* is from a Greek word meaning to separate. In hydrolysis, a large, chemically complex molecule is broken apart with the addition of water. Because the original molecule becomes hydrated, this reaction is also called a *hydration* reaction. Notice that the general formula for hydrolysis reactions is opposite that of dehydration synthesis reactions:

$$A{-}B + H_2O \rightarrow A{-}OH + H{-}B$$

One example of hydrolysis is the catabolism or breakdown of the disaccharide sucrose to its smaller and chemically simpler monosaccharides (glucose and fructose). This process is illustrated in Figure 7.4b.

dehydration synthesis An anabolic process by which smaller, chemically simple compounds are joined and a molecule of water is released; also called *condensation*.

hydrolysis A catabolic process by which a large, chemically complex compound is broken apart with the addition of water.

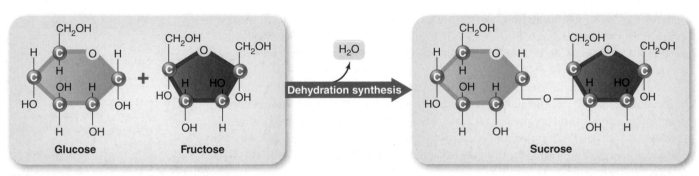

(a) Dehydration synthesis of glucose and fructose

(b) Hydrolysis of sucrose

FIGURE 7.4 (a) Dehydration synthesis of glucose and fructose. Glucose and fructose react and, with the release of water, combine to form sucrose. (b) Hydrolysis of sucrose. Sucrose undergoes hydrolysis, with the addition of water, to form glucose and fructose.

In Phosphorylation Reactions, Molecules Exchange Phosphate

The process by which phosphate is transferred from one molecule to another is called **phosphorylation.** For example, glucose undergoes phosphorylation when it first enters a cell:

$$C_6H_{12}O_6 \quad + \quad A—P—P—P \quad \rightarrow \quad C_6H_{12}O_6—P \quad\quad + \quad A—P—P$$

Glucose   ATP   Phosphorylated glucose   ADP

The newly phosphorylated glucose can either be stored as glycogen or be oxidized for immediate energy (discussed shortly). Another example of phosphorylation is the synthesis of ATP from ADP plus a free phosphate group (see Figure 7.2c). As you may have guessed, removal of phosphate groups, as in the breakdown of ATP (see Figure 7.2b), is called *dephosphorylation.*

In Oxidation–Reduction Reactions, Molecules Exchange Electrons

In **oxidation–reduction reactions,** the molecules involved exchange electrons, often in the form of hydrogen (which has just one electron). These reactions always occur together, as electrons gained by one molecule must be donated by another. The molecule that gives up an electron is said to be *oxidized,* because typically its electron has been removed by an oxygen atom. The molecule that has acquired an electron is said to be reduced, because, in gaining an electron (e^-), it becomes more negatively charged. In the human body, the oxygen needed for oxidation reactions is obtained from the air we breathe. Because they involve the exchange of electrons, oxidation–reduction (*redox*) reactions are classified as *exchange reactions.*

One example of a redox reaction important to metabolism involves **FAD (flavin adenine dinucleotide)** and $FADH_2$, two forms of riboflavin, one of the B-vitamins involved in energy metabolism. These compounds are required by several of the enzymes active in the electron transport chain, a key step in the production of your body's energy. $FADH_2$ is easily oxidized, losing electrons as hydrogen, and forming FAD (**Figure 7.5**). In contrast, FAD is easily reduced back to $FADH_2$ by the simple addition of hydrogen.

The production of energy from the energy-containing nutrients occurs through a series of oxidation–reduction reactions that ultimately yield carbon dioxide (CO_2) and water (H_2O). The oxidation of glucose and of fatty acids through this process is illustrated later in this chapter.

Enzymes Mediate Metabolic Reactions

As you know, chemical reactions in cells are typically influenced (mediated) by enzymes. During metabolism, one function of enzymes is to channel the energy-containing nutrients into useful metabolic pathways. For example, by increasing or decreasing the activity of one particular enzyme, the body can channel fatty acids either toward breakdown for energy or, if energy needs have already been met, toward storage as adipose tissue. Thus, enzymes are essential to the coordinated metabolism of the energy-containing nutrients.

phosphorylation The addition of one or more phosphate groups to a chemical compound.

oxidation–reduction reactions Reactions in which electrons are lost by one compound (it is oxidized) and simultaneously gained by another compound (it is reduced).

FAD (flavin adenine dinucleotide) A coenzyme derived from the B-vitamin riboflavin; FAD readily accepts electrons (hydrogen) from various donors.

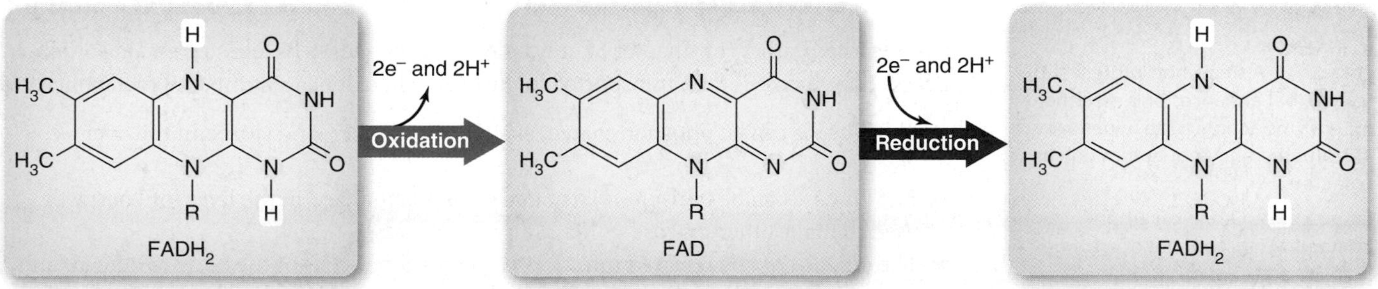

FIGURE 7.5 Oxidation and reduction of FAD and $FADH_2$. $FADH_2$ is easily oxidized to FAD, which can easily be reduced back to $FADH_2$.

FIGURE 7.6 Cofactors combine with enzymes to activate them, ensuring that the chemical reactions that depend upon these enzymes occur.

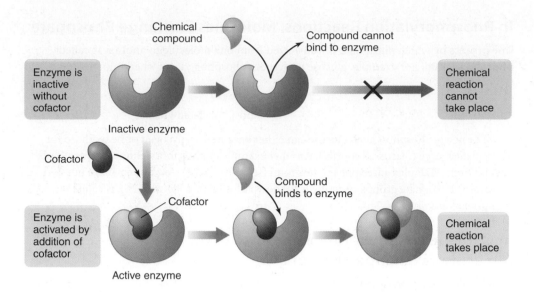

In order to function, enzymes generally require substances called **cofactors.** These small, non-protein substances (**Figure 7.6**) either enhance or are essential for the action of the enzyme. Many cofactors are minerals, such as iron or zinc, which may help bind different parts of an enzyme together, thereby speeding up the reaction.[1] If the cofactor is organic (contains carbon), it is termed a **coenzyme.** Many coenzymes are derived from vitamins, particularly B-vitamins. For example, FAD and $FADH_2$, derivatives of the B-vitamin ribo-flavin, function as coenzymes.[1,2] In short, minerals and vitamins functioning as cofactors or coenzymes are essential to ensure that metabolic pathways are as efficient as possible.

An example of an enzyme-driven metabolic reaction is the phosphorylation of glucose, mentioned earlier. The enzyme that activates this process is **glucokinase.** When glucose concentrations in the liver rise after a meal, the activity of this enzyme increases to handle the increased load, allowing for efficient metabolism of the glucose. Not every metabolic enzyme is as responsive, however. As discussed shortly, the liver enzyme that typically oxidizes alcohol does not increase in response to a sudden increase in alcohol consumption.

RECAP

Dehydration synthesis and hydrolysis are chemical reactions involving water. The reaction in which phosphate is transferred is called phosphorylation. In oxidation–reduction reactions, the molecules involved exchange electrons. Enzymes, coenzymes, and cofactors increase the efficiency of metabolism. ■

How Is Energy Extracted from Carbohydrates?

As you learned earlier (in Chapter 3), most dietary carbohydrate is digested and absorbed as glucose. The glucose is then transported to the liver, where it has a number of metabolic fates:

- The glucose can be phosphorylated, as described earlier, and stored in the liver as glycogen.
- The glucose can be phosphorylated and then metabolized in the liver for energy or used to make other glucose-containing compounds.
- The glucose can be released into circulation for other cells of the body to take up and use as a fuel or, in the case of muscle tissue, store as glycogen.
- The glucose, if consumed in excess of total energy needs, can be converted to fatty acids and stored as triglycerides, primarily in the adipose tissue.

cofactor A small, non-protein substance that enhances or is essential for enzyme action; trace minerals such as iron, zinc, and copper function as cofactors.

coenzyme Organic (carbon-containing) component of enzymes; many coenzymes are B-vitamins.

glucokinase An enzyme that adds a phosphate group to a molecule of glucose.

What happens to fructose and galactose, the other dietary monosaccharides? Although there are many other metabolic options for each, both can be (a) converted into glucose through a series of reactions or (b) channeled into the glycolysis pathway (discussed shortly) for energy production. For that reason, and because glucose is the dominant monosaccharide in the human diet, this discussion will explore how the body uses glucose as an energy source.

The oxidation of glucose for the production of energy progresses through three distinct stages, each of which takes place in a different part of the cell. The three stages are

1. Glycolysis
2. The tricarboxylic acid (TCA) cycle (also known as the Krebs cycle or citric acid cycle)
3. The electron transport chain, which is where the process of oxidative phosphorylation occurs

Step by step, we will review these metabolic pathways.

In Glycolysis, Glucose Is Broken Down into Pyruvate

The metabolic pathway used by cells to produce energy from glucose begins with a sequence of reactions known as **glycolysis** (**Figure 7.7**). Because glycolysis occurs in the cytosol, even

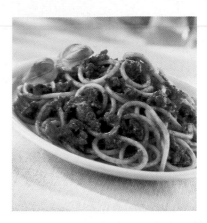

Most dietary carbohydrate is digested and absorbed as glucose.

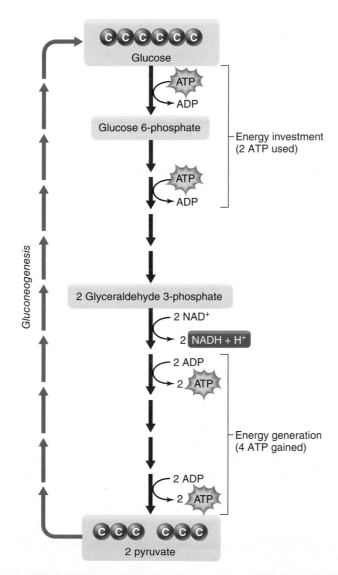

FIGURE 7.7 Overview of glycolysis. In the first stage of glucose oxidation, glucose is converted to pyruvate. A separate pathway provides for the regeneration of glucose via gluconeogenesis, which requires the input of ATP. Net production from glycolysis: two pyruvate molecules, two ATP, and two NADH 1 H⁺.

glycolysis   A sequence of chemical reactions that converts glucose to pyruvate.

cells without mitochondria can extract energy from this pathway. Also, because the reactions of glycolysis are anaerobic (that is, do not require oxygen), this short pathway can be completed even when tissues are in an oxygen-deprived state.

During glycolysis, six-carbon glucose is converted into two molecules of three-carbon pyruvate. The first step of glycolysis is the phosphorylation of glucose, which, as described earlier, yields glucose 6-phosphate and ADP. The ATP that fuels this reaction is stored in the cell. Then, several enzyme-driven reactions result in the formation of pyruvate. (These reactions are omitted from Figure 7.7 but included in the complete figure in Appendix B.) Initially, the process of glycolysis requires two ATP for the phosphorylation of glucose, but eventually this pathway produces a small amount (four molecules) of ATP, thus yielding a net of two ATP to be used as energy for the cell.

As shown in Figure 7.7, the process of glycolysis is one example of an oxidative pathway, because two hydrogen atoms (with their electrons) are released. These hydrogen atoms are picked up by two molecules of the coenzyme **NAD (nicotinamide adenine dinucleotide),** derived from the B-vitamin niacin, forming two molecules of NADH, the reduced form of NAD. The metabolic fate of the newly formed NADH will be explained shortly.

If the pyruvate molecules generated by glycolysis are to be used for the production of energy, they must go through a number of additional metabolic steps, which vary depending on whether oxygen is present (*aerobic* environment) or absent (*anaerobic* environment). If energy is not immediately needed by the cell, pyruvate can be used to resynthesize glucose, which can be stored as glycogen or used in the synthesis of other carbohydrate-containing substances (which will then be stored). The resynthesis of glucose from pyruvate can be thought of as "moving back up" this stage of the metabolic pathway, which occurs through a separate series of reactions (see Figure 7.7). This reverse process is known as gluconeogenesis and will be discussed later in this chapter.

In the Absence of Oxygen, Pyruvate Is Converted to Lactic Acid

In the absence of oxygen, the pyruvate produced through glycolysis is anaerobically converted to **lactate (lactic acid).** This one-step reaction involves a simple transfer of hydrogen. Both pyruvate and lactate are three-carbon compounds, so there is no loss or gain of carbon atoms. In a reversal of the hydrogen transfer that occurred in glycolysis (when NAD$^+$ accepted $2H^+ + 2e^-$ to form NADH + H$^+$), the conversion of pyruvate to lactate involves the transfer of $2e^- + 2H^+$ from NADH to lactate, leaving NAD$^+$ (**Figure 7.8a**). The production of lactate therefore regenerates the NAD$^+$ required for the continued functioning of the glycolysis pathway.

The anaerobic conversion of pyruvate to lactate occurs in cells with few or no mitochondria, such as the red blood cells and the lens and cornea of the eye. It also occurs in the muscle cells during high-intensity exercise, when oxygen delivery to the muscle is limited. Compared with the entire three-stage oxidation of glucose, the production of energy in this phase of anaerobic glycolysis is not very efficient. The short pathway from pyruvate to lactate does not yield any ATP; therefore, when one molecule of glucose is converted to lactate, the only ATP produced is the two (net) ATP units that were generated when the glucose was initially converted to pyruvate (see Figure 7.8). The anaerobic production of lactate is, however, a way of producing at least a small amount of energy when oxygen is absent or in those cells lacking mitochondria. The production of lactate, also known as lactic acid, also allows the regeneration of NAD$^+$, so that glycolysis can continue.

During intense exercise, lactic acid and other acids and metabolic by-products can build up in tissues, especially the muscle tissues, which some believe contributes to fatigue and soreness (see the **Nutrition Myth or Fact?** box in Chapter 14, page 574). The low production of energy as ATP through the anaerobic production of lactate is one of the many reasons individuals cannot sustain high-intensity exercise for long periods of time. After exercise, lactate can diffuse from the muscle cells into the blood, which transports it back to the liver. Then, when oxygen is readily available during the rest or recovery phase, it is reconverted to pyruvate, which can be used to synthesize glucose (Figure 7.8b). This process illustrates the

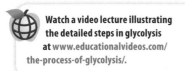

Watch a video lecture illustrating the detailed steps in glycolysis at www.educationalvideos.com/the-process-of-glycolysis/.

NAD (nicotinamide adenine dinucleotide) A coenzyme form of the B-vitamin niacin; NAD readily accepts electrons (hydrogen) from various donors.

lactate (lactic acid) A three-carbon compound produced from pyruvate in oxygen-deprived conditions.

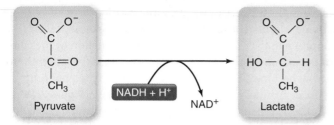

(a) Anaerobic conversion of pyruvate to lactate

FIGURE 7.8 (a) Anaerobic conversion of pyruvate to lactate. In the absence of oxygen, the body converts pyruvate to lactate. (b) Interconversion of lactate and glucose. After the anaerobic production and release of lactate by the muscle, when oxygen becomes available, the liver converts lactate back to glucose. (This process, known as the Cori cycle, is discussed in more detail in Chapter 14.)

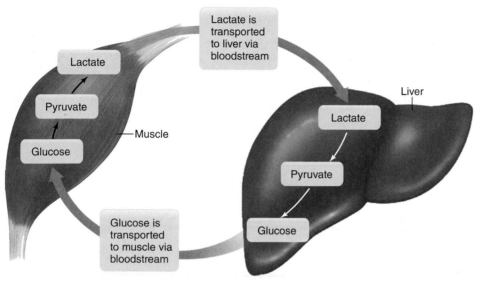

(b) Interconversion of lactate and glucose

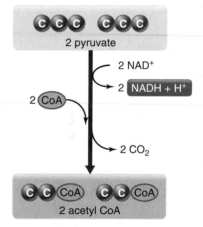

FIGURE 7.9 Aerobic conversion of pyruvate to acetyl CoA. In the presence of oxygen, the body converts pyruvate to acetyl CoA. This reaction links the first and second stages of glucose oxidation. The two pyruvate molecules were generated from glucose through glycolysis.

integration of metabolism between muscle tissues and the liver, as was mentioned earlier. (This cycle of glucose-to-lactate (during oxygen deprivation) followed by lactate-to-glucose (during oxygen availability) will be discussed in more detail in Chapter 14.)

In the Presence of Oxygen, Pyruvate Is Converted to Acetyl CoA

In an aerobic environment where oxygen is plentiful, pyruvate is converted to a two-carbon compound known as **acetyl CoA** (**Figure 7.9**). This reaction occurs in the mitochondria and therefore does not occur in red blood cells or other cells that lack mitochondria. *CoA* is shorthand for *coenzyme A*, a coenzyme derived from the B-vitamin pantothenic acid. As with the conversion of glucose to pyruvate, the metabolic pathway taking pyruvate to acetyl CoA generates NADH + H$^+$ from the niacin-derived coenzyme NAD$^+$. Pyruvate is a three-carbon compound, whereas acetyl CoA is a two-carbon metabolite. What happens to the other carbon? It ends up within the gas carbon dioxide (CO_2), which the lungs exhale as a waste product.

Unlike the metabolic option to convert lactate to glucose, once pyruvate is metabolized to acetyl CoA, there is no "going back" to glucose synthesis. In other words, there is no metabolic option for the conversion of acetyl CoA to glucose. Once acetyl CoA is produced, it can be further metabolized to produce energy (ATP) or, when the body has adequate ATP, redirected into fatty acid synthesis (discussed shortly).

The conversion of pyruvate to acetyl CoA is a critical step in the oxidation of glucose, because it links stage 1 (glycolysis) to stage 2 (the TCA cycle). This reaction also marks the transition of cytosol-based pathways to mitochondria-based pathways. To begin this step, pyruvate moves from the cytosol into the mitochondria, where it is converted to acetyl

acetyl CoA Coenzyme A (CoA) is derived from the B-vitamin pantothenic acid; it readily reacts with two-carbon acetate to form the metabolic intermediate acetyl CoA; sometimes referred to as *acetyl coenzyme A*.

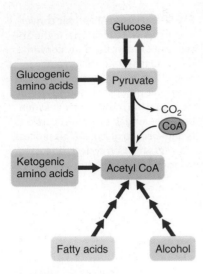

CoA. Once acetyl CoA is produced in the mitochondria, it cannot be transferred back across the mitochondrial membrane without conversion to another compound, called citrate. Thus, acetyl CoA is committed to the TCA cycle for energy production or the conversion to citrate, in which form it can move back out of the mitochondria for fat synthesis.

As this chapter proceeds, it will become clear that acetyl CoA is generated not only from glucose oxidation but also from fatty acid and amino acid catabolism (**Figure 7.10**). You may be familiar with the phrase "All roads lead to Rome." In metabolism, most "roads" (metabolic pathways) lead to acetyl CoA!

The TCA Cycle Begins with the Entry of Acetyl CoA

The process of glycolysis has a clear starting point (glucose) and a clear ending point (pyruvate). The linking step (pyruvate to acetyl CoA) also has distinct start and end points. In contrast, the **TCA cycle** is a continuous circle of eight metabolic reactions (**Figure 7.11**). The complete TCA cycle is illustrated in Appendix B, and a condensed version will be used here for simplicity.

The TCA cycle is located in the mitochondria of the cell, which is where all of the necessary metabolic enzymes can be found. The mitochondria are also the location of stage 3

FIGURE 7.10 Metabolic crossroads. Acetyl CoA is generated as a result of carbohydrate, fatty acid, amino acid, and alcohol metabolism.

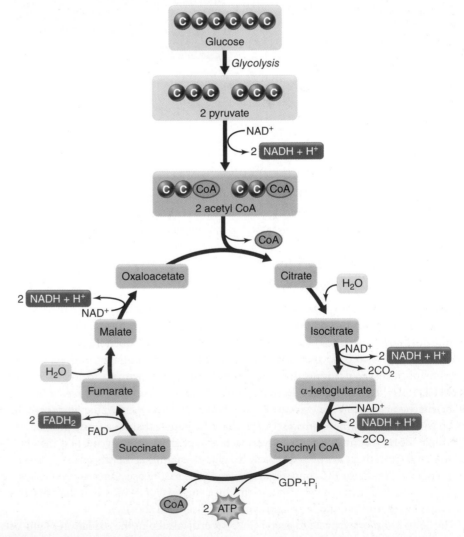

TCA cycle The tricarboxylic acid (TCA) cycle is a repetitive series of eight metabolic reactions, located in cell mitochondria, that metabolizes acetyl CoA for the production of carbon dioxide, high-energy GTP, and reduced coenzymes NADH and FADH$_2$.

FIGURE 7.11 Overview of the TCA cycle. In the second stage of glucose oxidation, acetyl CoA enters the TCA cycle, resulting in the release of carbon dioxide, GTP (ATP), and reduced coenzymes NADH and FADH$_2$.

of glucose oxidation (involving the electron transport chain) and ATP synthesis; thus, the transition between stages 2 and 3 is highly efficient.

We think of cycles as self-regenerative, but the acetyl CoA within the TCA cycle does not regenerate. As will be seen, the two carbons that form acetyl CoA end up within two molecules of carbon dioxide. In contrast, the fate of the four-carbon compound oxaloacetate does illustrate the cyclical nature of this stage of glucose oxidation: as shown in Figure 7.11, it is "used up" in the first step of the TCA cycle, where it is converted into citrate, and is regenerated from malate in the final step of the cycle.

Oxaloacetate and other metabolic intermediates within the TCA cycle are necessary for continued functioning of the TCA cycle; when these compounds are limited, the TCA cycle decreases in activity, and energy production sharply declines.[1] There are several situations in which lack of oxaloacetate causes a significant decrease in energy production. One is consumption of a diet very low in carbohydrates. Although oxaloacetate can be made from some amino acids, dietary carbohydrate is the primary source. The glucose that is derived from dietary carbohydrate can be converted to acetyl CoA (stage 1, Figure 7.11), which can enter the TCA cycle and be converted to oxaloacetate. In contrast, oxaloacetate cannot be synthesized from fatty acids. If a person is following a very-low-carbohydrate diet, such as the Atkins Diet, he or she will have limited ability to produce oxaloacetate, resulting in a slowdown of the TCA cycle.

The first step of the TCA cycle begins with the entry of acetyl CoA into the cycle. As previously explained, pyruvate crosses from the cytosol into the mitochondria, where it is converted into acetyl CoA. The two-carbon acetyl CoA reacts with four-carbon oxaloacetate to form six-carbon citrate (hence the term *citric acid cycle*), and the metabolic cycle begins. By the time all eight metabolic steps are completed, the cycle has produced two molecules of carbon dioxide; this is in addition to the one carbon dioxide produced in the earlier "linking" step.

In addition to the release of carbon dioxide, a high-energy compound known as GTP (guanosine triphosphate), equivalent to one ATP, is produced. Finally, a total of eight hydrogens, with their electrons, are transferred to two coenzymes—NAD^+ and FAD—producing NADH and $FADH_2$. These newly formed, hydrogen-rich coenzymes serve as the transition to stage 3, transporting the hydrogen atoms, with their electrons, to the electron transport chain.

For every molecule of glucose that goes through glycolysis, two pyruvate molecules are generated, leading to two molecules of acetyl CoA. Thus, the TCA cycle must complete two "rotations" for each molecule of glucose. From glycolysis through the TCA cycle, one molecule of glucose produces the following: six molecules of carbon dioxide (including those produced in the "linking step"), two ATP, two GTP, and ten reduced coenzymes (including the NADH from the linking step) as sources of hydrogen and electrons. Note, however, the low energy output: this small amount will not do much to fuel the activities of the body. It is not until the final stage of glucose oxidation that energy production as ATP assumes a major role.

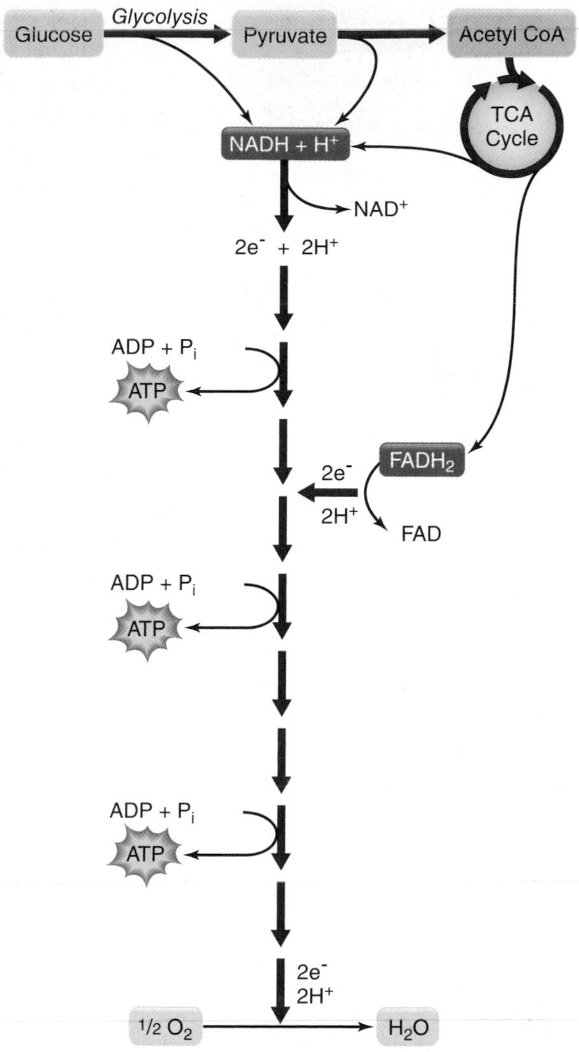

FIGURE 7.12 Overview of the electron transport chain. In the third and final stage of glucose oxidation, called *oxidative phosphorylation*, additional ATP and water are produced as electrons from NADH and $FADH_2$ and are passed from one carrier to the next along the electron transport chain.

Oxidative Phosphorylation Captures Energy as ATP

The third and final stage of glucose oxidation, termed *oxidative phosphorylation,* occurs in the **electron transport chain** and takes place in the inner membrane of the mitochondria (**Figure 7.12**). The electron transport chain is a series of enzyme-driven reactions or couplings; various proteins, called electron carriers, alternately accept, then donate, electrons.

electron transport chain A series of metabolic reactions that transports electrons from NAHD or $FADH_2$ through a series of carriers, resulting in ATP production.

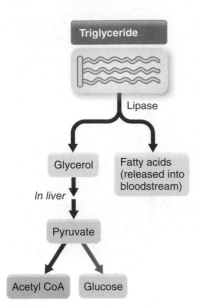

FIGURE 7.13 Conversion of glycerol to pyruvate. The glycerol derived from the catabolism of fatty acids is readily converted to pyruvate, which can be used for glucose synthesis or be converted to acetyl CoA.

The electrons come from the NADH and FADH$_2$ generated during glycolysis, the linking step, and the TCA cycle.

As summarized in Figure 7.12, as the electrons are passed from one carrier to the next, energy is released as ATP. In this process, NADH and FADH$_2$ are oxidized (lose electrons) and their electrons are eventually donated to O$_2$, which is reduced to H$_2$O (water). The energy released from the reduction of O$_2$ to water is used to phosphorylate mitochondrial ADP to ATP, thereby capturing the metabolic energy in ATP's high-energy phosphate bonds. Once formed, the ATP can exit the mitochondria for use by all components of the cell.

As mentioned, the final step in the electron transport chain occurs when oxygen accepts the low-energy electrons, reacts with hydrogen, and forms water. If the cell lacks adequate oxygen for this final step, the entire electron transport chain comes to a halt. Oxygen is essential for cellular energy production; without oxygen, cell metabolism stops.

This brings the process of glucose oxidation to a close. The complete process started with glucose and resulted in the production of carbon dioxide, water, and ATP. The carbon dioxide was produced in the linking step (pyruvate to acetyl CoA) and the TCA cycle. The water was produced in the final step of the electron transport chain. ATP was produced in various amounts during the three stages. It might surprise you to know that the amount of ATP produced by NADH and FADH$_2$ is not exact (about two to three ATP per NADH and one to two for FADH$_2$); thus, different researchers calculate different values for ATP production. Many biochemistry textbooks report a net of 30 to 32 ATP produced by the complete oxidation of one glucose molecule. Other references (including Appendix B of this textbook) use the range of 36 to 38 ATP per glucose molecule. This may seem confusing, but the study of nutrient metabolism is rarely an exact science.

RECAP

Glucose oxidation occurs in three well-defined stages: glycolysis, the TCA cycle, and oxidative phosphorylation. The conversion of pyruvate to acetyl CoA is a critical link between glycolysis and the TCA cycle. In the absence of oxygen, the pyruvate is converted to lactate, which can then be "recycled" by liver cells back into glucose. The end products of glucose oxidation are carbon dioxide, water, and ATP. ■

How Is Energy Extracted from Fats?

The fatty acids used for cellular energy can come from the triglycerides circulating in serum lipoproteins, including the dietary fat in chylomicrons, or from the triglycerides stored in body tissues, including adipose tissue. Because the triglyceride molecule is more complex than that of glucose, there are more steps involved in converting it into energy. Of course, the first step requires that each fatty acid be removed from the glycerol backbone. Through a process called **lipolysis,** dietary and adipocyte triglycerides are broken down by lipases to yield glycerol and three fatty acids. Triglycerides in lipoproteins are broken down through the action of *lipoprotein lipase,* whereas triglycerides in adipose cells are catabolized by the enzyme **hormone-sensitive lipase.** Whether the glycerol and fatty acids have come from dietary fat or stored body fat, they feed into the same metabolic pathways.

Glycerol Is Converted to Pyruvate

Glycerol, the small, three-carbon backbone of triglycerides, does not produce much energy but does serve other important metabolic functions. The liver readily converts glycerol into pyruvate, another three-carbon compound (**Figure 7.13**). As previously discussed, pyruvate can be converted into acetyl CoA for entry into the TCA cycle (see Figure 7.9), or it can be used for the regeneration of glucose (see Figure 7.7). Thus, in times of low energy or carbohydrate intake, the body can use the glycerol component of triglycerides as a source of glucose.

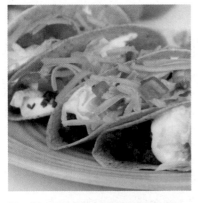

The first step in breaking down fats, such as fats in the meat and cheese of a taco, is lipolysis.

lipolysis The enzyme-driven catabolism of triglycerides into free fatty acids and glycerol.

hormone-sensitive lipase The enzyme that breaks down the triglycerides stored in adipose tissue.

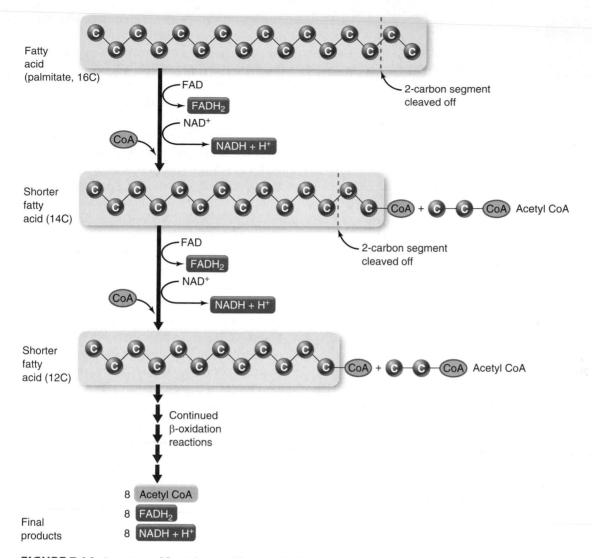

FIGURE 7.14 Overview of β-oxidation of fatty acids. Fatty acids are sequentially broken down into two-carbon segments that result in the formation of one additional acetyl CoA during each step of the process. A 16-carbon fatty acid yields 8 acetyl CoA units.

Fatty Acids Are Converted to Acetyl CoA

In yet another example of the integration of metabolism across different body organs, fatty acids released from adipose cells are attached to **albumin,** a blood protein, and transported to working cells in need of energy, such as muscle or liver cells. They are catabolized for energy through a process known as **β-oxidation,** or **fatty acid oxidation.** This metabolic pathway takes place in the mitochondria, which means that fatty acids must move from the cytosol across the mitochondrial membrane. Before the fatty acids can be transported into the mitochondria, however, they must be activated by the addition of co-enzyme A (CoA), the same coenzyme used in the synthesis of acetyl CoA from pyruvate. This reaction requires an "investment" of energy from ATP. The activated fatty acids are then shuttled across the mitochondrial membrane by a compound known as **carnitine.**

Once in the mitochondria, β-oxidation proceeds, systematically breaking down long-chain fatty acids into two-carbon segments that lead to the formation of acetyl-CoA units (**Figure 7.14**). Thus, a sixteen-carbon fatty acid is converted to eight acetyl-CoA units. As the two-carbon segments are cleaved off the fatty acid, high-energy electrons are trans-ferred to the coenzymes NAD^+ and FAD, forming $NADH + H^+$ and $FADH_2$, which feed into the electron transport chain. As with glucose oxidation, the acetyl CoA generated

albumin A serum protein, made in the liver, that transports free fatty acids from one body tissue to another.

β-oxidation (fatty acid oxidation) A series of metabolic reactions that oxidize free fatty acids, leading to the end products of water, carbon dioxide, and ATP.

carnitine A small, organic com-pound that transports free fatty acids from the cytosol into the mitochondria for oxidation.

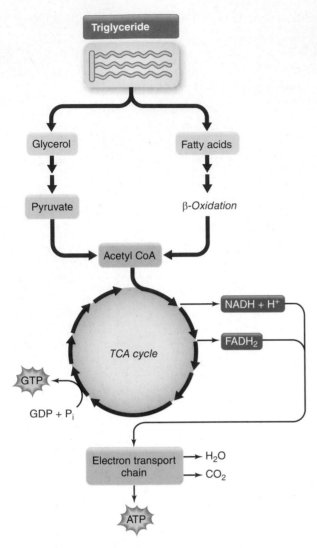

from fatty acid oxidation feeds into the TCA cycle for the production of ATP. The electron-rich coenzymes produced in the TCA cycle also feed into the electron transport chain and produce additional ATP. (See Appendix B for a more detailed view of β-oxidation.)

As previously described, the glycerol component of triglycerides can be used to synthesize glucose. Otherwise, it can feed into the TCA cycle after its conversion to pyruvate and acetyl CoA.

In summary, the process of extracting energy from triglycerides starts with fatty acids and glycerol and ends with the production of carbon dioxide, water, and ATP (**Figure 7.15**). These are the same three compounds produced during the oxidation of glucose.

As noted, because fatty acids almost always have more carbons than the six found in glucose, more acetyl CoA and more ATP are produced during β-oxidation of one long-chain fatty acid than during oxidation of glucose. A single eighteen-carbon fatty acid yields nearly 3.5 times the ATP than that derived from one six-carbon molecule of glucose. More importantly, fatty acids have relatively few oxygen atoms compared with oxygen-rich glucose (**Figure 7.16**). Fatty acids thus offer numerous opportunities for oxidation, which results in a higher output of NADH and $FADH_2$ and a higher number of electrons, leading to greater production of ATP through the electron transport chain. The result is that, on a per gram basis, fatty acids have a much higher energy potential compared with carbohydrates, approximately 9 kcal/g versus approximately 4 kcal/g.

Fatty Acids Cannot Be Converted to Glucose

Earlier, we noted that glycerol can be converted to pyruvate, which the liver is then able to convert to glucose. In contrast, there is no metabolic pathway to convert fatty acid–derived acetyl CoA into pyruvate for glucose synthesis. Because cells cannot convert acetyl CoA into glucose, it is impossible for fatty acids to feed into glucose production. Again, there is no metabolic pathway that allows for the conversion of fatty acids to glucose.

FIGURE 7.15 Extraction of energy from triglycerides. Glycerol and fatty acids can be metabolized to yield energy as ATP.

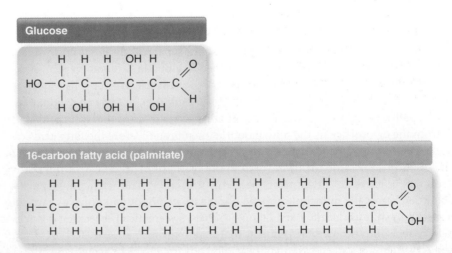

FIGURE 7.16 A comparison of glucose and fatty acid structures. In contrast with glucose, where each carbon is attached to an oxygen, there are many opportunities for oxidation of the carbon-to-hydrogen bonds of a fatty acid.

Nutrition Myth OR Fact?

Carnitine Supplements: A Fat-Burning Miracle?

Product labels, Internet advertisements, and TV infomercials practically shout the term "fat burner" in trying to convince consumers of the value of carnitine supplements; for years, carnitine has been included in many so-called weight-loss, fat-burning supplements.[1] The appeal of their claim is undeniable: use this product, and body fat will "melt" away.

Carnitine shuttles fatty acids across the mitochondrial membrane. Fatty acids are oxidized along the inside of the mitochondrial membrane, because that is where the enzymes of the β-oxidation pathway are found. If fatty acids can't get across the mitochondrial membrane, they will not be oxidized as a fuel and will accumulate. It seems logical, then, that carnitine supplements will increase fat oxidation and decrease body fat stores. But do they? There are two arguments often used in marketing carnitine supplements: (1) many people are low in carnitine and, so, would benefit from carnitine supplements, and (2) even healthy people with normal carnitine levels could lower their body fat by taking extra carnitine. How do these arguments hold up?

Looking at the first issue, are many people low in carnitine? Two important pieces of information are often left out of advertisements for carnitine supplements: (1) carnitine is widely available from a large number of foods, and (2) humans synthesize carnitine in amounts that fully meet the needs of healthy people. Food sources of carnitine include meat, poultry, fish, and dairy products; healthy children and adults on a mixed diet get all the carnitine needed from their normal diet. What about vegetarians and vegans? It is true that they *eat* much less dietary carnitine than nonvegetarians, but the body can easily synthesize it from the amino acids lysine and methionine. Lysine is found in legumes, including soybeans, whereas methionine is plentiful in grains, nuts, and seeds. Vegetarians commonly consume these foods in abundant amounts. As long as their diet provides enough of these foods, as well as the iron, niacin, vitamin B_6, and vitamin C used as cofactors, healthy vegetarians and vegans can meet their need for carnitine through endogenous (internal) synthesis. So, well-nourished, healthy people—vegetarians and vegans included—are rarely, if ever, low in carnitine.

What about the second claim? Do high doses of carnitine supplements benefit overweight or obese people? Manufacturers promote carnitine supplements as "fat burners" by implying that high intakes will increase blood levels, then muscle levels, of carnitine. Once in the muscle, the advertisements suggest, the carnitine would trigger fat oxidation and "burn up" body fat. Most studies have shown that taking large doses of carnitine, for up to 2 weeks, does not increase muscle carnitine levels and, so, would have no effect on body fat oxidation.[2] In addition, in one study, carnitine supplementation had no impact on weight loss in obese women.[3] Thus, well-controlled research has failed to support either of these claims.

Are there any situations when carnitine supplements are useful? Yes, but they are rare. People with certain genetic metabolic defects must be provided with supplementary carnitine, because they are unable to synthesize or utilize it;[4] patients with chronic kidney failure and those on dialysis treatment for kidney failure are often supplemented with carnitine as well.[5] In general, however, there is no evidence to support the claims that carnitine supplements increase the body's rate of fat oxidation or reduce body fat. The only "burning" you might experience when buying carnitine supplements is that of the money in your wallet!

References

1. Kreider, R. G., A. L. Almada, J. Antonio, C. Broeder, C. Earnest, M. Greenwood, T. Incledon, D. S. Kalman, S. M. Kleiner, B. Leutholtz, L. M. Lowery, R. Mendel, J. R. Stout, D. S. Willoughby, and T. N. Ziegenfuss. 2004. ISSN exercise and sport nutrition review: Research and recommendations. *J. Int. Soc. Sports Nutr.* 1(1):1–44.
2. Brass, E. P. 2004. Carnitine and sports medicine: Use or abuse? *Ann. NY Acad. Sci.* 1033:67–78.
3. Villani R. G., J. Gannon, M. Self, and P. A. Rich. 2000. L-carnitine supplementation combined with aerobic training does not promote weight loss in moderately obese women. *Int. J. Sport. Nutr. Exerc. Metab.* 10:199–207.
4. Stephens, F. B., D. Constantin-Teodosiu, and P. L. Greenhaff. 2007. New insights concerning the role of carnitine in the regulation of fuel metabolism in skeletal muscle. *J. Physiol.* 581(2):431–444.
5. Calvani, M., P. Benatti, A. Mancinelli, S. D'Iddio, V. Giordano, A. Koverech, A. Amato, and E. P. Brass. 2004. Carnitine replacement in end-stage renal disease and hemodialysis. *NY Ann. Acad. Sci.* 1033:52–66.

Ketones Are a By-Product of Fat Catabolism

Recall that the acetyl CoA that enters the TCA cycle can come from glucose or fatty acid catabolism. But the TCA cycle functions only when there is adequate oxaloacetate, a carbohydrate derivative (see Figure 7.11). In another science class, you may have heard the saying "Fat burns in the flame of carbohydrate": this need for oxaloacetate is what "the flame" refers to. Thus, if a person is following a very-low-carbohydrate diet or has too little functioning insulin to allow glucose to enter cells, oxaloacetate production falls and TCA cycle activity decreases. As fat catabolism continues during this carbohydrate-depleted state, acetyl CoA builds up, exceeding the ability of the TCA cycle to metabolize it, and accumulates in the liver cells.

As the acetyl CoA builds up, liver cells divert it into an alternative metabolic pathway leading to the synthesis of one or more **ketone bodies** (acetoacetate, acetone, and β-hydroxybutyrate or 3-hydroxybutyrate) (**Figure 7.17**). The liver constantly produces low levels of ketone bodies; however, production increases dramatically during times of very low carbohydrate intake, whether from prolonged fasting, starvation, or very-low-carbohydrate diets, as well as in people with type 1 diabetes who require external insulin for glucose transport into the cell. If someone with type 1 diabetes cannot obtain insulin, the body will be unable to maintain oxaloacetate production, the TCA cycle will shut down, and ketone production will increase. Ketone bodies are released from the liver into the bloodstream, where they can be taken up and used as an alternative fuel by the brain, certain kidney cells, and other body cells when their normal fuel source (glucose) is not available.

The production of energy from ketones is metabolically inefficient, because the total number of ATP produced will be lower than what would have been produced through β-oxidation of fatty acids. A little energy, however, is better than none; thus, ketone synthesis provides a backup energy system for carbohydrate-deprived cells.

When the rate of ketone production increases above its use by cells, blood and urine ketone levels rise, a condition known as *ketosis.* Typical blood levels of ketones are 3 mg/dL in a healthy individual eating a mixed diet but can rise to 90 mg/dL in severe ketosis, as seen in a person with type 1 diabetes without insulin. Ketones are acidic and inappropriately lower blood pH (increasing its acidity); thus, the body attempts to eliminate them by excreting them in the urine. This process, however, also causes dehydration, as fluid is lost in the urine. As the pH of the blood falls further and dehydration becomes more severe, *ketoacidosis* occurs. If allowed to persist unchecked, ketoacidosis can result in coma or death. A classic symptom of diabetic ketoacidosis is a fruity odor on the breath, which results from increased production of the specific ketone body acetone.

Although high levels of ketone bodies are normally harmful to the body, some medical conditions are treated with ketogenic diets. These medically supervised diets are high in protein and fat and extremely low in carbohydrates (10–20 g/d). See the **You Do the Math** box to get a better idea of the strict limitations of this medical ketogenic diet. One medical condition that seems to respond to a ketogenic diet is epilepsy, specifically childhood epilepsy that has not responded to other treatments. The ketones produced on this diet appear

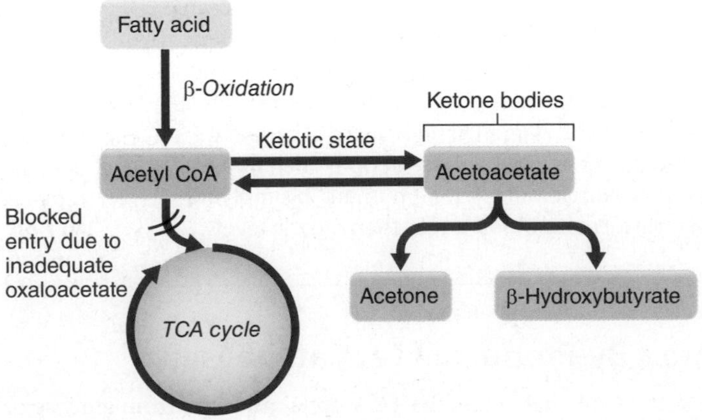

Read a father's story about the "miraculous" effect of a ketogenic diet on his son's epilepsy at www.nytimes.com/2010/11/21/magazine/21Epilepsy-t.html?_r=2&pagewanted=1&hp.

FIGURE 7.17 Overview of ketone synthesis. Ketones are produced when acetyl CoA is blocked from entering the TCA cycle. Two molecules of acetyl CoA combine to form acetoacetate, which can be converted to acetone or β-hydroxybutyrate. These three compounds are collectively called ketone bodies. Energy is later extracted from ketones when acetoacetate is reconverted back to acetyl CoA for entry into the TCA cycle.

ketone bodies   Three- and four-carbon compounds (acetoacetate, acetone, and β- or 3-hydroxybutyrate) derived when acetyl CoA levels become elevated.

Designing a Ketogenic Diet

As noted in our discussion on ketosis, some children with epilepsy are prescribed a ketogenic diet, in addition to their medication, to reduce the number or severity of their seizures. The benefits of the ketogenic diet for the reduction of epileptic seizures have been known for centuries; accounts of the beneficial effect of fasting on epilepsy are long-standing. American physicians have been using ketogenic diets to treat epilepsy for the past 80 years; however, we still do not know the specific mechanism of how ketones alter brain chemistry to reduce seizures.[1,2] A medical ketogenic diet is very high in fat and low in both protein and carbohydrate. Although the diet should always be developed and monitored by a registered dietitian and/or physician, you can work through these calculations to get a general idea of the diet plan.

Most children are prescribed a diet providing 4 g of fat (36 kcal) for every 1 g of protein/carbohydrate (4 kcal). A child needing 1,500 kcal/day would be fed 150 g of fat and about 38 g of protein/carbohydrate combined. Estimating the protein requirement at about 20 g per day, that means the child could eat 18 g of carbohydrates each day. In summary, the child's diet would be as follows:

1,500 kcal/day	
150 g of fat	1,350 fat kcal
20 g of protein	80 protein kcal
18 g of carbohydrate	72 carbohydrate kcal

Using the nutrient data from the food composition tables, develop a 1-day menu for this child. High-fat, low-protein/carbohydrate foods include cream, butter, bacon, oils, and so forth. Small amounts of fried chicken or fish would provide fat plus protein, as would nuts and peanut butter.

Obviously, children on a medical ketogenic diet eat very few fruits and vegetables, very little milk/dairy, and few grains/cereals. The dietitian develops a strict plan describing exactly how much of which foods are allowed; a nutrient supplement is also prescribed. Usually, the diet is tried for about 3 months to see how well it works. If there is little or no improvement, the dietitian will usually recommend a return to the normal diet.

References

1. Zupec-Kania, B. A., and E. Spellman. 2008. An overview of the ketogenic diet for pediatric epilepsy. *Nutr. Clinic. Pract.* 23(6):589–596.
2. Freeman, J. M., E. H. Kossoff, and A. L. Hartman. 2007. The ketogenic diet: One decade later. *Pediatrics* 119(3):535–543.

to reduce the number of severe seizures experienced. The exact mechanism by which the ketogenic diet exerts its anti-seizure action is not yet fully understood.[3,4]

RECAP

Triglycerides are broken down into glycerol and free fatty acids. Glycerol can be (a) converted to glucose via pyruvate or (b) oxidized for energy. Free fatty acids are oxidized to produce acetyl CoA and electron-rich coenzymes, which can enter the TCA cycle and electron transport chain. The end products of fatty acid oxidation are carbon dioxide, water, and ATP. Fatty acids cannot be converted into glucose. When cells face an inadequate supply of carbohydrate, fat catabolism increases and the excess acetyl CoA is diverted to ketone formation. ■

How Is Energy Extracted from Proteins?

As you read earlier in this text (in Chapter 6), the body's priority use of protein is for the building and repair of body tissues; however, small amounts of protein can be and are used for energy. The exact amount of protein used for energy will depend on the total energy in the diet and the amount of fat and carbohydrate consumed. The body preferentially uses

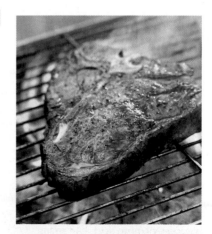

Dietary proteins are broken down into single amino acids or small peptides.

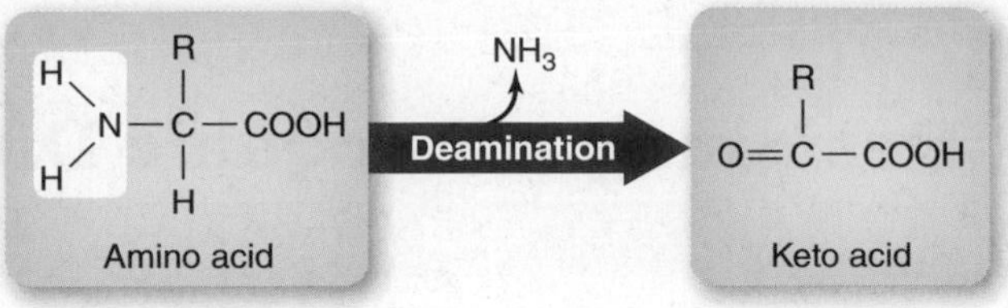

FIGURE 7.18 The process of oxidative deamination. Amino acids are deaminated when the amine group is removed; the remaining structure is known as a keto acid or carbon skeleton.

fat and carbohydrate as fuel sources and prefers to save protein for metabolic functions that cannot be performed by other compounds. Proteins are used as fuel sources primarily when total energy or carbohydrate intake is low.

In Proteolysis, Proteins Are Broken Down to Amino Acids

During protein breakdown, called **proteolysis,** dietary proteins are digested into single amino acids or small peptides that are absorbed into the body; eventually, the small peptides are further catabolized into single amino acids. These amino acids are absorbed, then transported to the liver, where they can be made into various proteins or released into the bloodstream for uptake by other cells for their unique building and repair functions. If protein is consumed in excess of what is needed by the cells, some of this protein can be used for energy or converted into fatty acids for storage as triglycerides. Additionally, if we don't eat enough total energy or carbohydrate, the tissues can break down some of the proteins in their cells for energy. This process is explained shortly.

In Oxidative Deamination, the Amino Group Is Removed

Under conditions of starvation or extreme dieting, the body must turn to its own tissues for energy, including protein. Amino acids are unique from other energy-containing nutrients in that they contain nitrogen, which must be removed, so that the remaining carbon skeleton can be used for energy. Thus, the utilization of amino acids for energy begins with oxidative *deamination* of the amino acids, which removes their amine (NH_2), or nitrogen, group and leaves a **carbon skeleton** (**Figure 7.18**). The end products of deamination are ammonia (NH_3), derived from the amine group, and the remaining carbon skeleton, often classified as a **keto acid.** (*Note:* Even though the terms *ketone* and *keto acid* appear very similar, they are produced from completely different metabolic pathways and have very different metabolic roles. Be careful not to get the two terms confused!)

After Oxidative Deamination, the Carbon Skeleton Feeds into Energy Production

The carbon skeleton produced through oxidative deamination can be channeled into glycolysis or the TCA pathway to produce energy (**Figure 7.19**). Each of the twenty amino acids (identified in Chapter 6) has a different carbon skeleton and is classified into a number of different groups, many of which overlap. For this discussion, there are two groups of interest:

- The carbon skeletons of **glucogenic amino acids** are converted to pyruvate, which can then be used to synthesize glucose or converted to acetyl CoA for entry into the TCA cycle. The primary glucogenic amino acids are alanine, glycine, serine, cysteine, and tryptophan.
- The carbon skeletons of **ketogenic amino acids** are converted directly to acetyl CoA for entry into the TCA cycle or for use in synthesizing fatty acids. The only totally ketogenic amino acids are leucine and lysine.

proteolysis The breakdown of dietary proteins into single amino acids or small peptides that are absorbed by the body.

carbon skeleton The unique "side group" that remains after deamination of an amino acid; also referred to as a *keto acid*.

keto acid The chemical structure that remains after deamination of an amino acid.

glucogenic amino acid An amino acid that can be converted to glucose via gluconeogenesis.

ketogenic amino acid An amino acid that can be converted to acetyl CoA for the synthesis of free fatty acids.

Many of the amino acids can feed into the TCA cycle at various entry points. For example, some amino acids can have both ketogenic and gluconeogenic functions. These include tyrosine, phenylalanine, tryptophan, lysine, and leucine. Because amino acids can have multiple functions, it is difficult to fit them into groups. Appendix B shows how the carbon skeletons of the various amino acids can contribute to TCA cycle intermediates, glucose production, fatty acid production, and/or ketone body production.

The amount of energy, or ATP, produced from the catabolism of amino acids depends on where in the metabolic pathway the carbon skeleton enters. The "higher up" the point of entry, such as conversion to pyruvate, the greater the ATP production. No amino acid, however, generates as much ATP as one molecule of glucose or one free fatty acid.

If Consumed in Excess, the Carbon Skeleton Feeds into Fatty Acid Synthesis

When proteins are consumed in excess of cells' immediate needs for protein and energy, both glucogenic and ketogenic amino acids feed into the production of acetyl CoA, which is then used to synthesize fatty acids for storage as triglycerides. Although many body-builders believe that high protein intakes lead to an increase in the synthesis of muscle mass, the reality is that excess protein leads to the same outcome as excess carbohydrate or fat: an increase in the synthesis of fatty acids and an increased deposition of triglycerides in adipose tissue.

Ammonia Is a By-Product of Protein Catabolism

Whereas some ammonia is useful as a nitrogen source for the synthesis of nonessential amino acids, high levels of ammonia are toxic to the body. Thus, the ammonia generated as a result of the deamination of amino acids must be quickly eliminated. To protect against ammonia toxicity, liver cells combine two molecules of ammonia together with carbon dioxide to form urea, which is much less toxic. **Figure 7.20** illustrates a simplified pathway for urea synthesis; the complete metabolic pathway can be found in Appendix B. The urea produced from amino acid catabolism is released from the liver into the bloodstream, then eliminated by the kidneys in the urine. When the body has to make and excrete a large amount of urea, as occurs with a very high protein intake, the kidney excretes a large

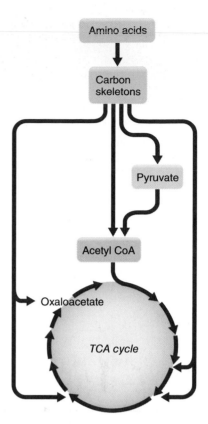

FIGURE 7.19 Extraction of energy from amino acids. The carbon skeletons of amino acids can be converted into pyruvate or acetyl CoA or can feed into the TCA cycle at various entry points. The point of entry into the catabolic pathway determines how much energy is extracted from that particular carbon skeleton.

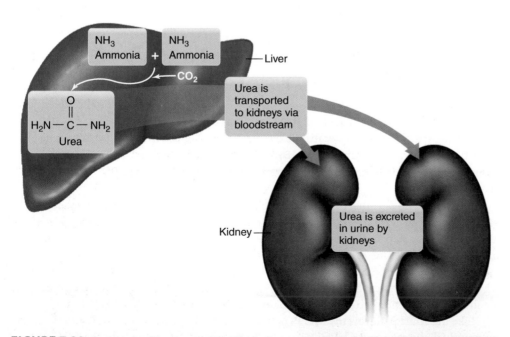

FIGURE 7.20 Overview of urea synthesis. The liver converts highly toxic ammonia, derived from deamination of amino acids, into urea. The urea is then released into the bloodstream for urinary excretion by the kidney.

TABLE 7.1 Extraction of Energy from Carbohydrate, Triglycerides, Protein, and Alcohol

Nutrient	Yields Energy as ATP?	Oxidative End Products?	Feeds into Glucose Production?	Feeds into Nonessential Amino Acid Production?	Feeds into Fatty Acid Production and Storage as Triglycerides?
Carbohydrate (glucose)	Yes	CO_2, H_2O	Yes	Yes, if source of nitrogen is available	Yes, although process is inefficient
Triglycerides: fatty acids	Yes	CO_2, H_2O	No	No	Yes
Triglycerides: glycerol	Yes	CO_2, H_2O	Yes, if carbohydrate is unavailable to cells	Yes, if source of nitrogen is available	Yes
Protein (amino acids)	Yes	CO_2, H_2O, N as urea	Yes, if carbohydrate is unavailable to cells	Yes	Yes
Alcohol	Yes	CO_2, H_2O	No	No	Yes

volume of urine. This in turn increases the risk for dehydration unless the individual drinks a large amount of water or other fluids.

The processes by which energy is extracted from carbohydrates, triglycerides, and proteins are summarized in **Table 7.1**.

RECAP

After deamination, the carbon skeletons of amino acids can be used as sources of energy. Glucogenic amino acids are converted into pyruvate, whereas ketogenic amino acids are converted into acetyl CoA. Some amino acids feed into the TCA cycle as various metabolic intermediates. The amine group released as a result of deamination can be transferred onto a keto acid for the synthesis of nonessential amino acids or, via ammonia, converted to and excreted as urea. ■

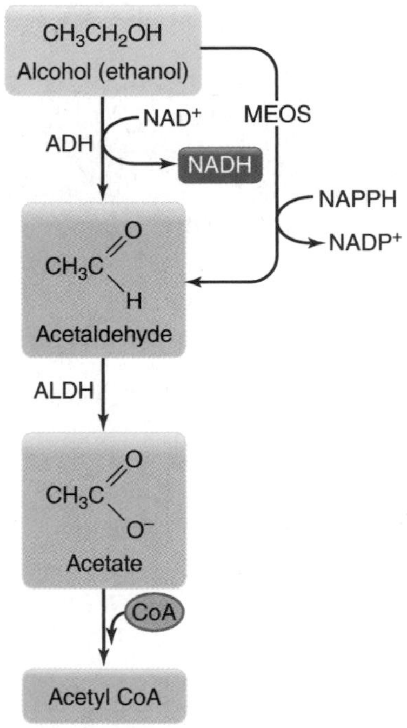

How Is Alcohol Metabolized?

We already took an In Depth look at alcohol (pages 160–171). Now we're ready to explore how the body metabolizes alcohol. Are there ways to speed up the process? These and other topics are explored here.

Alcohol Is Metabolized Through Oxidation

As with glucose and fatty acids, alcohol is metabolized in a stepwise fashion through a series of oxidation reactions. These differ according to a person's intake.

In people with low to moderate intakes, alcohol is oxidized first into acetaldehyde by the action of **alcohol dehydrogenase (ADH);** then the acetaldehyde is oxidized by **aldehyde dehydrogenase (ALDH)** into acetate (**Figure 7.21**). Finally, acetate is readily converted into acetyl CoA.

In people who chronically abuse alcohol, an alternative pathway, the **microsomal ethanol oxidizing system (MEOS),** becomes important for oxidizing the increased levels of alcohol. The *M* refers to the location of this enzyme group in microsomes, which are fragments of the membrane of endoplasmic reticulum. *EOS* refers to ethanol oxidizing enzymes that are part of a larger family termed P450 enzymes. These enzymes are inducible, which means the higher the intake of alcohol, the greater the activity of these enzymes. As alcohol intake continues to increase in alcohol abusers, the MEOS increases in response.

Like the ADH pathway, the MEOS pathway results in the formation of acetyl CoA. As previously discussed (pages 269–271), acetyl CoA is the primary "fuel" for the TCA cycle and is generated from the catabolism of carbohydrates, lipids, and amino acids. The oxidation of alcohol into acetaldehyde creates imbalances in two key pairs of coenzymes,

FIGURE 7.21 Pathways of alcohol metabolism. The primary metabolic by-product of alcohol oxidation is acetyl CoA.

alcohol dehydrogenase (ADH) An enzyme that converts ethanol to acetaldehyde in the first step of alcohol oxidation.

aldehyde dehydrogenase (ALDH) An enzyme that oxidizes acetaldehyde to acetate.

microsomal ethanol oxidizing system (MEOS) A liver enzyme system that oxidizes ethanol to acetaldehyde; its activity predominates at higher levels of alcohol intake.

$NAD^+/NADH$ and $NADP^+/NADPH$, which contribute to some of the metabolic and health problems associated with chronic alcohol abuse.

The Oxidation of Alcohol Begins in the Stomach

Although the oxidation of alcohol occurs primarily in the liver, a small but important amount of alcohol is actually oxidized in the stomach, before it is even absorbed into the bloodstream. This is known as *first-pass metabolism* and occurs via the ADH pathway. The action of gastric (stomach) ADH reduces, rather than simply delaying, the absorption of alcohol by as much as 20%. This enzyme is less active in young women than men; thus, women do not oxidize as much alcohol in their stomach, leaving more alcohol to be absorbed.[5] As a result of this biological difference, women absorb an average of 30% to 35% more alcohol than a similar-sized man consuming the same amount of alcohol. Gastric ADH activity decreases with age in men but apparently not in women, and there appear to be genetic differences in the amount or activity of this enzyme.[6] Fasting for as little as 1 day prior to alcohol consumption lowers gastric ADH activity, increasing the percentage of alcohol absorbed into the bloodstream for a given intake.

The Oxidation of Alcohol Continues in the Liver

Although a small amount is oxidized in the stomach, most of the alcohol consumed by an individual is rapidly absorbed into the bloodstream and transported to the liver, the primary site of alcohol oxidation. In the liver, the ADH pathway dominates at low to moderate intakes of alcohol, whereas the MEOS pathway becomes more important as the amount of alcohol consumed increases. The liver typically oxidizes alcohol at a fairly constant rate, equivalent to approximately one drink per hour. This rate varies somewhat with the individual's genetic profile, state of health, body size, use of medication, and nutritional status. If a person drinks more alcohol than the liver can oxidize over the same period of time, the excess is released back into the bloodstream. The greater the difference between rate of alcohol intake and rate of alcohol oxidation, the higher the blood alcohol level (**Figure 7.22**).

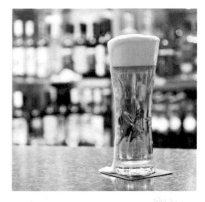

Alcohol is metabolized in the stomach and liver.

ALCOHOL IMPAIRMENT CHART

FEMALE											MALE									
Approximate blood alcohol concentration											Approximate blood alcohol concentration									
Drinks	Body Weight in Pounds										Drinks	Body Weight in Pounds								
	90	100	120	140	160	180	200	220	240			100	120	140	160	180	200	220	240	
0	.00	.00	.00	.00	.00	.00	.00	.00	.00	ONLY SAFE DRIVING LIMIT	0	.00	.00	.00	.00	.00	.00	.00	.00	ONLY SAFE DRIVING LIMIT
1	.05	.05	.04	.03	.03	.03	.02	.02	.02	Impairment Begins	1	.04	.03	.03	.02	.02	.02	.02	.02	Impairment Begins
2	.10	.09	.08	.07	.06	.05	.05	.04	.04	Driving Skills Affected	2	.08	.06	.05	.05	.04	.04	.03	.03	Driving Skills Affected
3	.15	.14	.11	.10	.09	.08	.07	.06	.06	Possible Criminal Penalties	3	.11	.09	.08	.07	.06	.06	.05	.05	Possible Criminal Penalties
4	.20	.18	.15	.13	.11	.10	.09	.08	.08		4	.15	.12	.11	.09	.08	.08	.07	.06	
5	.25	.23	.19	.16	.14	.13	.11	.10	.09		5	.19	.16	.13	.12	.11	.09	.09	.08	
6	.30	.27	.23	.19	.17	.15	.14	.12	.11	Legally Intoxicated Criminal Penalties	6	.23	.19	.16	.14	.13	.11	.10	.09	Legally Intoxicated Criminal Penalties
7	.35	.32	.27	.23	.20	.18	.16	.14	.13		7	.26	.22	.19	.16	.15	.13	.12	.11	
8	.40	.36	.30	.26	.23	.20	.18	.17	.15		8	.30	.25	.21	.19	.17	.15	.14	.13	
9	.45	.41	.34	.29	.26	.23	.20	.19	.17		9	.34	.28	.24	.21	.19	.17	.15	.14	
10	.51	.45	.38	.32	.28	.25	.23	.21†	.19		10	.38	.31	.27	.23	.21	.19	.17	.16	

Your body can get rid of one drink per hour. Each 1.5 oz of 80 proof liquor, 12 oz of beer or 5 oz of table wine = 1 drink.

FIGURE 7.22 Effect of alcohol intake on blood alcohol concentration (BAC) and driving behavior. A 180-lb male will experience a BAC of .08 and a significant decline in driving skills after only three drinks. (*Sources:* Female figure adapted from "BAC Chart Female" from Pennsylvania Liquor Control Board Website, Copyright © 2012 by Pennsylvania Liquor Control Board. Reprinted with permission. Male figure adapted from "BAC Chart Male" from Pennsylvania Liquor Control Board Website, Copyright © 2012 by Pennsylvania Liquor Control Board. Reprinted with permission.)

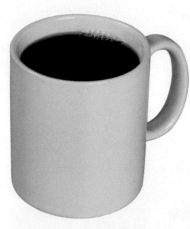

Black coffee will not speed the breakdown of alcohol.

Despite popular theories, there isn't much that can be done to speed up the breakdown of alcohol: it doesn't help to walk around (skeletal muscles don't oxidize alcohol), consume coffee or caffeinated beverages (caffeine doesn't increase rates of ADH or ALDH activity), or use commercial herbal or nutrient supplements (they have no impact on rates of ADH or ALDH activity). The key to avoiding the unwanted behavioral and physiologic consequences of alcohol is to consume alcohol at the rate of about one drink per hour, which then allows the liver to metabolize the alcohol at the same rate as it is taken in.

Although alcohol itself is a cellular toxin, acetaldehyde also produces specific and damaging effects. The amount of acetaldehyde that accumulates depends on the relative rates of activity for ADH and ALDH. In some ethnic groups, including certain Asian populations, the rate of ADH activity is normal or high and the activity of ALDH is relatively low. When a person with this genetic profile drinks alcohol, acetaldehyde accumulates. This typically leads to facial flushing, headaches, nausea, tachycardia (rapid heartbeat), and hyperventilation (rapid breathing), which are often unpleasant enough to inhibit future intake of alcohol. Researchers have long known that people with this type of enzyme imbalance are at low risk for alcohol abuse because the downside of alcohol intake typically outweighs any pleasurable effect, even at low levels of consumption.

As an individual's alcohol intake increases over time, the liver's ADH pathway for alcohol oxidation becomes less efficient, and the MEOS pathway becomes more active. As a result of increased MEOS activity, the liver metabolizes alcohol more efficiently, and blood alcohol levels rise more slowly for a given intake of alcohol. In other words, a heavy drinker who used to reach a blood alcohol concentration of 0.05 after only two drinks may not reach the same BAC until he has consumed four drinks. This condition reflects a metabolic tolerance to alcohol. Compared with light or moderate drinkers, people who chronically abuse alcohol must consume increasingly larger amounts before reaching a state of intoxication. Over time, they may need to consume twice as much alcohol as when they first started to drink in order to reach the same state of euphoria.

People who chronically consume alcohol in more-than-moderate amounts are at significant risk of dangerous drug–alcohol interactions. Thus, a number of pain relievers, antidepressants, and other drugs are clearly labeled "not to be consumed with alcohol." What accounts for this risk? The liver's MEOS system is used to metabolize not only alcohol but also many other drugs. When an individual is consuming alcohol, however, the MEOS enzymes prioritize alcohol metabolism, leaving the drugs to accumulate. This "metabolic diversion" away from drug detoxification means the medication remains intact, continues to circulate in the blood, and leads to an exaggerated or intensified drug effect. The combination of drugs and alcohol can be fatal, and drug label warnings must be taken very seriously.

Although the majority of ingested alcohol is oxidized by enzymatic pathways in the stomach and liver, a small amount, typically less than 10% of intake, is excreted through the urine, breath, and sweat. Alcohol is distributed throughout all body fluids and water-based tissue spaces in roughly equivalent concentrations. Increases in blood alcohol concentration are paralleled by increases in breath vapor alcohol levels; this relationship forms the basis of the common Breathalyzer testing done by law enforcement agencies. Some people try to rid themselves of alcohol through saunas and steam rooms, but the amount of alcohol lost through the increased sweat is negligible.

RECAP

The majority of ingested alcohol is oxidized in the stomach and liver by pathways involving ADH and ALDH. As an individual's alcohol intake increases over time, these pathways for alcohol oxidation become less efficient and the MEOS pathway becomes more active. The liver oxidizes alcohol at a steady rate of approximately one drink per hour; there is no effective way to speed up the liver's oxidation of alcohol. ■

How Is Energy Stored?

The body needs stored energy it can use during times of sleep, fasting, or exercise, when energy demands persist but food is not being consumed. The body typically stores extra energy as either fat, in the form of triglycerides, or carbohydrate, in the form of glycogen (discussed in the next section). Although humans appear to have an unlimited ability to store fat, only a limited amount of carbohydrate can be stored as glycogen (**Table 7.2**). The body has no storage mechanism for amino acids or nitrogen, and the pool of free amino acids in the blood is small. Thus, most of the body's amino acids are bound up in protein molecules. These factors make triglycerides the most useful form of stored energy.

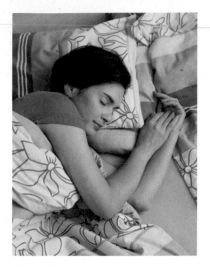

The body needs stored energy during sleep.

The Energy of Dietary Glucose Is Stored as Muscle and Liver Glycogen

Recall (from Chapter 4) that limited amounts of carbohydrate are stored in the body as glycogen, the storage form of glucose synthesized primarily in the liver and muscles. Glucose can easily be stored as glycogen within these tissues, and after an overnight fast, much of the carbohydrate consumed at breakfast is used to replenish the liver glycogen depleted during the night to maintain blood glucose levels.

Overall, the body stores approximately 250 to 500 kcal of carbohydrate as liver glycogen and approximately 800 to 2,000 kcal as muscle glycogen.[7] Of course, the amount of stored glycogen will depend on the adequacy of dietary carbohydrate and the size of the individual: people on a low-carbohydrate diet store very little glycogen, and larger individuals, assuming an adequate dietary carbohydrate intake, can store more glycogen because of the larger size of their muscle tissues and livers. But even in larger individuals, typical body stores of glycogen can be quickly depleted if dietary intake of carbohydrate is low and utilization of glucose as fuel is high. Individuals who participate in endurance exercise are heavy glycogen users; therefore, they need to make sure their glycogen stores are replenished after each workout or competitive event. (Chapter 14 explores the process of carbohydrate loading for endurance athletes in detail.)

The Energy of Dietary Triglycerides Is Stored as Adipose Tissue

Whenever we eat in excess of energy needs, the body uses the dietary carbohydrate for energy and preferentially stores the dietary fat as body fat. A number of factors contribute to this preference:

- The conversion of dietary fat to body fat is very efficient and requires little energy.
- Dietary fatty acids can be taken up by adipose tissue cells and converted into stored triglycerides without dramatic changes to the fatty acid structures from their original (dietary) form.
- The conversion of dietary carbohydrates to fatty acids that can be stored within the adipose cells requires a greater number of metabolic steps and is energy inefficient.
- When dietary carbohydrate is consumed in excess of the body's need, there is an increase in the oxidation of carbohydrate (glucose) over fat for energy, leaving more of the dietary fat available for storage in the adipose tissue.

TABLE 7.2 Body Energy Reserves of a Well-Nourished 70-kg* Male

	Triglycerides	Glycogen	Protein
Weight	15 kg	0.2 kg	6 kg
Kilocalories	135,000	800	24,000
*70 kg equals about 154 lb.			

Thus, when you overeat and consume a large meal, the fat within that meal will probably be converted to body fat and stored, whereas the carbohydrate in the meal will be used preferentially to fuel your body for the next 4 to 5 hours and to replenish glycogen stores.

The Energy of Dietary Proteins Is Found as Circulating Amino Acids

Although the body has no designated storage place for extra protein, some free amino acids circulating within the blood can be quickly broken down for energy if necessary. These free amino acids are either derived from dietary protein or are produced when tissue proteins are broken down. During protein catabolism, cells recycle as many of the amino acids as possible, using them to make new proteins or releasing them into the blood for uptake by other tissues. This process efficiently recycles many of the amino acids within the body, reducing the amount of protein required from food.

RECAP

The body is able to convert glucose into muscle and liver glycogen, the body's storage form of carbohydrate. Free fatty acids and glycerol are readily reassembled into triglycerides for storage in the adipose tissue, the body's largest energy depot. Technically, there are no protein stores in the human body; a small circulating pool of free amino acids can be used for energy if needed. ■

How Are Macronutrients Synthesized?

During the process of anabolism, a relatively small number of chemically simple components, including glucose, fatty acids, and amino acids, is used to synthesize a very large number of more complex body proteins, lipids, carbohydrates, and other compounds (recall Figure 7.1). The body also has the ability to synthesize glucose, fatty acids, and some amino acids. The following discussion will explore some of these common anabolic pathways.

Gluconeogenesis Is the Synthesis of Glucose

Glucose is the preferred source of energy for most body tissues and the sole or primary energy source for the brain and other nerve cells. If the supply of glucose is interrupted, loss of consciousness and even death may occur. In the absence of adequate dietary carbohydrate, liver glycogen can sustain blood glucose levels for several hours. Beyond that time, however, if dietary carbohydrate intake is not restored, the body must synthesize glucose from noncarbohydrate substances.

The process of making new glucose from noncarbohydrate substrates is called **gluconeogenesis** (**Figure 7.23**). The primary substrates for gluconeogenesis are the glucogenic amino acids derived from the catabolism of body proteins or free glucogenic amino acids circulating in the blood. Although the body cannot make glucose from free fatty acids, a small amount of glucose can be produced from the glycerol found in triglycerides.

The body relies on gluconeogenesis to maintain blood glucose levels at night when we are sleeping and during times of fasting, trauma, and exercise. Normally, the amount of body protein used for gluconeogenesis is low, but it increases dramatically during times of prolonged or severe illness, long-term fasting, or starvation. Protein catabolism for glucose production can lead to the destruction of vital tissue proteins, such as skeletal and heart muscles and organ proteins. The deadly consequences of this metabolic pathway are described in more detail in the section on starvation.

gluconeogenesis The synthesis of glucose from noncarbohydrate precursors, such as glucogenic amino acids and glycerol.

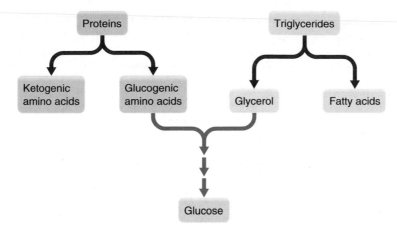

FIGURE 7.23 Overview of gluconeogenesis. In the absence of dietary carbohydrate and adequate glycogen stores, the body is able to convert glycerol and glucogenic amino acids into glucose.

Lipogenesis Is the Synthesis of Fatty Acids

Lipogenesis is the production of fat from nonfat substances, such as carbohydrates, ketogenic amino acids, and alcohol. This process is also called *de novo* **synthesis** of fatty acids, because it is the synthesis of new fatty acids from nonfat compounds. Lipogenesis typically occurs when individuals consume any energy-producing nutrient in excess of energy needs: excess dietary carbohydrate, protein, and alcohol all contribute to lipogenesis.

Most lipogenesis occurs in liver cells. How does the liver convert the six-carbon ring of glucose or the carbon skeleton of an amino acid to a long-chain fatty acid with many carbons? Not surprisingly, the process involves many steps. As shown in **Figure 7.24**, the two-carbon acetyl CoA units derived from glucose, amino acid, and alcohol metabolism are "reassembled" into fatty acid chains. The newly synthesized fatty acids are then combined with glycerol to form triglycerides. The liver releases these triglycerides as VLDLs,

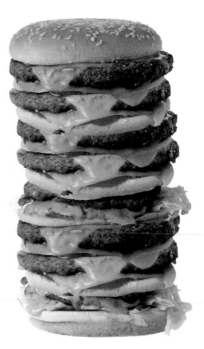

Consuming an excess amount of carbohydrate, protein, or alcohol will contribute to lipogenesis.

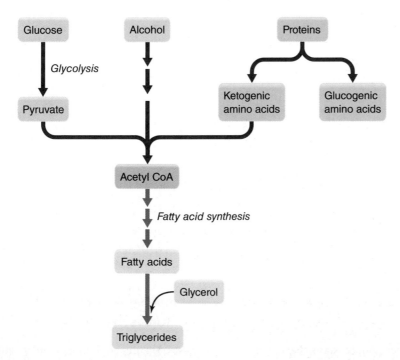

FIGURE 7.24 Overview of lipogenesis. Acetyl CoA, derived from glucose, ketogenic amino acids, or alcohol, can be converted into fatty acids for eventual storage as adipocyte triglycerides.

lipogenesis The synthesis of free fatty acids from nonlipid precursors, such as ketogenic amino acids or ethanol.

***de novo* synthesis** The process of synthesizing a compound "from scratch."

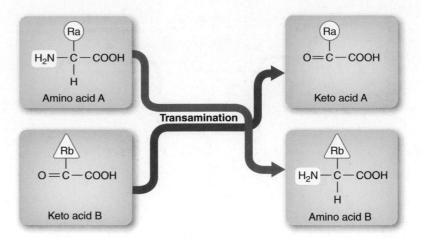

FIGURE 7.25 Transamination and the synthesis of nonessential amino acids. The amine group of amino acid A is transferred onto keto acid B, resulting in the formation of keto acid A and nonessential amino acid B.

which then circulate in the bloodstream. Eventually, the fatty acids are removed from the VLDLs, taken up into adipose tissue cells, and reassembled into triglycerides for storage as body fat. This is another example of the integration of metabolism that occurs between the liver and the adipose tissue.

The Synthesis of Nonessential Amino Acids

As discussed previously (in Chapter 6), the human body is capable of synthesizing as many as eleven nonessential amino acids (NEAAs). The body typically makes the carbon skeleton of NEAAs from carbohydrate- or fat-derived metabolites. The amine group can be provided through the process of transamination, where it is donated by one amino acid and accepted by a keto acid (**Figure 7.25**). When the keto acid accepts the donated amine group, it becomes a newly formed amino acid. The synthesis of nonessential amino acids occurs only when the body has enough energy and nitrogen to complete the necessary anabolic steps. During starvation, for example, energy intake is so low that the body stops the production of NEAAs.

Essential amino acids (EAAs) are distinguished from NEAAs by their carbon skeletons. The carbon skeletons of EAAs cannot be derived from carbohydrate or fat metabolic intermediates; therefore, EAAs must be consumed in their existing form from dietary proteins. Essential amino acids can be degraded or catabolized through several metabolic reactions, but they cannot be synthesized by cellular pathways.

RECAP

The dietary intake of carbohydrates, fats, and protein supplies the body with glucose, fatty acids, and amino acids. If nutrient intake is interrupted or inadequate, the body has the ability to endogenously (internally) synthesize glucose, almost all fatty acids, and eleven nonessential amino acids from readily available metabolic intermediates, including pyruvate and acetyl CoA. ■

What Hormones Regulate Metabolism?

To maintain homeostasis (balanced internal conditions), the body must regulate energy storage and breakdown as needed. Several anabolic and catabolic hormones work to regulate metabolism (**Table 7.3**).

TABLE 7.3 Hormonal Regulation of Metabolism

Metabolic State	Hormone	Site of Secretion	Role in Carbohydrate Metabolism	Role in Lipid Metabolism	Role in Protein Metabolism	Overall Metabolic Effect
Fed	Insulin	Pancreatic beta cells	Increases cell uptake of glucose Increases glycogen synthesis	Increases synthesis and storage of triglycerides	Increases cell uptake of amino acids and protein synthesis	Anabolic
Fasted	Glucagon	Pancreatic alpha cells	Increases glycogen degradation Increases gluconeogenesis	Increases lipolysis	Increases degradation of proteins	Catabolic
Exercise	Epinephrine	Adrenal medulla	Increases glycogen degradation	Increases lipolysis	No significant effect	Catabolic
Stress	Cortisol	Adrenal cortex	Decreases cell uptake of glucose Increases gluconeogenesis	Increases lipolysis	Decreases cell uptake of amino acids Increases degradation of proteins	Catabolic

The primary anabolic hormone is **insulin,** which increases in the blood after a meal, especially when protein and carbohydrate are consumed. Insulin activates enzymes that promote the storage of nutrients in the body and enables cells to take up glucose (in addition to fatty acids and amino acids). These compounds are then converted into glycogen, triglycerides, and body protein. Thus, insulin increases the uptake of substrates into cells, emphasizes macronutrient storage, and turns off catabolic processes within the body (see Table 7.3). If endogenous insulin production is inhibited in any way, then exogenous insulin must be provided through insulin injections or an insulin pump.

Conversely, **glucagon, epinephrine,** and **cortisol** are catabolic hormones that trigger the breakdown of stored triglycerides, glycogen, and body proteins for energy. They also turn off the anabolic pathways that store energy (see Table 7.3). As blood glucose drops, glucagon concentrations increase, prompting the body to release glucose from stored glycogen. During exercise, blood levels of epinephrine increase quickly, stimulating the breakdown of stored energy reserves. Cortisol, which rises during times of energy deprivation and physical stress, such as injury or exercise, also triggers the catabolism of stored energy.

A rise in blood cortisol levels also occurs during times of emotional stress and is considered a hallmark of the primitive "fight-or-flight" response. Catabolism of stored energy prepares the body to either fight or flee from an enemy, two situations that typically demand high energy. In today's world, however, we do not typically physically fight or flee from our enemies, so the fatty acids and glucose that are dumped into the bloodstream in response to stress are not utilized as physiologically intended. When day-to-day stresses chronically trigger elevations in blood cortisol levels during physically inactive periods, these metabolically inappropriate responses can increase a person's risk for excessive abdominal fat storage and/or glucose intolerance.

As you can see, a number of catabolic hormones regulate substrate breakdown, and insulin is the major anabolic hormone. Homeostasis requires a balance among these hormones. If one or more of them ceases to regulate properly, normal metabolic controls fail. For example, most people with type 2 diabetes make plenty of insulin, sometimes too much. As described (in Chapter 4), however, when the cells of people with type 2 diabetes become insensitive to insulin, they fail to take up glucose for fuel and must turn to glucogenic amino acids. Normally, insulin promotes amino acid uptake and protein synthesis; in people with type 2 diabetes, however, the ineffective insulin response triggers protein catabolism. Thus, normal metabolic controls are lost, and the balance between anabolism and catabolism is disrupted.

RECAP

To maintain homeostasis, the body must regulate energy storage and breakdown as needed. The primary anabolic hormone is insulin, whereas glucagon, epinephrine, and cortisol are catabolic hormones. ■

insulin   A hormone produced by the beta cells of the pancreas in response to increased blood levels of glucose that facilitates uptake of glucose by body cells.

glucagon   A hormone secreted by the alpha cells of the pancreas in response to decreased blood levels of glucose; it stimulates the liver to convert stored glycogen into glucose, which is released into the bloodstream and transported to cells for energy.

epinephrine   A hormone produced mainly by the adrenal medulla that stimulates the release of glucose from liver glycogen and the release of free fatty acids from stored triglycerides.

cortisol   A hormone produced by the adrenal cortex that increases rates of gluconeogenesis and lipolysis.

How Do Feeding and Fasting Affect Metabolism?

Although the need for energy is constant, most people eat or fuel their body on an intermittent basis. Every night, while we sleep, the body continues its metabolic processes, drawing upon stored energy. In the morning, when we "break our fast," the body receives an infusion of new energy sources. How does the body take advantage of energy when it is available, even if not needed at that moment? And how does it remain metabolically active even in the absence of food intake? The metabolic responses to the cycles of feeding and fasting are explored here.

Metabolic Responses to Feeding

For several hours after the consumption of a meal, food is digested and nutrients are absorbed. The bloodstream is enriched with glucose, fatty acids, and amino acids. Most cells are able to meet their immediate energy needs through glucose oxidation. Only if the meal was very low in carbohydrate would body cells break down fatty acids or amino acids for fuel.

The fed state (**Figure 7.26a**) is generally an anabolic state; after absorption, the end products of digestion are converted into larger, more chemically complex compounds. Glucose in excess of energy needs is converted to and stored as liver and muscle glycogen. Once glycogen stores are saturated, any remaining glucose is converted to fatty acids and eventually stored as triglycerides. Dietary fatty acids are combined with glycerol to form and be stored as triglycerides, largely in the adipose tissue. The liver takes up newly absorbed amino acids and converts some of them to needed proteins. The remaining amino acids are deaminated, and the carbon skeletons are converted to fatty acids for eventual storage as triglycerides.

Metabolic Responses to Short-Term Fasting

As the gap between meals lengthens beyond 3 hours or so, the body shifts from its previous anabolic state to a catabolic profile. Without a readily available supply of dietary carbohydrate, the body must turn inward in order to maintain normal blood glucose levels. Figure 7.26b (page 290) summarizes the interrelated metabolic responses to both short- and long-term fasting.

Recall (from Chapter 4) that muscle glycogen is "reserved" for muscle tissue alone and is not available for normalization of blood glucose levels. Liver glycogen is broken down and glucose is released into the bloodstream; however, the supply of liver glycogen is limited. Most body cells, including muscle cells, are able to switch to the use of fatty acids as fuel, conserving the remaining blood glucose for brain and other cells that rely very heavily on glucose as fuel. As the carbohydrate-deprived state continues, ketone bodies accumulate as fatty acid–derived acetyl CoA is blocked from entering the TCA cycle. The longer a person remains in a fasted state, the greater the rate of gluconeogenesis. Glucose is synthesized from glucogenic amino acids (drawn initially from free amino acids in the blood, then largely from the breakdown of muscle protein) and glycerol (derived from the catabolism of triglycerides). These short-term adaptations will provide the glucose and energy needed to meet the body's needs for a few days.

Metabolic Responses to Prolonged Starvation

After 2 to 3 days of fasting, the body senses an approaching crisis and responds with dramatic changes in its metabolic profile. Whether the starvation is the result of a voluntary action (for example, political protest, religious ritual, or self-defined act) or involuntary circumstances (such as a severe illness, famine, war, or extreme poverty), the body shifts into survival mode. There are two overriding problems to be solved: the problem of meeting energy requirements and the problem of maintaining blood glucose levels in support of glucose-dependent cells, such as brain and red blood cells. The body must solve these problems while maintaining the integrity of its essential functions, including preservation

Metabolic Response to Feeding

The fed state is generally an anabolic state: After digestion, absorption, and transport in the body, the end products of digestion can be synthesized into important biological compounds, used for energy, or converted to storage forms of energy.

■ Catabolism
■ Anabolism

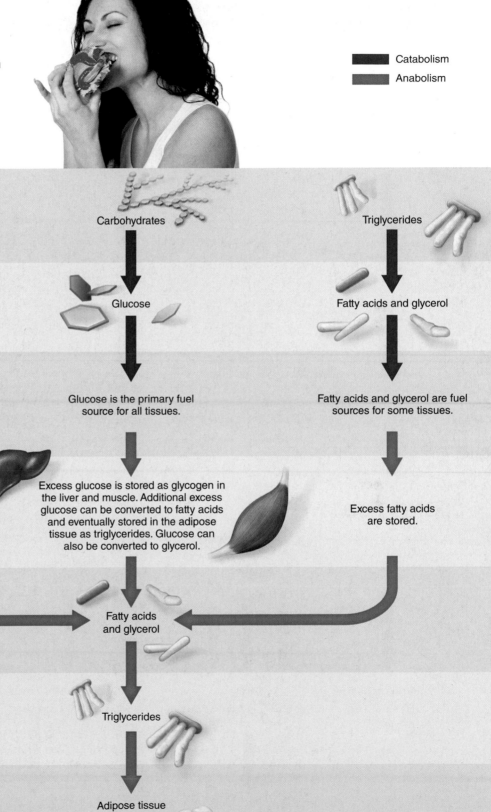

Proteins

Amino acids

Amino acids are used to synthesize body proteins for tissues such as muscle.

Excess amino acids can be used for energy or converted to fatty acids, which can be stored as triglycerides.

Carbohydrates

Glucose

Glucose is the primary fuel source for all tissues.

Excess glucose is stored as glycogen in the liver and muscle. Additional excess glucose can be converted to fatty acids and eventually stored in the adipose tissue as triglycerides. Glucose can also be converted to glycerol.

Triglycerides

Fatty acids and glycerol

Fatty acids and glycerol are fuel sources for some tissues.

Excess fatty acids are stored.

Fatty acids and glycerol

Triglycerides

Adipose tissue

Metabolic Response to Fasting

The fasting state is generally a catabolic state: After a period of fasting, when the body glycogen stores are reduced, the body increases its use of stored fatty acids.

■ Catabolism
■ Anabolism
■ Nutrient Transport

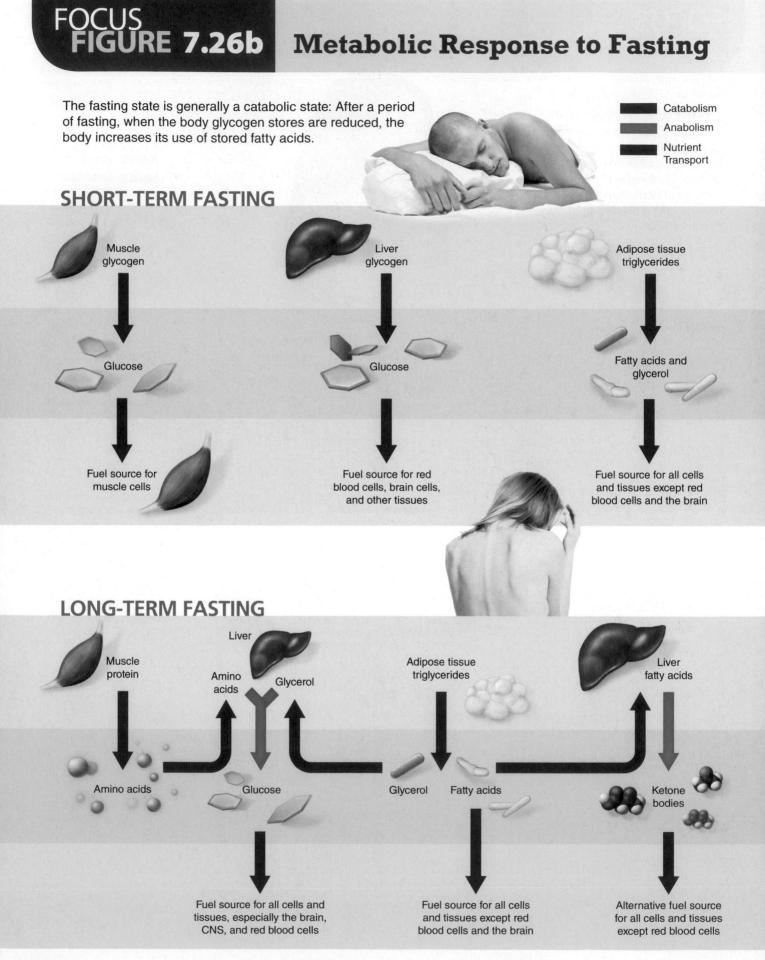

SHORT-TERM FASTING

Muscle glycogen

↓

Glucose

↓

Fuel source for muscle cells

Liver glycogen

↓

Glucose

↓

Fuel source for red blood cells, brain cells, and other tissues

Adipose tissue triglycerides

↓

Fatty acids and glycerol

↓

Fuel source for all cells and tissues except red blood cells and the brain

LONG-TERM FASTING

Muscle protein

↓

Amino acids

↑

Liver

Amino acids   Glycerol

↓

Glucose

↓

Fuel source for all cells and tissues, especially the brain, CNS, and red blood cells

Adipose tissue triglycerides

↓

Glycerol   Fatty acids

↓

Fuel source for all cells and tissues except red blood cells and the brain

Liver fatty acids

↓

Ketone bodies

↓

Alternative fuel source for all cells and tissues except red blood cells of skeletal and cardiac muscle, maintenance of the immune system, and continuation of brain function for as long as possible. How, then, does the body meet these challenges?

To solve the "energy problem," the body initiates several energy-conserving tactics: as fatigue sets in, there is a sharp decline in voluntary physical activity, core body temperature drops, and resting metabolic rate declines. Overall, the energy needs of the body drop dramatically. In order to meet the remaining energy needs, most cells further increase their use of fatty acids as primary fuel, conserving the limited supply of glucose. Plasma levels of free fatty acids increase sharply as they move from adipose stores to the tissues and cells in need of energy. Plasma ketone levels increase to an even greater extent as they are released from the liver and circulate throughout the body. Yet, even with these adaptations, the need by brain cells for a certain amount of glucose remains.

There are very few options available for solving the body's "glucose problem." As stored triglycerides are broken down to provide fatty acids for fuel, the glycerol component is used to provide small amounts of glucose. Glucogenic amino acids, however, remain the major source of glucose for use by the brain. Although the brain does shift away from its normal reliance on glucose and adapts to the use of ketone bodies for fuel, day after day, the body sacrifices muscle protein in order to maintain a small but essential supply of glucose.

Over time, after weeks to even months of starvation, a new crisis arises: adipose stores become depleted, depriving the body of its most efficient source of fuel. Now, not only the brain, but the entire body must survive on protein. With no other option available, the body begins to break down skeletal muscle, cardiac muscle, protein in organs such as the liver and kidney, and serum proteins, such as immune factors and transport proteins. As discussed (in Chapter 6), children with marasmus illustrate this final stage of depletion. They have no visible fat stores, their muscles are atrophied, and they lack the reserves to sustain the synthesis of immune, hair, skin, and other proteins. During this advanced stage of starvation, many die of heart failure as the cardiac muscle becomes too wasted to function properly. Others die of infections, lacking normal immune responses.

How long can a person survive complete starvation? Obviously, the need for water is critical; a person will die of dehydration long before reaching these final stages of prolonged starvation. Prior health and nutritional status play an important role: if a person enters starvation with large stores of body fat, his or her survival will be prolonged. If a person has good muscle mass and adequate nutrient stores, he or she is also at a slight advantage. The elderly and young children are more susceptible to the effects of starvation. Most previously healthy adults can survive without food for 1 to 3 months, assuming no illness or trauma and an adequate supply of water. Extreme environmental conditions and increased physical activity shorten survival time.

Nutrition
MILESTONE

It would seem obvious that the solution to prolonged starvation is simply to provide food—any food. However, over 65 years ago, a severe and often fatal condition called *refeeding syndrome* was identified among newly freed prisoners of war (POWs).

During World War II, more than 140,000 Allied POWs were held under conditions of extreme deprivation. In **1945**, the war ended, and POWs returned home to comprehensive medical care and plentiful American food. Shortly thereafter, researchers began describing the onset of heart failure following refeeding of previously starved POWs, often within 4 days of the reintroduction of food.

We now understand that rapid refeeding of a previously starved individual severely disrupts the metabolic equilibrium that had allowed the person to survive during starvation. Loss of muscle and fat stores leads to a loss of intracellular electrolytes, particularly phosphate, while serum electrolyte levels remain relatively stable. Rapid reintroduction of foods high in carbohydrate forces serum phosphate into cells to support the metabolism of glucose. As serum phosphate levels plunge (often along with magnesium and potassium), the person can experience respiratory failure, heart failure, seizures, and sudden death.

Clinicians now recognize the need to gradually reintroduce food to a starved person and to carefully monitor serum electrolytes, supplementing as needed. But even today, the risk for refeeding syndrome still exists among severe anorexics, chronic alcoholics, and patients with late-stage cancer, AIDS, or severe gastrointestinal disease.

RECAP

In the fed state, the body assumes an anabolic profile, converting newly absorbed glucose, fatty acids, and amino acids into stored glycogen and triglycerides and synthesizing some proteins. During short-term fasts, the body mobilizes stored glycogen and triglycerides to meet its need for glucose and energy. If the fasted state persists, more extreme adaptations to glucose and energy deficits occur. The body relies heavily on fatty acids and ketones as fuel sources and catabolizes proteins for gluconeogenesis. Over time, body fat and protein stores are so depleted that death occurs. ■

Nutri-Case

Hannah

"I was walking through the Student Union this morning, minding my own business, when this really attractive guy from biology class comes up to me all friendly, like I'm his long-lost sister or something. 'Hannah! Can I walk with you to class?' Now, I hardly know this guy, so I just shrugged, 'Sure, whatever . . .' Well, before you know it, he's trying to sell me this 'awesome'—that's what he kept calling it—weight-loss supplement. He tells me it's full of pyruvate, some kind of chemical that we need to burn fat. He says that, if I take it, my body will burn a lot more fat, so I'll use up my fat stores and lose weight. By the time we got to class, he had me half-convinced, but the supplements cost $30 a bottle, and I didn't even have that much on me. So I said I'd think about it and maybe buy some next week. But I'm not sure. My mom always says if it sounds too good to be true, it is."

Should Hannah buy the pyruvate supplements? Review the metabolic pathway of β-oxidation and consider whether or not it seems logical that consuming pyruvate supplements would increase the burning of the body's fat stores. Why or why not?

Chapter Review

TEST YOURSELF | ANSWERS

1 **T** All cells are metabolically active, but liver, muscle, and adipose cells are key locations for integration of metabolic pathways.

2 **T** Two vitamins that help produce energy from the macronutrients are riboflavin and niacin.

3 **F** Carbohydrate is also stored in the liver and in muscle as glycogen.

4 **F** There is no effective way to speed up the liver's breakdown of alcohol.

5 **T** During periods of starvation, body proteins are catabolized and their glucogenic amino acids are used in gluconeogenesis.

Summary

- Metabolism is the sum of all the chemical and physical processes by which the body breaks down and builds up molecules.

- All forms of life maintain a balance between anabolic and catabolic reactions, which determines if the body achieves growth and repair or if it persists in a state of loss.

- Metabolic pathways are clusters of chemical reactions that occur sequentially and achieve a particular goal, such as the breakdown of glucose for energy. These pathways are carefully controlled, either turned on or off, by hormones released within the body.

- Dehydration synthesis and hydrolysis are chemical reactions involving water, whereas phosphorylation is a chemical reaction in which phosphate is transferred. In oxidation–reduction reactions, the molecules involved exchange electrons.

- Enzymes, cofactors, and coenzymes increase the efficiency of metabolism.

- Glucose oxidation occurs in three well-defined stages: glycolysis, the TCA cycle, and oxidative phosphorylation via the electron transport chain. The end products of glucose oxidation are carbon dioxide, water, and ATP.

- During glycolysis, six-carbon glucose is converted into two molecules of three-carbon pyruvate. If glycolysis is anaerobic, pyruvate is converted to lactic acid. If glycolysis is aerobic, pyruvate is converted to acetyl CoA and enters the TCA cycle.

- During the TCA cycle, acetyl CoA, produced during carbohydrate, fat, or protein catabolism, results in the production of GTP or ATP, NADH, and $FADH_2$. The two final electron-rich compounds go through oxidative phosphorylation (as part of the electron transport chain) to produce energy as ATP.

- During oxidative phosphorylation, NADH and $FADH_2$ enter the electron transport chain, where, through a series of reactions, ATP is produced.

- Triglycerides are broken down into glycerol and free fatty acids. Glycerol can be (a) converted to glucose or (b) oxidized for energy. Free fatty acids are oxidized for energy but cannot be converted into glucose. In a carbohydrate-depleted state, fatty acids are diverted to ketone formation. The end products of fatty acid oxidation are carbon dioxide, water, and ATP.

- After deamination, the carbon skeletons of amino acids can be oxidized for energy. The carbon skeletons of glucogenic amino acids are converted into pyruvate, whereas those of ketogenic amino acids are converted into acetyl CoA. Some amino acids feed into the TCA cycle as various metabolic intermediates. The end products of amino acid oxidation are carbon dioxide, water, ATP, and urea.

- The amine group released as a result of deamination can be transferred onto a keto acid for the synthesis of nonessential amino acids or, via ammonia, converted to and excreted as urea.

- Alcohol metabolism begins in the stomach, where up to 20% of the alcohol consumed is oxidized. The remainder is oxidized in the liver. At high intakes, some alcohol continues to circulate in the blood, because the liver oxidizes alcohol at a steady rate of approximately one drink per hour.

- The body extracts energy from glucose, fatty acids, glycerol, and amino acids. Glycogen is the body's storage form of carbohydrate. Triglycerides in the adipose tissue form the body's largest energy depot. Technically, there are no protein stores in the human body.

- The dietary intake of carbohydrates, fats, and protein supplies the body with glucose, fatty acids, and amino acids. If intake is inadequate, the body synthesizes glucose, almost all fatty acids, and eleven nonessential amino acids from readily available metabolic intermediates.

- The primary substrates for gluconeogenesis are the glucogenic amino acids. A small amount of glucose can be produced from glycerol, but the body cannot make glucose from fatty acids.

- Excess dietary carbohydrate, protein, and alcohol all contribute to lipogenesis and triglyceride storage; excess dietary fat further increases triglyceride storage.

- The body can make the carbon skeletons of NEAAs from carbohydrate- or fat-derived metabolites. The amine group can be provided through the process of transamination. The carbon skeletons of EAAs cannot be derived from carbohydrate or fat metabolic intermediates; therefore, EAAs must be consumed in their existing form from dietary proteins.

- To maintain homeostasis, the body must regulate energy storage and breakdown as needed. The primary anabolic hormone is insulin, whereas glucagon, epinephrine, and cortisol are catabolic hormones.

- In the fed state, the body converts newly absorbed glucose, fatty acids, and amino acids into stored glycogen and triglycerides.

- During short-term fasts, the body uses stored glycogen and triglycerides to meet its need for glucose and energy. If the fast persists, the body relies heavily on fatty acids and ketones for fuel and initiates gluconeogenesis from glycerol and glucogenic amino acids to meet its glucose requirements. Over time, body fat and protein stores are so depleted that death occurs.

MasteringNutrition™

To further your understanding, go online and apply what you've learned to real-life case studies that will help you master the content!

Review Questions

1. One by-product of anaerobic glucose metabolism is
   a. lactic acid.
   b. acetyl CoA.
   c. oxaloacetate.
   d. six molecules of NADH.

2. Mitochondria are often called the cell's
   a. energy currency.
   b. power plant.
   c. fat producer.
   d. fat storage center.

3. In which of the following types of chemical reactions is a molecule catabolized by the addition of a molecule of water?
   a. hydrolysis
   b. dehydration synthesis
   c. oxidation
   d. phosphorylation

4. Anya skipped breakfast this morning. It is now midafternoon, and she has joined a friend for a late lunch. Although she rarely drinks alcohol, while waiting for her food to arrive, she enjoys a glass of wine. Which of the following statements best describes Anya's body's response to the alcohol?
   a. Gastric ADH oxidizes about 30% to 35% of the alcohol Anya consumes; the rest is absorbed into her bloodstream.
   b. When the alcohol enters Anya's bloodstream, her muscles quickly take it up for oxidation before her blood alcohol level increases.
   c. The microsomal ethanol oxidizing system breaks down about 20% of the alcohol Anya consumes before it is absorbed into her bloodstream.
   d. None of the above statements is true.

5. Glucogon, epinephrine, and cortisol are
   a. coenzymes.
   b. cofactors.
   c. anabolic hormones.
   d. catabolic hormones.

6. **True or false?** Liver synthesis of urea increases as dietary protein intake increases.

7. **True or false?** The body stores enough glycogen to last about 5 to 7 days.

8. **True or false?** Glucogenic amino acids can be converted into glucose during prolonged starvation.

9. **True or false?** The body requires energy to catabolize larger molecules into smaller molecules.

10. **True or false?** During glycolysis, glucose, a six-carbon compound, is converted to two molecules of pyruvate, a three-carbon compound.

11. Explain the statement that, within the electron transport chain, energy is captured in ATP.

12. Describe the process of fatty acid oxidation.

13. An elderly patient who has type 1 diabetes is admitted to the hospital in a state of severe ketoacidosis. The patient is comatose, but an elderly friend tells the admitting staff that he thinks his companion is sick because recently she has not had enough money to buy insulin. Describe a possible series of physiologic events that might have led to her ketoacidosis.

14. Review the information you learned about phenylketonuria (PKU) in Chapter 4; then describe the physiologic events likely to occur in a child with phenylketonuria who, unknown to his parents, goes off his diet every day at school and eats whatever his friends are eating.

15. Your Aunt Winifred has been overweight her entire life. Recently, she began a very strict semistarvation diet because it promises that "all the weight you lose will be fat." What information could you share with her that would explain why her weight loss will include loss of body protein, not just body fat?

Math Review

16. Your close friend Chris has just started using a "high-protein" supplement. Each serving provides a total of 1,800 mg of mixed amino acids, and the directions say to use three servings per day. If Chris weighs 170 lb, calculate (a) how much protein Chris needs, using the standard 0.8 g/kg body weight guideline, and (b) what percentage of Chris's total protein needs is met by the three servings. If three servings of this product costs $1.50, calculate how many eggs you could buy for $1.50 and how many grams of protein those eggs would provide. How would Chris feel if you shared your results?

Answers to Review Questions and Math Review are located in the MasteringNutrition Study Area.

Web Links

www.nutritionandmetabolism.com
Nutrition and Metabolism
An online, peer-reviewed journal with articles concerning the integration of nutrition, exercise physiology, clinical investigations, and metabolism.

www.msud-support.org
MSUD Family Support Group
This site offers practical advice for families with a child diagnosed with maple syrup urine disease (MSUD). There are updates on dietary products, treatment options, and research projects, as well as links to local networks.

www.pkuparents.org
California Coalition for PKU and Allied Disorders
This website directs users to support groups within their home state and provides updates on newly developed nutritional products for persons with PKU.

References

1. Champe, P. C., R. A. Harvey, and D. R. Ferrier. 2008. *Lippincott's Illustrated Reviews: Biochemistry*. 4th edn. Philadelphia: Lippincott Williams & Wilkins.

2. Shiel, W. C., and M. C. Stöppler (Eds.). 2008. *Webster's New World ™ Medical Dictionary*. 3rd edn. Hoboken, NJ: Wiley.

3. Patel, A., P. L. Pyzik, Z. Turner, J. E. Rubenstein, and E. H. Kossoff. 2010. Long-term outcomes of children treated with the ketogenic diet in the past. *Epilepsia* 51(7):1277–1282.

4. Freeman, J. M., and E. H. Kossoff. 2010. Ketosis and the ketogenic diet, 2010: advances in treating epilepsy and other disorders. *Advances in Pediatrics* 57(1):315–329.

5. Caballeria, J. 2003. Current concepts in alcohol metabolism. *Annals Hepatology* 2(2):60–68.

6. Anderson, P., and E. Scafato. 2010. *Alcohol and Older People— A Public Health Perspective*. Report for the Vintage Project. www.iss.it/binary/pres/cont/alcohol_and_older_people_vintage_project_report.pdf.

7. Karagounis, L. G., and J. A. Hawley. 2011. Genes, exercise, and glucose and insulin metabolism. In: Bouchard, C., and E. P Hoffman, eds. *Genetic and Molecular Aspects of Sport Performance* Oxford, UK: Wiley-Blackwell. DOI: 10.1002/9781444327335.ch21.

8. Jeukendrup, A. E., and R. Randell. 2011. Fat burners: nutrition supplements that increase fat metabolism. *Obesity Reviews* 12:841–851.

9. Nasser, M., H. Javaheri, Z. Fedorowicz, and Z. Noorani. 2012. Carnitine supplementation for inborn errors of metabolism (review). *The Cochrane Library*, Issue 2. www.thecochranelibrary.com.

10. Caló, L. A., U. Vertolli, P. A. Davis, and V. Savica. 2012. L carnitine in hemodialysis patients. *Hemodialysis International*. DOI: 10.1111/j.1542-4758.2012.00679.x.

"Speed Up Your Metabolism!" Is It Just a Dream?

The claims sound like a dream come true—consuming a particular food, supplement, or diet will rev up your metabolism and cause the pounds to melt away! Is there any truth to such claims? Are the recommendations safe? Let's examine the research evidence.

Claims for Single Foods or Food Components

A number of single foods or food ingredients have been promoted as *thermogenic,* having the ability to increase our metabolic rate through the production of heat. Calories expended as heat are not available for storage as body fat or additional body weight; thus, the theory is that so-called thermogenic foods promote weight loss (or at least reduce the individual's rate of weight gain). What foods are promoted as thermogenic, and what is their effect on metabolism and body weight?

Caffeine

One of the most researched and highly promoted food components is caffeine. About 90% of US adults consume caffeine every day from coffee, tea, soft drinks, and, to an increasing extent, energy drinks. A recent review of the research confirmed that caffeine increases metabolism, sometimes in a dose-response manner, where higher intakes of caffeine led to greater increases in energy expenditure. Caffeine is also known to specifically increase rates of fat oxidation, again with a dose-response relationship.[1]

The effect of caffeine on metabolic rate seems to be influenced by typical or habitual caffeine intake. Individuals who usually maintain high caffeine intakes will see less of a bump in metabolic rate with additional caffeine compared to those with lower typical intakes. High caffeine intakes may also increase blood pressure, interfere with normal sleep patterns, or lead to an irregular heartbeat.

One increasingly popular source of caffeine is green tea. In addition to caffeine, green tea contains high levels of physiologically active polyphenols, including several catechins, which have been shown to increase energy expenditure in a number of short- and long-term studies.[2, 3] Most researchers agree that the caffeine and catechins act in a synergistic manner (their combined effect on metabolic rate is greater than simply adding their individual effects together). In agreement with other research, the beneficial effect of green tea on metabolic rate is greater when one's usual intake of caffeine is relatively low. It is important to remember that increases in metabolic rate don't always lead to loss of weight or body fat. A recent review of the effects of green tea and green tea extracts concluded that, overall, consumption of green tea as a beverage or concentrated extract did not result in loss of body weight or reduction in waist circumference (a cardiometabolic risk factor).[4] Green tea is safe, widely available, widely consumed, and inexpensive. Some, but not all, researchers note a slight increase in blood pressure with green tea consumption.

The bottom line? Green tea is a great Calorie-free source of fluid and antioxidant-rich polyphenols. It may temporarily increase metabolic rate, but its effect on body weight is minimal at best.

Capsaicin

A compound found in hot (chili) peppers, capsaicin has been shown to increase energy expenditure in several human studies.[3] It has been estimated that an additional 15 Calories are burned for every teaspoon of cayenne pepper added to a meal. Serving meals with whole chili or hot peppers of any color will lead to a similar increase in metabolic rate and energy expenditure. While some people have a low tolerance for spicy foods, those who enjoy the taste of hot peppers can slightly increase their metabolic rate with little or no risk. Even better, additional research suggests that milder sweet peppers can also increase energy expenditure, although, again, only to a small extent.[5] Either way, adding hot or sweet peppers to your regular diet is safe and nutritious (peppers are rich in vitamin C, beta-carotene, and many other phytochemicals) and may provide a short-term boost in energy expenditure.

Cold Water

Believe it or not, consumption of cold water has also been shown to speed up your metabolism through a process known as *water-induced thermogenesis.*[6] Studies in adults have shown that drinking 500 mL (about 2 cups) of room-temperature water increased *resting energy expenditure* (*REE*) by as much as 30% within half an hour. When children were given 10 mL/kg of cold water (about 1½ cups for a child weighing 80 pounds), REE increased by 25%. This increase persisted for over 40 minutes.[6]

Let's do some math to see how this might translate into weight loss. Many children consume a large portion of their daily fluids as sweetened soft drinks. If children were to replace one 12-ounce soft drink per day with cold water, they would decrease their Calorie intake by about 180 kcal/day, which translates into about 19 pounds per year (at about 3,500 kcal per pound):

$$180 \text{ kcal/day} \times 365 \text{ days} = 65,700 \text{ kcal}/3,500 \text{ kcal per pound}$$
$$= \text{about 19 pounds}$$

In addition, the increased energy expenditure from drinking 12 ounces of cold water per day could theoretically amount to about 22 Calories per day, translating to a potential weight loss of just over 2 additional pounds per year:[6]

$$22 \text{ kcal/day} \times 365 \text{ days} = \text{about 8,000 kcal}/3,500 \text{ kcal per pound}$$
$$= \text{about 2 pounds}$$

From this simple calculation, you can see that replacing a beverage high in empty Calories with a Calorie-free beverage is a smart strategy for anyone trying to lose weight. Choosing cold water specifically is a healthful, cost-free, risk-free approach to boost one's metabolic rate and energy expenditure just a bit higher.

Fish Oil

Fish oil has also been promoted as a dietary component that may increase metabolic rate. Early studies reported that daily intake of 6 g of fish oil for 3 weeks increased resting metabolic rate, perhaps through its effect on lean body mass (the fish oil was found to increase lean body mass, which has a higher metabolic rate than fat mass). A more recent and longer (6-week) study, however, found no increase in metabolic rate with daily consumption of a 4-g fish oil supplement despite an increase in lean body mass.[7] Although fish oil has been shown to lower serum triglycerides, reduce the risk for heart attack and stroke in people with known cardiovascular disease, and reduce the buildup of atherosclerotic plaque, it does not appear to have much, if any, impact on metabolic rate.

Grapefruit

The so-called Grapefruit Diet has been a popular weight-loss plan for decades, but is there any evidence to support it? A study published several years ago reported that, among adults, eating one-half of a grapefruit at each meal led to a weight loss of about 3½ pounds over 12 weeks.[8] Although that may not sound like much progress toward weight control, some people lost as much as 10 pounds! Drinking 8 fl. oz of grapefruit juice also triggered a weight loss that was greater than what was measured in the control or placebo group, but not as great as among those eating the fruit. Daily eating habits otherwise remained unchanged and activity levels increased only slightly. It may be that the bulk of the fruit or its highly acidic taste led to a slight decrease in food intake at each meal, or it may be that grapefruit does, in fact, have some compound that increases energy expenditure. One thing we can say for sure is that anyone who follows this diet will certainly meet his or her need for vitamin C!

Diet Claims

In addition to these single food or food component claims, many diet programs claim that consumption of a high-protein diet (in which protein accounts for approximately 25% to 30% of total Calories) revs up metabolism. Research has consistently shown that this is true. When compared to diets of the same caloric intake but with lower levels of protein, high-protein diets increase metabolic rate and energy expenditure through thermogenesis.[7, 9] This is thought to be due to the fact that the thermic effect of dietary protein (the energy required to metabolize the food) is about 20% to 30%, a level much higher than that of carbohydrate (5% to 15%) or fat (0% to 3%).[7] In addition, high-protein diets are associated with higher levels of satiety, so people following such diets may stop eating sooner or wait longer before eating again. Finally, a high intake of protein helps maintain lean body mass during times of energy restriction, and lean body mass burns energy at a higher rate than adipose tissue. In total, these metabolic responses help explain why adopting a high-protein diet can support weight-loss efforts.

Physical Activity

If there is a single "magic bullet" for increasing metabolic rate, most researchers would agree it is physical activity. Many research studies have reported that purposeful physical activity not only increases metabolic rate during the period of activity but also increases resting metabolic rate for a variable period of time afterwards:

- Short bouts (15–30 minutes) of physical activity may increase metabolic rate for only 30 minutes or so, burning an extra 10–15 Calories.[10]
- Longer and more intense exercise can increase metabolic rate for up to 14 hours, burning an extra 200–300 Calories.[10]
- Endurance exercise (such as running, cycling, rowing, or swimming) is often, but not always, associated with increases in resting metabolic rate (RMR),[11] particularly at high intensities.[12]

- Interval training (that is, cycling or running at a high rate of speed for several minutes, followed by a recovery period at a lower intensity or rate) produces a post-exercise increase in energy expenditure that is greater in both magnitude and duration than that experienced with continuous aerobic activity, such as running or cycling at the same moderate speed.[13]
- Very-high-intensity resistance training (such as lifting extremely heavy weights at a rapid rate) has also been shown to increase metabolic rate above baseline measures.[14]

In addition to post-exercise increases in metabolic rate, physical activity (of adequate duration and intensity) also increases lean body mass, which itself speeds up metabolic rate. In healthy people, increased physical activity carries virtually no risks but offers multiple benefits.

If you are looking to boost your metabolism and lose weight, adding single foods or food components won't hurt if the foods are readily available and part of a healthful diet, but it probably won't make much of a difference, either. Consuming a lower proportion of carbohydrates and fats, and a higher proportion of protein, may help if you also reduce your total Calorie intake. Overall, however, regular, purposeful physical activity appears to be the most effective method for speeding up your metabolic rate and supporting weight loss.

CRITICAL THINKING QUESTIONS

- What would you say to your roommate if he told you he has decided to add hot chili powder to each meal? Are there any negative side effects he would need to be aware of? Are there other lifestyle changes he could make that would be more effective?

- Is it realistic for an obese teenage to "drink her fat away" by consuming large amounts of ice-cold water? Is it possible to drink too much water (see Chapter 9, page 361)?

- Would you be willing and able to modify your lifestyle using any of the approaches described? Pick three of the changes reviewed and describe the impact it would have on your day-to-activities. How realistic would it be for you to make all three changes at once?

REFERENCES

1. Hursel, R., W. Viechtbauer, A. G. Dulloo, A. Tremblay, L. Tappy, W. Rumpler, and M. S. Westerterp-Plantega. 2011. The effects of catechin rich teas and caffeine on energy expenditure and fat oxidation: a meta-analysis. *Obesity Rev.* 12:e573–e581.

2. Westerterp-Plantenga, M. S. 2010. Green tea catechins, caffeine and body-weight regulation. *Physiology & Behavior* 100:42–46.

3. Westerterp-Plantenga, M., K. Diepvens, A. M. C. P. Joosen, S. Bérubé-Parent, and A. Tremblay. 2006. Metabolic effects of spices, teas, and caffeine. *Physiology & Behavior* 89:85–91.

4. Phung, O. J., W. L. Baker, L. J. Matthews, M. Lanosa, A. Thorne, and C. I. Coleman. 2010. Effect of green tea catechins with or without caffeine on anthropometric measures: a systematic review and meta-analysis. *Am. J. Clin. Nutr.* 91:73–81.

5. Ludy, M. J., G. E. Moore, and R. D. Mattes. 2011. The effects of capsaicin and capsiate on energy balance: critical review and meta-analyses of studies in humans. *Chemical Senses.* Doi:10.1093/chemse/bjr1000.

6. Dubnov-Raz, G., N. W. Constantini, H. Yariv, S. Nice, and N. Shapira. 2011. Influence of water drinking on resting energy expenditure in overweight children. *Intnl. J. Obesity.* 35:1295–1300.

7. Abete, I., A. Astrup, J.A. Marti'nez, I. Thorsdottir, and M. A. Zulet. 2010. Obesity and the metabolic syndrome: role of different dietary macronutrient distribution patterns and specific nutritional components on weight loss and maintenance. *Nutr. Rev.* 68(4):214–231.

8. Fujioka, K., F. Greenway, J. Sheard, and Y. Ying. 2006. The effects of grapefruit on weight and insulin resistance: relationship to the metabolic syndrome. *J. Med. Food.* 9(1):49–54.

9. Bray, G. A., S. R. Smith, L. de Jonge, H. Xie, J. Rood, C. K. Martin, M. Most, C. Brock, S. Mancuso, and L. M. Redman. 2012. Effect of dietary protein content on weight gain, energy expenditure, and body composition during overeating. A randomized controlled trial. *JAMA.* 307(1):47–55.

10. Knab, A. M., R. A. Shanely, K. D. Corbin, F. Jin, W. Sha, and D. C. Nieman. 2011. A 45-minute vigorous exercise bout increases metabolic rate for 14 hours. *Med. Sci. Sports. Exerc.* 43(9):1643–1648.

11. Speakman, J. R., and C. Selman. 2003. Physical activity and resting metabolic rate. *Proc. Nutr. Soc.* 62:621–634.

12. Campbell, L., K. Wallman, and D. Green. 2010. The effects of intermittent exercise on physiological outcomes in an obese population: continuous versus interval walking. *J. Sport. Sci. Med.* 9:24–30.

13. King, J., C. Broeder, K. Browder, and L. Panton. A comparison of interval vs. steady-state exercise on substrate utilization in overweight women. *Med. Sci. Sports Exerc.* 34:S130.

14. Abboud, G. J. 2009. A comparison of the effects of two acute resistance training bouts on post exercise oxygen consumption. Florida State University Dissertation Publication No. 3373962.

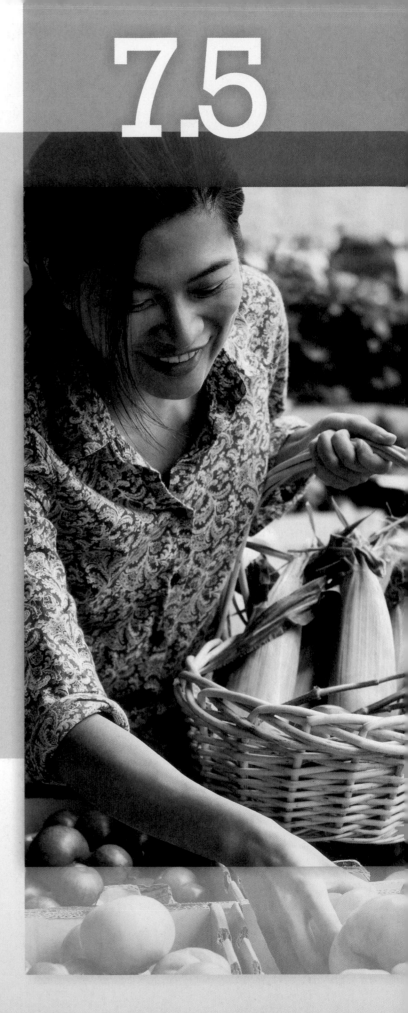

IN DEPTH

Vitamins and Minerals: Micronutrients with Macro Powers

Want to find out ...

- how a few fortunate accidents led to the discovery of micronutrients?

- where vitamins and minerals come from?

- why large doses of certain micronutrients— and which ones—could kill you?

- whether taking supplements provides the same health benefits you get from eating whole foods?

READ ON.

Have you ever heard about the college student on a junk-food diet who developed scurvy, a disease caused by inadequate intake of vitamin C? This urban legend seems to circulate on many college campuses every year, but that might be because there's some truth behind it. Away from their families, many college students adopt diets that are deficient in one or more micronutrients. For instance, some students adopt a vegan diet with insufficient iron, while others stop or cut back on eating foods rich in calcium and vitamin D. Why is it important to consume adequate levels of the micronutrients, and exactly what constitutes a micronutrient, anyway? This In Depth explores the discovery of micronutrients, their classification and naming, and their impact on our health.

Discovering the "Hidden" Nutrients

As you recall from earlier in this text (Chapter 1), there are three general classes of nutrients. Fluids provide water, which is essential for our survival and helps regulate many body functions. Macronutrients, which include carbohydrates, fats, and proteins, provide energy; thus, we need to consume them in relatively large amounts. **Micronutrients,** which include vitamins and minerals, are needed in much smaller amounts. They assist body functions such as energy metabolism and the formation and maintenance of healthy cells and tissues.

Much of our knowledge of vitamins and minerals comes from accidental observations of animals and humans. For instance, in the 1890s, a Dutch physician named C. Eijkman noticed that chickens fed polished rice developed paralysis, which could be reversed by feeding them whole-grain rice. Noting the high incidence of *beriberi*—a disease that results in extensive nerve damage—among hospital patients fed polished rice, Eijkman hypothesized that a highly refined diet was the primary cause of beriberi. We now know that whole-grain rice, with its nutrient-rich bran layer, contains the vitamin thiamin and that thiamin deficiency results in beriberi.

Similarly, in the early 1900s, it was observed that Japanese children living in fishing villages rarely developed a type of blindness that was common among Japanese children who did not eat fish. Experiments soon showed that cod liver oil, chicken liver, and eel fat prevented the disorder. We now know that each of these foods contains vitamin A, which is essential for healthy vision.

Such observations were followed by years of laboratory research before nutritionists came to fully accept the idea that very small amounts of substances present in food are critical to good health. In 1906, English scientist F. G. Hopkins coined the term *accessory factors* for those substances; we now call them vitamins and minerals.

How Are Vitamins Classified?

Vitamins are organic compounds that regulate a wide range of body processes. Of the thirteen vitamins recognized as essential, humans can synthesize only small amounts of vitamins D

and K, so we must consume virtually all of the vitamins in our diet. Most people who eat a varied and healthful diet can readily meet their vitamin needs from foods alone. The exceptions to this will be discussed shortly.

Fat-Soluble Vitamins

Vitamins A, D, E, and K are **fat-soluble vitamins (Table 1).** They are found in the fatty portions of foods (butterfat, cod liver oil, corn oil, and so on) and are absorbed along with dietary fat. Fat-containing meats, dairy products, nuts, seeds, vegetable oils, and avocados are all sources of one or more fat-soluble vitamins.

In general, the fat-soluble vitamins are readily stored in the body's adipose tissue; thus, we don't need to consume them every day. While this may simplify day-to-day menu planning, there is also a disadvantage to our ability to store these nutrients. When we consume more of them than we can use, they build up in the adipose tissue, liver, and other tissues and can reach toxic levels. Symptoms of fat-soluble vitamin toxicity, described in Table 1, include damage to our hair, skin, bones, eyes, and nervous system. Overconsumption of vitamin supplements is the most common cause of vitamin toxicity in the United States; rarely do our dietary choices lead to toxicity. Of the four fat-soluble vitamins, vitamins A and D are the most toxic; **megadosing** with ten or more times the recommended intake of either can result in irreversible organ damage and even death.

Even though we can store the fat-soluble vitamins, deficiencies can occur, especially in people who have a malabsorption disorder, such as celiac disease, that reduces their ability to absorb dietary fat. In addition, people who are "fat phobic," or eat very small amounts of dietary fat, are at risk for a deficiency. The consequences of fat-soluble vitamin deficiencies, described in Table 1, include osteoporosis, the loss of night vision, and even death in the most severe cases.

Water-Soluble Vitamins

Vitamin C (ascorbic acid) and the B-vitamins (thiamin, riboflavin, niacin, vitamin B_6, vitamin B_{12}, folate,

Avocados are a source of fat-soluble vitamins.

micronutrients Nutrients needed in relatively small amounts to support normal health and body functions. Vitamins and minerals are micronutrients.

vitamins Micronutrients that contain carbon and assist us in regulating our body's processes; classified as water soluble or fat soluble.

fat-soluble vitamins Vitamins that are not soluble in water but are soluble in fat; these include vitamins A, D, E, and K.

megadosing Taking a dose of a nutrient that is ten or more times greater than the recommended amount.

TABLE 1 Fat-Soluble Vitamins

Vitamin Name	Primary Functions	Recommended Intake*	Reliable Food Sources	Toxicity/Deficiency Symptoms
A (retinol, retinal, retinoic acid)	Required for ability of eyes to adjust to changes in light Protects color vision Assists cell differentiation Required for sperm production in men and fertilization in women Contributes to healthy bone Contributes to healthy immune system	RDA: Men: 900 µg/day Women: 700 µg/day UL: 3,000 µg/day	Preformed retinol: beef and chicken liver, egg yolks, milk Carotenoid precursors: spinach, carrots, mango, apricots, cantaloupe, pumpkin, yams	*Toxicity:* Fatigue, bone and joint pain, spontaneous abortion and birth defects of fetuses in pregnant women, nausea and diarrhea, liver damage, nervous system damage, blurred vision, hair loss, skin disorders *Deficiency:* Night blindness and xerophthalmia; impaired growth, immunity, and reproductive function
D (cholecalciferol)	Regulates blood calcium levels Maintains bone health Assists cell differentiation	RDA: Adults aged 19 to 70: 600 IU/day Adults aged >70: 800 IU/day UL 4,000 IU/day	Canned salmon and mackerel, milk, fortified cereals	*Toxicity:* Hypercalcemia *Deficiency:* Rickets in children, osteomalacia and/or osteoporosis in adults
E (tocopherol)	As a powerful antioxidant, protects cell membranes, polyunsaturated fatty acids, and vitamin A from oxidation Protects white blood cells Enhances immune function Improves absorption of vitamin A	RDA: Men: 15 mg/day Women: 15 mg/day UL: 1,000 mg/day	Sunflower seeds, almonds, vegetable oils, fortified cereals	*Toxicity:* Rare *Deficiency:* Hemolytic anemia; impairment of nerve, muscle, and immune function
K (phylloquinone, menaquinone, menadione)	Serves as a coenzyme during production of specific proteins that assist in blood coagulation and bone metabolism	AI: Men: 120 µg/day Women: 90 µg/day	Kale, spinach, turnip greens, brussels sprouts	*Toxicity:* None known *Deficiency:* Impaired blood clotting, possible effect on bone health

*RDA: Recommended Dietary Allowance; UL: upper limit; AI: Adequate Intake.

pantothenic acid, and biotin) are all **water-soluble vitamins** (**Table 2**). They are found in a wide variety of foods, including whole grains, fruits, vegetables, meats, and dairy products. They are easily absorbed through the intestinal tract directly into the bloodstream, where they then travel to target cells.

With the exception of vitamin B_{12}, we do not store large amounts of water-soluble vitamins. Instead, our kidneys filter from our bloodstream any excess amounts, and they are excreted in urine. Because we do not maintain stores of these vitamins in our tissues, toxicity is rare. When it does occur, however, it is often from the overuse of high-potency vitamin supplements. Toxicity can cause nerve damage and skin lesions.

Because most water-soluble vitamins are not stored in large amounts, they need to be consumed on a daily or weekly basis. Deficiency symptoms, including diseases or syndromes, can arise fairly quickly, especially during fetal development and in growing infants and children. The signs of water-soluble vitamin deficiency vary widely and are identified in Table 2.

water-soluble vitamins Vitamins that are soluble in water; these include vitamin C and the B-vitamins.

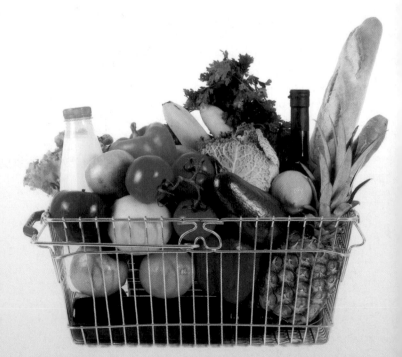

Water-soluble vitamins can be found in a variety of foods.

TABLE 2 Water-Soluble Vitamins

Vitamin Name	Primary Functions	Recommended Intake*	Reliable Food Sources	Toxicity/Deficiency Symptoms
Thiamin (vitamin B_1)	Required as enzyme cofactor for carbohydrate and amino acid metabolism	RDA: Men: 1.2 mg/day Women: 1.1 mg/day	Pork, fortified cereals, enriched rice and pasta, peas, tuna, legumes	*Toxicity:* None known *Deficiency:* Beriberi; fatigue, apathy, decreased memory, confusion, irritability, muscle weakness
Riboflavin (vitamin B_2)	Required as enzyme cofactor for carbohydrate and fat metabolism	RDA: Men: 1.3 mg/day Women: 1.1 mg/day	Beef liver, shrimp, milk and other dairy foods, fortified cereals, enriched breads and grains	*Toxicity:* None known *Deficiency:* Ariboflavinosis; swollen mouth and throat; seborrheic dermatitis; anemia
Niacin, nicotinamide, nicotinic acid	Required for carbohydrate and fat metabolism Plays role in DNA replication and repair and cell differentiation	RDA: Men: 16 mg/day Women: 14 mg/day UL: 35 mg/day	Beef liver, most cuts of meat/fish/poultry, fortified cereals, enriched breads and grains, canned tomato products	*Toxicity:* Flushing, liver damage, glucose intolerance, blurred vision differentiation *Deficiency:* Pellagra; vomiting, constipation, or diarrhea; apathy
Pyridoxine, pyridoxal, pyridoxamine (vitamin B_6)	Required as enzyme cofactor for carbohydrate and amino acid metabolism Assists synthesis of blood cells	RDA: Men and women aged 19 to 50: 1.3 mg/day Men aged >50: 1.7 mg/day Women aged >50:1.5 mg/day UL: 100 mg/day	Chickpeas (garbanzo beans), most cuts of meat/fish/poultry, fortified cereals, white potatoes	*Toxicity:* Nerve damage, skin lesions *Deficiency:* Anemia; seborrheic dermatitis; depression, confusion, and convulsions
Folate (folic acid)	Required as enzyme cofactor for amino acid metabolism Required for DNA synthesis Involved in metabolism of homocysteine	RDA: Men: 400 μg/day Women: 400 μg/day UL: 1,000 μg/day	Fortified cereals, enriched breads and grains, spinach, legumes (lentils, chickpeas, pinto beans), greens (spinach, romaine lettuce), liver	*Toxicity:* Masks symptoms of vitamin B_{12} deficiency, specifically signs of nerve damage *Deficiency:* Macrocytic anemia, neural tube defects in a developing fetus, elevated homocysteine levels
Cobalamin (vitamin B_{12})	Assists with formation of blood Required for healthy nervous system function Involved as enzyme cofactor in metabolism of homocysteine	RDA: Men: 2.4 μg/day Women: 2.4 μg/day	Shellfish, all cuts of meat/fish/poultry, milk and other dairy foods, fortified cereals	*Toxicity:* None known *Deficiency:* Pernicious anemia; tingling and numbness of extremities; nerve damage; memory loss, disorientation, and dementia
Pantothenic acid	Assists with fat metabolism	AI: Men: 5 mg/day Women: 5 mg/day	Meat/fish/poultry, shiitake mushrooms, fortified cereals, egg yolk	*Toxicity:* None known *Deficiency:* Rare
Biotin	Involved as enzyme cofactor in carbohydrate, fat, and protein metabolism	RDA: Men: 30 μg/day Women: 30 μg/day	Nuts, egg yolk	*Toxicity:* None known *Deficiency:* Rare
Ascorbic acid (vitamin C)	Antioxidant in extracellular fluid and lungs Regenerates oxidized vitamin E Assists with collagen synthesis Enhances immune function Assists in synthesis of hormones, neurotransmitters, and DNA Enhances iron absorption	RDA: Men: 90 mg/day Women: 75 mg/day Smokers: 35 mg more per day than RDA UL: 2,000 mg	Sweet peppers, citrus fruits and juices, broccoli, strawberries, kiwi	*Toxicity:* Nausea and diarrhea, nosebleeds, increased oxidative damage, increased formation of kidney stones in people with kidney disease *Deficiency:* Scurvy, bone pain and fractures, depression, anemia

* RDA: Recommended Dietary Allowance; UL: upper limit; AI: Adequate Intake.

Same Vitamin, Different Names and Forms

Food and supplement labels, magazine articles, and even nutrition textbooks often use simple, alphabetic (A, D, E, K) names for the fat-soluble vitamins. The letters reflect their order of discovery: vitamin A was discovered in 1916, whereas vitamin K was not isolated until 1939. These lay terms, however, are more appropriately viewed as "umbrellas" that unify a small cluster of chemically related compounds. For example, the term *vitamin A* refers to the specific compounds retinol, retinal, and retinoic acid. Similarly, *vitamin E* occurs naturally in eight forms, known as tocopherols, of which the primary form is alpha-tocopherol. Compounds with *vitamin D* activity include cholecalciferol and ergocalciferol, and the *vitamin K* "umbrella" includes phylloquinone and menaquinone. As you can see, most of the individual compounds making up a fat-soluble vitamin cluster have similar chemical designations (tocopherols, calciferols, and so on). Table 1 lists both the alphabetic and the chemical terms for the fat-soluble vitamins.

Similarly, there are both alphabetic and chemical designations for water-soluble vitamins. In some cases, such

What's the Best Way to Retain the Vitamins in Foods?

After selecting foods for their micronutrient value, it is important to store and prepare the foods properly. Minerals such as iron, calcium, and zinc are less affected by food-storage and -preparation techniques, but losses of both fat- and water-soluble vitamins can be very high if food is not properly handled. Here are a few tips:

- Use as little water as possible when rinsing, storing, or cooking foods to minimize the loss of water-soluble vitamins. For maximal retention of these vitamins, steam or microwave vegetables.

- Avoid high temperatures for long periods of time to maximize retention of vitamin C, thiamin, and riboflavin.

- Store foods in tightly sealed containers. Exposure to air dramatically reduces the amount of vitamins A, C, E, and K, as well as B-vitamins. Whenever possible, eat raw fruits and vegetables as soon as they are prepared.

- Keep milk and other dairy foods out of direct light. When exposed to light, the riboflavin in these and other foods is rapidly destroyed. Using coated cardboard cartons or opaque plastic bottles will protect the riboflavin in milk.

- Don't sacrifice nutrient value for appearance. Although the addition of baking soda to certain vegetables enhances their color, it also increases the pH of the cooking water (makes it more alkaline), destroying thiamin, riboflavin, vitamin K and vitamin C.

---

as *vitamin C* and *ascorbic acid*, you may be familiar with both terms. But few people would recognize *cobalamin* as *vitamin B$_{12}$*. Some of the water-soluble vitamins, such as niacin and vitamin B$_6$, mimic the "umbrella" clustering seen with vitamins A, E, D, and K: the term *vitamin B$_6$* includes pyridoxal, pyridoxine, and pyridoxamine. If you read any of these three terms on a supplement label, you'll know it refers to vitamin B$_6$.

Some vitamins exist in only one form. For example, thiamin is the only chemical compound known as *vitamin B$_1$*. There are no other related chemical compounds. Table 2 lists both the alphabetic and chemical terms for the water-soluble vitamins.

Since all vitamins are organic compounds, they are all more or less vulnerable to decay from exposure to heat, oxygen, or other factors. For tips on preserving the vitamins in the foods you eat, see the **Highlight** box (above) for details.

How Are Minerals Classified?

Minerals—naturally occurring inorganic substances, such as calcium, iron, and zinc—are solid, crystalline substances that do not contain carbon. All minerals are elements; that is, they are already in the simplest chemical form possible, and the body does not digest or break them down prior to absorption. For the same reason, they cannot be degraded on exposure to heat or any other natural process, so the minerals in foods remain intact during storage and cooking. Furthermore, unlike vitamins, they cannot be synthesized in the laboratory or by any plant or animal, including humans. Minerals are the same wherever they are found—in soil, a car part, or the

human body. The minerals in our foods ultimately come from the environment; for example, the selenium in soil and water is taken up into plants and then incorporated into the animals that eat the plants. Whether humans eat the plant foods directly or eat the animal products, all of the minerals in our food supply originate from Mother Earth!

Major Minerals

Major minerals are those the body requires in amounts of at least 100 mg per day. In addition, these minerals are found in the body in amounts of 5 g (5,000 mg) or higher. There are seven major minerals: sodium, potassium, phosphorus, chloride, calcium, magnesium, and sulfur. **Table 3** summarizes the primary functions, recommended intakes, food sources, and toxicity/deficiency symptoms of these minerals.

Trace Minerals

Trace minerals are those we need to consume in amounts of less than 100 mg per day. They are found in the human body in

---

minerals Naturally occurring inorganic substances that are not changed by natural or body processes, including digestion.

major minerals Minerals we need to consume in amounts of at least 100 mg per day and of which the total amount present in the body is at least 5 g (5,000 mg).

trace minerals Minerals we need to consume in amounts less than 100 mg per day and of which the total amount present in the body is less than 5 g (5,000 mg).

TABLE 3 Major Minerals

Mineral Name	Primary Functions	Recommended Intake*	Reliable Food Sources	Toxicity/Deficiency Symptoms
Sodium	Fluid balance Acid–base balance Transmission of nerve impulses Muscle contraction	AI: Adults: 1.5 g/day (1,500 mg/day)	Table salt, pickles, most canned soups, snack foods, cured luncheon meats, canned tomato products	*Toxicity:* Water retention, high blood pressure, loss of calcium in urine *Deficiency:* Muscle cramps, dizziness, fatigue, nausea, vomiting, mental confusion
Potassium	Fluid balance Transmission of nerve impulses Muscle contraction	AI: Adults: 4.7 g/day (4,700 mg/day)	Most fresh fruits and vegetables: potatoes, bananas, tomato juice, orange juice, melons	*Toxicity:* Muscle weakness, vomiting, irregular heartbeat *Deficiency:* Muscle weakness, paralysis, mental confusion, irregular heartbeat
Phosphorus	Fluid balance Bone formation Component of ATP, which provides energy for our bodies	RDA: Adults: 700 mg/day	Milk/cheese/yogurt, soy milk and tofu, legumes (lentils, black beans), nuts (almonds, peanuts and peanut butter), poultry	*Toxicity:* Muscle spasms, convulsions, low blood calcium *Deficiency:* Muscle weakness, muscle damage, bone pain, dizziness
Chloride	Fluid balance Transmission of nerve impulses Component of stomach acid (HCl) Antibacterial	AI: Adults: 2.3 g/day (2,300 mg/day)	Table salt	*Toxicity:* None known *Deficiency:* dangerous blood acid–base imbalances, irregular heartbeat
Calcium	Primary component of bone Acid–base balance Transmission of nerve impulses Muscle contraction	RDA: Adults aged 19 to 50 and men aged 51–70: 1,000 mg/day Women aged 51–70 and adults aged >70: 1,200 mg/day UL for adults 19–50: 2,500 mg/day UL for adults aged 51 and above: 2,000 mg/day	Milk/yogurt/cheese (best-absorbed form of calcium), sardines, collard greens and spinach, calcium-fortified juices	*Toxicity:* Mineral imbalances, shock, kidney failure, fatigue, mental confusion *Deficiency:* Osteoporosis, convulsions, heart failure
Magnesium	Component of bone Muscle contraction Assists more than 300 enzyme systems	RDA: Men aged 19 to 30: 400 mg/day Men aged: .30 420 mg/day Women aged 19 to 30: 310 mg/day Women aged >30: 320 mg/day UL: 350 mg/day	Greens (spinach, kale, collard greens), whole grains, seeds, nuts, legumes (navy and black beans)	*Toxicity:* None known *Deficiency:* Low blood calcium, muscle spasms or seizures, nausea, weakness, increased risk for chronic diseases (such as heart disease, hypertension, osteoporosis, and type 2 diabetes)
Sulfur	Component of certain B-vitamins and amino acids Acid–base balance Detoxification in liver	No DRI	Protein-rich foods	*Toxicity:* None known *Deficiency:* None known

* RDA: Recommended Dietary Allowance; UL: upper limit; AI: Adequate Intake; DRI: Dietary Reference Intake.

amounts of less than 5 g (5,000 mg). Currently, the Dietary Reference Intake (DRI) Committee recognizes eight trace minerals as essential for human health: selenium, fluoride, iodine, chromium, manganese, iron, zinc, and copper.[1] **Table 4** identifies the primary functions, recommended intakes, food sources, and toxicity/deficiency symptoms of these minerals.

Same Mineral, Different Forms

Unlike most vitamins, which can be identified by either alphabetic designations or the more complicated chemical terms, minerals are known by one name only. Iron, calcium, sodium, and all other minerals are simply referred to by their chemical name. That said, minerals do often exist within different chemical compounds; for example, a supplement label might identify calcium as calcium lactate, calcium gluconate, or calcium citrate. As we will discuss shortly, these different chemical compounds, while all containing the same elemental mineral, may differ in their ability to be absorbed by the body.

How Do Our Bodies Use Micronutrients?

Previously (in Chapter 3), we investigated the truth behind the claim "You are what you eat." We found out that the body must alter the composition of food in order to utilize it. This is

TABLE 4 Trace Minerals

Mineral Name	Primary Functions	Recommended Intake*	Reliable Food Sources	Toxicity/Deficiency Symptoms
Selenium	Required for carbohydrate and fat metabolism	RDA: Adults: 55 µg/day UL: 5 400 µg/day	Nuts, shellfish, meat/fish/poultry, whole grains	*Toxicity:* Brittle hair and nails, skin rashes, nausea and vomiting, weakness, liver disease *Deficiency:* Specific forms of heart disease and arthritis, impaired immune function, muscle pain and wasting, depression, hostility
Fluoride	Development and maintenance of healthy teeth and bones	RDA: Men: 4 mg/day Women: 3 mg/day UL: 2.2 mg/day for children aged 4 to 8; 10 mg/day for children aged > 8	Fish, seafood, legumes, whole grains, drinking water (variable)	*Toxicity:* Fluorosis of teeth and bones *Deficiency:* Dental caries, low bone density
Iodine	Synthesis of thyroid hormones Temperature regulation Reproduction and growth	RDA: Adults: 150 µg/day UL: 1,100 µg/day	Iodized salt, saltwater seafood	*Toxicity:* Goiter *Deficiency:* Goiter, hypothyroidism, cretinism in infant of mother who is iodine deficient
Chromium	Glucose transport Metabolism of DNA and RNA Immune function and growth	AI: Men aged 19 to 50: 35 µg/day Men aged >50: 30 µg/day Women aged 19 to 50: 25 µg/day Women aged >50: 20 µg/day	Whole grains, brewers yeast	*Toxicity:* None known *Deficiency:* Elevated blood glucose and blood lipids, damage to brain and nervous system
Manganese	Assists many enzyme systems Synthesis of protein found in bone and cartilage	AI: Men: 2.3 mg/day Women: 1.8 mg/day UL: 11 mg/day for adults	Whole grains, nuts, leafy vegetables, tea	*Toxicity:* impairment of neuromuscular system *Deficiency:* Impaired growth and reproductive function, reduced bone density, impaired glucose and lipid metabolism, skin rash
Iron	Component of hemoglobin in blood cells Component of myoglobin in muscle cells Assists many enzyme systems	RDA: Adult men: 8 mg/day Women aged 19 to 50: 18 mg/day Women aged >50: 8 mg/day	Meat/fish/poultry (best-absorbed form of iron), fortified cereals, legumes, spinach	*Toxicity:* Nausea, vomiting, and diarrhea; dizziness and confusion; rapid heartbeat; organ damage; death *Deficiency:* Iron-deficiency microcytic anemia (small red blood cells), hypochromic anemia
Zinc	Assists more than 100 enzyme systems Immune system function Growth and sexual maturation Gene regulation	RDA: Men: 11 mg/day Women: 8 mg/day UL: 40 mg/day	Meat/fish/poultry (best-absorbed form of zinc), fortified cereals, legumes	*Toxicity:* Nausea, vomiting, and diarrhea; headaches; depressed immune function; reduced absorption of copper *Deficiency:* Growth retardation, delayed sexual maturation, eye and skin lesions, hair loss, increased incidence of illness and infection
Copper	Assists many enzyme systems Iron transport	RDA: Adults: 900 µg/day UL: 10 mg/day	Shellfish, organ meats, nuts, legumes	*Toxicity:* Nausea, vomiting, and diarrhea; liver damage *Deficiency:* Anemia, reduced levels of white blood cells, osteoporosis in infants and growing children

* RDA: Recommended Dietary Allowance; UL: upper limit; AI: Adequate Intake.

also true for foods containing vitamins and minerals, because the micronutrients found in foods and supplements are not always in a chemical form that our cells can use. This discussion will highlight some of the ways in which our bodies modify the food forms of vitamins and minerals to maximize their absorption and utilization.

What We Eat Differs from What We Absorb

The most healthful diet is of no value to our bodies unless the nutrients can be absorbed and transported to the cells that need them. Unlike carbohydrates, fats, and proteins, which are efficiently absorbed (85–99% of what is eaten makes it into the blood), some micronutrients are so poorly absorbed that only 3–10% of what is eaten ever enters the bloodstream.

The absorption of many vitamins and minerals depends on their chemical form. Dietary iron, for example, can be in the form of *heme iron* (found only in meats, fish, and poultry) or *non-heme iron* (found in plant and animal foods, as well as iron-fortified foods and supplements). Healthy adults absorb about 25% of heme iron but as little as 3–5% of non-heme iron.

In addition, the presence of other factors within the same food influences mineral absorption. For example, approximately 30–45% of the calcium found in milk and dairy products is absorbed, but the calcium in spinach, Swiss chard, seeds, and nuts is absorbed at a much lower rate because factors in these foods bind the calcium and prevent its absorption. Non-heme iron, zinc, vitamin E, and vitamin B$_6$ are other micronutrients whose absorption can be reduced by various binding factors in foods.

The absorption of many vitamins and minerals is also influenced by other foods within the meal. For example, the fat-soluble vitamins are much better absorbed when the meal contains some dietary fat. Calcium absorption is increased by the presence of lactose, found in milk, and non-heme iron absorption can be doubled if the meal includes vitamin C–rich foods, such as red peppers, oranges, or tomatoes. On the other hand, high-fiber foods, such as whole grains and foods high in oxalic acid, such as tea, spinach, and rhubarb, can decrease the absorption of zinc and iron. It may seem an impossible task to correctly balance your food choices to optimize micronutrient

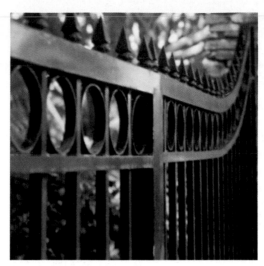

The iron in foods is chemically identical to that in a wrought iron fence.

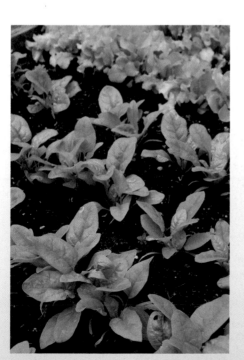

Plants absorb minerals from soil and water.

absorption, but the best approach, as always, is to eat a variety of healthful foods every day.

What We Eat Differs from What Our Cells Use

Many vitamins undergo one or more chemical transformations after they are eaten and absorbed into our bodies. For example, before they can go to work for our bodies, the B-vitamins must combine with other substances. For thiamin and vitamin B$_6$, a phosphate group is added. Vitamin D is another example: before cells can use it, the food form of vitamin D must have two hydroxyl (OH) groups added to its structure. These transformations activate the vitamin; because the reactions don't occur randomly, but only when the active vitamin is needed, they help the body maintain control over its metabolic pathways.

While the basic nature of minerals does not change, they can undergo minor modifications that change their atomic structure. Iron (Fe) may alternate between Fe^{2+} (ferrous) and Fe^{3+} (ferric); copper (Cu) may exist as Cu^{1+} or Cu^{2+}. These are just two examples of how micronutrients can be modified from one form to another to help the body make the best use of dietary nutrients.

Controversies in Micronutrient Metabolism

The science of nutrition continues to evolve, and our current understanding of vitamins and minerals will no doubt change over the next several years or decades. While some people interpret the term *controversy* as negative, nutrition controversies are exciting developments, proof of new information, and a sign of continued growth in the field.

Are Supplements Healthful Sources of Micronutrients?

For millions of years, humans relied solely on natural foodstuffs as their source of nutrients. Only within the past 60 years or so has a second option become available: nutrient supplements, including those added to fortified foods. Are the micronutrients in supplements any better or worse than those in foods? Do our bodies use the nutrients from these two sources any differently? These are issues that nutrition scientists and consumers continue to discuss.

As previously noted, the availability, or "usefulness," of micronutrients in foods depends in part on the food itself. The iron and calcium in spinach are poorly absorbed, whereas the iron in beef and the calcium in milk are absorbed efficiently. Because of these and other differences in the availability of micronutrients from different sources, it is difficult to generalize about the usefulness of supplements. Nevertheless, we can say a few things about this issue:

- In general, it is much easier to develop a toxic overload of nutrients from supplements than it is from foods. It is very difficult, if not impossible, to develop a vitamin or mineral toxicity through diet (food) alone.

- Some micronutrients consumed as supplements appear to be harmful to the health of certain subgroups of consumers. For example, recent research has shown that the use of common supplements, particularly iron, may actually increase the rates of death in older women.[2] Earlier, it was shown that high-potency beta-carotene supplements increase death rates among male smokers. Alcoholics are more susceptible to the potentially toxic effects of vitamin A supplements and should avoid their use unless prescribed by a healthcare provider. There is also some evidence that a high intake of vitamin A, including supplement use, increases the risk for osteoporosis and bone fractures in older women with low intakes of vitamin D.[3]

- Most minerals are better absorbed from animal food sources than they are from supplements. The one exception might be calcium citrate-malate, used in calcium-fortified juices. The body uses this form as effectively as the calcium from milk or yogurt.

- Enriching a low-nutrient food with a few vitamins and/or minerals does not turn it into a healthful food. For example, soda that has been fortified with selected micronutrients is still basically soda.

- Eating a variety of healthful foods provides you with many more nutrients, phytochemicals, and other dietary factors than supplements alone. Nutritionists are not even sure they have identified all the essential nutrients; it is possible that the list of essential micronutrients will expand in the future. Supplements provide only those nutrients that the manufacturer puts in; foods provide the nutrients that have been identified as well as yet-unknown factors.

- Many foods provide a balance of micronutrients and other factors, which work in concert with one another. The whole food is more healthful than its individual nutrients, providing benefits not always seen with purified supplements or highly refined, highly enriched food products. Two useful guidelines are "Eat food. Don't eat anything your great-great-grandmother wouldn't recognize as food"[4] and "Eat food, not too much, mostly plants."[5]

- A healthful diet, built from a wide variety of foods, offers social, emotional, and other benefits that are absent from supplements. Humans eat food, not nutrients.

On the other hand, micronutrient supplements can play an important role in promoting good health in some populations, such as pregnant women, children with poor eating habits, and people with certain illnesses. The risks and benefits of specific supplements versus whole foods are discussed later in this text (see Chapters 8 through 12 for specific nutrient details, and the **Nutrition Debate** box at the end of Chapter 10).

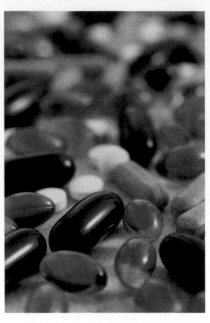

Thousands of supplements are marketed to consumers.

Can Micronutrients Prevent or Treat Chronic Disease?

Nutritionists and other healthcare professionals clearly accept the role that dietary fat plays in the prevention and treatment of heart disease. The relationship between total carbohydrate intake and the management of diabetes is also firmly established. Less clear, however, are the links between individual vitamins and minerals and certain chronic diseases.

A number of research studies have suggested, but not proven, links between the following micronutrients and disease states. In each case, adequate intake of the nutrient has been associated with lower disease risk.

- Vitamin D and colon cancer
- Vitamin E and complications of diabetes
- Vitamin K and osteoporosis
- Calcium and high blood pressure (hypertension)
- Chromium and type 2 diabetes in older adults
- Magnesium and muscle wasting (sarcopenia) in older adults
- Selenium and certain types of cancer

As consumers, it's important to critically evaluate any claim about the protective or disease-preventing ability of a specific vitamin or mineral. Supplements that provide megadoses of micronutrients are potentially harmful, and vitamin/mineral therapies should never replace more traditional, proven methods of disease treatment. Current, reputable information can provide updates as the research into micronutrients continues.

Do More Essential Micronutrients Exist?

Nutrition researchers continue to explore the potential of a variety of substances to qualify as essential micronutrients. Vitamin-like factors such as carnitine and trace minerals such as boron, nickel, and silicon seem to have beneficial roles in human health, yet additional information is needed to fully define their metabolic roles. Until more research is done, such substances can't be classified as essential micronutrients.

Another subject of controversy is the question "What is the appropriate intake of each micronutrient?" Contemporary research suggests that the answer is to be found in each individual's genetic profile. As you've learned (in Chapter 1), the science of *nutrigenomics* blends the study of human nutrition with that of genetics. It is becoming clear that some individuals require much higher or lower intakes of micronutrients to achieve optimal health. For example, researchers have identified a genetic variation in a subset of the population that increases their need for dietary folate.[6] Future studies may identify other examples of how a person's genetic profile influences his or her unique need for vitamins and minerals.

As the science of nutrition continues to evolve, the next 50 years will be an exciting time for micronutrient research. Who knows? Within a few decades, we all might have personalized micronutrient prescriptions matched to our gender, age, and DNA!

Nutri-Case — Liz

"I used to have dinner in the campus dining hall, but not anymore. It's too tempting to see everyone eating all that fattening food and then topping it off with a big dessert. My weight would balloon up in a week if I ate like that! So instead I stay in my dorm room and have a bowl of cereal with nonfat milk. The cereal box says it provides a full day's supply of all the vitamins and minerals, so I know it's nutritious. And when I eat cereal for dinner, it doesn't matter if I didn't eat all the right things earlier in the day!"

What do you think of Liz's "cereal suppers"? If the cereal provides 100% of the DRI for all vitamins and minerals, then is Liz correct that it doesn't matter what else she eats during the day? If not, why not? What factors besides the percentage of DRI does Liz need to consider?

Web Links

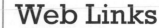

www.fda.gov
US Food and Drug Administration
Select "Food" and then "Dietary Supplements" for information on how to evaluate dietary supplements.

www.nal.usda.gov/fnic
Food and Nutrition Information Center
Click on "Dietary Supplements" to obtain information on vitamin and mineral supplements.

www.dietary-supplements.info.nih.gov
Office of Dietary Supplements
This site provides summaries of current research results and helpful information about the use of dietary supplements.

www.lpi.oregonstate.edu
Linus Pauling Institute of Oregon State University
This site provides information on vitamins and minerals that promote health and lower disease risk. You can search for individual nutrients (for example, vitamin C) as well as types of nutrients (for example, antioxidants).

References

1. Institute of Medicine, Food and Nutrition Board. 2001. *Dietary Reference Intakes for Vitamin A, Vitamin K, Arsenic, Boron, Chromium, Copper, Iodine, Iron, Manganese, Molybdenum, Nickel, Silicon, Vanadium, and Zinc.* Washington, DC: National Academies Press.
2. Mursu, J., K. Robien, L. J. Harnack, K. Park, and D. R. Jacobs Jr. 2011. Less is more: Dietary supplements and mortality rate in older women: the Iowa Women's Health Study. *Arch. Intern. Med.* 171:1625–1633.
3. Caire-Juvera, G., C. Ritenbaugh, J. Wactawski-Wende, L. G. Snetselaar, and Z. Chen. 2009. Vitamin A and retinol intakes and the risk of fractures among participants of the Women's Health Initiative Observational Study. *Am. J. Clin. Nutr.* 89:323–330.
4. Pollan, M. 2007. The age of nutritionism. *New York Times Magazine,* January 28.
5. Pollan, M. 2008. *In Defense of Foods.* New York: Penguin Press.
6. Solis, C., K. Veenema, A. A. Ivanov, S. Tran, R. Li, W. Wang, D. J. Moriarty, C. V. Maletz, and M. A. Caudill. 2008. Folate intake at RDA levels is inadequate for Mexican American men with the methylenetetrahydrofolate reductase 677TT genotype. *J. Nutr.* 138:67–72.

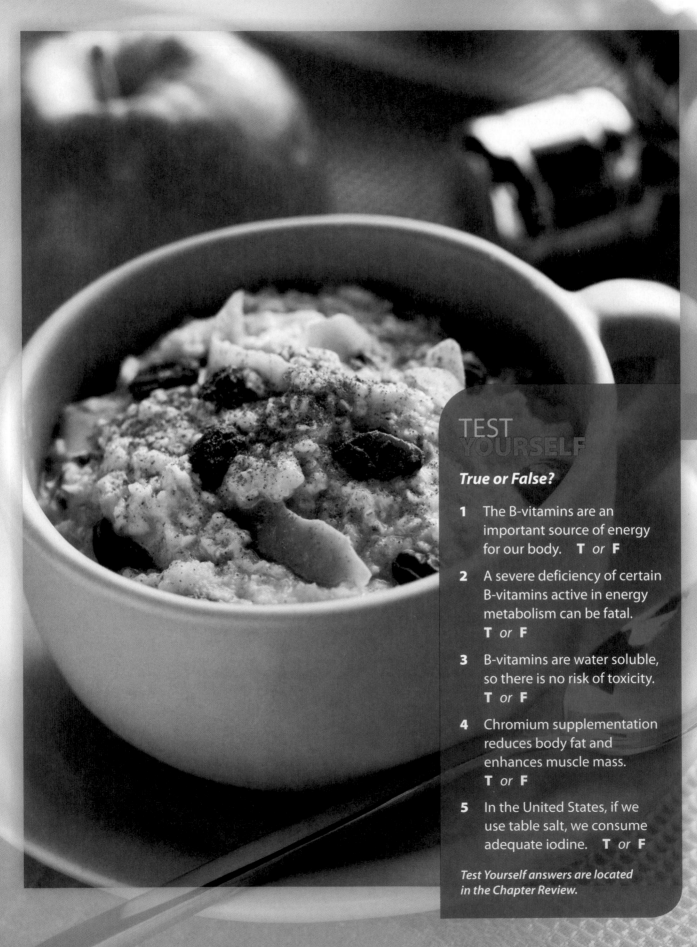

True or False?

1. The B-vitamins are an important source of energy for our body. **T** *or* **F**

2. A severe deficiency of certain B-vitamins active in energy metabolism can be fatal. **T** *or* **F**

3. B-vitamins are water soluble, so there is no risk of toxicity. **T** *or* **F**

4. Chromium supplementation reduces body fat and enhances muscle mass. **T** *or* **F**

5. In the United States, if we use table salt, we consume adequate iodine. **T** *or* **F**

Test Yourself answers are located in the Chapter Review.

8 Nutrients Involved in Energy Metabolism

Learning Objectives

After studying this chapter, you should be able to:

1. Describe how coenzymes enhance the activities of enzymes, *pp. 312–313*.

2. Name the B-vitamins that are primarily involved in energy metabolism and describe their function, *pp. 314–323*.

3. Identify the deficiency disorders associated with thiamin, niacin, and riboflavin, *pp. 316–318*.

4. Describe the toxic effects of high doses of niacin and vitamin B_6, *pp. 320–323*.

5. Discuss the association between vitamin B_6 and vascular disease, *pp. 323*.

6. Describe the sources, properties, and functions of folate, vitamin B_{12}, pantothenic acid, biotin, and choline, *pp. 323–331*

7. Describe the actions of at least two minerals that function as cofactors in energy metabolism, *pp. 330–333*.

8. Identify the deficiency disorders associated with poor iodine intake, *pp. 332–333*.

9. Explain why poor B-vitamin intake decreases the ability to do physical activity, *pp. 336–338*.

MasteringNutrition™

Go online for chapter quizzes, pre-tests, Interactive Activities and more!

D r. Leslie Bernstein looked in astonishment at the 80-year-old man in his office. A leading gastroenterologist and professor of medicine at Albert Einstein College of Medicine in New York City, he had admired Pop Katz for years as one of his most healthy patients, a strict vegan and athlete who just weeks before had been accomplishing 3-mile runs as if he were 40 years younger. Now he could barely stand. He was confused, cried easily, was wandering away from the house partially clothed, and had lost control of his bladder. Tests showed that he was not suffering from Alzheimer's disease, had not had a stroke, did not have a tumor or an infection, and had no evidence of exposure to pesticides, metals, drugs, or other toxins. Blood tests were normal, except that his red blood cells were slightly enlarged. Bernstein consulted with a neurologist, who diagnosed "rapidly progressive dementia of unknown origin."

Bernstein was unconvinced: "In a matter of weeks, a man who hadn't been sick for 80 years suddenly became demented . . . 'Holy smoke!' I thought, 'I'm an idiot! The man's been a vegetarian for 38 years. No meat. No fish. No eggs. No milk. He hasn't had any animal protein for decades. He has to be B_{12} deficient!'" Bernstein immediately tested Katz's blood, then gave him an injection of B_{12}. The blood test confirmed Bernstein's hunch: the level of B_{12} in Katz's blood was too low to measure. The morning after his injection, Katz could sit up without help. Within a week of ongoing treatment, he could read, play card games, and hold his own in conversations. Unfortunately, the delay in diagnosis left some permanent neurologic damage, including alterations in his personality and an inability to concentrate. Bernstein notes, "A diet free of animal protein can be healthful and safe, but it should be supplemented periodically with B_{12} by mouth or by injection."[1]

In this chapter, we explore the reasons certain B-vitamins, including vitamin B_{12}, are essential to the body's breakdown and use of the macronutrients and why severe deficiency of these vitamins is incompatible with life. We also discuss the role of the minerals iodine, chromium, manganese, and sulfur in energy metabolism; and we conclude the chapter with a look at the impact of low B-vitamin intake on our ability to work, play, and exercise.

How Does the Body Regulate Energy Metabolism?

We've explored the digestion and metabolism of carbohydrates, lipids, proteins, and alcohol (in Chapters 3 through 7). In those chapters, you learned that the regulation of energy metabolism is a complex process involving numerous biological substances and chemical pathways. Here, we describe how certain micronutrients we consume in our diet assist us in generating energy from the carbohydrates, lipids, and proteins we eat along with them.

The Body Requires Vitamins and Minerals to Produce Energy

Although vitamins and minerals do not contain Calories and thus do not directly provide energy, the body is unable to generate energy from the macronutrients without them. The B-vitamins are particularly important in assisting energy metabolism. They include thiamin, riboflavin, vitamin B_6, niacin, folate, vitamin B_{12}, pantothenic acid, and biotin. Except for vitamin B_{12}, these water-soluble vitamins need to be consumed regularly, because the body has no storage reservoir for them. Conversely, excess amounts of these vitamins, either from food or supplementation, are easily lost in the urine.

The primary role of six of the B-vitamins (thiamin, riboflavin, vitamin B_6, niacin, pantothenic acid, and biotin) is to act as coenzymes in a number of metabolic processes. As you previously learned (in Chapter 7), a coenzyme is an organic molecule that combines with an enzyme to activate it and help it do its job. The other two B-vitamins (folate and vitamin B_{12}) function secondarily in energy metabolism, and primarily in cell regeneration and the synthesis of red blood cells. We discuss their roles as blood nutrients later in this text (in Chapter 12).

Figure 8.1 provides a simple overview of how some of the B-vitamins act as coenzymes to promote energy metabolism, and **Figure 8.2** shows how these coenzymes participate in the energy metabolism pathways. For instance, thiamin is part of the coenzyme thiamin

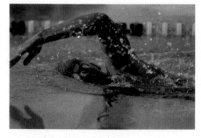

Vitamins do not provide energy directly, but the B-vitamins help the body create the energy that it needs from the foods we eat.

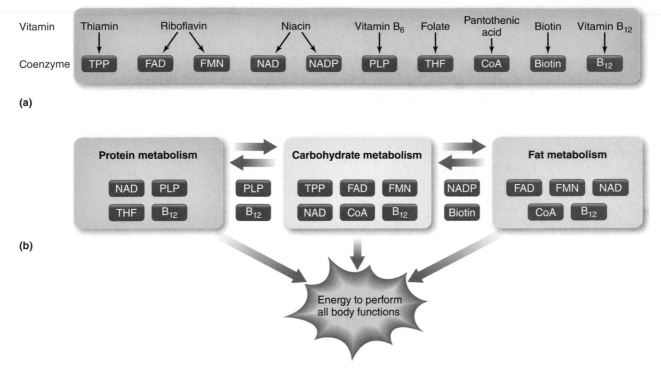

FIGURE 8.1 The B-vitamins play many important roles in the reactions involved in energy metabolism. **(a)** B-vitamins and the coenzymes they are a part of. **(b)** This chart illustrates many of the coenzymes essential for various metabolic functions; however, this is only a small sample of the thousands of roles that the B-vitamins play in our body. TPP, thiamin pyrophosphate; FAD, flavin adenine dinucleotide; FMN, flavin mononucleotide; NAD, nicotinamide adenine dinucleotide; NADP, nicotinamide adenine dinucleotide phosphate; PLP, pyridoxal phosphate; CoA, coenzyme A.

pyrophosphate, or TPP, which is required for the breakdown of glucose. Riboflavin is a part of two coenzymes, flavin mononucleotide (FMN) and flavin adenine dinucleotide (FAD), which help break down glucose and fatty acids.

Four minerals also function in energy metabolism: the trace minerals iodine, chromium, and manganese and the major mineral sulfur. A brief overview of the nutrients involved in energy metabolism is provided in **Table 8.1** (page 315). The specific functions of each B-vitamin and mineral involved in energy metabolism are described in this chapter.

Some Micronutrients Assist with Nutrient Transport and Hormone Production

Some micronutrients promote energy metabolism by facilitating the transport of nutrients into the cells. For instance, the mineral chromium helps improve glucose uptake into cells. Other micronutrients assist in the production of hormones that regulate metabolic processes; the mineral iodine, for example, is necessary for the synthesis of thyroid hormones, which regulate our metabolic rate and promote growth and development. The details of these processes and their related nutrients are discussed ahead.

RECAP

Vitamins and minerals are not direct sources of energy, but they help generate energy from carbohydrates, fats, proteins, and alcohol. Acting as coenzymes, micronutrients such as the B-vitamins assist enzymes in metabolizing macronutrients to produce energy. Minerals such as chromium and iodine assist with nutrient uptake into the cells and with regulating energy production and cell growth. ■

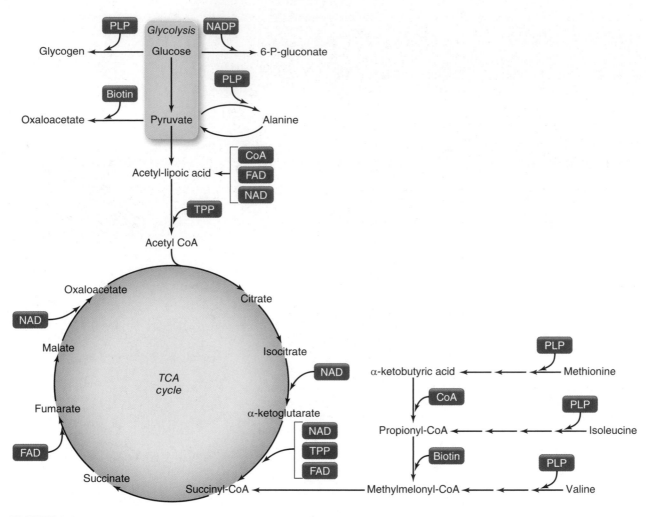

FIGURE 8.2 Example of some metabolic pathways that require B-vitamins for energy production.

Nutrition
MILESTONE

Thiamin deficiency results in a disease called *beriberi*, which causes paralysis of the lower limbs. Although beriberi has been known throughout recorded history, it was not until the 19th century, when steam-powered mills began removing the outer shell of rice and other grains, that the disease became widespread, especially in Southeast Asia. At the time, it was not known that the outer layer of the grain contains the highest concentrations of B-vitamins, including thiamin.

In **1906**, Drs. Christiaan Eijkman and Gerrit Grijns, Dutch physicians living in Java, described how they could produce beriberi in chickens or pigeons by feeding them polished rice and could cure them by feeding back the rice bran that had been removed during polishing. In 1911, Polish chemist Casimir Funk was able to isolate the water-soluble, nitrogen-containing compound in rice bran that was responsible for the cure. He referred to this compound as a "vital amine" and called it thiamin.

A Profile of Vitamins Involved in Energy Metabolism

As we have stated, the B-vitamins facilitate the production of energy in the body. A vitamin-like substance called choline also assists energy metabolism. In this section, we discuss the functions, recommended intakes, toxicity, and deficiency symptoms for the B-vitamins and choline.

Thiamin (Vitamin B_1)

Thiamin was the first B-vitamin discovered, hence its designation as vitamin B_1. Because this compound was recognized as vital to health and has a functional amine group, it was initially called "vitamine."[2] Later, this term was applied to several other nonmineral compounds that are essential for health, and the spelling was changed to *vitamin*. Thiamin was given a new name reflecting both its thiazole and amine groups. Thiamin is required for the formation of its coenzyme thiamin pyrophosphate, or TPP. The structures of thiamin and TPP are shown in **Figure 8.3**. The body converts dietary thiamin to TPP.

Functions of Thiamin

Thiamin is important in a number of energy-producing metabolic pathways within the body. As a part of TPP, thiamin plays a critical role in the breakdown of glucose for energy. For example, TPP is required for pyruvate dehydrogenase, the enzyme responsible for the conversion of pyruvate to acetyl-CoA (see Figure 8.2). This is a critical step in the conversion of glucose into a smaller molecule that can enter the TCA cycle for energy production. Thus, when dietary thiamin is inadequate, the body's ability to metabolize carbohydrate is diminished.

Another primary role of TPP is to act as a coenzyme in the metabolism of the branched-chain amino acids, which include leucine, isoleucine, and valine. TPP is a coenzyme for two α-keto acid dehydrogenase complexes. One of these enzyme complexes helps convert the carbon skeletons of the branched-chain amino acids into products that can enter the TCA cycle, whereas the other converts α-ketoglutarate to succinate in the TCA cycle (see Figure 8.2). The highest concentrations of the branched-chain amino acids are found in the muscle, where they make up approximately 25% of the content of the average protein. Thus, these amino acids play a significant role in providing fuel for the working muscle, especially during high-intensity exercise.[3]

TPP also assists in the production of DNA and RNA, making it important for cell regeneration and protein synthesis. Finally, it plays a role in the synthesis of neurotransmitters—chemicals that transmit messages throughout the central nervous system.

How Much Thiamin Should We Consume?

The RDA for thiamin for adults aged 19 years and older is 1.2 mg/day for men and 1.1 mg/day for women. According to NHANES III data, the average dietary intake of thiamin for men and women between the ages of 19 and 70 years is approximately 2 mg/day and approximately 1.5 mg/day, respectively.[4] Thus, it appears that the average adult in the United States gets adequate amounts of thiamin in the diet.

Those at greatest risk for poor thiamin status are the elderly, who typically have reduced total energy intakes; anyone with malabsorption syndrome; and patients on renal dialysis, since thiamin is easily cleared from the blood during dialysis. Also, people who eat a diet high in unenriched processed grains and simple sugars may be at risk for poor thiamin status.

TABLE 8.1 Overview of Nutrients Involved in Energy Metabolism

To see the full profile of nutrients involved in energy metabolism, turn to Chapter 7.5, In Depth: Vitamins and Minerals, pages 300–309.

Nutrient	Recommended Intake
Thiamin (vitamin B$_1$)	RDA for 19 years and older: Women = 1.1 mg/day Men = 1.2 mg/day
Riboflavin (vitamin B$_2$)	RDA for 19 years and older: Women = 1.1 mg/day Men = 1.3 mg/day
Niacin (nicotinamide and nicotinic acid)	RDA for 19 years and older: Women = 14 mg/day Men = 16 mg/day
Nutrient	**Recommended Intake**
Vitamin B$_6$ (pyridoxine)	RDA for 19 to 50 years of age: Women and men = 1.3 mg/day RDA for 51 years and older: Women = 1.5 mg/day Men = 1.7 mg/day
Folate (folic acid)	RDA for 19 years and older: Women and men = 400 µg/day
Vitamin B$_{12}$ (cobalamin)	RDA for 19 years and older: Women and men = 2.4 µg/day
Pantothenic acid	AI for 19 years and older: Women and men = 5 mg/day
Biotin	AI for 19 years and older: Women and men = 30 µg/day
Choline	AI for 19 years and older: Women = 425 mg/day Men = 550 mg/day

(a) Thiamin

(b) Thiamin pyrophosphate

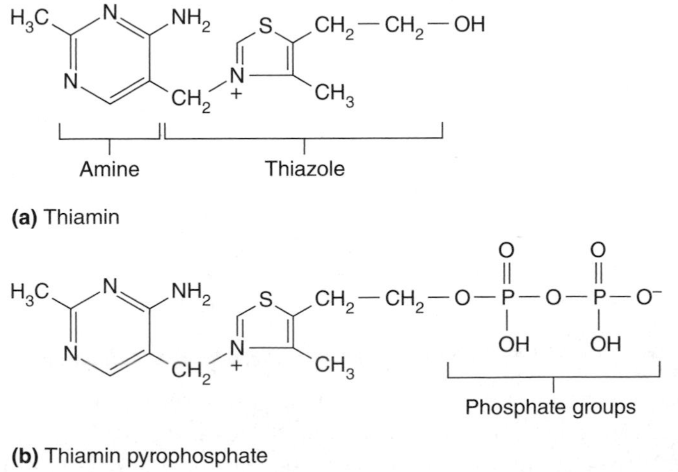

FIGURE 8.3 Structure of **(a)** thiamin and **(b)** thiamin pyrophosphate (TPP).

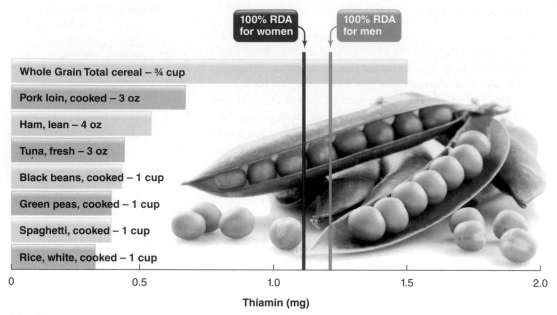

FIGURE 8.4 Common food sources of thiamin. The RDA for thiamin is 1.2 mg/day for men and 1.1 mg/day for women 19 years and older. (*Source:* Data from US Department of Agriculture, Agricultural Research Service. 2009. USDA Nutrient Database for Standard Reference, Release 22. Nutrient Data Laboratory Home Page. www.ars.usda.gov.)

Physically active individuals, especially those who consume high amounts of simple carbohydrate, such as candy, soda, and sport gels, may be at risk for poor B-vitamin status, including thiamin. Research indicates that depletion of the B-vitamins can reduce the ability to perform physical activity.[5] This is discussed in more detail at the end of the chapter.

Food Sources of Thiamin

Thiamin is found abundantly in ham and other pork products (**Figure 8.4**). Sunflower seeds, beans, oat bran, mixed dishes that contain whole or enriched grains and meat, tuna fish, soy milk, and soy-based meat substitutes are also good sources. Enriched and whole-grain foods, including fortified ready-to-eat cereals, are rich in several B-vitamins, including thiamin.

What Happens If We Consume Too Much Thiamin?

Excess thiamin is readily cleared by the kidneys, and to date there have been no reports of adverse effects from consuming high amounts of thiamin from either food or supplements. Thus, the Institute of Medicine (IOM) has not been able to set a tolerable upper intake level (UL) for thiamin.[4]

What Happens If We Don't Consume Enough Thiamin?

As the B-vitamins are involved in most energy-generating processes, the deficiency symptoms include a combination of fatigue, apathy, muscle weakness, and reduced cognitive function. Thiamin-deficiency disease is called **beriberi.** In this disease, the body's inability to metabolize energy leads to muscle wasting and nerve damage; in later stages, patients may be unable to move at all. The heart muscle may also be affected, and the patient may die of heart failure. Beriberi is seen in countries in which unenriched, processed grains are a primary food source; for instance, beriberi was widespread in Asia when rice was processed and refined, and it still occurs in refugee camps and other settlements dependent on poor-quality food supplies.

Thiamin deficiency is also seen in industrialized countries in people with chronic heavy alcohol consumption and limited food intake. This alcohol-related thiamin deficiency is called Wernicke–Korsakoff syndrome. High alcohol intake contributes to thiamin deficiency in three ways: it is generally accompanied by low thiamin intake; at the same time, it increases the need for thiamin to metabolize the alcohol; and it reduces thiamin

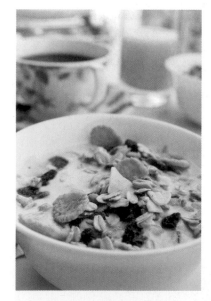

Ready-to-eat cereals are a good source of thiamin and other B-vitamins.

beriberi A disease caused by thiamin deficiency, characterized by muscle wasting and nerve damage.

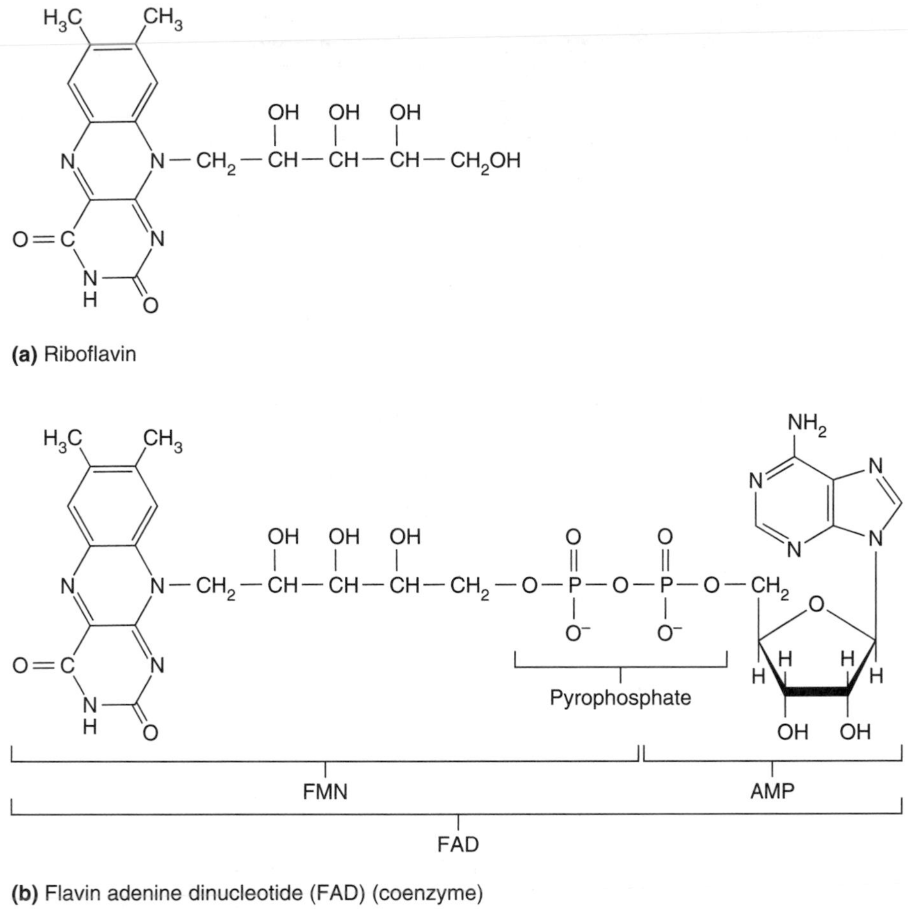

(a) Riboflavin

(b) Flavin adenine dinucleotide (FAD) (coenzyme)

absorption. Together, these factors contribute to thiamin deficiency.[6, 7] The symptoms of Wernicke–Korsakoff syndrome are tremors, confusion, and memory impairment.[7]

Riboflavin (Vitamin B$_2$)

In 1917, riboflavin became the second B-vitamin discovered; thus, it was designated vitamin B$_2$. The term *riboflavin* reflects its structure and color; *ribo* refers to the carbon-rich ribityl side chain, and *flavin*, which is associated with the multi-ring portion of the vitamin, refers to the yellow color this vitamin produces when dissolved in water (*flavus* means "yellow" in Latin) (**Figure 8.5a**). Riboflavin is relatively heat stable but sensitive to light: when exposed to light, the ribityl side chain is cleaved off and the vitamin loses its activity.

Functions of Riboflavin

Riboflavin is an important component of two coenzymes that are involved in oxidation–reduction reactions occurring within the energy-producing metabolic pathways, including the electron transport chain. These coenzymes, flavin mononucleotide (FMN) and flavin adenine dinucleotide (FAD), are involved in the metabolism of carbohydrates, fatty acids, and amino acids for energy. The structures of FMN and FAD are shown in Figure 8.5b: notice that FMN combines with adenosine monophosphate to produce FAD. For example, you will recall (from Chapter 7) that FAD and FMN function as electron acceptors in the electron transport chain, which eventually results in the production of ATP.

FAD is also a part of the α-ketoglutarate dehydrogenase complex, which converts α-ketoglutarate to succinate in one step of the TCA cycle (see Figure 8.2). It is also a coenzyme for succinate dehydrogenase, the enzyme involved in the conversion of succinate to fumarate in the next step of the TCA cycle. Finally, riboflavin is a part of the coenzyme required by glutathione peroxidase, which assists in the fight against oxidative damage. (Antioxidants are discussed in detail in Chapter 10, page 391.)

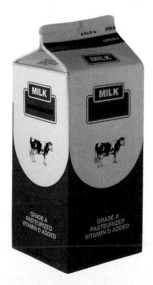

Milk is a significant source of riboflavin and is stored in opaque containers to prevent the destruction of riboflavin by light.

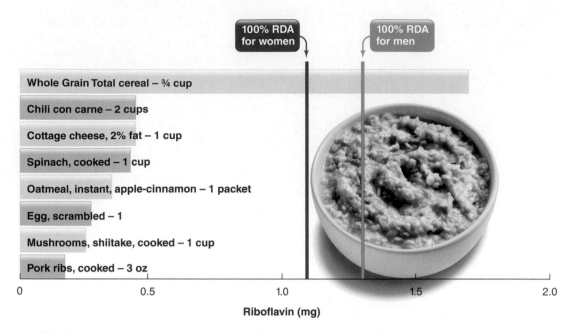

Whole Grain Total cereal – ¾ cup

Chili con carne – 2 cups

Cottage cheese, 2% fat – 1 cup

Spinach, cooked – 1 cup

Oatmeal, instant, apple-cinnamon – 1 packet

Egg, scrambled – 1

Mushrooms, shiitake, cooked – 1 cup

Pork ribs, cooked – 3 oz

| 0 | 0.5 | 1.0 | 1.5 | 2.0 |

Riboflavin (mg)

FIGURE 8.6 Common food sources of riboflavin. The RDA for riboflavin is 1.3 mg/day for men and 1.1 mg/day for women. (*Source:* Data from US Department of Agriculture, Agricultural Research Service. 2009. Nutrient Data Laboratory Home Page. www.ars.usda.gov.)

How Much Riboflavin Should We Consume?

The RDA for riboflavin for adults aged 19 years and older is 1.3 mg/day for men and 1.1 mg/day for women. Based on NHANES III data, the dietary intake of riboflavin from food for men between the ages of 19 and 70 years averages 2.0 to 2.3 mg/day (median = 2 mg/day) and for women of the same age 1.7 to 1.9 mg/day (median = 1.5 mg/day).[4] Thus, it appears that most adults in the United States get adequate amounts of riboflavin in their diet.

As with thiamin, those at greatest risk for low riboflavin intakes are the elderly, who may have reduced total energy intake; individuals who make poor food selections; those with malabsorption problems; and patients on renal dialysis.[8] Approximately one-third of the RDA for riboflavin is supplied in the American diet by milk and milk products; thus, it is easy to see how people who eliminate milk and milk products from their diet may also be at risk.[6]

Riboflavin is destroyed when it is exposed to light; thus, milk is generally stored in opaque containers. In addition to milk and other dairy products, good sources of riboflavin include eggs, meats (including organ meats), broccoli, enriched bread and grain products, and ready-to-eat cereals (**Figure 8.6**).

As with thiamin, there are no reports of adverse effects from consuming high amounts of riboflavin from either food or supplements; thus, the IOM has not been able to set a UL for riboflavin.[4]

Riboflavin deficiency is referred to as **ariboflavinosis.** Symptoms of ariboflavinosis include sore throat; swelling of the mucous membranes in the mouth and throat; lips that are dry and scaly; a purple-colored tongue; and inflamed, irritated patches on the skin. Severe riboflavin deficiency can impair the metabolism of vitamin B_6 (pyridoxine) and niacin.[4]

Niacin

Niacin is a generic name for two specific vitamin compounds, nicotinic acid and nicotinamide, which are shown in **Figure 8.7**. This B-vitamin was previously designated as vitamin B_3, a name you will sometimes still see on vitamin supplement labels. Niacin was first established as an essential nutrient in the treatment of pellagra in 1937. **Pellagra,** the deficiency of niacin, was first described in the 1700s and was common in the United States until the early 20th century. (For more information on the history of pellagra, see the **Highlight** box in Chapter 1, page 6.)

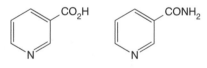

(a) Nicotinic acid   **(b)** Nicotinamide

FIGURE 8.7 Forms of niacin. **(a)** Structure of nicotinic acid. **(b)** Structure of nicotinamide. The generic term *niacin* is used to refer to these two compounds.

ariboflavinosis A condition caused by riboflavin deficiency.

pellagra A disease that results from severe niacin deficiency.

Functions of Niacin

The two forms of niacin, nicotinic acid and nicotinamide, are essential for the formation of the two coenzymes nicotinamide adenine dinucleotide (NAD) and nicotinamide adenine dinucleotide phosphate (NADP). These coenzymes, like those formed from riboflavin and thiamin, are required for the oxidation–reduction reactions involved in the catabolism of carbohydrate, fat, and protein for energy. For example, NADP-dependent dehydrogenase enzymes catalyze steps in the β-oxidation of fatty acids, the oxidation of ketone bodies, the degradation of carbohydrates, and the catabolism of amino acids.[6] Some metabolic pathways in which niacin functions are illustrated in Figure 8.2. Niacin is also an important coenzyme in DNA replication and repair and in the process of cell differentiation. Pharmaceutical preparations of niacin are sometimes prescribed for the treatment of abnormal blood lipids.[9]

How Much Niacin Should We Consume?

Niacin is a unique vitamin in that the body can synthesize a limited amount from the amino acid tryptophan. However, the ratio reflecting the conversion of tryptophan to niacin is 60:1; thus, the body relies on the diet to provide the majority of niacin necessary for functioning. The term *niacin equivalents (NE)* is used to express niacin intake recommendations, and it reflects the amount of niacin in our diet and the amount synthesized from tryptophan within the body. Recall that people consuming limited, corn-based diets are at significant risk for pellagra. This is not surprising, since corn is low in both niacin and the amino acid tryptophan.

The RDA for niacin for adults aged 19 and older is 16 mg/day of NE for men and 14 mg/day of NE for women. Based on NHANES III data, the average dietary intake of niacin from food for men and women between the ages of 19 and 70 years is approximately 27 mg/day and 21 mg/day, respectively.[4]

Good food sources of niacin include meat, fish, poultry, enriched bread products, and ready-to-eat cereals; however, the availability of this niacin for absorption varies. For example, the niacin in cereal grains is bound to other substances and is only 30% available for absorption, whereas the niacin found in meats is much more available.[4] To calculate the NE in your own diet, see **You Do the Math** (page 320). See **Figure 8.8** for the niacin content of commonly consumed foods.

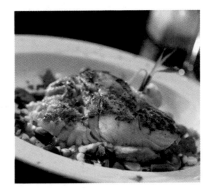

Halibut is a good source of niacin.

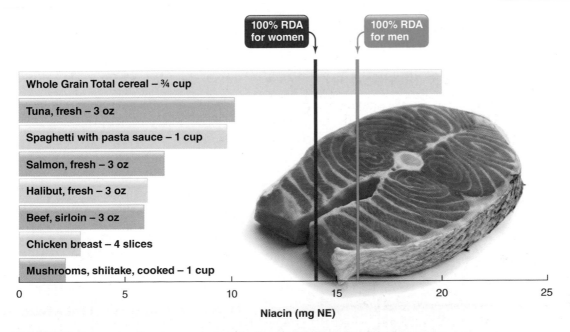

FIGURE 8.8 Common food sources of niacin. The RDA for niacin is 16 mg NE/day for men and 14 mg NE/day for women. (*Source:* Data from US Department of Agriculture, Agricultural Research Service. 2009. USDA Nutrient Database for Standard Reference, Release 22. Nutrient Data Laboratory Home Page. www.ars.usda.gov.)

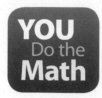

Calculating Niacin Equivalents

When you analyze your diet using the nutrient analysis program provided with this book, you will notice that the program calculates your total niacin equivalents (NE). How is this calculation done? How would you calculate your own intake of NE if the computer program was not doing this for you?

To calculate NE, you first need to determine the amount of two components of your diet: (1) total niacin intake from food in mg/day and (2) total intake of tryptophan in mg/day. Now you are ready to do the calculation, using the following formula.

Just keep in mind that 1 NE = either 60 mg of tryptophan or 1 mg of niacin.

Total NE = niacin intake from food + (tryptophan intake/60)

Now calculate the NE intake of an adult male who consumes 18.9 mg/day of niacin and 630 mg/day of tryptophan. What percentage of his total NE intake is coming from tryptophan? Is this person meeting his RDA?

There seem to be no adverse effects from the consumption of naturally occurring niacin in foods; however, niacin can cause toxicity symptoms when taken in supplement form.[4] These symptoms include *flushing,* which is burning, tingling, and itching sensations accompanied by a reddened flush, primarily on the face, arms, and chest. Liver damage, glucose intolerance, blurred vision, and edema of the eyes can be seen with very large doses of niacin taken over long periods of time. The UL for niacin is 35 mg/day and was determined based on the level of niacin below which flushing is typically not observed.

As mentioned, severe niacin deficiency causes pellagra, which is rarely seen in industrialized countries, except in cases of chronic alcoholism. Initial symptoms of pellagra include functional changes in the gastrointestinal tract, which decrease the amount of HCl produced and the absorption of nutrients, and lesions in the central nervous system, causing weakness, fatigue, and anorexia. These initial symptoms are followed by what have been identified as the "three Ds"—dermatitis, diarrhea, and dementia.[6] The word *pellagra* literally means "rough skin": dermatitis occurs on the parts of the body more exposed to the elements, such as the face, neck, hands, and feet. The diarrhea and dementia develop as the disease worsens, and they further affect the gastrointestinal tract and central nervous system.

Vitamin B$_6$ (Pyridoxine)

Vitamin B$_6$ is actually a group of three related compounds—pyridoxine (PN), pyridoxal (PL), and pyridoxamine (PM)—and their phosphate forms, which include pyridoxine phosphate (PNP), pyridoxal phosphate (PLP), and pyridoxamine phosphate (PMP), respectively. The structures of these compounds are shown in **Figure 8.9.**

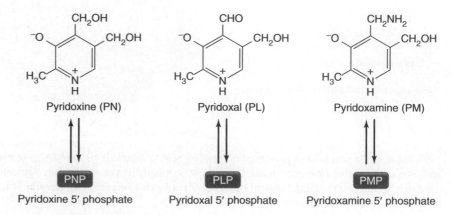

FIGURE 8.9 Structure of the vitamin B$_6$ compounds and their interconversions to the phosphorylated forms.

Functions of Vitamin B₆

Some of the metabolic pathways in which vitamin B_6 functions are illustrated in Figure 8.2. In the form of PLP, vitamin B_6 is a coenzyme for more than 100 enzymes involved in the metabolism of amino acids. Some of the critical roles of vitamin B_6 are listed here:

- *Amino acid metabolism.* Vitamin B_6 plays a critical role in transamination, which is a key process in making nonessential amino acids (see Chapter 6). Without adequate vitamin B_6, all amino acids become essential, as our body cannot make them in sufficient quantities.
- *Neurotransmitter synthesis.* Vitamin B_6 is a coenzyme involved in the synthesis of several neurotransmitters, a process that involves transamination. Neurotransmitters are chemicals necessary for the transmission of nerve impulses across synapses. Because of this, vitamin B_6 is important in cognitive function and normal brain activity. Abnormal brain waves have been observed in both infants and adults in vitamin B_6–deficient states.[10]
- *Carbohydrate metabolism.* Vitamin B_6 is a coenzyme assisting in the breakdown of stored glycogen into glucose. Thus, vitamin B_6 plays an important role in maintaining blood glucose during exercise. It is also important for the conversion of amino acids to glucose.
- *Heme synthesis.* The synthesis of heme, required for the production of hemoglobin and thus the transport of oxygen in red blood cells, requires vitamin B_6. Chronic vitamin B_6 deficiency can lead to small red blood cells with inadequate amounts of hemoglobin, which is called *microcytic, hypochromic anemia*.[10] (This is discussed in more detail in Chapter 12.)
- *Immune function.* Vitamin B_6 plays a role in maintaining the health and activity of lymphocytes and in producing adequate levels of antibodies in response to an immune challenge. The depression of immune function seen in vitamin B_6 deficiency may also be due to a reduction in vitamin B_6–dependent enzymes involved in DNA synthesis.
- *Metabolism of other nutrients.* Vitamin B_6 also plays a role in the metabolism of other nutrients, including niacin, folate, and carnitine.[10]
- *Reduction in cardiovascular disease (CVD) risk.* Vitamin B_6, folate, and vitamin B_{12} are closely interrelated in some metabolic functions, including the metabolism of methionine, an essential amino acid. The body metabolizes methionine to another amino acid, called **homocysteine.** In the presence of sufficient levels of vitamin B_6, homocysteine can then be converted to the nonessential amino acid cysteine (**Figure 8.10**). In the presence of sufficient levels of folate and vitamin B_{12}, homocysteine can also be converted back to methionine if the body's level of methionine becomes deficient. If these nutrients are not available, these conversion reactions cannot occur and homocysteine will accumulate in the blood. High levels of homocysteine have been associated with an increased risk for cardiovascular disease and as a measure of poor dietary intakes of vitamin B_6, folate, and vitamin B_{12}.

homocysteine An amino acid that requires adequate levels of folate, vitamin B_6 and vitamin B_{12} for its metabolism. High levels of homocysteine in the blood are associated with an increased risk for cardiovascular disease.

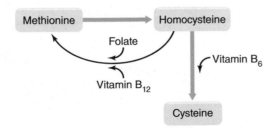

FIGURE 8.10 The body metabolizes methionine, an essential amino acid, to homocysteine. Notice, however, that homocysteine can then be converted back to methionine through a vitamin B_{12}– and folate–dependent reaction, or to cysteine through a vitamin B_6–dependent reaction. Cysteine is a nonessential amino acid important for making other biological compounds. Without these B-vitamins, blood levels of homocysteine can increase. High levels of homocysteine are a risk factor for cardiovascular disease.

How Much Vitamin B₆ Should We Consume?

The RDA for vitamin B₆ for adult men and women aged 19 to 50 years is 1.3 mg/day. For adults 51 years of age and older, the RDA increases to 1.7 mg/day for men and 1.5 mg/day for women. The increased requirement with aging is based on data indicating that more vitamin B₆ is required to maintain normal vitamin B₆ status, using blood PLP concentrations as a status indicator, in older individuals. Based on NHANES III data, the average dietary intake of vitamin B₆ from food for men and women between the ages of 19 and 70 years averages 2 mg/day and 1.5 to 1.6 mg/day, respectively.[4]

Because of the role vitamin B₆ plays in protein metabolism, it has been proposed that the requirement for vitamin B₆ be based on protein intake. Although the RDAs did not define vitamin B₆ intake in terms of protein intake, we do know that as protein intake increases more vitamin B₆ is required.[4] Fortunately, nature has combined vitamin B₆ with protein in many foods, so food sources high in protein are also typically high in vitamin B₆.

Food Sources of Vitamin B₆

Good sources of vitamin B₆ include meat, fish (especially tuna), poultry, and organ meats, which are also high in protein (**Figure 8.11**). Thus, protein and vitamin B₆ are provided together in the same food, which ensures adequate protein metabolism. Besides meat and fish, good food sources of vitamin B₆ include enriched ready-to-eat cereals, white potatoes and other starchy vegetables, bananas, and fortified soy-based meat substitutes. In the typical American diet, approximately 40% of the dietary vitamin B₆ comes from animal sources, while 60% comes from plants. For this reason, individuals who eliminate animal foods from their diet need to make sure they select plant foods high in vitamin B₆.

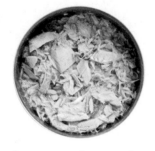

Tuna is a very good source of vitamin B₆.

What Happens If We Consume Too Much Vitamin B₆?

There are no adverse effects associated with high intakes of vitamin B₆ from food sources. Vitamin B₆ supplements have been used to treat conditions such as premenstrual syndrome

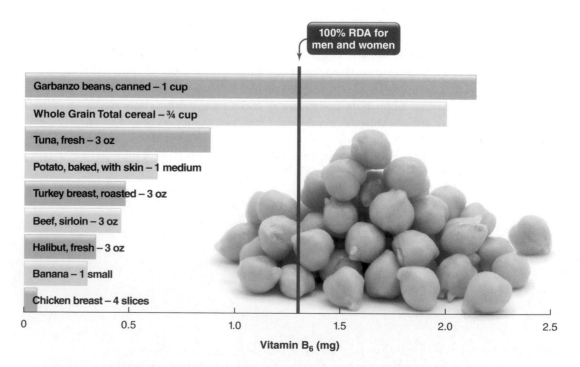

FIGURE 8.11 Common food sources of vitamin B₆. The RDA for vitamin B₆ is 1.3 mg/day for men and women aged 19 to 50 years. (*Source:* Data from US Department of Agriculture, Agricultural Research Service. 2009. USDA Nutrient Database for Standard Reference, Release 22. Nutrient Data Laboratory Home Page. www.ars.usda.gov.)

and carpal tunnel syndrome. Caution is required, however, when using such supplements. High doses of supplemental vitamin B_6 have been associated with sensory neuropathy and dermatological lesions.[4] Thus, the UL for vitamin B_6 is set at 100 mg/day. See the **Nutrition Debate** at the end of this chapter for more discussion of the potential relationship between high intakes of vitamin B_6 and premenstrual syndrome.

What Happens If We Don't Consume Enough Vitamin B_6?

A number of conditions appear to increase the need for vitamin B_6: alcoholism, certain prescription medications, intense physical activity, and chronic diseases, such as arthritis and vascular disease.[3, 4, 11] If we don't get enough vitamin B_6 in the diet, the symptoms of vitamin B_6 deficiency can develop. These include anemia, convulsions, depression, confusion, and inflamed, irritated patches on the skin. Notice that the symptoms associated with vitamin B_6 deficiency involve three tissues: skin, blood, and the nervous system. This fact reflects the role of vitamin B_6 in protein metabolism, red blood cell development, and the synthesis of neurotransmitters.

No specific disease is solely attributed to vitamin B_6 deficiency. However, recall that, if intakes of vitamin B_6, folate, and vitamin B_{12} are low, blood levels of homocysteine increase. High blood homocysteine concentrations are an independent risk factor for cardiovascular disease.

If you're wondering whether you're getting enough vitamin B_6—or too much!—see the **You Do the Math** box (page 324) and calculate your daily intake.

Folate

Folate was originally identified as a growth factor in green, leafy vegetables (foliage), hence the name.[12] The generic term *folate* is used for all the various forms of food folate that demonstrate biological activity. Folic acid (pteroylglutamate; see **Figure 8.12**) is the form of folate found in most supplements and used in the enrichment and fortification of foods.

Functions of Folate and Folic Acid

Within the body, folate functions primarily in association with folate-dependent coenzymes that act as acceptors and donors of one-carbon units. These enzymes are critical for DNA synthesis, cell differentiation, and amino acid metabolism, which occur within the cytosol, nucleus, and mitochondria of the cells. Folate's role in assisting with cell division makes it a critical nutrient during the first few weeks of pregnancy, when the combined sperm–egg cell multiplies rapidly to form the primitive tissues and structures of the human body. Without adequate folate, the embryo cannot develop properly. In particular, a group of nervous system malformations called *neural tube defects* are associated with low maternal folate intake. Folate is also essential in the synthesis of new cells, such as the red blood cells, and for the repair of damaged cells. (We will discuss the role of folate in red blood cell development more in Chapter 12.)

As already discussed, folate and vitamin B_{12} are needed for the regeneration of methionine from homocysteine. High levels of homocysteine have been associated with an increased risk for cardiovascular disease.

What Factors Alter Folate Digestion, Absorption, and Balance?

Dietary folates are hydrolyzed by the brush border of the lumen and then absorbed into the enterocytes. This process is typically achieved through a carrier-mediated process, but some folates can cross the mucosal cell membrane by diffusion. Folates are then released from the enterocytes into the portal circulation, in which they are transported to the liver.[12]

The bioavailability of folate varies, depending on its source. When folic acid is taken as a supplement or in a fortified food, such as breakfast cereal, the amount absorbed is high—nearly

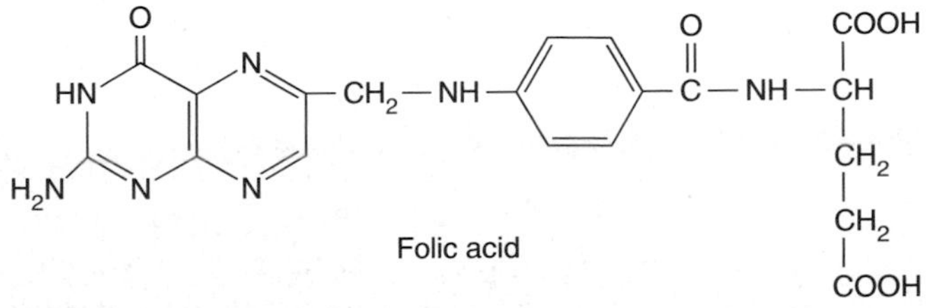

Folic acid

FIGURE 8.12 Structure of folate.

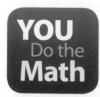

Calculating Your Daily Intake of Vitamin B₆

Open up your cupboard and take a look inside. How many processed foods providing B-vitamins do you consume on a typical day? Pull out all such foods, including breads, ready-to-eat cereals, pasta, energy bars, meal replacement drinks, and so forth. Then, if you take any supplements, including vitamins, protein powders, weight-loss supplements, and so forth, line those up too.

Now, let's see if we can determine whether you are meeting or exceeding your RDA for vitamin B_6. We'll limit our analysis to B_6 because it is one of the B-vitamins with a UL. Use the template provided below to document your vitamin B_6 intake for a typical day. On food labels, the amount of the vitamin will be given as a percentage of the daily value (%DV). Thus, you will first have to write down the %DV for each serving. Be sure to look at the serving size! If you eat two servings, you will need to multiply this value by 2, and so on. Finally, convert the %DV to the amount that you ate. For vitamin B_6, 100% of the DV is 2 mg. Notice that we have filled in one line of the template as an example; now you fill in the rest.

Meal	Food	%DV for B_6	Servings	%DV per Serving	B_6 Consumed (mg)
Breakfast	Wheaties	50%	2	100%	2 mg
Lunch					
Snack					
Dinner					
Supplements					
Total mg B_6/day:					

How much vitamin B_6 did you get each day from processed foods and supplements alone? How much additional vitamin B_6 would you estimate you get in whole foods, such as meat, fish, poultry, starchy vegetables, and bananas? Are you close to the UL for vitamin B_6 (100 mg for adults aged 19–70)? Although this assignment was designed to look at vitamin B_6, you can look at other micronutrients in your diet that have a UL.

85% to 100%.[4] However, the bioavailability of food folate is less than 50%.[12] When large doses of folic acid are taken as supplements, they are well absorbed, but the body has no mechanism for retaining this folate, so it is easily lost in the urine.

Because dietary folate is only half as bioavailable as synthetic folic acid, the amount of food folate in the diet is expressed as dietary folate equivalents, or DFE. In order to calculate the amount of DFE, you need to know that 1 µg of food folate is equal to 0.5 µg of folic acid taken on an empty stomach or 0.6 µg of folic acid taken with a meal.[4] Thus, to calculate the total DFE in an individual's diet, use the following equation:

µg of DFE provided in diet = µg of food folate per day + (1.7 × µg of synthetic folic acid/day)

Because this calculation can be time consuming, most nutrient databases calculate the DFE automatically, so that the total micrograms per day of folate provided in the nutrient analysis printout has already taken into account the bioavailability of the different types of folate in the diet.

Much of the folate circulating in the blood is attached to transport proteins, especially albumin, for delivery to the cells of the body. The red blood cells also contain folate attached to hemoglobin. Because this folate is not transferred out of the red blood cells to other tissues, it may be a good measure of folate status over the past 3 months—the life of red blood cells.[12] If red blood cell folate levels begin to drop, this indicates that, when the red blood cells were being formed, folate was inadequate in the body.

How Much Folate Should We Consume?

Folate is so important for good health and the prevention of birth defects that in 1998 the US Department of Agriculture (USDA) mandated the fortification with folic acid of enriched breads, flours, corn meals, rice, pastas, and other grain products. Because folic acid is highly available for absorption, the goal of this fortification was to increase folate intake among all Americans and thus decrease the risk for birth defects and chronic diseases associated with low folate intakes.

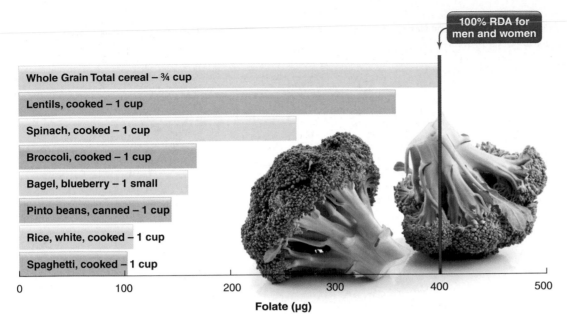

FIGURE 8.13 Common food sources of folate and folic acid. The RDA for folate is 400 µg/day for men and women. (*Source:* Data from US Dept of Agriculture, Agriculture Research Services. 2009. USDA Nutrient Database for Standard Reference, Release 22. Nutrient Data Laboratory Home Page. www.ars.usda.gov.)

The RDA for folate for adult men and women aged 19 years and older is 400 µg/day, with 600 µg/day required for pregnant women.[4] These higher levels of folate were set to minimize the risk for birth defects. The UL for folate is 1,000 µg/day.

Ready-to-eat cereals, bread, and other grain products are among the primary sources of folate in the United States; however, you need to read the label of processed grain products to make sure they contain folate. Other good food sources include liver, spinach, lentils, oatmeal, asparagus, and romaine lettuce. **Figure 8.13** shows some foods relatively high in folate. Losses of folate can occur when food is heated or when folate leaches out of cooked foods and the liquid from these foods is discarded. For this reason, cook green vegetables in a minimal amount of water and limit the time foods are exposed to high temperatures. These actions will help preserve the folate in the food.

What Happens If We Consume Too Much Folate?

There have been no studies suggesting toxic effects of consuming high amounts of folate in food; however; toxicity can occur with high amounts of supplemental folate.[12] One especially frustrating problem with folate toxicity is that it can mask a simultaneous vitamin B_{12} deficiency. This often results in a failure to detect the B_{12} deficiency and, as described in the chapter-opening case, a delay in diagnosis of B_{12} deficiency can contribute to severe damage to the nervous system. There do not appear to be any clear symptoms of folate toxicity independent from its interaction with vitamin B_{12} deficiency. However, as discussed in the Nutrition Debate at the end of this chapter, researchers are becoming concerned about some possible health risks, such as increased risk for cancer and allergies, now being associated with high supplemental doses of folic acid.

What Happens If We Consume Too Little Folate?

A folate deficiency can cause many adverse health effects, including *macrocytic anemia* (discussed in Chapter 12). Again, deficiencies in folate, vitamin B_6, and vitamin B_{12} can cause elevated levels of homocysteine in the blood, a condition that is associated with heart disease. When folate intake is inadequate in pregnant women, neural tube defects can occur. (Neural tube defects are discussed in more detail in Chapter 16.)

FIGURE 8.14 Structure of vitamin B_{12} (cyanocobalamin). As you can see, this is a highly complex molecule, and the Nobel Prize was awarded for the delineation of its structure.

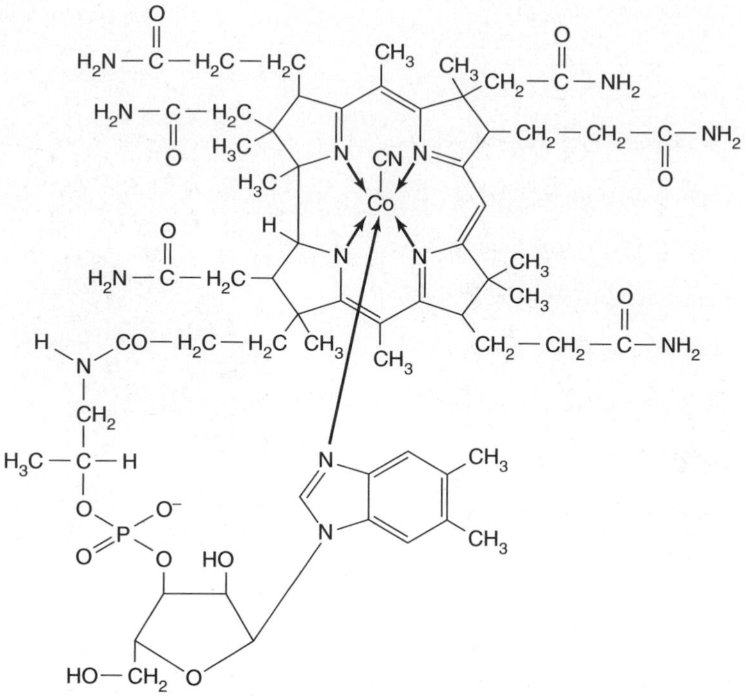

Vitamin B_{12} (Cyanocobalamin)

As with folate, the generic terms *vitamin B_{12}* and *cyanocobalamin* are used to describe a number of compounds that exhibit vitamin B_{12} biological activity. These compounds have cobalt in their center and are surrounded by ring structures. See **Figure 8.14** for a diagram of the structure of cyanocobalamin, which is derived when vitamin B_{12} is purified from natural sources.[12] As you can see, vitamin B_{12} is a complex molecule, and the Nobel Prize was awarded for the delineation of its structure.

Functions of Vitamin B_{12}

Vitamin B_{12} is part of coenzymes that assist with DNA synthesis, which is necessary for the proper formation of red blood cells.[13] As described in the chapter-opening scenario, vitamin B_{12} is essential for healthy functioning of the nervous system, because it helps maintain the myelin sheath that coats nerve fibers. When this sheath is damaged or absent, the conduction of nerve signals is altered, causing numerous neurologic problems.

Adequate levels of vitamin B_{12} and folate, as well as B_6, are also necessary for the metabolism of the amino acid homocysteine, which we discussed earlier.

What Factors Alter Vitamin B_{12} Absorption, Metabolism, and Balance?

Vitamin B_{12} is synthesized almost entirely by bacteria in animals. For this reason, plant sources generally do not contain vitamin B_{12}. Thus, the vitamin B_{12} in our diet comes almost exclusively from meat, eggs, dairy products, and some seafood and is approximately 50% bioavailable.[12]

The absorption of vitamin B_{12} is complex (**Figure 8.15**). In food, vitamin B_{12} is bound to protein. It is released from this protein in the acidic environment of the stomach, where it is then attached to another group of proteins called R-binders. The stomach also secretes **intrinsic factor,** a protein necessary for vitamin B_{12} absorption in the small intestine. The intrinsic factor and vitamin B_{12}–R-binder complexes formed in the stomach pass into the small intestine, where the R-binder protein is hydrolyzed by pancreatic proteolytic enzymes, after which free vitamin B_{12} binds to the intrinsic factor. The vitamin B_{12}–intrinsic factor complexes are then recognized by receptors on the enterocytes and

intrinsinc factor A protein secreted by cells of the stomach that binds to vitamin B_{12} and aids its absorption in the small intestine.

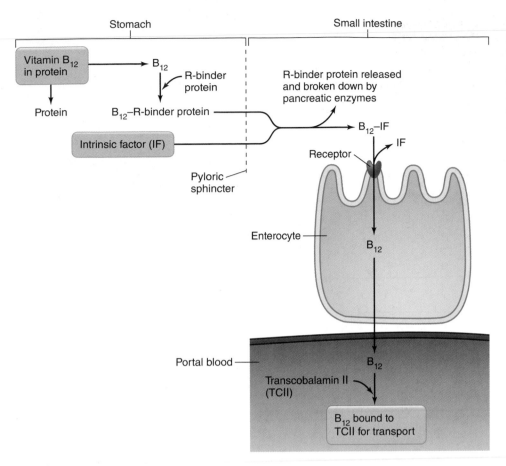

FIGURE 8.15 Digestion and absorption of vitamin B_{12}. (*Source:* "Advanced Nutrition and Human Metabolism (with InfoTrac®) 4e," by Gropper; Smith; Groff, 2005. Copyright © 2005 by Brooks/Cole, a part of Cengage Learning, Inc. Reproduced by permission.)

internalized. These receptors do not recognize vitamin B_{12} alone but only when it is bound to intrinsic factor. Within the enterocytes, vitamin B_{12} is released into the cytosol. The vitamin B_{12} is then released from the enterocyte, bound to a protein called transcobalamin II, and then transported to the cells of the body. The body stores vitamin B_{12} in the liver, approximately 2 to 3 mg, which means we can probably survive for months without vitamin B_{12} in our diet.[4] Vitamin B_{12} is lost from the system in the urine and bile.

How Much Vitamin B_{12} Should We Consume?

Vitamin B_{12} has two unique features. First, it is found almost exclusively in animal foods; thus, the elimination of animal foods from the diet increases the risk for deficiency. Second, it is a water-soluble vitamin that is stored in the liver. This storage is important for anyone consuming very little dietary vitamin B_{12}.

The RDA for vitamin B_{12} for adult men and women aged 19 and older is 2.4 µg/day. Vitamin B_{12} is found primarily in dairy products, eggs, meats, and poultry. **Figure 8.16** displays some foods relatively high in vitamin B_{12}. Individuals consuming a vegan diet need to eat vegetable-based foods that are fortified with vitamin B_{12} or take vitamin B_{12} supplements or injections to ensure that they maintain adequate blood levels of this nutrient.

As we age, our sources of vitamin B_{12} may need to change. Non-vegans younger than 51 years of age are generally able to meet the RDA for vitamin B_{12} by consuming it in foods. However, it is estimated that about 10% to 30% of adults older than 50 years have a condition referred to as **atrophic gastritis,** which results in low stomach-acid secretion. Because stomach acid separates foodbound vitamin B_{12} from dietary proteins, if the acid content of the stomach is inadequate, then we cannot free up enough vitamin B_{12} from food sources alone.[4] Because atrophic gastritis can affect almost one-third of the older adult population, it is recommended that people older than 50 years of age consume foods fortified with vitamin B_{12}, take a vitamin B_{12}–containing supplement, or have periodic vitamin B_{12} injections.

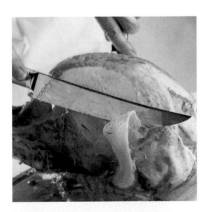

Turkey contains vitamin B_{12}.

atrophic gastritis A condition, frequently seen in people over the age of 50, in which stomach-acid secretions are low.

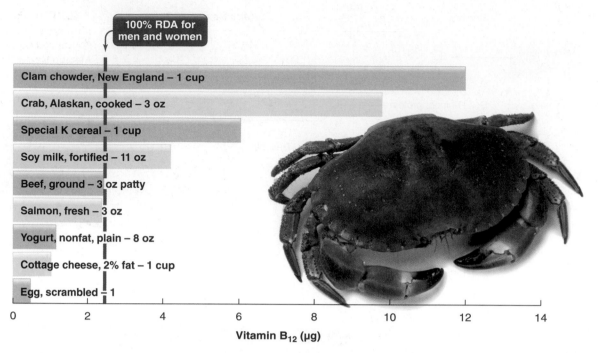

FIGURE 8.16 Common food sources of vitamin B_{12}. The RDA for vitamin B_{12} is 2.4 µg/day for men and women. (*Source:* Data from US Department of Agriculture, Agriculture Research Services. 2009. USDA Nutrient Data Base for Standard Reference, Release 22. Nutrient Data Laboratory Home Page. www.ars.usda.gov.)

There are no known adverse effects from consuming excess amounts of vitamin B_{12} from food. However, data are not available on the effects of excess amounts of vitamin B_{12} from supplements.

Vitamin B_{12} deficiency is rare but is generally associated with either dietary insufficiency or reduced absorption. Deficiency symptoms generally include those associated with anemia, as well as gastrointestinal and neurologic effects.[12, 13] The symptoms of anemia include pale skin, diminished energy and exercise tolerance, fatigue, and shortness of breath. Gastrointestinal symptoms include loss of appetite, constipation, excessive gas, and changes in the tongue.[13] Neurologic symptoms include tingling and numbness of extremities, abnormal gait, memory loss, dementia, disorientation, visual disturbances, insomnia, and impaired bladder and bowel control.[12] A deficiency of vitamin B_{12}, as with vitamin B_6 and folate, has been linked to cardiovascular disease due to high levels of homocysteine.

As noted, an important cause of vitamin B_{12} deficiency is reduced absorption. A common culprit in reduced absorption is a condition called pernicious anemia, which is caused by inadequate secretion of intrinsic factor by parietal cells of the stomach. (Pernicious anemia is discussed in more detail in Chapter 12.)

Pantothenic Acid

Pantothenic acid is an essential vitamin that is metabolized into two major coenzymes: coenzyme A (CoA) and acyl carrier protein (ACP), which are shown in **Figure 8.17**. Both are essential in the synthesis of fatty acids, while CoA is essential for fatty acid oxidation, ketone metabolism, and the metabolism of carbohydrate and protein.[14] For example, in the conversion of pyruvate to acetyl-CoA, the enzyme pyruvate dehydrogenase requires CoA. Many of the metabolic reactions that require pantothenic acid for energy production are illustrated in Figure 8.2. Besides its role in energy metabolism, pantothenic acid is required in the synthesis of cholesterol and steroids and in the detoxification of drugs.

The AI for pantothenic acid for adult men and women aged 19 years and older is 5 mg/day. Pantothenic acid is widely distributed in foods, with the average daily intake at

Shiitake mushrooms contain ten to twenty times more pantothenic acid than other types of mushrooms.

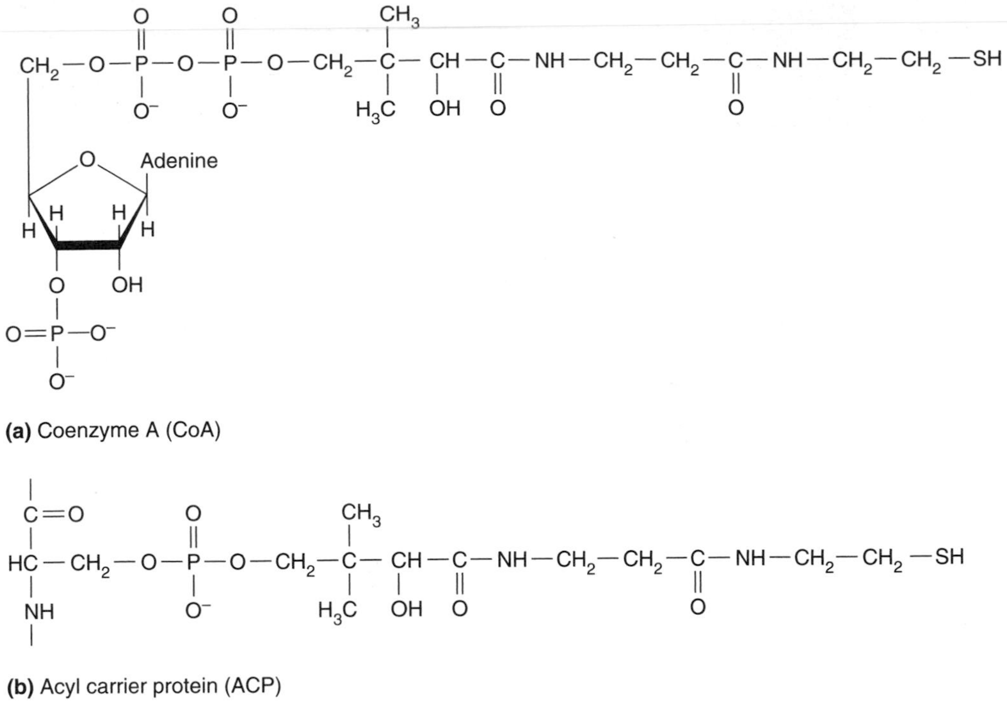

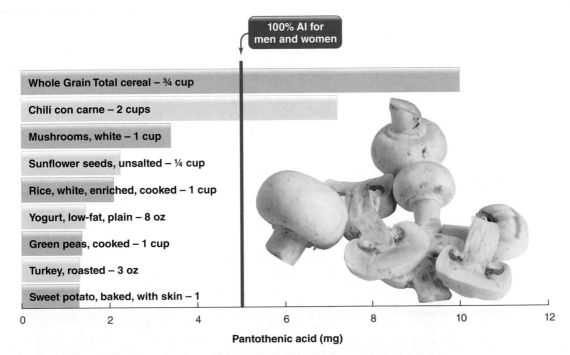

FIGURE 8.17 Structure of co-enzymes containing pantothenic acid. **(a)** Coenzyme A (CoA). **(b)** Acyl carrier protein (ACP).

(a) Coenzyme A (CoA)

(b) Acyl carrier protein (ACP)

approximately 5 mg/day and usual intakes ranging from 4 to 7 mg/day.[4, 14] Thus, the AI for pantothenic acid and the average dietary intake are similar. As mentioned, pantothenic acid is available from a variety of foods, including chicken, beef, egg yolk, potatoes, oat cereals, tomato products, whole grains, certain mushrooms, and organ meats (**Figure 8.18**). There are no known adverse effects from consuming excess amounts of pantothenic acid, and deficiencies of pantothenic acid are very rare.

100% AI for men and women

Whole Grain Total cereal – ¾ cup	
Chili con carne – 2 cups	
Mushrooms, white – 1 cup	
Sunflower seeds, unsalted – ¼ cup	
Rice, white, enriched, cooked – 1 cup	
Yogurt, low-fat, plain – 8 oz	
Green peas, cooked – 1 cup	
Turkey, roasted – 3 oz	
Sweet potato, baked, with skin – 1	

0   2   4   6   8   10   12

Pantothenic acid (mg)

FIGURE 8.18 Common food sources of pantothenic acid. The AI for pantothenic acid is 5 mg/day for men and women. (*Source:* Data from US Dept of Agriculture, Agriculture Research Services. 2009. USDA Nutrient Data Base for Standard Reference, Release 22. Nutrient Data Laboratory Home Page. www.ars.usda.gov.)

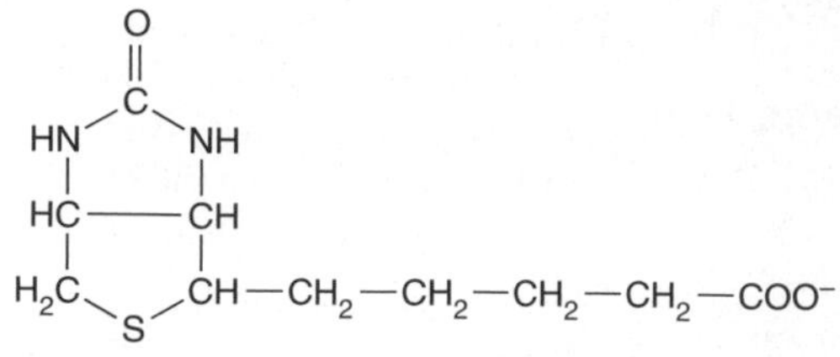

FIGURE 8.19 Structure of biotin.

Biotin

Biotin is a component of four carboxylase enzymes that are present in humans. These enzymes serve as the CO_2 (carbon dioxide) carrier and the carboxyl donor for substrates.[14] **Figure 8.19** shows the structure of biotin.

The enzymes that require biotin as a coenzyme are involved in fatty acid synthesis (for example, lipogenesis), gluconeogenesis, and carbohydrate, fat, and protein metabolism. For example, pyruvate carboxylase catalyzes the synthesis of oxaloacetate from pyruvate in the TCA cycle. Many of the enzyme reactions that require biotin for energy production are illustrated in Figure 8.2.

The AI for biotin for adult men and women aged 19 and older is 30 µg/day. The biotin content has been determined for very few foods, and these values are not reported in food composition tables or dietary analysis programs. In food, biotin exists as free biotin or bound to protein as biocytin, both of which appear to be widespread in foods. The free form of biotin is shown in Figure 8.19; the structure of biocytin is similar to that of free biotin but has an amino acid attached to the carboxyl end.

There are no known adverse effects from consuming excess amounts of biotin. Biotin deficiencies are typically seen only in people who consume a large number of raw egg whites over long periods of time. This is because raw egg whites contain a protein that binds with biotin and prevents its absorption. Biotin deficiencies are also seen in people fed total parenteral nutrition (nutrients administered by a route other than the GI tract) that is not supplemented with biotin. Symptoms include thinning of hair; loss of hair color; development of a red, scaly rash around the eyes, nose, and mouth; depression; lethargy; and hallucinations.

Choline

Choline is a vitamin-like substance that is important for metabolism, the structural integrity of cell membranes, and neurotransmission. It is typically grouped with the B-vitamins because of its role in fat digestion and transport and homocysteine metabolism.

Specifically, choline plays an important role in the metabolism and transport of fats and cholesterol. High amounts of the choline-containing compound phosphatidylcholine are found in bile, which aids fat digestion, and in the formation of lipoproteins, which transport endogenous and dietary fat and cholesterol in the blood to the cells. Choline is also necessary for the synthesis of phospholipids and other components of cell membranes; thus, choline plays a critical role in the structural integrity of cell membranes. Finally, choline accelerates the synthesis and release of **acetylcholine,** a neurotransmitter that is involved in many functions, including muscle movement and memory storage.

Nutri-Case

Judy

"Ever since my doctor put me on this crazy diet, I've been feeling hungry and exhausted. This morning I'm sitting in the lunch room on my break, and I actually doze off and start dreaming about food! Maureen, one of the girls I work with, comes in and has to wake me up! I told her what's been going on with me, and she thinks I should start taking some B-vitamins so I stay healthy while I'm on the diet. She says B-vitamins are the most important because they give you energy. Maybe after work I'll stop off at the mall and buy some. If they give you energy, maybe they'll make it easier to stick to my diet too."

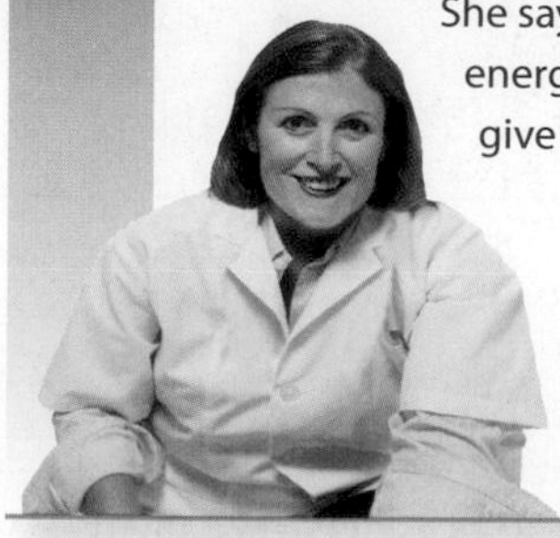

Is Judy's co-worker correct when she asserts that B-vitamins "give you energy"? Either way, do you think it's likely that Judy needs to take B-vitamin supplements to ensure that she "stays healthy" while she is on her prescribed diet? Why or why not? Finally, could taking B-vitamins help Judy stick to her diet?

acetylcholine A neurotransmitter that is involved in many functions, including muscle movement and memory storage.

Although small amounts of choline can be synthesized within the body, the amount made is insufficient for our needs; thus, choline is considered an essential dietary nutrient. Choline has an AI of 550 mg/day for men aged 19 and older and an AI of 425 mg/day for women aged 19 and older. There are limited data on the choline intake of North Americans, because choline intake is not reported in the NHANES or other large surveys. In addition, it is not reported in major nutrient databases. However, it is estimated that choline intakes in the United States and Canada range from 730 to 1,040 mg/day[4] based on the typical choline content of foods.

Choline is widespread in foods, typically in the form of phosphatidylcholine (see Figure 5.6 on page 182) in the cell membranes of the food. Foods that are high in choline include milk, liver, eggs, soybeans, cauliflower, and peanuts.[4, 12] Lecithin (a more common term for phosphatidylcholine) is added to foods during processing as an emulsifying agent, which also increases choline intakes in the diet. Inadequate intakes of choline can lead to increased fat accumulation in the liver, which eventually leads to liver damage. Excessive intake of supplemental choline results in various toxicity symptoms, including a fishy body odor, vomiting, excess salivation, sweating, diarrhea, and low blood pressure. The UL for choline for adults 19 years of age and older is 3.5 g/day.

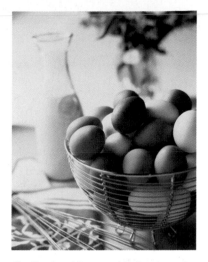

Choline is widespread in foods and can be found in eggs and milk.

RECAP

The B-vitamins include thiamin, riboflavin, niacin, vitamin B_6 (pyridoxine), folate, vitamin B_{12} (cobalamin), pantothenic acid, and biotin. The B-vitamins assist in the metabolism of carbohydrates, fats, protein, and alcohol. They are commonly found in whole grains, enriched breads, ready-to-eat cereals, meats, dairy products, and some fruits and vegetables. B-vitamin toxicity is rare unless a person consumes large doses as supplements. Choline is a vitamin-like substance that is required for the production of phosphatidylcholine. ■

A Profile of Minerals Involved in Energy Metabolism

In addition to the B-vitamins and choline, several minerals facilitate energy metabolism. These include iodine, chromium, manganese, and sulfur.

Iodine

Iodine is the heaviest trace element required for human health and a necessary component of the thyroid hormones, which help regulate human metabolism. In nature, this element is found primarily as inorganic salts in rocks, soil, plants, animals, and water as either iodine or iodide, but once it enters the GI tract, it is broken down to iodide, which is the negative ion of iodine, designated I^-. Upon absorption, the majority of this iodide is taken up by the thyroid gland.[15]

Functions of Iodine

As just noted, iodine is responsible for a single function within the body: the synthesis of thyroid hormones.[16] Although iodine's function is singular, the multiple actions of thyroid hormones mean that it affects the whole body. Thyroid hormones regulate key metabolic reactions associated with body temperature, resting metabolic rate, macronutrient metabolism, and reproduction and growth.[16]

The structure of the thyroid hormones, thyroxine (T_4) and 3, 5, 3′-triiodothyronine (T_3), illustrates the placement of iodine (I) in these two hormones (**Figure 8.20**). Both are derived from the iodination of the amino acid tyrosine, shown in Figure 8.20c. Notice that thyroxine has four iodine

(a) Thyroxine (T_4)

(b) 3, 5, 3′–Triiodothyronine (T_3)

(c) Tyrosine

FIGURE 8.20 Thyroid hormones contain iodine (I). **(a)** Structure of the thyroid hormone T_4. **(b)** Structure of the thyroid hormone T_3. Both are derived from the iodination of **(c)** tyrosine, an amino acid.

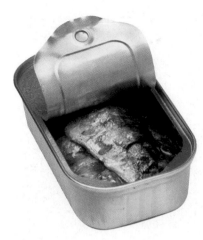

Saltwater fish, fresh or canned, contain iodine.

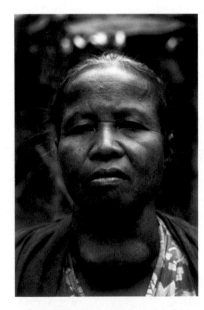

FIGURE 8.21 Goiter, or enlargement of the thyroid gland, occurs with both iodine toxicity and deficiency.

goiter Enlargement of the thyroid gland; can be caused by iodine toxicity or deficiency.

cretinism A unique form of mental retardation that occurs in infants when the mother experiences iodine deficiency during pregnancy.

hypothyroidism A condition characterized by low blood levels of thyroid hormone.

molecules as part of its structure, whereas triiodothyronine has three—thus, the abbreviated designations T_4 and T_3. Thyroxine (T_4) is the primary circulating thyroid hormone. The removal of one iodine group is required to generate the active form of T_3.[16]

How Much Iodine Should We Consume?

The body needs relatively little iodine to maintain health. The RDA for adults 19 years of age and older is 150 µg/day. It is estimated that the iodine intake from food in the United States is approximately 200 to 300 µg/day for men and 190 to 210 µg/day for women.[4]

Very few foods are reliable sources of iodine, because the amount of iodine in foods varies according to the soil, irrigation, and fertilizers used. Saltwater foods, both fish and plants, tend to have higher amounts, because marine species concentrate iodine from seawater. Good food sources include saltwater fish, shrimp, seaweed, iodized salt, and white and whole-wheat breads made with iodized salt and bread conditioners. In addition, iodine is added to dairy cattle feed and used in sanitizing solutions in the dairy industry, making dairy foods an important source of iodine.

Iodine has been voluntarily added to salt in the United States since 1924 to combat iodine deficiency resulting from the poor iodine content of soils in this country. For many people, iodized salt is their primary source of iodine, and approximately ½ teaspoon of iodized salt meets the entire adult RDA for iodine. When you buy salt, look carefully at the package label, because stores carry both iodized and non-iodized salt. Most specialty salts, such as kosher salt or sea salt, do not have iodine added. If iodine has been added to the salt, it will be clearly marked on the label.

Excess iodine intakes can cause a number of health-related problems, especially related to thyroid gland function. Too much iodine blocks the synthesis of thyroid hormones. As the thyroid gland attempts to produce more hormones, it may enlarge, a condition known as **goiter** (**Figure 8.21**). (Goiter refers to the enlargement of the thyroid gland, regardless of its cause.) Iodine toxicity generally occurs as a result of excessive supplementation. Thus, the UL for iodine is 1,100 µg/day.

Paradoxically, goiter is also the most classic disorder of iodine deficiency. An insufficient supply of iodine means there is less iodine for the production of thyroid hormones. The body responds by stimulating the thyroid gland, including increasing the size of the gland, in an attempt to capture more iodine from the blood.

The development of a goiter is only one of many problems that result when iodine is insufficient in the diet. A broader term applied to the disorders associated with poor iodine intakes is *iodine deficiency disorders,* or *IDDs,* which include cretinism, growth and developmental disorders, mental deficiencies, neurologic disorders, decreased fertility, congenital abnormalities, and prenatal and infant death.[16, 17, 18] The World Health Organization (WHO) considers iodine deficiency to be the "greatest single cause of preventable brain damage and mental retardation" in the world.[18] If a woman experiences iodine deficiency during pregnancy, her infant has a high risk of being born with a unique form of mental impairment referred to as **cretinism.** In addition to mental impairment, the infant may suffer from stunted growth, deafness, and muteness. Among pregnant women, iodine deficiency may also increase the occurrence of spontaneous abortion, stillbirths and congenital abnormalities, and infant mortality.[16] The impact of mild iodine deficiency on the development of the brain and neurologic system of a child is more difficult to determine. Iodine deficiency can also cause **hypothyroidism** (low blood levels of thyroid hormone), which is characterized by decreased body temperature, an inability to tolerate cold environmental temperatures, weight gain, fatigue, and sluggishness.

According to the International Council for the Control of IDDs,[19] 2.2 billion people live in areas subject to iodine deficiency and are at increased risk for its health complications and consequences.[19] A recent global assessment of iodine status showed that 30% of the world's 241 million school-age children remain iodine deficient.[20] In the United States, large areas of crop-producing lands are low in iodine, and thus foods grown on these lands are low in iodine. As recently as the beginning of the 20th century, IDDs and goiter were considered endemic in the United States. However, the problem was not fully addressed until World War I, when many conscripted men were barred from military service because they had goiters. At that time, the treatment of goiters with sodium iodine was shown to be effective, and the search was on for a method of increasing iodine in the food supply by fortifying processed foods, increasing the level of iodine in the soil through fertilizers, or adding iodine to the feed of animals. After much debate, it was determined that the fortification of salt with iodine was the best solution. This action reduced the incidence of goiter to <2.8% of individuals in developed countries.[16, 18]

Hyperthyroidism (high blood levels of thyroid hormone) is most commonly caused by Graves' disease, which is an autoimmune disease that causes an overproduction of thyroid hormones. The symptoms include weight loss, increased heat production, muscular tremors, nervousness, a racing heartbeat, and protrusion of the eyes.

Chromium

Chromium is a trace mineral that plays an important role in carbohydrate metabolism. You may be surprised to learn that the chromium in your body is the same metal used in the chrome plating for cars. Chromium enhances the ability of insulin to transport glucose from the bloodstream into cells.[17] Chromium also plays important roles in the metabolism of RNA and DNA, in immune function, and in growth.

Chromium supplements are marketed to reduce body fat and enhance muscle mass and have become popular with bodybuilders and other athletes interested in improving their body composition. The **Nutrition: Myth or Fact?** box (page 334) investigates whether taking supplemental chromium is effective in improving body composition.

The body needs only small amounts of chromium. The AI for adults aged 19 to 50 years is 35 μg/day for men and 25 μg/day for women. For adults 51 years of age and older, the AI decreases to 30 μg/day and 20 μg/day for men and women, respectively.[17] The AI for individuals over 50 years was based on the energy intake of older adults, which is typically lower than that of younger individuals.

The question of whether the average diet provides adequate chromium is controversial. Chromium is widely distributed in foods, but concentrations in any particular food are not typically high. In addition, determining the chromium content of food is difficult because contamination can easily occur during laboratory analysis. Thus, we cannot determine average chromium intake from any currently existing nutrient database.

Foods identified as good sources of chromium include mushrooms, prunes, dark chocolate, nuts, whole grains, cereals, asparagus, brewer's yeast, some beers, red wine, and meats, especially processed meats. Dairy products are typically poor sources of chromium. Food-processing methods can also add chromium to foods, especially if the food is processed in stainless steel containers. For example, it is assumed that wine and beer derive some of their chromium content from processing.[17]

There appears to be no toxicity related to consuming chromium in the diet, but there are insufficient data to establish a UL for chromium. Because chromium supplements are widely used in the United States, the Institute of Medicine (IOM) has recommended more research to determine the safety of high-dose chromium supplements. Until this research is available, supplementation with high amounts of chromium is discouraged. Chromium deficiency appears to be uncommon in the United States. When chromium deficiency is induced in a research setting, glucose uptake into the cells is inhibited, causing a rise in blood glucose and insulin levels. Chromium deficiency can also result in elevated blood lipid levels and in damage to the brain and nervous system.[17]

Manganese

A trace mineral, manganese is a cofactor involved in protein, fat, and carbohydrate metabolism, gluconeogenesis, cholesterol synthesis, and the formation of urea, the primary component of urine.[21] It also assists in the synthesis of the protein matrix found in bone tissue and in building cartilage, a tissue supporting joints. Manganese is also an integral component of superoxide dismutase, an antioxidant enzyme. Thus, it assists in the conversion of

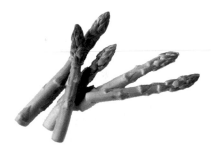

Our body contains very little chromium. Asparagus is a good dietary source of this trace mineral.

hyperthyroidism A condition characterized by high blood levels of thyroid hormone.

Can Chromium Supplements Enhance Body Composition?

Chromium supplements, predominantly in the form of chromium picolinate, are popular with bodybuilders, weight lifters, and overweight individuals who want to lose body fat. This popularity stems from claims that chromium increases muscle mass and muscle strength and decreases body fat. But are these claims myth or fact?

An early study of chromium supplementation was promising, in that chromium use in both untrained men and football players was found to decrease body fat and increase muscle mass.[1] These findings caused a surge in the popularity of chromium supplements and motivated many scientists across the United States to test the reproducibility of these early findings. The next study of chromium supplementation found no effects of chromium on muscle mass, body fat, or muscle strength.[2]

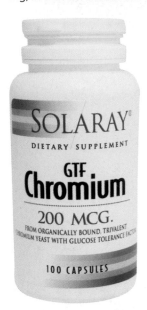

These contradictory reports led experts to closely examine the two studies. When they did so, they found a number of flaws in the methodology of both. One major concern with the first study was that the chromium status of the research participants prior to the study was not measured or controlled.[1] It was possible that the participants had started the study deficient in chromium; this deficiency could have caused a more positive reaction to chromium than would be expected in people with normal chromium status. Thus, subsequent studies were designed to control for participants' pre-study chromium status.

A second major concern was that body composition was measured in these studies using the skinfold technique, in which calipers are used to measure the thickness of the skin and fat at various sites on the body. Although this method gives a good general estimate of body fat in young, lean, healthy people, it is not sensitive to small changes in muscle mass. Thus, subsequent studies of chromium used more sophisticated methods of measuring body composition.

The results of research studies conducted over the past 10 years consistently show that chromium supplementation has no effect on muscle mass, body fat, or muscle strength in a variety of groups, including untrained college males and females, overweight and obese females, collegiate wrestlers, and older men and women.[3, 4, 5, 6, 7, 8, 9] Neither have scientists found an effect of chromium on body composition when different types of experimental designs have been used, with varying energy intakes and exercise expenditure.[10, 11] Despite this overwhelming evidence to the contrary,[12, 13] many supplement companies still claim that chromium supplements enhance strength and muscle mass and reduce body fat. These claims result in millions of dollars of sales of supplements to consumers each year. Before you decide to purchase chromium supplements, read some of the studies cited here. The information they provide may help you avoid being one of the many consumers fooled by this costly nutrition myth.

References

1. Evans, G. W. 1989. The effect of chromium picolinate on insulin controlled parameters in humans. *Int. J. Biosoc. Med. Res.* 11:163–180.
2. Hasten, D. L., E. P. Rome, D. B. Franks, and M. Hegsted. 1992. Effects of chromium picolinate on beginning weight training students. *Int. J. Sports Nutr.* 2:343–350.
3. Lukaski, H. C., W. W. Bolonchuk, W. A. Siders, and D. B. Milne. 1996. Chromium supplementation and resistance training: effects on body composition, strength, and trace element status of men. *Am. J. Clin. Nutr.* 63:954–965.
4. Hallmark, M. A., T. H. Reynolds, C. A. DeSouza, C. O. Dotson, R. A. Anderson, and M. A. Rogers. 1996. Effects of chromium and resistive training on muscle strength and body composition. *Med. Sci. Sports. Exerc.* 28:139–144.
5. Pasman, W. J., M. S. Westerterp-Plantenga, and W. H. Saris. 1997. The effectiveness of long-term supplementation of carbohydrate, chromium, fiber and caffeine on weight maintenance. *Int. J. Obes. Relat. Metab. Disord.* 21:1143–1151.
6. Walker, L. S., M. G. Bemben, D. A. Bemben, and A. W. Knehans. 1998. Chromium picolinate effects on body composition and muscular performance in wrestlers. *Med. Sci. Sports Exerc.* 30:1730–1737.
7. Campbell, W. W., L. J. Joseph, S. L. Davey, D. Cyr-Campbell, R. A. Anderson, and W. J. Evans. 1999. Effects of resistance training and chromium picolinate on body composition and skeletal muscle in older men. *J. Appl. Physiol.* 86:29–39.
8. Volpe, S. L., H. W. Huang, K. Larpadisorn, and I. I. Lesser. 2001. Effect of chromium supplementation and exercise on body composition, resting metabolic rate and selected biochemical parameters in moderately obese women following an exercise program. *J. Am. Coll. Nutr.* 20:293–306.
9. Campbell, W. W., L. J. O. Joseph, R. A. Anderson, S. L. Davey, J. Hinton, and W. J. Evans. 2002. Effects of resistive training and chromium picolinate on body composition and skeletal muscle size in older women. *Int. J. Sports Nutr. Exerc. Metab.* 12:125–135.
10. Diaz, L. D., B. A. Watkin, Y. Li, R. A. Anderson, and W. W. Campbell. 2008. Chromium picolinate and conjugated linoleic acid do not synergistically influence diet- and exercise-induced changes in body composition and health indexes in overweight women. *J. Nutr. Biochem.* 19:61–68.
11. Lukaski, H. C., W. A. Siders, and J. G. Penland. 2007. Chromium picolinate supplementation in women: effects on body weight, composition and iron status. *Nutr.* 23:187–195.
12. Arbor Nutrition Clinical Nutrition Updates. 2007, October. Chromium, body building and weight loss. 284:1–3.
13. Manore, M. M. 2012. Dietary supplements for improving body composition and reducing body weight. Where is the evidence? *International Journal of Sport Nutrition and Exercise Metabolism* (prepublication, 2012).

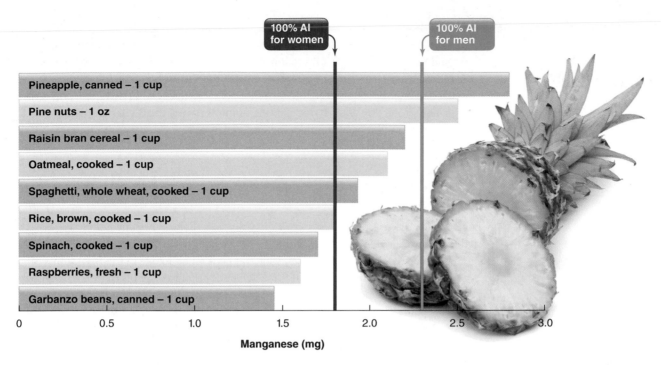

100% AI for women

100% AI for men

Pineapple, canned – 1 cup

Pine nuts – 1 oz

Raisin bran cereal – 1 cup

Oatmeal, cooked – 1 cup

Spaghetti, whole wheat, cooked – 1 cup

Rice, brown, cooked – 1 cup

Spinach, cooked – 1 cup

Raspberries, fresh – 1 cup

Garbanzo beans, canned – 1 cup

0   0.5   1.0   1.5   2.0   2.5   3.0

Manganese (mg)

FIGURE 8.22 Common food sources of manganese. The AI for manganese is 2.3 mg/day for men and 1.8 mg/day for women. (*Source:* Data from US Department of Agriculture, Agriculture Research Service. 2009. USDA Nutrient Data Base for Standard Reference, Release 22. Nutrient Data Laboratory Home Page. www.ars.usda.gov.)

free radicals to less damaging substances, protecting the body from oxidative damage (see Chapter 10).

The AI for manganese for adults 19 years of age and older is 2.3 mg/day for men and 1.8 mg/day for women. Manganese requirements are easily met, as this mineral is widespread in foods and is readily available in a varied diet. Whole-grain foods, such as oat bran, wheat flour, whole-wheat spaghetti, and brown rice, are good sources of manganese (**Figure 8.22**). Other sources include pineapple, pine nuts, okra, spinach, and raspberries. Overall, grain products contribute approximately 37% of dietary manganese, and vegetables and beverages, primarily tea, contribute another 18% to 20%.[17]

Manganese toxicity can occur in occupational environments, such as mines, in which workers inhale manganese dust. It can also result from drinking water high in manganese. Toxicity results in impairment of the neuromuscular system, causing symptoms similar to those seen in Parkinson's disease, such as muscle spasms and tremors. Elevated blood manganese concentrations and neurotoxicity were the criteria used to determine the UL for manganese, which is 11 mg/day for adults 19 years of age and older.[17]

Manganese deficiency is rare in humans. Symptoms include impaired growth and reproductive function, reduced bone density and impaired skeletal growth, impaired glucose and lipid metabolism, and skin rash.

Sulfur

Sulfur is a major mineral and a component of the B-vitamins thiamin and biotin. As such, it is essential for macronutrient metabolism. In addition, as part of the amino acids methionine and cysteine, sulfur helps stabilize the three-dimensional shapes of proteins in the body. The liver requires sulfur to assist in the detoxification of alcohol and various drugs, and sulfur helps to maintain acid–base balance.

The body is able to obtain ample amounts of sulfur from our consumption of protein-containing foods; as a result, there is no DRI specifically for sulfur. There are no known toxicity or deficiency symptoms associated with sulfur.

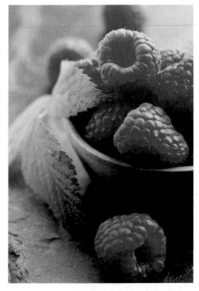

Raspberries are one of the many foods that contain manganese.

RECAP

Iodine is necessary for the synthesis of thyroid hormones, which regulate metabolic rate and body temperature. Chromium assists the transport of glucose into the cell, the metabolism of RNA and DNA, and immune function and growth. Manganese is involved in energy metabolism, the formation of urea, the synthesis of bone and cartilage, and protection against free radicals. Sulfur is part of the B-vitamins thiamin and biotin and the amino acids methionine and cysteine. ■

What Disorders Can Result from Inadequate B-Vitamin Intake?

We have already discussed the classic deficiency diseases that can result when intake of selected B-vitamins is significantly inadequate, such as beriberi with thiamin deficiency and pellagra with niacin deficiency. However, what happens when intake of the B-vitamins is low, but not low enough to cause one of these deficiency diseases? In other words, what happens when the diet provides a minimum level of B-vitamins, but not enough to fully supply the metabolic pathways of the body with the coenzymes they need? Now we'll discuss how a low intake of the B-vitamins can affect an individual's ability to perform physical activity.

How Do Researchers Compare Vitamin Status in Active and Sedentary Populations?

As you have learned in this chapter, the B-vitamins are coenzymes for many metabolic reactions that produce energy. Thus, it is not surprising that researchers would ask the question, Do individuals who engage in regular physical activity have higher needs for B-vitamins than sedentary adults? Researchers have attempted to answer this question in a number of ways.

First, researchers have designed studies in which they identify individuals with poor B-vitamin status and then determine the impact of the low status on the individuals' ability to perform exercise. They can then compare the average performance of low-status individuals to the average performance of those with good B-vitamin status.

Second, they have performed controlled metabolic diet studies to determine if athletes need higher levels of B-vitamins than sedentary adults to maintain their vitamin status. For more information on this type of study, see the box: **Highlight: How Do Scientists Determine Vitamin Requirements?** (page 337).

Third, researchers have conducted cross-sectional studies that compare the nutritional status of trained athletes to sedentary individuals to determine the frequency of poor B-vitamin status in each group. A drawback of cross-sectional studies is that the two groups of people they compare may have other differences besides their fitness level that contribute to their differences in nutritional status. Cross-sectional studies help determine whether differences exist between two groups, but more detailed studies are needed to determine if those differences are due to level of physical activity alone.

Perhaps the ideal study of the effect of physical activity on B-vitamin status would be longitudinal, controlling B-vitamin intake over several months in a study group of athletes, while varying their activity level from low to high. Researchers would then be able to monitor any changes in nutritional status and determine whether these changes affect an individual's ability to perform physical activity. Unfortunately, such studies are difficult and expensive to conduct.

What Evidence Links Exercise Performance and B-Vitamin Status?

Because of the role B-vitamins play in energy production during exercise, researchers generally assume that individuals with poor B-vitamin status will have a reduced ability to perform physical activity. This hypothesis has been supported in classic studies examining the effect of thiamin, riboflavin, and vitamin B_6 deficiency on work performance.[22, 23]

How Do Scientists Determine Vitamin Requirements?

HIGHLIGHT

Throughout this book, we identify the precise amounts of the different vitamins you need to consume each day to maintain good health. But have you ever wondered how researchers determine these recommendations? Of the several methods used, one of the most rigorous is the metabolic diet study.

The goal of a metabolic diet study is to determine how vitamin assessment parameters in the blood, urine, and feces change as the dietary intake of a nutrient, such as vitamin B_6, is closely controlled. In a metabolic diet study, which may last for weeks or months, all foods eaten by study participants are carefully prepared, weighed to within 0.1 g, and recorded. Subjects are usually required to either live at the research facility (where all physical activity is monitored) or go to the research facility for all their meals. Depending on the nutrient being studied, all fluids, even water, may also be provided to the participant. Throughout the study, each participant's body weight is measured daily to prevent any increase or decrease in weight. If weight does change, energy intake is altered so that the subject returns to the baseline weight. This must be done without altering the intake of the vitamin being studied. Because many of the vitamins we talked about in this chapter help metabolize protein, fat, and/or carbohydrate, it is important that the body stores of these macronutrients do not change during the metabolic study. This is why monitoring weight and physical activity is so important. At different times during the study, vitamin assessment parameters are measured in the blood, urine, and feces. This may require that the subject collect all urine and feces throughout the study.

For example, let's say you want to determine whether active and sedentary men have different requirements for vitamin B_6. You know that, during physical activity, carbohydrate is burned for fuel and that protein is necessary for the building and repair of muscle tissue. You also know that vitamin B_6 is very important for glucose and protein metabolism; thus, physical activity might increase the body's need for this B-vitamin.

To compare vitamin B_6 requirements, you might design a study as follows. First, you would recruit active young men between the ages of 20 and 35 years (all of equal fitness

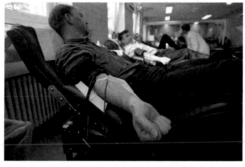

levels and exercising the same number of hours/week), as well as sedentary males of the same age. You would then feed the participants a succession of three different diets, each lasting 3 weeks, and each providing a different level of vitamin B_6. The diets would consist of the following:

1. Vitamin B_6 below the RDA (1.0 mg/day)
2. Vitamin B_6 at the level of the RDA (1.3 mg/day)
3. Vitamin B_6 above the RDA (1.6 mg/day)

Ideally, you would randomly assign these diets, so that one individual might be fed diet number 1 while another individual is on diet number 2 and another is on diet number 3. By randomly assigning the diets, you ensure that you do not dictate the order in which they are fed. Because you don't want the effect of one diet to carry over to the next diet you are feeding, you would need to include a "washout" period between diets. How long this washout period lasted would depend on the vitamin you were researching, but for our example, 6 weeks should be long enough, because vitamin B_6 is a water-soluble vitamin. During the washout period, all participants would be fed a diet providing the RDA for vitamin B_6 for normal, healthy men.

During the study period, you would need to ensure that the subjects did not eat any foods except what you fed them. In addition, study participants must be monitored to *make sure they eat all the food*. Throughout the study, the amount of vitamin B_6 in the foods would need to be determined via chemical analysis in a lab, as would the amount of vitamin B_6 in the participants' blood, urine, and fecal samples. You would also need to make sure all subjects maintained baseline body weights.

You would then determine the nutritional status of the men when they were on each of the three test diets to determine which diet was able to keep assessment parameters within normal range. You would also compare vitamin status between groups for each of the diets. If the active men had poor status on 1.3 mg/day of vitamin B_6, while the sedentary subjects had adequate status on this level, you would conclude that the RDA was not adequate for the active individuals and they would need more vitamin B_6 to maintain good status.

For example, a team of Dutch researchers depleted 24 healthy, active men of thiamin, riboflavin, and vitamin B_6 over an 11-week period by feeding them a diet high in unenriched processed foods, such as white bread, white rice, margarine, and soft drinks.[22] Specifically, the diet contained only 50% of the RDA for thiamin, riboflavin, and vitamin B_6. Researchers then examined the effect of this B-vitamin deficiency on the men's ability to perform physical activity. They found that B-vitamin depletion significantly decreased the ability to perform maximal work by 7% to 12%, depending on the testing method used. Thus, it took only 11 weeks of eating a low-B-vitamin diet before these men were unable to exercise at the same intensity and duration as they had when they were consuming adequate amounts of these vitamins.

Notice that, in the Dutch study, the diet the participants ate was high in unenriched processed foods. In the United States, the Food and Drug Administration mandated the enrichment of foods made with refined grains, such as wheat, corn, and rice, in the 1940s. The micronutrients added back include thiamin, riboflavin, niacin, and iron. Thus, some of the nutrients lost in the milling process are replaced by the enrichment process. Moreover, as mentioned earlier, the enrichment of breads and cereals with folic acid began in 1996.

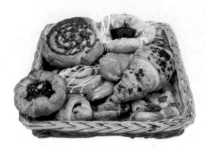

Diets high in processed foods and simple carbohydrates are low in B-vitamins.

RECAP

The hypothesis that individuals with poor B-vitamin status will have a reduced ability to perform physical activity has been supported in studies examining the effect of thiamin, riboflavin, and vitamin B_6 deficiency on work performance. Consuming a diet high in whole grains, fruits, vegetables, and lean meats and dairy will ensure that your body has adequate B-vitamins to fuel physical activity. In the United States, some of the nutrients lost in the milling of grains are replaced by the enrichment process. ■

Chapter Review

TEST YOURSELF | ANSWERS

1 **F** B-vitamins do not directly provide energy. However, they play critical roles in ensuring that the body is able to generate energy from carbohydrates, fats, and proteins.

2 **T** A severe niacin deficiency can cause pellagra, which once killed thousands of people in the United States alone each year; and thiamin deficiency causes beriberi, which can result in heart failure.

3 **F** The IOM has set ULs for both niacin and vitamin B_6. High intakes of these nutrients can cause adverse effects.

4 **F** Research studies have failed to show any consistent effects of chromium supplements on reducing body fat or enhancing muscle mass.

5 **F** Not necessarily! Although much of the salt sold in the United States is iodized, you need to read the label carefully. Some brands of table salt, kosher salt, sea salt, and other specialty salts do not provide iodine.

Summary

- The B-vitamins include thiamin, riboflavin, vitamin B_6, niacin, folate, vitamin B_{12}, pantothenic acid, and biotin.

- The B-vitamins act as coenzymes. In this role, they activate enzymes and assist them in the metabolism of carbohydrates, fats, amino acids, and alcohol for energy; the synthesis of fatty acids and cholesterol; and gluconeogenesis.

- Food sources of the B-vitamins include whole grains, enriched breads, ready-to-eat cereals, meats, dairy products, and some fruits and vegetables.

- A deficiency of thiamin can cause beriberi, and a deficiency of niacin can cause pellagra.

- Vitamin B_6 plays a critical role in transamination; without adequate B_6, all amino acids become essential.

- Folate deficiency in the early weeks of pregnancy significantly increases the risk of having a baby with a neural tube defect.

- Vitamin B_{12} is found exclusively in animal-based foods and fortified foods.

- Inadequate intakes of vitamin B_6, folate, and vitamin B_{12} are associated with elevated blood levels of the amino acid homocysteine. This, in turn, is associated with an increased risk for cardiovascular disease.

- Toxicity is possible with megadoses of some B-vitamins from supplements.

- Choline is a vitamin-like substance that assists with homocysteine metabolism. Choline also accelerates the synthesis and release of acetylcholine, a neurotransmitter.

- Iodine is a trace mineral needed for the synthesis of thyroid hormones. Thyroid hormones are integral to the regulation of body temperature, the maintenance of resting metabolic rate, and healthy reproduction and growth.

- Chromium is a trace mineral that enhances the ability of insulin to transport glucose from the bloodstream into the cell. Chromium is also necessary for the metabolism of RNA and DNA, and it supports normal growth and immune function.

- Manganese is a trace mineral that acts as a cofactor in energy metabolism and the formation of urea.

- Sulfur is a major mineral that is a component of thiamin and biotin and the amino acids methionine and cysteine.

- Inadequate levels of the B-vitamins can reduce an individual's ability to perform physical activity. A diet high in unenriched processed foods typically provides inadequate levels of the B-vitamins.

MasteringNutrition™

To further your understanding, go online and apply what you've learned to real-life case studies that will help you master the content!

Review Questions

1. The B-vitamins include
   a. niacin, folate, and iodine.
   b. cobalamin, iodine, and chromium.
   c. manganese, riboflavin, and pyridoxine.
   d. thiamin, pantothenic acid, and biotin.

2. Which of the following statements about choline is true?
   a. Choline is found exclusively in foods of animal origin.
   b. Choline is a B-vitamin that assists in carbohydrate metabolism.
   c. Choline is a neurotransmitter that is involved in muscle movement and memory storage.
   d. Choline is necessary for the synthesis of phospholipids and other components of cell membranes.

3. According to the World Health Organization (WHO), the greatest single cause of preventable brain damage and mental retardation in the world is
   a. iodine deficiency.
   b. chromium deficiency.
   c. manganese deficiency.
   d. sulfur deficiency.

4. Which of the following lunches provides the highest levels of thiamin, riboflavin, niacin, and vitamin B_6?
   a. cheeseburger on a white bun, french fries, applesauce, diet soda
   b. tuna sandwich on whole-wheat bread, green peas, banana, 1 cup of low-fat milk
   c. yogurt parfait (made with plain low-fat yogurt, canned peaches, and raw, unprocessed oats), fresh-squeezed orange juice
   d. green salad with olive oil and vinegar dressing, low-fat cottage cheese, slice of sourdough bread with butter, water

5. Which of the following statements is true of vitamin B_{12}?
   a. It is critical to transamination.
   b. It is found naturally only in animal-based foods.
   c. Its primary function in the body is to act as a coenzyme in protein metabolism.
   d. Deficiency during the early weeks of pregnancy can result in a newborn with a neural tube defect.

6. **True or false?** There is no DRI for sulfur.

7. **True or false?** Biotin is a B-vitamin.

8. **True or false?** Iodine is necessary for the synthesis of thyroid hormones.

9. **True or false?** Wernicke–Korsakoff syndrome is a thiamin deficiency related to chronic alcohol abuse.

10. **True or false?** In the United States, milk is fortified with riboflavin to prevent pellagra.

11. Would you expect goiter to be more common in coastal regions or inland? Explain your answer.

12. Explain the statement that, without vitamin B_6, all amino acids become essential.

13. Aaron eats only whole, unprocessed foods and beverages. He asserts that "we would all be better off if we ate foods fresh off the farm" instead of allowing our food industry to "spray" foods with factory-produced vitamins and minerals. Do you agree with Aaron's position? Why or why not?

14. Your great-aunt is on renal dialysis. Explain the implications, if any, for her B-vitamin status.

15. In the chapter-opening story, Mr. Katz was given an injection of vitamin B_{12}. Why didn't his physician simply give him the vitamin in pill form?

Math Review

16. Calculate the DFE in the diet of an individual who consumes the following:

   ■ Food folate = 70 µg/day; synthetic folic acid from fortified foods = 224 µg/day

   How many DFE is this person getting per day? What percentage of this person's total DFE is coming from synthetic vs. food folate?

Answers to Review Questions and Math Review can be found online in the MasteringNutrition Study Area.

Web Links

www.ars.usda.gov/ba/bhnrc/ndl
Nutrient Data Laboratory Home Page
Click on "Reports for Single Nutrients" to find reports listing food sources for selected nutrients.

www.unicef.org/nutrition/
UNICEF: Nutrition
This site provides information about micronutrient deficiencies in developing countries and UNICEF's efforts and programs to combat them.

www.euro.who.int/en/home
World Health Organization (WHO)
This site provides information on nutrient deficiencies throughout the world, including iodine-deficiency disorders (IDDs).

www.ods.od.nih.gov
National Institutes of Health (NIH) Office of Dietary Supplements
This site provides information on vitamins and minerals, the safe use of supplements, and the research available on the treatment of health problems and disease with various supplements.

www.lpi.oregonstate.edu
Linus Pauling Institute at Oregon State University
This site provides accurate and current information on vitamins, minerals, and phytochemicals that promote health and prevent disease. Search for information on a micronutrient using the micronutrient information center.

References

1. Bernstein, L. 2000, February. Dementia without a cause: lack of vitamin B_{12} can cause dementia. *Discover.* www.discover.com/issues/feb–00/departments/featdementia. (Accessed March 2004.)

2. Butterworth R. F. 2006. Thiamin. In: M. E. Shils, M. Shike, A. C. Ross, B. Caballero, and R. J. Cousins, eds. *Modern Nutrition in Health and Disease,* 10th edn. Philadelphia: Lippincott Williams & Wilkins, pp. 426–433.

3. Manore, M. N., N. A. Meyer, and J. T. Thompson. 2009. *Sport Nutrition for Health and Performance,* 2nd edn. Champaign, IL: Human Kinetics, pp. 109–131.

4. Institute of Medicine, Food and Nutrition Board. 1998. *Dietary Reference Intakes for Thiamin, Riboflavin, Niacin, Vitamin B_6, Folate, Vitamin B_{12}, Pantothenic Acid, Biotin, and Choline.* Washington, DC: National Academy Press.

5. Woolf, K., D. L. LoBuono, and M. M. Manore. 2012. B-vitamins and physical activity: is need increased? In: Beals, K. A., ed. *Nutrition and the Female Athlete: From Research to Practice.* Baton Rouge, FL: CRC Press.

6. McCormick, D. B. 2006. Niacin, riboflavin, and thiamin. In: M. H. Stipanuk, ed. *Biochemical and Physiological Aspects of Human Nutrition,* 2nd edn. Philadelphia: W. B. Saunders, pp. 665–691.

7. Bates, C. J. 2006. Thiamin. In: Bowman, B. A. and R. M. Russel, eds., *Present Knowledge in Nutrition,* 9th edn. Washington, DC: ILSI Press, pp. 242–249.

8. Wilken, K. G., and V. Juneja. 2008. Medical nutrition therapy for renal disorders. In: Mahan, K. L., and S. Escott-Stump, eds. *Krause's Food and Nutrition Therapy.* Philadelphia: W. B. Saunders, pp. 921–958.

9. Hochholzer, W., D. D. Berg, and R. P. Giugliano. 2011. The facts behind niacin. *Therapeutic Advances in Cardiovascular Disease* 5(5):227–240.

10. Mackey, A. D., S. R. Davis, and J. F. Gregory III. 2006. Vitamin B_6. In: M. E. Shils, M. Shike, A. C. Ross, B. Caballero, and R. Cousins, eds. *Modern Nutrition in Health and Disease,* 10th edn. Philadelphia: Lippincott Williams & Wilkins, pp. 452–461.

11. Huang, S. C., J. C. Wei, D. J. Wu, and Y. C. Huang. 2010. Vitamin B_6 supplementation improves pro-inflammatory responses in patients with rheumatoid arthritis. *European Journal of Clinical Nutrition* 64(9):1007–1013.

12. Shane, B. 2006. Folic acid, vitamin B_{12}, and vitamin B_6. In: M. H. Stipanuk, ed. *Biochemical, Physiological, and Molecular Aspects of Human Nutrition.* Philadelphia: W. B. Saunders, pp. 693–732.

13. Gibson, S. R. 2005. *Principles of Nutritional Assessment,* 2nd edn. New York: Oxford University Press.

14. Sweetman, L. 2006. Pantothenic acid and biotin. In: M. H. Stipanuk, ed. *Biochemical and Physiological Aspects of Human Nutrition.* Philadelphia: W. B. Saunders, pp. 733–759.

15. Dunn, J. T. 2006. Iodine. In: M. E. Shils, M. Shike, A. C. Ross, B. Caballero, and R. Cousins, eds. *Modern Nutrition in Health and Disease,* 10th edn. Philadelphia: Lippincott Williams & Wilkins, pp. 300–311.

16. Freake, H. C. 2006. Iodine. In: M. H. Stipanuk, ed. *Biochemical and Physiological Aspects of Human Nutrition.* Philadelphia: W. B. Saunders, pp. 1068–1090.

17. Institute of Medicine, Food and Nutrition Board. 2001. *Dietary Reference Intakes for Vitamin A, Vitamin K, Arsenic, Boron, Chromium, Copper, Iodine, Iron, Manganese, Molybdenum, Nickel, Silicon, Vanadium, and Zinc.* Washington, DC: National Academy Press.

18. World Health Organization. 2004. Nutrition. Micronutrient deficiencies. International Council of Control of Iodine Deficiency Disorders. www.euro.who.int/en/what-we-do/health-topics/disease-prevention/nutrition/activities/technical-support-to-member-states/micronutrient-deficiencies. (Accessed March 2012.)

19. International Council for the Control of Iodine Deficiency Disorders (ICCIDD). 2009. Iodine deficiency. www.iccidd.org/pages/iodine-deficiency.php. (Accessed February 2012.)

20. Andersson, M., V. Karumbunathan, and M. B. Zimmerman. 2012. Global iodine status in 2011 and trends over the past decade. *J. Nutr.* DOI:10.3945/jn.111.149393.

21. Grider, A. 2006. Zinc, copper and manganese. In: M. H. Stipanuk, ed. *Biochemical and Physiological Aspects of Human Nutrition.* Philadelphia: W. B. Saunders, pp. 1043–1067.

22. van der Beek, E. J., W. van Dokkum, J. Schrijver, M. Wedel, A. W. K. Gaillard, A. Wesstra, H. van de Weerd, and R. J. J. Hermus. 1988. Thiamin, riboflavin, and vitamins B_6 and C: impact of combined restricted intake on functional performance in man. *Am. J. Clin. Nutr.* 48:1451–1462.

23. van der Beek, E. J., W. van Dokkum, M. Wedel, J. Schrijver, and H. van den Berg. 1994. Thiamin, riboflavin and vitamin B_6: impact of restricted intake on physical performance in man. *J. Am. Coll. Nutr.* 13:629–640.

Treating Premenstrual Syndrome with Vitamin B$_6$ and Folic Acid: Does It Work? Is It Risky?

Perform an Internet search for treatments for premenstrual syndrome (PMS) and you are likely to find many recommendations for supplementing with magnesium, calcium, vitamin E, folic acid, and vitamin B$_6$. Many PMS supplements sold in pharmacy or health food stores contain 50 to 200 mg of vitamin B$_6$ per capsule or tablet and/or 400 µg of folate, with the recommendation that the consumer take at least two capsules per day. As you learned in this chapter, the UL of vitamin B$_6$ is 100 mg/day, and high doses of vitamin B$_6$ over an extended period of time can cause neurologic disorders. The UL for folate is 1,000 µg per day. There is concern that higher doses can mask B$_{12}$ deficiency and contribute to cancer, allergies, and other diseases.[1, 2] Is there research to support recommending high levels of folic acid and vitamin B$_6$ for PMS? Do the benefits of supplementing outweigh the risks for adverse effects or toxicity?

What Is PMS?

PMS is a disorder characterized by a cluster of symptoms triggered by hormonal changes that occur 1 to 2 weeks prior to the start of menstruation. These symptoms typically fall into the two general categories in the following lists, which the American College of Obstetricians and Gynecologists uses in the diagnosis of PMS.[3]

- *Emotional symptoms:* depression, angry outbursts, irritability, crying spells, anxiety, confusion, social withdrawal, poor concentration, insomnia, increased napping, and changes in sexual desire
- *Physical symptoms:* thirst and appetite changes (food cravings), breast tenderness, bloating and weight gain, swelling of hands and feet, abdominal pain, headache, aches and pain, fatigue, skin problems, and gastrointestinal distress

For a woman to be diagnosed with PMS, she typically has to report a pattern of symptoms meeting the following criteria.[3] The pattern must

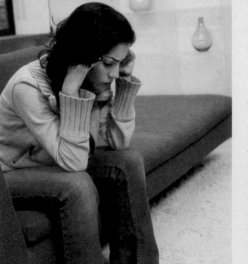

Headaches, anxiety, irritability, tension, and depression are common symptoms of PMS.

- be present in the 5 days before her period for atleast three menstrual cycles in a row
- end within 4 days after her period starts
- interfere with some of her normal activities

Currently, there is no universally accepted medical treatment for PMS. Not surprisingly, given the diversity of its associated symptoms, a wide variety of clinical and alternative therapies are used:

- *Antidepressants* to help relieve the emotional symptoms of PMS
- *Hormonal contraceptives*, which can stabilize shifts in reproductive hormones
- *Diuretics* to help ease the fluid retention associated with PMS in some women
- *Nonsteroidal anti-inflammatory drugs*, such as ibuprofen or naproxen, to relieve cramping and aches and pain
- *Vitamins*, especially folic acid, vitamin B$_6$, and vitamin E
- *Minerals*, especially calcium and magnesium
- *Amino acid supplements*, such as L-tryptophan
- *Various herbs*, including ginkgo biloba, St. John's wort, kava-kava, chaste tree fruit, and *dong quai*[3, 4, 5, 6]

Unfortunately, some of these remedies have the potential for negative health consequences if taken in excess. Here, we discuss vitamin B$_6$ and folic acid.

Vitamin B$_6$ Toxicity

The *New England Journal of Medicine* first reported concerns about the use of vitamin B$_6$ for PMS in 1983. Researchers described the development of sensory neuropathy (a disorder affecting the sensory nerves) in seven women, 20 to 43 years of age, taking high doses of pyridoxine, the most common form of vitamin B$_6$ in supplements.[7]

Five of the women began with 50 to 100 mg/day of vitamin B_6 before steadily increasing their dose in an attempt to derive a benefit. In one case, a 27-year-old woman began taking 500 mg/day of vitamin B_6 to treat premenstrual edema. Over the course of a year, she gradually increased her dose to 5,000 mg/day (5 g/day), which is fifty times higher than the UL for vitamin B_6. She reported a tingling sensation in her neck, legs, and feet; numbness in her hands and feet; impaired walking; and impairment in handling small objects. She also noticed changes in the feeling in her lips and tongue. Within 2 months of stopping her supplement, she began to see improvement in her gait and sensation, but it was 7 months before she could walk without a cane. At the time the report was written, the numbness in her legs and hands had still not improved.

A total of four of the seven women became so severely disabled they could not walk or could walk only with a cane. The others experienced less severe symptoms, including "lightning-like" pains in their calves and shins, especially after exercise. Unfortunately, none of the women reported that the supplements had improved their premenstrual edema, made them feel better, or improved their mood, the reasons they gave for taking the supplement in the first place.

In summary, four of the seven women began feeling better within 6 months after stopping supplementation but still had diminished sensory perception. Two of them did not experience recovery until 2 to 3 years after supplementation had stopped.

Adverse Effects of High Folic Acid Intake

It has long been recognized that high doses of folic acid can mask vitamin B_{12} deficiency and contribute to neurologic complications; however, there is now evidence that high doses of supplemental folic acid over a period of time may have other adverse health outcomes.[1,2] The amount of folic acid associated with these adverse outcomes varies greatly, ranging from 400 to over 1,000 μg/day. The following are a few of these adverse effects:

- Increased multiple births
- Predisposition to allergies[8]

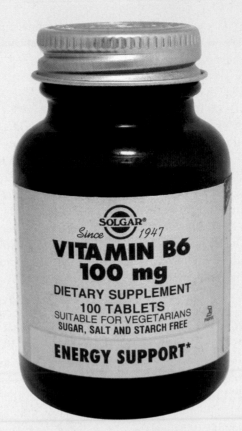

Vitamin B_6: do the potential benefits outweigh the risk of toxicity?

- Interference with zinc absorption
- Promotion of cancer; adequate amounts of folate might protect against cancer, but high doses of supplemental folic acid might stimulate the growth of precancerous or cancerous cells[9]

Since commercial breads and cereals are fortified with folic acid, some researchers are concerned that women might be getting too much folic acid if they supplement with high doses and consume significant amounts of these fortified foods daily.

Does Research Support the Treatment of PMS with Vitamin B_6 and Folic Acid?

Does a review of the research literature support the use of high doses of folic acid and vitamin B_6 for the treatment of PMS? To date, there have been nine randomized clinical trials testing whether vitamin B_6 supplementation improves PMS symptoms. These nine trials, including 940 subjects, were systematically reviewed by researchers in the United Kingdom to determine if there was enough evidence to recommend using vitamin B_6 as a treatment for PMS.[10] Unfortunately, none of the clinical trials met the highest criteria set for research quality. The results show that about half of the studies reported some positive effects of vitamin B_6 supplements on PMS symptoms when compared to the placebo group, but frequently the improvement was only for some of the symptoms. The authors concluded that "there was insufficient evidence of high enough quality to give a confident recommendation for using vitamin B_6 in the treatment of PMS."[10] A more recent research trial with 94 women found that 80 mg of vitamin B_6 daily for 3 months was associated with a statistically significant reduction in some PMS symptoms.[11] If vitamin B_6 is to have a positive effect on PMS, it needs to be taken daily, not just when symptoms appear.[3]

Research has reported an association between folic acid deficiency and depression,[12] but the research supporting a recommendation of folic acid for PMS treatment is weak. The Office of Women's Health has listed folic acid supplementation as an alternative treatment for PMS,[13] but The American

College of Obstetricians and Gynecologists does not make the same recommendation.[3] Currently, there are no studies that have specifically examined the use of folic acid supplementation for the reduction of PMS symptoms.

Researchers have, however, examined whether dietary B-vitamin intake in general is associated with increased or decreased PMS diagnosis.[14] In the Nurses' Health Study II Cohort, at baseline in 1991, all women were PMS free. After 10 years, 1,057 women were confirmed with PMS and 1,968 were confirmed as PMS free. Researchers then examined their B-vitamin intake over this decade to determine if those with higher B-vitamin intake were more or less likely to be diagnosed with PMS. They found no significant associations between the incidence of PMS and dietary intakes of B-vitamins, including vitamin B_6 and folate; neither did they see an association between supplemental B_6 and PMS.

At this time, there does not appear to be strong enough evidence to recommend vitamin B_6 or folic acid supplements for the treatment of PMS, especially in the high doses typically found in PMS supplements. Some of the problems observed when reviewing these studies reveal why the authors could not give definitive recommendations. For example, one study showed that 58% of the individuals taking vitamin B_6 felt better, but so did 59% of the individuals taking the placebo; thus, there were no differences between the groups. Many of the studies showed improvement in only some of the symptoms of PMS, such as anxiety and food cravings but not headaches and depression. Finally, the level of treatment in the studies varied greatly, from 50 to 600 mg/day of vitamin B_6. Thus, although some studies suggest a benefit, the evidence for the efficacy of treating PMS with vitamin B_6 is not convincing and further research is needed.[4, 6, 10]

CRITICAL THINKING QUESTIONS

- Do you think the limited benefits of treating PMS with vitamin B_6 or folic acid outweigh the risks of toxicity or negative health effects?

- What would you do if a friend told you she was taking 100 mg/day of vitamin B_6 for PMS?

- What if she told you she was taking twice that amount and had been doing so for several months?

For more information on the use of vitamins and minerals for PMS, see the National Institutes of Health (NIH) Office of Dietary Supplements in Web Links (page 340).

REFERENCES

1. Arbor Clinical Nutrition Upates. 2010, December. Can folate supplements be dangerous? Part 2. 327:1–5.

2. Institute of Medicine, Food and Nutrition Board. 1998. *Dietary Reference Intakes for Thiamin, Riboflavin, Niacin, Vitamin B$_6$, Folate, Vitamin B$_{12}$, Pantothenic Acid, Biotin, and Choline*. Washington, DC: National Academy Press.

3. American College of Obstetricians and Gynecologists. 2011. Premenstrual Syndrome Fact Sheet. www.acog.org/Search?Keyword=premenstrual+syndrome. (Accessed March 2012.)

4. Rapkin, A. 2003. The review of treatment of premenstrual syndrome & premenstrual dysphoric disorder. *Psychoneuroendocrinology* 28:39–53.

5. Canning, S., M. Waterman, and L. Dye. 2006. Dietary supplements and herbal remedies for premenstrual syndrome (PMS): a meta-analysis of randomized controlled trials. *J. Reproductive and Infant Psychol.* 24:363–378.

6. Whalen, A. M., T. M. Jurgen, and H. Naylor. 2009. Herbs, vitamins and minerals in the treatment of premenstrual syndrome: a systemic review. 16(3):e407–429.

7. Schaumburg, H., J. Kaplan, A. Winderbank, N. Vick, S. Rasmus, D. Pleasure, and M. J. Brown. 1983. Sensory neuropathy from pyridoxine abuse: a new megavitamin syndrome. *N. Engl. J. Med.* 309:445–448.

8. Withrow, M. J., et al. 2009. Effect of supplemental folic acid in pregnancy on childhood asthma: a prospective birth cohort study. *Am. J. Epidemiol.* 170(12):1486–1493.

9. Ebbing, M., et al. 2009. Cancer incidence and mortality after treatment with folic acid and vitamin B$_{12}$. *JAMA* 203(19):2119–20026.

10. Connolly, M. 2001. Premenstrual syndrome: an update on definitions, diagnosis and management. *Advances in Psychiatric Treatment* 7:469–477.

11. Kashanian, M., R. Mazinani, and S. Jalalmanesh. 2007. Pyridoxine (vitamin B$_6$) therapy for premenstrual syndrome. *Int. J. Gynaecol. Obstet.* 96:43–44.

12. Cho, Y. J., J. Y. Han, J. S. Choi, H. K. Ahn, H. M. Ryu, M. M. Y. Kim, J. H. Yang, A. A. Nava-Ocampo, and G. Koren. 2008. Prenatal multivitamins containing folic acid do not decrease prevalence of depression among pregnant women. *J. Obstetrics and Gynaecology.* 28(5):482–484.

13. Department of Health and Human Services, Office of Women's Health. 2010. Premenstrual Syndrome Fact Sheet. www.womenshealth.gov/publications/our-publications/fact-sheet/premenstrual-syndrome.cfm. (Accessed March 2012.)

14. Chocano-Bedoya, P. O., J. E. Manson, S. E. Hankinson, W. C. Willett, S. R. Johnson, L. Chasan-Taber, A. G. Ronnenberg, C. Bigelow, and E. R. Berthone-Johnson. 2011. Dietary B vitamin intake and incident premenstrual syndrome. *American Journal of Clinical Nutrition* 93(5):1080–1086.

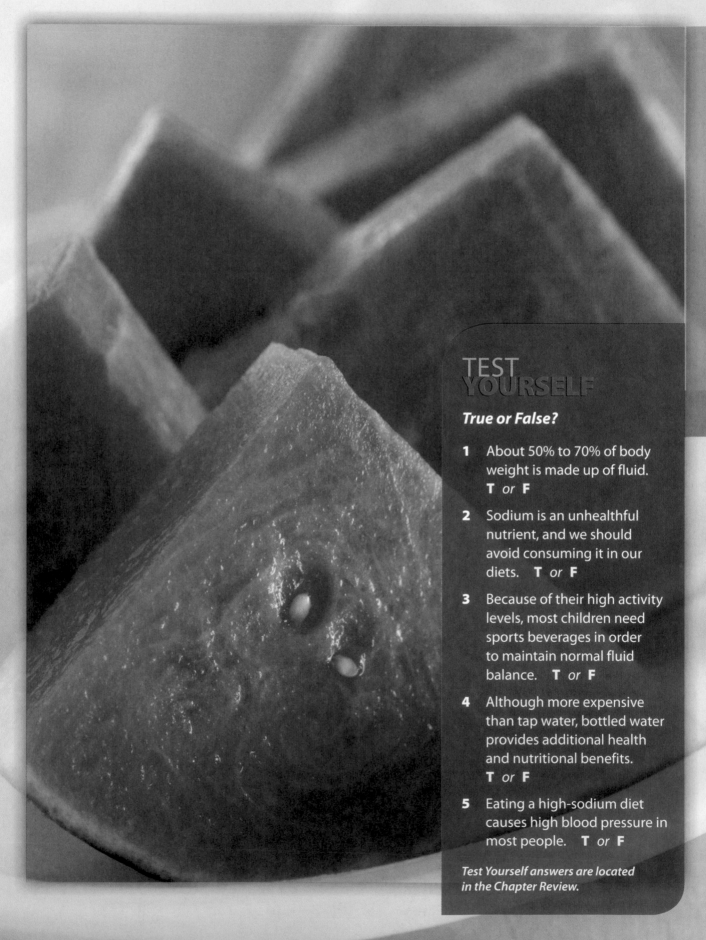

True or False?

1 About 50% to 70% of body weight is made up of fluid. **T** *or* **F**

2 Sodium is an unhealthful nutrient, and we should avoid consuming it in our diets. **T** *or* **F**

3 Because of their high activity levels, most children need sports beverages in order to maintain normal fluid balance. **T** *or* **F**

4 Although more expensive than tap water, bottled water provides additional health and nutritional benefits. **T** *or* **F**

5 Eating a high-sodium diet causes high blood pressure in most people. **T** *or* **F**

Test Yourself answers are located in the Chapter Review.

9 Nutrients Involved in Fluid and Electrolyte Balance

Learning Objectives

After studying this chapter, you should be able to:

1. Distinguish among extracellular fluid, intracellular fluid, interstitial fluid, and intravascular fluid, *p. 348.*

2. Identify four nutrients that function as electrolytes in our bodies, *pp. 349–350.*

3. Discuss how the kidneys regulate blood pressure and blood volume, *pp. 350–351.*

4. List three functions of water in our bodies, *pp. 350–352.*

5. Describe how electrolytes assist in the regulation of healthful fluid balance, *pp. 352–355.*

6. Describe the avenues of fluid intake and excretion in our bodies, and explain how the body maintains acid–base balance, *p. 355–358.*

7. Identify and describe the functions of the four minerals involved in electrolyte balance, *pp. 365-371.*

8. Define *hypernatremia* and *hyponatremia* and identify factors that can cause these conditions, *pp. 366–367.*

9. Describe the disorders related to fluid and electrolyte imbalance and identify their symptoms, *pp. 372–373.*

10. Define *hypertension* and list three lifestyle changes that can reduce it, *pp. 373–376.*

MasteringNutrition™

Go online for chapter quizzes, pre-tests, Interactive Activities and more!

When reading or hearing the words "hazing death" and "drinking too much," most of us immediately think of alcohol poisoning. Over the past decade, however, there have been several hazing deaths caused by the overconsumption of water. That's right—pure, "wholesome" water. In 2003, for example, when a fraternity pledge at State University of New York at Plattsburg was forced to drink too much water, he fell into a coma caused by swelling of the brain and died. A similar fraternity "prank" known as water chugging nearly killed a 21-year-old student at Southern Methodist University in Texas the same year. In 2005, a fraternity hazing at California State University—Chico, left 21-year-old Matthew Carrington dead after he was forced to consume gallons of water while performing calisthenics in a cold basement.[1] The official cause of his death was hyponatremia, or "low blood sodium." This condition is also known as water intoxication or water poisoning.

What is hyponatremia, and how does it differ from dehydration? Are you at risk for either condition? Do sports beverages confer any protection against these fluid imbalances? If at the start of cross-country practice on a hot, humid afternoon a friend confided to you about a drinking binge the night before and admitted having vomited twice that morning, what would you say? Would you urge your friend to tell your coach, and if so, why?

In this chapter, we explore the role of fluids and electrolytes in keeping the body properly hydrated and maintaining the functions of nerves and muscles. We also discuss how blood pressure is maintained and take a look at some disorders that occur when fluids and electrolytes are out of balance.

What Are Fluids and Electrolytes, and What Are Their Functions?

You know, of course, that orange juice, blood, and shampoo are all fluids, but what makes them so? A **fluid** is a substance characterized by its ability to move freely and changeably, adapting to the shape of the container that holds it. This may not seem very important, but as you'll learn in this chapter, the fluid composition of cells and tissues is critical to the body's ability to function.

Body Fluid Is the Liquid Portion of Cells and Tissues

Between about 50% and 70% of a healthy adult's body weight is fluid. When we cut a finger, we can see some of this fluid dripping out as blood, but the fluid in the bloodstream can't account for such a large percentage of one's total body weight. So where is all this fluid hiding?

About two-thirds of the body's fluid is held within the walls of cells and is therefore called **intracellular fluid** (**Figure 9.1a**). Every cell in the body contains fluid. When cells lose their fluid, they quickly shrink and die. On the other hand, when cells take in too much fluid, they swell and burst apart. This is why appropriate fluid balance—which we'll discuss throughout this chapter—is so critical to life.

The remaining third of the body's fluid is referred to as **extracellular fluid** because it flows outside of the cells (see Figure 9.1a). There are two types of extracellular fluid:

1. **Interstitial fluid** flows between the cells that make up a particular tissue or organ, such as muscle fibers or the liver (Figure 9.1b).
2. **Intravascular fluid** is the water in the bloodstream and lymph. *Plasma* is specifically the extracellular fluid portion of blood that transports blood cells within the body's arteries, veins, and capillaries (Figure 9.1c).

Not every tissue in the body contains the same amount of fluid. Lean tissues, such as muscle, are more than 70% fluid, whereas fat tissue is between only 10% and 20% fluid. This is not surprising, considering the hydrophobic nature of lipid cells (which was discussed in Chapter 5).

fluid A substance composed of molecules that move past one another freely. Fluids are characterized by their ability to conform to the shape of whatever container holds them.

intracellular fluid The fluid held at any given time within the walls of the body's cells.

extracellular fluid The fluid outside of the body's cells, either in the body's tissues (interstitial fluid) or as the liquid portion of the blood or lymph (intravascular fluid).

interstitial fluid The fluid that flows between the cells that make up a particular tissue or organ, such as muscle fibers or the liver.

intravascular fluid The fluid in the bloodstream and lymph.

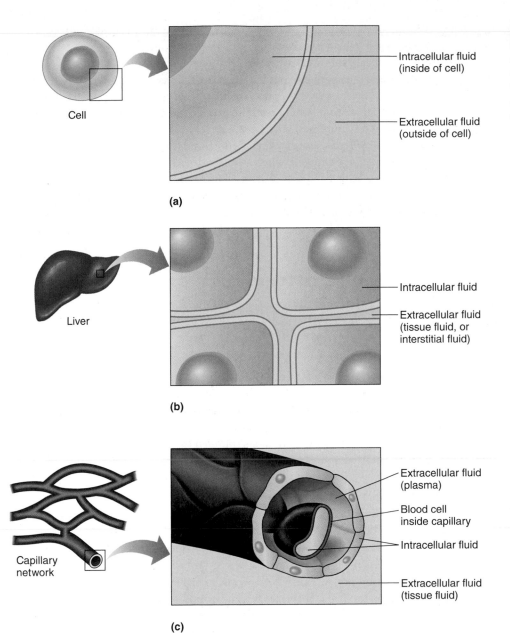

FIGURE 9.1 The components of body fluid. **(a)** Intracellular fluid is contained within the cells that make up our body tissues. Extracellular fluid is external to cells. **(b)** Interstitial fluid is external to tissue cells, and **(c)** plasma is external to blood cells.

Body fluid levels also vary according to gender and age. Males have more lean tissue than females and thus a higher percentage of body weight as fluid. The amount of body fluid as a percentage of total weight decreases with age. About 75% of an infant's body weight is water, whereas the total body water of an elderly person is generally less than 50% of body weight. This decrease in total body water is, in part, a result of the loss of lean tissue that commonly occurs as people age.

Body Fluid Is Composed of Water and Dissolved Substances Called Electrolytes

Water is made up of molecules consisting of two hydrogen atoms bound to one oxygen atom (H_2O). Although water is essential to maintain life, we would quickly die if our cell and tissue fluids contained only water. Instead, within the body fluids are a variety of dissolved substances (called *solutes*) critical to life. These include four major minerals: sodium,

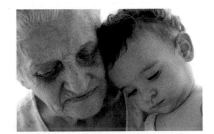

As we age, our body water content decreases: approximately 75% of an infant's body weight is composed of water, whereas an elderly adult's is only 50% or less.

potassium, chloride, and phosphorus. We consume these minerals in compounds called *salts,* including table salt, which is made of sodium and chloride.

These mineral salts are called **electrolytes,** because when they dissolve in water, the two component minerals separate into electrically charged **ions,** which are themselves commonly referred to as electrolytes. An ion's electrical charge, which can be positive or negative, is the "spark" that stimulates nerves and causes muscles to contract, making electrolytes critical to body function.

Of the four major minerals just mentioned, the ionic forms of sodium (Na^+) and potassium (K^+) are positively charged, whereas chloride (Cl^-) and phosphorus (in the form of hydrogen phosphate, or HPO_4^{2-}) are negatively charged. In the intracellular fluid, potassium and phosphate are the predominant ions. In the extracellular fluid, sodium and chloride predominate. There is a slight difference in electrical charge on either side of the cell's membrane that is needed in order for the cell to perform its normal functions.

Fluids Serve Many Critical Functions

Water not only quenches our thirst; it performs a number of functions that are critical to support life.

Fluids Dissolve and Transport Substances

Water is an excellent **solvent,** which means it is capable of dissolving a wide variety of substances. All water-soluble substances—such as amino acids, glucose, the water-soluble vitamins, minerals, and some medications—are readily transported via the bloodstream. In contrast, lipids do not dissolve in water. To overcome this incompatibility, lipids and the fat-soluble vitamins are either attached to or surrounded by water-soluble proteins, so that they, too, can be transported in the blood to the cells.

Fluids Account for Blood Volume

Blood volume is the amount of fluid in blood; thus, appropriate body fluid levels are essential to maintaining healthful blood volume. When blood volume rises inappropriately, blood pressure increases; when blood volume decreases inappropriately, blood pressure decreases. As you know, high blood pressure is an important risk factor for heart disease and stroke, whereas low blood pressure can cause people to feel tired, confused, or dizzy. We discuss high blood pressure (called *hypertension*) later in this chapter.

The kidneys play a central role in the regulation of blood volume and blood pressure. While filtering the blood, they reabsorb (retain) water and other nutrients that the body needs and excrete waste products and excess water in the urine. Changes in blood volume, blood pressure, and concentration of solutes in the blood signal the kidneys to adjust the volume and concentration of urine.

Imagine that you have just finished working out for an hour, during which time you did not drink any fluids but you lost fluid through sweat. In response to the increased concentration of solutes in your blood, **antidiuretic hormone (ADH)** is released from the pituitary gland (**Figure 9.2**). The action of ADH is appropriately described by its name: a **diuretic** is a substance that increases fluid loss via the urine. In contrast, ADH has an antidiuretic effect, stimulating the kidneys to reabsorb water and to reduce the production of urine.

Simultaneously, your reduced blood volume has resulted in a decrease in blood pressure. This drop in blood pressure stimulates pressure receptors in the kidney, which signal the kidney to secrete the enzyme **renin.** Renin then activates a blood protein called angiotensinogen, which is produced in the liver. Angiotensinogen is the precursor of another blood protein, angiotensin I. Angiotensin I is converted to **angiotensin II,** which is a powerful vasoconstrictor; this means it works to constrict the diameter of blood vessels, which results in an increase in blood pressure.

electrolyte A compound that disassociates in solution into positively and negatively charged ions and is thus capable of conducting an electrical current; the ions in such a solution.

ion Any electrically charged particle, either positively or negatively charged.

solvent A substance that is capable of mixing with and breaking apart a variety of compounds. Water is an excellent solvent.

blood volume The amount of fluid in blood.

antidiuretic hormone (ADH) A hormone released from the pituitary gland in response to an increase in blood solute concentration. ADH stimulates the kidneys to reabsorb water and to reduce the production of urine.

diuretic A substance that increases fluid loss via the urine. Common diuretics include alcohol and prescription medications for high blood pressure and other disorders.

renin An enzyme secreted by the kidneys in response to a decrease in blood pressure. Renin converts the blood protein angiotensinogen to angiotensin I, which eventually results in an increase in sodium reabsorption.

angiotensin II A potent vasoconstrictor that constricts the diameter of blood vessels and increases blood pressure; it also signals the release of the hormone aldosterone from the adrenal glands.

FIGURE 9.2 Regulation of blood volume and blood pressure by the kidneys.

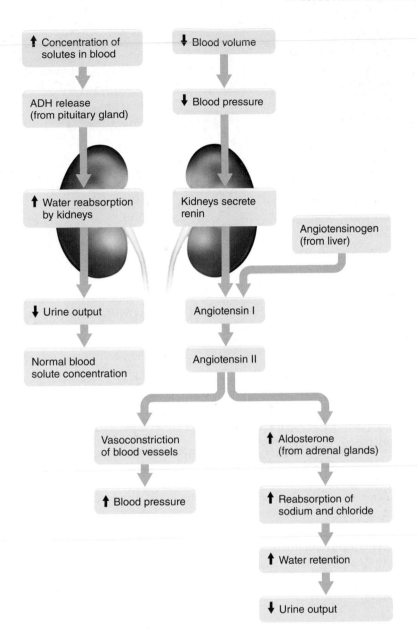

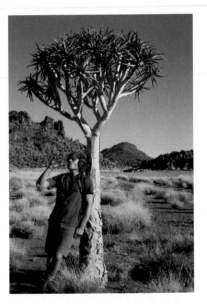

To prevent heat-related illness, a hiker needs to adjust his or her fluid intake according to the humidity level and temperature of the environment.

Angiotensin II also signals the release of the hormone **aldosterone** from the adrenal glands. Aldosterone signals the kidneys to retain sodium and chloride. Because water travels with the ionic form of these two minerals, this results in water retention, which increases blood pressure and decreases urine output. These responses help regulate fluid balance and blood pressure.

Fluids Help Maintain Body Temperature

Just as overheating is disastrous to a car engine, a high internal temperature can cause the body to stop functioning. Fluids are vital to the body's ability to maintain its temperature within a safe range. Two factors account for the cooling power of fluids. First, water has a high capacity for heat: it takes a lot of energy to raise its temperature. Because the body contains a lot of water, only sustained high heat can increase body temperature.

Second, body fluids are our primary coolant. When heat needs to be released from the body, there is an increase in the flow of blood from the warm body core to the vessels lying just under the skin. This action transports heat out to the body periphery, where it can be released from the skin. When we are hot, the sweat glands secrete more sweat from

aldosterone A hormone released from the adrenal glands that signals the kidneys to retain sodium and chloride, which in turn results in the retention of water.

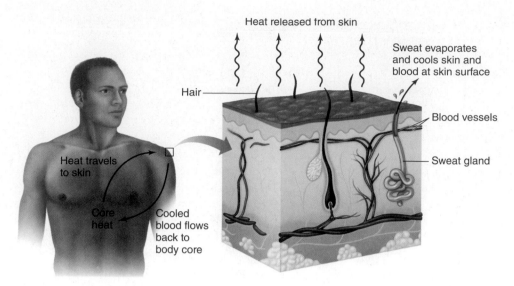

FIGURE 9.3 Evaporative cooling occurs when heat is transported from the body core through the bloodstream to the surface of the skin. The water evaporates into the air and carries away heat. This cools the blood, which circulates back to the body core, reducing body temperature.

Would the proteins in your body tissues "cook" at the same temperature that would fry an egg? For a short, fun video from NPR on the experiment that answered this question, go to www.youtube.com/watch?v=IqwPS6wJN-c.

the skin. As this sweat evaporates off of the skin's surface, heat is released into the environment. As a result, the skin and underlying blood are cooled. This process, called *evaporative cooling*, is illustrated in **Figure 9.3**. This cooler blood flows back to the body's core and reduces internal body temperature.

Fluids Protect and Lubricate the Tissues

Water is a major part of the fluids that protect and lubricate tissues. The cerebrospinal fluid that surrounds the brain and spinal column protects these vital tissues from damage, and a fetus in a mother's womb is protected by amniotic fluid. Synovial fluid lubricates joints, and tears cleanse and lubricate the eyes. Saliva moistens the food we eat, and the mucus lining the walls of the GI tract helps the food move smoothly along. Finally, the pleural fluid covering the lungs allows their friction-free expansion and retraction behind the chest wall.

RECAP

Body fluid consists of water plus a variety of dissolved substances, including electrically charged minerals called electrolytes. Water serves many important functions, including dissolving and transporting substances, accounting for blood volume, regulating body temperature, and cushioning and lubricating body tissues. ■

Electrolytes Support Many Body Functions

Now that you know why fluid is so essential to the body's functioning, we're ready to explore the critical role of the minerals within it.

Electrolytes Help Regulate Fluid Balance

Cell membranes are *permeable* to water. This means that water flows easily through them. Cells cannot voluntarily regulate this flow of water and thus have no active control over the balance of fluid between the intracellular and extracellular compartments. In contrast, cell membranes are *not* freely permeable to electrolytes. Sodium, potassium, and the other electrolytes stay where they are, either inside or outside of a cell, unless they are actively transported elsewhere by special proteins. So how do electrolytes help the cells maintain their fluid balance? To answer this question, we need to review a bit of chemistry.

Imagine that you have a special filter that has the same properties as cell membranes; in other words, this filter is freely permeable to water but not permeable to electrolytes. Now imagine that you insert this filter into a glass of dilute salt water to divide the glass into two chambers (**Figure 9.4a**). The water levels on both sides of the filter would, of course, be identical, because it is freely permeable to water. Now imagine that you add a full teaspoon of salt to the water on one side of the filter only (Figure 9.4b). In solution, the salt would immediately dissociate into sodium and chloride ions. You would therefore see the water on the "dilute salt water" side of the glass suddenly begin to flow through the filter to the "concentrated salt water" side of the glass (Figure 9.4c). Why would this mysterious movement of water occur? The answer is that water always moves from areas where solutes, such as sodium and chloride, are in low concentrations to areas where they are highly concentrated. This movement is referred to as **osmosis.** To put it another way, electrolytes attract water toward areas where they are concentrated. This movement of water toward solutes continues until the concentration of solutes is equal on both sides of the cell membrane.

Water follows the movement of electrolytes; this action provides a means to control movement of water into and out of the cells. The pressure that is needed to keep the particles in a solution from drawing liquid toward them across a semipermeable membrane is referred to as **osmotic pressure.** Cells can regulate the osmotic pressure, and thus the balance of fluids between their internal and extracellular environments, by using special transport proteins to actively pump electrolytes across their membranes. (For an example of how transport proteins pump sodium and potassium across the cell membrane, see Chapter 6, Figure 6.14.)

By maintaining the appropriate movement of electrolytes into and out of the cell, the body maintains a healthful balance of fluid and electrolytes between the intracellular and extracellular compartments (**Figure 9.5a**). If the concentration of electrolytes is much

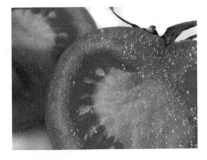

By sprinkling salt on a slice of tomato, you can see for yourself the effects of osmotic pressure.

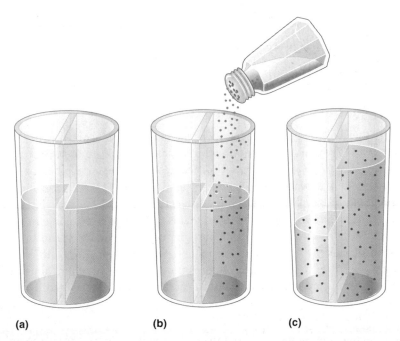

(a)   (b)   (c)

FIGURE 9.4 Osmosis. **(a)** A filter that is freely permeable to water only is placed in a glass of dilute salt water. **(b)** Additional salt is added to only one side of the glass. **(c)** Drawn by the high concentration of electrolytes, water flows to the "concentrated salt water" side of the filter. This flow of water into the concentrated solution will continue until the concentration of electrolytes on both sides of the membrane is equal.

osmosis The movement of water (or any solvent) through a semipermeable membrane from an area where solutes are less concentrated to areas where they are highly concentrated.

osmotic pressure The pressure that is needed to keep the particles in a solution from drawing liquid toward them across a semipermeable membrane.

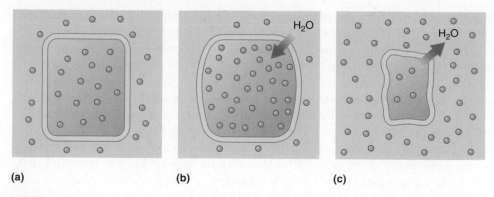

(a) (b) (c)

FIGURE 9.5 The health of our bodies' cells depends on maintaining the proper balance of fluids and electrolytes on both sides of the cell membrane. **(a)** The concentration of electrolytes is the same on both sides of the cell membrane. **(b)** The concentration of electrolytes is much greater inside the cell, drawing water into the cell and making it swell. **(c)** The concentration of electrolytes is much greater outside the cell, drawing water out of the cell and making it shrink.

higher inside of the cells as compared with outside, water will flow into the cells in such large amounts that the cells can burst (Figure 9.5b). On the other hand, if the extracellular environment contains too high a concentration of electrolytes, water flows out of the cells, and they can dry up (Figure 9.5c).

Certain illnesses can threaten the delicate balance of fluid inside and outside of the cells. You may have heard of someone being hospitalized because of excessive diarrhea or vomiting. When this happens, the body loses a great deal of fluid from the intestinal tract and extracellular compartment. This causes the loss of both water and electrolytes. In some cases, the relative loss of water is greater than the loss of electrolytes, and the body's extracellular electrolyte concentration then becomes very high. In response, a great deal of intracellular fluid leaves the cells to try to balance the high electrolyte concentration in the extracellular fluid. These imbalances in fluid and electrolytes change the flow of electrical impulses through the heart, causing an irregular heart rate that can be fatal if left untreated. Food poisoning and eating disorders involving repeated vomiting and diarrhea can also result in death from life-threatening fluid and electrolyte imbalances, including disorders that create an excessive loss of electrolytes versus an excessive loss of fluid.

Electrolytes Enable Nerves to Respond to Stimuli

In addition to their role in maintaining fluid balance, electrolytes are critical in enabling nerves to respond to stimuli. Nerve impulses are initiated at the membrane of a nerve cell in response to a change in the degree of electrical charge across the membrane. An influx of sodium into a nerve cell causes the cell to become slightly less negatively charged. This is called *depolarization* (**Figure 9.6**). If enough sodium enters the cell, the change in electrical charge triggers an *action potential*, an electrical signal that is then propagated along the length of the cell. Once the signal is transmitted, that portion of cell membrane returns to its normal electrical state through the release of potassium to the outside of the cell. This return of the cell to its initial electrical state is termed *repolarization*. Thus, both sodium and potassium play critical roles in ensuring that nerve impulses are generated, transmitted, and completed.

Electrolytes Signal Muscles to Contract

Muscles contract because of a series of complex physiologic changes that we will not describe in detail here. Simply stated, muscles are stimulated to contract in response to stimulation of nerve cells. As described earlier, sodium and potassium play a key role in the generation of nerve impulses, or electrical signals. When a muscle fiber is stimulated by an electrical signal, changes occur in the cell membrane that lead to an increased flow of calcium into the muscle from the extracellular fluid. This release of calcium into the muscle

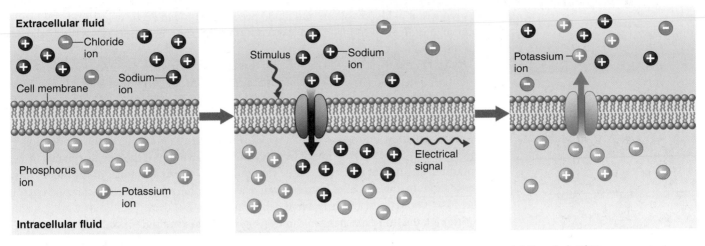

(a) Resting state   **(b) Depolarization**   **(c) Repolarization**

FIGURE 9.6 The role of electrolytes in conduction of a nerve impulse. **(a)** In the resting state, the intracellular fluid has slightly more ions with a negative charge. **(b)** A stimulus causes changes to occur that prompt the influx of sodium into the interior of the cell. Sodium has a positive charge, so when this happens, the charge inside the cell becomes slightly positive. This is called depolarization. If enough sodium enters the cell, an action potential is transmitted to adjacent regions of the cell membrane. **(c)** Release of potassium to the exterior of the cell allows the first portion of the membrane to return to the resting state almost immediately. This is called repolarization.

stimulates muscle contraction. The muscles can relax after a contraction once the electrical signal is complete and calcium has been pumped out of the muscle cell.

RECAP

Electrolytes help regulate fluid balance by controlling the movement of fluid into and out of cells. Electrolytes, specifically sodium and potassium, play a key role in generating nerve impulses in response to stimuli. Calcium is an electrolyte that stimulates muscle contraction. ■

How Does the Body Maintain Fluid Balance?

The proper balance of fluid is maintained in the body by a series of mechanisms that prompt us to drink and retain fluid when we are dehydrated and to excrete fluid as urine when we consume more than we need.

The Thirst Mechanism Prompts Us to Drink Fluids

Imagine that, at lunch, you ate a ham sandwich and a bag of salted potato chips. Now it's almost time for your afternoon seminar to end and you are very thirsty. When the instructor dismisses class, you dash to the nearest drinking fountain. What prompted you to suddenly feel so thirsty?

The body's command center for fluid intake is a cluster of nerve cells in the same part of the brain we studied in relation to food intake; that is, the *hypothalamus*. Within the hypothalamus is a group of cells, collectively referred to as the **thirst mechanism,** that causes us to consciously desire fluids. The thirst mechanism prompts us to feel thirsty when it is stimulated by the following:

- Increased concentration of salt and other dissolved substances in the blood. Remember that ham sandwich and those potato chips? Both of these foods are salty, and eating them increased the blood's sodium concentration.

thirst mechanism A cluster of nerve cells in the hypothalamus that stimulates our conscious desire to drink fluids in response to an increase in the concentration of salt in our blood or a decrease in blood pressure and blood volume.

- A reduction in blood volume and blood pressure. This can occur when fluids are lost through profuse sweating, blood loss, vomiting, diarrhea, or simply when fluid intake is too low.
- Dryness in the tissues of the mouth and throat. Tissue dryness reflects a lower amount of fluid in the bloodstream, which causes a reduced production of saliva.

Once the hypothalamus detects such changes, it stimulates the release of ADH to signal the kidneys to reduce urine flow and return more water to the bloodstream. As previously discussed, the kidneys also secrete renin, which eventually results in the production of angiotensin II and the retention of water. Water is drawn out of the salivary glands in the mouth in an attempt to further dilute the concentration of substances in the blood; this causes the mouth and throat to become even drier. Together, these mechanisms prevent a further loss of body fluid and help avoid dehydration.

Although the thirst mechanism can trigger an increase in fluid intake, this mechanism alone is not always sufficient: people tend to drink until they are no longer thirsty, but the amount of fluid consumed may not be enough to achieve fluid balance. This is particularly true when body water is rapidly lost, such as during intense exercise in the heat or high humidity. Because the thirst mechanism has some limitations, it is important that you drink regularly throughout the day and not wait to drink until you become thirsty, especially if you are active.

We Gain Fluids through Intake and Metabolism

The fluid needed each day is obtained from two primary sources: consumption of beverages and foods and the production of metabolic water by the body. Of course, you know that beverages are mostly water, but it isn't as easy to see the water content in foods. For example, iceberg lettuce is almost 96% water, and even almonds contain a small amount of water (**Figure 9.7**).

Metabolic water is the water formed from the body's metabolic reactions. In the breakdown of fat, carbohydrate, and protein, adenosine triphosphate (ATP), carbon dioxide, and water are produced. The water that is formed during metabolic reactions contributes about 10% to 14% of the water the body needs each day.

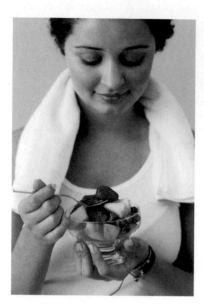
Fruits and vegetables are delicious sources of dietary water.

metabolic water   The water formed as a by-product of the body's metabolic reactions.

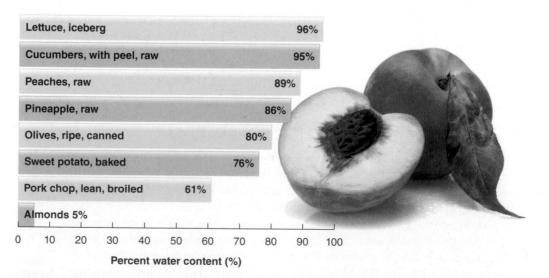

FIGURE 9.7 Water content of different foods. Much of your daily water intake comes from the foods you eat. (*Source:* Data from US Department of Agriculture, Agricultural Research Service. 2009. USDA Nutrient Database for Standard Reference, Release 22. Nutrient Data Laboratory Home Page. www.ars.usda.gov/ba/bhnrc/ndl.)

We Lose Fluids through Urine, Sweat, Evaporation, Exhalation, and Feces

Water loss that is noticeable, such as through urine output and sweating, is referred to as **sensible water loss.** Most of the water we consume is excreted through the kidneys in the form of urine. When we consume more water than we need, the kidneys process and excrete it in the form of dilute urine.

The second type of sensible water loss is via sweat. The sweat glands produce more sweat during exercise or when a person is in a hot environment. The evaporation of sweat from the skin releases heat, which cools the skin and reduces the body's core temperature.

Water is continuously evaporated from the skin even when a person is not consciously sweating, and water is continuously exhaled from the lungs. Water loss through these avenues is referred to as **insensible water loss,** as it is not perceived by the person. Under normal resting conditions, insensible water loss is less than 1 liter (L) of fluid each day; during heavy exercise or in hot weather, a person can lose up to 2 L of water per hour from insensible water loss.

Under normal conditions, only about 150 to 200 mL of water is lost each day in the feces. The gastrointestinal tract typically reabsorbs much of the large amounts of fluids that pass through it each day. However, when someone suffers from extreme diarrhea due to illness or from consuming excess laxatives, water loss in the feces can be as high as several liters per day.

In addition to these five common routes of fluid loss, certain situations can cause a significant loss of fluid from the body:

- Illnesses that involve fever, coughing, vomiting, diarrhea, and a runny nose significantly increase fluid loss. This is why doctors advise people to drink plenty of fluids when they are ill.
- Traumatic injury, internal hemorrhaging, blood donation, and surgery also increase loss of fluid because of the blood loss involved.
- Exercise increases fluid loss via sweat and respiration; although urine production typically decreases during exercise, fluid losses increase through the skin and lungs.
- Environmental conditions that increase fluid loss include high altitudes, cold and hot temperatures, and low humidity, such as in a desert or on an airplane. Because the water content of these environments is low, water from the body readily evaporates into the atmosphere. We also breathe faster at higher altitudes due to the lower oxygen pressure; this results in greater fluid loss via the lungs. We sweat more in the heat, thus losing more water. Cold temperatures can trigger hormonal changes that result in an increased fluid loss.
- Pregnancy increases fluid loss for the mother, because fluids are continually diverted to the fetus and amniotic fluid.
- Breastfeeding requires a significant increase in fluid intake to make up for the loss of fluid as breast milk.
- Consumption of diuretics can result in dangerously excessive fluid loss. Diuretics include certain prescription medications and alcohol. Many over-the-counter weight-loss remedies are really just diuretics. In the past, it was believed that the caffeine in beverages such as coffee, tea, and cola could cause serious dehydration, but recent research suggests that caffeinated drinks do not have a significant impact on the hydration status of adults.[2] The caffeine content of numerous beverages and foods is listed in Appendix F.

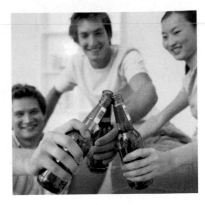

Drinking alcoholic beverages causes an increase in water loss because alcohol is a diuretic.

RECAP

A healthy fluid level is maintained in the body by balancing intake with excretion. Primary sources of fluids include water and other beverages, foods, and the production of metabolic water in the body. Fluid losses occur through urination, sweating, the feces, evaporation, and exhalation from the lungs. ■

sensible water loss   Water loss that is noticeable, such as through urine output and sweating.

insensible water loss   The unperceived loss of water, such as through evaporation from the skin and exhalation from the lungs during breathing.

How Does the Body Maintain Acid–Base Balance?

Recall (from Chapter 3) that an acid is a compound that releases hydrogen ions in solution, whereas a base is a substance that takes up hydrogen ions. The body's cellular processes, including energy metabolism, result in the constant production of both acids and bases. These substances are neutralized through the addition of buffers or through actions of the lungs or the kidneys. These homeostatic mechanisms (detailed later in this chapter) enable the body to maintain control over the pH—or acid–base balance—of the blood, which normally is slightly alkaline, ranging from about 7.35 to 7.45. (For a review of the pH scale, see **You Do The Math**, Chapter 3, page 85.)

If the blood pH moves beyond this narrow range, life-threatening complications develop. The body goes into a state called *acidosis* when the blood pH drops below 7.35. *Alkalosis* results if the blood pH rises above 7.45. Both acidosis and alkalosis can be caused by disorders affecting metabolism, respiration, or kidney function. For example, uncontrolled diabetes can result in a buildup of ketones, which are weak acids, and prompt acidosis, whereas the loss of gastric acid following repeated episodes of vomiting can cause alkalosis. Acidosis and alkalosis can cause coma and death by denaturing vital body proteins, such as enzymes and hemoglobin.

Three major systems account for the body's ability to regulate acid–base balance: blood buffers, the lungs, and the kidneys.

- *Blood buffers.* The blood transports many natural buffers. Proteins are excellent buffers, having the ability to take up excess hydrogen ions during acidosis and the ability to release hydrogen ions when the blood becomes too basic. Another blood buffer is the bicarbonate-carbonic acid system. Carbon dioxide (CO_2), one of the end products of energy metabolism, dissolves in the bloodstream to form carbonic acid (H_2CO_3), which itself dissociates into hydrogen (H^+) and bicarbonate ions (HCO_3^-):

$$CO_2 + H_2O \leftrightarrow H_2CO_3 \leftrightarrow H^+ + HCO_3^-$$

  Notice that this reaction is reversible: the bicarbonate ions are able to take up excess hydrogen ions or release hydrogen ions as needed in order to maintain acid–base balance.
- *Respiratory compensation.* Although fast acting, blood buffers don't have enough buffering capacity to correct large or long-term acid–base imbalances. The second line of defense is the lungs. By increasing or decreasing the rate of respiration, the lungs regulate the amount of carbonic acid in the blood. High levels of carbonic acid (acidosis) trigger hyperventilation. Excess carbon dioxide is forced out, helping to increase blood pH. In a state of alkalosis, with high blood levels of bicarbonate, respiration slows, carbon dioxide is retained, and more carbonic acid is formed, decreasing blood pH.
- *Renal compensation.* Since there is a limit to how fast or slow a person can breathe, the ability of the lungs to regulate acid–base balance is also limited. The last line of defense is the kidneys. Healthy kidneys have the capacity to either secrete into blood or excrete into urine significant bicarbonate to correct acid–base imbalances. They can also use non-bicarbonate buffers, such as ammonia or hydrogen phosphate, to excrete excess hydrogen ions.

By working together, blood buffers, the lungs, and the kidneys are usually able to maintain blood pH in a homeostatic range. When these mechanisms fail, clinical intervention, such as the intravenous administration of bicarbonate to a patient with diabetic ketoacidosis, may be necessary to save the patient's life.

A Profile of Nutrients Involved in Hydration and Neuromuscular Function

Nutrients that assist in maintaining hydration and neuromuscular function include water and the minerals sodium, potassium, chloride, and phosphorus (**Table 9.1**). As previously discussed (in Chapter 1), these minerals are classified as *major minerals,* as the body needs more than 100 mg of each per day.

TABLE 9.1 Overview of Nutrients Involved in Hydration and Neuromuscular Function

To see the full profile of micronutrients, turn to Chapter 7.5, In Depth, Vitamins and Minerals: Micronutrients with Macro Powers, *pages 300–309.*	

Nutrient	Recommended Intake
Sodium	1.5 g/day*
Potassium	4.7 g/day*
Chloride	2.3 g/day*
Phosphorus	700 mg/day[†]

*Adequate Intake (AI).
[†]RDA.

Calcium and magnesium also function as electrolytes and influence the body's fluid balance and neuromuscular function; however, because of their critical importance to bone health, they are discussed later in this text (in Chapter 11).

Water

Water is essential for life. Although we can live for weeks without food, we can survive only a few days without water, depending on environmental temperature. We do not have the capacity to store water, so we must continuously replace the water lost each day.

How Much Water Should We Drink?

The need for water varies greatly depending on age, body size, health status, physical activity level, and exposure to environmental conditions. It is important to pay attention to how much the need for water changes under various conditions, so that dehydration can be avoided.

Fluid requirements are very individualized. For example, a highly active male athlete training in a hot environment may require up to 10 L of fluid per day to maintain healthy fluid balance, whereas an inactive, petite woman who lives in a mild climate and works in a temperature-controlled office building may require only about 3 L of fluid per day. The DRI for adult men aged 19 to 50 years is 3.7 L of total water per day. This includes approximately 3.0 L (13 cups) as total water, other beverages, and food.[3] The DRI for adult women aged 19 to 50 is 2.7 L of total water per day. This includes about 2.2 L (9 cups) as total water, other beverages, and food.[4]

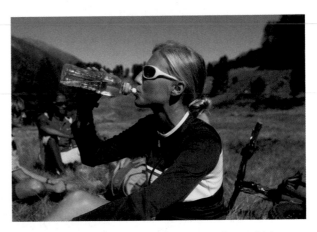

Vigorous exercise causes significant water loss, which must be replenished to optimize performance and health.

Figure 9.8 shows the amount and sources of water intake and output for a woman expending 2,500 kcal per day. Based on current recommendations, this woman needs about 3,000 mL of water per day:

- Water from metabolism provides 300 mL of water.
- The foods she eats provides her with an additional 500 mL of water each day.
- The beverages she drinks provide the remainder of water needed, which is equal to 2,200 mL.

An 8-oz glass of water is equal to 240 mL. In this example, the woman would need to drink nine glasses of fluid to meet her needs. You may have read or heard that drinking eight glasses of fluid each day is recommended for most people.[4] Drinking this amount will provide most people with enough fluid to maintain proper fluid balance. Remember, however, that this recommendation of eight glasses of fluid each day is a general guideline. For some people, that amount of fluid may be too high, or it may fluctuate with certain environmental conditions or changes in physical activities.

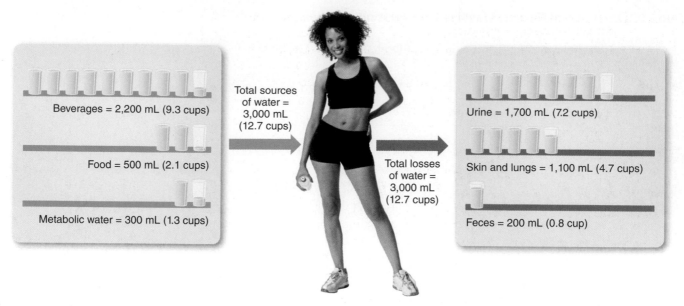

FIGURE 9.8 Amounts and categories of water sources and losses for a woman expending 2,500 kcal per day.

In contrast, athletes and others who are highly active, especially those working in very hot environments, may require more fluid than the current recommendations. The amount of sweat lost during strenuous activity is very individualized and depends on body size, activity intensity, level of fitness, environmental temperature, and humidity. We do know that some people can lose as much as 10% of body weight or mass during a marathon held in extreme heat[5] and that professional and collegiate football players can lose up to 10 L of sweat per day.[6] Thus, these individuals need to drink more to replace the fluid they lose. Sodium is the major electrolyte lost in sweat; we also lose some potassium and small amounts of iron and calcium in sweat.

Because of fluid and electrolyte losses during exercise, some athletes drink sports beverages instead of plain water to help them maintain fluid balance. Recently, sports beverages have also become popular with recreationally active people and non-athletes, including an increasing number of children and adolescents.[7] Is there a health benefit to consuming these beverages instead of plain water? See the **Nutrition Debate** on sports beverages at the end of this chapter to find out.

Sources of Drinking Water

So many types of drinking water are available in the United States, how can we distinguish among them? Carbonated water contains carbon dioxide gas that either occurs naturally or is added to the water. Mineral water contains 250 to 500 parts per million (ppm) of minerals. Many people prefer the unique taste of mineral water; however, a number of brands contain high amounts of sodium and so should be avoided by people who are trying to reduce their sodium intake. Distilled water is processed in such a way that all dissolved minerals are removed; this type of water is sometimes recommended for use in steam irons, as it will not clog the iron with mineral buildup, but it has a flat taste. Purified water has been treated so that all dissolved minerals and contaminants are removed, making this type of water useful in research and medical procedures. Of course, we can also drink the tap water found in our homes and in public places.

One of the major changes in the beverage industry during the past two decades has been the growth in sales of bottled water. Americans now consume about 28 gallons of bottled water per person, per year.[8] This meteoric rise in bottled water production and consumption is most likely due to the convenience of drinking bottled water, to the health messages related to drinking more water, to the recognition that water is more beneficial than other packaged beverages, and to the public's fears related to the safety of tap water. While recent environmental concerns related to disposal of water bottles blunted the use of bottled water to some extent, the bottled water industry has responded to these concerns with several environmental initiatives, such as smaller bottle caps, thinner bottles, and greater use of recyclable containers.[8] Is bottled water safer or more healthful than tap water? Refer to the **Nutrition Myth or Fact?** box to find the answer.

What Happens If We Drink Too Much Water?

Drinking too much water and becoming overhydrated is very rare. Even individuals who regularly consume large quantities of water do not develop major health problems because healthy kidneys are able to excrete the excess water.

Certain illnesses can cause excessive reabsorption or retention of water by the kidneys. When this occurs, overhydration and dilution of blood sodium result. Also, as described in the introductory story on water-related hazing, it is possible to overhydrate and dangerously dilute serum sodium concentration. This condition, called *hyponatremia,* is discussed in more detail in the next section.

What Happens If We Don't Drink Enough Water?

Dehydration results when we do not drink enough water or are unable to retain the water we drink. It is one of the leading causes of death around the world. Because an understanding of the physiology of dehydration requires familiarity with the roles of and requirements for the major electrolytes, we discuss this condition, along with a related illness called *heat stroke,* later in this chapter.

All Beverages Are Not Created Equal

Many commercial beverages contain several important nutrients in addition to their water content, whereas others provide water and refined sugar but very little else. Let's review the health benefits of and potential concerns about some of the most popular beverages on the market.

Milk and Milk Substitutes

Low-fat and skim milk are healthful beverage choices for many people, because they provide protein, calcium, phosphorus, vitamin D, and usually vitamin A. Many brands of fluid milk are now "specialized" and provide additional calcium, vitamin E, essential fatty acids, and/or plant sterols (to lower serum cholesterol). Kefir, a blended yogurt drink, is also a good source of most of these nutrients. Calcium-fortified soy milk provides protein and calcium, and many brands provide vitamin D. In contrast, almond and rice milks are low in protein, with only 1 gram per cup.

When purchasing flavored milk, kefir, or milk substitutes, check the Nutrition Facts Panel for the sugar content. Some brands of chocolate milk, for example, can contain 6 or more teaspoons of refined sugar in a single cup.

Hot Beverages

Coffee made without cream or non-dairy creamer can be a healthful beverage choice if consumed in moderation. As mentioned earlier, recent research suggests that its caffeine content does not significantly decrease the body's hydration status, and the calcium in coffee drinks made with milk, such as café con leche and café latte, can be significant. Coffee is known to provide several types of phytochemicals (beneficial plant chemicals) that may actually lower the risk for certain chronic diseases, such as type 2 diabetes.[9] There is also growing evidence that people who drink coffee have a lower risk for stroke, although not all research supports that theory.[10] While some people are sensitive to the caffeine in coffee, moderate consumption is safe and potentially healthful.

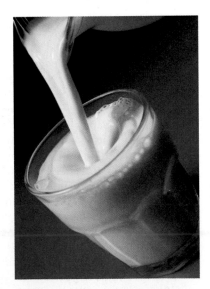

Low-fat and skim milk are healthful beverage choices for many people.

Nutrition Myth OR Fact?

Is Bottled Water Safer or More Healthful Than Tap Water?

Bottled water has become increasingly popular during the past 20 years. It is estimated that Americans drank almost 9 billion gallons of bottled water in 2010.[1] Many people, including children and adolescents, prefer the taste of bottled water to that of tap water. They also feel that bottled water is safer and better for them. Is this true?

The water we drink in the United States generally comes from two sources: surface water and groundwater. *Surface water* comes from lakes, rivers, and reservoirs. Common contaminants of surface water include runoff from highways, pesticides, animal wastes, and industrial wastes. Many of the cities across the United States obtain their water from surface-water sources. *Groundwater* comes from underground rock formations called *aquifers*. People who live in rural areas generally pump groundwater from a well as their water source. Hazardous substances leaking from waste sites, dumps, landfills, and oil and gas pipelines can contaminate groundwater. Groundwater can also be contaminated by naturally occurring substances, such as arsenic or high levels of iron.

Water treatment plants treat and purify community water supplies, typically with either chlorine or ozone. These chemicals are effective in killing many contaminants. Water treatment plants routinely check our water supplies for hazardous chemicals, minerals, and other contaminants. Because of these efforts, the United States has one of the safest water systems in the world. In addition, many water treatment plants fluoridate the water to prevent dental decay and optimize oral health.

The Environmental Protection Agency (EPA) sets and monitors the standards for our city water systems. The EPA does not monitor water from private wells, but it publishes recommendations for well owners to help them maintain a safe water supply. Local water regulatory agencies must provide an annual report on specific water contaminants to all households served by that agency.

In contrast, the Food and Drug Administration (FDA) regulates bottled water. It does not require that bottled water meet quality standards higher than those for public water. As with tap water, bottled water is taken from either surface water or groundwater sources. Bottled water is often treated and filtered by different methods than those used for tap water, and thus its taste and appearance may differ. For instance, most bottling plants use an ozone treatment instead of chlorine to disinfect water, and many people feel this process leaves the water tasting better than water treated with chlorine.

Although bottled water may or may not taste better than tap water, there is no evidence that it is safer to drink. For example, there is no strong research to support the use of bottled water by most persons with compromised immune systems. On the other hand, some people do not have access to safe tap water where they live. Mining by-products, lead, and other contaminants are major concerns in some parts of the United States.[2] For these people, bottled water may be the safer choice.

Is bottled water more healthful? While some brands may contain more minerals than tap water, bottled water has no other nutritional advantages over tap water. In fact, many bottled waters are labeled "from a public water source," which means the bottles are filled from the tap! In addition, most bottled waters

fail to provide optimal levels of fluoride, increasing the risk for dental decay in children.[3]

As the popularity of bottled water has increased, there are growing concerns about the potential burden drinking bottled water can have on the environment.[2] Specifically, many people have become concerned that the world will be inundated with billions of plastic bottles, since it has been estimated that fewer than 30% of plastic water bottles are recycled and the remainder end up in landfills.[3] Although plastic bottles can be reused, they do not last forever, and bacterial growth becomes a concern with repeated use. Many environmentally conscious consumers have begun using stainless steel, aluminum, glass, or plastic reusable bottles.

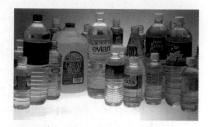

Many varieties of bottled water are available to consumers.

Should you spend money on bottled water? Before you decide, consider this simple calculation: let's say you purchase one bottle of water 5 days a week from the vending machine at the gym when you finish your workout. It costs you $1.00. Over the course of a single year, you'll have spent over $250 and will have added over 250 bottles to recycling centers or landfills! Some brands of bottled water cost as much as 10,000 times more than tap water on a per ounce basis![4]

If, after reading this discussion, you still choose to drink bottled water, look for brands that carry the trademark of the International Bottled Water Association (IBWA). This association follows the regulations of the FDA. If you get your water from a water cooler, make sure the cooler is cleaned once per month by running half a gallon of white vinegar through it, then rinsing thoroughly with about 5 gallons of clean water. For more information on drinking water safety, go to the EPA website at www.epa.gov; for information on bottled water, go to www.bottledwater.org.

References

1. International Bottled Water Association. 2011. U.S. Bottled Water Volume Grew 3.5% in 2010 as Economic Conditions Begin to Improve. www.bottledwater.org/news/us-bottled-water-volume-grew-35-2010-economic-conditions-begin-improve. (Accessed June 2012.)
2. Merkel, L., C. Bicking, and D. Sekhar. 2012. Parents' perceptions of water safety and quality. *J. Community Health.* 37:195–201.
3. Huerta-Saenz, L., M. Irigoyen, J. Benavides, and M. Mendoza. 2012. Tap or bottled water: drinking preferences among urban minority children and adolescents. *J. Community Health.* 37:54–58.
4. Saylor, A., L. S. Prokopy, and S. Amberg. 2011. What's wrong with the tap? Examining perceptions of tap water and bottled water at Purdue University. *Environmental Management* 48:588–601.

Tea is second only to water as the most commonly consumed beverage in the world. With the exception of red tea and herbal teas, which do not contain caffeine, all forms of tea come from the same plant, *Camellia sinesis*. Black tea is the most highly processed (the tea leaves are fully fermented), while oolong tea leaves are only partially fermented. Green tea leaves have been dried and steamed but not fermented. White tea is made only from the buds or first leaves of the tea plant; like green tea, white tea leaves are dried but not fermented. White and green teas have much higher levels of phytochemicals than black and oolong teas. These phytochemicals are thought to contribute to the health-promoting qualities of tea, including decreased risk for heart disease, diabetes, and certain cancers; decreased levels of LDL-cholesterol; and increased levels of HDL-cholesterol.[11] Some research suggests that green and white tea may have antibacterial and antiviral effects. All teas derived from *Camellia sinesis* provide caffeine and related stimulants. The amount of caffeine in brewed tea is usually half the amount in most brewed coffee. The longer tea leaves are fermented, the higher the caffeine level. Black tea has the most caffeine, followed by oolong and green teas; white tea has the least caffeine of all nonherbal teas. If consumed without added sugar, tea is an excellent source of fluid that may have unexpected long-term health benefits.

Chocolate and cocoa-based beverages provide small amounts of a compound called theobromine, which has effects similar to but milder than those of caffeine and is present in amounts lower than those found in coffee, tea, or colas. Dark chocolate is rich in phytochemicals known as flavanols, which may lower risk for heart attack and stroke.[12] Hot chocolate made with dark cocoa powder and skim or low-fat milk is a nutritious and satisfying drink.

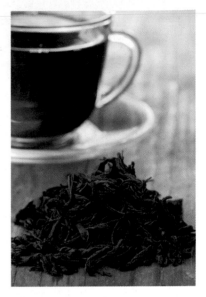

After water, tea is the most commonly consumed beverage in the world.

Soft Drinks and Other Sweet Beverages

Most soft drinks, juice drinks, flavored waters, and bottled teas and coffee drinks are loaded with added sugars. As discussed earlier (in Chapter 3), the potential health consequences of widespread use of high-fructose corn syrup (HFCS) are the subject of debate. As a result, many beverage manufacturers are switching to "pure cane sugar" to sweeten their products; however, sugars provide the same number of Calories per gram, no matter their molecular structure. Similarly, some beverage producers have begun to use "fruit juice concentrate" as a source of added sugar. Although it sounds like a healthy option, the concentrate is little more than pure sugar, with none of the fiber or other nutrients that make fruit a nutritious food. Honey is another popular source of added sugar, but it is also Calorie dense and low in nutrient value.

As many package sizes increase, the Calorie count for sweetened drinks can be unexpectedly high. For example, you might think of cranberry juice cocktail as a healthful beverage, but did you know that one 8-oz serving contains more than 7 teaspoons of added sugar, providing 112 Calories? Even 100% fruit juice with no added sugar is high in Calories. For instance, an 8-ounce serving of a popular brand of premium orange juice provides the same number of Calories as cranberry juice cocktail.

Energy Drinks

Energy drinks are another popular beverage option, with over $9 billion in sales in 2011. These products advertise their ability to provide a boost, jump start, buzz, punch, or rocket-powered blast! As many as half of all adolescents and young adults consume these products, although nutrition experts and consumer groups have raised significant concerns.[7,13] Many of these beverages contain more than three times the amount of caffeine in a comparable serving of cola, and a few contain up to ten times the caffeine in cola. In addition, many energy drinks contain guarana seed extract: guarana seeds contain more caffeine than coffee beans, so their "extract" is simply a potent source of additional caffeine. Some also contain *taurine*, an amino acid associated with muscle contraction.

There is little research on the effects of these ingredients, either alone or in combination with one another, particularly in children and adolescents. We do know that these

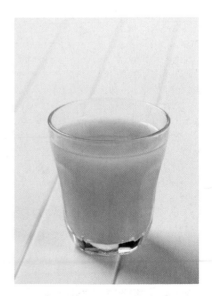

Many fruit juices are made from juice concentrate that is little more than pure sugar and, thus, are Calorie dense.

substances can significantly increase blood pressure and heart rate. Moreover, mood swings, behavioral disorders, insomnia, dizziness, tremors, seizures, caffeine dependency, dehydration, and other problems have been linked to consumption of energy drinks. Over 5,000 cases of caffeine overdose were reported in 2007; nearly half of those affected were younger than 19 years of age.[13] Although the FDA limits the amount of caffeine in soft drinks, it has no legal authority to regulate the ingredients, including caffeine, in energy drinks, since they are classified as dietary supplements, not food.

Energy drinks are also a source of significant added sugar. For example, a 16-ounce bottle of Rockstar Original contains 62 grams—more than 15 teaspoons—of sugar and 248 empty Calories. In short, as a source of fluid, energy drinks have a high potential for undesirable side effects and should be avoided by children and adolescents and used sparingly by adults.

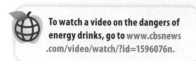

To watch a video on the dangers of energy drinks, go to www.cbsnews.com/video/watch/?id=1596076n.

Designer Waters

So-called designer waters are made with added nutrients and/or herbs that supposedly enhance memory, delay aging, boost energy levels, or strengthen the immune response. Many of these products are labeled with disclaimers such as "This statement has not been evaluated by the FDA. This product is not intended to diagnose, treat, cure, or prevent any disease." This disclaimer is required by the FDA whenever a food manufacturer makes a structure-function claim (see Chapter 2). In other words, manufacturers must acknowledge that the statements made on the labels of these designer waters are not based on research!

In fact, the amounts of nutrients or other substances added to these waters are usually so low, compared to what can be obtained from foods, that they rarely make much of an impact on the consumer's health or well-being. In contrast, if these designer waters are made with high-fructose corn syrup, cane sugar, honey, or other sweetener, they can add more than 300 Calories to the day's intake.

Sports Beverages and Coconut Water

We noted earlier that, because of the potential for fluid and electrolyte imbalances during rigorous exercise, many endurance athletes drink sports beverages, which provide water, electrolytes, and a source of carbohydrate, before, during, and after workouts. Others are turning to coconut water, marketed as a good source of electrolytes and "natural sugars." Coconut water, while growing in popularity, is still viewed primarily as a specialty product. If you drink sports beverages, you may want to check out the **Nutrition Debate** at the end of this chapter to learn whether they're right for you.

*Nutri-*Case

Theo

"Our basketball coach keeps reminding us how important it is to drink at least 8 cups of fluid a day, even on days when we don't have practice or a game. At first that seemed like an awful lot, but after keeping track of what I drank yesterday, I figure I'm good. I had a 16-ounce energy drink on my way to classes, a 12-ounce coffee mocha on my morning break, a 16-ounce Coca-Cola with lunch, and a 12-ounce bottle of Gatorade when I finished working out at the gym. With dinner in the cafeteria, I had an 8-ounce carton of chocolate milk. Then while I was studying in the dorm, I got a 12-ounce Mountain Dew from the vending machine. I'm not sure what all that adds up to, but I know it's more than 8 cups. It's not as hard as I thought to get enough fluid!"

How many ounces are in 8 cups of fluid? How many ounces of fluid did Theo drink? Did he meet, or exceed, the recommended fluid intake? What do you think of the nutritional quality of his fluid choices?

Answers are located in the MasteringNutrition Study Area.

As you can see, American consumers have a wide range of beverage choices available to them. Poor choices can increase total caloric intake and lower daily nutrient intake. Over the past 40 years, the caloric contribution of beverages to our total energy intake has almost doubled. Plain drinking water is available free of charge, contributes no Calories, contains no additives, is highly effective in quenching thirst and maintaining hydration status, and poses no health threat. For most of us, most of the time, water really is the perfect beverage choice.

Sodium

Virtually all of the dietary sodium consumed is absorbed by the body. Most dietary sodium is absorbed from the small intestine, although some can be absorbed in the large intestine. As discussed earlier in this chapter, the kidneys reabsorb sodium when it needs to be retained by the body and excrete excess sodium in the urine.

Over the past 20 years, researchers have linked high sodium intake to an increased risk for high blood pressure in some individuals. Because of this link, many people have come to believe that sodium is harmful to the body. That oversimplification, however, is just not true: sodium is essential for survival.

Functions of Sodium

Sodium has a variety of functions. As discussed earlier in this chapter, it is the major positively charged electrolyte in the extracellular fluid. Its exchange with potassium across cell membranes allows cells to maintain proper fluid balance; it also helps regulate blood pressure and acid–base balance.

Sodium also assists with the transmission of nerve signals and aids in muscle contraction and relaxation. Finally, sodium assists in the absorption of glucose from the small intestine. Glucose is absorbed via active transport that involves sodium-dependent glucose transporters.

How Much Sodium Should We Consume?

Although many people are concerned about consuming too much sodium, it should not be completely eliminated from the diet.

Recommended Dietary Intake for Sodium   The AI for sodium is 1.5 g/day (1,500 mg/day) for adult men and women aged 19 to 50 years, which is equivalent to just over half a teaspoon of salt.[4] The AI drops to 1.3 g/day for those 51 to 70 years of age and 1.2 g/d for persons over the age of 70 years. Most people in the United States greatly exceed this guideline, consuming between 3 and 6 g of sodium per day. Most health organizations recommend a daily sodium intake of no more than 2.3 g per day. The 2010 Dietary Guidelines recommend that African Americans (who have a higher risk for hypertension), people with hypertension or diabetes, and adults over the age of 51 years limit their daily sodium intake to no more than 1.5 g.[14]

Food Sources of Sodium   Sodium is found naturally in many common foods, and many processed foods contain large amounts of added sodium. Thus, it is easy to consume excess amounts in our daily diets. Try to guess which of the following foods contains the most sodium: 1 cup of tomato juice, 1 oz of potato chips, or 4 saltine crackers. Now look at **Table 9.2** (page 366) to find the answer. This table shows foods that are high in sodium and gives lower-sodium alternatives. Are you surprised to find out that, of all these food items, the tomato juice has the most sodium? When eating processed foods, such as lunch meats, canned soups and beans, vegetable juices, and prepackaged rice and pasta dishes, look for labels with the words "low-sodium" or "no added salt," as these foods are lower in sodium than the original versions.

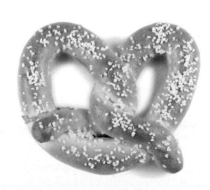

Many popular snack foods, such as pretzels, are high in sodium.

TABLE 9.2 High-Sodium Foods and Lower-Sodium Alternatives

High-Sodium Food	Sodium (mg)	Lower-Sodium Food	Sodium (mg)
Dill pickle (1 large, 4 in.)	1,731	Low-sodium dill pickle (1 large, 4 in.)	25
Ham, cured, roasted (3 oz)	1,177	Pork, loin roast (3 oz)	54
Chipped beef (3 oz)	913	Beef chuck roast, cooked (3 oz)	53
Tomato juice, regular (1 cup)	654	Tomato juice, lower sodium (1 cup)	24
Tomato sauce, canned (½ cup)	741	Fresh tomato (1 medium)	11
Canned cream corn (1 cup)	730	Cooked corn, fresh (1 cup)	28
Tomato soup, canned (1 cup)	695	Lower-sodium tomato soup, canned (1 cup)	480
Potato chips, salted (1 oz)	168	Baked potato, unsalted (1 medium)	14
Saltine crackers (4 each)	156	Saltine crackers, unsalted (4 each)	100

Source: Data from US Department of Agriculture. 2005. USDA National Nutrient Database for Standard Reference, Release 18. Nutrient Data Laboratory Home Page. www.ars.usda.gov/ba/bhnrc/ndl.

What Happens If We Consume Too Much Sodium?

People who consume high-sodium diets are at increased risk for high blood pressure, especially if their potassium intake is low.[15] This strong relationship has prompted many health organizations to recommend lowering sodium intakes. The National Salt Reduction Initiative (NSRI) is a voluntary collaboration among more than eighty organizations, with the goal of reducing sodium in restaurant and packaged foods 25% by the year 2014. A similar program in Finland led to a 30% decrease in sodium intake over several decades, with a concurrent drop in hypertension, stroke, and coronary heart disease deaths.[16] Whether high-sodium diets actually cause high blood pressure is the subject of some controversy; many researchers believe a high sodium to potassium ratio is the primary dietary pattern leading to increased risk.[16]

Also controversial is the effect of high sodium intake on bone loss: high urinary losses of sodium, which reflect high sodium intakes, have been associated with increased urinary excretion of calcium and lower bone density in young women.[17] Sodium-induced losses of calcium were greatest in those women with relatively low calcium intakes. In contrast, other research has shown that a high sodium intake did not negatively impact bone health in older women with adequate calcium intake.[18]

Hypernatremia refers to an abnormally high blood sodium concentration. It is usually caused by a rapid intake of high amounts of sodium, such as when a shipwrecked sailor drinks seawater. Eating a high-sodium diet does not usually cause hypernatremia in a healthy person, as the kidneys are able to excrete excess sodium in the urine. But people with congestive heart failure or kidney disease are not able to excrete sodium effectively, making them more prone to the condition. Hypernatremia is dangerous, because it causes an abnormally high blood volume, leading to edema (swelling) of tissues and raising blood pressure to unhealthy levels.

What Happens If We Don't Consume Enough Sodium?

Because dietary sodium intake is so high in the United States, deficiencies are extremely rare, except in individuals who sweat heavily or consume little or no sodium in the diet. Nevertheless, certain conditions can cause dangerously low blood sodium levels. **Hyponatremia,** abnormally low blood sodium concentration, can occur in active people who drink large volumes of water and fail to replace sodium. This was the subject of the

hypernatremia A condition in which blood sodium levels are dangerously high.

hyponatremia A condition in which blood sodium levels are dangerously low.

Can Water Be Too Much of a Good Thing? Hyponatremia in Marathon Runners

The 2002 death of Boston Marathon runner Cynthia Lucero, the 2007 death of London Marathon runner David Rogers, and several similar deaths have gained attention in recent years. How can seemingly healthy, highly fit individuals competing in marathons collapse and even die during or after a race? One common challenge faced by these athletes is maintaining a proper balance of fluid and electrolytes during the race.

It is well known that people participating in distance events, such as marathons (26.2 miles), need to drink enough fluid to ensure proper fluid balance. But how much is enough? The winner of the women's marathon in the Athens Olympics, running in 97-degree heat, drank for just 30 seconds of the entire race. Surprisingly, recent research has suggested that some runners, particularly novices, may be at greater risk from drinking too much water than from drinking too little.[1]

Risk factors for exercise-associated hyponatremia among marathon runners include a longer race time (slower pace), female gender, low BMI, lower rate of sweating, and intake of large amounts of fluid during the race.[1,2] Experts observe that elite runners complete a race more quickly and drink as they run; thus, they simply don't have time to overdo the fluids. In contrast, less experienced athletes run more slowly, increasing the total time that they are competing; at the same time, they consume very large amounts of fluid to avoid potential dehydration. The slower and longer these individuals run, the more they drink and the more diluted their blood sodium levels become. One recent study found that 12% of participants in a marathon developed hyponatremia,[3] although other studies report rates as high as 20%. As many as half of hyponatremic runners require hospitalization.

Hyponatremia is a dangerous and potentially fatal condition, but it can be prevented. There is now greater emphasis on appropriate hydration, as compared to what had typically been a one-sided promotion emphasizing the need to drink. Having said that, the fear of hyponatremia should not cause athletes to avoid drinking adequate fluids during long-distance activities, as dehydration and subsequent heat

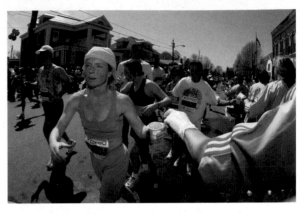

Consuming too much water can deplete blood sodium levels.

illness are as important to prevent as hyponatremia. The key to staying safe during competitive events is to match fluid and sodium intake with sweat loss. Athletes should weigh themselves regularly before and after training to determine average sweat loss and then consume enough fluid to minimize loss of body weight but not enough to cause weight gain. Drinking sports beverages, which contain electrolytes (particularly sodium), and moderating fluid intake during marathons and other long-distance events can also help prevent hyponatremia.

References

1. American College of Sports Medicine, American Dietetic Association, and Dietitians of Canada. 2009. Joint position statement: nutrition and athletic performance. *Med. Sci. Sports Exercise.* 41:709–731.
2. Potter, V. J. V. 2011. Eat your water for health, sport performance, and weight control. *Am. J. Lifestyle Med.* 5:316–319.
3. Kipps, C., S. Sharma, and D. T. Pedoe. 2011. The incidence of exercise-associated hyponatremia in the London Marathon. *Brit. J. Sports Med.* 45:14–19.

chapter-opening vignette and is discussed in the **Highlight** box (above). Severe diarrhea, vomiting, or excessive, prolonged sweating can also cause hyponatremia.

Symptoms of hyponatremia include headaches, dizziness, fatigue, nausea, vomiting, and muscle cramps. If hyponatremia is left untreated, it can lead to seizures, coma, and death. Treatment for hyponatremia includes the ingestion of liquids and foods high in sodium and may even require the administration of electrolyte-rich solutions intravenously if the person has lost consciousness or is not able to consume beverages and foods by mouth.[12–15]

RECAP

Sodium is the primary positively charged electrolyte in the extracellular fluid. It works to maintain fluid balance and blood pressure, assists in acid–base balance and transmission of nerve signals, aids muscle contraction, and assists in the absorption of some nutrients. The AI for sodium is 1.5 g per day. Deficiencies are rare, because the typical American diet is high in sodium. Excessive sodium intake, particularly when potassium intake is low, has been related to high blood pressure and, on low-calcium diets, loss of bone density. ■

Potassium

As we discussed previously, potassium is the major positively charged electrolyte in the intracellular fluid. It is a major constituent of all living cells and is found in both plants and animals. About 85% of dietary potassium is absorbed, and, as with sodium, the kidneys regulate reabsorption and urinary excretion of potassium.

Functions of Potassium

Potassium and sodium work together to maintain proper fluid balance and to regulate the contraction of muscles and transmission of nerve impulses. Potassium also assists in maintaining blood pressure. In contrast with a high-sodium diet, eating a diet high in potassium actually helps maintain a lower blood pressure.

How Much Potassium Should We Consume?

We can reduce our risk for high blood pressure by consuming adequate potassium in our diets. The AI for potassium for adult men and women aged 19 to 50 years is 4.7 g/day (4,700 mg/day).[3] Unlike sodium, which is abundant in the typical American diet, potassium is abundant in foods that many Americans fail to consume in adequate amounts, particularly fresh fruits and vegetables. **Figure 9.9** identifies foods that are high

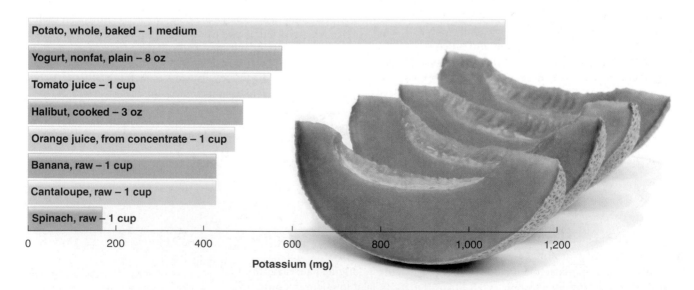

FIGURE 9.9 Common food sources of potassium. The AI for potassium is 4.7 g/day. (*Source:* Data from US Department of Agriculture, Agricultural Research Service. 2009. USDA Nutrient Database for Standard Reference, Release 22. Nutrient Data Laboratory Home Page. www.ars.usda.gov/ba/bhnrc/ndl.)

in potassium. Processing foods generally increases their amount of sodium and decreases their amount of potassium. Thus, you can optimize your potassium intake and reduce your sodium intake by avoiding processed foods and eating more fresh fruits, vegetables, legumes, and whole grains. Following these tips can also help you increase your consumption of potassium:

- For breakfast, look for cereals containing bran and/or wheat germ, or sprinkle fruit and yogurt with wheat germ.
- Toss a banana, some dried apricots, or a bag of sunflower seeds into your backpack for a mid-morning snack.
- Instead of soft drinks, choose low-fat milk, kefir, soy milk, or low-sodium vegetable juice, or blend low-fat vanilla yogurt with ice cubes and a banana.
- Serve avocado or bean dip with veggie slices.
- Make a tropical salad with avocado, papaya, and grapefruit.
- Make sweet potato fries (toss potato slices in olive oil and bake at 400° for 15–20 minutes), or bake a wedge of acorn squash.

Salmon and other fish, lean cuts of beef, and tomato juice are other foods that can boost your potassium intake. As discussed ahead, the DASH (Dietary Approaches to Stop Hypertension) diet is designed to provide an optimal intake of potassium.

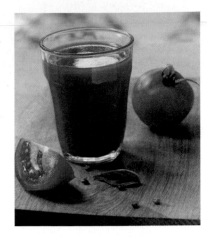

Low-sodium tomato juice is an excellent source of potassium.

What Happens If We Consume Too Much Potassium?

People with healthy kidneys are able to excrete excess potassium effectively. However, people with kidney disease are not able to regulate their blood potassium levels. **Hyperkalemia,** or high blood potassium concentration, occurs when potassium is not efficiently excreted from the body. Because of potassium's role in cardiac muscle contraction, severe hyperkalemia can alter the normal rhythm of the heart, resulting in heart attack and death. People with kidney disease must monitor their potassium intake very carefully and should avoid consuming salt substitutes, as these products are high in potassium.

What Happens If We Don't Consume Enough Potassium?

Because potassium is widespread in many foods, a dietary potassium deficiency is rare. However, potassium deficiency is not uncommon among people who have serious medical disorders. Kidney disease, diabetic ketoacidosis, and other illnesses can lead to potassium deficiency.

In addition, people with high blood pressure who are prescribed certain diuretic medications to treat their disease are at risk for potassium deficiency. As we noted earlier, diuretics promote the excretion of fluid as urine through the kidneys. Some diuretics also increase the body's urinary excretion of potassium. People who are taking diuretic medications should have their blood potassium monitored regularly and should eat foods that are high in potassium to prevent **hypokalemia,** or low blood potassium concentration. This is not a universal recommendation, however, because some diuretics are specially formulated to spare or retain potassium; therefore, people taking diuretics should consult their physician regarding dietary potassium intake.

Extreme dehydration, vomiting, and diarrhea can also cause hypokalemia, as can long-term consumption of natural licorice, which contains glycyrrhizic acid (GZA), a substance that increases urinary excretion of potassium. Because the majority of foods that contain licorice flavoring in the United States do not contain GZA, licorice-induced hypokalemia is rarely seen here. People who abuse alcohol or laxatives can suffer from hypokalemia. Symptoms include confusion, loss of appetite, and muscle weakness. Severe cases of hypokalemia result in fatal changes in heart rate; many deaths attributed to extreme dehydration or an eating disorder are caused by abnormal heart rhythms due to hypokalemia.

hyperkalemia A condition in which blood potassium levels are dangerously high.

hypokalemia A condition in which blood potassium levels are dangerously low.

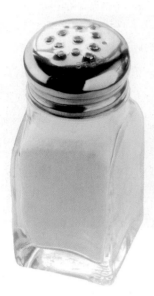

Almost all dietary chloride is consumed through table salt.

RECAP

Potassium is the major positively charged electrolyte inside of the cell. It regulates fluid balance, blood pressure, and muscle contraction, and it helps in the transmission of nerve impulses. The AI for potassium is 4.7 g per day. Potassium is found in abundance in fresh foods, particularly fruits and vegetables. Both hyperkalemia and hypokalemia can result in heart failure and death. ■

Chloride

Chloride is a negatively charged ion that is obtained almost exclusively from sodium chloride, or table salt. It should not be confused with *chlorine,* which is a poisonous gas used to kill germs in our water supply. As with sodium, the majority of dietary chloride is absorbed in the small intestine. The kidneys regulate urinary excretion of chloride.

Functions of Chloride

Coupled with sodium in the extracellular fluid, chloride assists with the maintenance of fluid balance. Chloride is also a part of hydrochloric acid (HCl) in the stomach. Chloride also works with the white blood cells during an immune response to help kill bacteria, and it assists in the transmission of nerve impulses.

How Much Chloride Should We Consume?

The AI for chloride for adult men and women aged 19 to 50 years is 2.3 g/day (2,300 mg/day).[3] As chloride is coupled with sodium to form table salt, our primary dietary source of chloride is salt in our foods. Chloride is also found in some fruits and vegetables. Keep in mind that salt is composed of about 60% chloride; thus, you can calculate the content of chloride in processed foods by multiplying its salt content by 0.60 (60%). For instance, a food that contains 500 mg of salt would contain 300 mg of chloride (500 mg $\times$ 0.60 = 300 mg).

Because we consume virtually all of our dietary chloride in the form of sodium chloride, there is no known toxicity symptom for chloride alone, although consuming excess amounts of sodium chloride over a prolonged period leads to hypertension in salt-sensitive individuals. Chloride deficiency is rare, even in people who consume a low-sodium diet. It can occur, however, during conditions of severe dehydration and frequent vomiting. This is sometimes seen in people with eating disorders who regularly vomit to rid their bodies of unwanted energy.

Phosphorus

Phosphorus is the major intracellular negatively charged electrolyte. In the body, phosphorus is most commonly found combined with oxygen in the form of phosphate, PO_4^{-3}. Phosphorus is an essential constituent of all cells and is found in both plants and animals. Adults absorb about 55% to 70% of dietary phosphorus, primarily in the small intestine. The active form of vitamin D (1,25-dihydroxyvitamin D, or calcitriol) facilitates the absorption of phosphorus, whereas consumption of aluminum-containing antacids and high doses of calcium carbonate reduce its absorption. The kidneys regulate reabsorption and urinary excretion of phosphorus.

Functions of Phosphorus

Phosphorus works with potassium inside the cell to maintain proper fluid balance. It also plays a critical role in bone formation, as it is a part of the mineral complex of bone. In fact, about 85% of the body's phosphorus is stored in the bones.

As a primary component of ATP, phosphorus plays a key role in creating energy for the body through the reactions in glycolysis and oxidative phosphorylation. It also helps regulate many biochemical reactions by activating and deactivating enzymes during phosphorylation. Phosphorus is a part of both DNA and RNA, and it is a component of cell membranes (as phospholipids) and of lipoproteins.

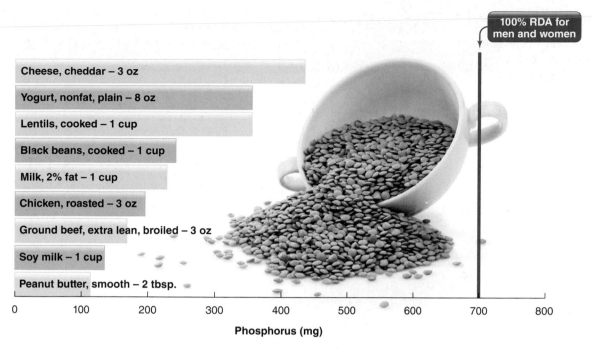

FIGURE 9.10 Common food sources of phosphorus. The RDA for phosphorus is 700 mg/day. (*Source:* Data from US Department of Agriculture, Agricultural Research Service. 2009. USDA Nutrient Database for Standard Reference, Release 22. Nutrient Data Laboratory Home Page. www.ars.usda.gov/ba/bhnrc/ndl.)

How Much Phosphorus Should We Consume?

The RDA for phosphorus is 700 mg per day.[19] The average U.S. adult consumes about twice this amount each day; thus, phosphorus deficiencies are rare. Phosphorus is widespread in many foods and is found in high amounts in foods that contain protein. Milk, meats, and eggs are good sources of phosphorus (**Figure 9.10**).

It is important to note that phosphorus from animal sources is absorbed more readily than phosphorus from plant sources. Much of the phosphorus in plant foods such as beans, whole-grain cereals, and nuts is found in the form of **phytic acid,** a plant storage form of phosphorus. Our bodies do not produce enzymes that can break down phytic acid, but we are still able to absorb up to 50% of the phosphorus found in plant foods because the bacteria in the large intestine can break down phytic acid. Soft drinks are another common source of phosphorus in the American diet.

People suffering from kidney disease and people taking too many vitamin D supplements or too many phosphorus-containing antacids can suffer from high blood phosphorus levels. Severely high levels of blood phosphorus cause muscle spasms and convulsions.

As previously noted, deficiencies of phosphorus are rare. People who may suffer from low blood phosphorus levels include premature infants, elderly people with poor diets, and people who abuse alcohol. People with vitamin D deficiency—hyperparathyroidism (oversecretion of parathyroid hormone)—and those who overuse antacids that bind with phosphorus may also have low blood phosphorus levels.

RECAP

Chloride is the major negatively charged electrolyte outside the cell, and phosphorus is the major negatively charged electrolyte inside the cell. Both are important for fluid balance. The AI for chloride is 2.3 g per day. Our main dietary source of chloride is sodium chloride. The RDA for phosphorus is 700 mg per day, and it is commonly found in high-protein foods. ■

phytic acid The form of phosphorus stored in plants.

TABLE 9.3 Percentages of Body Fluid Loss Correlated with Weight Loss and Symptoms

% Body Water Loss	Weight Lost If You Weigh 160 lb	Weight Lost If You Weigh 130 lb	Symptoms
1–2	1.6 lb–3.2 lb	1.3 lb–2.6 lb	Strong thirst, loss of appetite, feeling uncomfortable
3–5	4.8 lb–8.0 lb	3.9 lb–6.5 lb	Dry mouth, reduced urine output, greater difficulty working and concentrating, flushed skin, tingling extremities, impatience, sleepiness, nausea, emotional instability
6–8	9.6 lb–12.8 lb	7.8 lb–10.4 lb	Increased body temperature that doesn't decrease, increased heart rate and breathing rate, dizziness, difficulty breathing, slurred speech, mental confusion, muscle weakness, blue lips
9–11	14.4 lb–17.6 lb	11.7 lb–14.3 lb	Muscle spasms, delirium, swollen tongue, poor balance and circulation, kidney failure, decreased blood volume and blood pressure

What Disorders Are Related to Fluid and Electrolyte Imbalances?

A number of serious, and potentially fatal, disorders can result from an imbalance of fluid and electrolytes in the body, while other disorders contribute to fluid and electrolyte imbalance. We review some of these here.

Dehydration

Dehydration is a serious health problem that results when fluid losses exceed fluid intake. It can occur as a result of heavy exercise or exposure to high environmental temperatures, when the body loses significant amounts of water through increased sweating and breathing. However, elderly people and infants can get dehydrated even when inactive, as their risk for dehydration is much higher than that of healthy young and middle-aged adults. The elderly are at increased risk because they have a lower total amount of body water and their thirst mechanism is less effective than that of a younger person; they are therefore less likely to meet their fluid needs. Infants, on the other hand, excrete urine at a higher rate, cannot tell us when they are thirsty, and have a greater ratio of body surface area to body core, causing their bodies to respond more dramatically to heat and cold and to lose more body water than older children.

Dehydration is classified in terms of the percentage of weight loss that is exclusively due to the loss of fluid. As indicated in **Table 9.3**, relatively small losses in body water result in symptoms such as thirst, discomfort, and loss of appetite. More severe water losses result in symptoms that include sleepiness, nausea, flushed skin, and problems with mental concentration. Severe losses of body water can result in delirium, coma, cardiac arrest, and death.

We discussed earlier the importance of fluid replacement when you are exercising. How can you tell whether you are drinking enough fluid before, during, and after your exercise sessions? First, you can measure your body weight before and after each session. If you weighed in at 160 lb before basketball practice, and immediately afterward you weigh 158 lb, then you have lost 2 lb of body weight. This is equal to 1.3% of your body weight prior to practice. As you can see in Table 9.3, you are most likely feeling strong thirst, diminished appetite, and even general discomfort. Your goal is to consume enough water and other fluids to fully rehydrate prior to your next exercise session. This would require drinking about 1.5 times as much fluid as was lost (1 pound of weight loss equals 2 cups of fluid).[20]

A simpler method of monitoring your fluid levels is to observe the color of your urine (**Figure 9.11**). If you are properly hydrated, your urine should be clear to pale

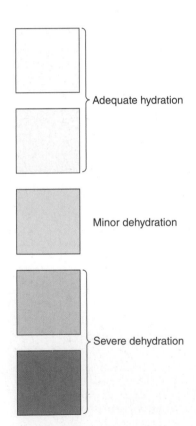

FIGURE 9.11 Urine color chart. Color variations indicate levels of hydration.

- Adequate hydration
- Minor dehydration
- Severe dehydration

dehydration The depletion of body fluid, which results when fluid excretion exceeds fluid intake.

yellow in color, similar to diluted lemonade. Urine that is medium to dark yellow in color, similar to apple juice, indicates an inadequate fluid intake. Very dark or brown-colored urine, such as the color of a cola beverage, is a sign of severe dehydration and indicates potential muscle breakdown and kidney damage. People should strive to maintain a urine color that is clear or pale yellow.

Heat Stroke

Heat stroke is a potentially fatal heat illness characterized by failure of the body's heat-regulating mechanisms. Symptoms include rapid pulse; hot, dry skin; high temperature; vomiting; diarrhea; hallucinations; and loss of consciousness (coma).

Recall that evaporative cooling is less efficient in a humid environment, because the sweat is less able to evaporate. Therefore, athletes who work out in hot, humid weather are particularly vulnerable to heat stroke. Over a 1-week period in 2011, one coach and three high school football players died from heat-related complications.[21] These deaths are more common in overweight or obese athletes for two reasons. Significant muscle mass produces a lot of body heat, while excess body fat adds an extra layer of insulation that makes it more difficult to dissipate that heat. Tight-fitting uniforms and helmets also trap warm air and blunt the body's ability to cool itself.

Heat-related deaths also occur among collegiate and professional athletes. These deaths have prompted national attention and resulted in strict guidelines encouraging regular fluid breaks and cancellation of events or changing the time of the event to avoid high heat and humidity. In addition, people who are active in a hot environment should stop exercising if they feel dizzy, light-headed, disoriented, or nauseated. Heat illnesses can be avoided by following established guidelines for fluid intake before, during, and after exercise.

Water Intoxication

Recall that it is possible to drink too much water. **Overhydration,** or *water intoxication,* is rare. It generally occurs only in people with health problems that cause the kidneys to retain too much water, causing overhydration and hyponatremia, which were discussed earlier. However, in addition to the hazing rituals discussed in our chapter opening, individuals have died of overhydration while following a fad diet or participating in a competition encouraging excessive water intake. In a 2007 radio contest, staff members pressured contestants to consume very large amounts of water in a short period of time while preventing them from going to the bathroom. One contestant, a 28-year-old mother who wanted to win the contest prize, a video game console, for her three children, died a few hours after returning home. In 2012, a 12-year-old girl died after participating in a card game with friends in which the loser of each hand had to drink a glass of water. Thus, the overconsumption of water can be deadly and should never be thought of as a prank or a joke.

Hypertension

One of the major chronic diseases in the United States is high blood pressure, which healthcare professionals refer to as **hypertension.** A person with hypertension is unable to maintain blood pressure in a healthy range. It was recently estimated that nearly 32% of U.S. adults over the age of 20 have hypertension.[22] The prevalence is even higher (42%) among African American adults.[23]Although hypertension itself is often without symptoms, it increases a person's risk for many other serious conditions, including heart disease, stroke, and kidney disease; it can also reduce brain function, impair physical mobility, and cause death.

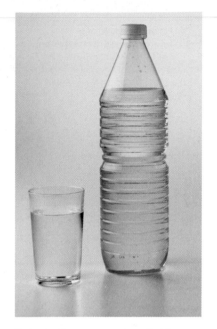

Dehydration occurs when fluid losses exceed fluid intake.

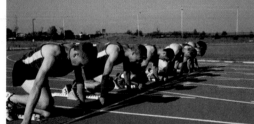

Athletes who train or compete in hot weather are vulnerable to heat stroke.

heat stroke   A potentially fatal heat illness characterized by hot, dry skin; rapid heart rate; vomiting; diarrhea; elevated body temperature; hallucinations; and coma.

overhydration   The dilution of body fluid. It results when water intake or retention is excessive.

hypertension   A chronic condition characterized by above-average blood pressure readings–specifically, systolic blood pressure over 140 mm Hg or diastolic blood pressure over 90 mm Hg.

For an informative video on hypertension and its consequences, visit http://www.thevisualmd.com/health_centers/cardiovascular_health/hypertension/what_is_hypertension_video

How Is Hypertension Defined?

Blood pressure is measured in two phases: systolic and diastolic. *Systolic blood pressure* represents the pressure exerted in the arteries at the moment that the heart contracts, sending blood into the blood vessels. *Diastolic blood pressure* represents the pressure in the arteries between contractions, when the heart is relaxed. You can also think of diastolic blood pressure as the resistance in the arteries that the heart must pump against every time it beats. Blood pressure is measured in millimeters of mercury (mm Hg). When your blood pressure is measured, the systolic pressure is given first, followed by the diastolic pressure. For example, your reading might be given as "115 (systolic) over 75 (diastolic)." Here are the clinical classifications of blood pressure measurements:

- Optimal blood pressure is a systolic blood pressure *less than* 120 mm Hg and a diastolic blood pressure *less than* 80 mm Hg.
- Pre-hypertension is defined as a systolic blood pressure between 120 and 139 mm Hg or a diastolic blood pressure between 80 and 89 mm Hg.
- Hypertension is a systolic blood pressure greater than or equal to 140 mm Hg or a diastolic blood pressure greater than or equal to 90 mm Hg.

What Causes Hypertension?

For about 90% to 95% of people who have hypertension, its causes are unknown. This type is referred to as *primary,* or *essential, hypertension.* For the other 5% to 10% of people with hypertension, the causes include kidney disease, sleep apnea (a sleep disorder that affects breathing), and chronic alcohol abuse. It is estimated that over half of all adults with hypertension have a condition known as **salt sensitivity.** These people respond to a high salt intake by experiencing an increase in blood pressure; they also experience a decrease in blood pressure when salt intake is low. People who do not experience changes in blood pressure with changes in salt intake are referred to as **salt resistant.**

Risk factors associated with hypertension include overweight and obesity, as increased blood volume leads to increased pressure on blood vessel walls. Low levels of physical activity also increase the risk. Tobacco use is a primary risk factor for hypertension, because it immediately raises blood pressure, and chronic use damages the lining of the blood vessels, increasing the likelihood of plaque deposition. Excessive alcohol intake and a poor diet are also risk factors.

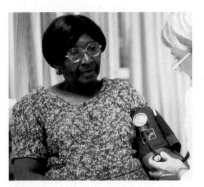

Hypertension is a major chronic disease in the United States, affecting more than 50% of adults over 65 years of age.

Lifestyle Changes Can Reduce Hypertension

Although we do not know what causes most cases of hypertension, certain lifestyle changes can help reduce it:[24]

- Lose weight. Systolic blood pressure values have been shown to decrease 5 to 20 points in people who were overweight or obese and lost an average of 22 lb of body weight.
- Increase your physical activity. The amount and intensity of exercise needed to improve blood pressure are easily achievable for most people. Regular physical activity, such as brisk walking, lasting at least 30 minutes per day most days of the week, can help lower blood pressure.
- Reduce your alcohol intake. Because alcohol consumption can worsen high blood pressure, it is suggested that people with this disease abstain from drinking alcohol or limit their intake to no more than one (women) or two (men) drinks per day.
- Reduce your sodium intake, especially if you are salt sensitive. Some people who are not salt sensitive also benefit from eating lower-sodium diets.
- Eat more whole grains, fruits, vegetables, and low-fat dairy foods.
- Stop smoking. If you currently use tobacco, quit.

Among nutrition and healthcare professionals, one area of controversy is the impact that sodium intake has on our blood pressure. For years it was believed that the high sodium intakes of the typical American diet led to hypertension. This is because people who

salt sensitivity   A condition in which certain people respond to a high salt intake by experiencing an increase in blood pressure; these people also experience a decrease in blood pressure when salt intake is low.

salt resistant   A condition in which certain people do not experience changes in blood pressure with changes in salt intake.

live in countries in which sodium intake is high have greater rates of hypertension than people from countries in which sodium intake is low. We have recently learned, however, that not everyone with hypertension is sensitive to sodium. Unfortunately, it is impossible to know who is, as there is no definitive test for the condition. Because lowering sodium intake does not reduce blood pressure in all people with hypertension, there is significant debate over whether everyone can benefit from eating a lower-sodium diet. Despite this debate, the leading health organizations, including the American Heart Association, the National High Blood Pressure Education Program, and the National Heart, Lung, and Blood Institute of the National Institutes of Health, continue to support a reduction in dietary sodium to 2,300 mg per day, as recommended in the Dietary Guidelines for Americans.[14] Currently, the average sodium intake in the United States is about 3,400 mg per day. As previously noted, these efforts are being increasingly supported by food manufacturers, the restaurant industry, and other corporate partners.[16]

The Role of the DASH Diet Plan

The **DASH diet** plan resulted from a large research study funded by the National Institutes of Health (NIH).[2, 25] DASH stands for Dietary Approaches to Stop Hypertension; thus, this study was designed to assess the effects of the DASH Diet on high blood pressure. **Figure 9.12** (page 376) shows the DASH eating plan for a 2,000-kcal-per-day diet. This plan is similar to the goals of the *Dietary Guidelines for Americans, 2010*[14] in that it is low in fat and high in fiber. The DASH Diet also emphasizes foods that are rich in potassium, calcium, and magnesium, including 10 servings of fruits and vegetables each day along with whole-grain foods and low-fat or nonfat milk and dairy products. The sodium content of the DASH Diet is about 3 g (or 3,000 mg) of sodium, which is slightly less than the average sodium intake in the United States.

Over the past several years, many research studies have convincingly illustrated that eating the DASH Diet has a positive impact on blood pressure, even among adolescents.[25] Decreases in blood pressure can occur within the first 2 weeks of following it. Researchers estimated that if all Americans followed the DASH diet plan, heart disease would be reduced by 15% and the number of strokes would be 27% lower.

Another study of the DASH Diet found that blood pressure continues to decrease if sodium intake is reduced below 3,000 mg per day.[26] Participants ate a DASH Diet that provided high, intermediate, and low levels of sodium. After 1 month on this diet, all people eating the DASH Diet saw a significant decrease in their blood pressure; however, those who ate the lowest-sodium version of the DASH Diet experienced the largest decrease. Additional research has shown that the benefits of the DASH Diet are also enhanced when combined with exercise or weight loss.[27] These results indicate that eating a diet low in sodium and high in fruits and vegetables, whole grains, and low/no-fat dairy reduces blood pressure and decreases the risk for heart disease and stroke.

In addition to its beneficial effects in reducing blood pressure, the DASH Diet has also been shown to lower risk for coronary heart disease and stroke,[28] as well as the risk for metabolic syndrome.[29] Finally, the DASH Diet has been shown to be particularly beneficial in hypertensive African Americans, a population group at very high risk for the disease and its complications.[30]

Medications

For some individuals, lifestyle changes are not completely effective in normalizing hypertension. When this is the case, a variety of medications can bring a person's blood pressure into the normal range. Individuals taking medications to control blood pressure should also continue to practice the healthful lifestyle changes identified earlier, as these changes will continue to benefit their long-term health.

Hypertension is called "the silent killer," because often there are no obvious symptoms of this disease. For this reason, it is important that people get their blood pressure checked

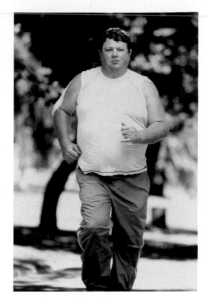

Losing weight and increasing physical activity can help fight hypertension.

DASH diet The Dietary Approaches to Stop Hypertension diet plan emphasizing fruits and vegetables, whole grains, low/no-fat milk and dairy, and lean meats.

FIGURE 9.12 The DASH diet plan. The plan is based on a 2,000-kcal-per-day diet. The number of servings in a food group may differ from the number listed here, depending on your own energy needs. (*Source:* "Healthier Eating with DASH," National Institutes of Health from National Heart, Lung and Blood Institute website.)

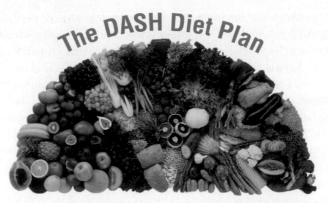

The DASH Diet Plan

Food Group	Daily Servings	Serving Size
Grains and grain products	7–8	1 slice bread 1 cup ready-to-eat cereal* ½ cup cooked rice, pasta, or cereal
Vegetables	4–5	1 cup raw leafy vegetables ½ cup cooked vegetable 6 fl. oz vegetable juice
Fruits	4–5	1 medium fruit ¼ cup dried fruit ½ cup fresh, frozen, or canned fruit 6 fl. oz fruit juice
Low-fat or fat-free dairy foods	2–3	8 fl. oz milk 1 cup yogurt 1½ oz cheese
Lean meats, poultry, and fish	2 or less	3 oz cooked lean meats, skinless poultry, or fish
Nuts, seeds, and dry beans	4–5 per week	⅓ cup or 1½ oz nuts 1 tbsp. or ½ oz seeds ½ cup cooked dry beans
Fats and oils†	2–3	1 tsp. soft margarine 1 tbsp. low-fat mayonnaise 2 tbsp. light salad dressing 1 tsp. vegetable oil
Sweets	5 per week	1 tbsp. sugar 1 tbsp. jelly or jam ½ oz jelly beans 8 fl. oz lemonade

*Serving sizes vary between ½ and 1¼ cups. Check the product's nutrition label.

†Fat content changes serving counts for fats and oils: for example, 1 tablespoon of regular salad dressing equals 1 serving; 1 tablespoon of a low-fat dressing equals ½ serving; 1 tablespoon of a fat-free dressing equals 0 servings.

seizures Uncontrollable muscle spasms caused by increased nervous system excitability that can result from electrolyte imbalances or a chronic disease, such as epilepsy.

muscle cramps Involuntary, spasmodic, and painful muscle contractions that last for many seconds or even minutes; electrolyte imbalances are often the cause of muscle cramps.

on a regular basis. Tragically, many people with hypertension fail to take their prescribed medication because they do not feel sick. Some of these people eventually suffer the consequences of their actions by experiencing a heart attack or stroke.

Neuromuscular Disorders

Because nerves synapse with muscles, electrolyte imbalances that alter nervous system function will in turn disturb muscle function. For example, **seizures** are uncontrollable muscle spasms that may be localized to one area of the body, such as the face, or can violently wrack a person's entire body. **Muscle cramps** are involuntary, spasmodic, and painful muscle contractions that last for many seconds or even minutes. Hypernatremia that occurs with dehydration is known to cause cramps, as are other electrolyte imbalances. Muscle weakness and paralysis can also occur with severe electrolyte imbalances, such as hypokalemia, hyperkalemia, and low blood phosphorus levels.

Kidney Disorders

The kidneys play a major role in the regulation of fluid, electrolyte, and acid–base balance, so it is not surprising that diseases of the kidneys result in abnormalities throughout the body. Many forms of kidney disease lead to edema and abnormal retention of body fluid, since the kidneys are no longer able to effectively excrete excess fluid. Similarly, blood levels of many electrolytes, such as sodium, potassium, and phosphorus, increase to dangerously high concentrations. High levels of potassium can lead to abnormal heart rhythms and heart failure, while increased levels of phosphorus can drive down serum calcium levels.

Congestive Heart Failure

Congestive heart failure (CHF) is a condition in which the heart can no longer pump an adequate supply of blood to the rest of the body. It can develop following an infection involving the heart or from coronary artery disease, heart valve disease, or other disorders. When the heart fails to adequately pump blood, fluids tend to accumulate in certain tissues and body spaces. If the right side of the heart fails, fluid accumulates in the legs and feet, as well as the abdominal area. Failure of the left side of the heart leads to accumulation of fluid in the lungs, causing shortness of breath and inability to maintain activity levels. Management of congestive heart failure often includes restriction of sodium and fluids. To calculate appropriate fluid restriction for a client with CHF, see the **You Do the Math** box (below).

Obesity

Among many Americans, inappropriate beverage choices contribute significantly to weight gain and obesity. Until about 50 years ago, beverage choices were fairly limited and serving sizes were small—the original bottles of Coca-Cola held just 6 to 7 ounces! The

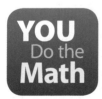

Calculating Fluid Restriction

Fluid restriction is often required in the management of congestive heart failure (CHF). A typical fluid "prescription" is 30 mL/ kg body weight/day. Suppose that one of your older relatives suffers from CHF and asks you to help figure out a day's worth of beverages. (In this example, we will ignore the water content of foods, although many dietitians include foods when calculating the fluid intake of seriously ill patients.) Your relative weighs 168 lb and enjoys drinking milk, orange juice, and plain water.

In order to calculate how many fluid ounces are permitted each day, you will first need to convert body weight from pounds to kilograms:

$$168 \text{ lb} \div 2.2 \text{ lb/kg} = 76.4 \text{ kg}$$

Next, multiply the fluid allowance of 30 mL/kg by body weight:

$$30 \text{ mL/kg} \times 76.4 \text{ kg} = 2,292 \text{ mL}$$

Finally, convert mL to fluid ounces. There are roughly 30 mL/fl. oz:

$$2,292 \text{ mL} \div 30 \text{ mL/fl. oz} = \text{around 76 fl. oz}$$

Your relative could drink 12 fl. oz of milk, 8 fl. oz of orange juice, and 56 fl. oz of water or other beverages.

Here is a similar problem for you to solve: a young woman is restricted to 25 mL/kg body weight/day. She weighs 122 lb. How much total fluid (in fluid ounces) is she allowed to drink each day?

Answers are located online in the MasteringNutrition Study Area.

introduction of a very cheap sweetener, high-fructose corn syrup, and dramatic changes in the sizing, marketing, and sales of beverages led to a surge in the popularity of super-size sodas and other sweetened drinks. Today, a convenience-store soda may hold 64 ounces, with 59 teaspoons of sugar and 800 Calories!

Although sales of sweetened beverages have dropped considerably over the past few years, Americans continue to take in approximately 21% of their Calories from beverages, mostly in the form of sweetened soft drinks and fruit juices. As we discussed earlier, sweetened bottled waters, bottled teas, energy drinks, and specialty coffee drinks have also contributed to the problem: a "frappucino" at one prominent national coffee chain provides 520 Calories, which is more than one-fourth of an average adult's total daily Calorie needs.

Beverages with a high Calorie content do little to curb appetite, so most people do not compensate for the extra Calories they drink by eating less. In addition, sweetened beverages displace more nutritious beverages, such as milk, which provides protein, calcium, vitamin D, and other nutrients important for bone health.

In the past, very few people realized how many Calories were in the sweetened beverages they drank, and how significantly such beverages were contributing to the growing problem of obesity. Recently, however, public health agencies have been raising awareness of the empty Calorie content of sweetened beverages, and some are advocating that a first step in any weight-loss program should be to entirely eliminate these products from the diet. Some municipalities have proposed taxing soft drinks and other sugary beverages, and in May 2012, the mayor of New York City announced a proposed ban on the sale of all sugary drinks larger than 16 ounces at city restaurants, delis, food kiosks, movie theaters, and stadiums. Members of the American Beverage Association have not committed to reducing the level of added sugars in their products; however, they have launched a "Clear on Calories" campaign, which clearly puts Calorie information on the front of the product. All beverages packaged in containers 20 fl. oz or smaller now display the total Calories per package, not just per serving. Thus, when consumers buy a 20-oz bottle of sweetened tea, they know they'll be consuming, for example, 250 Calories if they drink the whole bottle.

To watch a video of the American Beverage Association's Clear on Calories ad, go to www.ameribev.org/nutrition--science/clear-on-calories/ads--multimedia/.

RECAP

Dehydration, heat stroke, and even death can occur when water loss exceeds water intake. Hypertension is a major chronic illness in the United States; it can often be controlled by losing weight if overweight, increasing physical activity, avoiding smoking, decreasing alcohol intake, and making specific dietary changes, such as those in the DASH Diet. Electrolyte imbalances can lead to neuromuscular disorders. Fluid and electrolyte imbalances can result from diseases such as certain forms of kidney and heart failure. Excessive intake of sugary beverages can contribute significantly to obesity. ∎

Chapter Review

TEST YOURSELF | *ANSWERS*

1 **T** Between approximately 50% and 70% of our body weight consists of fluid.

2 **F** Sodium is a nutrient necessary for health, but we should not consume more than recommended amounts.

3 **F** Children rarely exercise to the point of needing the added sugar and electrolytes found in sports beverages. Pure water is almost always the best choice.

4 **F** There is no evidence that bottled water consistently offers any additional health or nutrition benefits compared to tap water.

5 **F** We do not know the precise cause of high blood pressure in most people. A high-sodium diet, however, can contribute to high blood pressure in a subset of people who are sensitive to sodium.

Summary

- Approximately 50% to 70% of a healthy adult's body weight is fluid. Two-thirds of this fluid is intracellular fluid, and the remainder is extracellular fluid.

- Electrolytes are electrically charged particles found in body fluid that assist in maintaining fluid balance and the normal functioning of cells and the nervous system.

- Water acts as a solvent, provides protection and lubrication for organs and tissues, and acts to maintain blood volume, blood pressure, and body temperature.

- The three primary sources of fluid intake are beverages, foods, and metabolic water produced by chemical reactions during metabolism.

- The primary avenues of fluid excretion are sensible water loss (urine and sweat), insensible water loss (via evaporation and exhalation), and feces.

- Conditions that significantly increase water loss from our bodies include fever, vomiting, diarrhea, hemorrhage, blood donation, heavy exercise, and exposure to heat, cold, and altitude.

- The body relies on blood buffers, the respiratory system, and the kidneys to maintain normal acid–base balance.

- Fluid intake needs are highly variable and depend on body size, age, physical activity, health status, and environmental conditions.

- Some beverages, such as milk and milk alternatives, provide important nutrients. Many others, from soft drinks to flavored waters, provide little more than empty Calories. Sports drinks are most appropriate for athletes. Energy drinks are inappropriate for children, adolescents, and young adults.

- Drinking too much water can lead to overhydration and hyponatremia, or dilution of blood sodium, whereas drinking too little water leads to dehydration, one of the leading causes of death around the world.

- Sodium assists in maintaining fluid balance, blood pressure, nervous function, and muscle contraction.

- Consuming excess sodium can cause high blood pressure or hypernatremia. Sodium deficiencies are rare, but hyponatremia can occur when excessive fluid intake is not accompanied by adequate sodium intake.

- Potassium assists in maintaining fluid balance, healthy blood pressure, transmission of nerve impulses, and muscle function.

- Hyperkalemia is excess blood potassium, which occurs due to kidney disease or malfunction. Hypokalemia is low blood potassium and can occur as a result of kidney disease, diabetic acidosis, and the use of some diuretic medications.

- Chloride assists in maintaining fluid balance, normal nerve transmission, and the digestion of food via the action of HCl.

- Phosphorus assists in maintaining fluid balance and transferring energy via ATP. It is also a component of bone, phospholipids, genetic material, and lipoproteins.

- Dehydration occurs when water excretion exceeds water intake. Individuals at risk include the elderly, infants, people exercising heavily for prolonged periods in the heat, and individuals suffering from prolonged vomiting and diarrhea.

- Heat stroke occurs when the body's core temperature rises above 100°F. Heat stroke can lead to death if left untreated.

- Overhydration, or water intoxication, is caused by consuming too much water. Hyponatremia can also result from water intoxication.

- Hypertension, or high blood pressure, increases the risk for heart disease, stroke, and kidney disease. Consuming excess sodium is associated with hypertension in some, but not all, people.

- Lifestyle changes such as normalization of body weight, regular physical activity, and dietary modifications, such as the DASH Diet, are effective and low-risk approaches that reduce a person's risk for hypertension.

- Certain forms of kidney and heart failure contribute to fluid and electrolyte imbalance and require specific dietary controls.

MasteringNutrition™

To further your understanding, go online and apply what you've learned to real-life case studies that will help you master the content!

Review Questions

1. Which of the following is a characteristic of potassium?
   a. It is the major positively charged electrolyte in the extracellular fluid.
   b. It can be found in fresh fruits and vegetables.
   c. It is a critical component of the mineral complex of bone.
   d. It is the major negatively charged electrolyte in the extracellular fluid.

2. Which of the following people probably has the greatest percentage of body fluid?
   a. a female adult who is slightly overweight and vomits nightly after eating dinner
   b. an elderly male of average weight who has low blood pressure
   c. an overweight football player who has just completed a practice session in high heat
   d. a healthy infant of average weight

3. Plasma is one example of
   a. extracellular fluid.
   b. intracellular fluid.
   c. tissue fluid.
   d. metabolic water.

4. Which of the following is true of the cell membrane?
   a. It is freely permeable to water and many solutes.
   b. It is freely permeable only to water.
   c. It is freely permeable only to water and fats.
   d. It is freely permeable only to water and proteins.

5. Which of the following lifestyle changes has been shown to reduce hypertension in all people with high blood pressure?
   a. consuming a low-sodium diet
   b. normalizing body weight
   c. getting at least 8 hours of sleep nightly
   d. consuming one to two glasses of red wine daily

6. **True or false?** Drinking lots of water throughout a marathon will prevent fluid and electrolyte imbalances.

7. **True or false?** A decreased concentration of electrolytes in our blood stimulates the thirst mechanism.

8. **True or false?** Hypernatremia is commonly caused by a rapid intake of plain water.

9. **True or false?** Absence of thirst is a reliable indicator of adequate hydration.

10. **True or false?** Conditions that increase fluid loss include constipation, blood transfusions, and high humidity.

11. Explain why severe diarrhea in a young child can lead to death from heart failure.

12. After winning a cross-country relay race, you and your teammates celebrate with a trip to the local tavern for a few beers. That evening, you feel shaky and disoriented, and you have a "pins and needles" feeling in your hands and feet. What could be going on that is contributing to these feelings?

13. For lunch today, your choices are (a) chicken soup, a ham sandwich, and a can of tomato juice or (b) potato salad, a tuna-fish sandwich, and a bottle of mineral water. You have hockey practice in mid-afternoon. Which lunch should you choose, and why?

14. Your cousin, who is breastfeeding her 3-month-old daughter, confesses to you that she has resorted to taking over-the-counter weight-loss pills to help her lose the weight she gained during pregnancy. What concerns might this raise?

15. While visiting your grandmother over the holidays, you notice that she avoids drinking any beverage with her evening meal or in the hours prior to bedtime. You ask her about it, and she explains that she avoids fluids so that she won't have to get up and go to the bathroom during the night. "Though I still don't get a good night's sleep," she sighs. "Many nights I wake up with cramps in my legs and have to get up and walk around, anyway!" Could there be a link here? If so, explain.

Math Review

16. Your roommate comes home after basketball practice and tells you he has lost 3 lb. Knowing that 1 pound of body weight loss represents the loss of 2 cups of fluid, how much fluid should he consume over the next few hours in order to fully rehydrate? (Recall that the goal of rehydration is to consume 1.5 times *more* fluid than is lost).

Answers to Review Questions and Math Review can be found online in the MasteringNutrition Study Area.

Web Links

www.epa.gov/OW
US Environmental Protection Agency (EPA)
Go to the EPA's water site for more information about drinking-water quality, standards, and safety.

www.bottledwater.org
International Bottled Water Association
Find current information about bottled water from this trade association that represents the bottled water industry.

www.mayoclinic.com/health/dehydration
Mayo Clinic
You can find a clear explanation of the causes and consequences of dehydration at this website link.

www.mayoclinic.com/health/hyponatremia
Mayo Clinic
Explore this link to learn more about how to avoid hyponatremia.

www.mayoclinic.com/health/water
Mayo Clinic
Review the major factors that determine your need for water.

www.nlm.nih.gov/medlineplus
MEDLINE Plus Health Information
Search for "dehydration" and "heat stroke" to obtain additional resources and the latest news about the dangers of these heat-related illnesses.

www.nhlbi.nih.gov
National Heart, Lung, and Blood Institute
Go to this site to learn more about heart disease, including how to prevent high blood pressure.

www.americanheart.org
American Heart Association
The American Heart Association provides plenty of tips on how to lower your blood pressure.

www.nih.gov
National Institutes of Health (NIH)
Search this site to learn more about the DASH Diet (Dietary Approaches to Stop Hypertension).

References

1. Ballantyne, C. 2007. Strange but true: drinking too much water can kill. *Scientific American* June 27, 2007. www .scientificamerican.com/article.cfm?id=strange-but-true-drinking-too-much-water-can-kill. (Accessed June 2012.)

2. Ruxton, C. H., and V. A. Hart. 2011. Black tea is not significantly different from water in the maintenance of normal hydration in human subjects: results from a randomized controlled trial. *Brit. J. Nutr.* 106:588–595.

3. Institute of Medicine. 2004. *Dietary Reference Intakes for Water, Potassium, Sodium, Chloride, and Sulfate.* Washington, DC: National Academies Press.

4. Potter, V. J. V. 2011. Eat your water for health, sport performance, and weight control. *Am. J. Lifestyle Med.* 5:316–319.

5. Beis, L. Y., M. Wright-Whyte, B. Fudge, T. Noakes, and Y. Pitsiladis. 2012. Drinking behaviors of elite male runners during marathon competition. *Clin. J. Sport Med.* 22:254–261.

6. Godek, S. F., C. Peduzzi, R. Burkholder, S. Condon, G. Dorshimer, and A. R. Bartolozzi. 2010. Sweat rates, sweat sodium concentrations, and sodium losses in 3 groups of professional football players. *J. Athletic Training.* 45:364–371.

7. Committee on Nutrition and The Council on Sports Medicine and Fitness. 2011. Clinical report-sports drinks and energy drinks for children and adolescents: are they appropriate? *Ped.* 127:1182–1189.

8. International Bottled Water Association. 2011. U.S. Bottled Water Volume Grew 3.5% in 2010 as Eeconomic Conditions Begin to Improve. www.bottledwater.org/news/us-bottled-water-volume-grew-35-2010-economic-conditions-begin-improve. (Accessed June 2012.)

9. Zhang, Y., E. T. Lee, L. D. Cowan, R. R. Fabsitz, and B. V. Howard. 2011. Coffee consumption and the incidence of type 2 diabetes in men and women with normal glucose tolerance: the Strong Heart Study. *Nutr., Metab., Cardiovasc. Dis.* 21:418–423.

10. Larsson, S. C., J. Virtamo, and A. Wolk. 2011. Coffee consumption and risk of stroke in women. *Stroke* 42:908–912.

11. Westerterp-Plantenga, M. S. 2010. Green tea catechins, caffeine and body-weight regulation. *Physiology & Behavior* 100:42–46.

12. Zomer, E., A. Owen, J. Magliano, D. Liew, and C. M. Reid. 2012. The effectiveness and cost effectiveness of dark chocolate consumption as prevention therapy in people at risk of cardiovascular disease: best case scenario analysis using a Markov model. *BMJ.* 344:e3657. DOI:10.1136/bmj.e3657.

13. Seifert, S. M., J. L. Schaechter, E. R. Hershorin, and S. E. Lipshultz. 2011. Health effects of energy drinks on children, adolescents, and young adults. *Pediatrics* 127:511–528.

14. US Department of Agriculture and US Department of Health and Human Services. 2010. *Dietary Guidelines for Americans,* 2010. 7th ed. Washington, DC: US Government Printing Office. www.dietaryguidelinesgov.

15. Yan, Q., T. Liu, E. V. Kuklina, W. D. Flanders, Y. Hong, C. Gillespie, M. Chang, M. Gwinn, N. Dowling, M. J. Khoury, and F. B. Hu. 2011. Sodium and potassium intake and mortality among US adults. *Arch. Internal Med.* 171:1183–1191.

16. Sliver, L. D., and T. A. Farley. 2011. Sodium and potassium intake: mortality effects and policy implications. *Arch. Internal Med.* 171:1191–1192.

17. Bedford, J. L., and S. I. Barr. 2011. Higher urinary sodium, a proxy for intake, is associated with increased calcium excretion and lower hip bone density in healthy young women with lower calcium intakes. *Nutrients* 3:951–961.

18. Ilich, J. Z., R. A. Brownbill, and D. C. Coster. 2010. Higher habitual sodium intake is not detrimental for bones in older women with adequate calcium intake. *Eur. J. Appl. Physiol.* 109: 745–755.

19. Institute of Medicine. Food and Nutrition Board. 1999. *Dietary Reference Intakes for Calcium, Phosphorus, Magnesium, Vitamin D, and Fluoride.* Washington, DC: National Academies Press.

20. Meyer, N. L., M. M. Manore, and J. Berning. 2012. Fueling for fitness: food and fluid recommendations for before, during, and after exercise. *ACSM's Health & Fitness J.* 16:7–12.

21. Roan, S. 2011. Scientists Study Surge in Heat-Related Football Deaths. *Los Angeles Times,* August 8, 2011. http://articles.latimes.com/print/2011/aug/08/health/la-he-football-heat-20110808. (Accessed June 2012.)

22. National Center for Health Statistics. 2012. *Health, United States, 2011: With special feature on socioeconomic status and health.* Hyattsville, MD.

23. Frieden, T. R., Centers for Disease Control and Prevention (CDC). 2011. CDC health disparities and inequalities report-United States 2011. *MMWR. Surveill. Summ.* 60(suppl.):1–2.

24. Mayo Clinic Staff. 2011. Ten Ways to Control Blood Pressure without Medication. hwww.mayoclinic.com/health/high-blood-pressure/HI00027. (Accessed June 2012.)

25. Moore, L. L., M. L. Bradless, M. R. Singer, M. M. Qureshi, J. R. Buendia, and S. R. Daniels. 2012. Dietary Approaches to Stop Hypertension (DASH) eating pattern and risk of elevated blood pressure in adolescent girls. *Brit. J.* Available on CJO 2012 DOI:10.1017/S000711451100715X.

26. Sacks, F. M., L. P. Svetkey, W. M. Vollmer, L. J. Appel, G. A. Bray, D. Harsha, E. Obarzanek, P. R. Conlin, E. R. Miller III, D. G. Simons-Morton, N. Karanja, P. Lin for the DASH-Sodium Collaborative Research Group. 2001. Effects on blood pressure of reduced dietary sodium and the Dietary Approaches to Stop Hypertension (DASH) Diet. *NEJM.* 344:3–10.

27. Smith, P. J., J. A. Blumenthal, M. A. Babyak, L. Craighead, K. A. Welsh Bohmer, J. N. Browndyke, T. A. Strauman, and A. Sherwood. 2010. Effects of the Dietary Approaches to Stop Hypertension Diet, exercise, and caloric restriction on neurocognition in overweight adults with high blood pressure. *Hypertension* 55:1331–1338.

28. Liese, A. D., A. Bortsov, A. L. B. Günther, D. Dabelea, K. Reynolds, D. A. Standiford, L. Liu, D. E. Williams, E. J. Mayer-Davis, R. B. D'Agostino, R. Bell, and S. Marcovina. 2011. Association of DASH Diet with cardiovascular risk factors in youth with diabetes mellitus: the SEARCH for diabetes in youth study. *Circulation* 123:1410–1417.

29. LaGuardia, H. A., L. L. Hamm, and J. Chen. 2012. The metabolic syndrome and risk of chronic kidney disease: pathophysiology and intervention strategies. *J. Nutr. Metab.* DOI:10.1155/2012652608.

30. Gertoni, A. G., C. G. Foy, J. C. Hunter, S. A. Quandt, M. Z. Vitolins, and M. C. Witt-Glover. 2011. A multilevel assessment of barriers to adoption of Dietary Approaches to Stop Hypertension (DASH) among African Americans of low socioeconomic status. *J. Health Care Poor Underserved.* 22:1205–1220.

Sports Beverages: Help or Hype?

Once considered specialty items used exclusively by elite athletes, sports beverages have become popular everyday beverage choices for both active and nonactive people. These drinks have become such reliable money makers that most large beverage companies now produce them. This surge in popularity leads us to ask four important questions:

- Do sports beverages benefit highly active athletes?
- Do sports beverages benefit recreationally active people?
- Do sedentary adults benefit from the consumption of sports beverages?
- Are sports beverages necessary or appropriate for children and adolescents?

The first question is relatively easy to answer. Sports beverages were originally developed to meet the unique fluid, electrolyte, and carbohydrate needs of competitive athletes. They are particularly beneficial for athletes who exercise in the heat and are thus at an even greater risk for loss of water and electrolytes through respiration and sweat. In addition, the carbohydrates in sports beverages provide critical fuel during relatively intense exercise bouts lasting more than 1 hour. Some athletes, such as endurance cyclists, regularly train or compete for 6 to 8 hours a day. With this schedule, it is almost impossible for them to eat enough solid foods to meet their energy needs, and sports beverages can help fill the caloric gap. For all these reasons, in response to the first question, the answer is yes: endurance athletes are able to exercise longer, maintain a higher intensity, and improve performance times when they drink a sports beverage during exercise.[1]

Do recreationally active people need to consume sports beverages? The short answer is that most probably do not. The few who exercise for periods longer than 1 hour at an intense level of effort probably can benefit from consuming the carbohydrate and electrolytes in sports beverages during exercise. In general, the duration and intensity of exercise, the environmental conditions, and the characteristics of the individual determine whether or not sports beverages can be more beneficial than plain

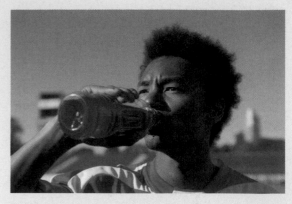

Sports beverages were originally designed to meet the needs of competitive athletes.

water. Here are some situations in which drinking a sports beverage is appropriate:[2]

- Before exercising in conditions when dehydration can occur, especially if someone is already dehydrated prior to exercise
- During exercise or physical work in high heat and/or high humidity, especially for those not accustomed to activity in the heat
- During exercise at high altitude and in cold environments
- After exercise when rapid rehydration is needed or desired
- Between exercise bouts when it is difficult to consume food, such as between multiple soccer matches during a tournament
- During exercise sessions that last longer than 60 minutes, when blood glucose levels get low and risk for dehydration increases
- During exercise in people who may have poor glycogen stores due to illness or inability to eat enough solid food prior to exercise

Interestingly, sports beverages have become very popular with people who do little or no regular exercise. Do these people benefit from drinking sports beverages? The response to this question is *no*: there does not appear to be any evidence that people who do not exercise or exercise very little derive any benefits from consuming sports beverages. Even if these individuals live in a hot environment, they should be able to replenish the fluid and electrolytes they lose during sweating by drinking water and other beverages and eating a normal diet.

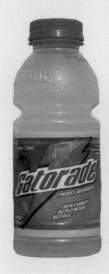

In addition, negative consequences can result when inactive people drink sports beverages. The primary consequence is weight gain, which could lead to obesity. As you can see in **Table 9.4**, sports beverages contain not only fluid and electrolytes but also energy. While some manufacturers are producing "light" sports beverages that are lower in Calories than the traditional product, drinking 12 fl. oz (1.5 cups) of a traditionally formulated Gatorade adds 90 kcal to a person's daily energy intake. Many inactive people consume two to three times this amount each day. Inactive people have much lower energy needs than athletes. With obesity rates at an all-time high, it is important that the foods and beverages consumed provide "Calories that count"—that is, Calories that support our health.

Finally, are sports beverages beneficial for children and adolescents? They have been increasingly marketed to these younger consumers, as well as to schools seeking alternatives to sugar-sweetened sodas, and their consumption is on the rise. However, the American Academy of Pediatrics has concluded that, "for the average child engaged in routine physical activity, the use of sports drinks in place of water is generally unnecessary."[3] Commercial sports beverages are most appropriate for children and adolescents who participate in vigorous, intensive exercise for prolonged periods of time; these products provide the carbohydrate necessary to maintain blood glucose, the electrolytes to replace sweat losses, and the fluid to prevent dehydration. Otherwise,

children and adolescents should view water as the "beverage of choice" on a routine basis and as the most appropriate rehydration fluid before, during, and after most routine periods of physical activity or exercise.[3]

Inappropriate use of sports beverages by children and youth not only adds empty Calories to their diet but also increases their risk for erosion of tooth enamel. Most sports drinks have a pH in the acidic range (pH 3–4) and many include citric acid, which rapidly demineralizes the tooth surface. The Institute of Medicine, in its policy-setting report *Nutrition Standards for Foods in Schools,* advised that schools "restrict sports drinks to use by athletes only during prolonged, vigorous sports activities."[4] Parents, coaches and teachers, healthcare providers, and school administrators need to join together to ensure appropriate use of sports beverages by children and adolescents.

CRITICAL THINKING QUESTIONS

■ Are sports beverages smart choices for you? Why or why not?

■ Why do you think sports drinks are so popular among inactive people?

■ Should registered dietitians and other healthcare professionals discourage overweight clients from consuming sports beverages? Why or why not?

■ As a volunteer coach for a youth soccer league, what would you suggest when parents ask you what types of drinks they should bring for their children?

TABLE 9.4 Nutrient Content of Sports Beverages and Other Common Beverages*

Beverage	Energy (kcal)	Carbohydrate (g)	Sodium (mg)	Potassium (mg)
Cola, regular	153	39	15	4
Ginger ale	124	32	26	4
Beer, regular	146	9	18	89
Gatorade	90	22.5	144	39
All Sport	80	22.5	55.5	55.5
Coconut Water	69	13.5[†]	378	375
Beer, light	8	<1	1	5
Coffee, brewed	7.5	1.5	7.5	192
Cola, diet	4	<1	21	0
Tea, brewed	3	<1	7	88
Water, bottled	0	0	2	0
Water, tap	0	0	7	0

*Amounts compared are 12 fl. oz (1.5 cups).
†Includes 9 g sugar, 4.5 g fiber

REFERENCES

1. Kreider, R. B., C. D. Wilborn, L. Taylor, B. Campbell, A. L. Almada, R. Collins, M. Cooke, C. P. Earnest, M. Greenwood, D. K. Kalman, C. M. Kerksick, S. M. Kleiner, B. Leutholtz, H. Lopez, L. M. Lowery, R. Mendel, A. Smith, M. Spano, R. Wildman, D. S. Willoughby, T. N. Ziegenfuss, and J. Antonio. 2010. ISSN exercise & sport nutrition review: research & recommendations. *J. Intern. Soc. Sports Nutr.* 7:7–51.

2. American College of Sports Medicine, American Dietetic Association, and Dietitians of Canada. 2009. Joint position statement: nutrition and athletic performance. *Med. Sci. Sports Exercise.* 41:709–731.

3. Committee on Nutrition and Council on Sports Medicine and Fitness. 2011. Clinical report—sports drinks and energy drinks for children and adolescents: are they appropriate? *Pediatrics* 127:1182–1189.

4. Institute of Medicine. *Nutrition Standards for Foods in Schools: Leading the Way Toward Healthier Youth.* Washington, DC: National Academies Press; 2007.

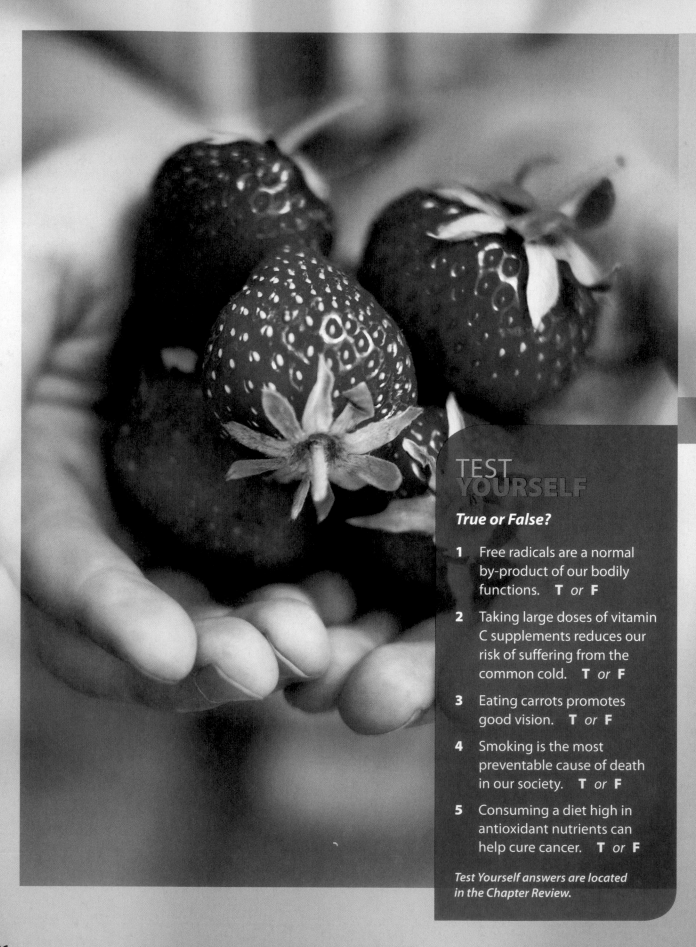

10 Nutrients Involved in Antioxidant Function and Vision

Learning Objectives

After studying this chapter, you should be able to:

1. Define *free radicals* and discuss how they can damage cells, *pp. 389–390.*

2. Describe how antioxidants protect cells from the oxidative damage caused by free radicals, *p. 390.*

3. List three antioxidant enzyme systems and describe how these systems help fight oxidative damage, *p. 390.*

4. Identify and describe the functions of three vitamins that have antioxidant properties, *pp. 391–399, 402–408.*

5. Identify and describe the key functions of a phytochemical with antioxidant properties, *pp. 399–402.*

6. Describe how vitamin A works to ensure healthy vision, *pp. 403–404.*

7. Identify food sources that are high in nutrients with antioxidant properties, *pp. 393, 397–398, 401–402, 406–407, 410.*

8. Identify three minerals with antioxidant properties, and describe the functions of one of them, *pp. 409–411.*

9. Describe the characteristics of cancer and the relationship between antioxidant nutrients and the risk for cancer, *pp. 411–417.*

10. Discuss how consuming foods with antioxidant nutrients can reduce the risk for cardiovascular disease, *pp. 417–418.*

MasteringNutrition™

Go online for chapter quizzes, pre-tests, Interactive Activities and more!

M ika, a first-year student at a university hundreds of miles from home, just opened another care package from her mom. As usual, it contained an assortment of healthful snacks, a box of chamomile tea, and several types of supplements: echinacea extract to ward off colds, powdered papaya for good digestion, and antioxidant vitamins. "Wow, Mika!" her roommate laughed. "Can you let your mom know I'm available for adoption?"

"I guess she just wants me to stay healthy," Mika sighed. She wondered what her mother would think if she ever found out how much junk food Mika had been eating since she'd started college, that she'd been binge drinking every weekend, or that she'd been smoking since high school. "Still," Mika reminded herself, "at least I take the vitamins she sends."

What do you think of Mika's current lifestyle? Can a poor diet, binge drinking, and smoking cause cancer or other health problems, and can the use of dietary supplements provide some protection? What are antioxidant vitamins, and why do you think Mika's mom included a bottle of these in her care package? If your health food store were promoting an antioxidant supplement, would you buy it?

It isn't easy to sort fact from fiction when it comes to antioxidants—especially when they're in the form of supplements. Internet ads and articles in fitness and health magazines tout their benefits, yet some researchers claim that they don't protect us from diseases and in some cases may even be harmful. In this chapter, you'll learn what antioxidants are and how they work in the body. We'll also discuss the multiple roles of vitamin A in promoting healthy vision, cell differentiation, and other key functions.

What Are Antioxidants and How Does the Body Use Them?

Antioxidants are compounds that protect cells from the damage caused by oxidation. *Anti* means "against," and antioxidants work *against,* or *prevent,* oxidation. Before we can go further in our discussion of antioxidants, we need to review what oxidation is and how it damages cells.

Oxidation Is a Chemical Reaction in Which Atoms Lose Electrons

As you recall (from Chapter 7), during metabolic reactions, atoms may lose electrons (**Figure 10.1a**). This loss of electrons is called **oxidation,** because it is fueled by oxygen. Atoms are also capable of gaining electrons, through a complementary process called *reduction* (Figure 10.1b). Because oxidation-reduction reactions typically result in an even exchange of electrons, scientists call them *exchange reactions.*

Stable atoms have an even number of electrons orbiting in pairs at successive distances (called *shells* or *rings*) from the nucleus. When a stable atom loses an electron during oxidation, it is left with an odd number of electrons in its outermost shell. In other words, it now has an *unpaired electron.* In most exchange reactions, two unpaired electrons immediately

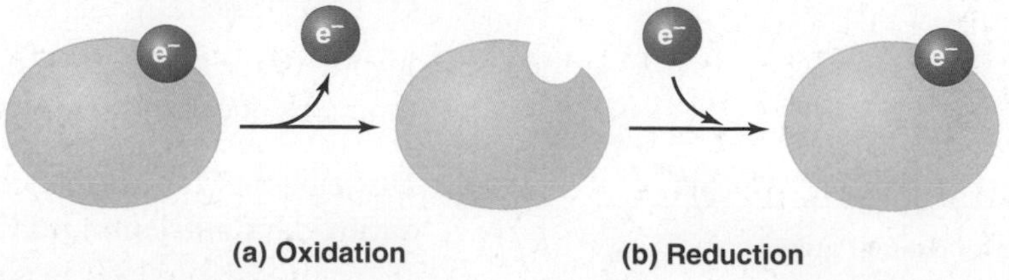

antioxidant A compound that has the ability to prevent or repair the damage caused by oxidation.

oxidation A chemical reaction in which molecules of a substance are broken down into their component atoms. During oxidation, the atoms involved lose electrons.

(a) Oxidation   **(b) Reduction**

FIGURE 10.1 Exchange reactions consist of two parts. **(a)** During oxidation, atoms *lose* electrons. **(b)** In the second part of the reaction, atoms *gain* electrons, which is called reduction.

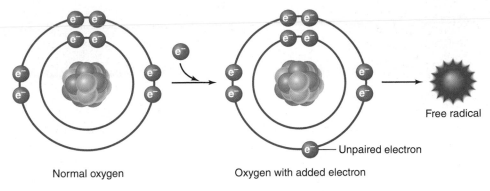

Normal oxygen   Oxygen with added electron   Free radical

Unpaired electron

FIGURE 10.2 Normally, an oxygen atom contains eight electrons. Occasionally, oxygen will accept an unpaired electron during the oxidation process. This acceptance of a single electron causes oxygen to become an unstable atom called a free radical.

pair up with other unpaired electrons, making newly stabilized molecules, but in some cases, atoms with unpaired electrons in their outermost shell remain unpaired. Such atoms are highly unstable and are called **free radicals.** When an oxygen molecule becomes a free radical, it is specifically referred to as a **reactive oxygen species (ROS).**

As you learned (in Chapter 7), the body uses oxygen and hydrogen to generate energy (ATP). The process of metabolism sometimes results in the release of single electrons. Occasionally, oxygen accepts one of these single electrons (**Figure 10.2**). When it does so, the newly unstable oxygen atom becomes a free radical because of the added unpaired electron. This type of free-radical production is common during metabolism. Free radicals are also formed from other metabolic processes, such as when our immune system produces inflammation to fight allergens or infections. Other factors that cause free-radical formation include exposure to air pollution, ultraviolet (UV) rays from the sun, other types of radiation, tobacco smoke, industrial chemicals, and asbestos. Continual exposure to these factors leads to uncontrollable free-radical formation, cell damage, and disease, as discussed next.

Free Radicals Can Destabilize Other Molecules and Damage Cells

Why are we concerned with the formation of free radicals? Simply put, it is because of their destabilizing power. If you were to think of paired electrons as a married couple, a free radical would be an extremely seductive outsider. Its unpaired electron exerts a powerful attraction toward all stable molecules around it. In an attempt to stabilize itself, a free radical will "steal" an electron from stable compounds, in turn generating more unstable free radicals. This is a dangerous chain reaction, because the free radicals generated can damage or destroy cells.

One of the most significant sites of free-radical damage is the cell membrane. As shown in **Figure 10.3a**, free radicals that form within the phospholipid bilayer of cell membranes steal electrons from the stable lipid heads. When the lipid heads, which are hydrophobic, are destroyed, they no longer repel water. With the cell membrane's integrity lost, its ability to regulate the movement of fluids and nutrients into and out of the cell is also lost. This loss of cell integrity causes damage to the cell and to all systems affected by the cell.

Other sites of free-radical damage include low-density lipoproteins (LDLs), cell proteins, and DNA. Damage to LDLs and cell proteins disrupts the transport of substances into and out of cells and alters cell function, whereas defective DNA results in faulty protein synthesis. These changes can also cause harmful changes (mutations) in cells or prompt cells to die prematurely. Free radicals also promote blood-vessel inflammation

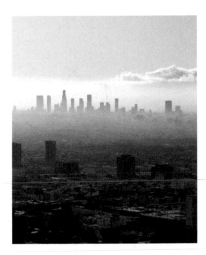

Exposure to pollution from car exhaust and industrial waste increases our production of free radicals.

free radical A highly unstable atom with an unpaired electron in its outermost shell.

reactive oxygen species (ROS) An oxygen molecule that has become a free radical.

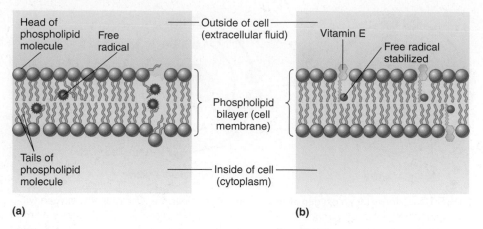

FIGURE 10.3 **(a)** The formation of free radicals in the lipid portion of our cell membranes can cause a dangerous chain reaction that damages the integrity of the membrane and can cause cell death. **(b)** Vitamin E is stored in the lipid portion of our cell membranes. By donating an electron to free radicals, it protects the lipid molecules in our cell membranes from being oxidized and stops the chain reaction of oxidative damage.

and the formation of clots, both of which are risk factors for cardiovascular disease. Not surprisingly, many diseases are linked with free-radical production, including cancer, heart disease, type 2 diabetes, arthritis, cataracts, and Alzheimer's and Parkinson's diseases.

Antioxidants Work by Stabilizing Free Radicals or Opposing Oxidation

How does the body fight free radicals and repair the damage they cause? These actions are performed by antioxidant vitamins, minerals, and phytochemicals and other compounds. These antioxidants perform their role in three ways:

1. Antioxidant vitamins work independently by donating their electrons or hydrogen atoms to free radicals to stabilize them and reduce the damage caused by oxidation (see Figure 10.3b).
2. Antioxidant minerals, including selenium, copper, iron, zinc, and manganese, act as cofactors within complex *antioxidant enzyme systems* that convert free radicals to less damaging substances that are excreted by the body. They also work to break down fatty acids that have become oxidized, thereby destroying the free radicals associated with them. Antioxidant enzyme systems also make more vitamin antioxidants available to fight other free radicals. The following are examples of antioxidant enzyme systems:
   - Superoxide dismutase converts free radicals to less damaging substances, such as hydrogen peroxide.
   - Catalase removes hydrogen peroxide from the body by converting it to water and oxygen.
   - Glutathione peroxidase also removes hydrogen peroxide from the body and stops the production of free radicals in lipids.
3. *Phytochemicals* (beneficial plant chemicals,) such as *beta-carotene* and other compounds, help stabilize free radicals and prevent damage to cells and tissues.

In summary, free-radical formation is generally kept safely under control by certain vitamins, minerals working within antioxidant systems, and phytochemicals. Next, we take a look at the specific vitamins and minerals involved. Phytochemicals are discussed in In Depth: Phytochemicals, immediately following this chapter.

RECAP

Free radicals are formed when a stable atom loses or gains an electron and this electron remains unpaired. They can be produced as a normal by-product of oxidation reactions, when our immune system fights allergens or infections, and when we are exposed to radiation or toxic substances. Free radicals can damage our cell membranes, low-density lipoproteins (LDLs), cell proteins, and DNA and are associated with many chronic diseases, including heart disease, various cancers, and type 2 diabetes. Antioxidant vitamins donate electrons or hydrogen atoms to free radicals to stabilize them. Antioxidant minerals function as part of antioxidant enzyme systems that convert free radicals to less damaging substances. Some phytochemicals also have antioxidant properties. ■

A Profile of Nutrients That Function As Antioxidants

The body cannot form antioxidants spontaneously. Instead, we must consume them in our diets. Nutrients that appear to have antioxidant properties or are part of our protective antioxidant enzyme systems include vitamins E, C, and A; beta-carotene (a phytochemical that is a precursor to vitamin A); and the mineral selenium (**Table 10.1**). The minerals copper, iron, zinc, and manganese play a peripheral role in fighting oxidation and are only mentioned in this chapter. Let's review each of these nutrients now and learn more about their functions in the body.

Vitamin E

Vitamin E is one of the fat-soluble vitamins. It is absorbed with dietary fat and incorporated into the chylomicrons. As the chylomicrons are broken down, most of the vitamin E remains in their remnants and is transported to the liver. There, vitamin E is incorporated into very-low-density lipoproteins (VLDLs) and released into the blood. As previously described (in Chapter 5), VLDLs are transport vehicles that ferry triglycerides from their source to the body's cells. After VLDLs release their triglyceride load, they become LDLs. Vitamin E is a part of both VLDLs and LDLs and is transported to the tissues and cells by both of these lipoproteins.

Vitamin E and the other fat-soluble vitamins are stored in the body. The liver serves as a storage site for vitamins A and D, and about 90% of the vitamin E in the body is stored in our adipose tissue. The remaining vitamin E is found in cell membranes.

TABLE 10.1 Nutrients Involved in Antioxidant Function and Vision

To see the full profile of all micronutrients, turn to Chapter 7.5, In Depth: Vitamins and Minerals: Micronutrients with Macro Powers, pages 300–309.

Nutrient	Recommended Intake
Vitamin E (fat soluble)	RDA: Women and men = 15 mg alpha-tocopheral
Vitamin C (water soluble)	RDA: Women = 75 mg Men = 90 mg Smokers = 35 mg more per day than RDA
Beta-carotene (fat-soluble provitamin for vitamin A)	None at this time
Vitamin A (fat soluble)	RDA: Women: 700 µg Men: 900 µg
Selenium (trace mineral)	RDA: Women and men = 55 µg

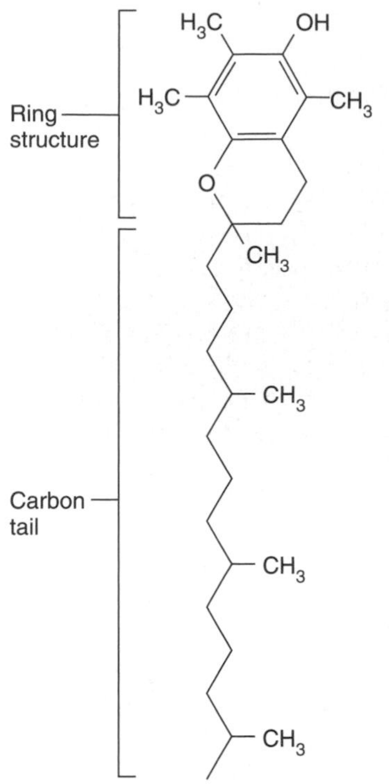

FIGURE 10.4 Chemical structure of α-tocopherol. Note that α-tocopherol is composed of a ring structure and a long carbon tail. Variations in the spatial orientation of the carbon atoms in this tail and in the composition of the tail itself are what result in forming the different tocopherol and tocotrienol compounds.

tocotrienols A family of vitamin E that does not play an important biological role in our bodies.

tocopherols A family of vitamin E that is the active form in our bodies.

erythrocyte hemolysis The rupturing or breakdown of red blood cells, or erythrocytes.

Forms of Vitamin E

Vitamin E is actually two separate families of compounds, **tocotrienols** and **tocopherols.** None of the four tocotrienol compounds—alpha, beta, gamma, and delta—appears to play an active role in the body. The tocopherol compounds are the biologically active forms. Four tocopherol compounds have been discovered; as with tocotrienol, these have been designated alpha, beta, gamma, and delta. Of them, the most active, or potent, vitamin E compound found in food and supplements is *alpha-tocopherol* (**Figure 10.4**). The RDA for vitamin E is expressed as alpha-tocopherol in milligrams per day (α-tocopherol, mg per day). Food labels and vitamin and mineral supplements may express vitamin E in units of alpha-tocopherol equivalents (α-TE), in milligrams, and as International Units (IU). Supplements may contain either the natural form of vitamin E (called d-alpha-tocopherol) or the synthetic form (dl-alpha-tocopherol). The following can be used for conversion purposes:

- In food, 1 α-TE is equal to 1 mg of active vitamin E.
- In supplements containing the natural form of vitamin E, 1 IU is equal to 0.67 mg α-TE.
- In supplements containing the synthetic form of vitamin E, 1 IU is equal to 0.45 mg α-TE.

Functions of Vitamin E

The primary function of vitamin E is as an antioxidant: it donates an electron to free radicals, stabilizing them and preventing them from destabilizing other molecules. Once vitamin E is oxidized, it is either excreted from the body or recycled back into active vitamin E through the help of other antioxidant nutrients, such as vitamin C.

Because vitamin E is prevalent in adipose tissue and cell membranes, its action specifically protects polyunsaturated fatty acids (PUFAs) and other fatty components of our cells and cell membranes from being oxidized (see Figure 10.3b). Vitamin E also protects LDLs from being oxidized, thereby lowering the risk for heart disease. (The relationship between antioxidants and heart disease is reviewed later in this chapter.) In addition to protecting PUFAs and LDLs, vitamin E protects the membranes of red blood cells from oxidation and plays a critical role in protecting the cells of our lungs, which are constantly exposed to oxygen and the potentially damaging effects of oxidation. Vitamin E's role in protecting PUFAs and other fatty components also explains why it is added to many oil-based foods and skin-care products—by preventing oxidation in these products, it reduces rancidity and spoilage.

Vitamin E serves many other roles essential to human health. It is critical for normal fetal and early childhood development of nerves and muscles, as well as for maintenance of their functions. It protects white blood cells and other components of the immune system, thereby helping the body defend against illness and disease. It also improves the absorption of vitamin A if the dietary intake of vitamin A is low.

How Much Vitamin E Should We Consume?

Considering the importance of vitamin E to our health, you might think that you need to consume a huge amount daily. In fact, the RDA is modest, and the food sources are plentiful.

Recommended Dietary Allowance for Vitamin E The RDA for vitamin E for men and women is 15 mg alpha-tocopherol per day. This is the amount determined to be sufficient to prevent **erythrocyte hemolysis,** or the rupturing (*lysis*) of red blood cells (*erythrocytes*). The Tolerable Upper Intake Level (UL) is 1,000 mg alpha-tocopherol per day. Remember that one of the primary roles of vitamin E is to protect PUFAs from oxidation. Thus, our need for vitamin E increases as we eat more oils and other foods that contain PUFAs. Fortunately, these foods also contain vitamin E, so we typically consume enough vitamin E within them to protect their PUFAs from oxidation.

Good Food Sources of Vitamin E Vitamin E is widespread in foods from plant sources (**Figure 10.5**). Much of the vitamin E that we consume comes from products such as spreads, salad dressings, and mayonnaise made from vegetable oils, including safflower oil, sunflower oil, canola oil, and soybean oil. Nuts, seeds, soybeans, and some vegetable—including spinach, broccoli, and avocados—also contribute vitamin E to our diets. Although no single fruit or vegetable contains very high amounts of vitamin E, eating the recommended amounts of fruits and vegetables each day will help ensure adequate intake of this nutrient. Cereals are often fortified with vitamin E, and other grain products contribute modest amounts to our diets. Animal and dairy products are poor sources. Here are some tips for eating more vitamin E:

- Eat cereals high in vitamin E for breakfast or as a snack.
- Add sunflower seeds to salads and trail mixes, or just have them as a snack.
- Add sliced almonds to salads, granola, and trail mixes to boost vitamin E intake.
- Pack a peanut butter sandwich for lunch.
- Eat veggies throughout the day—for snacks, for sides, and in main dishes.
- When dressing a salad, use vitamin E—rich oils, such as sunflower, safflower, or canola.
- Enjoy some fresh, homemade guacamole: mash a ripe avocado with a squeeze of lime juice and a sprinkle of garlic salt.

Vitamin E is destroyed by exposure to oxygen, metals, ultraviolet light, and heat. Although raw (uncooked) vegetable oils contain vitamin E, heating these oils destroys vitamin E. Thus, foods that are deep-fried and processed contain little vitamin E; this includes most fast foods.

Nutrition
MILESTONE

In **1922**, Herbert M. Evans from UC Berkeley and Katharine Scott Bishop from Johns Hopkins University School of Medicine published a landmark paper in the journal *Science* identifying the existence of "an unrecognized dietary factor essential for reproduction." Similar studies were being conducted by Henry Mattill and colleagues at the University of Iowa, who in 1923 discovered that wheat germ is a rich source of this dietary factor. In 1924, research scientist Bennet Sure named this factor vitamin E, as vitamins A, B, C, and D had already been identified.

For the next decade, the research teams of both Evans and Mattill worked independently to identify the antioxidant properties of vitamin E. In 1936, Evans' team isolated vitamin E from wheat germ oil and chemically characterized it, naming it *tocopherol* from the Greek words *phero* ("to bring") and *tocos* ("childbirth"). In 1937, collaboration between Mattill's and Evans' research groups confirmed that alpha-, beta-, and gamma-tocopherols are effective antioxidants. The antioxidant function of vitamin E is still recognized as one of its primary roles in human physiology and health.

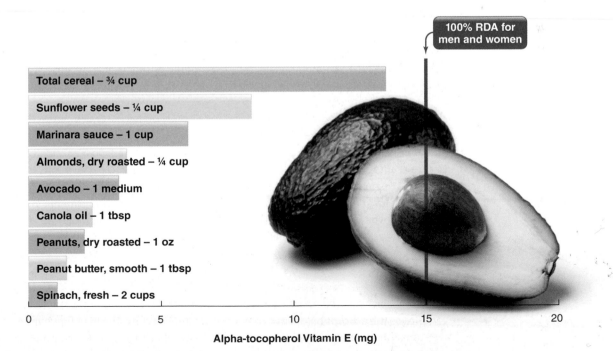

FIGURE 10.5 Common food sources of vitamin E. The RDA for vitamin E is 15 mg α-tocopherol per day for men and women. (*Source:* Data from U.S. Department of Agriculture, Agricultural Research Service, 2011. USDA National Nutrient Database for Standard Reference, Release 24. www.ars.usda.gov/ba/bhnrc/ndl

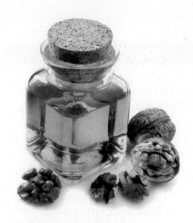

Vegetable oils, nuts, seeds, and avocados are good sources of vitamin E.

What Happens If We Consume Too Much Vitamin E?

Until recently, standard supplemental doses (one to eighteen times the RDA) of vitamin E were not associated with any adverse health effects. However, a 2005 study found that, among adults 55 years of age or older with vascular disease or diabetes, a daily intake of 268 mg of vitamin E per day (about eighteen times the RDA) for approximately 7 years resulted in a significant increase in heart failure.[1] Additional studies have also shown a significant increase in premature mortality in middle-aged or older adults with risk factors for chronic diseases as a result of taking vitamin E supplements in doses ranging from 10 IU to 5,000 IU per day.[2,3] It is currently unclear as to whether there are increased risks for healthy people who are taking vitamin E supplements. However, the Selenium and Vitamin E Cancer Prevention Trial (SELECT) found that taking 400 IU per day of vitamin E supplements increased the risk for prostate cancer by 17% in healthy U.S. men from the general population.[4]

Some individuals report side effects such as nausea, intestinal distress, and diarrhea with vitamin E supplementation. In addition, certain medications interact negatively with vitamin E. The most important of these are the *anticoagulants,* substances that stop blood from clotting excessively. Aspirin is an anticoagulant, as is the prescription drug Coumadin. Vitamin E supplements can augment the action of these substances, causing uncontrollable bleeding. In addition, evidence suggests that in some people, long-term use of standard vitamin E supplements may cause hemorrhaging in the brain, leading to a hemorrhagic stroke.[5]

What Happens If We Don't Consume Enough Vitamin E?

True vitamin E deficiencies are uncommon in humans. This is primarily because vitamin E is fat soluble, so we typically store adequate amounts in our fatty tissues, even when our current intakes are low. Vitamin E deficiencies are usually a result of diseases that cause malabsorption of fat, such as those that affect the small intestine, liver, gallbladder, and pancreas. As noted earlier (in Chapter 3), the liver makes bile, which is necessary for the absorption of fat. The gallbladder delivers the bile into our intestines, where it facilitates digestion of fat. The pancreas makes fat-digesting enzymes. Thus, when the liver, gallbladder, or pancreas is not functioning properly, fat and the fat-soluble vitamins, including vitamin E, cannot be absorbed, leading to their deficiency.

Results from three national surveys suggest that the diets of most Americans do not provide the RDA for vitamin E.[6,7] However, these intake estimates may be low, as the amounts and types of fat added during cooking are often not known and thus are not included in survey estimates.

Despite the rarity of true vitamin E deficiencies, they do occur. One vitamin E deficiency symptom is erythrocyte hemolysis. This rupturing of red blood cells leads to *anemia,* a condition in which the red blood cells cannot carry and transport enough oxygen to the tissues, leading to fatigue, weakness, and a diminished ability to perform physical and mental work. (Anemia is discussed in more detail in Chapter 12.) Vitamin E deficiency can also cause loss of muscle coordination and reflexes, leading to impairments in vision, speech, and movement. Vitamin E deficiency can also impair immune function, especially when body stores of the mineral selenium are low.

RECAP

Vitamin E protects cell membranes from oxidation, enhances immune function, and improves the absorption of vitamin A if dietary intake is low. The RDA for vitamin E is 15 mg alpha-tocopherol per day for men and women. Vitamin E is found primarily in vegetable oils and nuts. Toxicity is uncommon, but taking very high doses can cause excessive bleeding, and supplementation has been linked to premature mortality in some studies. A genuine deficiency is rare, but symptoms include anemia and impaired vision, speech, and movement. ■

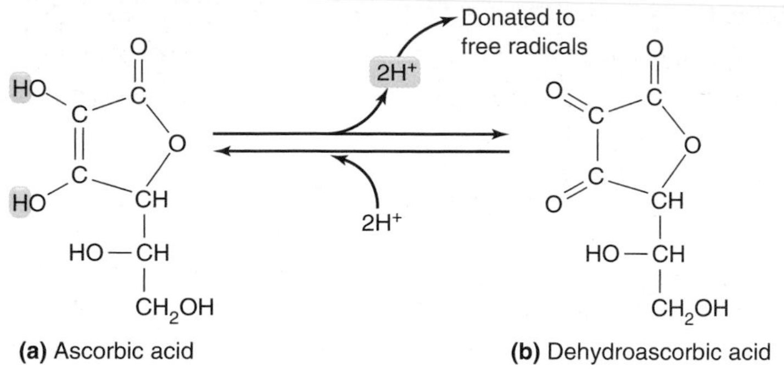

FIGURE 10.6 Chemical structures of ascorbic acid and dehydroascorbic acid. **(a)** By donating two of its hydrogens to free radicals, ascorbic acid protects against oxidative damage and becomes **(b)** dehydroascorbic acid. In turn, dehydroascorbic acid can accept two hydrogens to become ascorbic acid.

Vitamin C

Vitamin C is water soluble. We must therefore consume it on a regular basis, as any excess is excreted (primarily in the urine) rather than stored. There are two active forms of vitamin C: ascorbic acid and dehydroascorbic acid (**Figure 10.6**). Interestingly, most animals can make their own vitamin C from glucose. Humans and guinea pigs are two groups that cannot synthesize their own vitamin C and must consume it in the diet.

At low concentrations, vitamin C is absorbed in the intestines via active transport; at high concentrations, it is absorbed via simple diffusion. Between consumptions of 30 to 80 mg/day, about 70% to 90% of dietary vitamin C is absorbed, but absorption falls to less than 50% when more than 1 g per day is consumed.[8] The kidneys regulate excretion of vitamin C, with increased excretion occurring during periods of high dietary intake and decreased excretion when dietary intakes are low.

Functions of Vitamin C

Vitamin C is probably most well known for its role in preventing scurvy, a disease that ravaged sailors on long sea voyages centuries ago. In fact, the derivation of the term *ascorbic acid* means a ("without") *scorbic* ("having scurvy"). Scurvy was characterized by bleeding tissues, especially of the gums, and is thought to have caused more than half of the deaths that occurred at sea. During these long voyages, the crew ate all of the fruits and vegetables early in the trip, then had only grain and animal products available until they reached land to resupply. In 1740 in England, Dr. James Lind discovered that citrus fruits can prevent scurvy. This is due to their high vitamin C content. Fifty years after the discovery of the link between citrus fruits and prevention of scurvy, the British navy finally required all ships to provide daily lemon juice rations for each sailor to prevent the onset of scurvy. A century later, sailors were given lime juice rations, earning them the nickname "limeys." It wasn't until 1930 that vitamin C was discovered and identified as a nutrient.

One reason that vitamin C prevents scurvy is that it assists in the synthesis of **collagen.** Collagen, a protein, is a critical component of all connective tissues in the body, including bone, teeth, skin, tendons, and blood vessels. Collagen assists in preventing bruises, and it ensures proper wound healing, as it is a part of scar tissue and a component of the tissue that mends broken bones. Without adequate vitamin C, the body cannot form collagen, and tissue hemorrhage, or bleeding, occurs. Vitamin C may also be involved in the synthesis of other components of connective tissues, such as elastin and bone matrix.

In addition to connective tissues, vitamin C assists in the synthesis of DNA, bile, neurotransmitters such as serotonin (which helps regulate mood), and carnitine, which transports long-chain fatty acids from the cytosol into the mitochondria for energy production.

collagen A protein found in all connective tissues in the body.

Vitamin C also helps ensure appropriate levels of thyroxine, a hormone produced by the thyroid gland, to support basal metabolic rate and maintain body temperature. Other hormones that are synthesized with assistance from vitamin C include epinephrine, norepinephrine, and steroid hormones.

Vitamin C also acts as an antioxidant. Because it is water soluble, it is an important antioxidant in the extracellular fluid. Like vitamin E, it donates electrons to free radicals, thus preventing the damage of cells and tissues (see Figure 10.6a). It also protects LDL-cholesterol from oxidation, which may reduce the risk for cardiovascular disease. Vitamin C acts as an important antioxidant in the lungs, helping protect us from the damage caused by ozone and cigarette smoke. It also enhances immune function by protecting the white blood cells from the oxidative damage that occurs in response to fighting illness and infection. But contrary to popular belief, it is not a miracle cure (see the **Nutrition Myth or Fact?** box on page 397). In the stomach, vitamin C reduces the formation of *nitrosamines,* cancer-causing agents found in foods such as cured and processed meats. We discuss the role of vitamin C and other antioxidants in preventing some forms of cancer later in this chapter.

Vitamin C also regenerates vitamin E after it has been oxidized. This occurs when ascorbic acid donates electrons to vitamin E radicals, becoming dehydroascorbic acid (**Figure 10.7**). The regenerated vitamin E can then continue to protect cell membranes and other tissues. In turn, dehydroascorbic acid is regenerated as an antioxidant by gaining an electron from the reduced form of **glutathione (GSH),** which is a tripeptide composed of glycine, cysteine, and glutamic acid. Glutathione is then restored to its antioxidant form by the enzyme *glutathione reductase,* in a reaction (not shown in Figure 10.7) that is dependent on the mineral selenium, which is discussed later in this chapter.

Vitamin C also enhances the absorption of iron. It is recommended that people with low iron stores consume vitamin C–rich foods along with iron sources to improve

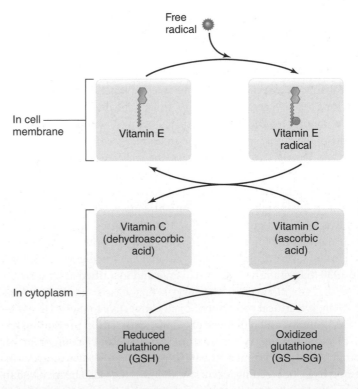

glutathione (GSH) A tripeptide composed of glycine, cysteine, and glutamic acid that assists in regenerating vitamin C into its antioxidant form.

FIGURE 10.7 Regeneration of vitamin E by vitamin C. Vitamin E neutralizes free radicals in the cell membrane, and vitamin C (in the form of ascorbic acid) regenerates vitamin E from the resulting vitamin E radical. Vitamin C (in the form of dehydroascorbic acid) is regenerated to ascorbic acid by the reduced form of glutathione (GSH).

Nutrition Myth OR Fact?

Can Vitamin C Prevent the Common Cold?

What do you do when you feel a cold coming on? If you are like many people, you drink a lot of orange juice or take vitamin C supplements to ward it off. Do these tactics really help prevent a cold?

It is well known that vitamin C is important for a healthy immune system. A deficiency of vitamin C can seriously weaken the immune cells' ability to detect and destroy invading microbes, increasing susceptibility to many diseases and illnesses—including the common cold. Many people have taken vitamin C supplements to prevent the common cold, basing their behavior on its actions of enhancing our immune function. Interestingly, scientific studies do not support this action. A recent review of many of the studies of vitamin C and the common cold found that people taking vitamin C regularly in an attempt to ward off the common cold experienced as many colds as people who took a placebo. However, the *duration* of their colds was significantly reduced—by 8% in adults and 13.6% in children.[1] Timing appears to be important, though: taking vitamin C after the onset of cold symptoms did not reduce either the duration or severity of the cold. Interestingly, taking vitamin C supplements regularly did reduce the number of colds experienced in marathon runners, skiers, and soldiers participating in exercises done under extreme environmental conditions.

The amount of vitamin C taken in these studies was at least 200 mg per day, with many using doses as high as 4,000 mg per day (more than forty times the RDA), with no harmful effects noted in those studies that reported adverse events.

In summary, it appears that, for most people, taking vitamin C supplements regularly will not prevent colds but may reduce their duration. Consuming a healthful diet that includes excellent sources of vitamin C will also help you maintain a strong immune system. Taking vitamin C after the onset of cold symptoms does not appear to help, so next time you feel a cold coming on, you may want to think twice before taking extra vitamin C.

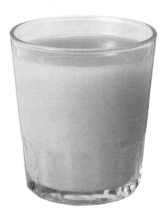

Reference

1. Hemilä, H., E. Chalker, B. Treacy, and B. Douglas. 2007. Vitamin C for preventing and treating the common cold. *Cochrane Database of Systematic Reviews*. Issue 3. Art. No. CD000980. DOI: 10.1002/14651858.CD000980.pub3.

---

absorption. For people with high iron stores, this practice can be dangerous and lead to iron toxicity (see Chapter 12, pages 479–480).

How Much Vitamin C Should We Consume?

Although popular opinion suggests that our needs for vitamin C are high, we really only require amounts that are easily obtained when we eat the recommended amounts of fruits and vegetables daily.

Recommended Dietary Allowance for Vitamin C   The RDA for vitamin C is 90 mg per day for men and 75 mg per day for women. The Tolerable Upper Intake Level (UL) is 2,000 mg per day for adults. Smoking increases a person's need for vitamin C; thus, the RDA for smokers is 35 mg more per day than for nonsmokers. This equals 125 mg per day for men and 110 mg per day for women. Other high-stress situations that may increase the need for vitamin C include healing from a traumatic injury, surgery, or burns and the use of oral contraceptives among women; there is no consensus as to how much extra vitamin C is needed in these circumstances.

Good Food Sources of Vitamin C   Fruits and vegetables are the best sources of vitamin C. Because heat and oxygen destroy vitamin C, fresh sources of these foods have the highest content. Cooking foods, especially boiling them, leaches their vitamin C, which is then lost when we strain them. The forms of cooking that are least likely to compromise the vitamin C content of foods are steaming, microwaving, and stir-frying.

As indicated in **Figure 10.8**, many fruits and vegetables are high in vitamin C. Citrus fruits (such as oranges, lemons, and limes), potatoes, strawberries, tomatoes, kiwifruit,

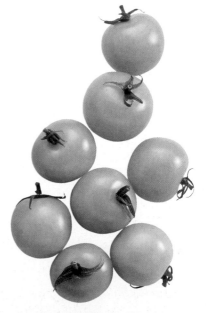

Many fruits, such as these yellow tomatoes, are high in vitamin C.

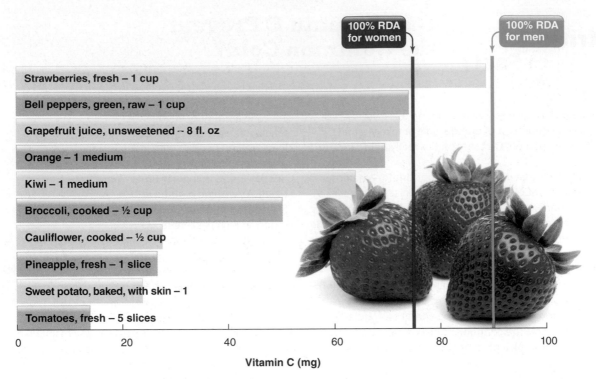

FIGURE 10.8 Common food sources of vitamin C. The RDA for vitamin C is 90 mg per day for men and 75 mg per day for women. (*Source:* Data from U.S. Department of Agriculture, Agricultural Research Service, 2011. USDA National Nutrient Database for Standard Reference, Release 24. http://www.ars.usda.gov/ba/bhnrc/ndl)

broccoli, spinach and other leafy greens, cabbage, green and red peppers, and cauliflower are excellent sources of vitamin C. Fortified beverages and cereals are also good sources. Dairy foods, meats, and nonfortified cereals and grains provide little or no vitamin C.

Here are some tips for selecting foods high in vitamin C:

- Mix strawberries, kiwifruit, cantaloupe, and oranges for a tasty fruit salad loaded with vitamin C.
- Include tomatoes on salads, wraps, and sandwiches for more vitamin C.
- Make your own fresh-squeezed orange or grapefruit juice.
- Add your favorite vitamin C–rich fruits, such as strawberries, to smoothies.
- Buy ready-to-eat vegetables, such as baby carrots and cherry tomatoes, and toss some in a zip-lock bag to take to school or work.
- Put a few slices of romaine lettuce on your sandwich.
- Throw a small container of orange slices, fresh pineapple chunks, or berries into your backpack for an afternoon snack.
- Store some 100% juice boxes in your freezer to pack with your lunch. They'll thaw slowly, keeping the rest of your lunch cool, and many brands contain a full day's supply of vitamin C in just 6 oz.
- Enjoy raw bell peppers with low-fat dip for a crunchy snack.

By eating the recommended amounts of fruits and vegetables daily, we can easily meet the body's requirement for vitamin C. A serving of vegetables is ½ cup of cooked or 1 cup of raw vegetables or 6 oz of vegetable juice, and a serving of fruit is one medium fruit, 1 cup of chopped or canned fruit, or 6 oz of 100% fruit juice.

What Happens If We Consume Too Much Vitamin C?

Because vitamin C is water soluble, we usually excrete any excess. Consuming excess amounts in food sources does not lead to toxicity, and only supplements can lead to toxic doses. Taking megadoses of vitamin C is not fatal; however, the side effects of doses exceeding 2,000 mg per day for a prolonged period include nausea, diarrhea, nosebleeds, and abdominal cramps.

There are rare instances in which consuming even moderately excessive doses of vitamin C can be harmful. As mentioned earlier, vitamin C enhances the absorption of iron. This action is beneficial to people who need to increase iron absorption. It can be harmful, however, to people with a disease called *hemochromatosis,* which causes an excess accumulation of iron in the body. Such iron toxicity can damage tissues and lead to a heart attack. In people who have preexisting kidney disease, taking excess vitamin C can lead to the formation of kidney stones. This does not appear to occur in healthy individuals.

Critics of vitamin C supplementation claim that taking the supplemental form of the vitamin is "unbalanced" nutrition and leads vitamin C to act as a prooxidant. A **prooxidant,** as you might guess, is a nutrient that promotes oxidation. It does this by pushing the balance of exchange reactions toward oxidation, which promotes the production of free radicals. Although the results of a few studies suggested that vitamin C acts as a prooxidant, these studies were found to be flawed or irrelevant for humans. At the present time, there appears to be no strong scientific evidence that vitamin C, either from food or dietary supplements, acts as a prooxidant in humans.

What Happens If We Don't Consume Enough Vitamin C?

Vitamin C deficiencies are rare in developed countries but can occur in developing countries. Scurvy is the most common vitamin C–deficiency disease. The symptoms of scurvy appear after about 1 month of a vitamin C–deficient diet and include bleeding gums, loose teeth, weakness, wounds that fail to heal, swollen ankles and wrists, bone pain and fractures, diarrhea, weakness, and depression. Anemia can also result from vitamin C deficiency. People most at risk are those who eat few fruits and vegetables, including impoverished or homebound individuals, and people who abuse alcohol and drugs.

RECAP

Vitamin C scavenges free radicals and regenerates vitamin E after it has been oxidized. Vitamin C prevents scurvy and assists in the synthesis of collagen, hormones, neurotransmitters, and DNA. Vitamin C also enhances iron absorption. The RDA for vitamin C is 90 mg per day for men and 75 mg per day for women. Many fruits and vegetables are high in vitamin C. Toxicity is uncommon with dietary intake; symptoms include nausea, diarrhea, and nosebleeds. Deficiency symptoms include scurvy, anemia, diarrhea, and depression. ■

Beta-Carotene

Although beta-carotene is not considered an essential nutrient, it is a *provitamin* found in many fruits and vegetables. **Provitamins** are inactive forms of vitamins that the body cannot use until they are converted to their active form. Our bodies convert beta-carotene to an active form of vitamin A, *retinol;* thus, beta-carotene is a precursor of retinol.

Beta-carotene is a phytochemical classified as a **carotenoid,** one of a group of plant pigments that are the basis for the red, orange, and deep-yellow colors of many fruits and vegetables. (Even dark-green, leafy vegetables contain plenty of carotenoids, but the green pigment, chlorophyll, masks their color.) Although there are more than 600 carotenoids in nature, only about 50 are found in the typical human diet. The 6 most common carotenoids found in human blood are alpha-carotene, beta-carotene, beta-cryptoxanthin, lutein, lycopene, and zeaxanthin. Of these, the body can convert only alpha-carotene, beta-carotene, and beta-cryptoxanthin to retinol. These are referred to as *provitamin A carotenoids.* We are just beginning to learn more about how carotenoids function in our bodies and how they may affect our health.

prooxidant A nutrient that promotes oxidation and oxidative cell and tissue damage.

provitamin An inactive form of a vitamin that the body can convert to an active form. An example is beta-carotene.

carotenoids Fat-soluble plant pigments that the body stores in the liver and adipose tissues. The body is able to convert certain carotenoids to vitamin A.

Cleavage here results
in two molecules of
vitamin A

Beta-carotene

Two molecules of
vitamin A (in the
form of retinol)

FIGURE 10.9 Chemical structure of beta-carotene. Cleavage of beta-carotene can result in the formation of two molecules of vitamin A.

One molecule of beta-carotene can be split to form two molecules of active vitamin A (**Figure 10.9**). So why are 12 g of beta-carotene considered equivalent to just 1 g of vitamin A? Several factors account for this. Sometimes a beta-carotene molecule is cleaved in such a way that only one molecule of vitamin A is produced. In addition, not all of the dietary beta-carotene that is consumed is converted to vitamin A, and the absorption of beta-carotene from the intestines is not as efficient as our absorption of vitamin A. Nutritionists express the units of beta-carotene in a food as Retinol Activity Equivalents, or RAE. This measurement indicates how much active vitamin A is available to the body after it has converted the beta-carotene in the food.

Functions of Beta-Carotene

Beta-carotene and some other carotenoids are recognized to have antioxidant properties. Like vitamin E, they are fat soluble and fight the harmful effects of oxidation in the lipid portions of the cell membranes and in LDLs; however, compared to vitamin E, beta-carotene is a relatively weak antioxidant. In fact, other carotenoids, such as lycopene and lutein, may be stronger antioxidants.

Carotenoids play other important roles in the body through their antioxidant actions:

- Enhance the immune system and boost the body's ability to fight illness and disease
- Protect skin from the damage caused by the sun's ultraviolet rays
- Protect our eyes from damage, preventing or delaying age-related vision impairment

Carotenoids are also associated with a decreased risk for certain types of cancer. We discuss the roles of carotenoids and other antioxidants in cancer later in this chapter.

How Much Beta-Carotene Should We Consume?

Nutritional scientists do not consider beta-carotene and other carotenoids to be essential nutrients, as they play no known essential roles in our bodies and are not associated with any deficiency symptoms. Thus, no RDA for these compounds has been established. Eating the recommended five servings of fruits and vegetables each provides approximately 6 to 8 mg of beta-carotene.[9]

Supplements containing beta-carotene are very popular, and supplementation studies have typically prescribed doses of 15 to 30 mg of beta-carotene. Do these studies support claims that beta-carotene supplementation can reduce our risk for chronic diseases, particularly cancer? Large, randomized, controlled trials, such as the Alpha-Tocopherol Beta-Carotene (ATBC) Cancer Prevention

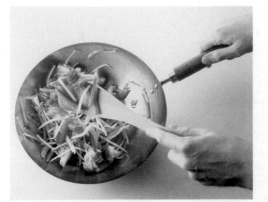

Fresh vegetables are good sources of vitamin C and beta-carotene.

Study and the Beta-Carotene and Retinol Efficacy Trial (CARET), have found that, contrary to expectations, taking beta-carotene supplements *increased* the rates of premature death from lung cancer, heart disease and stroke.[10,11] A recent systematic review of the available published studies reports that beta-carotene supplementation has no effect on the incidence of all cancers combined, pancreatic cancer, colorectal cancer, prostate cancer, breast cancer, melanoma, and nonmelanoma skin cancer. However, the incidence of lung and stomach cancers was significantly increased in those taking higher doses (20–30 mg per day), as well as in smokers and asbestos workers.[12]

Good Food Sources of Beta-Carotene

Fruits and vegetables that are red, orange, yellow, and deep green are generally high in beta-carotene and other carotenoids, such as lutein and lycopene. Eating the recommended amounts of fruits and vegetables each day ensures an adequate intake of carotenoids. Because of its color, beta-carotene is used as a natural coloring agent for many foods, including margarine, yellow cheddar cheese, cereal, cake mixes, gelatins, and soft drinks. However, these foods are not significant sources of beta-carotene. **Figure 10.10** identifies common foods that are high in beta-carotene. The following are some ways to boost your intake of dietary beta-carotene:

- Start your day with an orange, a grapefruit, a pear, a banana, an apple, or a slice of cantaloupe. All are good sources of beta-carotene.
- Pack a zip-lock bag of carrot slices or dried apricots in your lunch.
- Instead of french fries, think orange! Slice raw sweet potatoes, toss the slices in olive or canola oil, and bake.
- Add veggies to homemade pizza.
- Add shredded carrots to cake and muffin batters.
- Taking dessert to a potluck? Make a pumpkin pie! It's easy if you use canned pumpkin and follow the recipe on the can.
- Go green, too! The next time you have a salad, go for the dark-green, leafy vegetables instead of iceberg lettuce.
- Add raw spinach or other green, leafy vegetables to wraps and sandwiches.

We generally absorb only between 20% and 40% of the carotenoids present in the foods we eat. In contrast to vitamins E and C, carotenoids are better absorbed from cooked

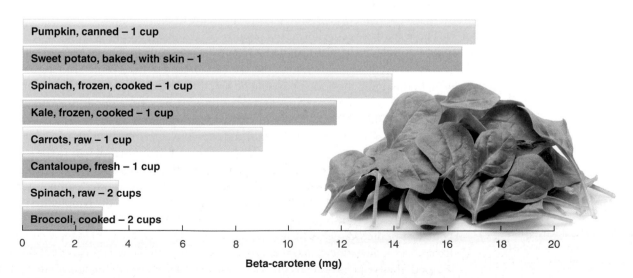

FIGURE 10.10 Common food sources of beta-carotene. There is no RDA for beta-carotene. (*Source:* Data from U.S. Department of Agriculture, Agricultural Research Service, 2011. USDA National Nutrient Database for Standard Reference, Release 24. www.ars.usda.gov/ba/bhnrc/ndl)

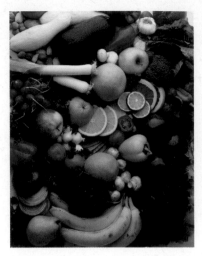

Foods that are high in carotenoids are easy to recognize by their bright colors.

foods. Carotenoids are bound in the cells of plants, and the process of lightly cooking these plants breaks chemical bonds and can rupture cell walls, which humans don't digest. These actions result in more of the carotenoids being released from the plant. For instance, 1 cup of raw carrots contains approximately 9 mg of beta-carotene, whereas the same amount of cooked frozen carrots contains approximately 12 mg.[13]

What Happens If We Consume Too Much Beta-Carotene?

Consuming large amounts of beta-carotene or other carotenoids in foods does not appear to cause toxic symptoms. However, your skin can turn yellow or orange if you consume large amounts of foods that are high in beta-carotene. This condition is referred to as *carotenosis* or *carotenodermia,* and it appears to be both reversible and harmless. Taking beta-carotene supplements is not generally recommended due to the risks just mentioned and because we can get adequate amounts of this nutrient by eating more fruits and vegetables.

What Happens If We Don't Consume Enough Beta-Carotene?

There are no known deficiency symptoms for beta-carotene or other carotenoids apart from beta-carotene's function as a precursor for vitamin A.

RECAP

Beta-carotene is a carotenoid and a provitamin of vitamin A. It protects the lipid portions of cell membranes and LDL-cholesterol from oxidative damage. It also enhances immune function and protects vision. There is no RDA for beta-carotene. Orange, red, and deep-green fruits and vegetables are good sources of beta-carotene. Taking beta-carotene supplements can increase the risk for death from lung and stomach cancers. There are no known toxicity or deficiency symptoms of beta-carotene when consumed from food, but yellowing of the skin can occur if too much beta-carotene is consumed. ■

Vitamin A

As early as AD 30, the Roman writer Aulus Cornelius Celsus described in his medical encyclopedia, *De Medicina,* a condition called *night blindness* and recommended as a cure the consumption of liver. We now know that night blindness is due to a deficiency of vitamin A, a fat-soluble vitamin stored primarily in the liver of animals.

There are three active forms of vitamin A in the body: **retinol** is the alcohol form, **retinal** is the aldehyde form, and **retinoic acid** is the acid form. These three forms are collectively referred to as the *retinoids* (**Figure 10.11**). Of the three, retinol has the starring role in maintaining the body's physiologic functions. Remember from the previous section that beta-carotene is a precursor to vitamin A. When we eat foods that contain beta-carotene, it is converted to retinol in the wall of the small intestine. Preformed vitamin A is present in foods in the form of retinol and as *retinyl ester-compounds,* in which retinol is attached to a fatty acid. These retinyl ester-compounds are hydrolyzed in the small intestine, leaving retinol in its free form. Free retinol is then absorbed into the wall of the small intestine, where a fatty acid is attached to form new retinyl ester-compounds. These compounds are then packaged into chylomicrons and enter into the lymphatic system. The chylomicrons transport vitamin A to the cells as needed or into the liver for storage. About 90% of the vitamin A we absorb is stored in the liver; the remainder is stored in adipose tissue, the kidneys, and the lungs. Because fat-soluble vitamins cannot dissolve in the blood, they require proteins that can bind with and transport them from their storage sites through the bloodstream to target tissues and cells. *Retinol-binding protein* is one such carrier protein for vitamin A. Retinol-binding protein carries retinol from the liver to the cells that require it.

retinol An active, alcohol form of vitamin A that plays an important role in healthy vision and immune function.

retinal An active, aldehyde form of vitamin A that plays an important role in healthy vision and immune function.

retinoic acid An active, acid form of vitamin A that plays an important role in cell growth and immune function.

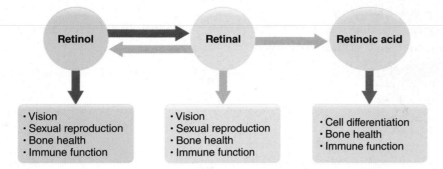

FIGURE 10.11 The three active forms of vitamin A in our bodies are retinol, retinal, and retinoic acid. Retinol and retinal can be converted interchangeably; retinoic acid is formed from retinal, and this process is irreversible. Each form of vitamin A contributes to many of our bodily processes.

The unit of expression for vitamin A is Retinol Activity Equivalents (RAE). You may still see the expression Retinol Equivalents (RE) or International Units (IU) for vitamin A on food labels or dietary supplements. The conversions to RAE from various dietary forms of retinol are as follows:

- 1 RAE = 1 microgram (μg) retinol
- 1 RAE = 12 μg beta-carotene
- 1 RAE = 24 μg alpha-carotene or beta-cryptoxanthin
- 1 RAE = 1 RE
- 1 RAE = 3.3 IU

Conversion rates from IU to μg RAE are as follows:

- 1 IU retinol from food or supplements = 0.3 μg RAE
- 1 IU beta-carotene from supplements = 0.15 μg RAE
- 1 IU beta-carotene from food = 0.05 μg RAE
- 1 IU alpha-carotene or beta-cryptoxanthin = 0.025 μg RAE

Functions of Vitamin A

The known functions of vitamin A are numerous, and researchers speculate that many are still to be discovered.

Vitamin A Is Essential to Sight A critical role of vitamin A in the body is the maintenance of healthy vision. Vitamin A affects our sight in two ways: it enables us to react to changes in the brightness of light, and it enables us to distinguish between different wavelengths of light—in other words, to see different colors. Let's take a closer look at this process.

Light enters the eyes through the cornea, travels through the lens, and then hits the **retina,** which is a delicate membrane lining the back of the inner eyeball (**Figure 10.12**). You might already have guessed how *retinal* got its name: it is found in—and is integral to—the retina. In the retina, retinal combines with a protein called **opsin** to form **rhodopsin,** a light-sensitive pigment. Rhodopsin is found in the **rod cells,** which are cells that react to dim light and interpret black-and-white images.

When light hits the retina, the rod cells go through a **bleaching process.** In this reaction, rhodopsin is split into retinal and opsin, and the rod cells lose their color. The retinal component also changes spatial orientation from a *cis* configuration, which is bent, into a *trans* configuration, which is straight. The opsin component also changes shape. These changes in retinal and opsin during the bleaching process generate a nerve impulse that travels to the brain, resulting in the perception of a black-and-white image. Most of the

retina The delicate, light-sensitive membrane lining the inner eyeball and connected to the optic nerve. It contains retinal.

opsin A protein that combines with retinal in the retina to form rhodopsin.

rhodopsin A light-sensitive pigment found in the rod cells that is formed by retinal and opsin.

rod cells Light-sensitive cells found in the retina that contain rhodopsin and react to dim light and interpret black-and-white images.

bleaching process A reaction in which the rod cells in the retina lose their color when rhodopsin is split into retinal and opsin.

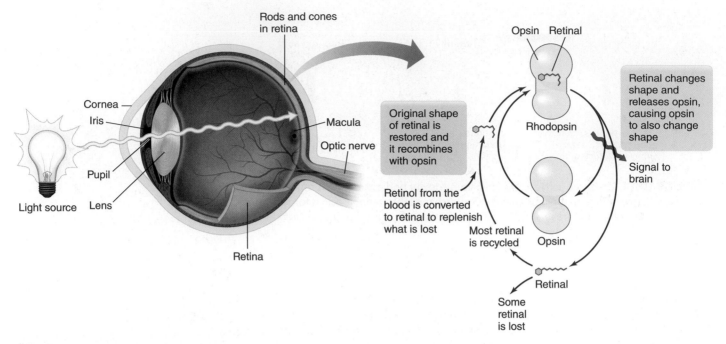

FIGURE 10.12 Vitamin A is necessary to maintain healthy vision. Light enters the eye through the cornea, travels through the lens, and hits the retina, located in the back of the eye. In the rod cells of the retina, retinal is combined with opsin to form rhodopsin. As light hits the rod cells, they lose color, and the components of rhodopsin, retinal and opsin, split and change shape. These changes cause transmission of the signal to the brain that enables us to see.

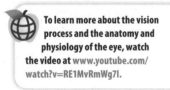

To learn more about the vision process and the anatomy and physiology of the eye, watch the video at www.youtube.com/watch?v=RE1MvRmWg7I.

night blindness A vitamin A–deficiency disorder that results in loss of the ability to see in dim light.

cone cells Light-sensitive cells found in the retina that contain the pigment iodopsin and react to bright light and interpret color images.

iodopsin A color-sensitive pigment found in the cone cells of the retina.

cell differentiation The process by which immature, undifferentiated stem cells develop into highly specialized functional cells of discrete organs and tissues.

retinal is converted back to its original *cis* form and binds with opsin to regenerate rhodopsin, allowing the visual cycle to begin again. However, some of the retinal is lost with each cycle and must be replaced by retinol from the bloodstream. This visual cycle goes on continually, allowing our eyes to adjust moment to moment to subtle changes in our surroundings or in the level of light.

When levels of vitamin A are deficient, people suffer from a condition referred to as night blindness. **Night blindness** results in the inability of the eyes to adjust to dim light. It can also result in the failure to regain sight quickly after a bright flash of light (**Figure 10.13**).

At the same time that we are interpreting black-and-white images, the **cone cells** of the retina, which are only effective in bright light, use retinal to interpret different wavelengths of light as different colors. The pigment involved in color vision is **iodopsin.** Iodopsin experiences similar changes during the color vision cycle as rhodopsin does during the black-and-white vision cycle. As with the rod cells, the cone cells can also be affected by a deficiency of vitamin A, resulting in color blindness.

In summary, the abilities to adjust to dim light, recover from a bright flash of light, and see in color are all critically dependent on adequate levels of retinal in the eyes.

Vitamin A Contributes to Cell Differentiation Another important role of vitamin A is its contribution to **cell differentiation,** the process by which stem cells mature into highly specialized cells that perform unique functions. The retinoic acid form of vitamin A interacts with the receptor sites on a cell's DNA. This interaction influences gene expression and the determination of the type of cells that the stem cells eventually become. Obviously, this process is critical to the development of healthy organs and effectively functioning body systems.

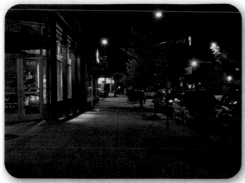
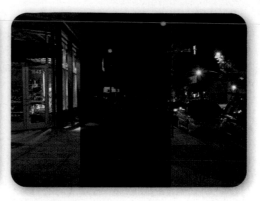

(a) Normal night vision   Poor night vision

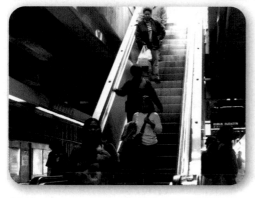
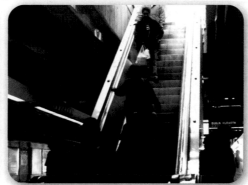

(b) Normal light adjustment   Slow light adjustment

FIGURE 10.13 A deficiency of vitamin A can result in night blindness. This condition results in **(a)** diminished side vision and overall poor night vision and **(b)** difficulty in adjusting from bright light to dim light.

An example of cell differentiation is the development of epithelial cells, such as skin cells, and mucus-producing cells of the protective linings of the lungs, vagina, intestines, stomach, bladder, urinary tract, and eyes. The mucus that epithelial cells produce lubricates the tissue and helps propel microbes, dust particles, foods, and fluids out of the body tissues (for example, when we cough up secretions or empty the bladder). When vitamin A levels are insufficient, the epithelial cells fail to differentiate appropriately, and we lose these protective barriers against infectious microbes and irritants.

Vitamin A is also critical to the differentiation of specialized immune cells called *T-lymphocytes,* or *T cells.* T cells assist in fighting infections. You can therefore see why vitamin A deficiency can lead to a breakdown of immune responses and to infections and other disorders of the lungs and respiratory tract, urinary tract, vagina, and eyes.

Other Functions of Vitamin A   Vitamin A is involved in reproduction. Although its exact role is unclear, it appears necessary for sperm production in men and for fertilization to occur in women. It also contributes to healthy bone growth by assisting in breaking down old bone, so that new, longer, and stronger bone can develop. As a result of a vitamin A deficiency, children suffer from stunted growth and wasting.

Past limited research indicated that vitamin A may act as an antioxidant by scavenging free radicals and protecting LDLs from oxidation. However, in the absence of recent research confirming this view, we can only say that it is unclear if vitamin A makes some minimal contribution to antioxidant function.

Search the Internet and you'll find plenty of sites claiming a direct link between vitamin A deficiency and acne and insisting that vitamin A supplements can successfully treat it. Should you believe the hype?

In 2006, a study reported an association between low blood levels of vitamin A and the presence of acne: the more severe the acne, the lower the levels of vitamin A.[14] Although these findings may seem suggestive, this study was conducted with a very small number of participants who were not randomly selected. Also, plasma levels of vitamin A were assessed to indicate vitamin A status; however, the Institute of Medicine states that plasma levels of vitamin A are not necessarily an indicator of vitamin A status.[15] To date, these results have not been replicated by other researchers, and there appears to be no evidence that vitamin A deficiency causes acne.

Interestingly, two effective treatments for acne are synthetic derivatives of vitamin A. Retin-A, or tretinoin, is a treatment applied to the skin. Accutane, or isotretinoin, is taken orally. These medications should be used carefully and only under the supervision of a licensed physician. Both medications increase a person's sensitivity to the sun, and it is recommended that exposure to sunlight be limited while using them. They also can cause birth defects in infants if used while a woman is pregnant and can lead to other toxicity problems, depression, and suicide in some individuals. Contrary to what you might read on the Internet, vitamin A itself has no effect on acne; thus, vitamin A supplements are not recommended in its treatment.

How Much Vitamin A Should We Consume?

Vitamin A toxicity can occur readily, because it is a fat-soluble vitamin, so it is important to consume only the amount recommended for your gender and age range.

Recommended Dietary Intake for Vitamin A The RDA for vitamin A is 900 μg per day for men and 700 μg per day for women. The UL is 3,000 μg per day of preformed vitamin A in women (including those pregnant and lactating) and men.

How can you determine the μg RAE when expressed as IU units that come from various food and supplement sources? Refer to the **You Do the Math** box (page 408) to learn how to apply these conversions.

Good Food Sources of Vitamin A Vitamin A is present in both animal and plant sources. To calculate the total RAE in a person's diet, you must take into consideration both the amount of retinol and the amount of provitamin A carotenoids that are present in the foods eaten. Remember that 12 μg of beta-carotene yields 1 μg of RAE, and 24 μg of alpha-carotene or beta-cryptoxanthin yields 1 μg of RAE. Thus, if a person consumes 400 μg retinol, 1,200 μg beta-carotene, and 3,000 μg alpha-carotene, the total RAE is equal to 400 μg + (1,200 μg ÷ 12) + (3,000 μg ÷ 24), or 625 μg RAE.

The most common sources of dietary preformed vitamin A are animal foods such as beef liver, chicken liver, eggs, and whole-fat dairy products. Vitamin A is also found in fortified reduced-fat milks, margarine, and some breakfast cereals (**Figure 10.14**). The other sources of the vitamin A we consume are foods high in beta-carotene and other carotenoids that can be converted to vitamin A. As discussed earlier in this chapter, dark-green, orange, and deep-yellow fruits and vegetables are good sources of beta-carotene and thus of vitamin A. Carrots, spinach, mango, cantaloupe, and tomato juice are excellent sources of vitamin A because they contain beta-carotene.

What Happens If We Consume Too Much Vitamin A?

Vitamin A is highly toxic, and toxicity symptoms develop after consuming only three to four times the RDA. Toxicity rarely results from food sources, but vitamin A supplementation is known to have caused severe illness and even death. In pregnant women, it can cause serious birth defects and spontaneous abortion. Other toxicity symptoms include fatigue, loss of appetite, blurred vision, hair loss, skin disorders, bone and joint pain, abdominal pain, nausea, diarrhea, and damage to the liver and nervous system. If caught in time, many of these symptoms are reversible once vitamin A supplementation is stopped. However, permanent damage can occur to the liver, eyes, and other organs. Because liver

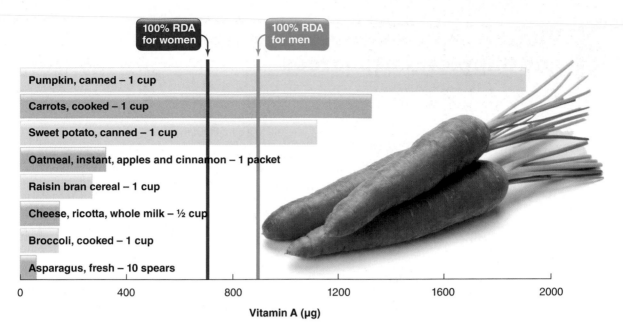

FIGURE 10.14 Common food sources of vitamin A. The RDA for vitamin A is 900 μg per day for men and 700 μg per day for women. (*Source:* Data from U.S. Department of Agriculture, Agricultural Research Service, 2011. USDA National Nutrient Database for Standard Reference, Release 24. www.ars.usda.gov/ba/bhnrc/ndl)

contains such a high amount of vitamin A, children and pregnant women should not consume liver on a daily or weekly basis.

What Happens If We Don't Consume Enough Vitamin A?

As discussed earlier, night blindness and color blindness can result from vitamin A deficiency. How severe a problem is night blindness? Although much less common among people of developed nations, vitamin A deficiency is a severe public health concern in developing countries. According to the World Health Organization, approximately 250 million preschool children suffer from vitamin A deficiency.[16] Of the children affected, 250,000 to 500,000 become permanently blinded every year. Because of their risky health status, at least half of these children are likely to die within 1 year of losing their sight. Death is often due to infections and illnesses, including measles and diarrhea, which are easily treated in more affluent countries. Vitamin A deficiency is also a tragedy for pregnant women in many developing countries. They often suffer from night blindness, are more likely to transmit HIV to their child if HIV-positive, and run a greater risk for maternal mortality. (Chapter 19 discusses what is being done to combat vitamin A deficiency and night blindness throughout the world.)

If vitamin A deficiency progresses, it can result in irreversible blindness due to hardening of the cornea (the transparent membrane covering the front of the eye), a condition called **xerophthalmia.** The prefix of this word, *xero-,* comes from a Greek word meaning "dry." Lack of vitamin A causes the epithelial cells of the cornea to lose their ability to produce mucus, causing the eye to become very dry. This leaves the cornea susceptible to damage, infection, and hardening. Once the cornea hardens in this way, the resulting blindness is irreversible. This is why it is critical to catch vitamin A deficiency in its early stages and treat it with either the regular consumption of fruits and vegetables that contain beta-carotene or vitamin A supplementation.

Vitamin A deficiency can also lead to follicular **hyperkeratosis,** a condition characterized by the excess accumulation of the protein keratin in the hair follicles. Keratin is usually found only on the outermost surface of skin, hair, nails, and tooth enamel. With hyperkeratosis, keratin clogs hair follicles, makes skin rough and bumpy; prevents

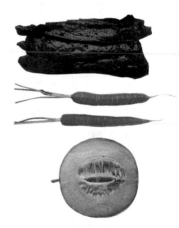

Liver, carrots, and cantaloupe all contain carotenoids that can be converted to vitamin A.

xerophthalmia An irreversible blindness due to hardening of the cornea and drying of the mucous membranes of the eye.

hyperkeratosis A condition resulting in the excess accumulation of the protein keratin in the follicles of the skin; this condition can also impair the ability of epithelial tissues to produce mucus.

YOU Do the Math

Vitamin A Unit Conversions from Food and Supplement Sources

Shaleen is a 24-year-old female who is neither pregnant nor lactating, and she wants to better understand how the various forms of vitamin A she may consume from food and supplements contribute to her RDA. The information she has available is in IU units, and she wants to calculate how these sources contribute to her RDA of 700 µg RAE. (To do the math, Shaleen refers to the conversion rates listed on page 403).

On the same page, she saw that the conversion rates from IU to µg RAE are as follows:

- 1 IU retinol from food or supplements = 0.3 µg RAE
- 1 IU beta-carotene from supplements = 0.15 µg RAE
- 1 IU beta-carotene from food = 0.05 µg RAE
- 1 IU alpha-carotene or beta-cryptoxanthin = 0.025 µg RAE

a. If Shaleen were to consume all of her vitamin A as retinol from food or supplements, how many IU units would she need to consume to meet her RDA?

As Shaleen's RDA is 700 µg RAE, and 1 IU retinol from food or supplements is equal to 0.3 µg RAE, this is equal to 700 µg RAE ÷ 0.3 µg RAE per 1 IU = 2333 IU of retinol.

b. If Shaleen consumed a vegetarian diet and consumed all of her vitamin A as beta-carotene from food, how many IU units would she need to consume to meet her RDA?

1 IU retinol from beta-carotene from food is equal to 0.05 µg RAE. Thus, 700 µg RAE ÷ 0.05 µg RAE per 1 IU = 14,000 IU of retinol.

c. In reality, Shaleen consumes a mixed diet in which she gets her vitamin A from a variety of food sources. She uses MyDietAnalysis to analyze her diet and finds she is currently consuming 600 µg RAE, which is 85.7% of the RDA, where (600 µg RAE ÷ 700 µg RAE) × 100 = 85.7%. She is considering taking a beta-carotene supplement to reach her RDA. She finds a supplement advertised on the Internet that contains 10,000 IU of beta-carotene and is enriched with carrots, parsley, and watercress. She knows that 1 IU of beta-carotene from supplements is equal to 0.15 µg RAE. Thus, the total amount of µg RAE she would get by taking this supplement is

10,000 IU × 0.15 µg RAE = 1500 µg RAE, which is well above the 100 µg RAE she needs to meet the RDA!

Shaleen would be much wiser to consume this 100 µg RAE from fruits and vegetables high in beta-carotene. As 1 µg RAE = 12 µg beta-carotene from food, she determines that she needs to consume 1,200 µg of beta-carotene from food (12 µg beta-carotene × 100 µg RAE needed to meet the RDA). She refers to the US Department of Agriculture Nutrient Database Standard Reference 24 on the Internet at www.ars.usda.gov/Services/docs.htm?docid=22114, looks at the report of food sources specifically for beta-carotene, and discovers she can simply and more safely consume 1 cup of cooked broccoli (1,449 µg beta-carotene) or one raw carrot (5,965 µg beta-carotene) to easily and inexpensively meet her RDA for vitamin A.

Now use your own diet assessment to determine *your* intake of vitamin A. What percentage of the RDA for vitamin A do you currently consume? If you were to consume the same beta-carotene supplement that Shaleen considered, how many could you take before exceeding the UL for vitamin A based on your current dietary intake of vitamin A?

Answers will vary depending on individual body criteria and intake levels.

---

proper sweating through the sweat glands; and causes skin to become very dry and thick. Hyperkeratosis can also affect the epithelial cells of various tissues, including the mouth, urinary tract, vagina, and eyes, reducing the production of mucus by these tissues and leading to an increased risk for infection. Hyperkeratosis can be reversed with vitamin A supplementation.

Other deficiency symptoms include impaired immunity, increased risk for illness and infections, reproductive system disorders, and failure of normal growth. Individuals who are at risk for vitamin A deficiency include elderly people with poor diets, newborn or premature infants (due to low liver stores of vitamin A), young children with inadequate vegetable and fruit intakes, and alcoholics. Any condition that results in fat malabsorption can also lead to vitamin A deficiency. Children with cystic fibrosis; individuals with Crohn's disease, celiac disease, or diseases of the liver, pancreas, or gallbladder; and people who consume large amounts of the fat substitute Olestra are at risk for vitamin A deficiency.

RECAP

Vitamin A is critical for maintaining our vision. It is also necessary for cell differentiation, reproduction, and growth. The role of vitamin A as an antioxidant is still under investigation. The RDA for vitamin A is 900 µg per day for men and 700 µg per day for women. Animal liver, dairy products, and eggs are good animal sources of vitamin A; fruits and vegetables are high in beta-carotene, which is used to synthesize vitamin A. Supplementation can be dangerous, as toxicity is reached at levels of only three to four times the RDA. Toxicity symptoms include birth defects, spontaneous abortion, blurred vision, and liver damage. Deficiency symptoms include night blindness, impaired immune function, and growth failure. ■

Selenium

Selenium is a trace mineral, and it is found in varying amounts in soil and thus in the food grown there. Keep in mind that, although we need only minute amounts of trace minerals, they are just as important to our health as the vitamins and the major minerals. Selenium is efficiently absorbed, with about 50% to 90% of dietary selenium absorbed from the small intestine.[8]

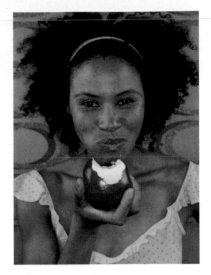

Eating plenty of fruits and vegetables can help prevent vitamin A deficiency.

Functions of Selenium

It is only recently that we have learned about the critical role of selenium as a nutrient in human health. In 1979, Chinese scientists reported an association between a heart disorder called **Keshan disease** and selenium deficiency. This disease occurs in children in the Keshan province of China, where the soil is depleted of selenium. The scientists found that Keshan disease can be prevented with selenium supplementation.

The selenium in our bodies is contained in amino acids. Two amino acid derivatives contain the majority of selenium in our bodies: **selenomethionine** is the storage form for selenium, and **selenocysteine** is the active form of selenium. Selenocysteine is a critical component of the glutathione peroxidase enzyme system, mentioned earlier. As shown in **Figure 10.15**, glutathione peroxidase breaks down the peroxides (such as hydrogen peroxide) that are formed by the body, so that they cannot form free radicals; this decrease in the

Keshan disease A heart disorder caused by selenium deficiency. It was first identified in children in the Keshan province of China.

selenomethionine An amino acid derivative that is the storage form for selenium in the body.

selenocysteine An amino acid derivative that is the active form of selenium in the body.

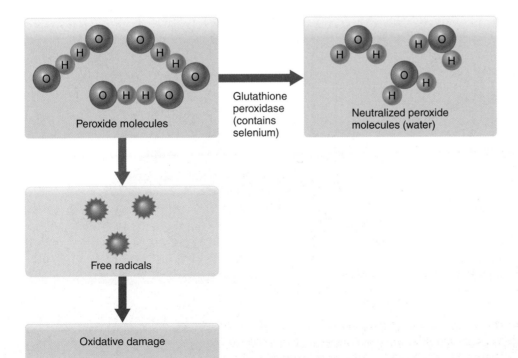

FIGURE 10.15 Selenium is part of glutathione peroxidase, which neutralizes peroxide molecules that are formed by the body, so that they cannot form free radicals; this decrease in the number of free radicals spares vitamin E and prevents oxidative damage.

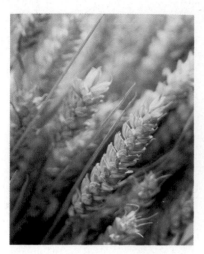

Wheat is a rich source of selenium.

number of free radicals spares vitamin E. Thus, selenium helps spare vitamin E and prevents oxidative damage to cell membranes.

Like vitamin C, selenium is needed for the production of *thyroxine,* or thyroid hormone. By this action, selenium is involved in the maintenance of basal metabolism and body temperature. Selenium appears to play a role in immune function, and poor selenium status is associated with higher rates of some forms of cancer.

How Much Selenium Should We Consume?

The content of selenium in foods is highly variable. As it is a trace mineral, we need only minute amounts to maintain health. The RDA for selenium is 55 μg per day for both men and women. The UL is 400 μg per day.

Selenium is present in both plant and animal food sources but in variable amounts. Because it is stored in the tissues of animals, selenium is found in reliably consistent amounts in animal foods. Organ meats, such as liver and kidney, as well as pork and seafood, are particularly good sources (**Figure 10.16**).

In contrast, the amount of selenium in plants is dependent on the selenium content of the soil in which the plant is grown. Many companies marketing selenium supplements warn that the agricultural soils in the United States are depleted of selenium and inform us that we need to take selenium supplements. In reality, the selenium content of soil varies greatly across North America, and because we obtain our food from a variety of geographic locations, few people in the United States suffer from selenium deficiency. This is especially true for people who eat even small quantities of meat or seafood.

What Happens If We Consume Too Much Selenium?

Selenium toxicity does not result from eating foods high in selenium. However, supplementation can cause toxicity. Toxicity symptoms include brittle hair and nails that can eventually break and fall off. Other symptoms include skin rashes, nausea, vomiting, weakness, and cirrhosis of the liver.

What Happens If We Don't Consume Enough Selenium?

As discussed previously, selenium deficiency is associated with a form of heart disease called Keshan disease. Selenium deficiency does not cause the disease, but selenium is

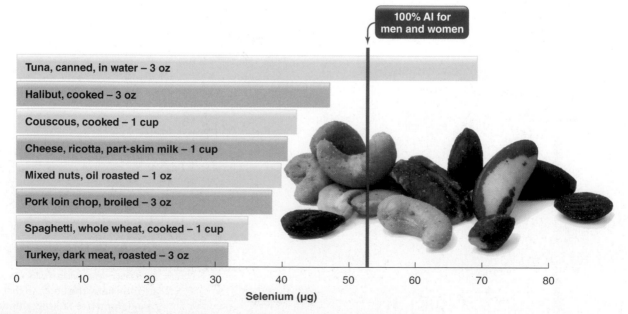

FIGURE 10.16 Common food sources of selenium. The RDA for selenium is 55 μg per day. (*Source:* Data from U.S. Department of Agriculture, Agricultural Research Service, 2011. USDA National Nutrient Database for Standard Reference, Release 24. www.ars.usda.gov/ba/bhnrc/ndl.)

necessary to help the immune system effectively fight the viral infection that causes the disease.[8] Selenium supplements significantly reduce the incidence of Keshan disease, but they cannot reduce the damage to the heart muscle once it occurs.

Another deficiency disorder is *Kashin-Beck disease,* a disease of the cartilage that results in deforming arthritis (**Figure 10.17**). Kashin-Beck disease is found in selenium-depleted areas in China and Tibet. Other deficiency symptoms include impaired immune responses, infertility, depression, impaired cognitive function, and muscle pain and wasting. Deficiencies of both selenium and iodine in pregnant women can cause a form of *cretinism* in the infant. (The condition of cretinism is discussed in Chapter 8.)

Copper, Iron, Zinc, and Manganese Assist in Antioxidant Function

As discussed earlier, there are numerous antioxidant enzyme systems in our bodies. Copper, zinc, and manganese are a part of the superoxide dismutase antioxidant enzyme system. Iron is part of the structure of catalase. In addition to their role in protecting against oxidative damage, these minerals play major roles in the optimal functioning of many other enzymes in the body. Copper, iron, and zinc help us maintain the health of our blood, and manganese is an important cofactor in carbohydrate metabolism (these nutrients are discussed in detail in Chapter 12).

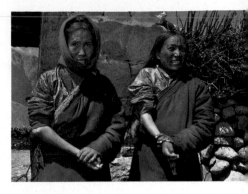

FIGURE 10.17 Selenium deficiency can lead to a type of deforming arthritis called Kashin-Beck disease.

RECAP

Selenium is part of the glutathione peroxidase enzyme system. It indirectly spares vitamin E from oxidative damage, and it assists with immune function and the production of thyroid hormone. Organ meats, pork, and seafood are good sources. The selenium content of plants is dependent on the amount of selenium in the soil in which they are grown. Toxicity symptoms include brittle hair and nails, nausea, vomiting, and liver cirrhosis. Deficiency can result in Keshan disease, Kashin-Beck disease, impaired immune function, infertility, and muscle wasting. Copper, zinc, and manganese are cofactors for the superoxide dismutase antioxidant enzyme system. Iron is a cofactor for the catalase antioxidant enzyme. These minerals play critical roles in blood health and energy metabolism. ■

What Disorders Are Related to Free-Radical Damage?

You've probably encountered a plethora of health claims related to the functions of antioxidants—for instance, that they slow the effects of aging or prevent heart disease and cancer. In opposition to these claims, there is some evidence that taking antioxidant supplements may be harmful (refer to the previous discussion on beta-carotene, pages 399–402.).

In this section, we will review what is currently known about the role of antioxidant nutrients in cancer and heart disease.

Cancer

Before we explore how antioxidants affect the risk for cancer, let's take a closer look at precisely what cancer is and how it spreads. **Cancer** is actually a group of diseases that are all characterized by cells that grow "out of control." By this we mean that cancer cells reproduce spontaneously and independently, and they are not inhibited by the boundaries of tissues and organs. Thus, they can aggressively invade tissues and organs far away from those in which they originally formed.

cancer A group of diseases characterized by cells that reproduce spontaneously and independently and may invade other tissues and organs.

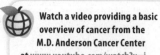

Watch a video providing a basic overview of cancer from the M.D. Anderson Cancer Center at www.youtube.com/watch?v=j_wRpa2b5Xl&feature=related.

Most forms of cancer result in one or more **tumors,** which are newly formed masses of undifferentiated cells that are immature and have no physiologic function. Although the word *tumor* sounds frightening, it is important to note that not every tumor is *malignant,* or cancerous. Many are *benign* (not harmful to us) and are made up of cells that will not spread widely.

Figure 10.18 shows how changes to normal cells prompt a series of other changes that can progress into cancer. There are three primary steps of cancer development: initiation, promotion, and progression. These steps occur as follows:

1. *Initiation:* The initiation of cancer occurs when a cell's DNA is *mutated* (changed). This mutation causes permanent changes in the cell that make it susceptible to promotion.
2. *Promotion:* During this phase, the genetically altered cell is stimulated to divide. A single mutated cell divides in two, and these double to four, and so on. The mutated DNA is locked into each new cell's genetic instructions. Because the enzymes that normally work to repair damaged cells cannot detect alterations in the DNA, the cells can continue to divide uninhibited. Typically, it takes many years for a mutated cell to double repeatedly into a tumor mass large enough to be detectable (about the size of a grape), and promotion is the longest stage in cancer development.[17]
3. *Progression:* During this phase, the cancerous cells grow out of control. They grow their own blood vessels, which supply them with blood and nutrients, and invade adjacent tissues. In this early stage of progression, the immune system can sometimes detect these cancerous cells and destroy them. However, if the cells continue to grow, they develop into malignant tumors, disrupting body functioning at their primary site and invading the circulatory and lymphatic systems to *metastasize* (spread) to distant sites in the body.

Although cancer is often fatal, a majority of people who develop cancer survive. In 2012 the American Cancer Society reported that the 5-year survival rate for all cancers was 67%.[18] Of course, cancers can be more or less aggressive, some are more readily detectable than others, and some tissues and organs are more vulnerable to cancer. All these factors influence the overall mortality rate associated with different cancers. The type of cancer with the highest mortality rate is lung cancer, with over 160,000 deaths in 2012. Even when it has not invaded regional tissues, the survival rate is just 52%, and with metastasis, this drops to just 4%. Cancer of the colon and/or rectum ranks second (more than 50,000 deaths in 2012), and breast cancer ranks third (almost 40,000 deaths).[18]

Nutri-Case

Gustavo

"Last night, there was an actress on TV talking about having colon cancer and saying everybody over age 50 should get tested. It brought back all the memories of my father's cancer, how thin and weak he got before he went to the doctor, so that by the time they found the cancer it had already spread too far. But I don't think I'm at risk. I only eat red meat two or three times a week, and I eat a piece of fruit or a vegetable at every meal. I don't smoke, and I get plenty of exercise, sunshine, and fresh air working in the vineyard."

What lifestyle factors reduce Gustavo's risk for cancer? What factors increase his risk? Think especially about possible occupational risk factors. Would you recommend he increase his consumption of fruits and vegetables? Why or why not? If Gustavo were your father, would you encourage him to have the screening test for colon cancer that the actress on television recommended?

tumor Any newly formed mass of immature, undifferentiated cells with no physiologic function.

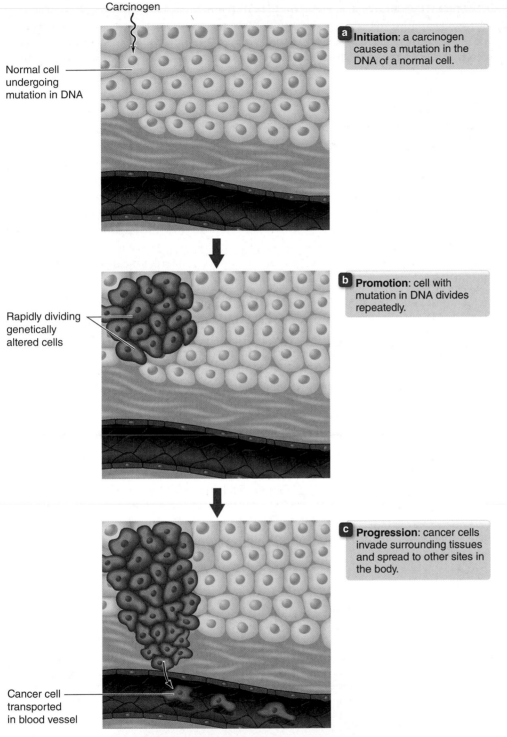

Carcinogen

Normal cell undergoing mutation in DNA

a **Initiation**: a carcinogen causes a mutation in the DNA of a normal cell.

Rapidly dividing genetically altered cells

b **Promotion**: cell with mutation in DNA divides repeatedly.

c **Progression**: cancer cells invade surrounding tissues and spread to other sites in the body.

Cancer cell transported in blood vessel

FIGURE 10.18 **(a)** Cancer cells develop as a result of a genetic mutation in the DNA of a normal cell. **(b)** The mutated cell replicates uncontrollably, eventually resulting in a tumor. **(c)** If not destroyed or removed, the cancerous tumor metastasizes to other parts of the body.

A Variety of Factors Influence Cancer Risk

Researchers estimate that about half of all men and one-third of all women will develop cancer during their lifetime.[18] But what factors cause cancer? Are you and your loved ones at risk? The answer depends on several factors, including your family history of cancer, your exposure to environmental agents, and various lifestyle choices.

Heredity can play a role in the development of cancer, because inherited "cancer genes," such as the *BRC* genes for breast cancer, increase the risk that an individual with those genes will develop cancer. However, only about 5% of all cancers are strongly

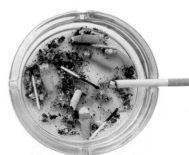

Using tobacco is a risk factor for cancer.

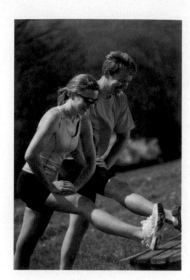

Staying physically active may help reduce our risk for some cancers.

hereditary.[18] In addition, it is important to bear in mind that a family history of cancer does not guarantee you will get cancer, too. It just means that you are at an increased risk and should take all preventive actions available to you. While some risk factors are out of your control, others are modifiable, which means that you can take positive steps to reduce your risk.

The American Cancer Society identifies six modifiable risk factors that have been shown to have the greatest impact on an individual's cancer risk; each is discussed next.[18]

Tobacco Use More than forty compounds in tobacco and tobacco smoke are *carcinogens,* or substances that can cause cancer. Smoking accounts for 30% of all cancer deaths and 80% of lung cancer deaths, and it increases the risk for acute myeloid leukemia and cancers of the nasopharynx, nasal cavity, paranasal sinus, lip, oral cavity, pharynx, larynx, lung, esophagus, pancreas, uterine cervix, ovaries, kidney, bladder, stomach, and colorectum (**Figure 10.19**).[18] Smoking can also cause heart disease, stroke, and emphysema. Overall, tobacco use accounts for about one in five deaths each year. (See the **Highlight** box on disorders linked to tobacco use.) The positive news is that tobacco use is a modifiable risk factor. If you smoke or use smokeless tobacco, you can reduce your risk for cancer considerably by quitting.

Weight, Diet, and Physical Activity Researchers estimate that one-third of cancer deaths are related to overweight or obesity, poor nutrition, and physical inactivity and thus could be prevented.[18] Nutritional factors that are protective against cancer include the consumption of foods rich in antioxidants, fiber, and phytochemicals. Diets high in saturated fats and low in fruits and vegetables increase the risk for cancers of the esophagus, colon, breast, and prostate.[19] Consumption of alcohol and compounds found in cured and charbroiled meats can also increase the risk for cancer.

A sedentary lifestyle increases the risk for colon cancer and possibly other forms of cancer. There is convincing evidence that regular physical activity decreases the risk for colon cancer, as well as probable evidence of a protective effect for endometrial cancer and postmenopausal breast cancer.[20] There is limited evidence that suggests physical activity may also be protective against cancers of the lung, pancreas, and breast (premenopausal). At this time, we do not know how exercise reduces the overall risk for cancer or for certain types of cancers. However, these findings have prompted the American Cancer Society and the National Cancer Institute to promote increased physical activity as a way to reduce our risk for cancer.

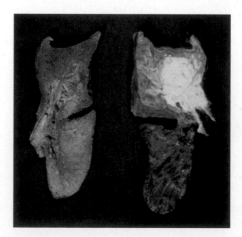

FIGURE 10.19 Cigarette smoking significantly increases our risk for lung and other types of cancer. The risk for lung cancer is twenty-three times higher in men who smoke and twelve times higher in women who smoke. **(a)** A normal, healthy lung; **(b)** the lung of a smoker. Notice the deposits of tar, as well as the areas of tumor growth.

Disorders Linked to Tobacco Use

HIGHLIGHT

Many people smoke cigarettes or cigars or use smokeless tobacco. The use of these products can lead to serious health consequences that together reduce life expectancy by more than 13 years in males and 14 years in females.[1] Tobacco use is a risk factor in development of all of the following diseases and health concerns:

1. Cancers
   - Lung
   - Larynx
   - Mouth (**Figure 10.20a**)
   - Pharynx
   - Esophagus
   - Bladder
   - Pancreas
   - Uterus
   - Kidney
   - Stomach
   - Some leukemias

2. Heart disease

3. Bronchitis

4. Emphysema

5. Stroke

6. Erectile dysfunction

7. Conditions related to maternal smoking
   - Miscarriage
   - Preterm delivery
   - Stillbirth
   - Infant death
   - Low birth weight

In addition, smoking causes a variety of other problems, such as the premature wrinkling and coarsening of the skin (shown in Figure 10.20b). Smoking also causes bad breath, yellowing of the fingernails and hair, and bad-smelling clothes, hair, and living quarters. Secondhand smoke is another concern, especially for those who live or work with smokers. Nonsmokers who are exposed to smoke at home or work increase their risk of developing heart disease by 25% to 30% and increase their risk of developing lung cancer by 20% to 30%. Research indicates that there is no risk-free level of exposure to secondhand smoke.[2]

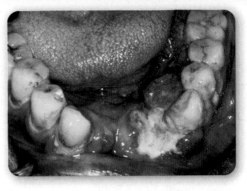

(a)

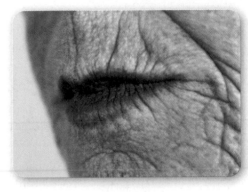

(b)

FIGURE 10.20 Effects of tobacco use. In addition to increasing your risk for lung cancer and cardiovascular disease, **(a)** using tobacco increases your risk for mouth cancer, and **(b)** smoking results in premature wrinkling of the skin, especially around the mouth.

References

1. American Cancer Society. 2012. ACS Guide to Quitting Smoking. www.cancer.org/docroot/PED/content/PED_10_13X_Guide_for_Quitting_Smoking.asp?sitearea5PED.
2. US Department of Health and Human Services (USDHHS). 2004. *The Health Consequences of Smoking: A Report of the Surgeon General.* Washington, DC: US Department of Health and Human Services, Centers for Disease Control and Prevention, National Center for Chronic Disease Prevention and Health Promotion, Office on Smoking and Health.

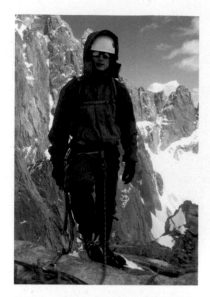

Arctic explorers wear special clothing to protect themselves from the cold, as well as from the high levels of ultraviolet rays from the sun.

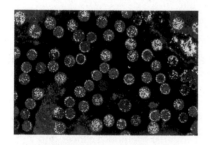

FIGURE 10.21 *Human papillomavirus* (HPV) is an infectious agent that can cause cancer.

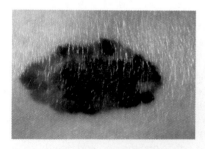

FIGURE 10.22 A lesion associated with malignant melanoma is characterized by asymmetry; uneven or blurred borders; mixed shades of tan, brown, black, and sometimes red or blue; and a diameter larger than a pencil eraser (6 mm).

Infectious Agents   Infectious agents account for 18% of cancers worldwide. For example, infection of the female cervix with the sexually transmitted virus *Human papillomavirus* is linked to cervical cancer (**Figure 10.21**), and infection with the bacterium *Helicobacter pylori* is linked not only to ulcers but also to stomach cancer. As microbial research advances, it is thought that more cancers will be linked to infectious agents.

Ultraviolet Radiation   Skin cancer is the most common form of cancer in the United States and accounts for over half of all cancers diagnosed each year. Most skin cancer cases are linked to exposure to ultraviolet (UV) rays from the sun and indoor tanning beds. UV rays damage the DNA of immature skin cells, which then reproduce uncontrollably. Research has shown that a person's risk for skin cancer doubles if he or she has had five or more sunburns; however, your risk for skin cancer still increases with UV exposure even if you do not get sunburned.[21] Exposure to tanning beds before age 35 increases by 75% your risk of developing the most invasive form of skin cancer.[22]

Skin cancer includes the nonmelanoma cancers (basal cell and squamous cell cancers), which are not typically invasive, and malignant melanoma, which is one of the most deadly of all types of cancer (**Figure 10.22**). Limiting exposure to sunlight to no more than 20 minutes between 10 AM and 4 PM can help reduce your risk for skin cancer while allowing your body to synthesize adequate vitamin D. After that, wear sunscreen with at least a 15 SPF (sun protection factor) rating and protective clothing.

Antioxidants Play a Role in Preventing Cancer

There is a large and growing body of evidence that antioxidants consumed in food play an important role in cancer prevention, but how? The following are some proposed mechanisms:

- Enhancing the immune system, which assists in the destruction and removal of precancerous cells from the body
- Inhibiting the growth of cancer cells and tumors
- Preventing oxidative damage to the cells' DNA by scavenging free radicals and stopping the formation and subsequent chain reaction of oxidized molecules

Eating whole foods that are high in antioxidants—especially fruits, vegetables, and whole grains—is linked with probable evidence of decreased risk for various cancers.[20] In addition, populations eating diets low in antioxidant nutrients have a higher risk for cancer. These studies show varying levels of association between consumption of dietary antioxidants and cancer risk, but they do not prove cause and effect. Nutrition experts agree that there are important interactions between antioxidant nutrients and other substances in foods, such as fiber and phytochemicals, which work together to reduce the risk for many types of cancers. Studies are now being conducted to determine whether eating foods high in antioxidants directly causes lower rates of cancer.

As discussed earlier in this chapter within the section on beta-carotene, the growing evidence over the past 20 years indicates that antioxidant supplementation does not reduce cancer risk; in fact, it may increase risks for various cancers and other chronic diseases.[10–12,23] Why have antioxidant supplements failed to bring the health benefits one might expect? It has been speculated that antioxidants taken in supplemental form may act as prooxidants in some situations, whereas antioxidants consumed in foods may be more balanced.

Thus, it appears that the best way to try to reduce our risks for cancer is to eat a diet with ample fruits and vegetables, maintain a healthy body weight, stay regularly physically active, quit smoking if applicable, and avoid exposure to infectious agents and UV radiation. Many studies are currently examining the impact of whole foods on the risk for various forms of cancer. The results of these studies will provide important insights into the link between whole foods and cancer. Refer to the **Nutrition Debate** at the end of the chapter to gain a better understanding of situations that may warrant vitamin and mineral supplementation.

Cardiovascular Disease

The details of *cardiovascular disease* (*CVD*) and its relationship to cholesterol and lipoproteins were presented earlier in this text (see Chapter 5). A brief review of CVD is presented here, focusing on the question of how antioxidants may reduce the risk for CVD.

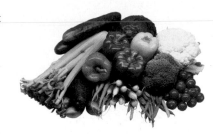

These vegetables provide antioxidant nutrients, fiber, and phytochemicals, all of which reduce the risk for some cancers.

Cardiovascular disease is the leading cause of death for adults in the United States. CVD encompasses all diseases of the heart and blood vessels, including coronary heart disease, hypertension (high blood pressure), and atherosclerosis (hardening of the arteries). The two primary manifestations of CVD are heart attack and stroke. Almost 750,000 people die each year from CVD, and it is estimated that CVD costs the United States $448 billion in healthcare costs and lost work revenue.[24,25]

Remember that the major risks for CVD are smoking, hypertension, high blood levels of LDL-cholesterol, obesity, and a sedentary lifestyle. Other risk factors include a low level of HDL-cholesterol, diabetes, family history (CVD in males younger than 55 years of age and females younger than 65 years of age), being a male older than 45 years of age, and being a postmenopausal woman. Although we cannot alter our gender, family history, or age, we can change our nutrition and physical activity habits to reduce our risk for CVD.

Research has recently identified a risk factor for CVD that may be even more important than elevated cholesterol levels: a condition called *low-grade inflammation.*[26] This condition weakens the atherosclerotic plaque in the blood vessels, making it more fragile. As the plaque becomes more fragile, it is more likely to burst, breaking away from the arterial lining and traveling freely in the bloodstream. It may then lodge in the blood vessels of the heart or brain, closing them off and leading to a heart attack or stroke, respectively.

In laboratory blood tests, the marker that indicates the degree of inflammation is C-reactive protein. Having higher levels of C-reactive protein increases the risk for a heart attack even if people do not have elevated cholesterol levels. For people with high levels of C-reactive protein and cholesterol, the risk for a heart attack is almost nine times higher than that for someone with normal cholesterol and C-reactive protein levels. These findings have prompted the medical community to develop standards for measuring C-reactive protein along with cholesterol as a test for CVD risk.

How can antioxidants decrease the risk for CVD? Laboratory studies suggest that some antioxidants, specifically vitamin E and lycopene, work in a variety of ways that reduce the damage to the vessels, which in turn reduces the risk for a heart attack or stroke. Some of the ways these nutrients might decrease the risk for CVD include scavenging free radicals, reducing low-grade inflammation, and reducing blood coagulation and the formation of blood clots.

Taking antioxidant supplements does not reduce the incidence of major cardiovascular events in men and women taking vitamins E or C.[5,27] In fact, a recently published systematic review and meta-analysis examining randomized, controlled trials on antioxidant supplements (including beta-carotene; vitamins A, C, and E; and selenium) found that taking beta-carotene and vitamin E supplements and relatively high doses of vitamin A *increases* the risk for premature mortality from all causes.[23] Vitamin C and selenium supplements have no effect of rates of premature mortality.

However epidemiological studies find consistent associations between consumption of foods high in antioxidants and decreased risks for CVD. It is important to note that other compounds (besides antioxidants) found in fruits, vegetables, and whole grains can reduce our risk for CVD. For instance, soluble fiber has been shown to reduce elevated LDL-cholesterol and total cholesterol. The most successful effects have been found in people eating oatmeal and oat-bran cereals. Dietary fiber in general has been shown to reduce blood pressure, lower total cholesterol levels, and improve blood glucose and insulin levels. Folate, a B-vitamin, is found in fortified cereals, bananas, legumes, orange juice, and green, leafy vegetables. Folate is known to reduce homocysteine levels in the blood, and a high concentration of homocysteine in the blood is a known risk factor for CVD. Thus, it appears that there are a plethora of nutrients and other components in fruits, vegetables, and whole-grain foods that may be protective against CVD.

RECAP

Cancer is a group of diseases in which genetically mutated cells grow out of control. Tobacco use, obesity, dietary factors, low physical activity levels, infectious agents, and UV radiation are related to a higher risk for some cancers. Eating foods high in antioxidants is associated with lower rates of cancer and cardiovascular disease (CVD), but studies of antioxidant supplements, cancer, and CVD indicate that taking these supplements can increase the risk for cancer and premature mortality. ■

Chapter Review

TEST YOURSELF | ANSWERS

1 **T** Free radicals are highly unstable atoms that can destabilize neighboring atoms or molecules and harm our cells; however, they are a normal by-product of human physiology.

2 **F** Overall, the research on vitamin C and colds does not show strong evidence that taking vitamin C supplements reduces our risk of suffering from the common cold.

3 **T** Carrots are an excellent source of beta-carotene, a precursor for vitamin A, which helps maintain good vision.

4 **T** According to the American Cancer Society, smoking is the most preventable cause of death in our society. In addition, tobacco use accounts for about 30% of all cancer deaths and is the primary modifiable risk factor for cancer. Among other factors known to significantly influence cancer risk are nutrition, sun exposure, and level of physical activity.

5 **F** Currently, there is no known dietary cure for cancer. However, eating a diet that is plentiful in fruits and vegetables and exercising regularly may help reduce our risk for some forms of cancer.

Summary

- Antioxidants are compounds that protect our cells from oxidative damage.

- Free radicals are produced under many situations, including when the body generates ATP, when the immune system fights infection, and when we are exposed to environmental toxins, such as pollution, radiation, and tobacco smoke.

- Free radicals are dangerous because they can damage the lipid portion of our cell membranes, destroying the integrity of our cell membranes. Free radicals also damage LDLs, cell proteins, and DNA.

- Antioxidant vitamins donate their electrons or hydrogen atoms to free radicals to neutralize them. Antioxidant minerals are cofactors in antioxidant enzyme systems, which convert free radicals to less damaging substances that our bodies excrete.

- Vitamin E is an antioxidant that protects the fatty components of cell membranes from oxidation. It also protects LDLs, vitamin A, and our lungs from oxidative damage. Other functions of vitamin E are the development of nerves and muscles, enhancement of the immune function, and improvement of the absorption of vitamin A if intake of vitamin A is low.

- Vitamin C is an antioxidant that is oxidized by free radicals and prevents the damage of cells and tissues. Vitamin C also regenerates vitamin E after it has been oxidized. Other functions of vitamin C include helping the synthesis of collagen, carnitine, various hormones, neurotransmitters, and DNA; enhancing immune function; and increasing the absorption of iron.

- Beta-carotene is one of about 600 carotenoids identified to date. Beta-carotene is a provitamin, or precursor, to vitamin A, meaning it is an inactive form of vitamin A that is converted to vitamin A in the body.

- Beta-carotene protects the lipid portions of our membranes and the LDL-cholesterol from oxidative damage. Other functions of beta-carotene include enhancing our immune systems, protecting our skin from sun damage, and protecting our eyes from oxidative damage. Eating foods high in carotenoids may help reduce our risk for some forms of cancer.

- Vitamin A is a fat-soluble vitamin. The three active forms of vitamin A are retinol, retinal, and retinoic acid. Beta-carotene is converted to vitamin A in the small intestine.

- Vitamin A is extremely important for healthy vision. It ensures our ability to adjust to changes in the brightness of light, and it helps us maintain color vision. Vitamin A was once considered an antioxidant, but this role is not supported by recent research evidence. Other functions of vitamin A include assistance in cell differentiation, maintenance of healthy immune function, sexual reproduction, and proper bone growth.

- Selenium is a trace mineral that is part of the structure of glutathione peroxidases, a family of antioxidant enzymes. Other functions of selenium include assisting in the production of thyroid hormone and enhancing immune function.

- Copper, iron, zinc, and manganese are minerals that act as cofactors for antioxidant enzyme systems. Copper, zinc, and manganese are part of the superoxide dismutase complex, whereas iron is part of catalase. These minerals also play critical roles in energy metabolism and blood formation.

- Antioxidants play a role in cancer and CVD prevention. Eating foods high in antioxidants results in lower rates of some cancers and risk for CVD, but taking antioxidant supplements can cause cancer and increase the risk for premature mortality.

MasteringNutrition™

To further your understanding, go online and apply what you've learned to real-life case studies that will help you master the content!

Review Questions

1. Which of the following is a characteristic of vitamin E?
   a. It enhances the absorption of iron.
   b. It can be manufactured from beta-carotene.
   c. It is a critical component of the glutathione peroxidase system.
   d. It is destroyed by exposure to high heat.

2. Oxidation is best described as a process in which
   a. a carcinogen causes a mutation in a stem cell's DNA.
   b. an atom loses an electron.
   c. an element loses an atom of oxygen.
   d. a compound loses a molecule of water.

3. Which of the following disorders is linked with the production of free radicals?
   a. cardiovascular disease
   b. carotenosis
   c. ulcers
   d. malaria

4. Which of the following are known carcinogens?
   a. phytochemicals
   b. antioxidants
   c. carotenoids
   d. nitrates

5. Taking daily doses of three to four times the RDA of which of the following nutrients may cause death?
   a. vitamin A
   b. vitamin C
   c. vitamin E
   d. selenium

6. **True or false?** Tocopherol is the biologically active form of vitamin E in our bodies.

7. **True or false?** Free-radical formation can occur as a result of normal cellular metabolism.

8. **True or false?** Vitamin C helps regenerate vitamin A.

9. **True or false?** Reliable food sources of selenium include beef liver, pork, and seafood.

10. **True or false?** Pregnant women are advised to consume plentiful quantities of beef liver.

11. Explain how free radicals damage cell membranes and lead to cell death.

12. Describe the process by which cancer occurs, beginning with initiation and ending with metastasis of the cancer to widespread body tissues.

13. Explain how vitamin E reduces our risk for heart disease.

14. Discuss the contribution of trace minerals, such as selenium, to the prevention of oxidation.

15. Your mother has a heart condition that requires her to take the prescription drug Coumadin, an anticoagulant. While chatting with you over lunch one day, she mentions that she has started taking an antioxidant supplement that is supposed to "boost cardiovascular health." You ask to see the supplement and note that it contains 500 mg vitamin E as alpha-tocopherol, 500 mg of vitamin C, and 100 µg of selenium. Should you be concerned? Why or why not?

Math Review

16. Joey is home, visiting his parents for the weekend, and he finds a bottle of vitamin E supplements in the medicine cabinet. He asks his parents about them, and his mother says that she is worried about having a weak immune system and read on the Internet that vitamin E can boost immunity. As Joey's mother eats plenty of plant foods and oils that are good sources of vitamin E, he is worried she may be consuming too much by adding these supplements to her diet. Each supplement capsule contains 400 IU of dl-alpha-tocopherol, and she takes one capsule each day. Answer the following questions:
    a. How much vitamin E in mg is Joey's mother consuming each day from these supplements?
    b. What percentage of the RDA for vitamin E do these supplements provide?
    c. Based on what you've learned in this chapter about vitamin E, should Joey's mother be worried about vitamin E toxicity? Would your answer be different if you learned that she is taking aspirin each day, as prescribed by her doctor?

Answers to Review Questions and Math Review can be found online in the MasteringNutrition Study Area.

Web Links

References

1. The HOPE and HOPE-TOO Trial Investigators. 2005. Effects of long-term vitamin E supplementation on cardiovascular events and cancer. A randomized controlled trial. *JAMA* 293:1338–1347.

2. Miller, E. R. 3rd, R. Pastor-Barriuso, D. Dalal, R. A. Riemersma, L. J. Appel, and E. Guallar. 2005. Meta-analysis: high-dosage vitamin E supplementation may increase all-cause mortality. *Ann. Intern. Med.* 142:37–46.

3. Bjelakovic, G., D. Nikolova, L. L. Gluud, R. G. Simonetti, and C. Gluud. 2007. Mortality in randomized trials of antioxidant supplements for primary and secondary prevention: systematic review and meta-analysis. *JAMA* 297:842–857.

4. Klein, E. A., I. M. Thompson Jr., C. M. Tangen, J. J. Crowley, M. S. Lucia, P. J. Goodman, L. M. Minasian, L. G. Ford, H. L. Parnes, J. M. Gaziano, D. D. Karp, M. M. Lieber, P. J. Walther, L. Klotz, J. K. Parsons, J. L. Chin, A. K. Darke, S. M. Lippman, G. E. Goodman, F. L. Meyskens Jr., and L. H. Baker. 2011. Vitamin E and the risk of prostate cancer: the Selenium and Vitamin E Cancer Prevention Trial (SELECT). *JAMA* 306:1549–1556.

5. Sesso, H. D., J. E. Buring, W. G. Christen, T. Kurth, C. Belanger, J. MacFadyn, V. Bubes, J. E. Manson, R. J. Glynn, and J. M. Gaziano. 2008. Vitamins E and C in the prevention of cardiovascular disease in men: The Physicians' Health Study II randomized controlled trial. *JAMA* 300(18):2123–2133.

6. Gao, X., P. E. Wilde, A. H. Lichtenstein, O. I. Bermudez, and K. L. Tucker. 2006. The maximal amount of dietary a-tocopherol intake in U.S. adults (NHANES 2001–2002). *J. Nutr.* 136:1021–1026.

7. Maras, J. E., O. I. Bermudez, N. Qiao, P. J. Bakun, E. L. Boody-Alter, and K. L. Tucker. 2004. Intake of alpha-tocopherol is limited among US adults. *J. Am. Diet. Assoc.* 104(4):567–575.

8. Institute of Medicine, Food and Nutrition Board. 2000. *Dietary Reference Intakes for Vitamin C, Vitamin E, Selenium, and Carotenoids.* Washington, DC: National Academy of Sciences, National Academies Press.

9. US National Library of Medicine. National Institutes of Health. 2011. MedlinePlus. Beta-carotene. www.nlm.nih.gov/medlineplus/druginfo/natural/999.html.

10. Albanes, D., O. P. Heinonen, J. K. Huttunen, P. R. Taylor, J. Virtamo, B. K. Edwards, J. Haapakoski, M. Rautalahti, A. M. Hartman, J. Palmgren, and P. Greenwald. 1995. Effects of a-tocopherol and a-carotene supplements on cancer incidence in the Alpha-Tocopherol Beta-Carotene Cancer Prevention Study. *Am. J. Clin. Nutr.* 62(suppl.):1427S–1430S.

11. Omenn, G. S., G. E. Goodman, M. D. Thornquist, J. Balmes, M. R. Cullen, A. Glass, J. P. Keogh, F. L. Meyskens Jr., B. Valanis, J. H. Williams Jr., S. Barnhart, and S. Hammar. 1996. Effects of a combination of beta carotene and vitamin A on lung cancer and cardiovascular disease. *N. Engl. J. Med.* 334:1150–1155.

12. Druesne-Pecollo, N., P. Latino-Martel, T. Norat, E. Barrandon, S. Bertrais, P. Galan, and S. Hercberg. 2010. Beta-carotene supplementation and cancer risk: a systematic risk and meta-analysis of randomized controlled trials. *Int. J. Cancer* 127(1):172–184.

13. US Department of Agriculture (USDA), Agricultural Research Service. 2011. USDA National Nutrient Database for Standard Reference, Release 24. http://www.ars.usda.gov/Services/docs .htm?docid=22114

14. El-akawi, Z., N. Abdel-Latif, and K. Abdul-Razzak. 2006. Does the plasma level of vitamins A and E affect acne condition? *Clin. Experimen. Dermatol.* 31:430–434.

15. Institute of Medicine. Food and Nutrition Board. 2001. *Dietary Reference Intakes for Vitamin A, Vitamin K, Arsenic, Boron, Chromium, Copper, Iodine, Iron, Manganese, Molybdenum, Nickel, Silicon, Vanadium, and Zinc.* Washington, DC: National Academy Press.

16. World Health Organization (WHO). 2012. Micronutrient Deficiencies. Vitamin A Deficiency. www.who.int/nutrition/topics/vad/en/.

17. McConnell, T. H. 2007. *The Nature of Disease: Pathology for the Health Professions.* Baltimore: Lippincott Williams & Wilkins.

18. American Cancer Society. 2012. *Cancer Facts and Figures, 2012.* Atlanta: American Cancer Society. www.cancer.org/acs/groups/content/@epidemiologysurveilance/documents/document/acspc-031941.pdf.

19. Garcia, M., A. Jemal, E. M. Ward, M. M. Center, Y. Hao, R. L. Siegel, and M. J. Thun. 2007. *Global Cancer Facts & Figures 2007.* Atlanta: American Cancer Society.

20. World Cancer Research Fund/American Institute for Cancer Research (AICR). 2007. *Food, Nutrition, Physical Activity and the Prevention of Cancer: A Global Perspective.* Washington, DC: AICR. www.dietandcancerreport.org/cancer_resource_center/second_expert_report.php.

21. Pfahlberg, A., K. F. Kolmel, and O. Gefeller. 2002. Adult vs. childhood susceptibility to melanoma. Is there a difference? *Arch. Dermatol.* 138:1234–1235.

22. Heinonen, O. P., D. Albanes, J. Virtamo, P. R. Taylor, J. K. Huttunen, A. M. Hartman, J. Haapakoski, N. Malila, M. Rautalahti, S. Ripatti, H. Maepaa, and International Agency for Research on Cancer (IARC). 2007. The association of use of sunbeds with cutaneous malignant melanoma and other skin cancers: a systematic review. *Intl. J. Cancer.* 120:1116–1122.

23. Bjelakovic, G., D. Nikolova, L. L. Gluud, R. G. Simonetti, and C. Gluud. 2012. Antioxidant supplements for prevention of mortality in healthy participants and patients with various diseases. *Cochrane Database of Systematic Reviews*, Issue 3. Art. No.: CD007176. DOI: 10.1002/14651858.CD007176.pub2.

24. National Center for Chronic Disease Prevention and Health Promotion (NCCDPHP). 2008. Chronic Disease Prevention. Chronic Disease Overview. www.cdc.gov/nccdphp/overview .htm.

25. Centers for Disease Control and Prevention. 2012. Injury Prevention & Control: Data & Statistics. Ten Leading Causes of Death and Injury. www.cdc.gov/injury/wisqars/LeadingCauses .html.

26. Ridker, P. M., and N. Cook. 2004. Clinical usefulness of very high and very low levels of c-reactive protein across the full range of Framingham risk scores. *Circulation* 109:1955–1959.

27. Lee, I. M., N. R. Cook, J. M. Gaziano, D. Gordon, P. M. Ridker, J. E. Manson, C. H. Hennekens, and J. E. Buring. 2005. Vitamin E in the primary prevention of cardiovascular disease and cancer: The Women's Health Study: a randomized controlled trial. *JAMA* 294(1):56–65.

Vitamin and Mineral Supplementation: Necessity or Waste?

Marcus has type 2 diabetes and high blood pressure and is worried about his health. After attending a seminar on vitamin and mineral supplements, Marcus was convinced that he needed to take a supplement providing 200–800% of the Daily Value for many vitamins and minerals, as well as an herbal preparation for "heart health." After a few months of taking these supplements on a daily basis, Marcus started to experience headaches, nausea, diarrhea, and tingling in his hands and feet. He decided to talk to his doctor about the supplements he was taking to determine whether they could be causing his symptoms.

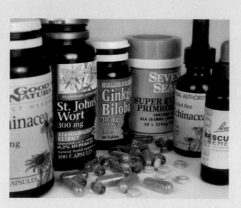

Supplements can take the form of powders, pills, or liquid.

Marcus's story is not unique. The use of dietary supplements in the United States has skyrocketed in recent years. One industry source cites annual sales of supplements in the United States at $25.5 billion.[1] A review of national opinion surveys found that a significant number of Americans regularly take dietary supplements, but they do not report the use of these products to their physicians because they feel their physicians have little knowledge of these products and may harbor a bias toward their use.[2] Interestingly, many supplement users state that they would continue to use these products even if scientific studies found them to be ineffective!

Why do so many people take dietary supplements? Many people believe they cannot consume adequate nutrients in their diet. Others have been advised by their healthcare provider to take a supplement to address a given health concern. There are people, like Marcus, who believe that they can use certain supplements to treat their disease. Others use supplements in the hope that they'll enhance their appearance or athletic performance.

Are such uses wise? A waste of money? Dangerous? Who *should* be taking supplements? These questions are not easy to answer. Before deciding whether you might benefit from taking dietary supplements, read on.

What Are Dietary Supplements?

According to the US Food and Drug Administration (FDA), a dietary supplement is "a product taken by mouth that contains a 'dietary ingredient' intended to supplement the diet."[3] Supplements may contain vitamins, minerals, herbs or other botanicals, amino acids, enzymes, tissues from animal organs or glands, or a concentrate, a metabolite, a constituent, or an extract. Supplements come in many forms, including pills, capsules, liquids, and powders.

How Are Dietary Supplements Regulated?

As presented in the Dietary Supplement Health and Education Act (DSHEA) of 1994, dietary supplements are categorized within the general group of foods, not drugs. This means that the regulation of supplements is much less rigorous than the regulation of drugs. Currently, the FDA is reconsidering how it regulates food and supplements that are marketed with health claims, but no changes have been finalized. As an informed consumer, you should know the following:

- Dietary supplements do not need approval from the FDA before they are marketed.
- The company that manufactures a supplement is responsible for determining that the supplement is safe; the FDA does not test any supplement for safety prior to marketing.
- Supplement companies do not have to provide the FDA with any evidence that their supplements are safe unless the company is marketing a new dietary ingredient that was not sold in the United States prior to 1994.
- There are at present no federal guidelines on practices to ensure the purity, quality, safety, and composition of dietary supplements.
- There are no rules to limit the serving size or amount of a nutrient in any dietary supplement.
- Once a supplement is marketed, the FDA must prove it unsafe before the product will be removed from the market.

Despite these limitations in supplement regulation, supplement manufacturers are required to follow dietary supplement labeling guidelines. There are specific requirements for the information that must be included on supplement labels. Federal advertising regulations also require that any claims on the label must be truthful and not misleading and that advertisers must be able to substantiate all label claims. In addition, labels bearing a claim must also include the disclaimer "This statement has not been evaluated by the FDA. This product is not intended to diagnose, cure, or prevent any disease." Any products not meeting these guidelines can be removed from the market.

How Can You Avoid Fraudulent or Dangerous Supplements?

Although many of the supplement products sold today are safe, some are not. In addition, some companies are less than forthright about the true content of the ingredients in their supplements. How can you avoid purchasing fraudulent or dangerous supplements? The FDA suggests that consumers do the following to protect themselves:[4]

1. Look for the US Pharmacopoeia (USP) symbol or notation on the label. This symbol indicates that the manufacturer followed the standards established by the USP for drugs for features such as purity, strength, quality, packaging, labeling, and acceptable length of storage.
2. Consider buying recognized brands of supplements. Although not guaranteed, products made by nationally recognized companies more likely have well-established manufacturing standards.
3. Do not assume that the word *natural* on the label means that the product is safe. Arsenic, lead, and mercury are all natural substances that can kill you if consumed in large enough quantities.
4. Do not hesitate to question a company about how it makes its products. Reputable companies have nothing to hide and are more than happy to inform their customers about the safety and quality of their products.

Many supplements are sold over the Internet. Keep these criteria in mind each time you consider buying a dietary supplement over the web:[5]

1. What is the purpose of the website? Is it trying to sell a product or educate the consumer? Keep in mind that the primary purpose of supplement companies is to make money. Look for sites that provide educational information about a specific nutrient or product and don't just focus on selling the products.
2. Does the site contain accurate information? This is the most difficult thing for a consumer to determine. Testimonials are *not* reliable and accurate; claims supported by scientific research are most desirable. If what the company claims about its product sounds too good to be true, it probably is.
3. Does the site contain reputable references? References should be from articles published in peer-reviewed scientific journals. References should be complete and contain author names, article title, journal title, date, volume, and page numbers. This information allows the consumer to check original research for the validity of a company's claims about its product. Be cautious of sites that refer to claims that are "proven by research studies" but fail to provide a complete reference.

4. Who owns or sponsors the site? Full disclosure regarding sponsorship and possible sources of bias or conflict of interest should be included in the site's information.
5. Who wrote the information? Websites should clearly identify the author of the article and include the credentials of the author. Recognized experts include individuals with relevant health-related credentials, such as RD, PhD, MD, or MS. Keep in mind that this person is responsible for the information posted in the article but may not be the creator of the website.
6. Is the information current and updated regularly? As information about supplements changes regularly, websites should be updated regularly, and the date should be clearly posted. All websites should also include contact information to allow consumers to ask questions about the information posted.

Should You Take a Dietary Supplement?

Contrary to what some people believe, not all people need to supplement their diets all of the time. In fact, foods contain a diverse combination of compounds that are critical to our health, and vitamin and mineral supplements do not contain the same amount or variety of substances found in foods. Thus, dietary supplements are not substitutes for whole foods. However, our nutritional needs change throughout our life spans, so you may benefit from taking a supplement at certain times for certain reasons. For instance, if you adopt a vegan diet in your college years, your healthcare provider might prescribe a supplement providing riboflavin, vitamin B12, vitamin D, calcium, iron, and zinc. Animal products are high in these nutrients, so if you eliminate these foods, you might not get enough of these nutrients in the other foods you are eating. Or if you're a member of your college soccer team, your team's sport dietitian might advise taking a supplement formulated to provide micronutrients that support intense physical activity.

Dietary supplements include hundreds of thousands of products sold for many purposes, and it is impossible to discuss here all of the various situations in which their use may be advisable. So to simplify this discussion, let's focus on identifying the groups of people who may or may not benefit from taking vitamin and mineral supplements.

Table 10.2 lists groups of people who may benefit from supplementation. But even if you fall within one of these groups, it's still important to analyze your total diet to determine whether you need to take the vitamin or mineral supplement indicated. It is also a good idea to check with your healthcare provider or a registered dietitian (RD) before taking any supplements, as supplements can interfere with some prescription and over-the-counter medications.

TABLE 10.2 Individuals Who May Benefit from Dietary Supplementation

Type of Individual	Specific Supplements That May Help
Newborns	Routinely given a single dose of vitamin K at birth
Infants	Depends on age and nutrition; may need iron, vitamin D, or other nutrients
Children not drinking fluoridated water	Fluoride supplements
Children on strict vegetarian diets	Vitamin B_{12}, iron, zinc, vitamin D (if not exposed to sunlight)
Children with poor eating habits or overweight children on an energy-restricted diet	Multivitamin/multimineral supplement that does not exceed the RDA for the nutrients it contains
Pregnant teenagers	Iron and folic acid; other nutrients may be necessary if diet is very poor
Women who may become pregnant	Multivitamin or multivitamin/multimineral supplement that contains 0.4 mg of folic acid
Pregnant or lactating women	Multivitamin/multimineral supplement that contains iron, folic acid, zinc, copper, calcium, vitamin B_6, vitamin C, vitamin D
People on prolonged weight-reduction diets	Multivitamin/multimineral supplement
People recovering from serious illness or surgery	Multivitamin/multimineral supplement
People with HIV/AIDS or other wasting diseases; people addicted to drugs or alcohol	Multivitamin/multimineral supplement or single-nutrient supplements
People who do not consume adequate calcium	Calcium supplements: for example, women need to consume 1,000 to 1,200 mg of dietary calcium per day; thus, supplements may be necessary
People whose exposure to sunlight is inadequate to allow synthesis of adequate vitamin D	Vitamin D
People eating a vegan diet	Vitamin B_{12}, riboflavin, calcium, vitamin D, iron, zinc
People who have had portions of the intestinal tract removed; people who have a malabsorptive disease	Depends on the exact condition; may include various fat-soluble and/or water-soluble vitamins and other nutrients
People with lactose intolerance	Calcium supplements
Elderly people	Multivitamin/multimineral supplement, vitamin B_{12}

Of course, many people who do not need to take supplements do so anyway. The following are instances in which taking vitamin and mineral supplements is unnecessary, or even harmful:

1. Providing fluoride supplements to children who already drink fluoridated water
2. Taking supplements in the belief that they will cure a disease, such as cancer, diabetes, or heart disease
3. Taking supplements with certain medications. For instance, people who take the blood-thinning drug Coumadin should not take vitamin E or K supplements, as this can cause excessive bleeding. People who take aspirin daily should check with their physicians before taking vitamin E or K supplements, as aspirin also thins the blood.
4. Taking nonprescribed supplements if you have liver or kidney disease. Physicians may prescribe vitamin and mineral supplements for their patients, because many nutrients are lost during treatment for these diseases. However, these individuals cannot properly metabolize

certain supplements and should not take any that are not prescribed by their physicians because of a high risk for toxicity.

5. Taking beta-carotene supplements, particularly if you are a smoker. As already mentioned, there is evidence that beta-carotene supplementation increases the risk for lung and other cancers and increases the risk for premature mortality.
6. Taking vitamins and minerals in an attempt to improve physical appearance or athletic performance. There is no evidence that vitamin and mineral supplements enhance appearance or athletic performance in healthy adults who consume a varied diet with adequate energy.
7. Taking supplements to increase energy level. Vitamin and mineral supplements do not provide energy, because they do not contain fat, carbohydrate, or protein (sources of Calories). Although many vitamins and minerals are necessary for us to produce energy, taking dietary supplements in place of eating food will not provide us with the energy necessary to live a healthy and productive life.

TABLE 10.3 Ingredients Found in Supplements That Are Associated with Illnesses and Injuries

Ingredient	Potential Risks
Herbal Ingredients	
Chaparral	Liver disease
Kava (also known as kava kava)	Severe liver toxicity
Comfrey	Obstruction of blood flow to liver, possible death
Slimming/dieters' teas	Nausea, diarrhea, vomiting, stomach cramps, constipation, fainting, possible death
Ephedra (also known as ma huang, Chinese ephedra, and epitonin)	High blood pressure, irregular heartbeat, nerve damage, insomnia, tremors, headaches, seizures, heart attack, stroke, possible death
Germander	Liver disease, possible death
Lobelia	Breathing problems, excessive sweating, rapid heartbeat, low blood pressure, coma, possible death
Magnolia-Stephania preparation	Kidney disease, can lead to permanent kidney failure
Willow bark	Reye's syndrome (a potentially fatal disease that may occur when children take aspirin), allergic reaction in adults
Wormwood	Numbness of legs and arms, loss of intellectual processing, delirium, paralysis
Vitamins and Essential Minerals	
Vitamin A (when taking 25,000 IU or more per day)	Birth defects, bone abnormalities, severe liver disease
Vitamin B$_6$ (when taking more than 100 mg per day)	Loss of balance, injuries to nerves that alter touch sensation
Niacin (when taking slow-release doses of 500 mg or more per day or when taking immediate-release doses of 750 mg or more per day)	Stomach pain; nausea; vomiting; bloating; cramping; diarrhea; liver disease; damage to the muscles, eyes, and heart
Selenium (when taking 800 to 1,000 μg per day)	Tissue damage
Other Ingredients	
Germanium (a nonessential mineral)	Kidney damage
L-tryptophan (an amino acid)	Eosinophilia-myalgia syndrome (a potentially fatal blood disorder that causes high fever)

Sources: Data from U.S. Food and Drug Administration. 2009. Dietary supplements. http://www.fda.gov/Food/DietarySupplements/Alerts/default.htm

8. Taking single-nutrient supplements, unless a qualified healthcare practitioner prescribes a single-nutrient supplement for a diagnosed medical condition (iron supplements for someone with anemia). These products contain very high amounts of the given nutrient, and taking them can quickly lead to toxicity.

The Academy of Nutrition and Dietetics advises that the ideal nutritional strategy for optimizing health is to eat a healthful diet that contains a variety of whole foods.[6] If you do use a supplement, select one that contains no more than 100% of the recommended levels for the nutrients it contains. Avoid taking single-nutrient supplements unless advised to do so by your healthcare practitioner. Finally, avoid taking supplements that contain substances known to cause illness or injuries. Some of these substances are listed in **Table 10.3**.

CRITICAL THINKING QUESTIONS

■ Do you think that the FDA should more closely regulate supplement manufacturers? If so, how?

■ Have you decided whether taking a supplement is right for you? Why or why not?

REFERENCES

1. Nutrition Business Journal. 2009. *2009 Nutrition Industry Overview.* Vol XIV, No 6/7, June/July. ©Penton Media, Inc.
2. Blendon, R. J., C. M. DesRoches, J. M. Benson, M. Brodie, and D. E. Altman. 2001. Americans' views on the use and regulation of dietary supplements. *Arch. Intern. Med.* 26:805–810.
3. US Food and Drug Administration (FDA). 2009. Overview of Dietary Supplements. http://www.fda.gov/Food/DietarySupplements/default.htm
4. US Food and Drug Administration (FDA). 2009. Dietary Supplements. Tips for the Savvy Supplement User: Making Informed Decisions and Evaluating Information. http://www.fda.gov/food/dietarysupplements/consumerinformation/ucm110567.htm.
5. Dancho, C., and M. M. Manore. 2001. Dietary supplement information on the World Wide Web. Sorting fact from fiction. *ACSM's Health and Fitness Journal* 5:7–12.
6. Academy of Nutrition and Dietetics. 2005. Dietary supplements. *J. Am. Diet. Assoc.* 102:460–470.

Phytochemicals

Want to find out . . .

- **what's behind all the fuss about phytochemicals?**

- **why stressing your cells can be a *good* thing?**

- **why you can't put fruits and vegetables into a pill?**

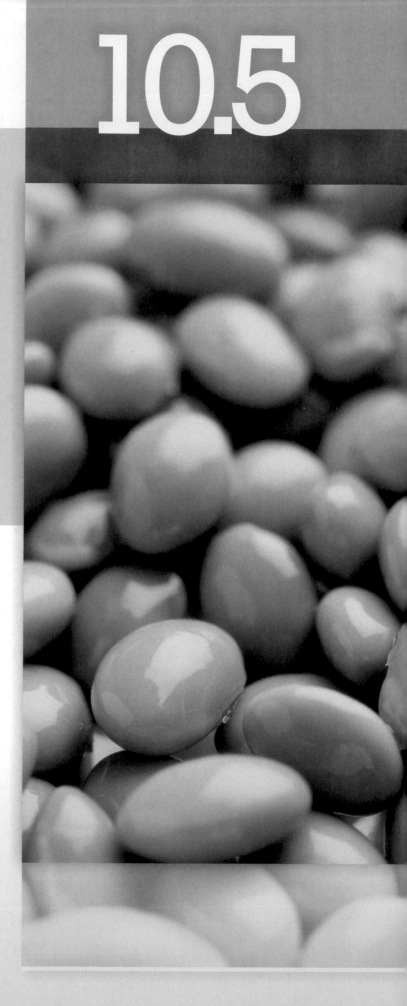

READ ON.

Imagine a patient seeing his physician for his annual physical exam. The physician measures his blood pressure and finds it slightly elevated. At the close of the visit, he hands the patient a prescription: *one apple; two servings of dark-green, leafy vegetables; ½ cup of oatmeal, and 2 cups of soy milk daily.* The patient accepts the prescription gratefully, assuring his physician as he says goodbye, "I'll stop at the market on my way home!"

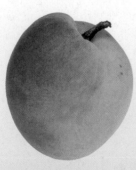

Apricots contain carotenoids, a type of phytochemical.

Sound unreal? As researchers provide more and more evidence on the link between plant foods and health, it's possible that scenarios like this might become familiar. Here, we explore *In Depth* some of the reasons why certain chemicals that occur naturally in plant foods are thought to promote our health. Who knows? When you finish reading, you might find yourself writing up your own health-promoting grocery list!

What Are Phytochemicals?

Phyto means "plant", so **phytochemicals** are literally plant chemicals. These naturally occurring compounds are believed to protect plants from a variety of injurious agents, including insects, microbes, the oxygen they produce, and the UV light they capture and transform into the nutrients we need. Although more than 10,000 different phytochemicals have already been identified, researchers believe there may be thousands more.[1] They are present in whole grains, fruits, mushrooms, legumes and other vegetables, coffee, tea, wine, beer, herbs, spices, and many other plant-based foods. Any one food can contain hundreds. **Figure 1** identifies a few of the most common phytochemical groups.

Phytochemicals are not considered nutrients—that is, substances necessary for sustaining life. Whereas a total lack of vitamin C or iron is incompatible with life, a total lack of lutein or allylic sulfur compounds is not known to be fatal. On the other hand, eating an abundance of phytochemical-rich foods has been shown to reduce the risk for cardiovascular disease, cancer, diabetes, Alzheimer's disease, cataracts, and age-related functional decline.[1, 2]

The evidence supporting this observation of a reduced disease risk stems mainly from large epidemiological studies in which people report their usual food intake to researchers, who then look for relationships between specific dietary patterns and common diseases. These large studies often find that the reduced disease risk from high intakes of plant foods cannot be attributed solely to differences in intake of macronutrients and micronutrients. This suggests that other compounds in plant foods may be reducing the risk for disease.

Bear in mind, however, that epidemiological studies can reveal only *associations* between general patterns of food intake and health conditions; they cannot prove that a food or dietary pattern directly *causes* a health outcome. Even well-controlled laboratory studies typically research only one phytochemical group—or sometimes just one food—at a time. When the results are published, we read about them in the popular press: one day we're advised to eat blueberries, another day pomegranates. (We explore one of these dietary recommendations in the **Highlight** box on page 429.)

Are news stories promoting phytochemicals hype—or science? To better understand how phytochemicals influence health and disease, let's review the current state of phytochemical research.

How Might Phytochemicals Help Prevent or Treat Disease?

For decades, laboratory experiments have shown that, at least in the test tube, many phytochemicals have antioxidant properties; that is, they have the capacity to neutralize the free radicals that damage our cells. Free radicals are not only an unavoidable by-product of normal metabolism but are also produced in response to radiation, air pollution, industrial chemicals, tobacco smoke, infections, and even intense exercise.

The health effects of this oxidative damage typically don't arise until later in life. Many **diseases of aging,** such as cardiovascular disease, cancer, cataracts, arthritis, and certain neurologic disorders, have been linked to oxidative damage that accumulates over years. It's no surprise, therefore, that antioxidant-rich foods reduce the risk for these conditions.

Unfortunately, biology is not fully explained by a few simple chemical reactions. In fact, some research into phytochemicals suggests that their health-promoting properties can be unrelated to their antioxidant activity.[3] This is in part because phytochemicals are modified during digestion and after absorption, so that cells are exposed to metabolites that are structurally different from the phytochemicals found in foods.[4] Moreover, phytochemicals are thought to work in synergy with one another and with other compounds in foods, in medications, and in the human body. Thus, the test tube can only hint at what is happening inside the body.

Fortunately, researchers have also employed cellular and animal studies, which reveal that phytochemicals have a broad range of health-promoting functions in addition to their antioxidant properties. For example, phytochemicals are thought to do the following:

- Reduce inflammation, which is linked to the development of cardiovascular disease, cancer, and Alzheimer's disease and is symptomatic of allergies and arthritis.[1, 5]
- Impede the initiation and progression of cancer by enhancing the activity of enzymes that detoxify carcinogens, slowing tumor cell growth, inhibiting signaling pathways among cancer cells, and instructing cancer cells to self-destruct.[1, 6]
- Combat infections by enhancing our immune function, reducing bacterial resistance to antibiotics, and acting as antibacterial and antiviral agents.[7]
- Protect against cardiovascular disease by modulating blood lipids and reducing platelet aggregation, blood clotting, and blockage of blood vessels.[8]
- Inhibit lipid synthesis and increase fatty acid oxidation, thereby potentially acting as an "antiobesity" agent.[9, 10]

In addition, research over the past decade has increasingly focused on the beneficial role of phytochemicals in increasing the effectiveness of medications used to treat disease. When administered in concentrated doses along with traditional medications, certain phytochemicals work synergistically to enhance or prolong the effectiveness of those

phytochemicals Compounds found in plants believed to have health-promoting effects in humans.

diseases of aging Conditions that typically occur later in life as a result of lifelong accumulated risk, such as from lack of physical activity or exposure to carcinogens.

Phytochemical	Health Claims	Food Source	
Carotenoids: alpha-carotene, beta-carotene, lutein, lycopene, zeaxanthin, etc.	Diets with foods rich in these phytochemicals may reduce the risk for cardiovascular disease, certain cancers (e.g., prostate), and age-related eye diseases (cataracts, macular degeneration).	Red, orange, and deep-green vegetables and fruits, such as carrots, cantaloupe, sweet potatoes, apricots, kale, spinach, pumpkin, and tomatoes	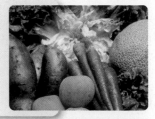
Flavonoids:[1] flavones, flavonols (e.g., quercetin), catechins (e.g., epigallocatechin gallate or EGCG), anthocyanidins, isoflavonoids, etc.	Diets with foods rich in these phytochemicals are associated with lower risk for cardiovascular disease and cancer, possibly because of reduced inflammation, blood clotting, and blood pressure and increased detoxification of carcinogens or reduction in replication of cancerous cells.	Berries, black and green tea, chocolate, purple grapes and juice, citrus fruits, olives, soybeans and soy products (soy milk, tofu, soy flour, textured vegetable protein), flaxseed, whole wheat, nuts	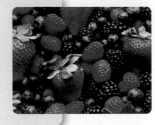
Phenolic acids:[1] ellagic acid, ferulic acid, caffeic acid, curcumin, etc.	Similar benefits as flavonoids.	Coffee beans, fruits (apples, pears, berries, grapes, oranges, prunes, strawberries), potatoes, mustard, oats, soy	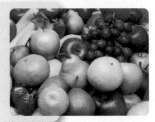
Phytoestrogens:[2] genistein, diadzein, lignans	Foods rich in these phytochemicals may provide benefits to bones and reduce the risk for cardiovascular disease and cancers of reproductive tissues (e.g., breast, prostate).	Soybeans and soy products (soy milk, tofu, soy flour, textured vegetable protein), flaxseed, whole grains	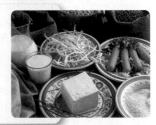
Organosulfur compounds: allylic sulfur compounds, indoles, isothiocyanates, etc.	Foods rich in these phytochemicals may protect against a wide variety of cancers.	Garlic, leeks, onions, chives, cruciferous vegetables (broccoli, cabbage, cauliflower), horseradish, mustard greens	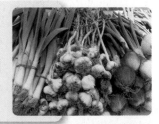

[1] Flavonoids, phenolic acids, and stilbenes are three groups of phytochemicals called phenolics. The phytochemical Resveratrol is a stilbene. Flavonoids and phenolic acids are the most abundant phenolics in our diet.

[2] Phytoestrogens include phytochemicals that have mild or anti-estrogenic action in our body. They are grouped together based on this similarity in biological function, but they also can be classified into other phytochemical groups, such as isoflavonoids.

FIGURE 1 Health claims and food sources of phytochemicals.

Will a PB&J Keep the Doctor Away?

Whole-grain bread, natural peanut butter, and grape jelly: how could a food that tastes so good be good for the body, too? We've known for decades about the fiber, micronutrients, and healthful unsaturated fats a PB&J sandwich provides. But recently, research has revealed that the comforting PB&J is a good source of phytochemicals, too, especially those in the phenolics group, which includes flavonoids, phenolic acids, and a small group called stilbenes.

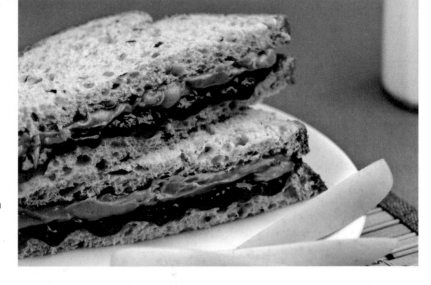

antimicrobial and anti-inflammatory properties, resveratrol is thought to have protective effects against cancer, heart disease, obesity, infections, and degenerative neurologic diseases.[3, 4]

Despite the host of phytochemicals in a PB&J, no one knows what an effective "dose" of any one of them might be, or whether the amounts in a PB&J would qualify as protective, even if you ate one every day. What we do know is that a PB&J makes a highly nutritious meal or snack, doesn't need refrigeration, is inexpensive, and tastes great.

Peanut butter, peanuts and other nuts, as well as grapes and whole-wheat bread, are all rich in flavonoids. In clinical studies, participants who added nuts to their diet experienced an improved lipid profile and blood vessel function, as well as reduced inflammation, all factors associated with reduced heart disease risk. They also experienced no weight gain![1]

Phenolic acids are also present in your sandwich. Grapes provide ellagic acid, which has anti-inflammatory properties, and peanuts and whole-wheat bread contain salicylic acid, which appears to induce self-destruction in cancer cells.[2]

Among the stilbenes, the most famous is probably resveratrol, which you may recall is found in wine. (See the **In Depth** on alcohol on pages 160–171.) Your PB&J provides resveratrol because it is also present in peanuts and grapes, including—in minute amounts—grape jelly. A chemical with

References

1. Vinson, J. A., and Y. Cal. 2012. Nuts, especially walnuts, have both antioxidant quantity and efficacy and exhibit significant potential health benefits. *Food Func.* 3(2):134–140.
2. Paterson, J., G. Baxter, J. Lawrence, and D. Duthie. 2006. Is there a role for dietary salicylates in health? *Proc. Nutr. Soc.* 65(1):93–96.
3. Whitlock, N. C., and S. J. Baek. 2012. The anti-cancer effects of resveratrol: modulation of transcription factors. *Nutr. Cancer.* 64(4):493–502.
4. Svajger, U., and M. Geras. 2012. Anti-inflammatory effects of resveratrol and its potential use in therapy of immune-mediated diseases. *Int. Rev. Immunol.* 31(3):202–222.

medications. Most such research is still in the stage of clinical trials, but this synergistic effect has been shown in the treatment of bacterial infections that have developed resistance to traditional antibiotics, as well as with chemotherapy drugs in the treatment of cancer.[1, 7, 11]

Why Is There No RDA for Phytochemicals?

There is no RDA for phytochemicals. Even for carotenoids, probably the most studied class, a 2011 update from the Institute of Medicine affirmed that there is not enough evidence to identify with confidence a possible impact of these compounds on chronic disease and thus establish a daily recommended intake.[12] Given the many benefits of phytochemicals in helping prevent and treat disease, why is there no RDA?

First, as noted earlier, phytochemicals interact with each other and with other substances in foods and in the body to produce a synergistic effect that is greater than the sum of the effects of individual phytochemicals. Teasing out the different contributions and determining precise therapeutic ratios would thus be essentially impossible. Moreover, phytochemicals can act in different ways under different circumstances in the body. For example, phytoestrogens in soy appear to reduce the incidence of breast cancer in healthy women, but they may enhance cancer development when the disease is already present.[13] For these reasons, no RDA for phytochemicals can safely be established for any life stage group. People with nutritional concerns related to specific disorders are advised to consult with their physician or a registered dietitian.

Although you might assume that the more phytochemicals you consume the better, that's somewhat simplistic. Their ability to promote your health may depend on your consuming them in foods. That is, phytochemicals appear to be beneficial in the low doses commonly provided by foods, but they may be ineffective or even harmful when consumed as supplements. This may be due to their mode of action: scientists now believe that, instead of *protecting* our cells, phytochemicals might benefit our health by *stressing* our cells, causing them to rev up their internal defense systems.[3] Cells are very well equipped to deal with minor stresses, but not with

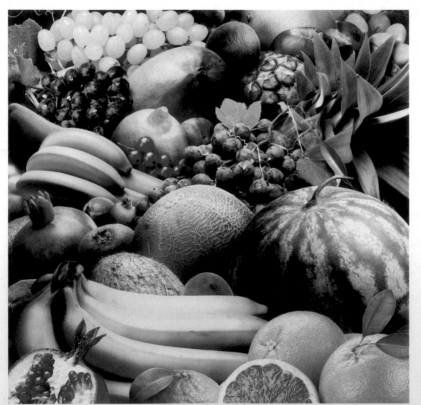

Avoid phytochemical supplements; instead, focus on consuming whole foods.

excessive stress, which may explain why clinical trials with phytochemical supplements may not show the same benefits as high intakes of plant foods.[3, 14]

So are phytochemical supplements harmful? Generally speaking, taking high doses of anything is risky. A basic principle of toxicology is that any compound can be toxic if the dose is high enough. Dietary supplements are no exception to this rule. For example, a classic study found that supplementing with 20 to 30 mg/day of beta-carotene for 4 to 6 years *increased* lung cancer risk by 16% to 28% in smokers.[15, 16] Based on these and other results, experts recommend against beta-carotene supplementation for chronic disease prevention or treatment.[17]

In short, whereas there is ample evidence to support the health benefits of diets rich in fruits, legumes and other vegetables, whole grains, and nuts, no recommendation for precise amounts can be given, and phytochemical supplements should be avoided. The best advice for optimal health is to consume a plant-based diet consisting of as many whole foods as possible.

Web Links

www.aicr.org
American Institute for Cancer Research (AICR)
Search for "phytochemicals" to learn about the AICR's position and recommendations on phytochemicals, and their role in cancer prevention.

www.lpi.oregonstate.edu
Linus Pauling Institute
This extensive website covers not only phytochemicals but also nutrients and other cutting-edge health and nutrition topics.

References

1. Russo, M., C. Spagnuolo, I. Tedesco, and G. L. Russo. 2010. Phytochemicals in cancer prevention and therapy: truth or dare? *Toxins* 2(4):517–551.

2. Chun, O. K., et al. 2007. Estimated dietary flavonoid intake and major food sources of US adults. *J. Nutr.* 137:1244–1252.

3. Melton, L. 2006. The antioxidant myth: a medical fairy tale. *New Sci.* 2563:40–43.

4. Manach, C., J. Hubert, R. Llorach, and A. Scalbert. 2009. The complex links between dietary phytochemicals and human health deciphered by metabolomics. *Mol. Nutr. Food Res.* 53(10):1303–1315.

5. Bellik, Y., S. M. Hammoudi, F. Abdellah, M. Iguer-Ouada, and L. Boukraa. 2012. Phytochemicals to prevent inflammation and allergy. *Recent Pat. Inflamm. Allergy Drug Discov.* 6(2):147–58.

6. Huang, W. Y., Y. A. Cal, and Y. Zhang. 2010. Natural phenolic compounds from medicinal herbs and dietary plants: potential use for cancer prevention. *Nutr. Cancer* 62(1):1–20.

7. Gibbons, S. 2008. Phytochemicals for bacterial resistance: strengths, weaknesses, and opportunities. *Planta. Med.* 74(6):594–602.

8. Vasanthi, H. R., N. Shrishrimal, and D. K. Das. 2012. Phytochemicals from plants to combat cardiovascular disease. *Curr. Med. Chem.* 19(14):2242–2251.

9. Ban, J. O., et al. 2012. Antiobesity effects of a sulfur compound thiacremenone mediated via down-regulation of serum triglyceride and glucose levels and lipid accumulation in the liver of db/db mice. *Phytother. Res.* doi 10.1002/ptr.3729[e-pub ahead of print].

10. Huang, B., H. D. Yuan, Y. Kim do, H. Y. Quan, and S. H. Chung. 2011. Cinnamaldehyde prevents adipocyte differentiation and adipogenesis via regulation of peroxisome proliferators-activated receptor-Y (PPARγ) and AMP-activated protein kinase (AMPK) pathways. *J. Agric. Food Chem.* 59(8):3666–3673.

11. Wenwen, X., J. J. Huang, and P. C. K. Cheung. 2012. Extract of *Pleurotus pulmonarius* suppresses liver cancer development and progression through inhibition of VEGF-induced P13K/AKT signaling pathway. *PLoS One* 7(3):e34406.

12. Panel on Dietary Antioxidants and Related Compounds. Food and Nutrition Board. Institute of Medicine. 2011, May 10. Antioxidants Panel: Activity. www.iom.edu/Activities/Nutrition/AntioxidantsPanel.aspx.

13. Rice S., and S. A. Whitehead. 2006. Phytoestrogens and breast cancer—promoters or protectors? *Endocr. Relat. Cancer* 13(4):995–1015.

14. Meyskens, F. L., and E. Szabo. 2005. Diet and cancer: the disconnect between epidemiology and randomized clinical trials. *Cancer Epidemiol. Biomarkers Prev.* 14(6):1366–1369.

15. The Alpha-Tocopherol, Beta-Carotene Cancer Prevention Study Group. 1994. The effect of vitamin E and beta carotene on the incidence of lung cancer and other cancers in male smokers. *N. Engl. J. Med.* 330(15):1029–1035.

16. Omenn, G. S., et al. 1996. Risk factors for lung cancer and for intervention effects in CARET, the Beta-Carotene and Retinol Efficacy Trial. *J. Natl. Cancer Inst.* 88(21):1550–1559.

17. US Preventive Services Task Force. 2006. Multivitamin/mineral supplements and prevention of chronic disease: evidence report and technology assessment number 139. AHRQ Publication No. 06-E012. www.ahrq.gov/downloads/pub/evidence/pdf/multivit/multivit.pdf.

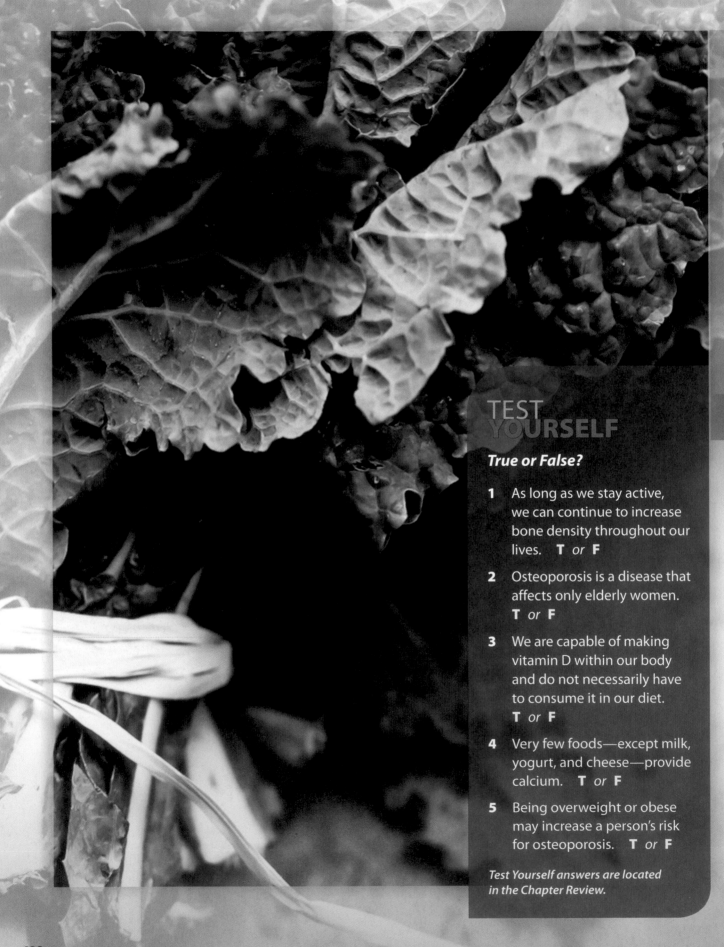

11
Nutrients Involved in Bone Health

Learning Objectives

After studying this chapter, you should be able to:

1. Identify the functions of bones in the human body and name four different bone types, *pp. 434–435*.

2. Describe the processes of bone growth, modeling, and remodeling, *pp. 435–437*.

3. Describe three methods used to assess bone health and density, *pp. 437–438*.

4. List and describe the functions of the key nutrients that play important roles in maintaining bone health, *pp. 438–457*.

5. Identify foods that are good sources of calcium, *pp. 441–443*.

6. Delineate the process by which the body synthesizes vitamin D from exposure to sunlight, and explain why the geographic region where people live affects their ability to do so, *pp. 445–448*.

7. Identify foods that are good sources of vitamin K, phosphorus, and magnesium, *pp. 451–455*.

8. Describe the main functions of fluoride in the development and maintenance of teeth and bones, and the results of consuming too much and too little fluoride, *pp. 455–457*.

9. Define *osteoporosis* and identify the factors that influence the risk for developing the disease, *pp. 458–461*.

10. Describe current treatments used to treat osteoporosis, *p. 461*.

MasteringNutrition™

Go online for chapter quizzes, pre-tests, Interactive Activities, and more!

433

In northern Maine, hockey is the local sport. So what's a poster of NBA star Chris Paul—who plays for the Los Angeles Clippers—doing on the cafeteria walls in local schools? Paul is one of many athletes participating in the "Body by Milk" ad campaign by the Milk Processor Education Program to teach kids about the benefits of drinking milk. On the campaign's TV commercials and website, athletes like Paul tell kids that the protein in milk helps build strong muscles and the calcium helps build strong bones.

Is the campaign working? Consumption of milk has plummeted from 31 gallons per person per year in 1970 to just 20.4 gallons in 2010, likely because of competition from other popular beverages. In 2010, the average American consumed less than 1 cup of milk each day, as opposed to more than 2.5 cups of carbonated soft drinks, fruit drinks, and sports beverages.[1] This trend concerns healthcare professionals, because milk is a convenient source of a form of calcium that's easily absorbed by the body, and calcium is required for kids and teens to build dense, compact bones. What's more, milk is fortified with vitamin D and is a good source of phosphorus, two more nutrients critical to bone health.

Still, milk is hardly the only food source of these nutrients. What other foods build bone? And how does bone grow—and break down? We'll begin this chapter with a quick look at the components and activities of bone tissue. Then we'll discuss the nutrients, dietary choices, and other lifestyle factors that play a critical role in maintaining bone health.

How Does the Body Maintain Bone Health?

Contrary to what most people think, the skeleton is not an inactive collection of bones that simply holds the body together. Bones are living organs that contain several tissues, including two types of bone tissue, cartilage, and connective tissue. Nerves and blood vessels run within channels in bone tissue, supporting its activities. Bones have many important functions in the body, some of which might surprise you (**Table 11.1**). For instance, did you know that most blood cells are formed deep within the bones?

Given the importance of bones, it is critical that we maintain their health. Bone health is achieved through complex interactions among nutrients, hormones, and environmental factors. To better understand these interactions, we first need to learn about how bone structure and the constant activity of bone tissue influence bone health throughout our lifetime.

The Composition of Bone Provides Strength and Flexibility

We tend to think of bones as totally rigid, but if they were, how could we twist and jump our way through a basketball game or even carry an armload of books up a flight of stairs? Bones need to be both strong and flexible, so that they can resist the compression, stretching, and twisting that occur throughout our daily activities. Fortunately, the composition of bone is ideally suited for its complex job: about 65% of bone tissue is made up of

TABLE 11.1 Functions of Bone in the Human Body

Functions Related to Structure and Support	Functions Related to Metabolic Processes
■ Bones provide physical support for organs and body segments. ■ Bones protect vital organs; for example, the rib cage protects the lungs, the skull protects the brain, and the vertebrae of the spine protect the spinal cord. ■ Bones work with muscles and tendons to allow movement—muscles attach to bones via tendons, and their contraction produces movement at the body's joints.	■ Bone tissue acts as a storage reservoir for many minerals, including calcium, phosphorus, and fluoride. The body draws on such deposits when these minerals are needed for various body processes; however, this can reduce bone mass. ■ Most blood cells are produced in the bone marrow.

an assortment of minerals (mostly calcium and phosphorus) that provide hardness, but the remaining 35% is a mixture of organic substances that provide strength, durability, and flexibility. The most important of these substances is a fibrous protein called **collagen.** You might be surprised to learn that collagen fibers are actually stronger than steel fibers of similar size! Within bones, the minerals form tiny crystals (called *hydroxyapatite*) that cluster around the collagen fibers. This design enables bones to bear weight while responding to our demands for movement.

If you examine a bone very closely, you will notice two distinct types of tissue (**Figure 11.1**): cortical bone and trabecular bone. **Cortical bone,** which is also called **compact bone,** is very dense. It constitutes approximately 80% of the skeleton. The outer surface of all bones is cortical; plus, many small bones of the body, such as the bones of the wrists, hands, and feet, are made entirely of cortical bone. Although cortical bone looks solid to the naked eye, it actually contains many microscopic openings, which serve as passageways for blood vessels and nerves.

In contrast, **trabecular bone** makes up only 20% of the skeleton. It is found within the ends of the long bones (such as the bones of the arms and legs), the spinal vertebrae, the sternum (breastbone), the ribs, most bones of the skull, and the pelvis. Trabecular bone is sometimes referred to as **spongy bone,** because to the naked eye it looks like a sponge, with cavities and no clear organization. The microscope reveals that trabecular bone is, in fact, aligned in a precise network of columns that protect the bone from stress. You can think of trabecular bone as the scaffolding of the inside of the bone that supports the outer cortical bone.

Cortical and trabecular bone also differ in their rate of turnover—that is, in how quickly the bone tissue is broken down and replenished. Trabecular bone has a faster turnover rate than cortical bone. This makes trabecular bone more sensitive to changes in hormones and nutritional deficiencies. It also accounts for the much higher rate of age-related fractures in the spine and pelvis (including the hip)—both of which contain a significant amount of trabecular bone. Let's investigate how bone turnover influences bone health.

The Constant Activity of Bone Tissue Promotes Bone Health

Bones develop through a series of three processes: bone growth, bone modeling, and bone remodeling (**Figure 11.2**). Bone growth and modeling begin during the early months of fetal life, when the skeleton is forming, and continue until early adulthood. Bone remodeling predominates during adulthood; this process helps us maintain a healthy skeleton as we age.

Bone Growth and Modeling Determine the Size and Shape of Our Bones

Through the process of *bone growth*, the size of bones increases. The first period of rapid bone growth is from birth to age 2, but growth continues in spurts throughout childhood

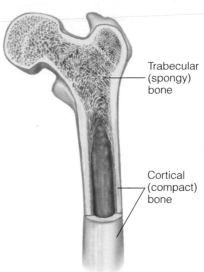

FIGURE 11.1 The structure of bone. Notice the difference in density between the trabecular (spongy) bone and the cortical (compact) bone.

collagen   A protein that forms strong fibers in bone and connective tissue.

cortical bone (compact bone) A dense bone tissue that makes up the outer surface of all bones, as well as the entirety of most small bones of the body.

trabecular bone (spongy bone) A porous bone tissue that makes up only 20% of the skeleton and is found within the ends of the long bones, inside the spinal vertebrae, inside the flat bones (sternum, ribs, and most bones of the skull), and inside the bones of the pelvis.

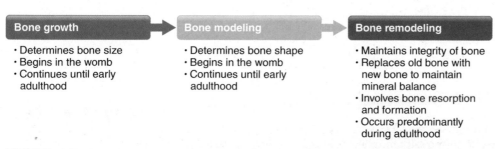

Bone growth	Bone modeling	Bone remodeling
• Determines bone size • Begins in the womb • Continues until early adulthood	• Determines bone shape • Begins in the womb • Continues until early adulthood	• Maintains integrity of bone • Replaces old bone with new bone to maintain mineral balance • Involves bone resorption and formation • Occurs predominantly during adulthood

FIGURE 11.2 Bone develops through three processes: bone growth, bone modeling, and bone remodeling.

and into adolescence. Most girls reach their adult height by age 14, and boys generally reach adult height by age 17.[2] In the later decades of life, some loss in height usually occurs because of decreased bone density in the spine.

Bone modeling is the process by which the shape of bones is determined, from the round "pebble" bones that make up the wrists to the uniquely shaped bones of the face to the long bones of the arms and legs. Even after bones stop growing in length, they can still increase in thickness if we stress them by engaging in repetitive exercise, such as weight training, or by being overweight or obese.

Although the size and shape of bones do not change significantly after puberty, our **bone density,** or compactness of our bones, continues to develop into early adulthood. *Peak bone density* is the point at which our bones are strongest because they are at their highest density. The following factors are associated with a lower peak bone density: [3–5]

- Late pubertal age in boys and late onset of menstruation in girls
- Inadequate calcium intake
- Low body weight
- Physical inactivity during adolescence

About 90% of a woman's bone density has been built by 17 years of age, whereas the majority of a man's bone density has been built by his twenties. However, male or female, before we reach the age of 30 years, our bodies have reached peak bone mass, and we can no longer significantly add to our bone density. In our thirties, our bone density remains relatively stable, but by age 40, it has begun its irreversible decline.

Bone Remodeling Maintains a Balance Between Breakdown and Repair

Although our bones cannot increase in density after our twenties, bone tissue still remains very active throughout adulthood, balancing the breakdown of older bone tissue and the formation of new bone tissue. This bone recycling process is called **remodeling**. Remodeling is also used to repair fractures and to strengthen bone regions that are exposed to higher physical stress. The process of remodeling involves two steps: resorption and formation.

Bone is broken down through the process of **resorption** (**Figure 11.3a**). During resorption, cells called **osteoclasts** erode the bone surface by secreting enzymes and acids that dig grooves into the bone matrix. One of the primary reasons the body regularly breaks down bone is to release calcium into the bloodstream. As discussed in more detail later in this chapter, calcium is critical for many physiologic processes, and bone is an important

bone density   The degree of compactness of bone tissue, reflecting the strength of the bones. *Peak bone density* is the point at which a bone is strongest.

remodeling   The two-step process by which bone tissue is recycled; includes the breakdown of existing bone and the formation of new bone.

resorption   The process by which the surface of bone is broken down by cells called osteoclasts.

osteoclasts   Cells that erode the surface of bones by secreting enzymes and acids that dig grooves into the bone matrix.

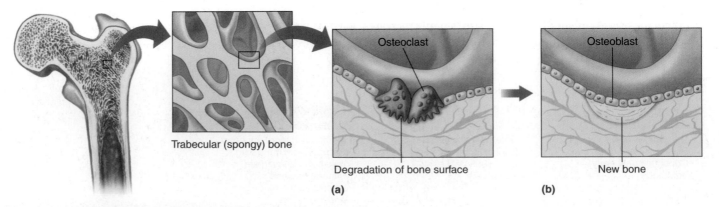

FIGURE 11.3 Bone remodeling involves resorption and formation. **(a)** Osteoclasts erode the bone surface by degrading its components, including calcium, other minerals, and collagen; these components are then transported to the bloodstream. **(b)** Osteoblasts work to build new bone by filling the pit formed by the resorption process with new bone.

calcium reservoir. The body also breaks down bone that is fractured and needs to be repaired. Resorption at the injury site smoothes the rough edges created by the break. Bone may also be broken down in areas away from the fracture site to obtain the minerals that are needed to repair the damage. Regardless of the reason, once bone is broken down, the resulting products are transported into the bloodstream and used for various body functions.

New bone is formed through the action of cells called **osteoblasts,** or "bone builders" (see Figure 11.3b). These cells work to synthesize new bone matrix by laying down the collagen-containing organic component of bone. Within this substance, the hydroxyapatite crystallizes and packs together to create new bone where it is needed.

In young, healthy adults, the processes of bone resorption and formation are equal, so that just as much bone is broken down as is built, maintaining bone mass. Around 40 years of age, bone resorption begins to occur more rapidly than bone formation, and this imbalance results in an overall loss in bone density. Because this affects the vertebrae of the spine, people tend to lose height as they age. As discussed shortly, achieving a high peak bone mass through proper nutrition and exercise when we are young provides us with a stronger skeleton before the loss of bone begins. It can therefore reduce our risk for *osteoporosis*, a disorder characterized by low-density bones that fracture easily. Osteoporosis is discussed later in this chapter.

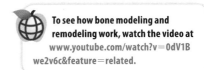

To see how bone modeling and remodeling work, watch the video at www.youtube.com/watch?v=0dV1B we2v6c&feature=related.

RECAP

Bones are organs that contain metabolically active tissues composed primarily of minerals and a fibrous protein called collagen. Of the two types of bone, cortical bone is more dense and trabecular bone is more porous. Trabecular bone is also more sensitive to hormonal and nutritional factors and turns over more rapidly than cortical bone. The three types of bone activity are growth, modeling, and remodeling. Bones reach their peak bone mass by the late teenage years into the twenties; bone mass begins to decline around age 40. ■

How Do We Assess Bone Health?

Over the past 40 years, technological advancements have led to the development of a number of affordable methods for measuring bone health. **Dual energy x-ray absorptiometry** (**DXA** or **DEXA**) is considered the most accurate assessment tool for measuring bone density. This method can measure the density of the bone mass over the entire body. Software is also available that provides an estimation of percentage of body fat.

The DXA procedure is simple, painless, and noninvasive and is considered to be of minimal risk. It takes just 15 to 30 minutes to complete. The person participating in the test remains fully clothed but must remove all jewelry or other metal objects. The participant lies quietly on a table, and bone density is assessed through the use of a very low level of x-ray (**Figure 11.4**, page 438).

DXA is a very important tool to determine a person's risk for osteoporosis. It generates a bone density score, which is compared to the average peak bone density of a healthy 30-year-old. Doctors use this comparison, which is known as a **T-score,** to assess the risk for fracture and to determine whether the person has osteoporosis. T-scores are interpreted as follows:

- A T score between +1 and −1 means that the individual's bone density is normal.
- A T-score between −1 and −2.5 indicates low bone mass and an increased risk for fractures.
- A T-score more negative than −2.5 indicates that the person has osteoporosis.

DXA tests are generally recommended for postmenopausal women, because they are at highest risk for osteoporosis and fracture. Men and younger women may also be recommended for a DXA test if they have significant risk factors for osteoporosis.

osteoblasts   Cells that prompt the formation of new bone matrix by laying down the collagen-containing component of bone, which is then mineralized.

dual energy x-ray absorptiometry (DXA, DEXA)   Currently the most accurate tool for measuring bone density.

T-score   A numerical score comparing an individual's bone density to the average peak bone density of a 30-year-old healthy adult, to determine the risk for osteoporosis.

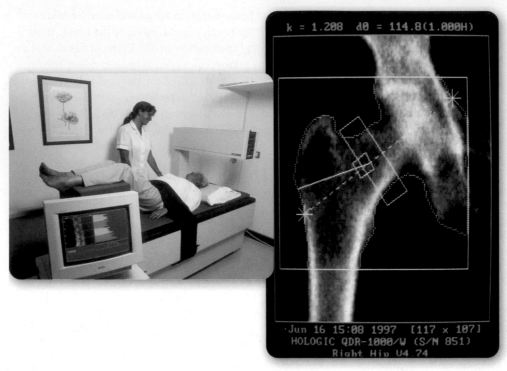

FIGURE 11.4 Dual energy x-ray absorptiometry is a safe and simple procedure that assesses bone density.

Other technologies have been developed to measure bone density. The quantitative ultrasound technique uses sound waves to measure the density of bone in the heel, shin, and kneecap. Peripheral dual energy x-ray absorptiometry, or pDXA, is a form of DXA that measures bone density in the peripheral regions of our bodies, including the wrist, heel, or finger. Single energy x-ray absorptiometry is a method that measures bone density at the wrist or heel. These technologies are frequently used at health fairs, because the machines are portable and provide scores faster than the traditional DXA.

RECAP

Dual energy x-ray absorptiometry (DXA or DEXA) is the gold-standard measurement of bone mass. It is a simple, painless, and minimal-risk procedure. The results of a DXA include a T-score, which is a comparison of the person's bone density to that of a 30-year-old healthy adult. A T-score lower than −1 indicates poor bone density. Quantitative ultrasound, peripheral dual energy x-ray absorptiometry, and single energy x-ray absorptiometry are additional methods that can be used to measure bone density. ■

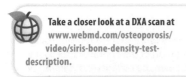
Take a closer look at a DXA scan at www.webmd.com/osteoporosis/video/siris-bone-density-test-description.

A Profile of Nutrients That Maintain Bone Health

Calcium is the most recognized nutrient associated with bone health; however, vitamins D and K, phosphorus, magnesium, and fluoride are also essential for strong bones, and the roles of other vitamins, minerals, and phytochemicals are currently being researched.

Calcium

Dietary calcium is absorbed in the intestines via active transport and passive diffusion across the intestinal mucosal membrane. The majority of the calcium consumed is absorbed from the duodenum, as this area of the small intestine is slightly more acidic than the more distal regions, and calcium absorption is enhanced in an acidic environment. Active transport of calcium is dependent on the active form of vitamin D, or 1,25-dihydroxyvitamin D; most of the absorption of calcium at low to moderate intake levels is accounted for by this vitamin D–enhanced active transport. Passive diffusion of calcium across the intestinal mucosal membrane is a function of the calcium concentration gradient in the intestines, and this mechanism becomes a more important means of calcium absorption at high calcium intakes.[6]

Recall (from Chapter 1) that the major minerals are those required in our diets in amounts greater than 100 mg per day. Calcium is by far the most abundant major mineral in the body, comprising about 2% of our entire body weight! Not surprisingly, it plays many critical roles in maintaining overall function and health.

Functions of Calcium

One of the primary functions of calcium is to provide structure to the bones and teeth. About 99% of the calcium in the body is stored in the hydroxyapatite crystals built up on the collagen foundation of bone. As noted earlier, the combination of crystals and collagen provides both the characteristic hardness of bone and the flexibility needed to support various activities.

The remaining 1% of calcium in the body is found in the blood and soft tissues. Calcium is alkaline, or basic, and plays a critical role in assisting with acid–base balance. We cannot survive for long if our blood calcium level rises above or falls below a very narrow range; therefore, the body maintains the appropriate blood calcium level at all costs.

Figure 11.5 illustrates how various organ systems and hormones work together to maintain blood calcium levels. When blood calcium levels fall (Figure 11.5a), the parathyroid glands are stimulated to produce **parathyroid hormone (PTH).** Also known as parathormone, PTH stimulates the activation of vitamin D. Together, PTH and vitamin D stimulate the kidneys to reabsorb calcium from the bloodstream. They also stimulate osteoclasts to break down bone, releasing more calcium into the bloodstream. In addition, vitamin D increases the absorption of calcium from the intestines. Through these three mechanisms, blood calcium levels increase.

When blood calcium levels are too high, the thyroid gland secretes a hormone called **calcitonin,** which inhibits the actions of vitamin D (Figure 11.5b). Thus, calcitonin prevents reabsorption of calcium in the kidneys, limits calcium absorption in the intestines, and inhibits the osteoclasts from breaking down bone.

As just noted, the body must maintain blood calcium levels within a very narrow range. Thus, when an individual does not consume or absorb enough calcium from the diet, osteoclasts erode bone, so that calcium can be released into the blood. To maintain healthy bone density, we need to consume and absorb enough calcium to balance the calcium taken from our bones.

Calcium is also critical for the normal transmission of nerve impulses. Calcium flows into nerve cells and stimulates the release of molecules called neurotransmitters, which transfer the nerve impulses from one nerve cell (neuron) to another. Without adequate calcium, the nerves' ability to transmit messages is inhibited. Not surprisingly, when blood calcium levels fall dangerously low, a person can experience convulsions.

A fourth role of calcium is to assist in muscle contraction, which is initiated when calcium flows into muscle cells. Conversely, muscles relax when calcium is pumped back outside of muscle cells. If calcium levels are inadequate, normal muscle contraction and

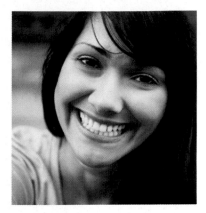

A major role of calcium is to form and maintain bones and teeth.

parathyroid hormone (PTH) A hormone secreted by the parathyroid gland when blood calcium levels fall. It is also known as parathormone, and it increases blood calcium levels by stimulating the activation of vitamin D, increasing reabsorption of calcium from the kidneys, and stimulating osteoclasts to break down bone, which releases more calcium into the bloodstream.

calcitonin A hormone secreted by the thyroid gland when blood calcium levels are too high. Calcitonin inhibits the actions of vitamin D, preventing reabsorption of calcium in the kidneys, limiting calcium absorption in the intestines, and inhibiting the osteoclasts from breaking down bone.

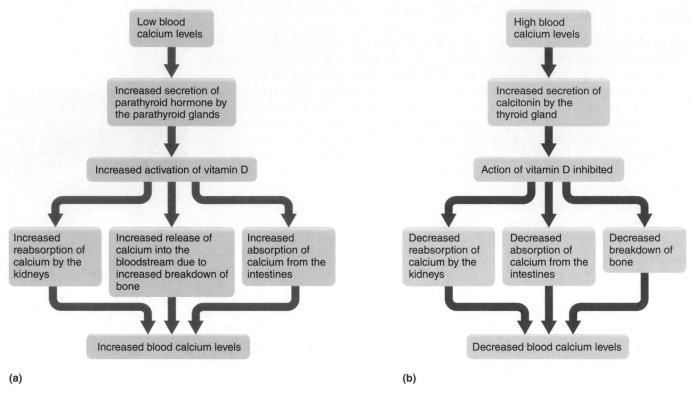

FIGURE 11.5 Regulation of blood calcium levels by various organs and hormones. **(a)** Low blood calcium levels stimulate the production of parathyroid hormone and activation of vitamin D, which in turn causes an increase in blood calcium levels. **(b)** High blood calcium levels stimulate the secretion of calcitonin, which in turn causes a decrease in blood calcium levels.

relaxation are inhibited, and the person may suffer from twitching and spasms. This is referred to as **calcium tetany.** High levels of blood calcium can cause **calcium rigor,** an inability of muscles to relax, which leads to a hardening or stiffening of the muscles. These problems affect the function not only of skeletal muscles but also of heart muscle and can cause heart failure.

Other functions of calcium include the maintenance of healthy blood pressure, the initiation of blood clotting, and the regulation of various hormones and enzymes.

How Much Calcium Should We Consume?

Calcium requirements, and thus recommended intakes, vary according to age and gender. Many people of all ages fail to consume enough calcium to maintain bone health.

Recommended Dietary Intake for Calcium   The RDA for adult men aged 19 to 70 years and women aged 19 to 50 years is 1,000 mg of calcium per day. For men older than 70 years of age and women older than 50 years of age, the RDA increases to 1,200 mg of calcium per day. At 1,300 mg per day, the RDA for boys and girls aged 9 to 18 years is even higher, reflecting their developing bone mass. The Upper Limit (UL) for calcium is 2,500 mg for all age groups (**Table 11.2**).

A nutrient's **bioavailability** is the degree to which the body can absorb and use any given nutrient. The bioavailability of calcium depends in part on a person's age and need for calcium. For example, infants, children, and adolescents can absorb more than 60% of the calcium they consume, as calcium needs are very high during these stages of life. In addition, pregnant and lactating women can absorb about 50% of dietary calcium. In

calcium tetany   A condition in which muscles experience twitching and spasms due to inadequate blood calcium levels.

calcium rigor   A failure of muscles to relax, which leads to a hardening or stiffening of the muscles; caused by high levels of blood calcium.

bioavailability   The degree to which the body can absorb and use any given nutrient.

TABLE 11.2 Overview of Nutrients Essential to Bone Health

To see the full profile of micronutrients, turn to Chapter 7.5, In Depth: Vitamins and Minerals: Micronutrients with Macro Powers, pages 300–309.

Nutrient	Recommended Intake
Calcium (major mineral)	RDA: Adults aged 19 to 50 years = 1,000 mg/day Men aged 51–70 = 1,000 mg/day; men aged >70 = 1,200 mg/day Women aged >50 = 1,200 mg/day UL = 2,500 mg/day
Vitamin D (fat-soluble vitamin)	RDA:* Adults aged 19 to 50 years = 600 IU/day Adults aged 50 to 70 years = 600 IU/day Adults aged >70 years = 800 IU/day
Vitamin K (fat-soluble vitamin)	AI: Women = 90 μg/day Men = 120 μg/day
Phosphorus (major mineral)	RDA: Adults = 700 mg/day
Magnesium (major mineral)	RDA: Women aged 19 to 30 years = 310 mg/day Women aged >30 years = 320 mg/day Men aged 19 to 30 years = 400 mg/day Men aged >30 years = 420 mg/day
Fluoride (trace mineral)	RDA: Women = 3 mg/day Men = 4 mg/day UL = 2.2 mg/day for children aged 4 to 8; children >8 = 10 mg/day

*Based on the assumption that a person does not get adequate sun exposure.

contrast, healthy, young adults absorb only about 30% of the calcium consumed in the diet. When calcium needs are high, the body can generally increase its absorption from the small intestine. Although older adults have a high need for calcium, their ability to absorb calcium from the small intestine diminishes with age and can be as low as 25%. These variations in bioavailability and absorption capacity were taken into account when calcium recommendations were determined.

The bioavailability of calcium also depends on how much calcium is consumed throughout the day or at any one time. When diets are generally high in calcium, absorption of calcium is reduced. In addition, the body cannot absorb more than 500 mg of calcium at any one time, and as the amount of calcium in a single meal or supplement goes up, the fraction that is absorbed goes down. This explains why it is critical to consume calcium-rich foods throughout the day, rather than relying on a single, high-dose supplement. Conversely, when dietary intake of calcium is low, the absorption of calcium is increased.

Dietary factors can also affect the absorption of calcium. Binding factors, such as phytates and oxalates, occur naturally in some calcium-rich seeds, nuts, grains, and vegetables, such as spinach and Swiss chard. Such factors bind to the calcium in these foods and prevent its absorption from the small intestine. Additionally, consuming calcium with iron, zinc, magnesium, or phosphorus can interfere with the absorption and utilization of all these minerals. Despite these potential interactions, the Institute of Medicine has concluded that there is not sufficient evidence to suggest that these interactions cause deficiencies of calcium or other minerals in healthy individuals.[6]

Finally, because vitamin D is necessary for the absorption of calcium, a lack of vitamin D severely limits the bioavailability of calcium. We'll discuss this and other contributions of vitamin D to bone health shortly.

Foods Rich in Calcium   Dairy products are among the most common sources of calcium in the U.S. diet. Skim milk, low-fat cheeses, and nonfat yogurt are nutritious sources of calcium (**Figure 11.6**, page 442). Ice cream, regular cheese, and whole milk also contain a relatively high amount of calcium, but these foods should be eaten in moderation because

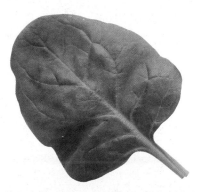

Although spinach contains high levels of calcium, binding factors in the plant prevent much of its absorption in the body.

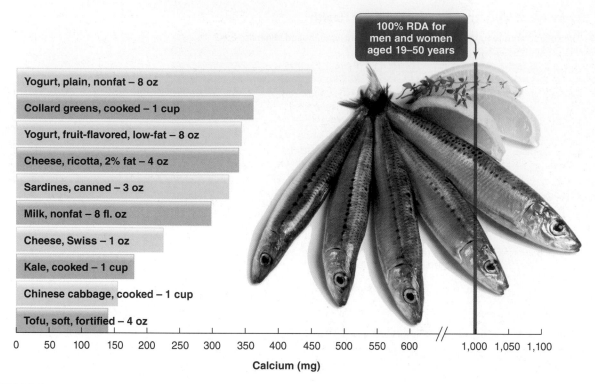

FIGURE 11.6 Common food sources of calcium. The RDA for calcium is 1,000 mg of calcium per day for men and women aged 19 to 50. (*Source:* Data from US Department of Agriculture, Agricultural Research Service, 2011, USDA Nutrient Database for Standard Reference, Release 24. Nutrient Data Laboratory Home Page, www.ars.usda.gov/ba/bhnrc/ndl.)

Kale is a good source of calcium.

To find out if you're getting enough calcium in your diet, take the calcium quiz at www.dairycouncilofca.org/Tools/CalciumQuiz.

of their high saturated fat and energy content. Cottage cheese is one dairy product that is a relatively poor source of calcium, as the processing of this food removes a great deal of the calcium. One cup of low-fat cottage cheese contains approximately 150 mg of calcium, whereas the same serving of low-fat milk contains almost 300 mg. However, calcium-fortified cottage cheese contains 400 mg of calcium.

Other good sources of calcium are green, leafy vegetables, such as kale, collard greens, turnip greens, broccoli, cauliflower, green cabbage, brussels sprouts, and Chinese cabbage (bok choy). The bioavailability of the calcium in these vegetables is relatively high compared to spinach, as these vegetables contain low levels of oxalates. Many packaged foods are now available fortified with calcium. For example, you can buy calcium-fortified orange juice, soy milk, rice milk, and tofu processed with calcium. Some dairies have even boosted the amount of calcium in their brand of milk!

Figure 11.7 illustrates serving sizes of various calcium-rich foods that contain the equivalent amount of calcium as one glass (8 fl. oz) of skim milk. As you can see from this figure, a wide variety of foods can be consumed each day to contribute to adequate calcium intakes. When you are selecting foods that are good sources of calcium, it is important to remember that we do not absorb 100% of the calcium contained in our foods. For example, although a serving of milk contains approximately 300 mg of calcium, we do not actually absorb this entire amount. To learn more about how calcium absorption rates vary for select foods, see the **Nutrition Label Activity** box (page 444).

In general, meats and fish are not good sources of calcium. An exception is canned fish with bones (for example, sardines or salmon), providing you eat the bones. Fruits (except dried figs) and nonfortified grain products are also poor sources of calcium.

As you can see, many foods are good sources of calcium. Nevertheless, many Americans do not have adequate intakes because they consume very few dairy-based foods and calcium-rich vegetables. At particular risk are women and young girls. For example, a large national survey conducted by the US Department of Agriculture found that teenage girls consumed less than 60% of the recommended amount of calcium.[7]

A variety of quick, simple tools are available on the Internet to assist individuals in determining their daily calcium intake. Most of these tools are designed to provide an estimated calcium intake score based on the types and amounts of calcium-rich foods a person consumes. Refer to the Nutrition Online link (page 442, margin) to access one of these tools. In addition, follow these tips to help you add more calcium to your bone bank:

- At the grocery store, stock up on calcium-fortified juices and milk replacements. Look for single-serving, portable "juice boxes" with calcium-fortified juice, milk, or chocolate milk.
- Purchase breakfast cereals and breads that are fortified with calcium.
- Add some crushed, unhulled sesame seeds, which are loaded with calcium, to recipes for baked goods, or toss some on salads, in yogurt, or on your breakfast cereal.
- For quick snacks, purchase single-serving cups of yogurt, individually wrapped "cheese sticks," or calcium-fortified protein bars.
- Keep on hand shredded Parmesan or any other hard cheese, and sprinkle it on hot soups, chili, salads, pasta, and other dishes.
- In any recipe, replace sour cream or mayonnaise with nonfat plain yogurt.
- Add nonfat dry milk powder to hot cereals, soups, chili, recipes for baked goods, coffee, and hot cocoa. One-third of a cup of nonfat dry milk powder provides the same amount of calcium as a whole cup of nonfat milk.
- Make a yogurt smoothie by blending nonfat plain or flavored yogurt with fresh or frozen fruit.
- At your favorite café, instead of black coffee, order a skim milk latte. Instead of black tea, order a cup of chai—spiced Indian tea brewed with milk.
- At home, brew a cup of strong coffee; then add half a cup of warm skim milk for a café au lait.
- When eating out, order skim milk instead of a soft drink with your meal.

If you do not consume enough dietary calcium, you will probably benefit from taking calcium supplements. Refer to the **Highlight** box "Calcium Supplements: Which Ones Are Best?" (page 445) to learn how to choose a calcium supplement that is right for you.

What Happens If We Consume Too Much Calcium?

In general, consuming too much calcium in the diet does not lead to significant toxicity symptoms in healthy individuals. Much of the excess calcium is excreted in feces. However, excessive intake of calcium from supplements can lead to health problems. As mentioned earlier, one concern with consuming too much calcium is that it can lead to various mineral imbalances, because calcium interferes with the absorption of other minerals, including iron, zinc, and magnesium. This interference may only be of major concern in individuals vulnerable to mineral imbalance, such as the elderly and people who consume very low amounts of minerals in their diets. Another potential problem is kidney stone formation: calcium from foods does not increase the risk for kidney stones, but some studies suggest that taking calcium supplements can.[8]

Various diseases and metabolic disorders can alter the body's ability to regulate blood calcium. **Hypercalcemia** is a condition in which blood calcium levels reach abnormally high concentrations. Hypercalcemia can be caused by cancer and by the overproduction of PTH. Recall that PTH stimulates the osteoclasts to break down bone and release more calcium into the bloodstream. Symptoms of hypercalcemia include fatigue, loss of appetite, constipation, and mental confusion, and it can lead to coma and possibly death. Hypercalcemia can also result in an accumulation of calcium deposits in the soft tissues, such as the liver and kidneys, causing failure of these organs.

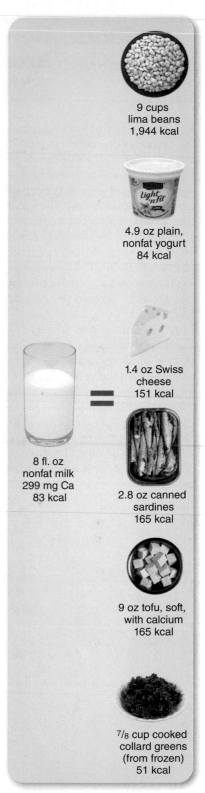

9 cups
lima beans
1,944 kcal

4.9 oz plain,
nonfat yogurt
84 kcal

1.4 oz Swiss
cheese
151 kcal

8 fl. oz
nonfat milk
299 mg Ca
83 kcal

2.8 oz canned
sardines
165 kcal

9 oz tofu, soft,
with calcium
165 kcal

7/8 cup cooked
collard greens
(from frozen)
51 kcal

FIGURE 11.7 Serving sizes and energy content of various foods that contain the same amount of calcium as an 8-fl. oz glass of skim milk.

hypercalcemia A condition characterized by an abnormally high concentration of calcium in the blood.

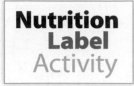

How Much Calcium Am I Really Consuming?

As you have learned in this chapter, we do not absorb 100% of the calcium contained in our foods. This is particularly true for individuals who eat a diet dominated by foods that are high in fiber, oxalates, and phytates, such as whole grains and certain vegetables. So if you want to design an eating plan that contains adequate calcium, it's important to understand how the rate of calcium absorption differs for the foods you include.

Estimates of the rate of calcium absorption have been established for a variety of common foods that are considered good sources of calcium. The following table shows some of these foods, their calcium content per serving, the calcium absorption rate, and the estimated amount of calcium absorbed from each food.

As you can see from this table, many dairy products have a similar calcium absorption rate, just over 30%. Interestingly, many green, leafy vegetables have a higher absorption rate of around 60%; however, because a typical serving of these foods contains less calcium than dairy foods, you would have to eat more vegetables to get the same calcium as you would from a standard serving of dairy foods. Note the relatively low calcium absorption rate for spinach, even though it contains a relatively high amount of calcium. This is due to the high levels of oxalates in spinach, which bind with calcium and reduce its bioavailability.

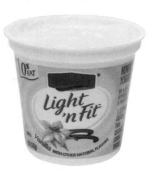

Remember that the RDA for calcium takes these differences in absorption rate into account. Thus, the 300 mg of calcium in a glass of milk counts as 300 mg toward your daily calcium goal. In general, you can trust that dairy products are good, absorbable sources of calcium, as are most dark-green, leafy vegetables. Other dietary sources of calcium

Food	Serving Size	Calcium per Serving (mg)*	Absorption Rate (%)†	Estimated Amount of Calcium Absorbed (mg)
Yogurt, plain skim milk	8 fl. oz	452	32	145
Milk, skim	1 cup	299	32	96
Milk, 2%	1 cup	244	32	78
Kale, frozen, cooked	1 cup	179	59	106
Turnip greens, boiled	1 cup	197	52	103
Broccoli, frozen, chopped, cooked	1 cup	61	61	37
Cauliflower, boiled	1 cup	20	69	14
Spinach, frozen, cooked	1 cup	291	5	14

*Data from US Department of Agriculture, Agricultural Research Service. 2011. USDA National Nutrient Database for Standard Reference, Release 24. www.ars .usda.gov/ba/bhnrc/ndl.
†Data from Weaver, C. M., W. R. Proulx, and R. Heaney. 1999. Choices for achieving adequate dietary calcium with a vegetarian diet. *Am. J. Clin. Nutr.* 70(suppl.):543S–548S; and Weaver, C. M., and K. L. Plawecki. 1994. Dietary calcium: adequacy of a vegetarian diet. *Am. J. Clin. Nutr.* 59(suppl.):1238S–1241S.

with good absorption rates include calcium-fortified orange juice, soy milk, and rice milk; tofu processed with calcium; and fortified breakfast cereals. Armed with this knowledge, you will be better able to select food sources that can optimize your calcium intake and support bone health.

What Happens If We Don't Consume Enough Calcium?

There are no short-term symptoms associated with consuming too little calcium. Even when a person does not consume enough dietary calcium, the body continues to tightly regulate blood calcium levels by taking the calcium from bone. A long-term repercussion of inadequate calcium intake is osteoporosis. But because other nutrients may be involved, we'll discuss this disease later in the chapter.

Hypocalcemia is the condition of having an abnormally low level of calcium in the blood. Hypocalcemia does not result from consuming too little dietary calcium, but is caused by various diseases, including kidney disease, vitamin D deficiency, and diseases that inhibit the production of PTH. Symptoms of hypocalcemia include muscle spasms and convulsions.

hypocalcemia A condition characterized by an abnormally low concentration of calcium in the blood.

HIGHLIGHT

Calcium Supplements: Which Ones Are Best?

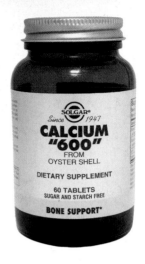

We know that calcium is a critical nutrient for bone health. Now that so many products are fortified with calcium, from cereals and energy bars to orange juice and soy milk, it is not difficult for many people, even vegans, to get sufficient calcium from the diet. Still, small or inactive people who eat less to maintain a healthful weight may not be able to consume enough food to provide adequate calcium, and elderly people may need more calcium than they can obtain in their normal diets. In these circumstances, calcium supplements may be warranted.

Numerous calcium supplements are available to consumers, but which are best? Most supplements come in the form of calcium carbonate, calcium citrate, calcium lactate, or calcium phosphate. Our bodies are able to absorb about 30% of the calcium from these various forms. Calcium citrate malate, which is the form of calcium used in fortified juices, is slightly more absorbable at 35%. Many antacids are also good sources of calcium, and it appears they are safe to take as long as you consume only enough to get the recommended level of calcium.

What is the most cost-effective form of calcium? In general, supplements that contain calcium carbonate tend to have more calcium per pill than other types. Thus, you are getting more calcium for your money when you buy this type. However, be sure to read the label of any calcium supplement you are considering taking to determine just how much calcium it contains. Some very expensive calcium supplements do not contain a lot of calcium per pill, and you could be wasting your money.

The lead content of calcium supplements is an important public health concern. Those made from "natural" sources, such as oyster shell, bone meal, and dolomite, are known to be higher in lead, and some of these products can contain dangerously high levels. The Food and Drug Administration (FDA) has set an Upper Limit of 7.5 µg of lead per 1,000 mg of calcium, but currently calcium supplements are not tested for lead content, and it is the manufacturer's responsibility to ensure that its supplements meet FDA standards. To avoid taking supplements that contain too much lead, look for supplements claiming to be lead-free, and make sure the word *purified* is on the label in addition to the US Pharmacopeia (USP) symbol.

If you decide to use a calcium supplement, how should you take it? Remember that the body cannot absorb more than 500 mg of calcium at any given time. Thus, taking a supplement that contains 1,000 mg calcium will be no more effective than taking one that contains 500 mg calcium. If at all possible, try to consume calcium supplements in small doses throughout the day. In addition, calcium is absorbed better with meals, as the calcium stays in the intestinal tract longer during a meal and more calcium can be absorbed.

By consuming foods high in calcium throughout the day, you can avoid the need for calcium supplements. But if you cannot consume enough calcium in your diet, many inexpensive, safe, and effective supplements are available. The best supplement for you is the one that you can tolerate and is affordable, lead-free, and readily available when you need it.

RECAP

Calcium is the most abundant mineral in the body and a significant component of bones. It is also necessary for normal nerve and muscle function. Blood calcium is maintained within a very narrow range, and bone calcium is used to maintain normal blood calcium if dietary intake is inadequate. The RDA for calcium is 1,000 mg per day for adults aged 19 to 50; the RDA increases to 1,200 mg per day for men older than 70 years of age and women older than 50 years of age, and goes up to 1,300 mg per day for adolescents. Dairy products, canned fish with bones, and some green, leafy vegetables are good sources of calcium. The most common long-term effect of inadequate calcium consumption is osteoporosis. ■

Vitamin D

Vitamin D is like other fat-soluble vitamins in that excess amounts are stored in the liver and adipose tissue. But vitamin D is different from other nutrients in two ways. First, vitamin D does not always need to come from the diet. This is because the body can synthesize

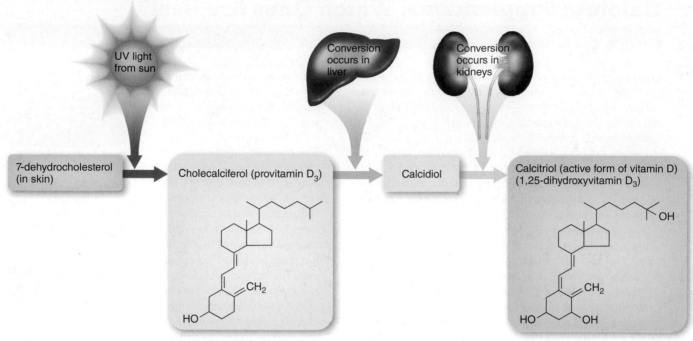

FIGURE 11.8 The process of converting sunlight into vitamin D in our skin. When the ultraviolet rays of the sun hit the skin, they react with 7-dehydrocholesterol. This compound is converted to cholecalciferol, an inactive form of vitamin D that is also called provitamin D_3. Cholecalciferol is then converted to calcidiol in the liver. Calcidiol travels to the kidneys, where it is converted into calcitriol, which is considered the primary active form of vitamin D in our bodies.

vitamin D using energy from exposure to sunlight. However, when we do not get enough sunlight, we must consume vitamin D in our diets. Second, in addition to being a nutrient, vitamin D is considered a *hormone,* because it is made in one part of the body yet regulates various activities in other parts of the body.

Figure 11.8 illustrates how the body makes vitamin D by converting a cholesterol compound in our skin to the active form of vitamin D that we need to function properly. When the ultraviolet rays of the sun hit the skin, they react with 7-dehydrocholesterol. This cholesterol compound is converted into a precursor of vitamin D, **cholecalciferol,** which is also called provitamin D_3. This inactive form is then converted to calcidiol in the liver, where it is stored. When needed, calcidiol travels to the kidneys, where it is converted into **calcitriol,** which is considered the primary active form of vitamin D in the body. Calcitriol then circulates to various parts of the body, performing its many functions. Excess calcitriol can also be stored in adipose tissue for later use.

Functions of Vitamin D

As you've learned, vitamin D, PTH, and calcitonin all work together continuously to regulate blood calcium levels, which in turn maintains bone health. They do this by regulating the absorption of calcium and phosphorus from the small intestine, causing more to be absorbed when the need for them is higher and less when the need is lower. They also decrease or increase blood calcium levels by signaling the kidneys to excrete more or less calcium in the urine. Finally, vitamin D works with PTH to stimulate osteoclasts to break down bone when calcium is needed elsewhere in the body.

Vitamin D is also necessary for the normal calcification of bone; this means it assists the process by which minerals such as calcium and phosphorus are crystallized. Vitamin D may also play a role in decreasing the formation of some cancerous tumors, as it can prevent certain types of cells from growing out of control. Like vitamin A, vitamin D appears to play a role in cell differentiation in various tissues.

cholecalciferol Vitamin D_3, a form of vitamin D found in animal foods and the form we synthesize from the sun.

calcitriol The primary active form of vitamin D in the body.

How Much Vitamin D Should We Consume?

If your exposure to the sun is adequate, then you do not need to consume any vitamin D in your diet. But how do you know whether you are getting enough sun?

Recommended Dietary Intake for Vitamin D   This RDA is based on the assumption that an individual does not get adequate sun exposure. Of the many factors that affect the ability to synthesize vitamin D from sunlight, latitude and time of year are most significant (**Table 11.3**). People living in very sunny climates relatively close to the equator, such as the southern United States and Mexico, may synthesize enough vitamin D from the sun to meet their needs throughout the year—as long as they spend time outdoors. However, vitamin D synthesis from the sun is not possible during most of the winter months for people living in places located at a latitude of more than 40°N or more than 40°S. At these latitudes in winter the sun never rises high enough in the sky to provide the amount of direct sunlight needed. The 40°N latitude runs like a belt across the United States from northern Pennsylvania in the East to northern California in the West (**Figure 11.9**). In addition, entire countries, such as Canada and the United Kingdom, are affected, as are countries and regions in the far Southern Hemisphere. Thus, many people around the world need to consume vitamin D in their diets, particularly during the winter months.

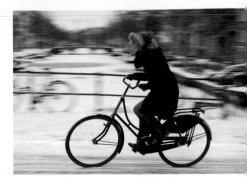

Vitamin D synthesis from the sun is not possible during most of the winter months for people living in high latitudes. Therefore, many people around the world need to consume vitamin D in their diets, particularly during the winter.

Other factors influencing vitamin D synthesis include the time of day, skin color, age, and body weight status:

- More vitamin D can be synthesized during the time of day when the sun's rays are strongest, generally between 10 AM and 3 PM. Vitamin D synthesis is severely limited or may be nonexistent on overcast days.
- Darker skin contains more melanin pigment, which reduces the penetration of sunlight. Thus, people with dark skin have a more difficult time synthesizing vitamin D from the sun than do light-skinned people.
- People 65 years of age or older experience a fourfold decrease in their capacity to synthesize vitamin D from the sun; they are also more likely to spend more time indoors and may have inadequate dietary intakes.[9]
- Obesity is associated with lower levels of circulating vitamin D, possibly because of lower bioavailability of cholecalciferol from adipose tissue, decreased exposure to sunlight due to limited mobility or time spent outdoors with skin exposed, and alterations in vitamin D metabolism in the liver.[10,11]

TABLE 11.3 Factors Affecting Sunlight-Mediated Synthesis of Vitamin D in the Skin

Factors That Enhance Synthesis of Vitamin D	Factors That Inhibit Synthesis of Vitamin D
Season—summer months, particularly June and July, during which most vitamin D is produced	Season—winter months (October through February), resulting in little or no vitamin D production
Latitude—locations closer to the equator, which get more sunlight throughout the year	Latitude—regions north of 40°N and south of 40°S, which get inadequate sunlight
Time of day—generally, between 9:00 AM and 3:00 PM (depending on latitude and time of year)	Time of day—early morning, late afternoon, and evening hours Age—older, due to reduced skin thickness with age
Age—younger	Use of sunscreen with SPF 8 or greater
Limited or no use of sunscreen	Cloudy weather
Sunny weather	Protective clothing
Exposed skin	Darker skin pigmentation
Lighter skin pigmentation	Glass and plastics—windows or other barriers made of glass or plastic (such as Plexiglas), which block the sun's rays Obesity—possible negative effect on metabolism and storage of vitamin D

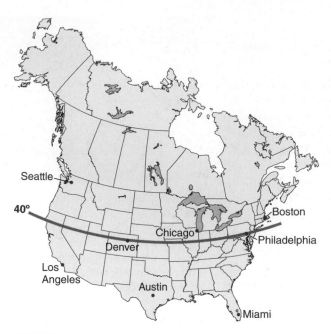

FIGURE 11.9 This map illustrates the geographic location of 40° latitude in the United States. In southern cities below 40° latitude, such as Los Angeles, Austin, and Miami, the sunlight is strong enough to allow for vitamin D synthesis throughout the year. In northern cities above 40° latitude, such as Seattle, Chicago, and Boston, the sunlight is too weak from about mid-October to mid-March to allow for adequate vitamin D synthesis.

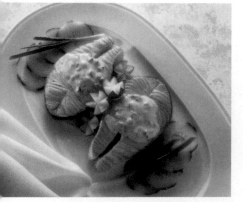

Fatty fish contain vitamin D.

ergocalciferol Vitamin D$_2$, a form of vitamin D found exclusively in plant foods.

Wearing protective clothing and sunscreen (with an SPF greater than 8) limits sun exposure, so it is suggested that we expose our hands, face, and arms to the sun two or three times per week for a period of time that is one-third to one-half of the amount it would take to get sunburned.[12] This means that, if you normally sunburn in 1 hour, you should expose yourself to the sun for 20 to 30 minutes two or three times per week to synthesize adequate amounts of vitamin D. Again, this guideline does not apply to people living in more northern climates during the winter months; they can get enough vitamin D only by consuming it in their diets.

Because not everyone is able to get adequate sun exposure throughout the year, an RDA has been established for vitamin D. For men and women aged 19 to 70 years, the RDA is 600 IU, and for adults older than 70 years, it is 800 IU. The UL for vitamin D is 4,000 IU for everyone 9 years of age and older. Recent evidence suggests that the current RDA for vitamin D is not sufficient to maintain optimal bone health and reduce the risks for diseases such as cancer; the controversy surrounding the current recommendations for vitamin D intake are discussed in more detail in the **Nutrition Debate** at the end of this chapter.

When reading labels, you will see the amount of vitamin D expressed on food and supplement labels in units of either μg or IU. For conversion purposes, 1 μg of vitamin D is equal to 40 IU of vitamin D. Refer to the **You Do the Math** box (page 449) to learn how to convert vitamin D units from food and supplement sources.

Vitamin D: Fish, Fortified Foods, Supplements, or Sunlight There are many forms of vitamin D, but only two can be converted into calcitriol. Vitamin D$_2$, also called **ergocalciferol**, is found exclusively in plant foods, whereas vitamin D$_3$, or cholecalciferol, is found in animal foods. As noted earlier, cholecalciferol also is the form of vitamin D we synthesize from the sun.

Most foods naturally contain very little vitamin D. The few exceptions are cod liver oil and fatty fish (such as salmon, mackerel, and sardines), foods that few Americans consume in adequate amounts. Egg yolks, beef liver, and cheese also provide small amounts of vitamin D, but we would have to eat very large amounts to consume enough vitamin D.

Thus, the primary source of vitamin D in the diet is from fortified foods, such as milk (**Figure 11.10**). In the United States, milk is fortified with 100 IU of vitamin D per cup.[13] Additional foods fortified with vitamin D include some breakfast cereals, margarine, orange juice, and yogurt. Because plants contain very little vitamin D, vegetarians who consume no fortified dairy products need to obtain their vitamin D from sun exposure, fortified soy or cereal products, or supplements.

What Happens If We Consume Too Much Vitamin D?

A person cannot get too much vitamin D from sun exposure, as the skin has the ability to limit its production. As noted, foods contain little natural vitamin D. Thus, the only way a person can consume too much vitamin D is through supplementation.

Consuming too much vitamin D causes hypercalcemia, or high blood calcium concentrations. As discussed in the section on calcium, symptoms of hypercalcemia include weakness, loss of appetite, constipation, mental confusion, vomiting, excessive urine output, and extreme thirst. Hypercalcemia also leads to the formation of calcium deposits in soft tissues, such as the kidney, liver, and heart. In addition, toxic levels of vitamin D lead to increased bone loss, because calcium is then pulled from the bones and excreted more readily from the kidneys.

Vitamin D Unit Conversions from Foods and Supplements

Labels on foods and supplements may express vitamin D content in units of either IU or µg. Judy's physician is concerned about her vitamin D intake, because Judy is obese, rarely drinks milk, and doesn't spend much time outdoors in the sun. He recommends that she increase her consumption of foods that are good sources of vitamin D. Judy's RDA for vitamin D is 600 IU per day. Recall that 1 µg of vitamin D is equal to 40 IU.

Judy enjoys tuna-fish sandwiches, and her doctor has explained that tuna is high in vitamin D. At the grocery store, she finds that 3 oz of canned tuna (packed in oil) contains 5 µg of vitamin D. Judy decides that she'll add a 1-oz slice of American cheese (fortified with vitamin D) to her sandwich. The cheese contains 2 µg of vitamin D.

a. How much vitamin D in IU units do these two foods contain?

Tuna: 5 µg × 40 IU = 200 IU of vitamin D

American cheese: 2 µg × 40 IU = 80 IU of vitamin D

Thus, these two foods contain a total of 280 IU of vitamin D.

b. Assuming Judy does not get adequate sun exposure and these two foods are the only sources of vitamin D she consumes today, how much of the RDA for vitamin D are these sources contributing to her diet?

Again, Judy's RDA for vitamin D is 600 IU per day:
(280 IU ÷ 600 IU) × 100 = 47% of the RDA is supplied by these foods.

c. If Judy decides to take a vitamin D supplement in addition to consuming these foods to meet her RDA, what amount of vitamin D (in µg) would be sufficient?

The amount of vitamin D not supplied by foods is 600 IU − 280 IU = 320 IU

320 IU ÷ 40 µg in 1 IU = 8 µg vitamin D in supplement form

Now use your own diet assessment to determine *your* intake of vitamin D. What percentage of the RDA for vitamin D do you currently consume? Do you get adequate sunlight to ensure you meet your needs for vitamin D? If not, what foods (and in what amounts) can you consume to meet your RDA for vitamin D?

Answers will vary depending on body type and individual nutrient needs.

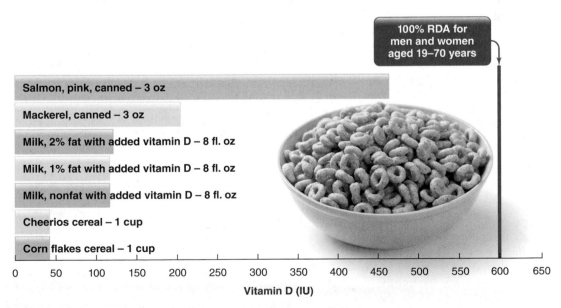

FIGURE 11.10 Common food sources of vitamin D. For men and women aged 19 to 70 years, the RDA for vitamin D is 600 IU per day. The RDA increases to 800 IU per day for adults over the age of 70 years. (*Source*: Data from US Department of Agriculture, Agricultural Research Service, 2011, USDA Nutrient Database for Standard Reference, Release 24. Nutrient Data Laboratory Home Page, www.ars.usda.gov/ba/bhnrc/ndl.)

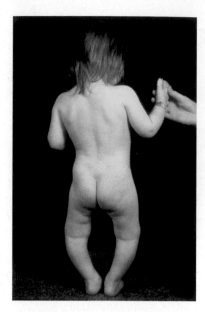

FIGURE 11.11 A vitamin D deficiency causes a bone-deforming disease in children called rickets.

What Happens If We Don't Consume Enough Vitamin D?

The primary deficiency associated with inadequate vitamin D is loss of bone mass. In fact, when vitamin D levels are inadequate, the intestines can absorb only 10% to 15% of the calcium consumed. Vitamin D deficiencies occur most often in individuals who have diseases that cause intestinal malabsorption of fat and thus the fat-soluble vitamins. People with liver disease, kidney disease, Crohn's disease, celiac disease, cystic fibrosis, or Whipple's disease may suffer from vitamin D deficiency and require supplements.

Vitamin D–deficiency disease in children, called **rickets,** results in inadequate mineralization (or *demineralization*) of the skeleton. The classic sign of rickets is deformity of the skeleton, such as bowed legs and knocked knees (**Figure 11.11**). However, severe cases can be fatal. Rickets is not common in the United States because of fortification of milk products with vitamin D, but children with illnesses that cause fat malabsorption, or who drink no milk and get limited sun exposure, are at increased risk. There is no national surveillance program for rickets, and thus it is not clear what the prevalence of rickets is in the United States. However, a review of reported cases of rickets among children in the United States found that approximately 83% were African American, and 95% had been breastfed.[14,15] Breast milk contains very little vitamin D, and less than 5% of the breast-fed children were reported to have received vitamin D supplementation. Thus, rickets appears to occur more commonly in children with darker skin (their need for adequate sun exposure is higher than that of light-skinned children) and in breast-fed children who do not receive adequate vitamin D supplementation. Rickets is still a significant nutritional problem for children living outside the United States.

Vitamin D–deficiency disease in adults is called **osteomalacia,** a term meaning "soft bones." With osteomalacia, bones become weak and prone to fractures. Osteoporosis, discussed in detail later in this chapter, can also result from a vitamin D deficiency.

Vitamin D deficiencies have recently been found to be more common among American adults than previously thought. This may be partly due to jobs and lifestyle choices that keep people indoors for most of the day. Not surprisingly, the population at greatest risk is older, institutionalized individuals who get little or no sun exposure.

Various medications can also alter the metabolism and activity of vitamin D. For instance, glucocorticoids, which are medications used to reduce inflammation, can cause bone loss by inhibiting the ability to absorb calcium through the actions of vitamin D. Anti-seizure medications, such as phenobarbital and Dilantin, alter vitamin D metabolism. Thus, people who are taking such medications may need to increase their vitamin D intake.

Nutrition
MILESTONE

The disease rickets has been reported throughout history, with the earliest descriptions in 1645 and 1650 credited to two English physicians, Daniel Whistler and Francis Glisson. In 1890, the British scientist T. A. Palm found a relationship between geographic distribution of rickets and sunlight, and he concluded that rickets is caused by inadequate exposure to sun. However, no major advances in the study and treatment of rickets were made until the early 20th century, when scientists began to explore how dietary factors might be used to treat rickets. Elmer McCollum, a nutritional biochemist at Johns Hopkins University, and his colleagues ran a series of experiments in rats in which cod liver oil was found to be an effective treatment for rickets.

In **1922**, McCollum and colleagues identified the effective *anti-rachitic* agent (an agent that cures rickets) in cod liver oil, which was named vitamin D, as it was the fourth vitamin to be discovered. By the 1930s, the use of cod liver oil to treat rickets was common throughout the United States, and the fortification of milk with vitamin D led to the almost complete eradication of rickets by the mid-1940s.

RECAP

Vitamin D is a fat-soluble vitamin and a hormone. It can be made in the skin using energy from sunlight. Vitamin D regulates blood calcium levels and maintains bone health. The RDA for vitamin D is 600 IU per day for adult men and women aged 19 to 70 years; the RDA increases to 800 IU per day for adults over the age of 70 years. Foods contain little vitamin D, with fortified milk being the primary source. Vitamin D toxicity causes hypercalcemia. Vitamin D deficiency can result in osteoporosis; rickets is vitamin D deficiency in children, whereas osteomalacia is vitamin D deficiency in adults. ■

Vitamin K

Vitamin K, a fat-soluble vitamin stored primarily in the liver, is actually a family of compounds known as quinones. **Phylloquinone,** which is the primary dietary form of vitamin K, is also the form found in plants; **menaquinone** is the animal form of vitamin K produced by bacteria in the large intestine (**Figure 11.12**).

The absorption of phylloquinone occurs in the jejunum and ileum of the small intestine, and its absorption is dependent on the normal flow of bile and pancreatic juice. Dietary fat enhances its absorption. The absorption of phylloquinone has been reported to be as low as 10% from boiled spinach eaten with butter to as high as 80% when given in its free form.[16] It is transported through the lymph as a component of chylomicrons, and it circulates to the liver, where most of the vitamin K in the body is stored. Small amounts of vitamin K are also stored in adipose tissue and bone.[16] The absorption of menaquinone is not well understood, and its contribution to the maintenance of vitamin K status has been difficult to assess.[17]

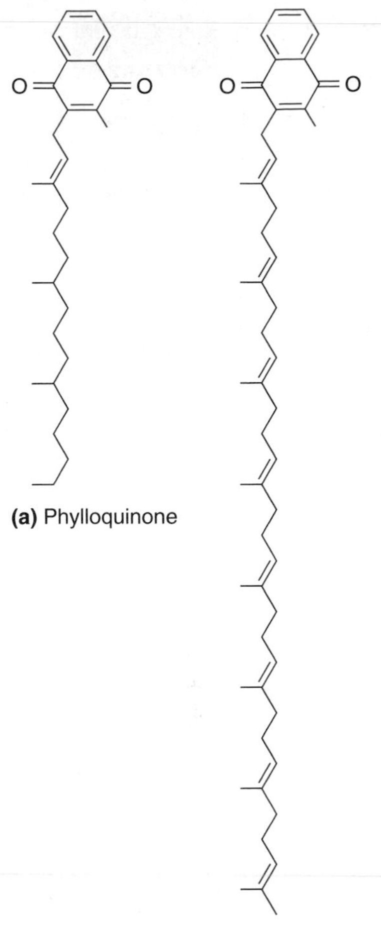

Functions of Vitamin K

The primary function of vitamin K is to serve as a coenzyme during the production of specific proteins that play important roles in the coagulation of blood and in bone metabolism. (Refer to Chapter 12 for an in-depth description of the role of vitamin K in maintaining blood health.) Here, we limit our discussion to vitamin K's role in the production of two bone proteins, referred to as "Gla" proteins: **Osteocalcin** is a Gla protein that is secreted by osteoblasts and is associated with bone remodeling. **Matrix Gla protein** is located in the protein matrix of bone and is found in cartilage, blood-vessel walls, and other soft tissues.[16] The specific role of vitamin K in maintaining bone health is unclear, with studies reporting conflicting results. A recent meta-analysis of randomized, controlled trials examining the effect of vitamin K on bone mineral density indicates that vitamin K has an overall modest effect, with gender, ethnicity, and type of vitamin K exerting variable effects on bone density.[18] Matrix Gla protein also appears to play a role in preventing the calcification of arteries, which may reduce the risk for cardiovascular disease.[19]

How Much Vitamin K Should We Consume?

We can obtain vitamin K from our diets, and we absorb the vitamin K produced by bacteria in the large intestine. These two sources of vitamin K usually provide adequate amounts of this nutrient to maintain health, and there is no RDA or UL for vitamin K. AI recommendations for adult men and adult women are 120 µg per day and 90 µg per day, respectively.

Only a few foods contribute substantially to our dietary intake of vitamin K. Green, leafy vegetables, including kale, spinach, collard greens, turnip greens, and lettuce, are good sources, as are broccoli, brussels sprouts, and cabbage. **Figure 11.13** (page 452) identifies the micrograms per serving for these foods.

What Happens If We Consume Too Much Vitamin K?

Based on our current knowledge, for healthy individuals there appear to be no side effects associated with consuming large amounts of vitamin K.[17] This seems to be true for both supplements and food sources. In the past, a synthetic form of vitamin K was used for therapeutic purposes and was shown to cause liver damage; thus, this form is no longer used.

What Happens If We Don't Consume Enough Vitamin K?

Vitamin K deficiency is associated with a reduced ability to form blood clots, leading to excessive bleeding; however, primary vitamin K deficiency is rare in humans. People with diseases that cause malabsorption of fat, such as celiac disease, Crohn's disease, and cystic fibrosis, can suffer secondarily from a deficiency of vitamin K. Long-term use of antibiotics,

(a) Phylloquinone

(b) Menaquinone

FIGURE 11.12 The chemical structure of **(a)** phylloquinone, the plant form of vitamin K, and **(b)** menaquinone, the animal form of vitamin K.

rickets A vitamin D–deficiency disease in children. Symptoms include deformities of the skeleton, such as bowed legs and knocked knees.

osteomalacia A vitamin D–deficiency disease in adults, in which bones become weak and prone to fractures.

phylloquinone The form of vitamin K found in plants.

menaquinone The form of vitamin K produced by bacteria in the large intestine.

osteocalcin A vitamin K–dependent protein that is secreted by osteoblasts and is associated with bone turnover.

matrix Gla protein A vitamin K–dependent protein located in the protein matrix of bone and in cartilage, blood-vessel walls, and other soft tissues.

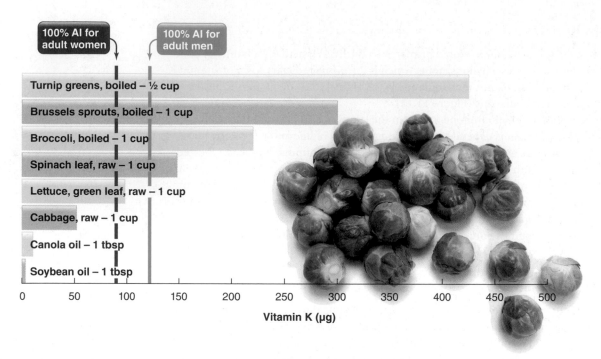

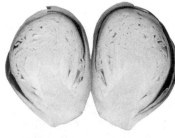

FIGURE 11.13 Common food sources of vitamin K. The AIs for adult men and adult women are 120 µg per day and 90 µg per day, respectively. (*Source:* Data from US Department of Agriculture, Agricultural Research Service, 2011, USDA Nutrient Database for Standard Reference, Release 24. Nutrient Data Laboratory Home Page, www.ars.usda.gov/ba/bhnrc/ndl.)

which typically reduce bacterial populations in the colon, combined with limited dietary intake of vitamin K–rich food sources, can also lead to vitamin K deficiency. Newborns are typically given an injection of vitamin K at birth, as they lack the intestinal bacteria necessary to produce this nutrient.

The impact of vitamin K deficiency on bone health is controversial. As recently described, the effect of vitamin K on bone mineral density appears to be modest, and studies report inconsistent results.[18] Thus, there is not enough scientific evidence to support the contention that vitamin K deficiency directly causes osteoporosis. In fact, there is no significant impact on overall bone density in people who take anticoagulant medications that result in a relative state of vitamin K deficiency.

RECAP

Vitamin K is a fat-soluble vitamin and coenzyme that is important for blood clotting and bone metabolism. We obtain vitamin K largely from bacteria in the large intestine. The AIs for adult men and adult women are 120 µg per day and 90 µg per day, respectively. Green, leafy vegetables and vegetable oils contain vitamin K. There are no known toxicity symptoms for vitamin K in healthy individuals. Vitamin K deficiency is rare and may lead to excessive bleeding. ■

Phosphorus

Phosphorus is the major negatively charged intracellular electrolyte (see Chapter 9). In the body, phosphorus is most commonly found combined with oxygen in the form of phosphate (PO_4^{3-}). Phosphorus is an essential constituent of all cells and is found in both plants and animals.

Functions of Phosphorus

Phosphorus plays a critical role in bone formation, as it is a part of the mineral complex of bone. As discussed earlier in this chapter, calcium and phosphorus crystallize

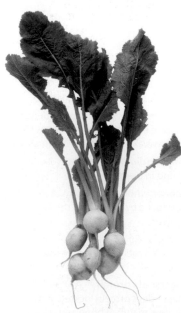

Green, leafy vegetables, including brussels sprouts and turnip greens, are good sources of vitamin K.

to form hydroxyapatite crystals, which provide the hardness of bone. About 85% of the body's phosphorus is stored in bones, with the rest stored in soft tissues, such as muscles and organs.

In addition to its role in fluid balance, phosphorus also helps activate and deactivate enzymes, and it is a component of lipoproteins, cell membranes, DNA and RNA, and several energy molecules, including adenosine triphosphate (ATP).

How Much Phosphorus Should We Consume?

The RDA for phosphorus is 700 mg for adults. In general, phosphorus is widespread in many foods and is found in high amounts in foods that contain protein. Milk, meats, and eggs are good sources.

Phosphorus is also found in many processed foods as a food additive, where it enhances smoothness, binding, and moisture retention. Moreover, in the form of phosphoric acid, it is added to soft drinks to give them a sharper, or more tart, flavor and to slow the growth of molds and bacteria. Our society has increased its consumption of processed foods and soft drinks substantially during the past 30 years, resulting in an estimated 10% to 15% increase in phosphorus consumption.[6,20]

In the past, some studies associated consumption of soft drinks with reduced bone mass or an increased risk for fractures in both youth and adults.[21-23] Some researchers proposed that the phosphoric acid content of soft drinks causes an increased loss of calcium—because calcium is drawn from bone into the blood to neutralize the excess acid. More recent evidence suggests that, in older women, it is specifically the intake of cola beverages, not carbonated beverages in general, that is associated with low bone mineral density.[24] This has contributed to speculation that it is the caffeine in colas that causes increased calcium loss through the urine. However, experts in this area of research have concluded that the most likely explanation for the link between soft drink consumption and poor bone health is the *milk-displacement effect*; that is, soft drinks take the place of milk in our diets, depriving us of calcium and vitamin D.[25]

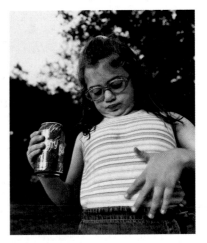

Phosphorus, in the form of phosphoric acid, is a major component of soft drinks.

What Happens If We Consume Too Much Phosphorus?

People with kidney disease and those who take too many vitamin D supplements or too many phosphorus-containing antacids can suffer from high blood phosphorus levels; severely high levels of blood phosphorus can cause muscle spasms and convulsions.

What Happens If We Don't Consume Enough Phosphorus?

Phosphorus deficiencies are rare but can occur in people who abuse alcohol, in premature infants, and in elderly people with poor diets. People with vitamin D deficiency, those who have hyperparathyroidism (oversecretion of parathyroid hormone), and those who overuse antacids that bind with phosphorus may also have low blood phosphorus levels.

RECAP

Phosphorus is the major negatively charged electrolyte inside the cell. It helps maintain fluid balance and bone health. It also assists in regulating chemical reactions, and it is a primary component of ATP, DNA, and RNA. Phosphorus is commonly found in high-protein foods. Excess phosphorus can lead to muscle spasms and convulsions, whereas phosphorus deficiencies are rare. ∎

Magnesium

Magnesium is a major mineral. Approximately 50% of dietary magnesium is absorbed via both passive and active transport mechanisms; maximal absorption of magnesium occurs in the distal jejunum and ileum of the small intestine. The absorption of magnesium decreases with higher dietary intakes. The kidneys are responsible for the regulation of blood magnesium levels. Two forms of vitamin D, 25-hydroxyvitamin D and 1,25-dihydroxyvitamin D, can enhance the intestinal absorption of magnesium to a limited extent. Excessive alcohol intake can cause magnesium depletion, and some diuretic medications can lead to increased excretion of magnesium in the urine. Dietary fiber and phytates decrease intestinal absorption of magnesium.

Total body magnesium content is approximately 25 g. About 50% to 60% of the magnesium in the body is found in bones, with the rest located in soft tissues.

Functions of Magnesium

Magnesium is one of the minerals that make up the structure of bone. It is also important in the regulation of bone and mineral status. Specifically, magnesium influences the formation of hydroxyapatite crystals through its regulation of calcium balance and its interactions with vitamin D and parathyroid hormone.

Magnesium is a critical cofactor for more than 300 enzyme systems. It is necessary for the production of ATP, and it plays an important role in DNA and protein synthesis and repair. Magnesium supplementation has been shown to improve insulin sensitivity, and there is epidemiological evidence that a high magnesium intake is associated with a decrease in the risk for colorectal cancer.[26,27] Magnesium supports normal vitamin D metabolism and action and is necessary for normal muscle contraction and blood clotting.

How Much Magnesium Should We Consume?

As magnesium is found in a wide variety of foods, people who are adequately nourished generally consume adequate magnesium in their diets. The RDA for magnesium changes across age groups and genders. For adult men 19 to 30 years of age, the RDA for magnesium is 400 mg per day; the RDA increases to 420 mg per day for men 31 years of age and older. For adult women 19 to 30 years of age, the RDA for magnesium is 310 mg per day; this value increases to 320 mg per day for women 31 years of age and older. There is no UL for magnesium consumed in food and water; the UL for magnesium from pharmacologic sources is 350 mg per day.

Magnesium is found in green, leafy vegetables, such as spinach; whole grains; seeds; and nuts. Other good food sources include seafood, beans, and some dairy products. Refined and processed foods are low in magnesium. **Figure 11.14** shows many foods that are good sources of magnesium.

The magnesium content of drinking water varies considerably. The "harder" the water, the higher its content of magnesium. This large variability in the magnesium content of water makes it impossible to estimate how much our drinking water contributes to the magnesium content of our diets.

The ability of the small intestine to absorb magnesium is reduced when one consumes a diet that is extremely high in fiber and phytates, because these substances bind with magnesium. Even though seeds and nuts are relatively high in fiber, they are excellent sources of absorbable magnesium. Overall, our absorption of magnesium should be sufficient if we consume the recommended amount of fiber (20 to 35 g per day). In contrast, higher dietary protein intakes enhance the absorption and retention of magnesium.

What Happens If We Consume Too Much Magnesium?

There are no known toxicity symptoms related to consuming excess magnesium in the diet. The toxicity symptoms that result from pharmacologic use of magnesium include diarrhea, nausea, and abdominal cramps. In extreme cases, large doses can result in acid–base imbalances, massive dehydration, cardiac arrest, and death. High blood magnesium, or **hypermagnesemia,** occurs in individuals with impaired kidney function who consume large amounts of nondietary magnesium, such as antacids. Side effects include impairment of nerve, muscle, and heart function.

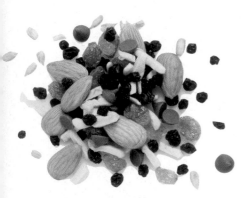

Trail mix with chocolate chips, nuts, and seeds is a common food source of magnesium.

hypermagnesemia A condition marked by an abnormally high concentration of magnesium in the blood.

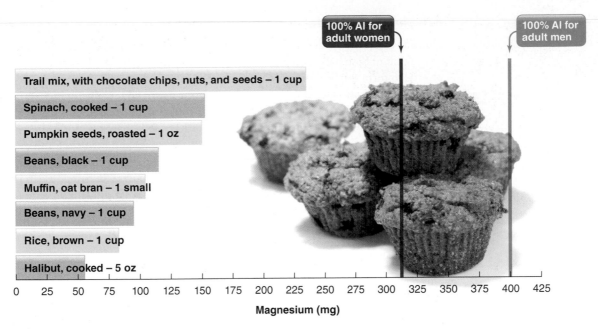

100% AI for adult women

100% AI for adult men

Trail mix, with chocolate chips, nuts, and seeds – 1 cup

Spinach, cooked – 1 cup

Pumpkin seeds, roasted – 1 oz

Beans, black – 1 cup

Muffin, oat bran – 1 small

Beans, navy – 1 cup

Rice, brown – 1 cup

Halibut, cooked – 5 oz

0   25   50   75   100   125   150   175   200   225   250   275   300   325   350   375   400   425

Magnesium (mg)

FIGURE 11.14 Common food sources of magnesium. For adult men 19 to 30 years of age, the RDA for magnesium is 400 mg per day; the RDA increases to 420 mg per day for men 31 years of age and older. For adult women 19 to 30 years of age, the RDA for magnesium is 310 mg per day; this value increases to 320 mg per day for women 31 years of age and older. (*Source:* Data from US Department of Agriculture, Agricultural Research Service, 2011, USDA Nutrient Database for Standard Reference, Release 24. Nutrient Data Laboratory Home Page, www.ars.usda.gov/ba/bhnrc/ndl.)

What Happens If We Don't Consume Enough Magnesium?

Hypomagnesemia, or low blood magnesium, results from magnesium deficiency. This condition may develop secondarily to kidney disease, chronic diarrhea, or chronic alcohol abuse. Elderly people seem to be at particularly high risk for low dietary intakes of magnesium and other micronutrients, because they have a reduced appetite and blunted senses of taste and smell. In addition, the elderly face challenges related to shopping and preparing micronutrient-dense meals, and their ability to absorb magnesium is reduced.

Low blood calcium levels are a side effect of hypomagnesemia. Other symptoms of magnesium deficiency include muscle cramps, spasms or seizures, nausea, weakness, irritability, and confusion. Considering magnesium's role in bone formation, it is not surprising that long-term magnesium deficiency is associated with osteoporosis. Magnesium deficiency is also associated with many other chronic diseases, including heart disease, high blood pressure, and type 2 diabetes.

RECAP

Magnesium is a major mineral found in fresh foods, including spinach, nuts, seeds, whole grains, and meats. Magnesium is important for bone health, energy production, and muscle function. The RDA for magnesium is a function of age and gender. Hypermagnesemia can result in diarrhea, muscle cramps, and cardiac arrest. Hypomagnesemia causes hypocalcemia, muscle cramps, spasms, and weakness. Magnesium deficiencies are also associated with osteoporosis, heart disease, high blood pressure, and type 2 diabetes. ■

Fluoride

Fluoride, a trace mineral, is the ionic form of the element fluorine. About 99% of the fluoride in the body is stored in teeth and bones.

hypomagnesemia A condition characterized by an abnormally low concentration of magnesium in the blood.

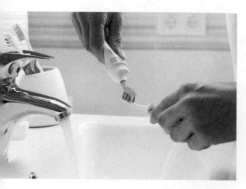

Fluoride is readily available in many communities in the United States through fluoridated water and dental products.

Functions of Fluoride

Fluoride assists in the development and maintenance of teeth and bones. During the development of both baby and permanent teeth, fluoride combines with calcium and phosphorus to form **fluorohydroxyapatite,** which is more resistant to destruction by acids and bacteria than hydroxyapatite. Even after all of our permanent teeth are in, treating them with fluoride, whether at the dentist's office or by using fluoridated toothpaste, gives them more protection against dental caries (cavities) than teeth that have not been treated. That's because fluoride enhances tooth mineralization, decreases and reverses tooth demineralization, and inhibits the metabolism of acid-producing bacteria that cause tooth decay.

Fluoride also stimulates new bone growth, and it is currently being researched as a potential treatment for osteoporosis both alone and in combination with other medications. While early results are promising, more research needs to be conducted to determine if fluoride is an effective treatment for osteoporosis.[28]

How Much Fluoride Should We Consume?

Our need for fluoride is relatively small. There is no RDA for fluoride. The AI for children aged 4 to 8 years is 1 mg per day; this value increases to 2 mg per day for boys and girls aged 9 to 13 years. The AI for boys and girls aged 14 to 18 years is 3 mg per day. The AI for adults is 4 mg per day for men and 3 mg per day for women. The UL for fluoride is 2.2 mg per day for children aged 4 to 8 years; the UL for everyone older than 8 years of age is 10 mg per day.

Fluoride is readily available in many communities in the United States through fluoridated water and dental products. In the mouth, fluoride is absorbed directly into the teeth and gums, and it can be absorbed from the gastrointestinal tract once it has been ingested.

In the early 1990s, there was considerable concern that our intake of fluoride was too high due to the consumption of fluoridated water and fluoride-containing toothpastes and mouthwashes; it was speculated that this high intake of fluoride could have been contributing to an increased risk for cancer, bone fractures, kidney and other organ damage, infertility, and Alzheimer's disease. After reviewing the potential health hazards of fluoride, the US Department of Health and Human Services and the National Cancer Institute found that there is no reliable scientific evidence available to indicate that fluoride increases our risks for these illnesses.[29,30]

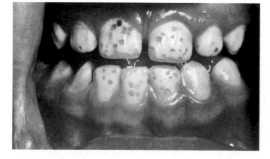

FIGURE 11.15 Consuming too much fluoride causes fluorosis, leading to staining and pitting of the teeth.

There are concerns that individuals who consume bottled water exclusively may be getting too little fluoride and increasing their risk for dental caries, as most bottled waters do not contain fluoride. However, these individuals may still consume fluoride through other beverages that contain fluoridated water and through fluoridated dental products. Toothpastes and mouthwashes that contain fluoride are widely marketed and used by most consumers in the United States, and these products can contribute as much, if not more, fluoride to our diets than fluoridated water. Fluoride supplements are available only by prescription, and these are generally given only to children who do not have access to fluoridated water. Incidentally, tea is a good source of fluoride: one 8-oz cup provides about 20% to 25% of the AI.

What Happens If We Consume Too Much Fluoride?

fluorohydroxyapatite A mineral compound in human teeth that contains fluoride, calcium, and phosphorus and is more resistant to destruction by acids and bacteria than hydroxyapatite.

fluorosis A condition characterized by staining and pitting of the teeth; caused by an abnormally high intake of fluoride.

Consuming too much fluoride increases the protein content of tooth enamel, resulting in a condition called **fluorosis.** Because increased protein makes the enamel more porous, the teeth become stained and pitted (**Figure 11.15**). Teeth seem to be at highest risk for fluorosis during the first 8 years of life, when the permanent teeth are developing. To reduce their risk, children should not swallow oral care products that are meant for topical use only, and children under the age of 6 years should be supervised while using fluoride-containing products. Mild fluorosis generally causes white patches on the teeth, but it has no effect on tooth function. Although moderate and severe fluorosis causes greater discoloration of the teeth, there appears to be no adverse effect on tooth function.[6]

Excess consumption of fluoride can also cause fluorosis of the skeleton. Mild skeletal fluorosis results in an increased bone mass and stiffness and pain in the joints. Moderate and severe skeletal fluorosis can be crippling, but it is extremely rare in the United States.[31]

What Happens If We Don't Consume Enough Fluoride?

The primary result of fluoride deficiency is dental caries. Adequate fluoride intake appears necessary at an early age and throughout adult life to reduce the risk for tooth decay. Inadequate fluoride intake may also be associated with lower bone density, but there is not enough research available to support the widespread use of fluoride to prevent osteoporosis. Studies are currently being done to determine the role fluoride might play in reducing the risk for osteoporosis and fractures.

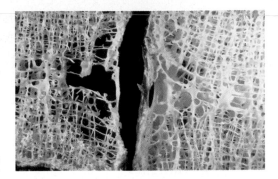

FIGURE 11.16 The vertebrae of a person with osteoporosis (left) are thinner and more collapsed than the vertebrae of a healthy person (right), in which the bone is more dense and uniform.

RECAP

Fluoride is a trace mineral whose primary function is to support the health of teeth and bones. The AI for fluoride is 4 mg and 3 mg per day for adult men and women, respectively. Primary sources of fluoride are fluoridated dental products and fluoridated water. Fluoride toxicity causes fluorosis of the teeth and skeleton, and fluoride deficiency causes an increase in tooth decay. ■

Osteoporosis Is the Most Prevalent Disorder Affecting Bone Health

Of the many disorders associated with poor bone health, the most prevalent in the United States is **osteoporosis,** a disease characterized by low bone mass. The bone tissue of a person with osteoporosis deteriorates over time, becoming thinner and more porous than that of a person with healthy bone. These structural changes weaken the bone, leading to a significantly reduced ability of the bone to bear weight (**Figure 11.16**). This greatly increases the person's risk for a fracture. In the United States, more than 2 million fractures each year are attributed to osteoporosis.[32]

Because the hip and the vertebrae of the spinal column are common sites of osteoporosis, it is not surprising that osteoporosis is the single most important cause of fractures of the hip and spine in older adults. These fractures are extremely painful and can be debilitating, with many individuals requiring nursing home care. In addition, they increase a person's risk for infection and other related illnesses, which can lead to premature death. In fact, about 24% of adults 50 years and older who suffer a hip fracture die within 1 year after the fracture occurs, and because men are typically older at the time of fracture, death rates are higher for men than for women.[32]

Osteoporosis of the spine also causes a generalized loss of height and can be disfiguring and painful: gradual compression fractures in the vertebrae of the upper back lead to a shortening and hunching of the spine called *kyphosis,* commonly referred to as *dowager's hump* (**Figure 11.17**). Moreover, back pain from collapsed or fractured vertebrae can be severe. However, especially in the early stages, osteoporosis can be a silent disease: the person may have no awareness of the condition until a fracture occurs.

Osteoporosis is a common disease: worldwide, one in three women and one in five men over the age of 50 are affected. In the United States, more than 10 million people have been diagnosed, and half of all women and one in four men over the age of 50 will suffer an osteoporosis-related fracture in their lifetime.[32,33]

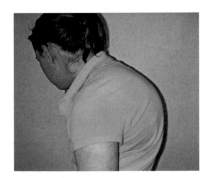

FIGURE 11.17 Gradual compression of the vertebrae in the upper back causes a shortening and rounding of the spine called *kyphosis*.

osteoporosis A disease characterized by low bone mass and deterioration of bone tissue, leading to increased bone fragility and fracture risk.

TABLE 11.4 Risk Factors for Osteoporosis

Modifiable Risk Factors	Nonmodifiable Risk Factors
Smoking	Older age (elderly)
Low body weight	Caucasian or Asian race
Low calcium intake	History of fractures as an adult
Low sun exposure	Family history of osteoporosis
Alcohol abuse	Gender (female)
History of amenorrhea (failure to menstruate) in women with inadequate nutrition	History of amenorrhea (failure to menstruate) in women, with no recognizable cause
Estrogen deficiency (females)	
Testosterone deficiency (males)	
Repeated falls	
Sedentary lifestyle	

Source: Table adapted from "Osteoporosis: Evaluation and Treatment" from *Comprehensive Therapy*, November 3, 2000, Volume 26 (3), Copyright © 2000 by Springer and Humana Press. Republished with kind permission from Springer Science & Business Media B.V.

What Influences Osteoporosis Risk?

The factors that influence the risk for osteoporosis are age, gender, genetics, substance use, nutrition, and physical activity (**Table 11.4**). Let's review these factors and identify lifestyle changes that reduce the risk for osteoporosis.

Aging Increases Osteoporosis Risk

Because bone density declines with age, low bone mass and osteoporosis are significant health concerns for older adults. The prevalence of osteoporosis and low bone mass is predicted to increase in the United States during the next 20 years, primarily because of increased longevity; as the U.S. population ages, more people will live long enough to suffer from osteoporosis.

Hormonal changes that occur with aging have a significant impact on bone loss. Average bone loss approximates 0.3% to 0.5% per year after 30 years of age; however, during menopause in women, levels of the hormone estrogen decrease dramatically and cause bone loss to increase to about 3% per year during the first 5 years of menopause. Both estrogen and testosterone play important roles in promoting the deposition of new bone and limiting the activity of osteoclasts. Thus, men can also suffer from osteoporosis, caused by age-related decreases in testosterone. In addition, reduced levels of physical activity in older people and a decreased ability to metabolize vitamin D with age exacerbate the hormone-related bone loss.

Gender and Genetics Affect Osteoporosis Risk

Approximately 80% of Americans with osteoporosis are women. There are three primary reasons for this:

- Women have a lower absolute bone density than men. From birth through puberty, bone mass is the same in girls as in boys. But during puberty, bone mass increases more in boys, probably because of their prolonged period of accelerated growth. This means that, when bone loss begins around age 40, women have less bone stored in their skeleton; thus, the loss of bone that occurs with aging causes osteoporosis sooner and to a greater extent in women.

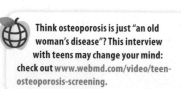

Think osteoporosis is just "an old woman's disease"? This interview with teens may change your mind: check out www.webmd.com/video/teen-osteoporosis-screening.

- The hormonal changes that occur in men as they age do not have as dramatic an effect on bone density as those in women.
- On average, women live longer than men, and because risk increases with age, more elderly women suffer from this disease.

A secondary factor that is gender-specific is the social pressure on girls to be thin. Extreme dieting is particularly harmful in adolescence, when bone mass is building and adequate consumption of calcium and other nutrients is critical. In many girls, weight loss causes both a loss of estrogen and reduced weight-bearing stress on the bones. In contrast, men experience pressure to "bulk up," typically by lifting weights. This puts healthful stress on the bones, resulting in increased density.

Some individuals have a family history of osteoporosis, which increases their risk for this disease. Particularly at risk are Caucasian women of low body weight who have a first-degree relative (mother or sister) with osteoporosis. Asian women are at higher risk than other non-Caucasian groups. Although we cannot change our gender or genetics, we can modify the lifestyle factors that affect our risk for osteoporosis.

Tobacco, Alcohol, and Caffeine Influence Osteoporosis Risk

Cigarette smoking is known to decrease bone density because of its effects on hormones that influence bone formation and resorption. For this reason, cigarette smoking increases the risk for osteoporosis and resulting fractures.

Chronic alcohol abuse is detrimental to bone health and is associated with high rates of fractures. In contrast, a meta-analysis of numerous research studies has shown that bone density is higher in people who are *moderate* drinkers.[34] Despite the fact that moderate alcohol intake may be protective for bone, the dangers of alcohol abuse for overall health warrant caution in considering any dietary recommendations. As is consistent with the alcohol intake recommendations related to heart disease, people should not start drinking if they are nondrinkers, and people who do drink should do so in moderation. That means no more than two drinks per day for men and one drink per day for women.

Some researchers consider excess caffeine consumption to be detrimental to bone health. Caffeine is known to increase calcium loss in the urine, at least over a brief period of time. Younger people are able to compensate for this calcium loss by increasing absorption of calcium from the intestine. However, older people are not always capable of compensating to the same degree. Although the findings have been inconsistent, recent research now indicates that the relative amounts of caffeine and calcium consumed are critical factors affecting bone health. In general, elderly women do not appear to be at risk for increased bone loss if they consume adequate amounts of calcium and moderate amounts of caffeine (equal to less than two cups of coffee, four cups of tea, or six 12-oz cans of caffeine-containing soft drinks per day).[35] Elderly women who consume high levels of caffeine (more than three cups of coffee per day) have much higher rates of bone loss than women with low intakes.[36] Thus, it appears important to bone health that we moderate our caffeine intake and consume an adequate amount of calcium.

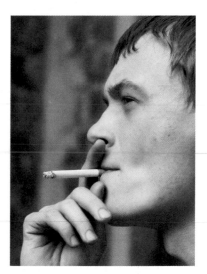

Smoking increases the risk for osteoporosis and resulting fractures.

Nutritional Factors Influence Osteoporosis Risk

In addition to their role in reducing the risk for heart disease and cancer, diets high in fruits and vegetables are also associated with improved bone health.[37,38] This is most likely due to the fact that fruits and vegetables are good sources of the nutrients that play a role in bone and collagen health, including magnesium, vitamin C, and vitamin K. The effects of protein, calcium, vitamin D, and sodium on bone health have been the subject of extensive research.

Protein   The effect of high dietary protein intake on bone health is controversial. High protein intakes have been shown to have both a negative and a positive impact on bone health. Although it is well established that high protein intakes increase calcium loss, protein is a critical component of bone tissue and is necessary for bone health. As for caffeine, the key to this mystery appears to be adequate calcium intake. In one study, older adults taking calcium and vitamin D supplements and eating higher-protein diets were able to significantly increase bone mass over a 3-year period, whereas those eating more protein and not taking supplements lost bone mass over the same time period.[39] Low protein intakes are also associated with bone loss and increased risk for osteoporosis and fractures in elderly people. Thus, there appears to be an interaction between dietary calcium and protein, in that adequate amounts of each nutrient are needed together to support bone health.

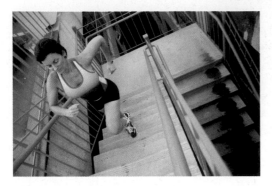

Regular weight-bearing exercises, such as jogging, can help increase and maintain bone mass.

Calcium and Vitamin D   Of the many nutrients that help maintain bone health, calcium and vitamin D have received the most attention for their role in the prevention of osteoporosis. Research studies conducted with older adults have shown that taking calcium and vitamin D supplements reduces bone loss and fracture risk. If people do not consume enough of these two nutrients over a prolonged period of time, their bone density is lower and they have a higher risk for bone fractures.

Because bones reach peak density when people are young, it is very important that children and adolescents consume a high-quality diet that contains the proper balance of calcium, vitamin D, protein, and other nutrients to allow for optimal bone growth. Young adults also require a proper balance of these nutrients to maintain bone mass. In older adults, diets rich in calcium and vitamin D can help minimize bone loss.

Sodium   Higher intakes of sodium are known to increase the kidneys' excretion of calcium in the urine. One study found that diets moderately high in salt increased excretion of urinary calcium and had a negative impact on bone calcium balance in postmenopausal women, particularly when calcium intakes were low.[40] However, there is no direct evidence that a high-sodium diet causes osteoporosis. At this time, the Institute of Medicine states that there is insufficient evidence to warrant different calcium recommendations based on dietary salt intake.[6]

Regular Physical Activity Reduces Osteoporosis Risk

Regular exercise is highly protective against bone loss and osteoporosis. Athletes are consistently shown to have more dense bones than non-athletes, and regular participation in weight-bearing exercises (such as walking, jogging, tennis, and strength training) can help increase and maintain bone mass. When we exercise, our muscles contract and pull on our bones; this stresses bone tissue in a healthful way that stimulates increases in bone density. In addition, carrying weight during activities such as walking and jogging stresses the bones of the legs, hips, and lower back, resulting in a healthier bone mass in these areas. It appears that people of all ages can improve and maintain bone health by consistent physical activity.

Can exercise ever be detrimental to bone health? Yes, exercise can be harmful when the body is not receiving the nutrients it needs to rebuild the hydroxyapatite and collagen broken

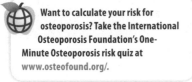

Want to calculate your risk for osteoporosis? Take the International Osteoporosis Foundation's One-Minute Osteoporosis risk quiz at www.osteofound.org/.

*Nutri-*Case

Gustavo

"When my wife, Antonia, fell and broke her hip, I was shocked. You see, the same thing happened to her mother, but she was an old lady by then! Antonia's only 68, and she still seems young and beautiful—at least to me! As soon as she's better, her doctor wants to do some kind of scan to see how thick her bones are. But I don't think she has that disease everyone talks about. She's always watched her weight and keeps active with our kids and grandchildren. It's true she likes her coffee and diet colas, and doesn't drink milk, but that's not enough to make a person's bones fall apart, is it?"

Review Table 11.4, page 458. Which risk factors apply to Antonia? Which risk factors do not? Given what Gustavo has said about his wife's nutrition and lifestyle, should he encourage her to have a DXA test? Why or why not?

down in response to physical activity. Thus, active people who are chronically malnourished, including people who are impoverished and those who suffer from eating disorders, are at increased fracture risk. Research has confirmed this association among nutrition, physical activity, and bone loss in the **female athlete triad,** a potentially serious condition characterized by the coexistence of three (a *triad* of) clinical conditions in some physically active females: low energy availability (with or without eating disorders), menstrual dysfunction, and low bone density. In the female athlete triad, inadequate food intake and regular strenuous exercise together result in a state of severe energy drain that causes a multitude of hormonal changes, including a reduction in estrogen production. Estrogen is important to maintaining healthy bone in women, so the loss of estrogen leads to low bone density and even osteoporosis in young women. (The female athlete triad is discussed *In Depth*, Chapter 13.5, on page 557.)

How Is Osteoporosis Treated?

Although there is no cure for osteoporosis, a variety of treatments can slow and even reverse bone loss. First, individuals with osteoporosis are encouraged to consume adequate calcium and vitamin D and to exercise regularly. Studies have shown that the most effective exercise programs include weight-bearing exercises, such as jogging, stair climbing, and resistance training.[41]

In addition, several medications are available:

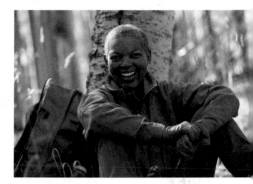

A healthy diet and regular physical activity can reduce your risk for osteoporosis.

- Bisphosphonates, such as alendronate (brand name Fosamax), which decrease bone loss and can increase bone density and reduce the risk of spinal and nonspinal fractures
- Selective estrogen receptor modulators, such as raloxifene (brand name Evista), which have an estrogen-like effect on bone tissue, slowing the rate of bone loss and prompting some increase in bone mass
- Calcitonin (brand name Calcimar or Miacalcin), a pharmacologic preparation of the same thyroid hormone mentioned earlier, which can reduce the rate of bone loss
- Hormone replacement therapy (HRT), which combines estrogen with a hormone called progestin and can reduce bone loss, increase bone density, and reduce the risk of hip and spinal fractures

All of these drugs can prompt side effects. For example, bisphosphonates are associated with several gastrointestinal side effects, including abdominal pain, constipation, diarrhea, heartburn, irritation of the esophagus, and difficulty swallowing. Although there has been some evidence that long-term use of bisphosphonates may increase the risk for "atypical" fractures, two recent studies have found that these fractures are still quite rare and that the relative benefits of taking the medication outweigh the potential risks.[42,43] Side effects of HRT include breast tenderness, changes in mood, vaginal bleeding, and an increased risk for gallbladder disease.

Until recently, it was believed that HRT protected women against heart disease. However, a landmark study published in 2002 found that one type of HRT actually increases a woman's risk for heart disease, stroke, and breast cancer.[44] As a result, hundreds of thousands of women in the United States have stopped taking HRT as a means to prevent or treat osteoporosis. However, despite the associated risks, it is recognized that HRT is still an effective treatment and prevention option for osteoporosis. It also reduces the risk for colorectal cancer. Thus, women should work with their physicians to weigh these benefits against the increased risks for breast cancer and heart disease when considering HRT as a treatment option for osteoporosis.

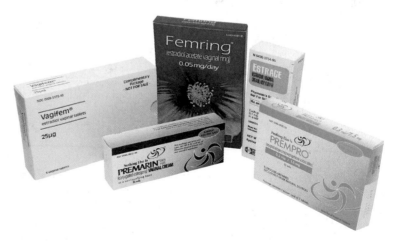

Hormone replacement medications come in a variety of forms.

female athlete triad A potentially serious condition characterized by the coexistence of three disorders: low energy availability, menstrual dysfunction, and low bone density.

RECAP

Osteoporosis is a major disease of concern for elderly men and women in the United States. Osteoporosis increases the risk for fractures and premature death from subsequent illness. Factors that increase the risk for osteoporosis include genetics, being female, being of the Caucasian or Asian race, low levels of estrogen, cigarette smoking, alcohol abuse, sedentary lifestyles, and diets low in calcium and vitamin D. Medications are available for the prevention and treatment of osteoporosis. ■

Chapter Review

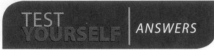

TEST YOURSELF | ANSWERS

1. **F** The majority of our bone mass and bone density is built by our late teens and early twenties. Thus, it's critical that we consume a healthy diet and participate in regular physical activity—behaviors that support bone development—during childhood and adolescence.

2. **F** Osteoporosis is more common among elderly women, but elderly men are also at increased risk for osteoporosis. Young women who suffer from an eating disorder and menstrual cycle irregularity, referred to as the female athlete triad, may also have osteoporosis.

3. **T** When exposed to sunlight, our bodies can convert a cholesterol compound in our skin to vitamin D.

4. **F** There are many good sources of calcium besides milk, yogurt, and cheese, including calcium-fortified juices and soy/rice beverages and green, leafy vegetables, such as kale, broccoli, and collard greens.

5. **T** Recent studies indicate that overweight and obese people are more likely to have poor vitamin D status than people of normal weight. Poor vitamin D status increases the risk for osteoporosis.

Summary

- Bone develops through three processes: growth, modeling, and remodeling. Bone size is determined during growth, bone shape is determined during modeling and remodeling, and bone remodeling also affects the density of bone.

- Dual energy x-ray absorptiometry (DEXA or DXA) is the most accurate tool for measuring bone density.

- Calcium is a major mineral that is an integral component of bones and teeth. Calcium levels are maintained in the blood at all times; calcium is also necessary for normal nerve impulse transmission, muscle contraction, healthy blood pressure, and blood clotting.

- The RDA for calcium is 1,000 mg per day for adult men and women aged 19 to 70 years, and 1,200 mg per day for adult men and women older than 70 years of age.

- Consuming excess calcium leads to mineral imbalance, and consuming inadequate calcium causes osteoporosis.

- Vitamin D is a fat-soluble vitamin that can be produced from a cholesterol compound in skin using energy from sunlight. Vitamin D regulates blood calcium levels, regulates absorption of calcium and phosphorus from the intestines, and helps maintain bone health.

- The RDA for vitamin D is 600 IU per day for adult men and women aged 19 to 70 years; the RDA increases to 800 IU per day for adults over the age of 70 years.

- Hypercalcemia results from consuming too much vitamin D, causing weakness, loss of appetite, diarrhea, vomiting, and formation of calcium deposits in soft tissues. Vitamin D deficiency leads to loss of bone mass, causing rickets in children or osteomalacia and osteoporosis in adults.

- Vitamin K is a fat-soluble vitamin that is obtained in the diet and is produced in the large intestine by normal bacteria. Vitamin K serves as a coenzyme for blood clotting and bone metabolism.

- Phosphorus is a major mineral that is an important part of the structure of bone; phosphorus is also a component of ATP, DNA, RNA, cell membranes, and lipoproteins.

- Magnesium is a major mineral. It is part of the structure of bone, it influences the formation of hydroxyapatite crystals and bone health through its regulation of calcium balance and the actions of vitamin D and parathyroid hormone, and it is a cofactor for more than 300 enzyme systems.

- Fluoride is a trace mineral that strengthens teeth and bones and reduces the risk for dental caries.

- Osteoporosis is a major bone disease in the United States, affecting more than 10 million Americans. About 80% of people with this disease are women, however men over the age of 50 are also at risk.

- Osteoporosis leads to increased risk for bone fractures and premature disability and death due to subsequent illness.

- Factors that increase the risk for osteoporosis include increased age, being female, being of the Caucasian or Asian race, cigarette smoking, alcohol abuse, low calcium and vitamin D intakes, and a sedentary lifestyle.

MasteringNutrition™

To further your understanding, go online and apply what you've learned to real-life case studies that will help you master the content!

Review Questions

1. Hydroxyapatite crystals are predominantly made up of
   a. calcium and phosphorus.
   b. hydrogen, oxygen, and titanium.
   c. calcium and vitamin D.
   d. calcium and magnesium.

2. On a DXA test, a T-score of +1.0 indicates that the patient
   a. has osteoporosis.
   b. is at greater risk for fractures than an average, healthy person of the same age.
   c. has normal bone density as compared to an average, healthy 30-year-old.
   d. has slightly lower bone density than an average, healthy person of the same age.

3. Which of the following statements about trabecular bone is true?
   a. It accounts for about 80% of the skeleton.
   b. It forms the core of all bones of the skeleton.
   c. It is also called compact bone.
   d. It provides the scaffolding for cortical bone.

4. Which of the following individuals is most likely to require vitamin D supplements?
   a. a dark-skinned child living in Hawaii
   b. a fair-skinned construction worker living in Florida
   c. a dark-skinned retiree living in Illinois
   d. a fair-skinned college student living in Oklahoma

5. Calcium is necessary for several body functions, including
   a. demineralization of bone, nerve transmission, and immune responses.
   b. cartilage structure, nerve transmission, and muscle contraction.
   c. structure of bone, nerve, and muscle tissue; immune responses; and muscle contraction.
   d. structure of bone, nerve transmission, and muscle contraction.

6. **True or false?** The process by which bone is formed through the action of osteoblasts and resorbed through the action of osteoclasts is called remodeling.

7. **True or false?** Moderate consumption of alcohol has been associated with increased bone density.

8. **True or false?** Although osteoporosis can lead to painful and debilitating fractures, it is not associated with an increased risk for premature death.

9. **True or false?** The amount of calcium we absorb depends on our age, our calcium intake, the types of calcium-rich foods we eat, and the body's supply of vitamin D.

10. **True or false?** The body synthesizes vitamin D from exposure to sunlight.

11. Explain why people with diseases that cause a malabsorption of fat may suffer from deficiency of vitamins D and K.

12. Most people reach their peak height by the end of adolescence, maintain that height for several decades, and then start to lose height in their later years. Describe the two processes behind this phenomenon.

13. The morning after reading this chapter, you are eating your usual breakfast cereal when you notice that the Nutrition Facts Panel on the box states that one serving contains 100% of your DRI for calcium. In addition, you're eating the cereal with about ½ cup of skim milk. Does this meal ensure that your calcium needs for the day are met? Why or why not?

14. Bert has light skin and lives in Buffalo, New York. How much time does Bert need to spend out of doors with exposed skin on winter days to avoid the need for consuming vitamin D in the diet or from supplements?

Math Review

15. Refer to the table in the **Nutrition Label Activity** (page 444) on calcium absorption rates for various food sources. How much broccoli would you need to consume to absorb the same amount of calcium as in 1 cup of skim milk?

Answers to Review Questions and Math Review can be found online in the MasteringNutrition Study Area.

Web Links

www.nlm.nih.gov/medlineplus
Medline Plus Health Information
Search for "rickets" or "osteomalacia" to learn more about these vitamin D–deficiency diseases.

www.ada.org
American Dental Association
Look under "Advocacy" and "Federal and State Issues" to learn more about the fluoridation of community water supplies and the use of fluoride-containing products.

www.nof.org
National Osteoporosis Foundation
Learn more about the causes, prevention, detection, and treatment of osteoporosis.

www.osteofound.org
International Osteoporosis Foundation
Find out more about this foundation and its mission to increase awareness and understanding of osteoporosis worldwide.

www.niams.nih.gov/Health_Info/Bone
National Institutes of Health
Osteoporosis and Related Bone Diseases—National Resource Center
Access this site for additional resources and information on metabolic bone diseases, including osteoporosis.

References

1. Zmuda, N. 2011. Bottoms up! A look at America's drinking habits. *AdvertisingAge*. http://adage.com/article/news/consumers-drink-soft-drinks-water-beer/228422/.

2. Ball, J. W., R. C. Bindler, and K. J. Cowen. 2011. *Pediatric Nursing: Caring for Children*. 5th edn. Upper Saddle River, NJ: Pearson.

3. Ho, A. Y. Y., and A. W. C. Kung. 2005. Determinants of peak bone mineral density and bone area in young women. *J. Bone Miner. Metab*. 23:470–475.

4. Chevalley, T., R. Rizzoli, D. Hans, S. Ferrari, and J. P. Bonjour. 2005. Interaction between calcium intake and menarcheal age on bone mass gain: an eight-year follow-up study from prepuberty to postmenarche. *J. Clin. Endocrinol. Metab*. 90:44–51.

5. Kindblom, J. M., M. Lorentzon, E. Norjavaara, A. Hellqvist, S. Nilsson, D. Mellström, and C. Ohlsson. 2006. Pubertal timing predicts previous fractures and BMD in young adult men: the GOOD Study. *J. Bone Min. Res*. 21:790–795.

6. Institute of Medicine, Food and Nutrition Board. 1997. *Dietary Reference Intakes for Calcium, Phosphorus, Magnesium, Vitamin D, and Fluoride*. Washington, DC: National Academy Press.

7. US Department of Agriculture, Economic Research Service. 2008. Dietary assessment of major trends in U.S. food consumption, 1970–2005. Economic Information Bulletin No. EIB-33, 1–27. www.ers.usda.gov/publications/eib33/.

8. US Department of Health and Human Services, National Kidney and Urologic Diseases Information Clearinghouse. 2010. Diet for kidney stone formation. NIH Publication No. 09-6425. http://kidney.niddk.nih.gov/kudiseases/pubs/kidneystonediet/index.aspx#how.

9. Institute of Medicine, Food and Nutrition Board. 2010. *Dietary Reference Intakes for Calcium and Vitamin D*. Washington, DC: National Academy Press.

10. Florez, H., R. Martinez, W. Chacra, N. Strickman-Stein, and S. Levis. 2007. Outdoor exercise reduces the risk of hypovitaminosis D in the obese. *J. Steroid Biochem. Mol. Biol*. 103:679–681.

11. Holick, M. F. 2005. The vitamin D epidemic and its health consequences. *J. Nutr*. 135:2739S–2748S.

12. Holick, M. F. 2007. Vitamin D deficiency. *N. Engl. J. Med*. 357:266–281.

13. Office of Dietary Supplements, National Institutes of Health. 2011. Dietary Supplement Fact Sheet: Vitamin D. http://ods.od.nih.gov/factsheets/VitaminD-HealthProfessional/.

14. Holick, M. F. 2006. Resurrection of vitamin D deficiency and rickets. *J. Clin. Invest*. 116:2062–2072.

15. Weisberg, P., K. S. Scanlon, R. Li, and M. E. Cogswell. 2004. Nutritional rickets among children in the United States: review of cases reported between 1986 and 2003. *Am. J. Clin. Nutr*. 80(suppl.):1697S–1705S.

16. Food and Agriculture Organization of the United Nations and World Health Organization. 2002. Vitamin K. In: *Human Vitamin and Mineral Requirements*. Report of a joint FAO/WHO expert consultation. www.micronutrient.org/idpas/pdf/846.10-CHAPTER10.pdf.

17. Institute of Medicine, Food and Nutrition Board. 2002. *Dietary Reference Intakes for Vitamin A, Vitamin K, Arsenic, Boron, Chromium, Copper, Iodine, Iron, Manganese, Molybdenum, Nickel, Silicon, Vanadium, and Zinc*. Washington, DC: National Academy Press.

18. Fang, Y., C. Hu, X. Tao, Y. Wan, and F. Tao. 2012. Effect of vitamin K on bone mineral density: a meta-analysis of randomized controlled trials. *J. Bone Miner. Metab*. 30(1):60–68.

19. Fodor, D., A. Albu, L. Poantä, and M. Porojan. 2010. Vitamin K and vascular calcifications. *Acta Physiol. Hung*. 97(3):256–266.

20. Briefel, R. R., and C. L. Johnson. 2004. Secular trends in dietary intake the United States. *Ann. Rev. Nutr*. 24:401–431.

21. Wyshak, G., R. E. Frisch, T. E. Albright, N. L. Albright, I. Schiff, and J. Witschi. 1989. Nonalcoholic carbonated beverage consumption and bone fractures among women former college athletes. *J. Orthop. Res*. 7:91–99.

22. Wyshak, G., and R. E. Frisch. 1994. Carbonated beverages, dietary calcium, the dietary calcium/phosphorus ratio, and bone fractures in girls and boys. *J. Adolesc. Health*. 15:210–215.

23. Wyshak, G. 2000. Teenaged girls, carbonated beverage consumption, and bone fractures. *Arch. Pediatr. Adolesc. Med*. 154:610–613.

24. Tucker, K. L., K. Morita, N. Qiao, M. T. Hannan, L. A. Cupples, and D. P. Kiel. 2006. Colas, but not other carbonated beverages, are associated with low bone mineral density in older women: The Framingham Osteoporosis Study. *Am. J. Clin. Nutr*. 84(4):936–942.

25. Fitzpatrick, L., and R. P. Heaney. 2003. Got soda? *J. Bone Miner. Res*. 18:1570–1572.

26. Rodríguez-Morán, M., and F. Guerrero-Romero. 2003. Oral magnesium supplementation improves insulin sensitivity and metabolic control in type 2 diabetic subjects. *Diab. Care*. 26(4):1147–1152.

27. Larsson, S. C., L. Bergkvist, and A. Wolk. 2005. Magnesium intake in relation to risk of colorectal cancer in women. *JAMA* 293:86–89.

28. American Dietetic Association. 2005. Position of the American Dietetic Association: the impact of fluoride on health. *J. Am. Diet. Assoc*. 105:1620–1628.

29. US Department of Health and Human Services. Public Health Service. 1991. Review of fluoride: benefits and risks. Report of the Ad Hoc Subcommittee on Fluoride of the Committee to Coordinate Environmental Health and Related Programs. www.health.gov/environment/ReviewofFluoride/default.htm.

30. National Cancer Institute, National Institutes of Health. 2012. National Cancer Institute FactSheet. Fluoridated Water. www.cancer.gov/cancertopics/factsheet/Risk/fluoridated-water.

31. Centers for Disease Control and Prevention. 2011. Community Water Fluoridation: Questions and Answers. www.cdc.gov/fluoridation/fact_sheets/cwf_qa.htm.

32. National Osteoporosis Foundation. 2011. Fast Facts on Osteoporosis. www.nof.org/node/40/.

33. International Osteoporosis Foundation. 2012. Osteoporosis & Musculoskeletal Disorders. Osteoporosis in Men. www.iofbonehealth.org/osteoporosis-men-0.

34. Berg, K. M., H. V. Kunins, J. L. Jackson, S. Nahvi, A. Chaudhry, K. A. Harris Jr., R. Malik, and J. H. Arnsten. 2008. Association between alcohol consumption and both osteoporotic fracture and bone density. *Am. J. Med*. 121(5):406–418.

35. Massey, L. K. 2001. Is caffeine a risk factor for bone loss in the elderly? *Am. J. Clin. Nutr*. 74:569–570.

36. Rapuri, P. B., J. C. Gallagher, H. K. Kinyamu, and K. L. Ryschon. 2001. Caffeine intake increases the rate of bone loss in elderly women and interacts with vitamin D receptor genotypes. *Am. J. Clin. Nutr.* 74:694–700.

37. New, S. A. 2004. Intake of fruit and vegetables: implications for bone health. *Proc. Nutr. Soc.* 62(4):889–899.

38. Prynne, C. J., G. D. Mishra, M. A. O'Connell, G. Muniz, M. A. Laskey, L. Yan, A. Prentice, and F. Ginty. 2006. Fruit and vegetable intakes and bone mineral status: a cross-sectional study in 5 age and sex cohorts. *Am. J. Clin. Nutr.* 83(6):1420–1428.

39. Dawson-Hughes, B., and S. S. Harris. 2002. Calcium intake influences the association of protein intake with rates of bone loss in elderly men and women. *Am. J. Clin. Nutr.* 75:773–779.

40. Teucher, B., J. R. Dainty, C. A. Spinks, G. Majsak-Newman, D. J. Berry, J. A. Hoogewerff, R. J. Foxall, J. Jakobsen, K. D. Cashman, A. Flynn, and S. J. Fairweather-Tait. 2008. Sodium and bone health: impact of moderately high and low salt intakes on calcium metabolism in postmenopausal women. *J. Bone Min. Res.* 23(9):1477–1485.

41. National Institute of Arthritis and Musculoskeletal and Skin Diseases. NIH Osteoporosis and Related Bone Diseases National Resource Center. 2012. Exercise for Your Bone Health. www.niams.nih.gov/Health_Info/bone/Bone_Health/Exercise /default.asp.

42. Black, D. M., M. P. Kelly, H. K. Genant, L. Palermo, R. Eastell, C. Bucci-Recthweg, J. Cauley, P. C. Leung, S. Boonen, A. Santora, A. de Papp, and D. C. Bauer for the Fracture Intervention Trial and HORIZON Pivotal Fracture Trial Steering Committees. 2010. Bisphosphonates and fractures of the subtrochanteric or diaphyseal femur. *N. Engl. J. Med.* 362:1761–1777.

43. Schilcher, J., K. Michaëlsson, and P. Aspenberg. 2011. Bisphosphonate use and atypical fractures of the femoral shaft. *N. Engl. J. Med.* 364:1728–1737.

44. Writing Group for the Women's Health Initiative Investigators. 2002. Risks and benefits of estrogen plus progestin in healthy postmenopausal women. Principal results from the Women's Health Initiative randomized control trial. *JAMA* 288:321–332.

Nutrition DEBATE

Vitamin D Deficiency: Why the Surge, and What Can Be Done?

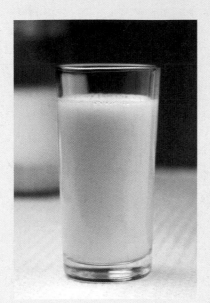

No doubt about it: unless you live at a latitude within 40° of the equator and spend time outdoors without sunscreen, it's tough to get enough vitamin D. That's because, as you learned in this chapter, there are very few natural food sources of vitamin D, and even fortified food sources are limited to milk and a handful of other products. But if meeting the Institute of Medicine's current RDA for vitamin D is already posing a challenge to many Americans, why are some researchers recommending even higher intakes?

Measurements of vitamin D status in a variety of population studies in recent years have led to a growing concern about widespread vitamin D deficiency and its associated diseases, including rickets in children and osteomalacia and osteoporosis in adults. Recent data from the National Health and Examination Survey (NHANES) indicate that, from 1994 to 2004, the prevalence of vitamin D deficiency in U.S. adults almost doubled, with over 90% of people with darker-pigmented skin (African Americans and Latinos) estimated to be vitamin D deficient.[1] In addition, since the Institute of Medicine set its vitamin D recommendations in 1997, new information has been published about vitamin D metabolism and its potential role in reducing the risks for diseases such as type 1 diabetes, some cancers, multiple sclerosis, and metabolic syndrome.[2,3] These discussions have resulted in some nutrition and bone health experts calling for a full review of the recent research on vitamin D and a reevaluation of the current recommendations.[4]

What is contributing to this dramatic increase in vitamin D insufficiency among Americans, and what can we do about it? Researchers have proposed the following three causative factors:[3,5]

- A downward trend in the consumption of vitamin D–fortified milk products
- A significant increase in sun avoidance and the use of sun protection products, such as sunscreen
- An increased rate of obesity, as obesity appears to alter the metabolism and storage of vitamin D such that vitamin D deficiency is more likely to occur

To address the first factor, people can increase their intake of vitamin D–fortified milk products; however, it is difficult to meet even the current RDA from consumption of milk alone. For instance, children and teens would have to drink a full quart each day to meet the recommendation![6] As a result, the use of vitamin D supplements is gaining wide support. Many healthcare providers now recommend that most children and adolescents who do not or cannot get adequate sun exposure take a supplement that provides up to 400 IU of vitamin D per day. Whether adults should consume a vitamin D supplement is currently under review by the Food and Nutrition Board, and its decision is expected to be published in the near future. Supplementation with vitamin D is efficient, inexpensive, and effective. Used correctly, it is also very safe. Although vitamin D toxicity is rare, supplementation should be monitored to ensure both a safe and an adequate intake.

What about the second factor—lack of sufficient exposure to sunlight? Responsible, safe exposure to sunlight offers many advantages: it will never lead to vitamin D toxicity, it is easy and virtually cost-free, and it may offer benefits beyond that of improved vitamin D status.[7] That's why many healthcare professionals advocate moderate sun exposure. They suggest that public health authorities soften the "sun avoidance" campaigns of recent years (**Figure 11.18**, page 468); they would like to see "well-balanced" recommendations that promote brief (15 minutes or so) periods of sun exposure—without sunscreen or sun-blocking clothing—two or three times a week, with avoidance of mid-day sun during summer months.[8]

To address the third factor in vitamin D deficiency—obesity—the only solution is to maintain a healthful weight. That means losing weight if you are overweight or obese. By doing so, you'll reduce your risk not only for vitamin D deficiency but also for cardiovascular disease, type 2 diabetes, and many forms of cancer.

Thus, although vitamin D deficiency is becoming a public health issue in the United States, there appear to be a number of strategies you can use to maintain a healthy vitamin D status.

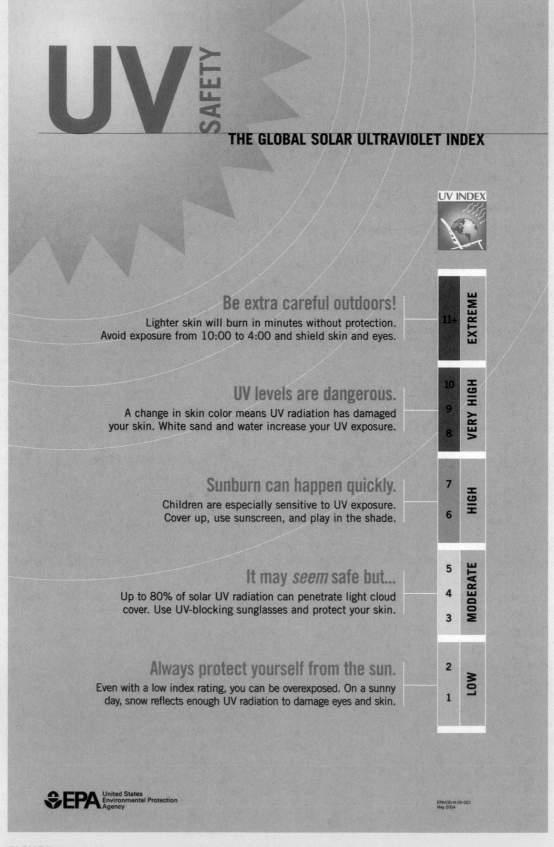

FIGURE 11.18 The Environmental Protection Agency is one of many public health agencies that warn Americans about the danger of exposure to even low levels of sun. (*Source:* UV Safety: The Global Solar Ultraviolet Index from the Environmental Protection Agency, May 2004.)

CRITICAL THINKING QUESTIONS

- Now that you've read this debate about what is presently known about vitamin D and its role in our health, do you think that the current recommendations are too low and should be increased?

- Do you think you would benefit from vitamin D supplementation? Why or why not?

- If you think you do need to improve your vitamin D status, what method(s) would you choose?

- Would you prefer to try to increase your circulating levels of vitamin D through natural foods, fortified foods, supplements, or increased sun exposure? State your reasoning.

REFERENCES

1. Ginde, A. A., M. C. Liu, and C. A. Camargo. 2009. Demographic differences and trends of vitamin D insufficiency in the U.S. population, 1988–2004. *Arch. Intern. Med.* 169:626–632.

2. Weaver, C. M., and J. C. Fleet. 2004. Vitamin D requirements: Current and future. *Am. J. Clin. Nutr.* 80(suppl.):1735S–1739S.

3. Adams, J. S., and M. Hewison. 2010. Update on vitamin D. *J. Clin. Endocrinol. Metab.* 95:471–478.

4. Yetley, E. A., B. Brulé, M. C. Cheney, C. D. Davis, K. A. Esslinger, P. W. F. Fischer, K. E. Friedl, L. S. Greene-Finestone, P. M. Guenther, D. M. Klurfeld, M. R. L'Abbe, and K. Y. McMurray. 2009. Dietary Reference Intakes for vitamin D: justification for a review of the 1997 values. *Am. J. Clin. Nutr.* 89:719–727.

5. Looker, A. C., C. M. Pfeiffer, D. A. Lacher, R. L. Schleicher, M. F. Picciano, and E. A. Yetley. 2008. Serum 25-hydroxyvitamin D status of the U.S. population: 1988–1994 compared with 2000–2004. *Am. J. Clin. Nutr.* 88:1519–1527.

6. Wolpowitz, D., and B. A. Gilchrest. 2006. The vitamin D questions: how much do we need and how should we get it? *J. Am. Acad. Dermatol.* 54(2):301–317.

7. Lucas, R. M., and A. L. Ponsonby. 2006. Considering the potential benefits as well as adverse effects of sun exposure: Can all the potential benefits be provided by oral vitamin D supplementation? *Prog. Biophys. Molec. Biol.* 92:140–149.

8. Reichrath, J. 2006. The challenge resulting from positive and negative effects of sunlight: how much solar UV exposure is appropriate to balance between risks of vitamin D deficiency and skin cancer? *Prog. Biophys. Molec. Biol.* 92:9–16.

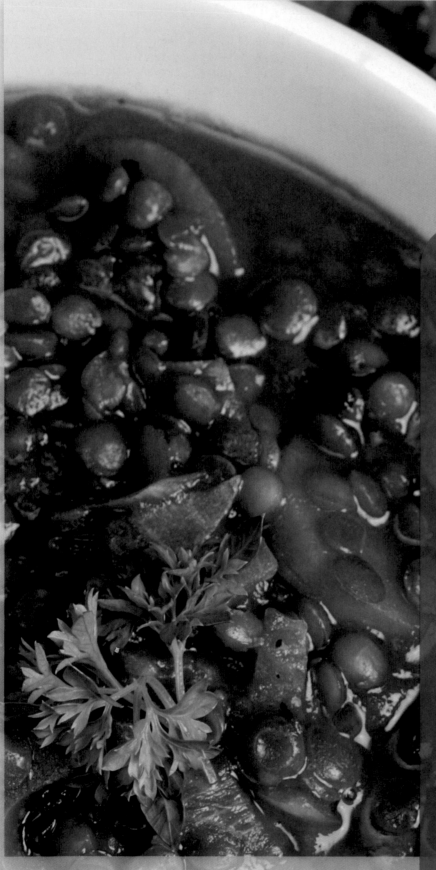

True or False?

1. Iron deficiency is the most common nutrient deficiency in the world.   **T** *or* **F**

2. To reduce their risk of having a baby with a serious central nervous system defect, women should begin taking folate supplements when they are planning a pregnancy or as soon as they learn they are pregnant.
T *or* **F**

3. People consuming a vegan diet are at greater risk for micronutrient deficiencies than are people who eat foods of animal origin.
T *or* **F**

4. *Anemia* is the clinical term for iron deficiency.   **T** *or* **F**

5. Fever, vomiting, and diarrhea all play a role in protecting the body from infectious disease.   **T** *or* **F**

Test Yourself answers are located in the Chapter Review.

12 Nutrients Involved in Blood Health and Immunity

Learning Objectives

After studying this chapter, you should be able to:

1. Identify the four components of blood, *p. 472.*

2. Discuss the role that iron plays in maintaining blood health overall, and specifically in oxygen transport, *pp. 472–482.*

3. Identify the three stages in the progression of iron deficiency, *pp. 480–482.*

4. Discuss the functions of zinc and copper and the contributions of these minerals to blood health, *pp. 483–487.*

5. Discuss the functions of vitamins K and B6 and their contributions to blood health, *pp. 488-489*

6. Describe the functions and contributions of folate and vitamin B_{12} to blood health, *pp. 489–492.*

7. Discuss the role of folate in preventing birth defects, supporting healthy pregnancies, and preventing anemia, *pp. 490–492.*

8. Describe the nonspecific and specific functions of the immune system, *pp. 493–494.*

9. Describe the effects of protein-energy malnutrition, obesity and essential fatty acids on immunity function, *pp. 494–496.*

10. Identify the key micronutrient deficiencies and excesses that are especially important for a strong immune response, *p. 496.*

MasteringNutrition™

Go online for chapter quizzes, pre-tests, Interactive Activities and more!

According to the World Health Organization, over 30% of the world's population is anemic. As a result, millions of children experience poor physical and cognitive development and an increased risk for infection and early death. Pregnant women are also at increased risk: in developing nations, half of all pregnant women are anemic, and anemia contributes to 20% of maternal deaths. Even in the United States, anemia is a major cause of behavioral and cognitive delays in children.

What is anemia, and what is the role of nutrition in causing or preventing it? Which micronutrients make the greatest contribution to the formation and maintenance of the red blood cells of our cardiovascular system, as well as the white blood cells of our immune system? How do they function? We explore these questions here.

Watch a video of red blood cell production from the National Library of Medicine at www.nlm.nih.gov/medlineplus/ency/anatomyvideos/000104.htm.

What Is the Role of Blood in Maintaining Health?

Blood transports to body cells virtually all the components necessary for life. No matter how much carbohydrate, fat, and protein we eat, we could not survive without healthy blood to transport these nutrients, and the oxygen to metabolize them, to our cells. In addition to transporting nutrients and oxygen, blood removes the waste products generated from metabolism, so that they can be properly excreted. Our health and our ability to perform daily activities are compromised if the quantity and quality of our blood is diminished.

Blood is actually a tissue, the only fluid tissue in the body. It has four components (**Figure 12.1**). **Erythrocytes,** or red blood cells, are the cells that transport oxygen. **Leukocytes,** or white blood cells, are the key to our immune function and protect us from infection and illness. **Platelets** are cell fragments that assist in the formation of blood clots and help stop bleeding. **Plasma** is the fluid portion of the blood, and it is needed to maintain adequate blood volume, so that blood can flow easily throughout the body.

Certain micronutrients play important roles in the maintenance of blood health through their actions as *coenzymes* and *cofactors* and as regulators of oxygen transport. These nutrients are discussed in detail in the following section.

erythrocytes Red blood cells; they transport oxygen in the blood.

leukocytes White blood cells; they protect the body from infection and illness.

platelets Cell fragments that assist in the formation of blood clots and help stop bleeding.

plasma The fluid portion of the blood; it is needed to maintain adequate blood volume, so that blood can flow easily throughout the body.

A Profile of Minerals That Maintain Blood Health

The minerals recognized as playing a critical role in maintaining blood health include iron, zinc, and copper (**Table 12.1**). Because blood is a tissue, adequate protein intake is also important for good blood health (see Chapter 6 for more on protein and its requirements).

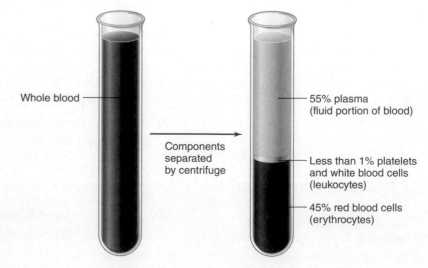

Whole blood

Components separated by centrifuge

55% plasma (fluid portion of blood)

Less than 1% platelets and white blood cells (leukocytes)

45% red blood cells (erythrocytes)

FIGURE 12.1 Blood has four components, which are visible when the blood is drawn into a test tube and spun in a centrifuge. The bottom layer is the erythrocytes, or red blood cells. The milky layer above the erythrocytes contains the leukocytes and platelets. The yellow fluid on top is the plasma.

TABLE 12.1 Overview of Nutrients Essential to Blood Health

To see the full profile of nutrients essential to bone health, turn to Chapter 7.5, In Depth: Vitamins and Minerals: Micronutrients with Macro Powers, pages 300–309.

Nutrient	Recommended Intake (RDA or AI and UL)
Iron	RDA: Women aged 19 to 50 years = 18 mg/day Men aged 19 to 50 years = 8 mg/day UL = 45 mg/day
Zinc	RDA: Women aged 19 to 50 years = 8 mg/day Men aged 19 to 50 years = 11 mg/day UL = 40 mg/day
Copper	RDA for all people 19–50 years = 90 µg/day UL = 10,000 µg/day
Vitamin K	AI: Women 19–50 years = 90 µg/day Men 19–50 years = 120 µg/day UL = none determined
Vitamin B_6 (pyridoxine)	RDA for all people 19–50 years = 1.3 mg/day RDA for people 51 and older: women = 1.5 mg/day; men = 1.7 mg/day
Folate (folic acid)	RDA for all people 19–50 years = 400 µg/day UL = 1,000 µg/day
Vitamin B_{12} (cyanocobalamin)	RDA for all people 19–50 years = 2.4 µg/day UL = not determined (ND)

Iron

Iron (Fe) is a trace mineral found in very small amounts in the body. Despite our relatively small need for iron, the World Health Organization lists iron deficiency as the most common nutrient deficiency in the world, including in industrialized countries.[1] Iron is a unique mineral with a positive charge that can easily give up and/or gain an electron, thereby changing its state from ferrous iron (Fe^{2+}) to ferric iron (Fe^{3+}) and back again. Although other forms of iron exist, ferrous and ferric iron are the two most common forms in our diet. Iron also binds easily to negatively charged elements, such as oxygen, nitrogen, and sulfur, a capacity that is important for the various functions iron plays in the body. We will discuss more about the various oxidative states of iron shortly.

Functions of Iron

Iron is a component of numerous proteins in the body, including enzymes and other proteins involved in energy production and both hemoglobin and myoglobin, the proteins involved in the transport and metabolism of oxygen. **Hemoglobin** is the oxygen-carrying protein found in the erythrocytes. It transports oxygen to tissues and accounts for almost two-thirds of all of the body's iron. Every day, within the bone marrow, the body produces approximately 200 billion erythrocytes, which require more than 24 mg of iron.[2] Thus, it is easy to see that hemoglobin synthesis for the formation of red blood cells is a primary factor in iron homeostasis. **Myoglobin,** another oxygen-carrying protein that is similar to hemoglobin, transports and stores oxygen within the muscles, accounting for approximately 10% of total iron in the body.

We cannot survive for more than a few minutes without oxygen; thus, hemoglobin's ability to transport oxygen throughout the body is critical to life. To carry oxygen, hemoglobin depends on the iron in its **heme** groups. As shown in **Figure 12.2**, the hemoglobin molecule consists of four polypeptide chains studded with four iron-containing heme groups. Iron is able to bind with and release oxygen easily. It does this by transferring electrons to and from the other atoms as it moves between various oxidation states. In the bloodstream, iron acts as a shuttle, picking up oxygen from the environment, binding it during its transport in the bloodstream, and then dropping it off again in our tissues.

hemoglobin The oxygen-carrying protein found in red blood cells; almost two-thirds of all of the iron in the body is found in hemoglobin.

myoglobin An iron-containing protein similar to hemoglobin except that it is found in muscle cells.

heme The iron-containing molecule found in hemoglobin.

FIGURE 12.2 Iron is contained in the heme portion of hemoglobin and myoglobin.

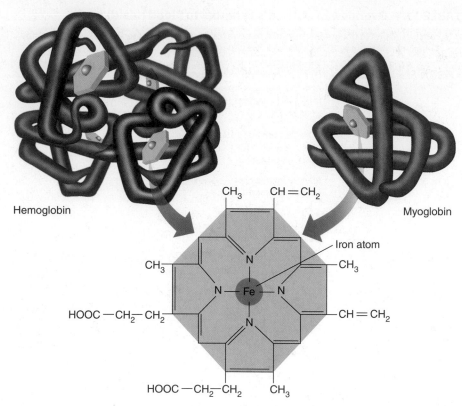

Heme portion containing iron (Fe)

As noted, iron is also important in energy metabolism. It is a component of the cytochromes, electron carriers within the metabolic pathways, which result in the production of energy from carbohydrates, fats, and protein. Cytochromes contain heme and thus require iron. If iron is not available to form them, the production of energy is limited, especially during times of high energy demand, such as during physical activity. Iron is also involved in some of the key enzymes in the tricarboxylic acid (TCA) cycle and for enzymes required in amino acid and lipid metabolism. As noted previously (in Chapter 10), iron is a part of the antioxidant enzyme system that assists in fighting free radicals. Interestingly, excess iron can also act as a prooxidant and promote the production of free radicals. Finally, iron is necessary for the enzymes involved in DNA synthesis and plays an important role in cognitive development and immune health (discussed later in this chapter).[2, 3]

How Does the Body Regulate Iron Homeostasis?

The body contains relatively little iron; men have less than 4 g of iron in their body, and women have just over 2 g. Iron is necessary for life, yet too much is toxic; therefore, the body maintains iron homeostasis primarily through regulating iron digestion, absorption, transport, storage, and excretion. **Figure 12.3** provides an overview of iron digestion, absorption, and transport.

Iron Digestion and Absorption The body's ability to digest and absorb dietary iron is influenced by a number of factors. The most important are the individual's iron status; the level of dietary iron consumption; the type of iron present in the foods consumed; the amount of stomach acid present to digest the foods; and the presence of the dietary factors that can either enhance or inhibit the absorption of iron.

Typically, the amount of iron absorbed from the diet is low, from 14% to 18%, depending on the way iron absorption is measured; however, if iron status is poor, absorption can increase to as high as 40%.[2, 3] Thus, people with poor iron status, such as those with iron deficiency, pregnant women, and people who have recently experienced blood loss (including menstruation) generally have the highest iron absorption rates. The typical Western

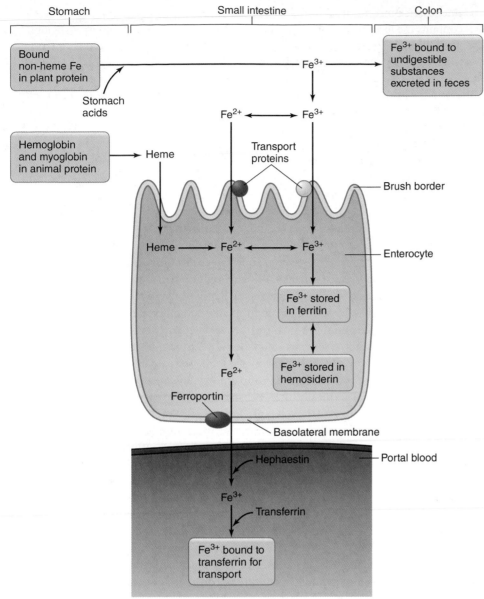

FIGURE 12.3 Overview of iron digestion, absorption, and transport. (*Source:* "Advance Nutrition and Human Metabolism (with InfoTrac®) 4e," by Gropper; Smith; Groff, 2005. Copyright © 2005 by Brooks/Cole, a part of Cengage Learning, Inc. Reproduced by permission. www.cengage.com/permissions)

diet of 2,000 kcal/day would contain about 12 mg of iron. In an individual with good iron status, only about 1.9 mg of this would be absorbed. However, in an individual with poor iron status, a maximum of 4.8 mg would be absorbed. By altering absorption rate, the body can improve iron status without dramatic increases in dietary iron intake.

Similarly, the total amount of iron consumed in the diet influences an individual's iron absorption rate. People who consume low levels of dietary iron absorb more iron from their foods than do those with higher dietary iron intakes. If the gut mucosal cells have a high iron pool, less iron is absorbed from the next meal.

The type of iron in foods is a major factor influencing iron absorption. There are two types:

- **Heme iron** is a part of hemoglobin and myoglobin and is found only in animal-based foods, such as meat, fish, and poultry.
- **Non-heme iron** is the form of iron that is not a part of hemoglobin or myoglobin. It is found in both plant-based and animal-based foods.

heme iron Iron that is a part of hemoglobin and myoglobin; it is found only in animal-based foods, such as meat, fish, and poultry.

non-heme iron The form of iron that is not a part of hemoglobin or myoglobin; it is found in animal-based and plant-based foods.

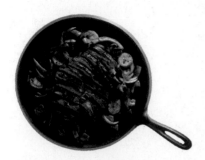

Cooking foods in cast-iron pans significantly increases their iron content.

meat factor A special factor found in meat, fish, and poultry that enhances the absorption of non-heme iron.

ferroportin An iron transporter that helps regulate intestinal iron absorption and the release of iron from the enterocyte into the general circulation.

hephaestin A copper-containing protein that oxidizes Fe^{2+} to Fe^{3+} once iron is transported across the basolateral membrane by ferroportin.

ceruloplasmin A copper-containing protein that transports copper in the body. It also plays a role in oxidizing ferric to ferrous iron (Fe^{2+} to Fe^{3+}).

transferrin The transport protein for iron.

ferritin A storage form of iron found primarily in the intestinal mucosa, spleen, bone marrow, and liver.

hemosiderin A storage form of iron found primarily in the intestinal mucosa, spleen, bone marrow, and liver.

Heme iron is more absorbable (15–35%) than non-heme iron (2–20%).[4] Once heme, which contains the ferrous form (Fe^{2+}), is released from either hemoglobin or myoglobin in the small intestine, it is rapidly bound to a specific receptor on the intestinal lumen and is taken into the enterocyte by endocytosis. Within the enterocyte, the heme group is broken down, and the iron that is released becomes part of a common iron pool within the cell. Because the iron in animal-based foods is about 40% heme iron (range 25–75%) and 60% non-heme iron, animal-based foods are good sources of absorbable iron.[5] Meat, fish, and poultry also contain a special **meat factor,** which enhances the absorption of non-heme iron in the diet.[2, 6]

In contrast, all of the iron found in plant-based foods is non-heme iron. Its absorption is significantly influenced by the individual's level of stomach acid. During digestion, non-heme iron–containing foods enter the stomach, where gastric juices containing pepsin and hydrocholic acid reduce the ferric iron (Fe^{3+}) to ferrous iron (Fe^{2+}), which is more soluble in the alkaline environment (higher pH) of the small intestine. Thus, adequate amounts of stomach acid are necessary for iron absorption. People with low levels of stomach acid, including many older adults, have a decreased ability to absorb iron. In addition, individuals who use medications that reduce stomach acid may reduce their iron absorption.

Once iron enters the duodenum, it is taken up by the enterocytes, with ferrous iron more rapidly absorbed than ferric iron. In addition, the solubility of non-heme iron in the small intestine is greatly modified by the presence of enhancing and inhibitory factors within the meal. Vitamin C enhances non-heme absorption from the gut by reducing dietary ferric to ferrous iron, which then forms a soluble iron–ascorbic acid complex in the stomach.[3] Conversely, iron absorption is impaired by phytates, polyphenols, vegetable proteins, fiber, and calcium. Typically, these substances bind to the ferric iron and form complexes that cannot be digested. Phytates are found in legumes, rice, and whole grains; and polyphenols are found in oregano, red wine, tea, and coffee. Soybean protein, fiber, and minerals such as calcium inhibit iron absorption. Because of the influence of these dietary factors on iron absorption, it is estimated that the bioavailability of iron from a vegan diet is approximately 1–10%,[5] compared with the 14–18% absorption of the typical Western diet.

To optimize absorption of the non-heme iron in plant foods, consume these foods either with foods rich in heme iron or in combination with foods high in vitamin C. For instance, eating meat with beans or vegetables enhances the absorption of the non-heme iron found in the beans and vegetables. Drinking a glass of orange juice with breakfast cereal will increase the absorption of the non-heme iron in the cereal. Avoid taking zinc or calcium supplements or drinking milk when eating iron-rich foods, as iron absorption will be impaired.

Finally, cooking foods in cast-iron pans will significantly increase the iron content of any meal. That's because the iron in the pan is released and combines with food during the cooking process.

Iron Transport Regardless of the form, iron taken into the enterocytes becomes part of the total iron pool. From this pool the iron can be stored within the enterocytes, or it can be transported across the membrane of the enterocytes by **ferroportin** into the interstitial fluid, from which it can enter the circulation. Ferroportin is an iron transporter that helps regulate intestinal iron absorption and release.[2] Iron crossing into the interstitial fluid is in the ferrous form (Fe^{2+}) but is quickly converted to ferric iron (Fe^{3+}) by either **hephaestin** in the intestinal basal cell membrane (see Figure 12.3) or **ceruloplasmin** in the blood, two copper-containing plasma proteins capable of oxidizing iron. This Fe^{3+} is rapidly bound to **transferrin,** the primary iron-transport protein in the blood, which transports the Fe^{3+} to the cells of the body. Transferrin receptors on the cells increase and decrease in number, depending on the cells' need for iron. In this way, cells can regulate the amount of iron they take in from the blood.

Iron Storage The body is capable of storing small amounts of iron in two storage forms: **ferritin** and **hemosiderin.** These storage forms of iron provide us with iron when our diet is inadequate or when our needs are high. Both ferritin and hemosiderin can be mobilized if the body needs iron.

Figure 12.3 shows iron storage in the enterocytes as ferritin or hemosiderin. Other common areas of iron storage are the liver, bone marrow, and spleen. Ferritin is the normal storage form, whereas hemosiderin storage occurs predominately in conditions of iron overload. However, if an iron overload occurs, and the excess iron is stored as hemosiderin in the heart and liver, organ damage can occur.

The amount of iron stored can vary dramatically between men and women, with women at greater risk of having low iron stores (from 300 to 1,000 mg). Average iron stores for men are estimated to be 500 to 1,500 mg. Women of childbearing age have one of the highest rates of iron deficiency, which is attributed to increased iron losses in menstrual blood, poor intakes of iron, and the additional iron requirements that accompany pregnancy. The iron "cost" of pregnancy is high; thus, a woman of childbearing age should have good iron stores prior to pregnancy and consume iron-rich foods during pregnancy. Iron supplements are routinely prescribed during the last two trimesters to ensure that there is adequate iron for the woman and her developing fetus. The iron needs of pregnancy are covered in more detail later in this text (see Chapter 16).

Regulation of Total Body Iron   The body regulates iron balance and homeostasis through three mechanisms:

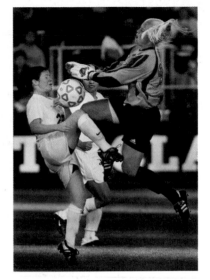

Athletes may have an increased need for iron.

- *Iron absorption.* As discussed earlier, the change in the iron absorption rate is based on the amount of iron consumed, the amount needed by the body, and the dietary factors that affect absorption.
- *Iron losses.* One of the major routes of iron loss is through the turnover of the gut enterocytes. Every 3 to 6 days, the gut cells are shed and lost into the lumen of the intestine. In this way, the iron stored as ferritin within the enterocytes is returned to the lumen, from which it is lost in the feces. The regulation of iron absorption in this way dramatically reduces the possibility of too much iron entering the system, regardless of the iron source. Iron can also be lost in blood (menses, blood donations, injury), sweat, and semen and passively from cells that are shed from the skin and urinary tract. The dietary recommendations for iron are based on an overall estimated daily iron turnover of 1.5 mg/d for menstruating women and 1.0 mg/d for sedentary men and postmenopausal women.[3] The typical menstruating female loses approximately 14 mg of iron per menstrual cycle; thus, the additional 0.5 mg/d would provide an extra 15 mg of iron per month to cover menstrual losses.[3] Women who experience heavy menstrual bleeding would have even greater iron losses, which would need to be covered by either dietary or supplemental iron. Active individuals can also have increased iron losses due to iron lost in urine, sweat, and increased red cell turnover.[3]
- *Storage and recycling of iron.* Stored iron gives the body access to iron to maintain health when intakes of dietary iron are low or losses are great. Conversely, once iron balance has been restored, the body will gradually increase the amount of iron stored, so that reserves are again available in times of need. The body is also efficient at recycling iron already within the system. The majority of the body's iron is bound to hemoglobin within the red blood cells, which have a life of 120 days. In order to prevent the body from losing this valuable source of iron, as old red cells are broken down, the iron is recycled and returned to the body's iron pool. The iron supplied through recycling is approximately twenty times greater than the amount of iron absorbed from the diet.[2] Thus, the body's ability to recycle iron is extremely important in maintaining iron homeostasis.

How Much Iron Should We Consume?

In determining the RDA for iron, researchers take into account the bioavailability of iron from food and absorption rates.

TABLE 12.2 Special Circumstances Affecting Iron Status

Circumstances That Improve Iron Status	Circumstances That Diminish Iron Status
Use of oral contraceptives—reduces menstrual blood loss in women.	**Use of hormone replacement therapy**—can cause uterine bleeding.
Breastfeeding—delays resumption of menstruation in new mothers and thereby reduces blood loss. It is therefore an important health measure, especially in developing nations.	**Eating a vegetarian diet**—reduces or eliminates sources of heme iron.
Consumption of iron-containing foods and supplements	**Intestinal parasite infection**—causes intestinal bleeding. Iron-deficiency anemia is common in people with intestinal parasite infection. **Blood donation**—reduces iron stores; people who donate frequently, particularly pre-menopausal women, may require iron supplementation. **Intense endurance exercise training**—appears to increase the risk for poor iron status because of many factors, including inflammation, suboptimal iron intake, and increased iron loss due to rupture of red blood cells and increased fecal losses.

Source: Data from Institute of Medicine, Food and Nutrition Board. 2002. *Dietary Reference Intakes for Vitamin A, Vitamin K, Arsenic, Boron, Chromium, Copper, Iodine, Iron, Manganese, Molybdenum, Nickel, Silicon, Vanadium, and Zinc.* Washington, DC: National Academies Press. © 2002 by the National Academy of Sciences.

Recommended Dietary Intakes for Iron The RDA for iron for men aged 19 years and older is 8 mg/day. The RDA for iron for women aged 19 to 50 years is 18 mg/day and decreases to 8 mg/day for women 51 years of age and older. The higher iron requirement for younger women is due to the excess iron and blood lost during menstruation. Pregnancy is a time of very high iron needs, and the RDA for pregnant women is 27 mg/day. The UL for iron for adults aged 19 and older is 45 mg/day. Although it is difficult to get too much iron from whole foods, it is easy to get high doses of iron from supplements and/or the use of highly fortified processed foods, such as breakfast cereals, meal-replacement drinks, energy bars, and protein powders. See the **You Do the Math** box to learn how to calculate your iron intake. Special circumstances that significantly affect iron status and may increase requirements are identified in **Table 12.2**.

Food Sources of Iron Foods rich in heme iron include meats, poultry, fish, and shellfish (**Figure 12.4**). Clams, oysters, and beef liver are particularly good sources, providing 5–11 mg of iron per serving. Many breakfast cereals and breads are enriched or fortified with iron; although this non-heme iron is less absorbable, it is still significant because these foods are a major part of the Western diet. Some vegetables and legumes, such as spinach,

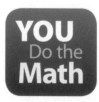

Calculating Daily Iron Intake

Determining whether you're getting the iron your body needs each day can be tricky, because the amount you consume may not be the amount that is absorbed. Food combinations, fortified foods, and supplements all make a difference. Determine the amount of iron available for absorption for Hannah, who is menstruating normally:

Foods with heme iron (15% available):

- Turkey, light meat (3 oz): 1.1 mg
- Tuna, light canned (3 oz): 1.3 mg

Foods with non-heme iron (5% available):

- Oatmeal, 1 instant packet: 11 mg
- Spinach, 1 cup raw: 6.4 mg
- Bread, whole-wheat, 2 slices: 1.4 mg

In addition, Hannah is taking a daily multivitamin/mineral supplement with 18 mg of Fe (5% available). This is the amount of iron in a typical 1-day multivitamin/mineral supplement designed for menstruating women.

What is the total available iron for absorption (mg/d)? Does it cover the amount of iron lost each day? If Hannah were not taking a daily supplement, would she still be getting adequate iron?

Answers are located online in the MasteringNutrition Study Area.

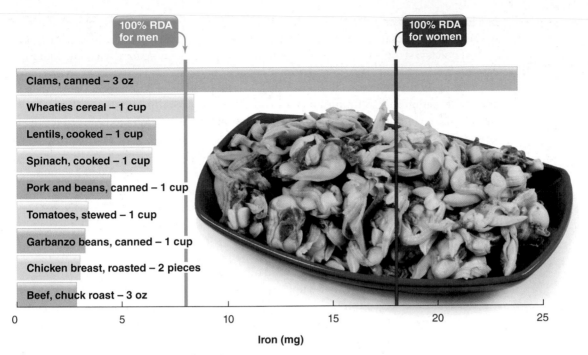

FIGURE 12.4 Common food sources of iron. The RDA for iron is 8 mg/day for men and 18 mg/day for women aged 19 to 50 years. (*Source:* Data from US Department of Agriculture, Agricultural Research Service, 2009, USDA Nutrient Database for Standard Reference, Release 22. Nutrient Data Laboratory Home Page, www.ars.usda.gov/ba/bhnrc/ndl.)

lentils, and beans, are also good sources of iron. The absorption of their non-heme iron can be enhanced by eating them with animal foods or vitamin C–rich foods. People who avoid animal products need to pay special attention to their diet to ensure adequate iron intake, because heme iron sources are eliminated.

Increasing Your Iron Intake Simple changes in your daily diet can help you increase your daily intake of iron and avoid deficiency. Here are a few:

- Shop for iron-fortified breads and breakfast cereals. Check the Nutrition Facts Panel!
- Consume a food or beverage that is high in vitamin C along with plant or animal sources of iron. For instance, drink a glass of orange juice with your morning toast to increase the absorption of the non-heme iron in the bread. Or add chopped tomatoes to beans or lentils. Or sprinkle lemon juice on fish.
- Add small amounts of meat, poultry, or fish to baked beans, vegetable soups, stir-fried vegetables, or salads to enhance the absorption of the non-heme iron in the plant-based foods.
- Cook foods in cast-iron pans to significantly increase the iron content of foods: the iron in the pan will be absorbed into the food during the cooking process.
- Avoid drinking red wine, coffee, or tea when eating iron-rich foods, as chemicals called polyphenols in these beverages will reduce iron absorption.
- Avoid drinking cow's milk or soymilk with iron-rich foods, as both calcium and soybean protein inhibit iron absorption.
- Avoid taking calcium supplements or zinc supplements with iron-rich foods, as these minerals decrease iron absorption.

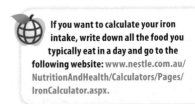

If you want to calculate your iron intake, write down all the food you typically eat in a day and go to the following website: www.nestle.com.au/NutritionAndHealth/Calculators/Pages/IronCalculator.aspx.

What Happens If We Consume Too Much Iron?

Accidental iron overdose is the most common cause of poisoning deaths in children younger than 6 years of age in the United States.[7] It is important for parents to take the same precautions with dietary supplements as they would with other drugs, keeping them in a locked cabinet or well out of reach of children. Symptoms of iron toxicity include nausea, vomiting, diarrhea, dizziness, confusion, and rapid heartbeat. If iron toxicity is not treated quickly, significant damage to the heart, central nervous system, liver, and kidneys can result in death.

Many adults who take iron supplements, even at prescribed doses, commonly experience constipation and gastrointestinal distress.[3] High doses of iron supplements can also cause nausea, vomiting, and diarrhea. Taking iron supplements with food can reduce these adverse effects in most, but not all, people.

As mentioned (in Chapter 10), some individuals suffer from a hereditary disorder called *hemochromatosis*. This disorder affects between 1-in-200 to 1-in-500 individuals, most of northern European origin.[8] Hemochromatosis is characterized by excessive absorption of dietary iron and altered iron storage. In this disease, the transport of iron from the enterocytes into the circulation is not regulated appropriately, and iron transport continues even when it is not needed.[9] Because the body has no homeostatic mechanism for eliminating high amounts of iron from the system, iron accumulates in body tissues over many years, causing organ damage and other disease. High levels of serum iron can also increase the risk for oxidative damage by stimulating the activity of free radicals, which are also associated with chronic diseases. Free radicals can damage coronary arteries and contribute to cardiovascular disease; they have also been associated with the oxidation of LDLs, which also can contribute to coronary artery damage.[4] Treatment includes reducing dietary intake of iron, avoiding high intakes of vitamin C, and blood removal, a process similar to the donation of blood except that the blood is not reused.

What Happens If We Don't Consume Enough Iron?

Iron deficiency is the most common nutrient deficiency in the world and can have a number of health consequences. People at particularly high risk for iron deficiency include infants and young children, menstruating girls and women, and pregnant women. Refer to the feature box **Highlight: Iron Deficiency Around the World** to learn more about the impact of iron deficiency on people around the world.

Many Factors Contribute to Iron Deficiency   For some individuals, iron deficiency is simply due to poor dietary intakes of iron. Other factors can include high iron losses in blood and sweat, a diet high in fiber or phytates that bind iron, low stomach acid, and poor iron absorption due to poor gut health or the consumption of dietary supplements containing high levels of minerals, such as calcium, that compete with iron absorption binding sites. Significant blood losses through blood donations, surgery, or heavy menstrual periods can contribute to poor iron status. Thus, the causes of iron deficiency and/or depletion can be numerous and may involve a number of issues that need to be addressed before iron status can be improved.

Iron Deficiency Progresses Through Three Stages   As shown in **Figure 12.5**, **stage I** of iron deficiency is called **iron depletion.**[10, 11] It is caused by a decrease in iron *stores*, resulting in reduced levels of circulating ferritin in the blood. As discussed earlier, ferritin is one form of stored iron. Small amounts of ferritin circulate in the blood, and these concentrations are highly correlated with iron stores.

During iron depletion, there are generally no physical symptoms because hemoglobin levels are not yet affected. However, when iron stores are low, the amount of iron available to mitochondrial proteins and enzymes appears to be depleted. This reduces the individual's ability to produce energy during periods of high demand. For example, research has shown that, when sedentary women with poor ferritin levels participated in an exercise-training program, they did not experience the same improvements in fitness as women who had adequate ferritin levels.[12]

The second stage of iron deficiency causes a decrease in the *transport* of iron and is called **iron-deficiency erythropoiesis (stage II)**. This stage is manifested by a reduction in the saturation of transferrin with iron. Transferrin, the transport protein for iron, has the ability to bind two iron molecules and transport them to the cells of the body. During this stage, the iron binding sites on transferrin are left empty, because there is no

iron depletion (stage I) The first phase of iron deficiency, characterized by a decrease in stored iron, which results in a decrease in blood ferritin levels.

iron-deficiency erythropoiesis (stage II) The second stage of iron deficiency, characterized by a decrease in the transport of iron in the blood.

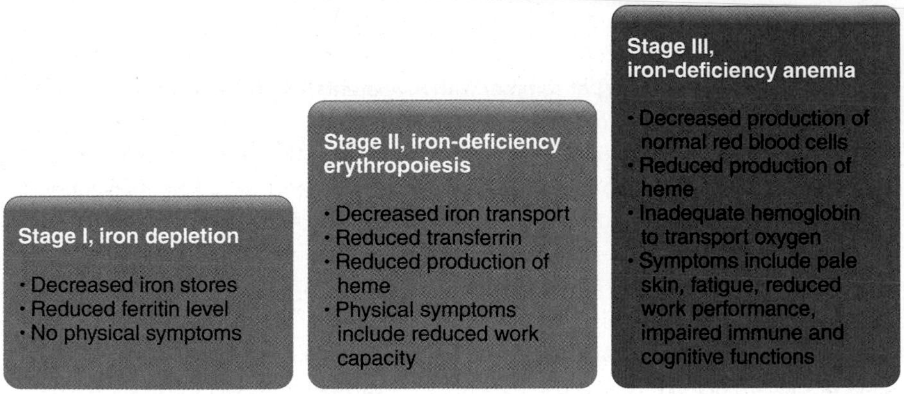

FIGURE 12.5 Iron deficiency passes through three stages. The first stage is identified by decreased iron stores and reduced ferritin levels. The second stage is identified by decreased iron transport and a reduction in transferrin. The final stage is iron-deficiency anemia, which is identified by decreased production of normal, healthy red blood cells and inadequate hemoglobin levels.

Stage I, iron depletion

- Decreased iron stores
- Reduced ferritin level
- No physical symptoms

Stage II, iron-deficiency erythropoiesis

- Decreased iron transport
- Reduced transferrin
- Reduced production of heme
- Physical symptoms include reduced work capacity

Stage III, iron-deficiency anemia

- Decreased production of normal red blood cells
- Reduced production of heme
- Inadequate hemoglobin to transport oxygen
- Symptoms include pale skin, fatigue, reduced work performance, impaired immune and cognitive functions

iron available for binding. This results in transferrin having an increased ability to bind iron, which is called *total iron binding capacity (TIBC)*. In addition, transferrin receptors on the cells increase to promote uptake of iron by the cell. Overall, then, individuals with iron-deficiency erythropoiesis have low serum ferritin and iron concentrations, a low level of iron saturation, and a high TIBC and transferrin receptors. The production of heme and the ability to make new red blood cells (for example, erythropoiesis) starts to decline during this stage, leading to symptoms of reduced work capacity, because fewer red blood cells are being made.

HIGHLIGHT

Iron Deficiency Around the World

Iron deficiency is the most common nutritional deficiency in the world. According to the World Health Organization, approximately 2 billion people, or 30% of the world's population, are anemic, many due to iron deficiency.[1] Because of its high prevalence worldwide, iron deficiency is considered an epidemic.

Those who are particularly susceptible to iron deficiency include people living in developing countries, pregnant women, and young children. But iron deficiency not only hurts individuals. Because it results in increased healthcare needs, premature death, resultant family breakdown, and lost work productivity, it also damages communities and entire nations.

Among children, the health consequences of iron-deficiency anemia are particularly devastating. They include

- Premature birth
- Low birth weight
- Increased risk for infections
- Increased risk for premature death
- Impaired cognitive and physical development
- Behavioral problems and poor school performance

Research is currently examining the role of iron supplementation in improving cognitive function. A meta-analysis of the current research literature suggests that iron supplementation in children suffering from iron-deficiency anemia can improve their intelligence quotient; however, the effect of supplementation on attention and concentration is not clear.[2]

The World Health Organization has developed a comprehensive plan to address all aspects of iron deficiency and anemia.[1, 3] This plan, which is being implemented in several developing countries, not only is restoring personal health but also is estimated to be capable of raising national productivity levels by 20 percent.

References

1. World Health Organization. 2012. Nutrition. Micronutrient Deficiencies: Iron Deficiency Anemia. www.who.int/nutrition/topics/ida/en/index.html.
2. Falkingham, M., A. Abdelhamid, P. Curtis, A. Fairweather-Tait, L. Dye, and L. Hooper. 2010. The effects of oral iron supplementation on cognition in older children and adults: a systemic review and meta-analysis. *J Nut.* 9:4.
3. Baltussen, R., C. Knai, and M. Sharan. 2004. Iron fortification and iron supplementation are cost-effective interventions to reduce iron deficiency in four subregions of the world. *J. Nut.* 134:2678–2684.

Liz

*Nutri-*Case

"It was really hard spending last summer with my parents, because we kept arguing over food! Even though I'd told them that I'm a vegetarian, they kept serving meals with meat! Then they'd get mad when I'd fix myself a hummus sandwich! When it was my turn to cook, I made lentils with brown rice, whole-wheat pasta primavera, vegetarian curries, and lots of other yummy meals, but my father still complained. He kept insisting, "You have to eat meat or you won't get enough iron!' I told him that plant foods have lots of iron, but he wouldn't listen. Was I ever glad to get back onto campus this fall!"

Recall that Liz is a ballet dancer who trains daily. If she eats a vegetarian diet, including meals such as the ones she describes here, will she be at risk for iron deficiency? Why or why not? Are there any other micronutrients that might be low in Liz's diet because she avoids meat? If so, what are they? Overall, will Liz get enough energy to support her high level of physical activity on a vegetarian diet? How would she know if she were low on energy?

During the third, and final, stage of iron deficiency, **iron-deficiency anemia (stage III)** results. In iron-deficiency anemia, the production of normal, healthy red blood cells has decreased, the cell size decreases by as much as a third, and hemoglobin levels are inadequate. Thus, too few red blood cells are made, and those that are made cannot bind and transport oxygen adequately. Individuals with stage III iron-deficiency anemia will still have abnormal values for all the assessment parameters measured in stages I and II.

Iron-Deficiency Anemia Is a Microcytic Anemia   The term *anemia* literally means "without blood"; it is used to refer to any condition in which hemoglobin levels are low, regardless of the cause.

Microcytic anemias are a group of anemias characterized by red blood cells that are smaller than normal (*micro-* means "small," and *–cyte* means "cell"). As just noted, red blood cells that are synthesized in an iron-deficient environment will be as much as a third smaller than normal and will not contain enough hemoglobin to transport adequate oxygen or to allow the proper transfer of electrons to produce energy. Microcytic anemia is sometimes referred to as *microcytic hypochromic anemia*, because reduced levels of hemoglobin deprive the cells of their bright red color (*hypo-* means "low," and *–chromic* refers to "color").

In iron-deficiency anemia, as normal red blood cell death occurs over time, more and more healthy red blood cells are replaced by microcytic cells. At the same time, fewer red blood cells are made. These changes prompt classic symptoms of oxygen and energy deprivation, including general fatigue, pale skin, depressed immune function, and impaired cognitive and nerve function, work performance, and memory. Pregnant women with severe anemia are at higher risk for low-birth-weight infants, premature delivery, and increased infant mortality.

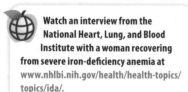

Watch an interview from the National Heart, Lung, and Blood Institute with a woman recovering from severe iron-deficiency anemia at www.nhlbi.nih.gov/health/health-topics/topics/ida/.

iron-deficiency anemia (stage III) A form of anemia that results from severe iron deficiency.

microcytic anemia   A form of anemia manifested as the production of smaller than normal red blood cells containing insufficient hemoglobin, which reduces the red blood cell's ability to transport oxygen; it can result from iron deficiency or vitamin B$_6$ deficiency.

RECAP

Iron is a trace mineral that, as part of the hemoglobin and myoglobin proteins, plays a major role in the transport of oxygen in the body. Iron is also a cofactor in many metabolic pathways involved in energy production. The RDA for adult men aged 19 years and older is 8 mg/day. The RDA for adult women aged 19 to 50 years is 18 mg/day. Meat, fish, and poultry are good sources of heme iron, which is more absorbable than non-heme iron. Toxicity symptoms for iron range from nausea and vomiting to organ damage and potentially death. If left untreated, iron depletion can eventually lead to iron-deficiency anemia. ■

Zinc

Zinc (Zn^{2+}) is a positively charged trace mineral that, like iron, is found in very small amounts in the body (1.5–2.5 g). Most of the zinc found in the body is concentrated in the muscles and bone. However, in contrast with iron and other minerals, zinc has no dedicated storage sites within the body. Instead a small, exchangeable pool of zinc is found in the bone, liver, and blood.[10] Loss of zinc from this pool, if not replaced, leads to zinc deficiency.

Functions of Zinc

Zinc has multiple functions within nearly every body system. As a component of various enzymes, zinc helps maintain the structural integrity of proteins and assists in the regulation of gene expression.[3] Without zinc, the body cannot grow, develop, or function properly. It is easiest to review the many roles of zinc in the body by dividing them into three categories: enzymatic, structural, and regulatory.

Enzymatic Functions   It is estimated that more than 100 different enzymes within the body require zinc for their functioning.[3] If zinc is not present, these enzymes cannot function properly and lose their activity. For example, we require zinc to metabolize alcohol (alcohol dehydrogenase), digest our food (carboxypeptidase C, aminopeptidase, phospholipase C), help form bone (collagenase), provide the body with energy through glycolysis, and synthesize the heme structure in hemoglobin. Thus, zinc, like iron, is required to make the oxygen-carrying component of hemoglobin. In this way, zinc contributes to the maintenance of blood health.

Structural Functions   Zinc helps maintain the structural integrity and shape of proteins. If proteins lose their shape, they lose their function, much like a plastic spoon that has melted into a ball. Zinc helps stabilize the structure of certain DNA-binding proteins, called *zinc fingers*, which help regulate gene expression by facilitating the folding of proteins into biologically active molecules used in gene regulation.[10] Zinc fingers also help stabilize vitamin A receptors in the retina of the eye, thereby facilitating night vision. Another function associated with zinc fingers is the sequencing of hormone receptors for vitamin D and thyroid hormone.

Zinc's ability to help maintain protein structures also includes maintaining the integrity of some enzymes. For example, zinc helps maintain the integrity of copper–zinc superoxide dismutase, which is important in helping prevent oxidative damage caused by free radicals. Zinc also helps maintain the integrity of enzymes involved in the development and activation of certain immune cells (discussed shortly). In fact, zinc has received so much attention for its contribution to immune system health that zinc lozenges have been formulated to fight the common cold. The **Nutrition Debate** box located at the end of this chapter explores the question of whether these lozenges are effective in combating the common cold.

Regulatory Functions   As a regulator of gene expression, zinc helps turn genes "on" and "off," thus regulating the body functions these genes control. For example, in humans, if zinc is not available to activate certain genes related to cellular growth during the development of the fetus and after the child is born, growth is stunted. Zinc also plays a role in cell signaling. For example, zinc helps maintain blood glucose levels by interacting with insulin and influencing the way fat cells take up glucose. Zinc also helps regulate the activity of a number of other hormones, such as human growth hormone, sex hormones, and corticosteroids.[10]

A number of biological actions require zinc in all three of the functions just covered. The major example of this is in reproduction. Zinc is critical for cell replication and normal growth. In fact, zinc deficiency was discovered in the early 1960s when researchers were trying to determine the cause of severe growth retardation, anemia, and poorly developed genitalia in some Middle Eastern males. These symptoms of zinc deficiency illustrate its critical role in normal growth and sexual maturation.

What Factors Alter Zinc Digestion, Absorption, and Balance?

Overall, zinc absorption is similar to that of iron, ranging from 10% to 35% of dietary zinc. People with poor zinc status absorb more zinc than individuals with optimal zinc status, and zinc absorption increases during times of growth, sexual development, and pregnancy. See **Figure 12.6** for an overview of zinc digestion, absorption, and transport.

Zinc is absorbed from the lumen of the intestine into the enterocytes through both active transport by carriers and simple diffusion, with the efficiency of absorption decreasing as the amount of zinc in the diet increases. Once inside the enterocytes, zinc can be released into the interstitial fluid (as discussed shortly) or bound to a protein called **metallothionein,** which prevents zinc from moving out of the enterocyte into the system. In this way, the body can regulate the amount of absorbed zinc that actually enters the total zinc pool of the body. When the enterocytes are sloughed off into the intestine, the zinc bound to metallothionein is lost in the feces. In this way, the body can maintain total zinc homeostasis.

Several dietary factors influence zinc absorption. High non-heme iron intakes can inhibit zinc absorption, which is a primary concern with iron supplementation, particularly during pregnancy and lactation. (Iron supplements contain non-heme iron.) High intakes of heme iron, however, appear to have no effect on zinc absorption. Although calcium is known to inhibit zinc absorption in animals, this effect has not been demonstrated in humans. The phytates and fiber found in whole grains and beans strongly inhibit zinc absorption. In contrast, dietary protein enhances zinc absorption, with animal-based proteins increasing the absorption of zinc to a much greater extent than plant-based proteins. It's not surprising, then, that the primary cause of the zinc deficiency in the Middle Eastern

metallothionein A zinc-containing protein within the enterocyte; it assists in the regulation of zinc homeostasis.

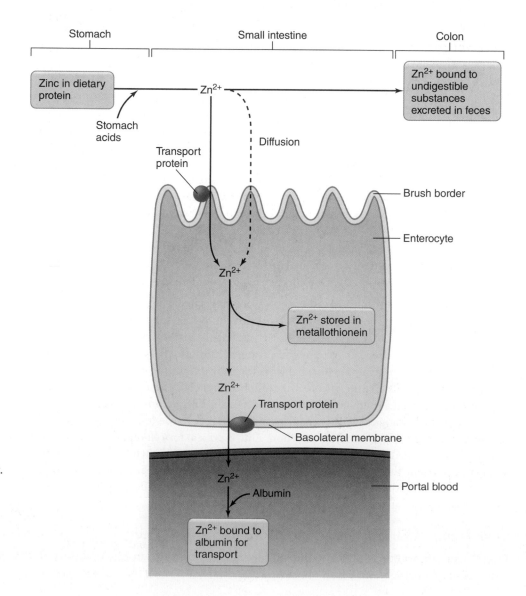

FIGURE 12.6 Overview of zinc digestion, absorption, and transport. (*Source:* "Advance Nutrition and Human Metabolism (with InfoTrac®) 4e," by Gropper; Smith; Groff, 2005. Copyright © 2005 by Brooks/Cole, a part of Cengage Learning, Inc. Reproduced by permission. www. cengage.com/permissions)

men mentioned earlier was their low consumption of meat and high consumption of beans and unleavened breads (also called *flat breads*). In leavening bread, the baker adds yeast to the dough. This not only makes the bread rise but also helps reduce the phytate content of the bread.

How Is Zinc Transported in the Body?

Zinc is absorbed from the lumen of the intestine and moves into the enterocyte. It then crosses the basolateral enterocyte membrane via a process of active transport using both a zinc transporter and energy (ATP). Upon reaching the interstitial fluid, zinc is picked up by albumin, a transport protein in the plasma, and carried via the portal vein to the liver. Once in the liver, some of the zinc is repackaged and released back into the blood, bound to either albumin (about 60%) or other transport proteins (about 40%). The bound zinc can then be delivered to the cells, where it is taken up by energy-dependent carriers.

How Much Zinc Should We Consume?

As with iron, our need for zinc is relatively small, but our dietary intakes and level of absorption are variable. Absorption factors were considered when the RDA for zinc was set.[3] The RDA values for zinc for adult men and women aged 19 and older are 11 mg/day and 8 mg/day, respectively. The UL for zinc for adults aged 19 and older is 40 mg/day.

Good food sources of zinc include red meats, some seafood, whole grains, and enriched grains and cereals. The dark meat of poultry has a higher content of zinc than white meat. As zinc is significantly more absorbable from animal-based foods, zinc deficiency is a concern for people eating a vegetarian or vegan diet. **Figure 12.7** shows various foods that are relatively high in zinc.

Nutrition
MILESTONE

In **1958**, Drs. James Halsted and Ananda Prasad, American physicians working in Iran, consulted together on the case of a 21-year-old Iranian man who looked like a 10-year-old boy.[13] In addition to his abnormally small size, he had underdeveloped genitalia; rough, dry skin; and cognitive deficits. Blood tests revealed that he was iron deficient. At first the physicians considered the possibility that the patient had a pituitary disorder, but when ten more such cases were brought to their attention within a short period of time, they discarded the hypothesis in favor of a dietary explanation. They noted that the bread the patients ate was unleavened, that their diet included almost no animal protein, and that they practiced geophagia—they ate clay. These factors were known to contribute to iron deficiency.

Although the effects of zinc deficiency in humans were unknown, they considered that the same factors might also have decreased the availability of zinc. Further experiments supported the hypothesis. The physicians found that patients administered supplemental zinc developed normal genitalia and secondary sexual characteristics within 6 months and an increase in height of 5–6 inches within 1 year. This research showed for the first time that zinc is essential to human health.

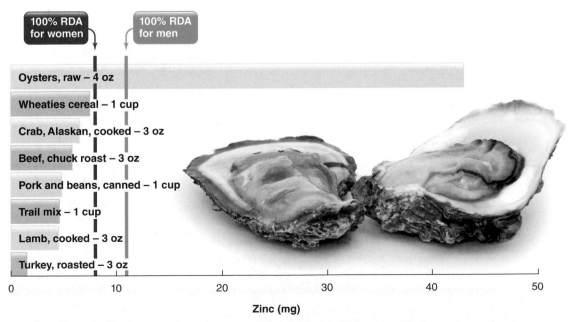

FIGURE 12.7 Common food sources of zinc. The RDA for zinc is 11 mg/day for men and 8 mg/day for women. (*Source:* Data from US Department of Agriculture, Agricultural Research Service, 2009, USDA Nutrient Database for Standard Reference, Release 22. Nutrient Data Laboratory Home Page, www.ars.usda.gov/ba/bhnrc/ndl.)

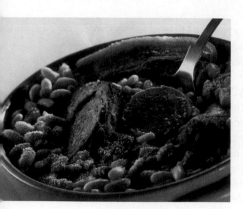

Zinc can be found in pork and beans.

Eating high amounts of dietary zinc does not appear to lead to toxicity; however, toxicity can occur from consuming high amounts of supplemental zinc. Toxicity symptoms include intestinal pain and cramps, nausea, vomiting, loss of appetite, diarrhea, and headaches. Excessive zinc supplementation has also been shown to depress immune function and decrease high-density lipoprotein concentrations. High intakes of zinc (five to six times the RDA) can also reduce copper and iron status, as zinc absorption interferes with the absorption of these minerals.[3]

Zinc deficiency is uncommon in the United States, occurring more often in countries in which people consume predominantly grain-based foods. When zinc deficiency does occur, it is primarily associated with growth retardation in children, in which the lack of zinc disrupts functions associated with growth hormone.[14] Other symptoms of zinc deficiency include diarrhea, delayed sexual maturation and impotence, eye and skin lesions, hair loss, and impaired appetite. As zinc is critical to a healthy immune system, zinc deficiency results in increased incidence of infections and illnesses.

Because we do not have good assessment parameters for zinc, we have no way of recognizing poor zinc status until deficiency symptoms occur. In developed countries, those at greatest risk for zinc deficiencies are individuals with malabsorption syndromes and adults and children who eliminate high-zinc foods from their diet while consuming diets high in fiber. For example, recent research has shown that low-income Hispanic children who are in lower growth percentiles than predicted respond to zinc supplementation by growing closer to the predicted rate.[14]

Copper

Copper is a trace mineral that is required for a number of enzymes that have oxidative functions. Fortunately, copper is widely distributed in foods and deficiency is rare.

Functions of Copper

In the body, copper is primarily found as a component of ceruloplasmin, a protein that is critical for its transport. Indeed, an individual's copper status is typically assessed by measuring plasma levels of ceruloplasmin. As we mentioned in the discussion of iron, ceruloplasmin is important for the oxidation of ferrous to ferric iron ($Fe^{2+} \rightarrow Fe^{3+}$), which is necessary before iron can bind to transferrin and be transported in the plasma.[3] Because of ceruloplasmin's role in iron metabolism, it is also called ferroxidase I. When ceruloplasmin is inadequate, the transport of iron for heme formation is impaired and anemia can result. Because iron cannot be transported properly, iron accumulates in the tissues, causing symptoms similar to those of the genetic disorder hemochromatosis (page 480).

Copper also functions as a cofactor in the metabolic pathways that produce energy, in the production of the connective tissues collagen and elastin, and as part of the superoxide dismutase enzyme system that fights the damage caused by free radicals. Copper is also necessary for the regulation of certain neurotransmitters, especially serotonin, important to brain function.

What Factors Alter Copper Absorption and Balance?

The major site of copper absorption is in the small intestine, with small amounts also absorbed in the stomach. As with zinc and iron, the amount of copper absorbed is related to the amount of copper in the diet, with absorption decreasing on high-copper diets and increasing on low-copper diets. Thus, regulation of copper absorption is one of the primary ways the body maintains good copper balance.

Copper is transported across the enterocytes by both carrier-mediated transport and simple diffusion.[14] Once absorbed, copper is bound to albumin (as with zinc), then transported in the portal blood to the liver. In the liver, about 60% to 95% of the copper is incorporated into ceruloplasmin, where it is then released into the plasma for general circulation and distribution to other tissues.[10] Copper is lost from the system in the feces when entero-cytes are sloughed off into the lumen. When the copper in bile is not reabsorbed, it, too, is lost in the feces.

How Much Copper Should We Consume?

As with iron and zinc, our need for copper is small, but our dietary intakes are variable and, as we have seen, absorption is influenced by a number of factors. People who eat a varied diet can easily meet their requirements for copper. High zinc intakes can reduce copper absorption and, subsequently, copper status. In fact, zinc supplementation is used as a treatment for a rare genetic disorder called Wilson's disease, in which copper toxicity occurs. High iron intakes can also interfere with copper absorption. The RDA for copper for men and women aged 19 years and older is 900 μg/day. The UL for adults aged 19 years and older is 10 mg/day.

Good food sources of copper include organ meats, seafood, nuts, and seeds. Whole-grain foods are also relatively good sources. **Figure 12.8** reviews some foods relatively high in copper.

The long-term effects of copper toxicity are not well studied in humans. However, accidental copper toxicity has occurred by drinking beverages that have come into contact with copper.[14] Toxicity symptoms include abdominal pain and cramps, nausea, diarrhea, and vomiting. Liver damage occurs in the extreme cases of copper toxicity seen with Wilson's disease and other health conditions associated with excessive copper levels. In Wilson's disease, the copper accumulates in the liver because the liver cells cannot incor-porate the copper into ceruloplasmin or eliminate it in the bile.[14]

Copper deficiency is rare but can occur in premature infants fed milk-based formulas and in adults fed prolonged formulated diets that are deficient in copper. Deficiency symptoms include anemia, reduced levels of white blood cells, and osteopo-rosis in infants and growing children, in whom the lack of copper contributes to bone demineralization.

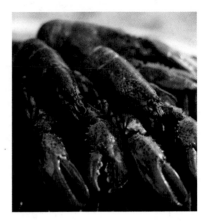

Lobster is a food that contains copper.

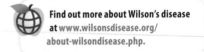

Find out more about Wilson's disease at www.wilsonsdisease.org/about-wilsondisease.php.

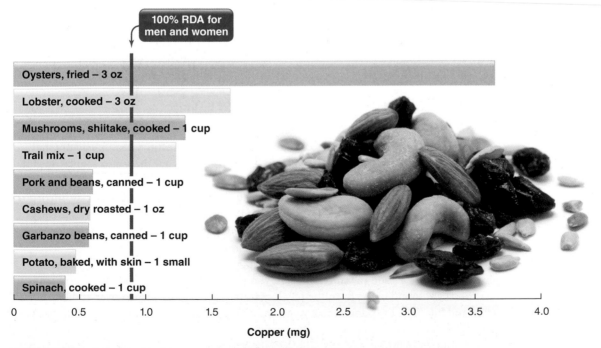

100% RDA for men and women

- Oysters, fried – 3 oz
- Lobster, cooked – 3 oz
- Mushrooms, shiitake, cooked – 1 cup
- Trail mix – 1 cup
- Pork and beans, canned – 1 cup
- Cashews, dry roasted – 1 oz
- Garbanzo beans, canned – 1 cup
- Potato, baked, with skin – 1 small
- Spinach, cooked – 1 cup

Copper (mg): 0   0.5   1.0   1.5   2.0   2.5   3.0   3.5   4.0

FIGURE 12.8 Common food sources of copper. The RDA for copper is 900 μg/day for men and women. (*Source:* Data from US Department of Agriculture, Agricultural Research Service. 2005. USDA Nutrient Database for Standard Reference, Release 21. www.ars.usda.gov/Services/docs.htm?docid=8964.)

RECAP

Zinc is a trace mineral that is a part of almost 100 enzymes that affect virtually every body system. It plays a critical role in hemoglobin synthesis, physical growth and sexual maturation, and immune function and assists in fighting oxidative damage. For adults, the RDA for zinc is 8 mg/d. Copper is a component of ceruloplasmin, a protein that is critical for the proper transport of iron. This trace mineral is also a cofactor in energy metabolism, in the production of the connective tissues collagen and elastin, and in the superoxide dismutase antioxidant enzyme system. For adults, the RDA for copper is 900 µg/day. ■

A Profile of Vitamins That Maintain Blood Health

The vitamins recognized as playing a critical role in maintaining blood health include vitamin K, vitamin B_6, folate, and vitamin B_{12} (see Table 12.1, page 473). Each of these vitamins has multiple functions, some of which were discussed in previous chapters. Here, we focus on their role in blood health.

Vitamin K

Vitamin K is a fat-soluble vitamin important for both bone and blood health. Although a number of compounds exhibit vitamin K activity, the primary forms are phylloquinones and menaquinones. Phylloquinones are the form of vitamin K found in green plants and the primary form of vitamin K in our diet, whereas menaquinones are synthesized in the intestine from bacteria. The role of vitamin K in the synthesis of proteins involved in maintaining bone density was discussed in detail earlier (see pp. 451–452, Chapter 11). In this section, we focus primarily on its role in blood health.

Functions of Vitamin K

Vitamin K acts as a coenzyme that assists in the synthesis of a number of proteins involved in the coagulation of blood, including *prothrombin* and the *procoagulants, factors VII, IX,* and *X*. Without adequate vitamin K, the blood does not clot properly: clotting time can be delayed or clotting may even fail to occur. The failure of the blood to clot can lead to increased bleeding from even minor wounds, as well as internal hemorrhaging.

What Factors Alter Vitamin K Absorption and Balance?

Vitamin K not only is found in food but also is synthesized in the intestine; thus, the amount of vitamin K needed from the diet will depend on intestinal health. Factors that reduce the ability of the gastrointestinal bacteria to produce vitamin K also reduce our total vitamin K status.

Because vitamin K is a fat-soluble vitamin, it is absorbed into the enterocyte, incorporated into chylomicrons, and then released into the lymphatic system with other dietary fats and fat-soluble vitamins. Any factors, either dietary or intestinal, that disrupt fat absorption will also disrupt vitamin K absorption.

Vitamin K is found in all the circulating lipoproteins, and assessment of plasma phylloquinone is a good measure of recent vitamin K intake.[15] Although both forms of vitamin K are found in the liver, the phylloquinones are rapidly turned over and lost in the urine and bile. The liver does not store vitamin K as it does other fat-soluble vitamins.

How Much Vitamin K Should We Consume?

Our needs for vitamin K are relatively small, but intakes of this nutrient in the United States are highly variable because vitamin K is found in relatively few foods.[3] Healthful

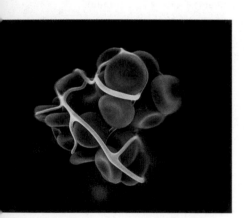

Blood clotting. Without enough vitamin K, the blood will not clot properly.

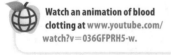

Watch an animation of blood clotting at www.youtube.com/ watch?v=036GFPRH5-w.

intestinal bacteria produce vitamin K in the large intestine, providing us with an important nondietary source. The AI for vitamin K for adults 19 years of age and older is 120 µg/day and 90 µg/day for men and women, respectively. There is no UL established for vitamin K at this time.[3]

In general, green, leafy vegetables are the major sources of vitamin K in our diet. Good sources include collard greens, kale, spinach, broccoli, brussels sprouts, and cabbage. Soybean and canola oils are also good sources.

There are no known side effects associated with consuming large amounts of vitamin K from supplements or from food.[3] In the past, a synthetic form of vitamin K was used for therapeutic purposes and was shown to cause liver damage; this form is no longer used.

Vitamin K deficiency inhibits the blood's ability to clot, resulting in excessive bleeding and even severe hemorrhaging in some cases. Fortunately, vitamin K deficiency is rare in humans. People with diseases that cause malabsorption of fat, such as celiac disease, Crohn's disease, and cystic fibrosis, can suffer secondarily from a deficiency of vitamin K. Newborns are typically given an injection of vitamin K at birth, as they lack the intestinal bacteria necessary to produce this nutrient.

As discussed previously (in Chapter 11), the impact of vitamin K deficiency on bone health is under investigation. Emerging research suggests that vitamin K may enhance the actions of vitamin D and calcium on bone.[16] Moreover, observational studies show that individuals with insufficient vitamin K have lower bone mass and increased hip fracture risk.[17]

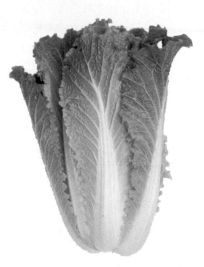

Green, leafy vegetables are a good source of vitamin K.

Vitamin B$_6$

Vitamin B$_6$ is essential for the synthesis of heme, the importance of which you learned about in the discussion of iron earlier in this chapter. It is required for the formation of the porphyrin rings that surround iron (see the lower portion of Figure 12.2) and therefore is an integral part of the heme complex. Without vitamin B$_6$, heme synthesis is impaired, just as it is with iron deficiency. For this reason, although we associate microcytic hypochromic anemia with iron deficiency, a deficiency in vitamin B$_6$ can also cause it. However, iron deficiency is the more common cause.

The RDA for vitamin B$_6$ for adult men and women aged 19 to 50 is 1.3 mg/day. In older adults, the RDA increases to 1.5 mg for women and 1.7 mg/day for men. The UL for vitamin B$_6$ is 100 mg/day.

Vitamin B$_6$ is abundant in meats, poultry, fish, and soy-based meat substitutes. Ready-to-eat cereals and starchy vegetables are also good sources. As discussed (in Chapter 8), high-dose supplements of vitamin B$_6$ can be toxic to nerves; however, toxicity is not seen with the consumption of B$_6$ in foods. Vitamin B$_6$ deficiency impairs red blood cell formation, as just discussed, and can result in microcytic anemia. It also impairs protein metabolism and the synthesis of neurotransmitters.

Folate

Folate is a water-soluble vitamin and one of the B-vitamins (discussed in Chapter 8). The generic term *folate* is used for all the various forms of food folate that demonstrate biological activity. Folic acid (pteroylglutamate; see Figure 8.12, page 323) is the form of folate found in most supplements and used in the enrichment and fortification of foods. Folate was originally identified as a growth factor in green, leafy vegetables (foliage), hence the name.[18]

Functions of Folate and Folic Acid in Blood Health

Much of the folate circulating in the blood is attached to transport proteins, especially albumin, for transport to cells of the body. The red blood cells also contain folate attached to hemoglobin. Because this folate is not transferred out of the red blood cells to other tissues, it may be a good measure of folate status over the past 3 months—the life of red blood cells.[18] If red blood cell folate levels begin to drop, this indicates that when the red blood cells were being formed, folate was inadequate in the body.

Alterations in total body folate status mimic those seen with iron.[10, 19] As the body has less and less folate available to it, the serum levels of folate begin to decline. This level of folate deficiency is called **negative folate balance (stage I)**. If folate is not increased in the diet or through supplementation, then **folate depletion (stage II)** occurs. This stage of folate deficiency is characterized by both low serum and red blood cell folate, with slightly elevated serum homocysteine concentrations. In **folate-deficiency erythropoiesis (stage III),** the folate levels in the body are low enough that the ability to synthesize new red blood cells is inhibited. Finally, in **folate-deficiency anemia (stage IV),** the number of red blood cells has declined because folate is not available for DNA synthesis, and macrocytic anemia develops. This condition is discussed in more detail shortly.

How Much Folate Should We Consume?

Folate is so important for good health and the prevention of birth defects that in 1998 the US Department of Agriculture (USDA) mandated the fortification with folic acid of enriched breads, flours, corn meals, rice, pastas, and other grain products. Because folic acid is highly available for absorption, the goal of this fortification was to increase folate intake in all Americans and thus decrease the risk for the birth defects and chronic diseases associated with low folate intakes.

The RDA for folate for adult men and women aged 19 years and older is 400 µg/day, with 600 µg/day required for pregnant women.[20] These higher levels of folate were set to minimize the risk for birth defects. The UL for folate is 1,000 µg/day.

Because of fortification, ready-to-eat cereals, bread, and other grain products are among the primary sources of folate in the United States; however, you need to read the label of processed grain products to make sure they contain folate. Other good food sources include liver, spinach, lentils, oatmeal, asparagus, and romaine lettuce.

Role of Folate in Neural Tube Defects

A woman's requirement for folate substantially increases during pregnancy. This is because of the high rate of cellular reproduction required to support the growing uterus, development of the placenta, expansion of the mother's red blood cells, and development of the embryo/fetus. Inadequate folate intake during pregnancy can cause macrocytic anemia. As noted previously (in Chapter 8), it also increases the risk for birth defects.

Neural tube defects (NTDs) are the most common malformations of the central nervous system that occur during embryonic and fetal development. The neural tube, which is formed by the fourth week of pregnancy, is a primitive structure that eventually develops into the brain and spinal cord of the fetus. In a folate-deficient environment, the tube will fail to fold and close properly. The resultant defect in the newborn depends on the degree of failure. The most common NTD is spina bifida (literally, "a cleft spine"), in which a portion of the spinal cord protrudes outside of the vertebral column.[21] Some neural tube defects are minor and can be surgically repaired; others result in paralysis, and still others are fatal. (The role of folate and NTDs during pregnancy are described in more detail in Chapter 16, pages 645-647.)

The nutritional challenge with NTDs is that they occur very early in a woman's pregnancy, almost always before a woman knows she is pregnant. Thus, adequate folate intake is extremely important for all sexually active women of childbearing age, whether or not they intend to become pregnant. To prevent NTDs, it is recommended that all women capable of becoming pregnant consume 400 µg of folate daily from supplements, fortified foods, or both in addition to the folate they consume in their standard diet.[20] The impact of folic acid fortification on the incidence of spina bifida in

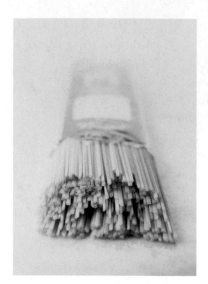

Ready-to-eat grain products, such as pasta, are often fortified with folic acid.

negative folate balance (stage I) The first stage of folate depletion, in which the body has less folate available to it and serum levels of folate begin to decline.

folate depletion (stage II) The second stage of folate depletion, in which both serum and red blood cell folate levels are low.

folate-deficiency erythropoiesis (stage III) The third stage of folate depletion, in which body levels of folate are so low that the ability to make new red blood cells is impaired.

folate-deficiency anemia (stage IV) A state of severe folate depletion in which there is inadequate folate for a long enough time that the number of red blood cells has declined.

neural tube defects (NTDs) The most common malformations of the central nervous system that occur during fetal development. A folate deficiency can cause neural tube defects.

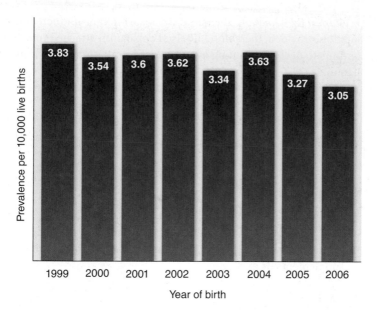

FIGURE 12.9 Prevalence of spina bifida in the years following mandatory folate fortification. (*Source:* Centers for Disease Control and Prevention, Spina bifida, data and statistics, 2011.)

the United States is shown in **Figure 12.9**. Notice the dramatic decrease after fortification was introduced in 1998.

Role of Folate in Macrocytic Anemia

Macrocytic anemias are characterized by the production of larger-than-normal red blood cells (macrocytes) containing insufficient hemoglobin, thus inhibiting adequate transport of oxygen. Symptoms of macrocytic anemia are similar to the symptoms that occur with microcytic anemias and include weakness, fatigue, difficulty concentrating, irritability, headache, shortness of breath, and reduced work tolerance. A severe folate deficiency is a common cause of macrocytic anemia. Folate deficiency impairs DNA synthesis, which impairs the normal production of red blood cells. Because vitamin B_{12} deficiency causes similar symptoms, it is important to determine if the macrocytic anemia observed is due to a folate or a vitamin B_{12} deficiency.

Vitamin B_{12} (Cyanocobalamin)

Vitamin B_{12} was introduced earlier (in Chapter 8). See Figure 8.14 (page 326) for a diagram of the structure of cyanocobalamin, which is derived when vitamin B_{12} is purified from natural sources.[18]

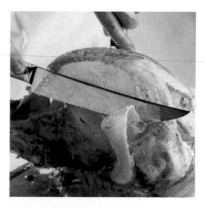

Turkey contains vitamin B_{12}.

Functions of Vitamin B_{12} in Blood Health

Vitamin B_{12} is part of coenzymes that assist with DNA synthesis, which is necessary for the proper formation of red blood cells.[10] It is also necessary for the regeneration of folic acid during red blood cell formation. As discussed (in Chapter 8), alterations in total body vitamin B_{12} status mimic those seen with iron and folate, with states of deficiency developing as the amount of vitamin B_{12} decreases in the body.[10] As vitamin B_{12} status decreases, the body's ability to synthesize new red blood cells decreases:

- *Stage I, or negative vitamin B_{12} balance:* a decline in the blood level of cobalamin attached to its transport protein. This occurs as vitamin B_{12} absorption declines, decreasing the amount of total vitamin B_{12} available to the body.

macrocytic anemia A form of anemia manifested as the production of larger than normal red blood cells containing insufficient hemoglobin, which inhibits adequate transport of oxygen; also called megaloblastic anemia. Macrocytic anemia can be caused by a severe folate deficiency or by vitamin B_{12} deficiency.

- *Stage II, or vitamin B_{12} depletion.* If vitamin B_{12} absorption is not increased or B_{12} supplementation provided, then blood levels of cobalamin attached to its transport protein continue to decline, resulting in a decreased saturation of the transport protein with cobalamin.
- *Stage III, or vitamin B_{12}–deficiency erythropoiesis.* The body's level of vitamin B_{12} is so low that the ability to synthesize new red blood cells is inhibited.
- *Stage IV, called vitamin B_{12}–deficiency anemia.* The number of red blood cells has declined because vitamin B_{12} is not available for DNA synthesis, and macrocytic anemia develops.

How Much Vitamin B_{12} Should We Consume?

The RDA for vitamin B_{12} for adult men and women aged 19 and older is 2.4 µg/day. Vitamin B_{12} is found primarily in dairy products, eggs, meats, poultry, fish, and shellfish. Individuals consuming a vegan diet need to eat foods that are fortified with vitamin B_{12} or take vitamin B_{12} supplements or injections.

Role of Vitamin B_{12} in Macrocytic Anemia

Pernicious anemia is classified as a type of macrocytic anemia and is associated with vitamin B_{12} deficiency. Pernicious anemia occurs at the end stage of an **autoimmune** disorder that causes the loss of various cells in the stomach, including the parietal cells that produce intrinsic factor. As you learned in Chapter 8, intrinsic factor binds to vitamin B_{12} in the small intestine and aids its absorption into the enterocyte. Without intrinsic factor, vitamin B_{12} cannot be absorbed from the gut. It is estimated that approximately 3% of elderly individuals test positive for intrinsic factor antibodies, suggesting that they do not make intrinsic factor.[18]

Macrocytic anemia can also occur in people who consume little or no vitamin B_{12} in their diet, such as people following a vegan diet. It is also commonly seen in people with malabsorption disorders, such as people with tapeworm infestation of the gut, as the worms take up the vitamin B_{12} before it can be absorbed by the intestines.

In addition to the symptoms associated with all anemias—such as pale skin, reduced energy and exercise tolerance, fatigue, and shortness of breath—lack of B_{12} also causes the destruction of the myelin sheath covering nerve cells, which facilitates impulse transmission. Thus, patients lose the ability to perform coordinated movements and to maintain body positioning. Central nervous system involvement can lead to irritability, confusion, depression, and even paranoia. As we saw in the scenario of Mr. Katz (in Chapter 8), after the onset of central nervous system–involved symptoms, even prompt intramuscular injections of vitamin B_{12} can only partially reverse the deficits.

As mentioned earlier, a deficiency of either folate or vitamin B_{12} causes similar symptoms, and high doses of folate supplements can mask the physical symptoms of vitamin B_{12} deficiency, so that this deficiency progresses unchecked and causes neurologic damage.[20] Thus, before treatment for macrocytic anemia can occur, the cause must be identified.

pernicious anemia A form of macrocytic anemia that is the primary cause of a vitamin B_{12} deficiency; occurs at the end stage of an autoimmune disorder that causes the loss of various cells in the stomach.

autoimmune A destructive immune response directed toward an individual's own tissues.

RECAP

Vitamin K is a fat-soluble vitamin and coenzyme that is important for blood clotting and bone metabolism. Bacteria manufacture vitamin K in the large intestine. Vitamin B_6, folate, and vitamin B_{12} are water-soluble vitamins essential in energy metabolism and blood health. All are involved in the synthesis of new red blood cells. Deficiency of vitamin B_6 can result in a form of microcytic anemia, whereas deficiency of folate or B_{12} can result in macrocytic anemia. ∎

What Is the Immune System, and How Does It Function?

A healthy immune system protects the body from infectious diseases, helps heal wounds, and guards against the development of cancers. Made up of cells and tissues throughout the body, the immune system acts as an integrated network to carry out surveillance against invaders and destroy them before they can cause significant tissue damage. Although immune cells communicate with one another extensively, each cell has a specialized protective function in either nonspecific or specific immunity.

Nonspecific Immune Function Protects Against All Potential Invaders

Nonspecific immune function is the body's primary defense against microbes, airborne particles, venom, and ingested toxins. Nonspecific immunity is active even if you are encountering the invader for the first time. Because even infants have all of the cells and tissues required for it to operate effectively, it is also called *innate immunity.*

Nonspecific defenses include intact skin and healthy mucous membranes, which block invaders from entering the blood, lungs, and other deeper tissues. Coughing, sneezing, vomiting, and diarrhea all expel harmful agents before they can take hold. Foodborne microbes can also be destroyed by stomach acid.

In addition, a variety of immune cells, including macrophages, neutrophils, and natural killer (NK) cells, work together to directly kill a wide variety of harmful microbes, or to kill infected body cells or cells with damaged DNA that otherwise could multiply to form a tumor.

Finally, our nonspecific defenses include the release of inflammatory chemicals that cause discomfort, loss of appetite, fatigue, and fever: most disease-causing microbes thrive at normal body temperature, whereas a high temperature inhibits their growth. Fever also facilitates the actions of cells and chemicals involved in repair.

Together, our nonspecific defenses can inhibit the penetration and reproduction of invaders until the slower-acting, but more effective, specific immune system is activated.

Specific Immune Function Protects Against Identified Antigens

Specific immune function is directed against recognized **antigens**—that is, portions of microbes or other foes that the immune system has encountered before and recognizes as foreign, or *non-self.* But how does this recognition occur?

The first time the immune system encounters a substance with an antigen that is detected as non-self, it produces a primary immune response. This response takes several days to peak, but eventually, in most cases, it destroys the invader. A key process within that primary immune response is the production of **memory cells** dedicated to the task of seeking out and destroying any substance bearing that particular antigen. Memory cells remain in circulation (in some cases, for life), so that any subsequent encounter with the same antigen causes a faster and stronger response. Often, the response is so fast that the person does not even feel sick.

Two Main Types of Cells Provide Specific Immunity

In specific immune responses, two primary types of immune cells are activated:

- **B cells** are a type of white blood cell. During a primary immune response, B cells differentiate into two types: the memory cells just described and **plasma cells.** The job of plasma cells is to produce thousands of *antibodies,* proteins that attach to recognized antigens on invaders and flag them for destruction.

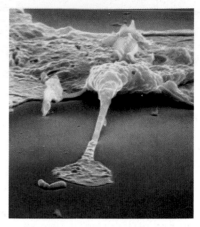

A macrophage is a type of nonspecific immune cell. The one shown here is about to engulf an invading microbe.

nonspecific immune function Generalized body defense mechanisms that protect against the entry of foreign agents, such as microbes and allergens; also called *innate immunity.*

specific immune function The strongest defense against pathogens. It requires adaptation of white blood cells that recognize antigens and that multiply to protect against the pathogens carrying those antigens; also called *adaptive immunity* or *acquired immunity.*

antigens Parts of a molecule, usually large proteins, from microbes, toxins, or other substances that are recognized by immune cells and activate an immune response.

memory cells White blood cells that recognize a particular antigen and circulate in the body, ready to respond if the antigen is encountered again. The purpose of vaccination is to create memory cells.

B cells White blood cells that can become either antibody-producing plasma cells or memory cells.

plasma cells White blood cells that have differentiated from activated B cells and produce millions of antibodies to an antigen during an infection.

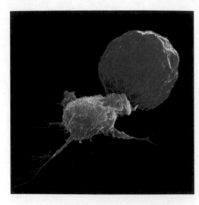

Natural killer (NK) cells are part of our nonspecific defenses. Here, an NK cell attacks two cancer cells.

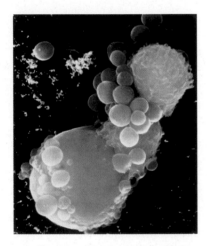

Two cytotoxic T cells (orange) killing another cell (mauve).

T cells White blood cells that are of several varieties, including cytotoxic T cells and helper T cells.

cytotoxic T cells Activated T cells that kill infected body cells.

helper T cells Activated T cells that secrete chemicals needed to activate other immune cells.

vaccination The method of administering a small amount of antigen to elicit an immune response for the purpose of developing memory cells that will protect against the disease at a later time.

antiserum Human or animal serum that contains antibodies to a particular antigen because of previous exposure to the disease or to a vaccine containing antigens from that infectious agent.

■ **T cells** are also white blood cells. They differentiate into several types, the most important of which are cytotoxic T cells and helper T cells. As their name suggests, **cytotoxic T cells** are toxic to body cells harboring microbes or any other non-self substances. For instance, by killing body cells that have been infected by a flu virus, they keep the virus from multiplying and spreading. **Helper T cells** don't kill directly. Rather, they manufacture chemicals that activate B cells and cytotoxic T cells.

Specific Immunity Can Be Acquired in a Variety of Ways

There are four primary ways in which humans acquire immunity to specific invaders:

■ One natural way is to have a disease once. For example, if you had mumps as a child, you will never get it again, because memory cells against mumps are continuously circulating throughout your body.

■ **Vaccinations** (also called *immunizations*) are another way to develop immunity. When you are vaccinated, a small amount of antigen from a particular microbe is injected into your body. Your plasma cells produce antibodies against the antigen, and memory cells begin to circulate. If you encounter the microbe later, your immune response will protect you from getting sick.

■ When a woman is pregnant, antibodies from her blood pass into the bloodstream of her fetus. These maternal antibodies protect a newborn during the first few months of life while the specific immune system is maturing. In addition, breast milk contains antibodies that protect the infant for as long as he or she nurses.

■ The injection of **antiserum** can provide immediate protection from a specific foe—for instance, to snake venom in the bloodstream of a victim of a snakebite. Antiserum is a pharmacologic preparation containing antibodies to specific antigens, such as those in snake venom. Injection of this antibody-rich serum provides immediate protection. Without it, the snake venom would be fatal before the victim's immune system could produce antibodies.

Immune System Malfunction Can Cause Chronic Inflammation and Infection

A malfunctioning immune system can damage body tissues or prevent the resolution of infection. For example, during allergic reactions, the immune system "interprets" harmless proteins that enter the body from the environment or food as dangerous and produces a hypersensitivity immune response. This can provoke a variety of symptoms, from a rash to wheezing to intestinal inflammation. Autoimmune responses occur when the body's own proteins are mistaken for pathogens. This occurs, for example, in rheumatoid arthritis and lupus and results in a chronic inflammatory state.

In some people, the immune system is compromised and cannot effectively quell infections. Chronic infection is commonly seen in malnourished individuals, as well as in people with immunodeficiency diseases. Cancer patients and transplant recipients also are more susceptible to infection when they are taking immunosuppressive drugs.

How Does Nutrition Affect the Immune System?

A nourishing diet provides all the nutrients the immune system needs to carry out its defense of the body. Single-nutrient deficiencies or subclinical deficiencies can cause subtle, but important, abnormalities in immune function, even in apparently healthy people. This type of malnutrition is common in hospitalized individuals and the elderly.[22] Recent studies have demonstrated that viruses multiplying in malnourished hosts actually become more infective and destructive than viruses multiplying in well-nourished hosts.[23]

Moreover, protein–energy malnutrition and severe deficiencies of several micronutrients reduce immune function. This problem is a leading cause of death in children in developing countries.[24]

Protein–Energy Malnutrition Impairs Immune Function

Malnutrition and infection participate in a vicious cycle: malnutrition increases the risk for infection; infection depresses appetite and often causes vomiting and diarrhea; decreased appetite, vomiting, and diarrhea cause malnutrition, which increases vulnerability to infection. Specifically, protein–energy malnutrition (see Chapter 6) is known to severely diminish the ability of the immune system to respond to antigens. Malnourished children show reduced production of antibodies and diminished capacity of their immune cells to kill bacteria.[25] In addition, a healthy immune response requires energy and amino acids, two things that are in short supply in a malnourished individual. The synergistic effect of protein–energy malnutrition and infection in diminishing both the capacity of the immune response and nutritional status is now widely recognized. Because even moderate nutrient deficiencies impair immune function, it has been suggested that decreased **immunocompetence** is a sensitive indicator of reduced nutritional status.

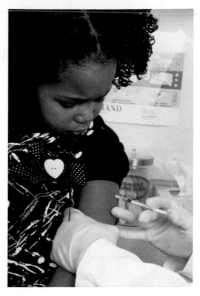

Vaccinations provide active immunity.

Obesity Increases the Incidence and Severity of Infections

Obesity has become a public health issue much more recently than the problem of protein–energy malnutrition. Therefore, fewer studies have been done on the effects of obesity on immune function. However, obesity has been associated with increased incidence of infection, delayed wound healing, and poor antibody response to vaccination.[26]

The mechanisms underlying lower immune function in obese individuals are unclear. Most, but not all, studies show a lower ability of B and T cells from obese individuals to multiply in response to stimulation. This inhibition is resolved after weight loss.[27] Short-term fasting by obese individuals appears to improve the killing capacity of macrophages and to increase serum concentrations of antibodies.[26] More consistent are the data documenting elevated levels of macrophages, inflammatory chemicals, and immune proteins in obese individuals, suggesting the existence of a low-grade inflammatory state.[28, 29] This inflammatory state is currently thought to increase the likelihood that obese individuals will develop asthma, hypertension, cardiovascular disease, and type 2 diabetes.[28, 29]

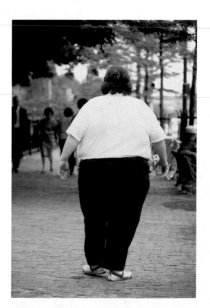

Obesity has been linked to disorders involving chronic inflammation, such as asthma, hypertension, heart disease, and type 2 diabetes.

Essential Fatty Acids Make Signaling Molecules for the Immune System

As previously noted (in Chapter 5), the essential fatty acids are precursors for important signaling molecules called eicosanoids. The immune system requires certain eicosanoids to respond appropriately to threatening agents. Experimental dietary deficiency of essential fatty acids impairs aspects of the immune response. On the other hand, excess amounts given by supplementation can also diminish immune function.[30]

This may be due in part to the importance of the *ratio* of omega-6 and omega-3 fatty acids in modulating the immune response. For example, omega-6 fatty acids are thought to promote the inflammatory response, which helps contain infection. In contrast, clinical trials have shown that omega-3 fatty acids diminish inflammation, including within blood vessels, and thus provide protection against heart disease. Indeed, the potential health benefits of omega-3 fatty acids in fish oils were first observed in Greenland Eskimos who had low levels of heart disease. However, their high incidence of tuberculosis raised the question of whether omega-3 fatty acids might diminish immune response to infections.

immunocompetence The body's ability to adequately produce an effective immune response to an antigen.

For these reasons, caution against both deficient and excessive intake of omega-3 fatty acids is prudent for maintaining appropriate immune response.[31] Both the absolute amount of omega-6 and omega-3 fatty acids and their ratio are considered important for health. The dietary reference intakes for adults over age 19 are 17 g omega-6 (linoleic acid) and 1.6 g omega-3 (linolenic acid) for men and 12 g omega-6 (linoleic acid) and 1.1 g omega-3 (linolenic acid) for women.[32]

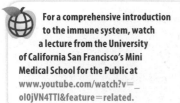

For a comprehensive introduction to the immune system, watch a lecture from the University of California San Francisco's Mini Medical School for the Public at www.youtube.com/watch?v=_ol0jVN4TTl&feature=related.

Certain Vitamins and Minerals Are Critical to a Strong Immune Response

Although all essential nutrients are likely needed in some measure for effective immune function, certain micronutrient deficiencies and excesses have been recognized as particularly important:

- *Vitamin A.* As early as the 1920s, vitamin A was called "the anti-infective vitamin" because it is needed to maintain the mucosal surfaces of the respiratory, gastrointestinal, and genitourinary tracts and for differentiation of immune system cells. More than 100 clinical trials have shown that vitamin A supplementation in populations with low vitamin A status reduces the incidence and fatality of infections of measles, malaria, and diarrheal diseases.[33] However, animal studies suggest that excessive vitamin A can actually suppress immune response and increase susceptibility to pathogens.[34] Thus, screening for vitamin A status before administering supplements has been recommended as part of public health efforts to combat deficiency.[35]
- *Vitamins C and E.* The immune activities of defensive cells such as macrophages require oxygen and generate a highly reactive molecule, called a *reactive oxygen species*, that can damage the cell membrane if there is insufficient antioxidant protection. Both vitamin C and vitamin E provide this protection.
- *Zinc.* The importance of zinc to immune function was suggested by the observation that Middle Easteners whose growth was stunted by zinc deficiency also died of infections by their early twenties.[36] Zinc is now known to be necessary for gene expression and enzyme activation for B and T cell proliferation. Even marginal zinc deficiency impairs immune response. However, excessive zinc supplementation depresses immunity, possibly by causing copper deficiency.
- *Copper.* Even a marginal copper deficiency reduces a growth factor needed for immune cells to multiply.[37] Lack of circulating neutrophils is a classic sign of copper deficiency in humans. Lack of copper also impairs the ability of both the neutrophils and macrophages to kill pathogens.
- *Iron.* Iron deficiency reduces the body's capacity to mount an effective immune response. The functions of B cells, T cells, and natural killer cells are clearly impaired in iron-deficiency anemia.[38] Macrophages take up and store iron during an infection and seem unaffected by deficiency. This storage is thought to be beneficial because it keeps iron away from invading microbes, which require iron to multiply. This may explain why some studies show that iron supplementation given to children during infection is detrimental, and why iron toxicity increases the rate of infections.[39] In addition, excessive iron is a potent oxidant that can damage immune-cell membranes.
- *Selenium.* In trace amounts, selenium is necessary for the synthesis of thirty-five body proteins, many of which are important enzymes.[40] Selenium has two roles in immune function. It is a required coenzyme for glutathione peroxidase, an important antioxidant enzyme in neutrophils and other immune cells. It also promotes proper B and T cell proliferation and antibody production. Selenium deficiency in an infected host also permits viruses to multiply over a longer time period and to mutate into more pathogenic strains.[23] However, selenium excess also impairs immune cell activity.[41] Thus, as with vitamin A and iron, both excess and deficiency of selenium compromise the ability to resolve infection.

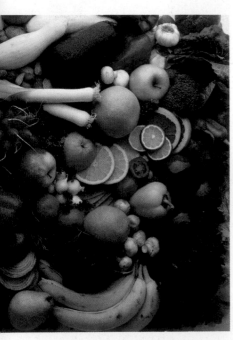

Vitamins E and C, found in fruits and vegetables, can contribute to immune system health.

RECAP

The main function of the immune system is to protect the body against foreign agents. Nonspecific defenses include skin, mucous membranes, enzymes, inflammatory chemicals, and certain defensive cells. Specific immunity is provided by B cells and T cells. B cells include plasma cells, which produce antibodies, and memory cells, which persist in the body, seeking the antigens to which they are sensitized. Cytotoxic T cells kill infected body cells, and helper T cells help B cells and cytotoxic T cells proliferate. A nourishing diet is important in optimizing immune response. Protein–energy malnutrition increases the frequency and severity of infection. Obesity compromises immune response, exacerbating infection and inflammation. Balanced consumption of omega-6 and omega-3 essential fatty acids is needed for the production of signaling molecules important in immune function. Vitamins A, C, and E and the minerals zinc, copper, iron, and selenium are all necessary for appropriate immune function. ■

Chapter Review

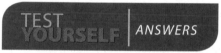

TEST YOURSELF | ANSWERS

1 **T** This deficiency is particularly common in infants, children, and women of childbearing age.

2 **F** To reduce their risk of having a baby with serious central nervous system defects, all women capable of becoming pregnant should take folate supplements. Beginning folate supplementation after recognizing a pregnancy, typically following the first missed menstrual period, may be too late to prevent a neural tube defect.

3 **T** People who consume a vegan diet need to pay particularly close attention to consuming enough vitamin B_{12}, iron, and zinc. In some cases, these individuals may need to take supplements to consume adequate amounts of these nutrients.

4 **F** The term *anemia* means "without blood" and can refer to any condition in which hemoglobin levels are low. Iron-deficiency anemia is just one type.

5 **T** Fever increases body temperature, making the internal environment inhospitable to microbes and increasing the rate of protective immune reactions. Vomiting and diarrhea expel microbes and toxins from the gastrointestinal tract before they can cause widespread tissue damage.

Summary

- Blood is the only fluid tissue in the body. It has four components: erythrocytes, or red blood cells; leukocytes, or white blood cells; platelets; and plasma, or the fluid portion of blood.

- Blood is critical for transporting oxygen and nutrients to cells and for removing waste products from cells so that these products can be properly excreted.

- Iron is a trace mineral. Almost two-thirds of the iron in the body is found in hemoglobin, the oxygen-carrying protein in blood. One of the primary functions of iron is to assist with the transportation of oxygen in blood. Iron is a cofactor for many of the enzymes involved in the metabolism of carbohydrates, fats, and protein. It is also a part of the antioxidant enzyme system that fights free radicals.

- *Anemia* is a term that means "without blood." Severe iron deficiency results in microcytic anemia, in which the production of normal, healthy red blood cells decreases and hemoglobin levels are inadequate. Deficiency of vitamin B_6 can also cause microcytic anemia.

- Zinc is a trace mineral that acts as a cofactor in the production of hemoglobin; in the superoxide dismutase antioxidant enzyme system; in the metabolism of carbohydrates, fats, and proteins; and in activating vitamin A in the retina. Zinc is also critical for cell reproduction and growth and for proper development and functioning of the immune system.

- Copper is a trace mineral that functions as a cofactor in the metabolic pathways that produce energy, in the production of collagen and elastin, and as part of the superoxide dismutase antioxidant enzyme system. Copper is also a component of ceruloplasmin, a protein needed for the proper transport of iron.

- Vitamin K is a fat-soluble vitamin that acts as a coenzyme assisting in the coagulation of blood. Vitamin K is also a coenzyme in the synthesis of proteins that assist in maintaining bone density.

- Three B-vitamins involved in the synthesis of red blood cells are vitamin B_6, folate, and vitamin B_{12}.

- Neural tube defects, which can result from inadequate folate intake during the first few weeks of pregnancy, are the most common malformations of the fetal central nervous system. Some neural tube defects are minor and can be treated with surgery; other neural tube defects are fatal.

- Macrocytic anemia results from folate or vitamin B_{12} deficiency and causes the formation of excessively large red blood cells that have reduced hemoglobin. Symptoms are similar to those of microcytic anemia. One form of macrocytic anemia, called pernicious anemia, is caused by a deficit of intrinsic factor, which in turn results in vitamin B_{12} deficiency.

- A healthy immune system is a network of cells and tissues that protects us from harmful agents.

- Nonspecific defenses include the skin and mucosal membranes as well as protective molecules, such as mucus, stomach acid, and enzymes, and immune cells, such as macrophages, neutrophils, and NK cells that destroy invaders.

- Specific immune function is directed against specific antigens. An initial encounter with a foreign agent triggers the development of immune cells that recognize that agent. On subsequent encounters with the same agent, these cells mount a faster, stronger immune response.

- The two primary types of cells involved in specific immunity are B cells and T cells.

- Plasma cells are B cells that produce antibodies that mark antigens for destruction. Memory cells are another type of B cell that, after becoming sensitized to a specific antigen, circulate in the body, seeking that antigen.

- Cytotoxic T cells destroy body cells harboring foreign agents, and helper T cells signal other immune cells to respond.

- Human beings can acquire immunity by experiencing an infection, being vaccinated, receiving maternal antibodies, or receiving an injection of antiserum.

- Malfunctions of the immune system include allergies, autoimmune diseases, chronic inflammation, and immunodeficiencies.

- Both protein–energy malnutrition and obesity impair immune responses.

- A balanced intake of omega-6 and omega-3 essential fatty acids is important for regulating immune function.

- Critical to immune function are vitamins A, C, and E and the minerals zinc, copper, iron, and selenium. In general, both deficiency and excess of these micronutrients can impair immune response.

MasteringNutrition™

To further your understanding, go online and apply what you've learned to real-life case studies that will help you master the content!

Review Questions

1. The micronutrient most closely associated with blood clotting is
   a. iron.
   b. vitamin K.
   c. zinc.
   d. vitamin B_{12}.

2. Which of the following statements about iron is true?
   a. Iron is stored primarily in the liver, the blood-vessel walls, and the heart muscle.
   b. Iron is a component of hemoglobin, myoglobin, and certain enzymes.
   c. Iron is a component of red blood cells, platelets, and plasma.
   d. Excess iron is stored primarily in the form of ferritin, cytochromes, and intrinsic factor.

3. Water-soluble vitamins essential for the formation of red blood cells include
   a. iron, vitamin K, and folate.
   b. vitamins K, B_6, and B_{12}.
   c. vitamins B_6, folate, and B_{12}.
   d. vitamins A, C, and E.

4. Which of the following cells produce antibodies?
   a. plasma cells
   b. antigens
   c. macrophages
   d. helper T cells

5. Breastfeeding promotes infant health because breast milk contains
   a. antiserum.
   b. ceruloplasmin.
   c. intrinsic factor.
   d. antibodies.

6. **True or false?** Blood has four components: erythrocytes, leukocytes, platelets, and plasma.

7. **True or false?** Iron deficiency causes pernicious anemia.

8. **True or false?** Wilson's disease occurs when copper deficiency allows the accumulation of iron in the body.

9. **True or false?** Studies suggest that excessive vitamin A, iron, or selenium can impair immune function.

10. **True or false?** Macrocytic anemias can result from deficiency of either folate or vitamin B_{12}.

11. Jessica is 11 years old and has just begun menstruating. She and her family members are vegans (that is, they consume only plant-based foods). Explain why Jessica's parents should be careful that their daughter consumes not only adequate iron and zinc but also adequate vitamin C.

12. Robert is a lacto-ovo-vegetarian. His typical daily diet includes milk, yogurt, cheese, eggs, nuts, seeds, legumes, whole grains, and a wide variety of fruits and vegetables. He does not take any supplements. What, if any, micronutrients are likely to be inadequate in his diet?

13. Janine is 23 years old and engaged to be married. She is 40 lb overweight, she has hypertension, and her mother suffered a mild stroke recently, at age 45. For all these reasons, Janine is highly motivated to lose weight and has put herself on a strict, low-carbohydrate diet recommended by a friend. She now scrupulously avoids breads, cereals, pastries, pasta, rice, and "starchy" fruits and vegetables. Identify two reasons Janine should begin taking a folate supplement.

14. What health risk do people who are emaciated and people who are obese have in common? Why?

Math Review

15. About 2 g of zinc are stored in the body of an average adult. An adult male consumes 20 mg of zinc each day. He thereby builds his total body store of zinc every 100 days. Is this statement true or false, and why?

Answers to Review Questions and Math Review can be found online in the MasteringNutrition Study Area.

Web Links

www.ars.usda.gov/ba/bhnrc/ndl
Nutrient Data Laboratory Home Page
Click on "Reports for Single Nutrients" to find reports listing food sources for selected nutrients.

www.bbc.co.uk/health/healthy_living/complementary_medicine/remedies_vitamins.shtml
BBC Healthy Living: Complementary Medicine: Vitamins
This page provides information on vitamins and minerals, signs of deficiency, therapeutic uses, and food sources.

www.anemia.com
Anemia Lifeline
Visit this site to learn about anemia and its various treatments.

www.unicef.org/nutrition/index.html
UNICEF—Nutrition
This site provides information about micronutrient deficiencies in developing countries and the efforts to combat them.

www.nlm.nih.gov/medlineplus/
Medline Plus, US National Library of Medicine, National Institutes of Health
Search this site for "neural tube defects" and find a wealth of information on the development and prevention of these conditions.

www.kidshealth.org/parent
Kidshealth.org
Search for "immune system" to find a good overview of the immune system.

www.fda.gov
US Food and Drug Administration (FDA)
Click on "Food" and then "Dietary Supplements" for a wealth of information about various dietary supplements and the FDA's regulation of them.

www.dietary-supplements.info.nih.gov
Office of Dietary Supplements (ODS)
Go to this site to obtain current research results and reliable information about dietary supplements.

References

1. World Health Organization. 2012. Nutrition. Micronutrient Deficiencies: Iron Deficiency Anemia. www.who.int/nutrition/topics/ida/en/index.html. (Accessed March 2012.)

2. Crichton, R. R. 2006. Iron. In: Stipanuk, M. H., ed. *Biochemical, Physiological, and Molecular Aspects of Human Nutrition.* Philadelphia: W. B. Saunders, pp. 1001–1042.

3. Institute of Medicine, Food and Nutrition Board. 2001. *Dietary Reference Intakes for Vitamin A, Vitamin K, Arsenic, Boron, Chromium, Copper, Iodine, Iron, Manganese, Molybdenum, Nickel, Silicon, Vanadium, and Zinc.* Washington, DC: National Academy Press.

4. National Institutes of Health, Office of Dietary Supplements. 2007. Iron fact sheet. http://ods.od.nih.gov/pdf/factsheets/iron.pdf. (Accessed March 2012.)

5. Sharp, P. A. 2010. Intestinal iron absorption: regulation by dietary and systemic factors. *Int. J. Vitam. Nutr. Res.* 80(4-5):231–242.

6. Hunt, J. R. 2010. Algorithms for iron and zinc bioavailability: are they accurate? *Int. J. Vitam. Nutr. Res.* 80(4-5):257–262.

7. Spanierman, C. S. 2011. Iron Toxicity in Emergency Medicine. Medscape Reference. Drugs, Diseases and Procedures. http://emedicine.medscape.com/article/815213-followup. (Accessed March 2012.)

8. Duchini, A. 2011. Hemochromatosis. Medscape Reference. Drugs, Disease and Procedures. http://emedicine.medscape.com/article/177216-overview. (Accessed March 2012.)

9. Ganz, T., and E. Nameth. 2011. Hepcidin and disorders of iron metabolism. *Annual Review of Medicine* 62:347–360.

10. Gibson, S. R. 2005. *Principles of Nutritional Assessment,* 2nd edn. New York: Oxford University Press.

11. Tussing-Humphreys, L., C. Pustacioglu, E. Nemeth, and C. Braunschweig. 2012. Rethinking iron regulation and assessment in iron deficiency, anemia of chronic disease, and obesity: introducing hepcidin. *J. Acad. Nutri. Diet.* 112:381–400.

12. Hinton, P. S., C. Giordano, T. Brownlie, and J. D. Hass. 2000. Iron supplementation improves endurance after training in iron-depleted, nonanemic women. *J. Appl. Physiol.* 88:1103–1111.

13. Prasad, A. S. 2009. Impact of the discovery of human zinc deficiency on health. *J. Am. Coll. Nutr.* 28(3):257–265.

14. Grider, A. 2006. Zinc, copper, and manganese. In: Stipanuk, M. H., ed. *Biochemical, Physiological, and Molecular Aspects of Human Nutrition.* Philadelphia: W. B. Saunders, pp. 1043–1067.

15. Wallin, R., and S. M. Huston. 2006. Vitamin K. In: Stipanuk, M. H., ed. *Biochemical, Physiological and Molecular Aspects of Human Nutrition.* Philadelphia: W. B. Saunders, pp. 797–818.

16. Bonjour, J. P., L. Gueguen, C. Palacios, M. J. Shearer, and C. M. Weaver. 2009. Minerals and vitamins in bone health: the potential value of dietary enhancement. *British J. Nutr.* 202(11):1581–1596.

17. Shea, M. K., and S. L. Booth. 2008. Update on the role of vitamin K in skeletal health. *Nutrition Reviews* 66(10):549–557.

18. Shane, B. 2006. Folic acid, vitamin B_{12}, and vitamin B_6. In: Stipanuk, M. H., ed. *Biochemical, Physiological, and Molecular Aspects of Human Nutrition.* Philadelphia: W. B. Saunders, pp. 693–732.

19. Carmel, R. 2006. Folic acid. In: Shils, M. E., M. Shike, A. C. Ross, B. Caballero, and R. J. Cousins, eds. *Modern Nutrition in Health and Disease,* 10th edn. Philadelphia: Lippincott Williams & Wilkins, pp. 470–481.

20. Institute of Medicine, Food and Nutrition Board. 1998. *Dietary Reference Intakes for Thiamin, Riboflavin, Niacin, Vitamin B_6, Folate, Vitamin B_{12}, Pantothenic Acid, Biotin, and Choline.* Washington, DC: National Academy Press.

21. Centers for Disease Control and Prevention. 2011. Spina Bifida, Data and Statistics. www.cdc.gov/ncbddd/spinabifida/data.html. (Accessed March 2012.)

22. Keusch, G. T. 2003. The history of nutrition: malnutrition, infection and immunity. *J. Nutr.* 133:336S–340S.

23. Beck, M. A., J. Handy, and O. A. Levander. 2004. Host nutritional status: the neglected virulence factor. *Trends Microbiol.* 12:417–423.

24. Brundtland, G. H. 2000. Nutrition and infection: malnutrition and mortality in public health. *Nutr. Rev.* 58:S1–4.

25. Scrimshaw, N. S. 2003. Historical concepts of interactions, synergism and antagonism between nutrition and infection. *J. Nutr.* 133:316S–321S.

26. Marti, A., A. Marcos, and J. A. Martinez. 2001. Obesity and immune function relationships. *Obesity Rev.* 2:131–140.

27. Lamas, O., A. Marti, and J. A. Martinez. 2002. Obesity and immunocompetence. *Eur. J. Cin. Nutr.* 56(suppl):S42–S45.

28. Fantuzzi, G. 2005. Adipose tissue, adipokines, and inflammation. *J. Allergy Clin. Immunol.* 115:911–919.

29. Lumeng, C. N., and A. R. Saltiel. 2011. Inflammatory links between obesity and metabolic disease. *Journal of Clinical Investigation* 121(6):2111–2117.

30. Calder, P. C., and C. J. Field. 2002. Fatty acids, inflammation and immunity. In: Calder, P. C., C. J. Field, and H. S. Gill, eds. *Nutrition and Immune Function.* New York: CABI, pp. 57–92.

31. Wu, D. 2004. Modulation of immune and inflammatory responses by dietary lipids. *Curr. Opin. Lipidol.* 15:43–47.

32. Institute of Medicine, Food and Nutrition Board. 2005. *Dietary Reference Intakes for Energy, Carbohydrate, Fiber, Fat, Fatty Acids, Cholesterol, Protein, and Amino Acids (Macronutrients).* Washington, DC: National Academy Press.

33. Semba, R. D. 2002. Vitamin A, infection and immune function. In: Calder, P. C., C. J. Field, and H. S. Gill, eds. *Nutrition and Immune Function.* New York: CABI, pp. 151–169.

34. Field, C. J., I. R. Johnson, and P. D. Schley. 2002. Nutrients and their role in host resistance to infection. *J. Leukoc. Biol.* 71:16–32.

35. Griffiths, J. K. 2000. The vitamin A paradox. *J. Pediatr.* 137:604–607.

36. Prasad, A. Zinc, infection and immune function. In: Calder, P. C., C. J. Field, and H. S. Gill, eds. *Nutrition and Immune Function.* New York: CABI, pp. 193–207.

37. Bonham, M., J. M. O'Connor, B. M. Hannigan, and J. J. Strain. 2002. The immune system as a physiological indicator of marginal copper status? *Br. J. Nutr.* 87:393–403.

38. Ekiz, C., L. Agaoglu, Z. Karakas, N. Gurel, and I. Yalsin. 2005. The effect of iron deficiency on the function of the immune system. *Hematology Journal* 5:579–583.

39. Kuvibidila, S., and B. S. Baliga. 2002. Role of iron in immunity and infection. In: Calder, P. C., C. J. Field, and H. S. Gill, eds. *Nutrition and Immune Function.* New York: CABI, pp. 209–228.

40. McKenzie, R. C., J. R. Arthur, S. M. Miller, T. S. Rafferty, and G. J. Beckett. 2002. Selenium and the immune system. In: Calder, P. C., C. J. Field, and H. S. Gill, eds. *Nutrition and Immune Function.* New York: CABI, pp. 229–250.

41. Nair, M. P., and S. A. Schwartz. 1990. Immunoregulation of natural and lymphokine-activated killer cells by selenium. *Immunopharmacology* 19:177–183.

Do Zinc Lozenges Help Fight the Common Cold?

The common cold has plagued human beings since the beginning of time. Approximately 62 million colds occur in the United States each year.[1] Children suffer from 6 to 10 colds each year, and adults average 2 to 4 per year. Although colds are typically benign, they cause discomfort and stress and result in approximately 20 million school days and 22 million work days lost each year.[1] Colds are also the most common reason people visit a medical professional, accounting for over 100 million primary care visits per year.[2] Finding a cure for the common cold has been at the forefront of modern medicine for many years.

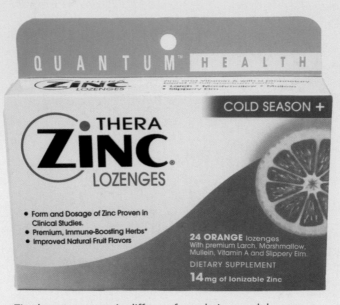

Zinc lozenges come in different formulations and dosages.

It is estimated that more than 200 different viruses can cause a cold. The most frequent causes of adult colds are a group of viruses called rhinoviruses, which account for approximately half of all colds.[2] Even within the rhinovirus category, there are over a 100 different distinct viruses; thus, finding treatments or potential cures for a cold is extremely challenging.

The role of zinc in the overall health of our immune system is well known, but zinc has also been shown to inhibit the replication of rhinoviruses and other viruses that cause the common cold. These specific findings have suggested that taking zinc supplements may reduce the length and severity of colds.[3, 4] Consequently, zinc lozenges were formulated as a means of providing potential relief from cold symptoms. These lozenges are readily found in a variety of formulations and dosages in most drugstores.

Does taking zinc in lozenge form actually reduce the length and severity of a cold? During the past 25 years, numerous research studies have been conducted to try to answer this question. Unfortunately, the results have been mixed.[4] Two recent reviews examined thirteen randomized controlled trials with over 966 participants.[5, 6] The first study found a reduction in the severity and duration of the common cold with zinc lozenges or syrups (30–160 mg/day) if administered within 24–48 hours of the onset of the cold.

Overall, the duration of the cold was reduced by about 1 day. Assessment of the severity of cold symptoms is more difficult, because there is no objective measure, but they did find that severity scores were very modestly reduced with supplementation. However, study participants reported significant negative effects from zinc supplementation as well, including a bad taste and nausea. The second review divided the studies by zinc dose. It found that, if 75 mg/day or less of zinc was given, no effect occurred; however, in three studies in which >75 mg/day of zinc acetate was given, there was a 42% reduction in cold duration. There were five studies that gave ≥75 mg/day of other zinc salts other than zinc acetate. In these studies there was a 20% reduction in cold duration.

Unfortunately, we will probably never know the true effect of zinc lozenges on colds for the following reasons:

- *It is difficult to truly "blind" participants to the treatment.* Because zinc lozenges have a unique taste, it may be difficult to truly "blind" the research participants as to whether they are getting zinc lozenges or a placebo. Knowledge of which lozenge they are taking would bias study participants.
- *Self-reported symptoms are subject to inaccuracy.* Many studies had the research participants self-report changes in symptoms, which may be inaccurate and influenced by mood and other emotional factors.
- *Subject compliance may be suspect.* Typically, participants are required to take the lozenges on a set schedule for 6 to 10 days. Unless they monitor all participants, researchers are forced to rely on the participants' self-reports of their compliance with the study protocol. Differences in compliance could lead to differences in outcomes.
- *A wide variety of viruses cause the common cold.* More than 200 viruses can cause a cold. It is highly unlikely

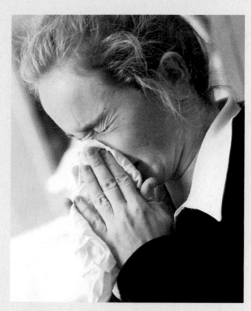

The congestion, fatigue, and other symptoms of the common cold cause absenteeism from work or school, as well as personal discomfort.

that zinc can combat all of them. It is possible that people who do not respond favorably to zinc lozenges are suffering from a cold virus that does not respond to zinc.

■ *Zinc formulations and dosages differ.* The type of zinc formulation and the dosages of zinc consumed by study participants differ across studies, which may determine how quickly the zinc ions are delivered to the tissues in the mouth. These differences most likely have contributed to various responses across studies. As mentioned, it is estimated that, for zinc to be effective, at least 75–80 mg of zinc should be consumed each day and that people should begin using the lozenges within 24 to 48 hours of the onset of cold symptoms. Also, the sweeteners and flavorings found in many zinc lozenges, such as citric acid, sorbitol, and mannitol, may bind the zinc and inhibit its ability to be absorbed into the body, limiting its effectiveness.

Because there is suggestive, but not conclusive, evidence supporting modest effectiveness of zinc lozenges in combating colds, the debate over whether people should take them will most likely continue.

CRITICAL THINKING QUESTIONS

■ Have you ever tried zinc lozenges for a cold? If so, did you find them effective? Were you bothered by any unpleasant side effects, such as a persistent bad taste, alteration in your sense of smell, or nausea?

■ Even if you have only about a 50/50 chance of reducing the length of your cold by 20–40% by taking zinc lozenges, do you think they're worth a try?

A word of caution: if you decide to use zinc lozenges, more is not necessarily better. Excessive or prolonged zinc supplementation can cause other mineral imbalances. Check the label of the product you are using, and do not exceed its recommended dosage or duration of use.

REFERENCES

1. National Institute of Allergy and Infectious Diseases. National Institutes of Health. 2011. The Common Cold. www.niaid.nih.gov/topics/commonCold/Pages/overview.aspx. (Accessed March 2012.)

2. Sigh, M., and R. R. Das. 2011. Zinc for the common cold. *Cochrane Database of Systemic Reviews.* Issue 2. Art. No. Cd001364. DOI: 10.1002/14651858.

3. Prasad, A. 1996. Zinc: the biology and therapeutics of an ion. *Ann. Intern. Med.* 125:142–143.

4. Jackson, J. L., E. Lesho, and C. Peterson. 2000. Zinc and the common cold: a meta-analysis revisited. *J. Nutr.* 130:1512S–1515S.

5. Sigh, M., and R. R. Das. 2011. Clinic potential of zinc in prophylaxis of the common cold. *Expert Rev. Respir Med.* 5(3):301–303.

6. Hemila, H. 2011. Zinc lozenges may shorten the duration of colds: a systematic review. *Open Respiratory Medicine Journal* 5:51–58.

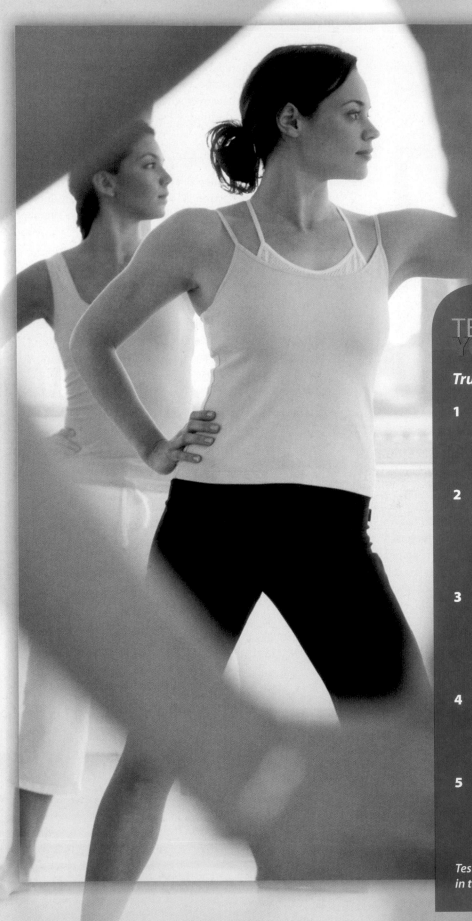

True or False?

1. Being underweight can be just as detrimental to our health as being obese. **T** *or* **F**

2. Obesity is a condition that is simply caused by people eating too much food and not getting enough exercise. **T** *or* **F**

3. Getting my body composition measured at the local fitness club will give me an accurate assessment of my body fat level. **T** *or* **F**

4. Although a majority of Americans are overweight, only about 20% of Americans are obese. **T** *or* **F**

5. People who are moderately overweight and physically active should be considered healthy. **T** *or* **F**

Test Yourself answers are located in the Chapter Review.

13

Achieving and Maintaining a Healthful Body Weight

Learning Objectives

After studying this chapter, you should be able to:

1. Define what is meant by a healthful weight, *p. 506.*

2. Define the terms *underweight, overweight, obesity,* and *morbid obesity* and discuss the potential health risks of each of these weight classifications, *pp. 507, 532–535.*

3. List at least three methods that can be used to assess your body composition or risk for obesity, *pp. 508–511.*

4. Define *direct calorimetry, indirect calorimetry,* and *doubly labeled water* and list one strength and one limitation of each of these methods, *pp. 513–514.*

5. Identify and discuss the three components of energy expenditure and explain the concept of energy balance, *pp. 511–518.*

6. Discuss three factors that can increase BMR and three factors that can decrease BMR, *pp. 514–515.*

7. List and describe at least two theories that link genetic influences to control of body weight, *pp. 518–519.*

8. Identify at least one example from each of the following factors that can influence body weight: metabolic, physiological, cultural, economic, psychological, and social, *pp. 520–525.*

9. Develop a diet plan for healthful weight loss, *pp. 528–532.*

10. List and describe three treatment options for obesity, *pp. 537–540.*

MasteringNutrition™

Go online for chapter quizzes, pre-tests, Interactive Activities and more!

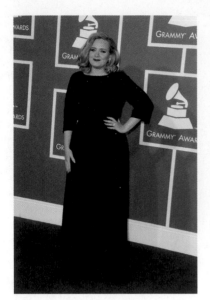

One's perception of a healthful body weight varies from person to person. British singer Adele is comfortable with her body weight.

In February of 2012, British pop singer Adele became only the second woman in history to win six Grammy Awards in one night. At age 24, she has won critical acclaim from musicians of various genres and the adoration of millions of fans worldwide. Still, some critics—perhaps most famously the fashion designer Karl Lagerfeld—focus not on her powerful, soulful voice but on her weight. Is Adele overweight? A size "14 to 16," she exudes supreme confidence in her large, curvy body and insists she's not interested in losing weight just because someone else thinks she should. Rather than worry about something as "petty" as what one looks like, Adele suggests, "The first thing to do is be happy with yourself and appreciate your body."[1]

Are you happy with your weight, shape, body composition, and fitness level? If not, what needs to change—your diet, your level of physical activity, or maybe just your attitude? What role do diet and physical activity play in maintaining a healthful body weight? How much of your body size and shape is due to genetics? What influence does society—including food advertising—have on your weight? And if you decide that you do need to lose weight, what's the best way to do it? In this chapter, we will explore these questions and provide some answers.

How Can You Evaluate Your Body Weight?

As you begin to think about achieving and maintaining a healthful weight, it's important to make sure you understand what a healthful body weight actually is and what methods you can use to figure out if your weight is healthful.

Understand What a Healthful Body Weight Really Is

We can define a healthful weight as all of the following:[2]

- A weight that is appropriate for your age and physical development
- A weight that you can achieve and sustain without severely curtailing your food intake or constantly dieting
- A weight that is compatible with normal blood pressure, lipid levels, and glucose tolerance
- A weight that is based on your genetic background and family history of body shape and weight
- A weight that promotes good eating habits and allows you to participate in regular physical activity
- A weight that is acceptable to you

As you can see, a healthful weight is one at which you don't have to be extremely thin or overly muscular. In addition, there is no one body type that can be defined as healthful. Thus, achieving a healthful body weight should not be dictated by the latest fad or current societal expectations of what is acceptable.

Various methods are available to help you determine whether you are currently maintaining a healthful body weight. Let's review a few of these methods.

Determine Your Body Mass Index (BMI)

Body mass index (BMI, or *Quetelet's index*) is a commonly used index representing the ratio of a person's body weight to the square of his or her height. A person's BMI can be calculated using the following equation:

$$\text{BMI (kg/m}^2) = \text{weight (kg)/height (m)}^2$$

For those less familiar with the metric system, there is an equation to calculate BMI using weight in pounds and height in inches:

$$\text{BMI (kg/m}^2) = [\text{weight (lb)/height (inches)}^2] \times 703$$

Watch an interview in which Adele talks with *60 Minutes* correspondent Anderson Cooper about her body image and weight at www.cbsnews .com/8301-504803_162-57376080-10391709/adele-talks-about-her-body-image-and-weight/. **(Link courtesy of CBS News.)**

body mass index (BMI) A measurement representing the ratio of a person's body weight to his or her height.

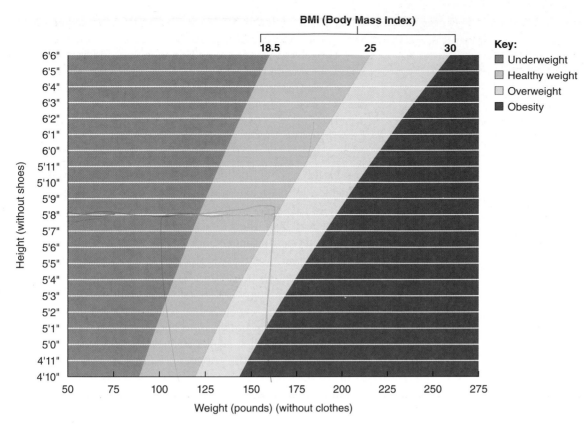

FIGURE 13.1 Measure your body mass index (BMI) using this graph. To determine your BMI, find the value for your height on the left and follow this line to the right until it intersects with the value for your weight on the bottom axis. The area on the graph where these two points intersect is your BMI.

A less exact but practical method is to use the graph in **Figure 13.1**, which shows approximate BMIs for a person's height and weight and whether a given BMI is in a healthful range.

Why Is BMI Important?

BMI provides an important clue to a person's overall health. Physicians, nutritionists, and other scientists define **underweight** as having too little body fat to maintain health, causing a person to have a weight that is below an acceptably defined standard for a given height. A person having a BMI less than 18.5 kg/m² is considered underweight. Normal weight ranges from 18.5 to 24.9 kg/m². **Overweight** is defined as having a moderate amount of excess body fat, resulting in a person having a weight that is greater than some accepted standard for a given height but is not considered obese. **Obesity** is defined as having an excess of body fat that adversely affects health, resulting in a person having a weight that is substantially greater than some accepted standard for a given height. A BMI value between 30 and 39.9 kg/m² is consistent with obesity. People can also suffer from **morbid obesity,** defined as a BMI greater than or equal to 40 kg/m²; in this case, the person's body weight exceeds 100% of normal, putting him or her at very high risk for serious health consequences.

Research studies show that a person's risk for type 2 diabetes, high blood pressure, heart disease, and many other diseases increases significantly when BMI is above a value of 30. On the other hand, being underweight and having a very low BMI, below 18.5, is also associated with increased risk for health problems.

Figure 13.2 shows how the *mortality rate,* or death rate, from all diseases increases significantly with a BMI value below 18.5 kg/m² or above 30 kg/m². Having a BMI value within the healthful range means that the risk of dying prematurely is within the expected average. For example, people with a BMI equal to or greater than 35 kg/m² have a risk of

 You can also calculate your BMI more precisely on the Internet using the BMI calculator found at www.nhlbisupport.com/bmi.

underweight Having too little body fat to maintain health, causing a person to have a weight that is below an acceptable defined standard for a given height; a BMI less than 18.5 kg/m².

overweight Having a moderate amount of excess body fat, resulting in a person having a weight that is greater than some accepted standard for a given height but is not considered obese; a BMI of 25 to 29.9 kg/m².

obesity Having an excess of body fat that adversely affects health, resulting in a person having a weight that is substantially greater than some accepted standard for a given height; a BMI of 30 to 39.9 kg/m².

morbid obesity A condition in which a person's body weight exceeds 100% of normal, putting him or her at very high risk for serious health consequences; a BMI ≥40 kg/m².

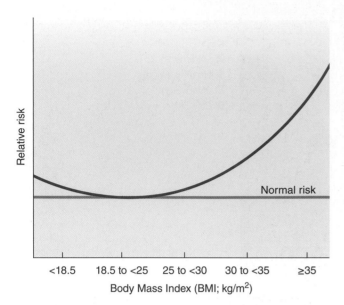

Relative risk

Normal risk

<18.5   18.5 to <25   25 to <30   30 to <35   ≥35
Body Mass Index (BMI; kg/m²)

FIGURE 13.2 Having a body mass index value below 18.5 kg/m² or above 30 kg/m² is significantly associated with an increased risk for premature mortality.

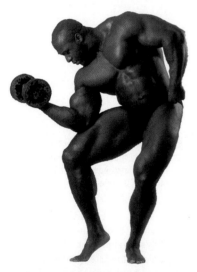

BMI is not an accurate indicator of overweight for certain populations, including heavily muscled people.

body composition The ratio of a person's body fat to lean body mass.

body fat mass The amount of body fat, or adipose tissue, a person has.

lean body mass The amount of fat-free tissue, or bone, muscle, and internal organs, a person has.

dying prematurely that is 50–100% higher than that of people with a BMI value in the range of 20–25 kg/m².

Theo always worries about being too thin, and he wonders if he is underweight. Theo calculates his BMI (see the calculations in the **You Do the Math** box, page 510) and is surprised to find that it is 22 kg/m² and falls within the normal range.

Limitations of BMI

While calculating your BMI can be very helpful in estimating your health risk, this method has a number of limitations that should be taken into consideration. BMI cannot tell us how much of a person's body mass is composed of fat, nor can it give us an indication of where on the body excess fat is stored. As we'll discuss shortly, upper-body fat stores increase the risk for chronic disease more than fat stores in the lower body. A person's age affects his or her BMI; BMI does not give a fair indication of overweight or obesity in people over the age of 65 years, as the BMI standards are based on data from younger people, and BMI does not accurately reflect the differential rates of bone and muscle loss in older people. BMI also cannot reflect differences in bone and muscle growth in children. Recent research indicates that BMI is more strongly associated with height in young people; thus, taller children are more likely to be identified as overweight or obese, even though they may not have higher levels of body fat.[3]

BMI also does not take into account physical and metabolic differences between people of different ethnic backgrounds. At the same BMI, people from different ethnic backgrounds will have different levels of body fat. For instance, African American and Polynesian people have less body fat than white people at the same BMI value, while Indonesian, Thai, and Ethiopian people have more body fat than white people at the same BMI value. There is also evidence that, even at the same BMI level, Asian, Hispanic, and African American women have a higher risk for diabetes than white women.[4] The same study also found that, when Asian and Hispanic women gained weight, their risk of developing diabetes over a 20-year period was approximately twice as high as it was for white and African American women who gained the same amount of weight.

Finally, BMI is limited when used with people who have a disproportionately higher muscle mass for a given height, such as certain types of athletes, and with pregnant and lactating women. For example, one of Theo's friends, Randy, is a 23-year-old weight lifter who is 5′7″ and weighs 210 pounds. According to our BMI calculations, Randy's BMI is 32.9, placing him in the obese category. Is Randy really obese? In cases such as his, an assessment of body composition is necessary.

Measure Your Body Composition

There are many methods available to assess your **body composition,** or the amount of **body fat mass** (*adipose tissue*) and **lean body mass** (*lean tissue*) you have. **Figure 13.3** lists and describes some of the more common methods. It is important to remember that measuring body composition provides only an *estimate* of your body fat and lean body mass; it cannot determine your exact level of these tissues. Because the range of error of these methods can be from 3% to more than 20%, body composition results should not be used as the only indicator of health status.

Let's return to Randy, whose BMI of 32.9 kg/m² places him in the obese category. Is he obese? Randy trains with weights 4 days per week, rides the exercise bike for about 30 minutes per session three times per week, and does not take drugs, smoke cigarettes, or drink alcohol. Through his local gym, Randy contacted a trained technician who

Method		Limitations

Underwater weighing:
Considered the most accurate method. Estimates body fat within a 2–3% margin of error. This means that if your underwater weighing test shows you have 20% body fat, this value could be no lower than 17% and no higher than 23%. Used primarily for research purposes.

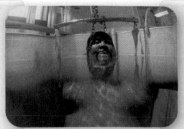

- Subject must be comfortable in water.
- Requires trained technician and specialized equipment.
- May not work well with extremely obese people.
- Must abstain from food for at least 8 hours and from exercise for at least 12 hours prior to testing.

Skinfolds:
Involves "pinching" a person's fold of skin (with its underlying layer of fat) at various locations of the body. The fold is measured using a specially designed caliper. When performed by a skilled technician, it can estimate body fat with an error of 3–4%. This means that if your skinfold test shows you have 20% body fat, your actual value could be as low as 16% or as high as 24%.

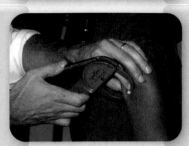

- Less accurate unless technician is well trained.
- Proper prediction equation must be used to improve accuracy.
- Person being measured may not want to be touched or to expose their skin.
- Cannot be used to measure obese people, as their skinfolds are too large for the caliper.

Bioelectrical impedance analysis (BIA):
Involves sending a very low level of electrical current through a person's body. As water is a good conductor of electricity and lean body mass is made up of mostly water, the rate at which the electricity is conducted gives an indication of a person's lean body mass and body fat. This method can be done while lying down, with electrodes attached to the feet, hands, and the BIA machine. Hand-held and standing models (which look like bathroom scales) are now available. Under the best of circumstances, BIA can estimate body fat with an error of 3–4%.

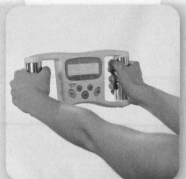

- Less accurate.
- Body fluid levels must be normal.
- Proper prediction equation must be used to improve accuracy.
- Should not eat for 4 hours and should not exercise for 12 hours prior to the test.
- No alcohol should be consumed within 48 hours of the test.
- Females should not be measured if they are retaining water due to menstrual cycle changes.

Dual-energy x-ray absorptiometry (DXA):
The technology is based on using very-low-level x-rays to differentiate among bone tissue, soft (or lean) tissue, and fat (or adipose) tissue. It involves lying for about 30 minutes on a specialized bed fully clothed, with all metal objects removed. The margin of error for predicting body fat ranges from 2% to 4%.

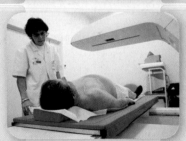

- Expensive; requires trained technician with specialized equipment.
- Cannot be used to measure extremely tall, short, or obese people, as they do not fit properly within the scanning area.

Bod Pod:
A machine that uses air displacement to measure body composition. This machine is a large, egg-shaped chamber made from fiberglass. The person being measured sits inside, wearing a swimsuit. The door is closed and the machine measures how much air is displaced. This value is used to calculate body composition. It appears promising as an easier and equally accurate alternative to underwater weighing in many populations, but it may overestimate body fat in some African American men.

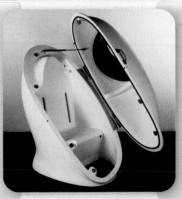

- Expensive.
- Less accurate in some populations.

FIGURE 13.3 Overview of various body composition assessment methods.

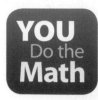

Calculating Your Body Mass Index

Calculate your personal BMI value based on your height and weight. Let's use Theo's values as an example:

$$BMI = weight\ (kg)/height\ (m)^2$$

1. Theo's weight is 200 lb. To convert his weight to kilograms, divide his weight in pounds by 2.2 lb per kg:

$$200\ lb/2.2\ lb\ per\ kg = 90.91\ kg$$

2. Theo's height is 6 feet 8 inches, or 80 inches. To convert his height to meters, multiply his height in inches by 0.0254 meters/inch:

$$80\ in. \times 0.0254\ m/in. = 2.03\ m$$

3. Find the square of his height in meters:

$$2.03\ m \times 2.03\ m = 4.13\ m^2$$

4. Then, divide his weight in kilograms by his height in square meters to get his BMI value:

$$90.91\ kg/4.13\ m^2 = 22.01\ kg/m^2$$

Is Theo underweight according to this BMI value? No. As you can see in Figure 13.1, this value shows that he is maintaining a normal, healthful weight!

---

assesses body composition. The results of his skinfold measurements show that his body fat is 9%. This value is within the healthful range for men. Randy is an example of a person whose BMI appears very high but who is not actually obese.

Assess Your Fat Distribution Patterns

To evaluate the health of your current body weight, it is also helpful to consider the way fat is distributed throughout your body. This is because your fat distribution pattern is known to affect your risk for various diseases. **Figure 13.4** shows two types of fat patterning. *Apple-shaped fat patterning*, or upper-body obesity, is known to significantly increase a person's risk for many chronic diseases, such as type 2 diabetes, heart disease, and high blood pressure. It is thought that the apple-shaped patterning causes problems with the metabolism of fat and carbohydrate, leading to unhealthful changes in blood cholesterol, insulin, glucose, and blood pressure. In contrast, *pear-shaped fat patterning*, or lower-body obesity, does not seem to significantly increase your risk for chronic diseases. Women tend to store fat in their lower body, and men in their abdominal region.

You can use the following three-step method to determine your type of fat patterning:

1. Ask a friend to measure the circumference of your natural waist, that is, the narrowest part of your torso as observed from the front (**Figure 13.5a**).
2. Then, have that friend measure your hip circumference at the maximal width of the buttocks as observed from the side (Figure 13.5b).
3. Then, divide the waist value by the hip value. This measurement is called your *waist-to-hip ratio*. For example, if your natural waist is 30 inches and your hips are 40 inches, then your waist-to-hip ratio is 30 divided by 40, which equals 0.75.

Once you figure out your ratio, how do you interpret it? An increased risk for chronic disease is associated with the following waist-to-hip ratios:

- In men, a ratio higher than 0.90
- In women, a ratio higher than 0.80

These ratios suggest an apple-shaped fat distribution pattern. In addition, waist circumference alone can indicate your risk for chronic disease. For males, your risk of chronic

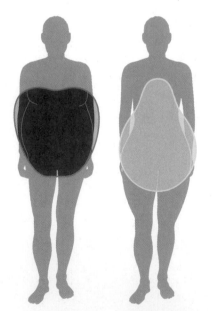

(a) Apple-shaped fat patterning **(b) Pear-shaped fat patterning**

FIGURE 13.4 Fat distribution patterns. **(a)** An apple-shaped fat distribution pattern increases an individual's risk for many chronic diseases. **(b)** A pear-shaped fat distribution pattern does not seem to be associated with an increased risk for chronic disease.

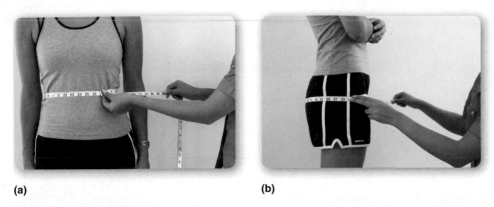

(a)   **(b)**

FIGURE 13.5 Determining your type of fat patterning. **(a)** Measure the circumference of your natural waist. **(b)** Measure the circumference of your hips at the maximal width of the buttocks as observed from the side. Dividing the waist value by the hip value gives you your waist-to-hip ratio.

disease is increased if your waist circumference is above 40 inches (102 cm). For females, your risk is increased at measurements above 35 inches (88 cm).

RECAP

Body mass index, body composition, and the waist-to-hip ratio and waist circumference are tools that can help you evaluate the health of your current body weight. None of these methods is completely accurate, but most may be used appropriately as general health indicators. ■

What Makes Us Gain and Lose Weight?

Have you ever wondered why some people are thin and others are overweight, even though they seem to eat about the same diet? If so, you're not alone. For hundreds of years, researchers have puzzled over what makes us gain and lose weight. In this section, we explore some information and current theories that may shed light on this complex question.

We Gain or Lose Weight When Energy Intake and Expenditure Are Out of Balance

Fluctuations in body weight are a result of changes in **energy intake** (the food and beverages consumed) and **energy expenditure** (the amount of energy expended at rest and during physical activity). This relationship between what we eat and what we do is defined by the energy balance equation:

Energy balance occurs when energy intake = Energy expenditure

Although the concept of energy balance appears simple, it is a dynamic process.[5] This means that, over time, factors that impact the energy intake side of the equation (including total energy consumed and the macronutrient composition of this energy) need to balance with the factors that impact the energy expenditure side of the equation. **Figure 13.6** shows how our weight changes when either side of this equation is altered. From this figure, you can see that, in order to lose body weight, we must expend more energy than we consume. In contrast, to gain weight, we must consume more energy than we expend. Unless we purposefully change one side of the equation, weight change is typically gradual and occurs over an extended period of time. Finding the proper balance between energy intake and expenditure allows someone to maintain a healthful body weight.

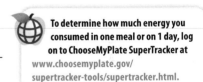
To determine how much energy you consumed in one meal or on 1 day, log on to ChooseMyPlate SuperTracker at www.choosemyplate.gov/supertracker-tools/supertracker.html.

energy intake The amount of energy a person consumes; in other words, the number of kcal consumed from food and beverages.

energy expenditure The energy the body expends to maintain its basic functions and to perform all levels of movement and activity.

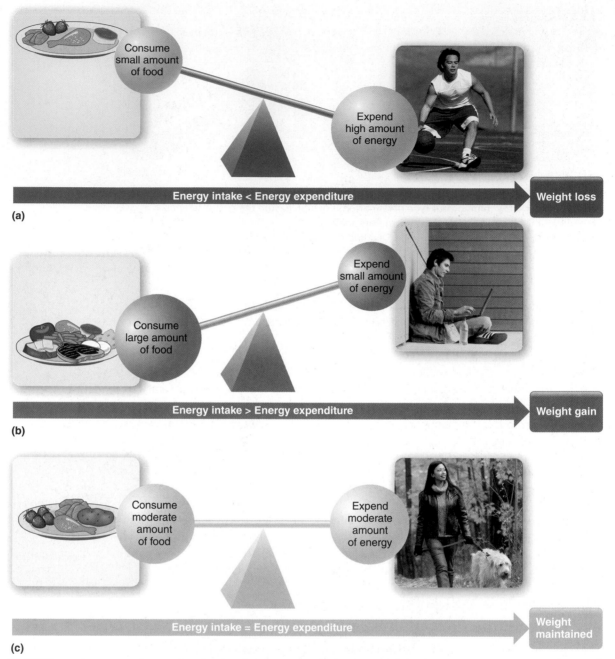

FIGURE 13.6 Energy balance describes the relationship between the food we eat and the energy we expend each day. **(a)** Weight loss occurs when food intake is less than energy output. **(b)** Weight gain occurs when food intake is greater than energy output. **(c)** We maintain our body weight when food intake equals energy output.

Energy Intake Is the Food We Eat Each Day

Energy intake is equal to the amount of energy in the food we eat each day. This value includes all foods and beverages. Daily energy intake is expressed as *kilocalories per day* (*kcal/day,* or *kcal/d*). Energy intake can be estimated manually by using food composition tables or computerized dietary analysis programs. The energy content of each food is a function of the amount of carbohydrate, fat, protein, and alcohol that each food contains; vitamins and minerals have no energy value, so they contribute zero kcal to our energy intake.

Remember that the energy value of carbohydrate and protein is 4 kcal/g and the energy value of fat is 9 kcal/g. The energy value of alcohol is 7 kcal/g. By multiplying the energy value (in kcal/g) by the amount of the nutrient (in g), you can calculate how much

energy is in a particular food. For instance, 1 cup of quick oatmeal has an energy value of
142 kcal. How is this energy value derived? One cup of oatmeal contains 6 g of protein, 25 g
of carbohydrate, and 2 g of fat. Using the energy values for each nutrient, you can calculate
the total energy content of oatmeal:

$$6 \text{ g protein} \times 4 \text{ kcal/g} = 24 \text{ kcal from protein}$$

$$25 \text{ g carbohydrate} \times 4 \text{ kcal/g} = 100 \text{ kcal from carbohydrate}$$

$$2 \text{ g fat} \times 9 \text{ kcal/g} = 18 \text{ kcal from fat}$$

$$\text{Total kcal for 1 cup oatmeal} = 24 \text{ kcal} + 100 \text{ kcal} + 18 \text{ kcal} = 142 \text{ kcal}$$

Over a period of time, when someone's total daily energy intake exceeds the amount of
energy that person expends, then weight gain results. Without exercise, this gain will likely
be fat. An excess intake of approximately 3,500 kcal will result in a gain of 1 pound. How is
this value derived?

- First, it is important to remember that there are 454 g in 1 pound and that the energy
  value of fat is 9 kcal/g.
- Second, you need to know that adipose tissue contains 87% fat (with the remainder
  being water).
- Finally, to calculate the amount of kcal that will result in a gain of 1 pound (454 g), you
  need to multiply the amount of weight, 454 g, by the proportion of fat in adipose tissue
  (87%, or 0.87) and then multiply this value by the energy value of fat (9 kcal/g):

$$454 \text{ g} \times 0.87 = 395 \text{ g of fat}$$

$$395 \text{ g} \times 9 \text{ kcal/g} = 3,555 \text{ kcal (which, for simplicity, is rounded to 3,500 kcal)}$$

Energy Expenditure Includes More Than Just Physical Activity

Energy expenditure (also known as energy output) is the energy the body expends to maintain its basic functions and to perform all levels of movement and activity. Total 24-hour
energy expenditure is calculated by estimating the energy used during rest and as a result
of physical activity. There are three components of energy expenditure: basal metabolic rate
(BMR), thermic effect of food (TEF), and energy cost of physical activity (**Figure 13.7**). We
discuss these components in detail shortly.

Energy Expenditure Can Be Measured Using Direct or Indirect Calorimetry Energy expenditure can be measured using direct or indirect calorimetry. **Direct calorimetry** is a method that
measures the amount of heat the body releases. This method is done using an air-tight chamber in which the heat produced by the body warms the water that surrounds the chamber.
The amount of energy a person expends is calculated from the changes in water temperature.
The minimum period of time that a person must stay in a direct calorimetry chamber is
24 hours; because of the burden to the individual, the high cost, and the complexity of this
method, it is rarely used to measure energy expenditure in humans.

Indirect calorimetry estimates energy expenditure by measuring oxygen consumption and carbon dioxide production. Because there is a predictable relationship between
the amount of heat produced (energy expended) by the body and the amount of oxygen
consumed and carbon dioxide produced, this method can be used to indirectly determine
energy expenditure. This method involves the use of a whole-body chamber, mask, hood,
or mouthpiece to collect expired air over a specified period of time. The expired air is
analyzed for oxygen and carbon dioxide content (**Figure 13.8**). This method is much less
expensive and more accessible than direct calorimetry, so it is most commonly used to
measure energy expenditure under both resting and physically active conditions.

Both direct and indirect calorimetry require a person to be confined to a laboratory setting or special metabolic chamber, which limits the ability to determine a person's energy expenditure in a free-living environment. This limitation is overcome in a
technique using **doubly labeled water,** that is, water labeled with isotopes of hydrogen

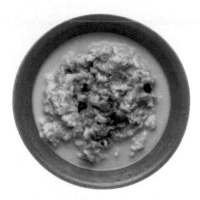

The energy provided by a bowl of
oatmeal is derived from its protein,
carbohydrate, and fat content.

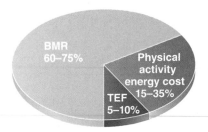

Components of energy expenditure

FIGURE 13.7 The components of
energy expenditure are basal metabolic rate (BMR), the thermic effect
of food (TEF), and the energy cost of
physical activity. BMR accounts for
60% to 75% of our total energy output, whereas TEF and physical activity
together account for 25% to 40%.

direct calorimetry A method used
to determine energy expenditure
by measuring the amount of heat
released by the body.

indirect calorimetry A method used
to estimate energy expenditure by
measuring oxygen consumption and
carbon dioxide production.

doubly labeled water A form of indirect calorimetry that measures total
daily energy expenditure through the
rate of carbon dioxide production. It
requires the consumption of water
that is labeled with nonradioactive
isotopes of hydrogen (deuterium,
or ^{2}H) and oxygen (^{18}O).

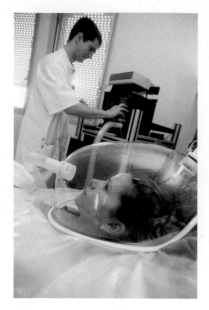

FIGURE 13.8 Indirect calorimetry can be used to measure the components of energy expenditure.

basal metabolic rate (BMR) The energy the body expends to maintain its fundamental physiologic functions.

(deuterium, or ^{2}H) and oxygen (^{18}O). In this method, the research subject consumes controlled amounts of doubly labeled water. Both the labeled hydrogen and oxygen are used during metabolism; the ^{2}H is eliminated in water, and the ^{18}O is eliminated in both water and carbon dioxide. Thus, the difference between the elimination rates of these labeled isotopes measures carbon dioxide production, which in turn can be used to estimate energy expenditure. The advantages of this method are that it measures energy expenditure in free-living situations over periods of 3 days to 3 weeks, requires only periodic collection of urine and requires little inconvenience to the person being measured. The primary disadvantages of the method are that it is expensive, the doubly labeled water is difficult to acquire, and it only measures total 24-hour energy expenditure. This method cannot separately measure the three components of energy expenditure discussed next: BMR, TEF, and the energy cost of physical activity.

Our Basal Metabolic Rate Is Our Energy Expenditure at Rest **Basal metabolic rate,** or **BMR,** is the energy expended just to maintain the body's *basal,* or *resting,* functions. These functions include respiration, circulation, body temperature, synthesis of new cells and tissues, secretion of hormones, and nervous system activity. The majority of our energy output each day (about 60% to 75%) is a result of our BMR. This means that 60% to 75% of our energy output goes to fuel the basic activities of staying alive, aside from any physical activity.

BMR varies widely among people. The primary determinant of our BMR is the amount of lean body mass we have. People with a higher lean body mass have a higher BMR, as lean body mass is more metabolically active than body fat. Thus, it takes more energy to support this active tissue. One common assumption is that obese people have a depressed BMR. This is usually not the case. Most studies of obese people show that the amount of energy they expend for every kilogram of lean body mass is similar to that of a non-obese person. Moreover, people who weigh more also have more lean body mass and consequently have a *higher* BMR. See **Figure 13.9** for an example of how lean body mass can vary for people with different body weights and body fat levels.

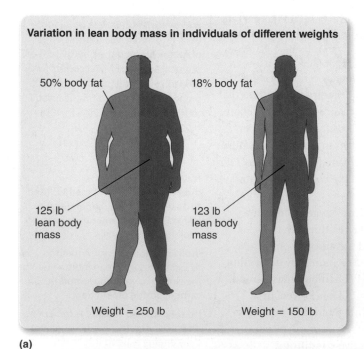

(a)

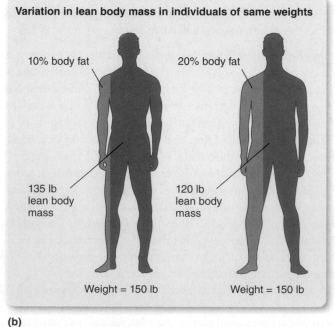

(b)

FIGURE 13.9 Lean body mass varies in people with different body weights and body fat levels. **(a)** The person on the left has a higher body weight, body fat, and lean body mass than the person on the right. **(b)** The two people are the same weight but the person on the right has more body fat and less lean body mass than the person on the left.

TABLE 13.1 Factors Affecting Basal Metabolic Rate (BMR)

Factors That Increase BMR	Factors That Decrease BMR
Higher lean body mass	Lower lean body mass
Greater height (more surface area)	Lower height
Younger age	Older age
Elevated levels of thyroid hormone	Depressed levels of thyroid hormone
Stress, fever, illness	Starvation or fasting
Male gender	Female gender
Pregnancy and lactation	
Certain drugs, such as stimulants, caffeine, and tobacco	

BMR decreases with age, approximately 3% to 5% per decade after age 30. This age-related decrease results partly from hormonal changes, but much of this change is due to the loss of lean body mass resulting from physical inactivity. Thus, a large proportion of this decrease may be prevented with regular physical activity. There are other factors that can affect a person's BMR, and some of them are listed in **Table 13.1**.

How can you estimate the amount of energy you expend for your BMR? Of the many methods that can be used, one of the simplest is to multiply your body weight in kilograms by 1.0 kcal per kilogram of body weight per hour for men or by 0.9 kcal per kilogram of body weight per hour for women. A little later in this chapter, you will have an opportunity to calculate your BMR and determine your total daily energy needs.

The Thermic Effect of Food Is the Energy Expended to Process Food   The **thermic effect of food (TEF)** is the energy we expend to digest, absorb, transport, metabolize, and store the nutrients we need. The TEF is equal to about 5% to 10% of the energy content of a meal, a relatively small amount. Thus, if a meal contains 500 kcal, the thermic effect of processing that meal is about 25 to 50 kcal. These values apply to eating what is referred to as a mixed diet, or a diet containing carbohydrate, fat, and protein. Individually, the processing of each nutrient takes a different amount of energy. Whereas fat requires very little energy to digest, transport, and store in our cells, protein and carbohydrate require relatively more energy to process.

The Energy Cost of Physical Activity Is Highly Variable   The **energy cost of physical activity** represents about 15% to 35% of our total energy output each day. This is the energy we expend in any movement or work above basal levels. This includes lower-intensity activities, such as sitting, standing, and walking, and higher-intensity activities, such as running, skiing, and bicycling. This also includes *spontaneous physical activity*, which includes subconscious activities such as fidgeting and shifting in one's seat. One of the most obvious ways to increase how much energy we expend as a result of physical activity is to do more activities for a longer period of time.

Table 13.2 lists the energy costs for certain activities. As you can see, activities such as running, swimming, and cross-country skiing, which involve moving our larger muscle groups (or more parts of the body) require more energy. The amount of energy we expend during activities is also affected by our body size, the intensity of the activity, and how long we perform the activity. This is why the values in Table 13.2 are expressed as kcal of energy per kilogram of body weight per minute.

Using the energy value for running at 6 miles per hour (a 10-minute-per-mile running pace) for 30 minutes, let's calculate how much energy Theo would expend doing this activity:

■ Theo's body weight (in kg) = 200 lb/2.2 lb/kg = 90.91 kg
■ Energy cost of running at 6 mph = 0.163 kcal/kg body weight/min

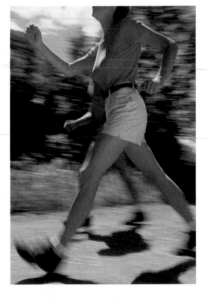

Brisk walking expends energy.

thermic effect of food (TEF)
The energy expended as a result of processing food consumed.

energy cost of physical activity
The energy that is expended on body movement and muscular work above basal levels.

TABLE 13.2 Energy Costs of Various Physical Activities

Activity	Intensity	Energy Cost (kcal/kg body weight/min)
Sitting, studying (including reading or writing)	Light	0.022
Cooking or food preparation (sitting or standing)	Light	0.033
Walking (to neighbor's house)	Light	0.042
Stretching—Hatha yoga	Moderate	0.042
Cleaning (dusting, straightening up, vacuuming, changing linen, carrying out trash)	Moderate	0.058
Weight lifting (free weights, Nautilus, or universal type)	Light or moderate	0.050
Bicycling, 10 mph	Leisure (work or pleasure)	0.067
Walking, 4 mph (brisk pace)	Moderate	0.083
Aerobics	Low impact	0.083
Weight lifting (free weights, Nautilus, or universal type)	Vigorous	0.100
Bicycling, 12 to 13.9 mph	Moderate	0.133
Running, 5 mph (12 minutes per mile)	Moderate	0.138
Running, 6 mph (10 minutes per mile)	Moderate	0.163
Running, 8.6 mph (7 minutes per mile)	Vigorous	0.205

Source: Data from The Compendium of Physical Activities Tracking Guide. Healthy Lifestyles Research Center, College of Nursing & Health Innovation, Arizona State University, website.

- At Theo's weight, the energy cost of running per minute = 0.163 kcal/kg body weight/min × 90.91 kg = 14.82 kcal/min
- If Theo runs at this pace for 30 minutes, his total energy output = 14.82 kcal/min × 30 min = 445 kcal

Given everything we've discussed so far, you're probably asking yourself, "How many kcal do I need each day to maintain my current weight?" This question is not always easy to answer, as our energy needs fluctuate from day to day according to our activity level, environmental conditions, and other factors, such as the amount and type of food we eat and our intake of caffeine, which temporarily increases our BMR. However, you can get a general estimate of how much energy your body needs to maintain your present weight. The **You Do the Math** box describes how you can estimate your total daily energy needs.

As researchers learn more about the factors that regulate body weight, it is clear that the accuracy and usefulness of the classic energy balance equation illustrated in Figure 13.6 do not reflect all the factors that impact body weight. This is because the equation in its current form is static—meaning it does not account for many factors that can alter energy intake and expenditure, nor does it help explain why people gain and lose weight differently. For example, if an individual consumed an additional 100 kcal each day above the energy needed to maintain weight (the energy content of 8 fl. oz of a cola beverage) for 10 years, he or she would consume an extra intake of 365,000 kcal! Based on the static energy balance equation, and assuming that no other changes occur in energy expenditure, this individual should gain 104 pounds. However, the static energy balance calculation does not take into account the increase in energy expenditure that would occur, including increased BMR and increased cost of moving a larger body, as weight increased. Thus, after a short period of positive energy balance, body weight would increase, resulting in an increase in energy expenditure, which will eventually balance the increased energy intake. The individual would then achieve energy balance and become weight stable at a higher body weight. Thus, the extra 100 kcal/d would actually result in a more realistic weight gain of a few pounds. To maintain this larger body size the individual would need to continue to eat these additional kcal. Of course, the amount of weight gained will depend on the

Calculating BMR and Total Daily Energy Needs

One potential way to estimate how much energy you need each day is to record your total food and beverage intake for a defined period of time, such as 3 or 7 days. You can then use a food composition table or computer dietary assessment program to estimate the amount of energy you eat each day. Assuming that your body weight is stable over this period of time, your average daily energy intake should represent how much energy you need to maintain your present weight.

Unfortunately, many studies of energy intake in humans have shown that dietary records estimating energy needs are not very accurate. Most studies show that humans underestimate the amount of energy they eat by 10% to 30%. Overweight people tend to underestimate by an even higher margin, at the same time overestimating the amount of activity they do. This means that someone who really eats about 2,000 kcal/day may record eating only 1,400 to 1,800 kcal/day. So one reason many people are confused about their ability to lose weight is that they are eating more than they realize.

A simpler and more accurate way to estimate your total daily energy needs is to calculate your BMR, then add the amount of energy you expend as a result of your activity level. Refer to the following example to learn how to do this. As the energy cost for the thermic effect of food is very small, you don't need to include it in your calculations.

1. *Calculate your BMR.* If you are a man, you will need to multiply your body weight in kilograms by 1 kcal per kilogram of body weight per hour. Assuming you weigh 175 pounds, your body weight in kilograms would be 175 lb/2.2 lb/kg = 79.5 kg. Next, multiply your weight in kilograms by 1 kcal per kilogram body weight per hour:

   1 kcal/kg body weight/hour × 79.5 kg = 79.5 kcal/hour

   Calculate your BMR for the total day (or 24 hours):

   79.5 kcal/hour × 24 hours/day = 1,909 kcal/day

   If you are a woman, multiply your body weight in kg by 0.9 kcal/kg body weight/hour.

2. *Estimate your activity level by selecting the description that most closely fits your general lifestyle.* The energy cost of activities is expressed as a percentage of your BMR. Refer to the values in the following table when estimating your own energy output.

3. *Multiply your BMR by the decimal equivalent of the lower and higher percentage values for your activity level.* Let's use the man referred to in step 1. He is a college student who lives on campus. He walks to classes located throughout campus,

carries his book bag, and spends most of his time reading and writing. He does not exercise on a regular basis. His lifestyle would be defined as lightly active, meaning he expends 50% to 70% of his BMR each day in activities. You want to calculate how much energy he expends at both ends of this activity level. How many kcal does this equal?

   1,909 kcal/day × 0.50 (50%) = 955 kcal/day
   1,909 kcal/day × 0.70 (70%) = 1,336 kcal/day

   These calculations show that this man expends about 955 to 1,336 kcal/day doing daily activities.

4. *Calculate total daily energy output by adding together BMR and the energy needed to perform daily activities.* In this man's case, his total daily energy output is

   1,909 kcal/day + 955 kcal/day = 2,864 kcal/day

   or

   1,909 kcal/day + 1,336 kcal/day = 3,245 kcal/day

   Assuming this man is maintaining his present weight, he requires between 2,864 and 3,245 kcal/day to stay in energy balance!

	Men	Women
Sedentary/Inactive	25–40%	25–35%
Involves mostly sitting, driving, or very low levels of activity		
Lightly Active	50–70%	40–60%
Involves a lot of sitting; may also involve some walking, moving around, and light lifting		
Moderately Active	65–80%	50–70%
Involves work plus intentional exercise, such as an hour of walking or walking 4 to 5 days per week; may have a job requiring some physical labor		
Heavily Active	90–120%	80–100%
Involves a great deal of physical labor, such as roofing, carpentry work, and/or regular heavy lifting and digging		
Exceptionally Active	130–145%	110–130%
Involves a lot of physical activities for work and intentional exercise; also applies to athletes who train for many hours each day, such as triathletes and marathon runners or other competitive athletes performing heavy, regular training		

Predict a more realistic time course for weight loss or weight gain for yourself based on a dynamic simulation model of human metabolism by going to http://bwsimulator.niddk.nih.gov.

number of extra kcal consumed, the macronutrient composition of these kcal (the amount of fat, carbohydrate, protein, or alcohol), and overall energy expenditure. The inadequacy of the classic energy balance equation has prompted experts to propose a dynamic equation of energy balance that takes into account the rates of energy intake and expenditure and their effect on rate of change of energy stores (including fat and lean tissues) in the body, not simply on body weight overall.[5]

RECAP

The energy balance equation relates food intake to energy expenditure. Eating more energy than you expend causes weight gain, while eating less energy than you expend causes weight loss. Energy expenditure can be measured using direct calorimetry, indirect calorimetry, and doubly labeled water. The three components of energy expenditure are basal metabolic rate, the thermic effect of food, and the energy cost of physical activity. ∎

Genetic Factors Affect Body Weight

Our genetic background influences our height, weight, body shape, and metabolic rate. A classic study shows that the body weights of adults who were adopted as children are similar to the weights of their biological parents, not their adoptive parents.[6] How much of our BMI can be accounted for by genetic influences remains controversial, however, with proposed values ranging from 50% to 90%.[7] This means that 10% to 50% of our BMI is accounted for by nongenetic, environmental factors and lifestyle choices, such as exposure to cheap, high-energy food and low levels of physical activity. This message that a relatively large proportion of our BMI is accounted for by genetic influences could prove to be detrimental to our efforts to convince people that they can reduce their weight by changing their lifestyle. Bloss and colleagues found that individuals who were genetically tested and found to have higher genetic risk for obesity were more likely to report a higher fat intake and lower levels of physical activity 6 months after they received these results.[8] We discuss here two theories linking genetics with our body weight: the thrifty gene theory and the set-point theory.

The Thrifty Gene Theory

The **thrifty gene theory** suggests that some people possess a gene (or genes) that causes them to be energetically thrifty. This means that at rest and even during active times these individuals expend less energy than people who do not possess this gene. The proposed purpose of this gene is to protect a person from starving to death during times of extreme food shortages. This theory has been applied to some Native American tribes, as these societies were exposed to centuries of feast and famine. Those with a thrifty metabolism survived when little food was available, and this trait was passed on to future generations. Although an actual thrifty gene (or genes) has not yet been identified, researchers continue to study this explanation as a potential cause of obesity.

If this theory is true, think about how people who possess this thrifty gene might respond to today's environment. Low levels of physical activity, inexpensive food sources that are high in fat and energy, and excessively large serving sizes are the norm in our society. People with a thrifty metabolism would experience a great amount of weight gain, and their body would be more resistant to weight loss. Theoretically, having thrifty genetics would be advantageous during times of minimal food resources; however, this state could lead to very high levels of obesity in times of plenty.

The existing evidence on genetics and obesity indicates that there is no one single "obesity gene." There are more than 120 genes currently identified that are associated with increasing a person's risk for obesity.[9] One gene that has received a great deal of attention is the fat mass and obesity-associated (*FTO*) gene. This gene is relatively common, with

thrifty gene theory A theory suggesting that some people possess a gene (or genes) that causes them to be energetically thrifty, resulting in their expending less energy at rest and during physical activity.

approximately 44% of Asian people and 65% of people from European and African descent having some form of the gene. A recent study indicates that physical activity can attenuate the influence of the *FTO* gene on obesity risk in adults and children by 27%; these results highlight the importance of regular physical activity in reducing risk for obesity in people who are genetically predisposed.[10]

The Set-Point Theory

The **set-point theory** suggests that our body is designed to maintain our weight within a narrow range, or at a "set point." In many cases, the body appears to respond in such a way as to maintain a person's current weight. When we dramatically reduce energy intake (such as with fasting or strict diets), the body responds with physiologic changes that cause BMR to drop. This results in a significant slowing of our energy output. In addition, being physically active while fasting or starving is difficult, because a person just doesn't have the energy for it. These two mechanisms of energy conservation may contribute to some of the rebound weight gain many dieters experience after they quit dieting.

Conversely, overeating in some people may cause an increase in BMR, thought to be due to an increased thermic effect of food as well as an increase in spontaneous physical activity. This in turn increases energy output and prevents weight gain. These changes may explain the limitations of the classic energy balance equation, mentioned earlier, in predicting how much weight people will gain from eating excess food.

In addition, we don't eat exactly the same amount of food each day; some days we overeat, and other days we eat less. When you think about how much our daily energy intake fluctuates (about 20% above and below our average monthly intake), our ability to maintain a certain weight over long periods of time suggests that there is some evidence to support the set-point theory.

Can we change our weight set point? It appears that, when we maintain changes in our diet and activity level over a long period of time, weight change does occur. This is obvious in the case of obesity, since many people who were normal weight as young adults become obese during middle adulthood. Also, many people do successfully lose weight and maintain that weight loss over long periods of time. Thus, the set-point theory cannot entirely account for the body's resistance to weight loss.

A classic study on weight gain in twins demonstrated how genetics may affect our tendency to maintain a set point.[11] Twelve pairs of male identical twins volunteered to stay in a dormitory, where they were supervised 24 hours a day for 120 consecutive days. Researchers measured how much energy each man needed to maintain his body weight at the beginning of the study. For 100 days, the subjects were fed 1,000 kcal more per day than they needed to maintain body weight. Daily physical activity was limited, but each person was allowed to walk outdoors for 30 minutes each day, read, watch television and videos, and play cards and video games. The research staff stayed with these men to ensure that they did not stray from the study protocol.

Although all these men were overfed enough energy to gain about 26 pounds, the average weight gain they experienced was only 18 pounds. They gained mostly fat but also about 6 pounds of lean body mass. Interestingly, while each twin gained an amount similar to that of his brother, there was a very wide range of weight gained overall: the lowest weight gain was 9.5 pounds, while the highest was more than 29 pounds! Keep in mind that the food these men ate and the activities they performed were tightly controlled.

This study shows that, when people overeat by the same amount of food, they can gain very different amounts of weight. Researchers theorize that those who are more resistant to weight gain when they overeat have the ability to increase BMR, store more excess energy as lean body mass instead of fat, and increase spontaneous physical activity. Thus, genetic differences may explain why some people are better able to maintain a certain weight set point.

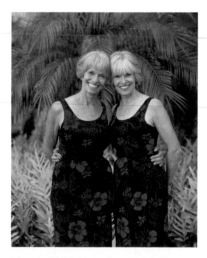

Identical twins tend to maintain a similar weight throughout life.

set-point theory A theory suggesting that the body raises or lowers energy expenditure in response to increased and decreased food intake and physical activity. This action maintains an individual's body weight within a narrow range.

RECAP

Many factors affect our ability to gain and lose weight. Our genetic background influences our height, weight, body shape, and metabolic rate. The thrifty gene theory suggests that some people possess a thrifty gene, or set of genes, that causes them to expend less energy at rest and during physical activity than people who do not have this gene (or genes). The set-point theory suggests that our body is designed to maintain weight within a narrow range, also called a set point. ■

Composition of the Diet Affects Fat Storage

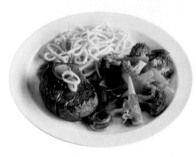

A balanced diet contains protein, carbohydrate, and fat.

As previously discussed, when we eat more energy than we expend, we gain weight. Most people eat a mixed diet, containing carbohydrate, fat, and protein. It is important to recognize that, if we avoided overeating, we would not gain weight. Scientists used to think that people would gain the same amount of weight if they ate too much food of any type, but now there is evidence to support the theory that, when we overeat, our body more readily stores the extra energy that comes from dietary fat, as this is the most efficient way to store excess energy. This may be due to the fact that eating fat doesn't cause much of an increase in metabolic rate, and the body stores fat in the form of adipose tissue quite easily. In contrast, when we consume excess energy by overeating protein or carbohydrate, our body's initial response is to use the energy from these macronutrients to fuel the body, with a smaller amount of the excess stored as fat. This does not mean, however, that you can eat as many low-fat foods as you want and not gain weight! Consistently overeating protein or carbohydrate can also lead to weight gain. Instead, maintain a balanced diet combining fat, carbohydrate, and protein, and reduce dietary fat to less than 35% of total energy. This strategy may help reduce the storage of fat energy as adipose tissue.

Metabolic Factors Influence Weight Loss and Gain

The following four metabolic factors have been identified as predictive of a person's risk for weight gain and resistance to weight loss:[5]

- *Relatively low metabolic rate.* As discussed previously, obese individuals weigh more and have a higher amount of lean tissue than people of normal weight and, thus, will have a higher absolute BMR. However at any given size, people vary in their relative BMR—it can be high, normal, or low. People who have a relatively low BMR are more at risk for weight gain and are resistant to weight loss.
- *Low level of spontaneous physical activity.* People who exhibit less spontaneous physical activity are at increased risk for weight gain.
- *Low sympathetic nervous system activity.* The sympathetic nervous system plays an important role in regulating all components of energy expenditure, and people with lower rates of sympathetic nervous system activity are more prone to obesity and more resistant to weight loss.
- *Low fat oxidation.* Some people oxidize relatively more carbohydrate for energy, which means that less fat will be oxidized and thus it will be stored in adipose tissue, so these people are at higher risk of gaining weight. People who oxidize relatively more fat for energy are more resistant to weight gain and are more successful at maintaining weight loss.

Physiologic Factors Influence Body Weight

Numerous physiologic factors affect body weight, including hypothalamic regulation of hunger and satiety, specific hormones, and other factors. Together, these contribute to the complexities of weight regulation.

Hunger and Satiety

As previously reviewed (in Chapter 3), *hunger* is the innate, physiologic drive or need to eat. Physical signals, such as a growling stomach and light-headedness, indicate when one is hungry. This drive for food is triggered by physiologic changes, such as low blood glucose, that affect chemicals in the brain. The hypothalamus plays an important role in hunger regulation. Special hypothalamic cells referred to as *feeding cells* respond to conditions of low blood glucose, causing hunger and driving a person to eat. Once one has eaten and the body has responded accordingly, other centers in the hypothalamus are triggered, and the desire to eat is reduced. The state reached in which there is no longer a desire to eat is referred to as *satiety*. Some people may have an insufficient satiety mechanism, which prevents them from feeling full after a meal, allowing them to overeat. It is important to recognize that people with a sufficient satiety mechanism can and do override these signals and overeat even when they are not hungry.

Energy-Regulating Hormones

Leptin is a protein; it is produced by adipose cells and functions as a hormone. First discovered in mice, leptin acts to reduce food intake and to cause a decrease in body weight and body fat. A gene called the obesity gene (*ob* gene) codes for the production of leptin. Obese mice were found to have a genetic mutation in the *ob* gene. This mutation reduces the ability of adipose cells to synthesize leptin in sufficient amounts; therefore, food intake increases dramatically, energy output is reduced, and weight gain occurs.

When these findings were first published, a great deal of excitement was generated about how leptin might decrease obesity in humans. Unfortunately, studies have shown that, although obese mice respond positively to leptin injections, obese humans do not. Instead, they tend to have very high amounts of leptin in their body and are insensitive to leptin's effects. In truth, researchers have just begun to learn about leptin and its role in the human body. They are currently studying its role in starvation and overeating, and it appears it might play a role in cardiovascular and kidney complications that result from obesity and related diseases.

In addition to leptin, numerous proteins affect the regulation of appetite and storage of body fat. Primary among these is **ghrelin,** a protein synthesized in the stomach. It acts as a hormone and plays an important role in appetite regulation through its actions in the hypothalamus. Ghrelin stimulates appetite and increases the amount of food one eats. Ghrelin levels increase before a meal and fall within about 1 hour after a meal. This action indicates that ghrelin may be a primary contributor to both hunger and satiety. Ghrelin levels appear to increase after weight loss, and researchers speculate that this factor could help explain why people who have lost weight have difficulty keeping it off.[12] We noted earlier that obese people seem to lose their sensitivity to leptin, but this is not true for ghrelin: obese people are just as sensitive to the effects of ghrelin as non-obese people.[13] For this reason, potential mechanisms that can block the actions of ghrelin are currently a prime target of research into the treatment of obesity.

Peptide YY, or **PYY,** is a protein produced in the gastrointestinal tract. It is released after a meal, in amounts proportional to the energy content of the meal. In contrast with ghrelin, PYY decreases appetite and inhibits food intake in animals and humans. Interestingly, obese individuals have lower levels of PYY when they are fasting and show less of an increase in PYY after a meal, compared with non-obese individuals, which suggests that PYY may be important in the manifestation and maintenance of obesity.[14]

Uncoupling proteins have recently become the focus of research into body weight. These proteins are found in the inner membrane of the mitochondria, which you may recall (from Chapter 7) are organelles present within cells that generate ATP, including skeletal muscle cells and adipose cells. Some research suggests that uncoupling proteins uncouple certain steps in ATP production; when this occurs, the process produces heat

leptin A hormone, produced by body fat, that acts to reduce food intake and to decrease body weight and body fat.

ghrelin A protein synthesized in the stomach that acts as a hormone and plays an important role in appetite regulation by stimulating appetite.

peptide YY (PYY) A protein produced in the gastrointestinal tract that is released after a meal in amounts proportional to the energy content of the meal; it decreases appetite and inhibits food intake.

instead of ATP. This production of heat increases energy expenditure and results in less storage of excess energy. Thus, a person with more uncoupling proteins or a higher activity of these proteins would be more resistant to weight gain and obesity.

Three forms of uncoupling proteins have been identified: UCP1 is found exclusively in **brown adipose tissue,** a type of adipose tissue that has more mitochondria than white adipose tissue. It is found in significant amounts in animals and newborn humans. It was traditionally thought that adult humans have very little brown adipose tissue. However, recent evidence suggests that humans may have substantially more brown adipose tissue than previously assumed,[15] and that people with higher BMI values have lower amounts of brown adipose tissue.[16] These findings suggest a possible role of brown adipose tissue in obesity. Two other uncoupling proteins, UCP2 and UCP3, are known to be important to energy expenditure and resistance to weight gain. These proteins are found in various tissues, including white adipose tissue and skeletal muscle. The roles of brown adipose tissue and uncoupling proteins in human obesity are currently being researched.

Other Physiologic Factors

The following other physiologic factors are known to increase satiety (or decrease food intake):

- The hormones serotonin and cholecystokinin (CCK); serotonin is made from the amino acid tryptophan, and CCK is produced by the intestinal cells and stimulates the gallbladder to secrete bile
- An increase in blood glucose levels, such as that normally seen after the consumption of a meal
- Stomach expansion
- Nutrient absorption from the small intestine

The following other physiologic factors can decrease satiety (or increase food intake):

- Beta-endorphins, which are hormones that enhance a sense of pleasure while eating, increasing food intake
- Neuropeptide Y, an amino-acid-containing compound produced in the hypothalamus; neuropeptide Y stimulates appetite
- Decreased blood glucose levels, such as the decrease that occurs after an overnight fast

Cultural and Economic Factors Affect Food Choices and Body Weight

Both cultural and economic factors can contribute to obesity. As previously discussed (in detail in Chapter 3), cultural factors (including religious beliefs and learned food preferences) affect our food choices and eating patterns. In addition, the customs of many cultures put food at the center of celebrations of festivals and holidays, and overeating is tacitly encouraged. In addition, as both parents now work outside the home in most American families, more people are embracing the "fast-food culture," eating highly processed and highly Caloric fast foods from restaurants and grocery stores rather than lower-kcal, home-cooked meals.

Coinciding with these cultural influences on food intake are cultural factors that promote an inactive life. These include the shift from manual labor to more sedentary jobs and increased access to labor-saving devices in all areas of our lives. Even seemingly minor changes—such as texting someone in your dorm instead of walking down the hall to chat or walking through an automated door instead of pushing a door open—add up to a lower expenditure of energy by the end of the day. Research with sedentary ethnic minority women in the United States indicates that other common barriers to increasing physical activity include lack of personal motivation, no physically active role models to emulate, acceptance of larger body size, exercise being considered culturally unacceptable, and fear for personal safety in both rural and urban settings.[17, 18] In short, cultural factors influence both food consumption and levels of physical activity and can contribute to weight gain.

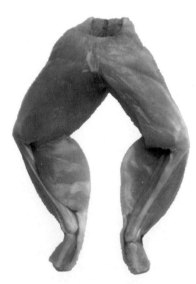

Food preferences often depend on culture. Some cultures enjoy foods such as frogs' legs, whereas others do not.

brown adipose tissue A type of adipose tissue that has more mitochondria than white adipose tissue and can increase energy expenditure by uncoupling oxidation from ATP production. It is found in significant amounts in animals and newborn humans.

Economic status is known to be related to health status, particularly in developed countries, such as the United States: people of lower economic status have higher rates of obesity and related chronic diseases than people of higher incomes.[19] In addition to the impact of one's income on access to healthcare, economic factors strongly impact our food choices and eating behaviors. It is a common belief that healthful foods are expensive, and that only wealthy people can afford to purchase them. While it is true that certain foods considered more healthful, such as organic foods, imported fruits and vegetables, many fish, and leaner selections of some meats, can be costly, does healthful eating always have to be expensive? Refer to the **Nutrition Myth or Fact?** box to learn more about whether a healthful diet can also be an affordable one.

Psychological and Social Factors Influence Behavior and Body Weight

Previously (in Chapter 3), we explored the concept that *appetite* can be experienced in the absence of hunger and therefore may be considered a psychological drive to eat, being stimulated by learned preferences for food and particular situations that promote eating. People may also follow social cues related to the timing and size of meals. Mood can also affect appetite, as some people will eat more or less if they feel depressed or happy. As you can imagine, appetite leads many people to overeat.

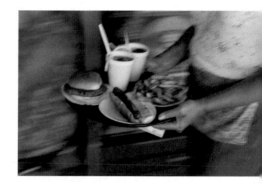

Easy-access and fast foods may be inexpensive and filling, but they are often also high in fat and sugar.

Some Social Factors Promote Overeating

Social factors—such as pressure from family and friends to eat the way they do—can encourage people to overeat. For example, the pressure to overeat on holidays is high, as family members or friends offer extra servings of favorite holiday foods and follow a very large meal with a rich dessert.

Americans also have numerous opportunities to overeat because of easy access throughout the day to foods high in fat and energy. Vending machines selling junk foods are everywhere: at some schools, in business offices, and even at fitness centers. Shopping malls are filled with fast-food restaurants, where inexpensive, large serving sizes are the norm. Food manufacturers are producing products in ever-larger serving sizes: Hardee's Monster Thickburger packs 1,290 kcal—which is 65% of the Calorie intake recommended for an average adult for an entire day! Even some foods traditionally considered healthful, such as some brands of peanut butter, yogurt, chicken soup, and flavored milks, are filled with added sugars and other ingredients that are high in energy. This easy access to large servings of high-energy meals and snacks leads many people to consume excess energy.

Some Social Factors Promote Inactivity

Social factors can also cause people to be less physically active. For instance, we don't even have to spend time or energy preparing food anymore, as everything is either ready-to-serve or requires just a few minutes to cook in a microwave oven. Other social factors restricting physical activity include living in an unsafe community; watching a lot of television; coping with family, community, and work responsibilities that do not involve physical activity; and living in an area with harsh weather conditions. Many overweight people identify such factors as major barriers to maintaining a healthful body weight, and research seems to confirm their influence.

Certainly, social factors are contributing to decreased physical activity among children. There was a time when children played outdoors regularly and physical education was offered daily in school. Today, many children cannot play outdoors due to safety concerns and lack of recreational facilities, and few schools have the resources to regularly offer physical education to children.

Another social factor promoting inactivity in both children and adults is the increasing dominance of technology in our choices of entertainment. Instead of participating in sports or gathering for a dance at the community hall, we go to the movies or stay at

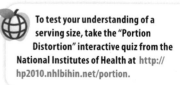

To test your understanding of a serving size, take the "Portion Distortion" interactive quiz from the National Institutes of Health at http:// hp2010.nhlbihin.net/portion.

Nutrition Myth OR Fact?

Does It Cost More to Eat Right?

The shelves of American supermarkets are filled with an abundance of healthful food options: organic meats and produce, exotic fish, out-of-season fresh fruits and vegetables flown in from warmer climates, whole-grain breads and cereals, and low-fat and low-sodium options of traditional foods. With all of this choice, it would seem easy for anyone to consume healthful foods throughout the year. But a closer look at the prices of these foods suggests that, for many, they simply are not affordable. This raises the question "Does eating right have to be expensive?"

It is a fact that organic foods are more expensive than non-organic options. However, as we'll explore in detail in Chapter 15, there is little evidence that organic foods are actually more nutritious than non-organic foods. In addition, some of the lowest-cost foods currently available in stores are also some of the most nutritious: these include beans, lentils, and other legumes; seasonal fruits; root vegetables, such as potatoes and winter squashes; frozen fruits and vegetables; and cooking oils high in mono- and polyunsaturated fats. In fact, frozen as well as canned fruits and vegetables are generally just as nutritious as fresh options, and they may be more so, depending on how long the fresh produce has been transported and stored and how long it has been sitting on the supermarket shelves. Thus, with some knowledge, skills, and focused attention, people can still eat healthfully on a tight budget.

Here are some more tips to help you save money when shopping for healthful foods:

- Buy whole grains such as cereals, brown rice, and pastas in bulk—they store well for longer periods and provide a good base for meals and snacks.
- Buy frozen vegetables on sale and stock up—these are just as healthful

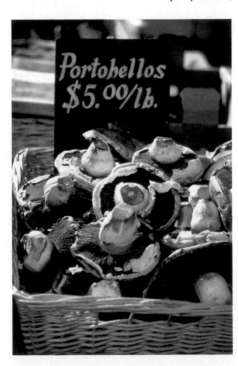

Although specialty foods (such as organic or imported products) can be expensive, lower-cost alternatives can be just as nutritious.

as fresh vegetables, require less preparation, and can be much cheaper.

- If lower-sodium options of canned vegetables are too expensive, buy the less expensive regular option and drain the juice from the vegetables before cooking.
- Consume smaller amounts of leaner meats—by eating less you'll not only save money but reduce your total intake of energy and fat while still providing the nutrients that support good health.
- Choose frozen fish or canned salmon or tuna packed in water as an alternative to fresh fish.
- Avoid frozen or dehydrated prepared meals. These are usually expensive; high in sodium, saturated fats, and energy; and low in fiber and other important nutrients.
- Buy generic or store brands of foods—be careful to check the labels to ensure the foods are similar in nutrient value to the higher-priced options.
- Cut coupons from local newspapers and magazines, and watch the sale circulars, so that you can stock up on healthful foods you can store.
- Consider cooking more meals at home; you'll have more control over what goes into your meals and will be able to cook larger amounts and freeze leftovers for future meals.

As you can see, eating healthfully does not have to be expensive. However, it helps to become a savvy consumer by reading food labels, comparing prices, and gaining the skills and confidence to cook at home. The information shared throughout this text should help you acquire these skills, so that you can eat healthfully, even on a limited budget!

home, watching television, surfing the Internet, and playing with video games and other hand-held devices. By reducing energy expenditure, these behaviors contribute to weight gain. For instance, a study of 11- to 13-year-old schoolchildren found that the children who watched more than 2 hours of television per night were more likely to be overweight or obese than the children who watched less than 2 hours of television per night. Similarly, television watching in adults has been shown to be associated with weight gain over a 4-year period.[20]

Social Pressures Can Promote Underweight

On the other hand, social pressures to maintain a lean body are great enough to encourage many people to undereat or to avoid foods that are perceived as "bad," especially fats. Our society ridicules and often ostracizes overweight people, many of whom face discrimination in housing, employment, and other areas of their lives. A recent study found that children who are obese are 60% more likely to experience bullying than children of normal weight.[21] Moreover, media images of waiflike fashion models and men in tight jeans with muscular chests and abdomens encourage many people—especially adolescents and young adults—to skip meals, resort to crash diets, and exercise obsessively. Even some people of normal body weight push themselves to achieve an unrealistic and unattainable weight goal, in the process threatening their health and even their lives (see Chapter 13.5, In Depth: Disordered Eating, immediately following this chapter, for information on the consequences of disordered eating).

It should be clear that how a person gains, loses, and maintains body weight is a complex matter. Most people who are overweight have tried several diet programs but have been unsuccessful in maintaining their weight loss. A significant number of these people have consequently given up all weight-loss attempts. Some even suffer from severe depression related to their body weight. Should we condemn these people as failures and continue to pressure them to lose weight? Should people who are overweight but otherwise healthy (for example, low blood pressure, cholesterol, triglycerides, and glucose levels) be advised to lose weight? As we continue to search for ways to help people achieve and maintain a healthful body weight, our society must take measures to reduce the social pressures facing people who are overweight or obese.

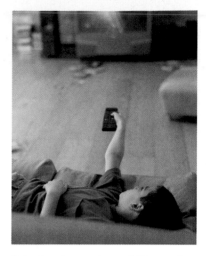

Behaviors learned as a child can affect adult weight and physical activity patterns.

RECAP

The macronutrient composition of the diet influences the storage of body fat, and metabolic factors, such as low relative resting metabolic rate, low spontaneous physical activity, low sympathetic nervous system activity, and low fat oxidation, increase the risk for weight gain. Physiologic factors, such as various energy-regulating hormones, impact body weight by their effects on satiety, appetite, and energy expenditure. Cultural and economic factors can significantly influence the amounts and types of food we eat. Psychological and social factors influencing weight include the ready availability of large portions of high-energy foods and lack of physical activity. Social pressures on those who are overweight can drive people to use harmful methods to achieve an unrealistic body weight. ■

*Nutri-*Case

Hannah

"I wonder what it would be like to be able to look in the mirror and not feel fat. Like my friend Kristi—she's been skinny since we were kids. I'm just the opposite: I've felt bad about my weight ever since I can remember. One of my worst memories is from the YMCA swim camp the summer I was 10 years old. Of course, we had to wear a swimsuit, and the other kids picked on me so bad I'll never forget it. One of the boys called me 'fatso,' and the girls were even meaner, especially when I was changing in the locker room. That was the last year I was in the swim camp, and I've never owned a swimsuit since."

Think back to your own childhood. Were you ever teased for some aspect of yourself that you felt unable to change? How might organizations that work with children, such as schools, YMCAs, scout troops, and church-based groups, increase their leaders' awareness of social stigmatization of overweight children and reduce incidents of teasing, bullying, and other insensitivity?

How Can You Achieve and Maintain a Healthful Body Weight?

Achieving and maintaining a healthful body weight involve three primary strategies:

- Gradual changes in energy intake
- Incorporation of regular and appropriate physical activity
- Application of behavior modification techniques

In this section, we first discuss popular diet plans, which may or may not incorporate these strategies. We then explain how to design a personalized weight-loss plan that includes all three of them. Finally, we review the use of prescribed medications and dietary supplements in losing weight.

If You Decide to Follow a Popular Diet Plan, Choose One Based on the Three Strategies

If you'd like to lose weight, the information ahead will help you design your own personalized diet plan. If you'd feel more comfortable following an established plan, however, many are available. How can you know whether it is based on sound dietary principles and whether its promise of long-term weight loss will prove true for *you*? Look to the three strategies just identified: Does the plan promote gradual reductions in energy intake? Does it advocate increased physical activity? Does it include strategies for modifying your eating and activity-related behaviors? Reputable diet plans incorporate all of these strategies. Unfortunately, many dieters are drawn to fad diets, which do not.

Avoid Fad Diets

Beware of fad diets! They are simply what their name implies—fads that do not result in long-term, healthful weight changes. To be precise, fad diets are programs that enjoy short-term popularity and are sold based on a marketing gimmick that appeals to the public's desires and fears. Of the hundreds of such diets on the market today, most will "die" within a year, only to be born again as a "new and improved" fad diet. The goal of the person or company designing and marketing a fad diet is to make money.

How can you tell if the program you are interested in qualifies as a fad diet? Here are some pointers to help you:

- The promoters of the diet claim that the program is new, improved, or based on some new discovery; however, no scientific data are available to support these claims.
- The program is touted for its ability to promote rapid weight loss or body fat loss, usually more than 2 pounds per week, and may include the claim that weight loss can be achieved with little or no physical exercise.
- The diet includes special foods and supplements, many of which are expensive and/or difficult to find or can be purchased only from the diet promoter. Common recommendations for these diets include avoiding certain foods, eating only a special combination of certain foods, and including "magic" foods in the diet that "burn fat" and "speed up metabolism."
- The diet may include a rigid menu that must be followed daily or may limit participants to eating a few select foods each day. Variety and balance are discouraged, and restriction of certain foods (such as fruits and vegetables) is encouraged.
- Many programs promote supplemental foods and/or nutritional supplements that are described as critical to the success of the diet. They usually include claims that these supplements can cure or prevent a variety of health ailments or that the diet can stop the aging process.

In a world where many of us feel we have to meet a certain physical standard to be attractive and "good enough," fad diets flourish, with millions of people trying one each year.[22] Unfortunately, the only people who usually benefit from them are their marketers, who can become very wealthy promoting programs that are highly ineffectual.

Diets Focusing on Macronutrient Composition May or May Not Work for You

It is well recognized that achieving a negative energy balance is the major factor in successful weight loss. The impact of the macronutrient composition of a diet is currently a topic of considerable debate. The three main types of weight-loss diets that have been most seriously and comprehensively researched all encourage increased consumption of certain macronutrients and restrict the consumption of others. Provided here is a brief review of these three main types and their general effects on weight loss and health parameters.

Diets High in Carbohydrate and Moderate in Fat and Protein   Nutritionally balanced high-carbohydrate, moderate-fat and -protein diets typically contain 55% to 60% of total energy intake as carbohydrate, 20% to 30% of total energy intake as fat, and 15% to 20% of energy intake as protein. These diets include Weight Watchers, Jenny Craig, and others that follow the general guidelines of the DASH diet and the USDA Food Guide. All of these diet plans emphasize that weight loss occurs when energy intake is lower than energy expenditure. The goal is gradual weight loss, or about 1 to 2 lb of body weight per week. Typical energy deficits are between 500 and 1,000 kcal/day. It is recommended that women eat no less than 1,000 to 1,200 kcal/day and that men consume no less than 1,200 to 1,400 kcal/day. Regular physical activity is encouraged.

To date, these types of low-energy diets have been researched more than any others. A substantial amount of high-quality scientific evidence (from randomized controlled trials) indicates that they may be effective in decreasing body weight—at least initially. In addition, the people who lose weight on these diets may also decrease their LDL-cholesterol, reduce their blood triglyceride levels, and decrease their blood pressure. However, recently published results from a randomized controlled trial following almost 50,000 US women for 7 years has caused considerable debate around whether these types of diets result in long-term weight loss or reduce the risk for chronic diseases. This study found that, contrary to established beliefs, this type of diet did not result in significant long-term weight loss or reduce the risks for breast and colorectal cancers or cardiovascular disease.[23–26] Is it possible that diets high in carbohydrate and moderate in fat and protein are not as effective as we'd come to believe? Refer to the **Nutrition Debate** at the end of this chapter (page 546) to learn more about this controversy.

Diets Low in Carbohydrate and High in Fat and Protein   Low-carbohydrate, high-fat and protein diets cycle in and out of popularity on a regular basis. By definition, these types of diets generally contain about 55% to 65% of total energy intake as fat and most of the remaining balance of daily energy intake as protein. Examples of these types of diets include Dr. Atkins' Diet Revolution, the Carbohydrate Addict's Diet, Life Without Bread, Sugar Busters, and Protein Power. These diets minimize the role of restricting total energy intake on weight loss. They instead advise participants to restrict carbohydrate intake, proposing that carbohydrates are addictive and that they cause significant overeating, insulin surges leading to excessive fat storage, and an overall metabolic imbalance that leads to obesity. The goal is to reduce carbohydrates enough to cause ketosis, which will decrease blood glucose and insulin levels and can reduce appetite.

Countless people claim to have lost substantial weight on these types of diets. Although quality scientific studies of these diets are just beginning to be conducted, the current limited evidence suggests that individuals following them, in both free-living and experimental conditions, do lose weight. In addition, it appears that those people who lose weight may also experience positive metabolic changes similar to those seen with higher-carbohydrate diets.

So are low-carb diets effective? A recent review of all of the published studies of these diets resulted in the conclusion that low-carb diets are just as effective, and possibly more effective, in regard to weight loss and reducing cardiovascular disease risk for a period of

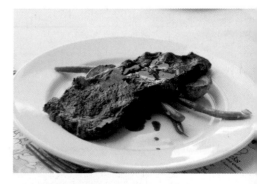

"Low-carb" diets may lead to weight loss but they can be nutritionally inadequate in some cases.

up to 1 year.[27] However, the authors conclude that the long-term health benefits of this type of a diet are unknown at this time, and more research must be conducted in this area.

Low-Fat and Very-Low-Fat Diets   Low-fat diets contain 11% to 19% of total energy as fat, whereas very-low-fat diets contain less than 10% of total energy as fat. Both of these types of diets are high in carbohydrate and moderate in protein. Examples include Dr. Dean Ornish's Program for Reversing Heart Disease and the New Pritikin Program. These programs were not originally designed for weight loss but, rather, were developed to decrease or reverse heart disease. They do not focus on total energy intake but emphasize eating foods higher in complex carbohydrates and fiber. Consumption of sugar and white flour is very limited. The Ornish diet is vegetarian, whereas the Pritikin diet allows 3.5 oz of lean meat per day. Regular physical activity is a key component of both.

These diets are not popular with consumers, who view them as too restrictive and difficult to follow. Thus, there are limited data on their effects. However, high-quality evidence suggests that people following these diets do lose weight, and some data suggest that they also experience decreased LDL-cholesterol, blood triglyceride, glucose, and insulin levels, as well as lower blood pressure. Few side effects have been reported on these diets; the most common is flatus, which typically decreases over time. Low-fat diets are low in vitamin B_{12}, and very-low-fat diets are low in essential fatty acids, vitamins B_{12} and E, and zinc. Thus, supplementation is needed. These types of diets are not considered safe for people with diabetes who are insulin dependent (either type 1 or type 2) or for people with carbohydrate-malabsorption illnesses.

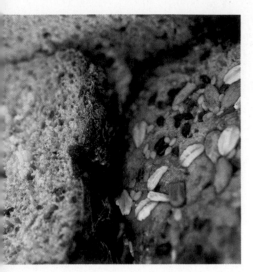

Low-fat and very-low-fat diets emphasize eating foods higher in complex carbohydrates and fiber.

If You Decide to Design Your Own Diet Plan, Include the Three Strategies

As we noted earlier, a healthful and effective weight-loss plan involves implementing a modest reduction in energy intake, incorporating physical activity into each day, and practicing changes in behavior that can assist you in reducing your energy intake and increasing your energy expenditure. Following are some guidelines for designing your own personalized diet plan that incorporates these strategies.

Set Realistic Goals

The first key to safe and effective weight loss is setting realistic goals related to how much weight to lose and how quickly to lose it. Although making gradual changes in body weight is frustrating for most people, this slower change is much more effective in maintaining weight loss over the long term. Ask yourself the question "How long did it take me to gain this extra weight?" If you are like most people, your answer is that it took 1 or more years, not just a few months. A fair expectation for weight loss is similarly gradual: experts recommend a pace of about 0.5 to 2 pounds per week. A weight-loss plan should never provide less than 1,200 kcal/day unless you are under a physician's supervision. Your weight-loss goals should also take into consideration any health-related concerns you have. After checking with your physician, you may decide initially to set a goal of simply maintaining your current weight and preventing additional weight gain. After your weight has remained stable for several weeks, you might then write down realistic goals for weight loss.

Goals that are more likely to be realistic and achievable share the following characteristics:

- *They are specific.* Telling yourself "I will eat less this week" is not helpful because the goal is not specific. An example of a specific goal is "I will eat only half of my restaurant entrée tonight and take the rest home and eat it tomorrow for lunch."
- *They are reasonable.* If you are not presently physically active, it would be unreasonable to set of a goal of exercising for 30 minutes every day. A more reasonable goal would be to exercise for 15 minutes per day, 3 days per week. Once you've achieved

that goal, you can increase the frequency, intensity, and time of exercise according to the improvements in fitness that you have experienced.

- *They are measurable.* Effective goals are ones you can measure. An example is "I will lose at least 1 pound by May 1st" or "I will substitute drinking water for my regular soft drink at lunch each day this week." Recording your specific, measurable goals will help you better determine whether you are achieving them.

By monitoring your progress regularly you can determine whether you are meeting your goals or whether you need to revise them based on accomplishments or challenges that arise.

Eat Smaller Portions of Lower-Fat Foods

The portion sizes of foods offered and sold in restaurants and grocery stores have expanded considerably over the past 40 years. One of the most challenging issues related to food is understanding what a healthful portion size is and knowing how to reduce the portion sizes of the foods we eat.

Studies indicate that, when children and adults are presented with large portion sizes of foods and beverages, they eat more energy overall and do not respond to cues of fullness.[28, 29] Thus, it has been suggested that effective weight-loss strategies include reducing both the portion size and the energy density of foods consumed, as well as replacing energy-dense beverages with low-Calorie or non-Calorie beverages.[29]

What specific changes can you make to reduce your energy intake and stay healthy? Here are some suggestions:

- Follow the serving sizes recommended in the USDA Food Patterns (ChooseMyPlate .gov). Making this change involves understanding what constitutes a portion and measuring foods to determine whether they meet or exceed the recommended amounts.
- To help increase your understanding of the portion sizes of packaged foods, measure out the amount of food that is identified as 1 serving on the Nutrition Facts Panel, and eat it from a plate or bowl instead of straight out of the box or bag.
- Try using smaller dishes, bowls, and glasses. This will make your portion appear larger, and you'll be eating or drinking less.
- When cooking at home, put a serving of the entrée on your plate; then freeze any leftovers in single-serving containers. This way, you won't be tempted to eat the whole batch before the food goes bad, and you'll have ready-made servings for future meals.
- To help fill you up, take second helpings of plain vegetables. That way, dessert may not seem so tempting!
- When buying snacks, go for single-serving, prepackaged items. If you buy larger bags or boxes, divide the snack into single-serving bags.
- When you have a treat, such as ice cream, measure out ½ cup, eat it slowly, and enjoy it!

Now that you have your portion sizes under control, what can you do to reduce the saturated fat and energy content of the portions you *do* eat? Remember that people trying to lose weight should aim for a total fat intake of 15% to 25% of total energy and a saturated fat intake of 10% or below. This goal can be achieved by eliminating extra fats, such as butter, margarine, and mayonnaise, and snack foods, such as ice cream, doughnuts, and cakes. Save these foods as occasional special treats. Select lower-fat versions of the foods listed in the USDA Food Patterns. This means selecting leaner cuts of meat (such as the white meat of poultry and extra-lean ground beef) and reduced-fat or skim dairy products and using lower-fat preparation methods (such as baking and broiling instead of frying). It also means switching from a sugar-filled beverage to a low-Calorie or non-Calorie beverage during and between meals.

In addition, try to increase the number of times each day that you choose foods that are relatively low in energy density. This includes salads (with low- or non-Calorie dressings), fruits, vegetables, low-fat and nonfat dairy products, and broth-based soups.

Research indicates that eating a diet low in energy density results in greater weight loss than simply reducing portion sizes.[30, 31] Because low energy-dense foods are relatively high in water and fiber than more energy-dense foods, they have a greater volume and occupy more space in the stomach, helping a person to feel full. In addition, low energy-dense foods are just as satiating as those higher in energy density, but they are lower in energy for every gram of food consumed. Thus, the energy content of an energy-dense eating plan is lower but equally as satisfying.

Figure 13.10 illustrates two sets of meals, one higher in energy density and one lower in energy density. You can see from this figure that simple changes to a meal, such as choosing lower-fat dairy products, skipping the high-fat condiments, and eating fresh fruit for dessert, can reduce energy intake without sacrificing taste, pleasure, or nutritional quality!

Participate in Regular Physical Activity

The Dietary Guidelines for Americans emphasize the role of physical activity in maintaining a healthful weight. Why? Of course, we expend extra energy during physical activity, but there's more to it than that, because exercise alone (without a reduction of energy intake) does not result in dramatic weight loss. Instead, one of the most important reasons for being regularly active is that it helps us maintain or increase our lean body mass and our BMR. In contrast, energy restriction alone causes us to lose lean body mass. As you've learned, the more lean body mass we have, the more energy we expend over the long term.

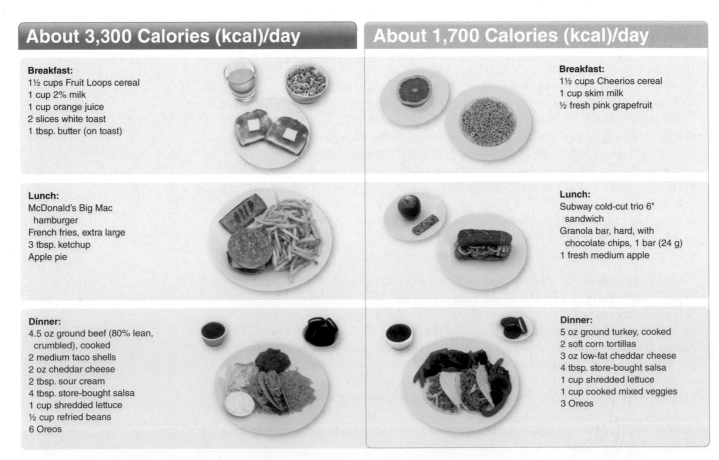

About 3,300 Calories (kcal)/day

Breakfast:
1½ cups Fruit Loops cereal
1 cup 2% milk
1 cup orange juice
2 slices white toast
1 tbsp. butter (on toast)

Lunch:
McDonald's Big Mac hamburger
French fries, extra large
3 tbsp. ketchup
Apple pie

Dinner:
4.5 oz ground beef (80% lean, crumbled), cooked
2 medium taco shells
2 oz cheddar cheese
2 tbsp. sour cream
4 tbsp. store-bought salsa
1 cup shredded lettuce
½ cup refried beans
6 Oreos

About 1,700 Calories (kcal)/day

Breakfast:
1½ cups Cheerios cereal
1 cup skim milk
½ fresh pink grapefruit

Lunch:
Subway cold-cut trio 6" sandwich
Granola bar, hard, with chocolate chips, 1 bar (24 g)
1 fresh medium apple

Dinner:
5 oz ground turkey, cooked
2 soft corn tortillas
3 oz low-fat cheddar cheese
4 tbsp. store-bought salsa
1 cup shredded lettuce
1 cup cooked mixed veggies
3 Oreos

FIGURE 13.10 The energy density of two sets of meals. The set on the left is higher in energy density, while the set on the right is lower in energy density and the preferred choice for a person trying to lose weight.

While very few weight-loss studies have documented long-term maintenance of weight loss, those that have find that only people who are regularly active are able to maintain most of their weight loss. The National Weight Control Registry is an ongoing project documenting the habits of people who have lost at least 30 pounds and kept their weight off for at least 1 year. Of the more than 4,000 people studied thus far, the average weight loss was 73 pounds over 5.7 years.[32] Almost all of the people (89%) reported changing both physical activity and dietary intake to lose weight and maintain weight loss. No one form of exercise seems to be most effective, but many people report doing some form of aerobic exercise (walking is the most commonly reported form of activity) for approximately 1 hour per day most days of the week. In fact, on average, this group expended more than 2,800 kcal each week through physical activity!

In addition to expending energy and maintaining lean body mass and BMR, regular physical activity improves our mood, results in a higher quality of sleep, increases self-esteem, and gives us a sense of accomplishment. All of these changes enhance our ability to engage in long-term healthful lifestyle behaviors.

What specific changes can you make to your level of physical activity? Although plenty of practical suggestions will be offered (in Chapter 14), here are some ideas that can help you start identifying—and overcoming—your barriers to an active life:

- "I don't have enough time!" An active lifestyle doesn't have to consume all your free time. Try to do a minimum of 30 minutes of moderate activity most—preferably all—days of the week. If you can, do 45 minutes. But remember, you don't have to get in all of your daily activity in one go! Be active for a few minutes at a time throughout your day. Walk from your dorm or apartment to classes, if possible. Instead of meeting friends for lunch, meet them for a lunchtime walk, jog, or workout. Break up study sessions with 3 minutes of jumping jacks. Skip the elevator and take the stairs. When you're talking on the phone, pace instead of sitting still.
- "I can't manage the details!" Bust this excuse by keeping clean clothes, shoes, water, and equipment for physical activity in a convenient place. If time management is an obstacle, enroll in a scheduled fitness class, yoga class, sports activity, walking group, or running club. Put it on your schedule of academic classes and make it part of your weekly routine.
- "I just don't like to work out!" You don't have to! Try dancing, roller blading, walking, hiking, swimming, tennis, or any other activity you enjoy.
- "I can't stay motivated!" Friends can help. Use the "buddy" system by exercising with a friend and calling each other when you need encouragement to stay motivated. Or keep a journal or log of your daily physical activity. Write your week's goal at the top of the page (such as "Walk to and from campus each day, and at least 10 minutes on campus at lunch").

Incorporate Appropriate Behavior Modifications into Daily Life

Successful weight loss and long-term maintenance of a healthful weight require people to modify their behaviors. Some of the behavior modifications related to food and physical activity were discussed in the previous sections. Here are a few more tips on modifying behavior that will assist you in losing weight and maintaining a healthful weight:

- Shop for food only when you're not hungry.
- Avoid buying problem foods—that is, foods that you may have difficulty eating in moderate amounts.
- Avoid purchasing high-fat, high-sugar foods from vending machines and convenience stores.
- Avoid feelings of deprivation by eating small, regular meals throughout the day.
- Eat only at set times in one location. Do not eat while studying, working, driving, watching television, and so forth.
- Slow down while eating.

- Keep a log of what you eat, when, and why. Try to identify social or emotional cues that cause you to overeat, such as getting a poor grade on an exam or feeling lonely. Then strategize about non-food-related ways to cope, such as phoning a sympathetic friend.
- Save high-fat, high-kcal snack foods, such as ice cream, doughnuts, and cakes, for occasional special treats.
- Whether at home or dining out, share food with others.
- Prepare healthful snacks to take along with you, so that you won't be tempted by foods from vending machines, fast-food restaurants, and so forth.
- Chew food slowly, taking at least 20 minutes to eat a full meal and stopping at once if you begin to feel full.
- Always use appropriate utensils.
- Leave food on your plate or store it for the next meal.
- Don't punish yourself for deviating from your plan (and you will—everyone does). Ask others to avoid responding to any slips you make.

RECAP

Achieving and maintaining a healthful weight involves gradual reductions in energy intake, such as by eating smaller portion sizes and limiting dietary fat; engaging in regular physical activity; and applying appropriate behavior modification techniques. Fad diets do not use these strategies and do not result in long-term, healthful weight change. Diets based on macronutrient composition may promote long-term weight loss, but some have unhealthful side effects. ■

What Disorders Are Related to Energy Intake?

At the beginning of this chapter, we provided some definitions of underweight, overweight, obesity, and morbid obesity. Let's take a closer look at these disorders.

Underweight

As defined earlier in this chapter, underweight occurs when a person has too little body fat to maintain health. People with a BMI of less than 18.5 kg/m² are typically considered underweight. Being underweight can be just as unhealthful as being obese, because it increases the risk for infections and illness and impairs the body's ability to recover. Some people are healthy but underweight because of their genetics and/or because they are very physically active and consume adequate energy to maintain their underweight status, but not enough to gain weight. In others, underweight is due to heavy smoking; an underlying disease, such as cancer or HIV infection; or an eating disorder, such as *anorexia nervosa* (see Chapter 13.5, In Depth: Disordered Eating).

Safe and Effective Weight Gain

With so much emphasis in the United States on obesity and weight loss, some find it surprising that many people are trying to gain weight. People looking to gain weight include those who are underweight to the extent that it is compromising their health and many athletes who are attempting to increase strength and power for competition.

To gain weight, people must eat more energy than they expend. While overeating large amounts of foods high in saturated fats (such as bacon, sausage, and cheese) can cause weight gain, doing this without exercising is not considered healthful because most of the weight gained is fat, and high-fat diets increase our risks for cardiovascular and other diseases. Unless there are medical reasons to eat a high-fat diet, it is recommended that people trying to gain weight eat a diet that is relatively low in dietary fat (less than 30% of total kcal) and relatively high in fiber-rich carbohydrates (55% of total kcal). Recommendations for weight gain include the following:

- Eat a diet that includes about 500 to 1,000 kcal/day more than is needed to maintain present body weight. Although we don't know exactly how much extra energy is needed to gain 1 pound, estimates range from 3,000 to 3,500 kcal. Thus, eating 500 to 1,000 kcal/day in excess should result in a gain of 1 to 2 pounds of weight each week.
- Eat frequently, including meals and numerous snacks throughout the day. Many underweight people do not take the time to eat often enough.
- Avoid the use of tobacco products, as they depress appetite and increase metabolic rate, and both of these effects oppose weight gain. Tobacco use also causes lung, mouth, and esophageal cancers and is a factor in cardiovascular disease.
- Exercise regularly and incorporate weight lifting or some other form of resistance training into your exercise routine. This form of exercise is most effective in increasing muscle mass. Performing aerobic exercise (such as walking, running, bicycling, or swimming) at least 30 minutes for 3 days per week will help maintain a healthy cardiovascular system.

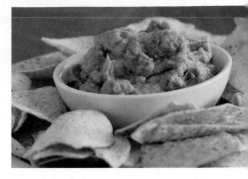

Eating frequent nutrient-dense snacks can help promote weight gain.

The key to gaining weight is to eat frequent meals throughout the day and to select energy-dense foods. When selecting foods that are higher in fat, make sure you select foods higher in polyunsaturated and monounsaturated fats (such as peanut butter, olive and canola oils, and avocados). For instance, smoothies and milkshakes made with low-fat milk or yogurt are a great way to take in a lot of energy. Eating peanut butter with fruit or celery and including salad dressings on your salad are other ways to increase the energy density of foods. The biggest challenge to weight gain is setting aside time to eat; by packing a lot of foods to take with you throughout the day, you can enhance your opportunities to eat more.

Amino Acid and Protein Supplements Do Not Increase Muscle Mass

As with weight loss, there are many products marketed for weight gain. Many of these products are said to be *anabolic*, that is, to increase muscle mass. The most common of these include amino acid and protein supplements, often powders used to make protein "shakes." Do these substances really work?

A growing body of evidence exists to show that amino acid and protein supplements are not necessary to enhance muscle gain; adequate intake of energy, protein from high-quality food sources, and resistance training promote healthy increases in muscle mass.[33] The health consequences of using them are unknown. Moreover, although they are legal to sell in the United States, all potentially anabolic substances are banned by the National Football League, the National Collegiate Athletic Association, and the International Olympic Committee. We also know that buying these substances can have a substantial slenderizing effect—on your wallet!

Overweight

Overweight is defined as having a moderate amount of excess body fat, resulting in a person having a weight for a given height that is greater than some accepted standard but is not considered obese. People with a BMI between 25 and 29.9 kg/m² are considered overweight. Being overweight does not appear to be as detrimental to our health as being obese, but some of the health risks of overweight include an increased risk for high blood pressure, heart disease, type 2 diabetes, sleep disorders, osteoarthritis, gallstones, and gynecological abnormalities. Overweight people also have a higher risk of becoming obese than people of normal weight, and obesity confers an even higher risk for these diseases and for premature death. Because of these concerns, health professionals recommend that overweight individuals adopt a lifestyle that incorporates healthful eating and regular

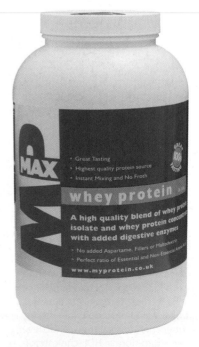

Protein powders or amino acid supplements will not enhance muscle growth or make you stronger.

physical activity in an attempt to prevent additional weight gain, to reduce body weight to a normal level, and/or to support long-term health even if body weight is not significantly reduced.

Obesity and Morbid Obesity

Obesity is defined as having an excess body fat that adversely affects health, resulting in a person having a weight for a given height that is substantially greater than some accepted standard. People with a BMI between 30 and 39.9 kg/m² are considered obese. Morbid obesity occurs when a person's body weight exceeds 100% of normal; people who are morbidly obese have a BMI greater than or equal to 40 kg/m².

Why Is Obesity Harmful?

Both overweight and obesity are considered an epidemic in the United States. Obesity rates have increased more than 50% during the past 20 years, and it is now estimated that about 35.7% of adults 20 years and older are obese.[34] This alarming rise in obesity is a major health concern because it is linked to many chronic diseases and complications:

- Hypertension
- Dyslipidemia, including elevated total cholesterol, triglycerides, and LDL-cholesterol and decreased HDL-cholesterol
- Type 2 diabetes
- Heart disease
- Stroke
- Gallbladder disease
- Osteoarthritis
- Sleep apnea
- Certain cancers, such as colon, breast, endometrial, and gallbladder cancer
- Menstrual irregularities and infertility
- Gestational diabetes, premature fetal deaths, neural tube defects, and complications during labor and delivery
- Depression
- Alzheimer's disease, dementia, and cognitive decline

Abdominal obesity, specifically a large amount of visceral fat that is stored deep within the abdomen (**Figure 13.11**), is one of five risk factors collectively referred to as **metabolic syndrome.** A diagnosis of metabolic syndrome—which is typically made if a person has three or more of the factors—increases one's risk for heart disease, type 2 diabetes, and stroke. These risk factors include the following:

- Abdominal obesity (defined as a waist circumference greater than or equal to 40 inches for men and 35 inches for women)
- Higher-than-normal triglyceride levels (greater than or equal to 150 mg/dL)
- Lower-than-normal HDL-cholesterol levels (less than 40 mg/dL in men and 50 mg/dL in women)
- Higher-than-normal blood pressure (greater than or equal to 130/85 mm Hg)
- Fasting blood glucose levels greater than or equal to 100 mg/dL, including people with diabetes[35]

Metabolic syndrome is one of a number of components of global cardiometabolic risk, which includes the factors of metabolic syndrome and the additional factors of elevated LDL-cholesterol (≥130 mg/dL), smoking, inflammation, and insulin resistance.[36, 37]

People with metabolic syndrome are twice as likely to develop heart disease and five times as likely to develop type 2 diabetes as people without metabolic syndrome. About 34% of adults in the United States have metabolic syndrome, and rising obesity rates are contributing to increased rates.[38]

metabolic syndrome A clustering of risk factors that increase one's risk for heart disease, type 2 diabetes, and stroke, including abdominal obesity, higher-than-normal triglyceride levels, lower-than-normal HDL-cholesterol levels, higher-than-normal blood pressure (greater than or equal to 130/85 mm Hg), and elevated fasting blood glucose levels.

Obesity is also associated with an increased risk for premature death: mortality rates for people with a BMI of 30 kg/m² or higher are 50% to 100% above the rates for those with a BMI between 20 and 25 kg/m². As discussed (in Chapter 1), several of the leading causes of death in the United States are associated with obesity.

Why Do People Become Obese?

Although it is certainly true that obesity, like overweight, is caused by eating more energy than is expended, it is also true that some people are more susceptible to becoming obese than others. As was seen with the twin study earlier in this chapter, different people consuming the same excessive energy and engaging in the same low level of physical activity will gain very different amounts of weight. Why? Research on the causes of obesity are ongoing, but let's explore some current theories.

Genetic and Physiologic Factors Influence Obesity Risk   Because a person's genetic background influences his or her height, weight, body shape, metabolic rate, and propensity to oxidize relatively more fat or carbohydrate, it can also affect a person's risk for obesity. Some obesity experts point out that, if proved, the existence of a thrifty gene or genes (discussed earlier) would show that obese people have a genetic tendency to expend less energy both at rest and during physical activity. Other researchers are working to determine whether the set-point theory can partially explain why many obese people are very resistant to weight loss. As we learn more about genetics, we will gain a greater understanding of the role it plays in the development and treatment of obesity.

We also discussed earlier several physiologic factors that may influence an individual's experience of hunger and satiation. These include the proteins leptin, ghrelin, PYY, and uncoupling proteins. Other physiologic factors, such as beta-endorphins, neuropeptide Y, and decreased blood glucose, can reduce satiety or increase hunger, theoretically promoting overeating and weight gain.

An abnormally low level of thyroid hormone, or an elevated level of the hormone cortisol, can lead to weight gain and obesity. A physician can check your blood for levels of these hormones. Certain prescription medications, including steroids used for asthma and other disorders, seizure medications, and some antidepressants, can slow basal metabolic rate or stimulate appetite, leading to weight gain.[39]

Childhood Obesity Is Linked to Adult Obesity   The prevalence of overweight and obesity in children and adolescents is increasing at an alarming rate in the United States (**Figure 13.12**). There was a time when having extra "baby fat" was considered good for the child. We assumed that childhood overweight was temporary and that the child would grow out of it. While it is important for children to have a certain minimum level of body fat to maintain health and to grow properly, researchers are now concerned that overweight and obesity are harming children's health and increasing their risk for overweight and obesity in adulthood.

Health data demonstrate that obese children are already showing signs of chronic disease while they are young, including elevated blood pressure, high cholesterol levels, and

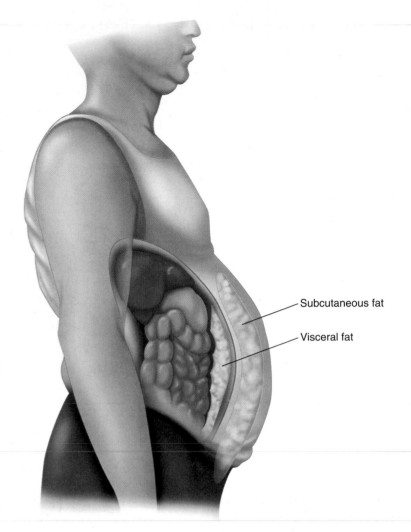

Subcutaneous fat

Visceral fat

FIGURE 13.11 Abdominal obesity, specifically a high amount of visceral fat stored deep within the abdomen, is one of the risk factors for metabolic syndrome.

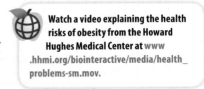

Watch a video explaining the health risks of obesity from the Howard Hughes Medical Center at www .hhmi.org/biointeractive/media/health_ problems-sm.mov.

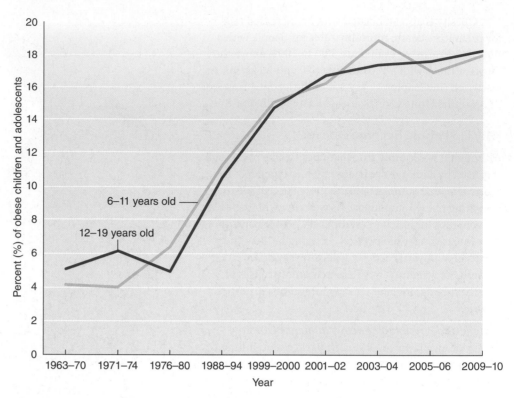

FIGURE 13.12 Increases in childhood and adolescent obesity from 1963 to 2010. (*Source:* Data from Centers for Disease Control and Prevention, National Center for Health Statistics. Prevalence of Obesity Among Children and Adolescents: United States, Trends 1963–1965 Through 2009–2010.)

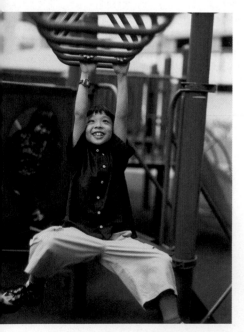

Adequate physical activity is instrumental in preventing childhood obesity.

changes in insulin and glucose metabolism that may increase the risk for type 2 diabetes (formerly known as *adult-onset diabetes*). In some communities, children as young as 5 years of age have been diagnosed with type 2 diabetes. Unfortunately, many of these children will maintain these disease risk factors into adulthood.

Does being an obese child guarantee that obesity will be maintained during adulthood? Although some children who are obese grow up to have a normal body weight, it has been estimated that about 70% of children who are obese maintain their higher weight as adults.[40]

Having either one or two overweight parents increases the risk for obesity two to four times. This may be explained in part by genetics or by unhealthful eating patterns or lack of physical activity within the family. We know that children who eat healthful diets that do not contain a lot of empty Calories and are very physically active are unlikely to become obese. In contrast, children who consume a lot of empty Calories and spend most of their time on the computer or watching television are more likely to be obese. When these patterns are carried into adolescence and adulthood, the obesity is likely to persist.

Social Factors Appear to Influence Obesity Risk We noted earlier that social factors influence body weight. In particular, poverty has been linked to obesity. One reason for this may be that high-Calorie processed foods cost less, are more satiating, and are easier to find and prepare than more healthful foods, such as fresh fruits and vegetables. Also, people living in poverty may not have access to safe places to walk, hike, or engage in other forms of physical activity, or to afford the cost of membership in a health club or commercial weight-loss program.

Our social ties may also have a subtle influence on our risk for obesity. Although their data have been challenged, researchers from Harvard Medical School evaluated a social network of more than 12,000 people and concluded that an individual's risk of becoming obese increases significantly—by 37–57%—if the person has a spouse, sibling, or friend who has become obese.[41]

Hence, obesity is a **multifactorial disease,** with genetics, physiology, and lifestyle choices all potentially contributing to the condition.

Does Obesity Respond to Treatment?

Ironically, up to 40% of women and 25% of men are dieting at any given time. How can obesity rates be so high when there are so many people dieting? Although relatively few studies have tracked maintenance of weight loss, existing evidence suggests that only about 20% of obese people are successful at long-term weight loss.[32] In this study, success was defined as losing at least 10% of initial body weight and maintaining the loss for at least 1 year. These results suggest that about 80% of obese people who are dieting are somehow failing to lose weight or to keep it off. Although these statistics might suggest that obesity somehow resists intervention, that's not the case. Bearing in mind that 20% of people do succeed in long-term maintenance of weight loss, the question becomes "How do they do it?"

Lifestyle Changes Can Help The first line of defense in treating obesity in adults is a low-energy diet and regular physical activity. Overweight and obese individuals should work with a healthcare practitioner to design and maintain a low-fat diet (less than 30% of total energy from fat) that has a deficit of 500 to 1,000 kcal/day. Physical activity should be increased gradually, so that the person can build a program in which he or she is exercising at least 30 minutes per day, five times per week. The Institute of Medicine[42] concurs that 30 minutes a day, five times a week is the minimum amount of physical activity needed, but up to 60 minutes per day may be necessary for many people to lose weight and to sustain a body weight in the healthy range over the long term.

Counseling and support groups, such as Overeaters Anonymous (OA), can help people maintain these dietary and activity changes. Psychotherapy can be particularly helpful in challenging clients to examine the underlying thought patterns, situations, and stressors that may be undermining their efforts at weight loss.

Weight Loss Can Be Enhanced with Prescribed Medications The biggest complaint about the lifestyle recommendations for healthful weight loss is that they are difficult to maintain. Many people have tried to follow them for years but have not been successful. In response to this challenge, prescription drugs have been developed to assist people with weight loss. These drugs typically act as appetite suppressants and may also increase satiety.

Weight-loss medications should be used only with proper supervision from a physician. Physician involvement is so critical because many drugs developed for weight loss have serious side effects. Some have even proven deadly. These life-threatening drugs were banned many years ago, yet they still serve as examples illustrating that the treatment of obesity through pharmacologic means is neither simple nor risk-free.

Two prescription weight-loss drugs are currently available: sibutramine and orlistat. Their long-term safety and efficacy are still being explored:

- Sibutramine (brand name Meridia) is an appetite suppressant that can cause increased heart rate and blood pressure in some people. Because many people who are overweight or obese have high blood pressure and are at increased risk for heart disease, these side effects could limit the widespread use of this drug. However, in one study, combining sibutramine therapy with medically supervised aerobic

Nutrition
MILESTONE

In **2007**, researchers from Harvard University and the University of California, San Diego, published evidence that obesity may be spread via social networks. Dr. Nicolas Christakis and Dr. James Fowler evaluated data involving over 12,000 people who participated in the Framingham Heart Study, a longitudinal cohort initiated in 1948. Data on BMI from 1971 to 2003 and statistical models were used to examine whether weight gain in participants was associated with weight gain in friends, siblings, spouses, or neighbors. The results showed that a person's chance of becoming obese was 57% higher if a friend became obese; 40% higher if a sibling became obese; and 37% higher if a spouse became obese. There was no evidence that neighbors had any effect on a person's obesity risk. Social distance was found to be much more important than geographic distance, suggesting that it was not exposure to the same environmental factors that caused people in close social networks to become obese. It may be that a person's perceptions of the acceptability of obesity changes when those close to him or her become obese. The researchers also theorized that, if social networks can increase obesity, they could be used as a means to spread positive health behaviors and reduce obesity.

multifactorial disease A disease that may be attributable to one or more of a variety of causes.

exercise and a low-fat diet resulted in significant weight loss and a significant decrease in heart rate and blood pressure.[43] In addition to increased blood pressure, the side effects of sibutramine include dry mouth, anorexia, constipation, insomnia, dizziness, and nausea.

■ Orlistat (brand name Xenical) inhibits the absorption of dietary fat from the intestinal tract, which can result in weight loss in some people. Recent research shows that taking orlistat results in significant weight loss in obese adolescents, and adults experience significant weight loss and improved blood lipid profiles when orlistat is combined with an energy-restricted diet.[44, 45] The side effects of orlistat include abdominal pain, fatty and loose stools, leaky stools, flatulence, and decreased absorption of fat-soluble nutrients, such as vitamins E and D.

Although the use of prescribed weight-loss medications is associated with side effects and a certain level of risk, they are justified for people who are obese. That's because the health risks of obesity override the risks of the medications. They are also advised for people who have a BMI greater than or equal to 27 kg/m² who also have other significant health risk factors, such as heart disease, high blood pressure, or type 2 diabetes.

Over-the-Counter Medications and Dietary Supplements Are Also Available Over-the-counter medications and dietary supplements are also marketed for weight loss. Alli is a lower dosage of Orlistat that is now sold over the counter. Due to side effects that have occurred with taking Alli, including pancreatitis, kidney stones, and liver damage, some consumer groups have called for its removal from the market. However, many medical experts and the pharmaceutical company that sells Alli state that the drug is safe and the benefits of the drug outweigh the risks.

It is important to remember that the Food and Drug Administration (FDA) requires prescription drugs and over-the-counter medications to undergo rigorous testing for safety and effectiveness before they can be released onto the market, but the FDA does not have a similar level of control over the sale of dietary supplements. Moreover, the FDA can pull a dietary supplement from the shelves only if it can prove that the supplement is dangerous. It cannot force the makers of an ineffective but harmless supplement to stop selling it. Two reviews of various supplements and alternative treatments for weight loss[46, 47] have concluded that there is insufficient evidence to support the use of the following products widely marketed to enhance weight loss: chromium, spirulina (blue-green algae), ginseng, chitosan (derived from the exoskeleton of crustaceans), green tea, and psyllium (a source of fiber). However, these products continue their brisk sales to people desperate to lose weight.

Many products marketed for weight loss do indeed increase metabolic rate and decrease appetite; however, they prompt these effects because they contain *stimulants*, substances that speed up physiologic processes. Use of these products may be dangerous, as abnormal increases in heart rate and blood pressure can occur. Stimulants commonly found in weight-loss supplements include caffeine, phenylpropanolamine (PPA), and ephedra:

■ *Caffeine.* In addition to being a stimulant, caffeine is addictive; nevertheless, it is legal and unregulated in most countries and is considered safe when consumed in moderate amounts (up to the equivalent of three to four cups of coffee). Adverse effects of high doses of caffeine include nervousness, irritability, anxiety, muscle twitching and tremors, headaches, elevated blood pressure, and irregular or rapid heartbeat. Long-term overuse of high doses of caffeine can lead to sleep and anxiety disorders that require clinical attention. Deaths due to caffeine toxicity have occurred primarily as a result of taking caffeine tablets.

■ *Phenylpropanolamine (PPA).* In the year 2000, in response to several deaths, the FDA banned over-the-counter medications containing phenylpropanolamine (PPA), an ingredient that had been used in many cough and cold medications as well as in weight-loss formulas. However, PPA may still be present in dietary supplements marketed for weight loss, as these are beyond FDA control.

- *Ephedra.* The use of ephedra has been associated with dangerous elevations in heart rate and blood pressure, and even death. The FDA has banned the manufacture and sale of ephedra in the United States; however, some weight-loss supplements still contain *ma huang*, the so-called herbal ephedra. *Ma huang* is simply the Chinese name for ephedra. Some weight-loss supplements contain a combination of *ma huang*, caffeine, and aspirin. As you can see, using weight-loss dietary supplements entails serious health risks.

Surgery Can Be Used to Treat Morbid Obesity For people who are morbidly obese, surgery may be recommended. Generally, surgery is advised for people with a BMI greater than or equal to 40 kg/m² or for people with a BMI greater than or equal to 35 kg/m² who have other life-threatening conditions, such as diabetes, hypertension, or elevated cholesterol levels. The three most common types of weight-loss surgery are gastroplasty, gastric bypass, and gastric banding (**Figure 13.13**).

Surgery is considered a last resort for morbidly obese people who have not been able to lose weight with energy restriction, exercise, and medications. This is because the risks of surgery in people with morbid obesity are extremely high. They include an increased rate of infections, formation of blood clots, and adverse reactions to anesthesia. After the surgery, many recipients face a lifetime of problems with chronic diarrhea, vomiting, intolerance to dairy products and other foods, dehydration, and nutritional deficiencies resulting from alterations in nutrient digestion and absorption that occur with bypass procedures. Thus, the potential benefits of the procedure must outweigh the risks. It is critical that each surgery candidate be carefully screened by a trained physician. If the immediate threat of serious disease and death is more dangerous than the risks associated with surgery, then the procedure is justified.

About one-third to one-half of people who receive obesity surgery lose significant amounts of weight and keep this weight off for at least 5 years. They also reduce their risk for type 2 diabetes and cardiovascular disease, and they may even improve their

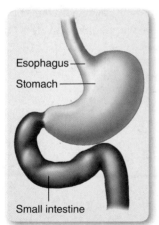 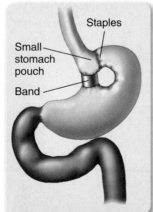 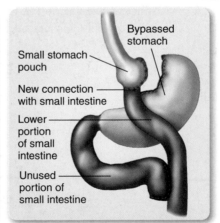 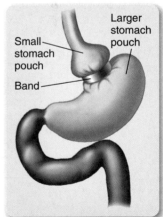

(a) Normal anatomy

(b) Vertical banded gastroplasty

(c) Gastric bypass

(d) Gastric banding

FIGURE 13.13 Three forms of surgery alter the **(a)** normal anatomy of the gastrointestinal tract to achieve weight loss in morbid obesity: **(b)** vertical banded gastroplasty, which involves partitioning or "stapling" a small section of the stomach to reduce total food intake; **(c)** gastric bypass, which involves attaching the lower part of the small intestine to the stomach, so that food bypasses most of the stomach and the duodenum of the small intestine, resulting in significantly less absorption of food in the intestine; and **(d)** gastric banding, a procedure in which stomach size is reduced using a constricting band, thus restricting food intake.

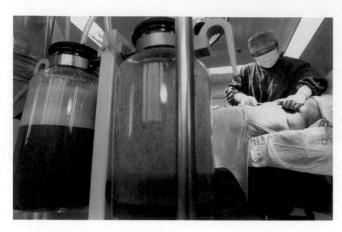

Liposuction removes fat cells from specific areas of the body.

ability to stay physically active over a prolonged period of time.[48] The reasons that one-half to two-thirds do not experience long-term success include the following:

- Inability to eat less over time, even with a smaller stomach
- Loosening of staples and gastric bands and enlargement of the stomach pouch
- Failure to survive the surgery or the postoperative recovery period

Liposuction is a cosmetic surgical procedure that removes fat cells from localized areas in the body. It is not recommended or typically used to treat obesity or morbid obesity. Instead, it is often used by normal or mildly overweight people to "spot reduce" fat from various areas of the body. This procedure is not without risks, however; blood clots, skin and nerve damage, adverse drug reactions, and perforation injuries can and do occur as a result of liposuction. It can also cause deformations in the area where the fat is removed. This procedure is not the solution to long-term weight loss, because the millions of fat cells that remain in the body after liposuction enlarge if the person continues to overeat. In addition, although liposuction may reduce the fat content of a localized area, it does not reduce a person's risk for the diseases that are more common among overweight or obese people. Only traditional weight loss with diet and exercise can reduce body fat and the risks for chronic diseases.

RECAP

Weight gain can be achieved by eating more and performing weight-lifting and aerobic exercise. Protein and amino acid supplements do not increase muscle mass, and their potential side effects are unknown. Obesity is a multifactorial disease, and genetics, physiology, and lifestyle choices are all thought to contribute. In addition, childhood obesity is strongly associated with adult obesity. Treatments for overweight and obesity include low-Calorie, low-fat diets in combination with regular physical activity. Prescription weight-loss medications and surgery are typically reserved for people who are obese. ■

Chapter Review

1 **F** Being underweight increases our risk for illness and premature death and in many cases can be just as unhealthful as being obese.

2 **F** Obesity is a multifactorial disease with many contributing factors. Although eating too much food and not getting enough exercise can lead to being overweight or obese, the disease of obesity is complex and is not simply caused by overeating.

3 **T** Body composition assessments can help give us a general idea of body fat levels, but most methods are not extremely accurate.

4 **F** According to the Centers for Disease Control and Prevention, in 2009–2010, approximately 35.7% of all adults in the United States were considered obese.

5 **T** Health can be defined in many ways. An individual who is overweight but who exercises regularly and has no additional risk factors for chronic diseases is considered a healthy person.

Summary

- Definitions of a healthful body weight include one that is appropriate for someone's age and level of development, promotes healthful blood lipids and glucose, can be achieved and sustained without constant dieting, promotes good eating habits, and allows for regular physical activity.

- Body mass index (BMI) is an index of weight per height squared. It is useful to indicate health risks associated with overweight and obesity in groups of people.

- Underweight is defined as having too little body fat to maintain health, causing a person to have a weight for a given height that is below an acceptably defined standard. A BMI below 18.5 is considered underweight.

- Overweight is defined as having a moderate amount of excess body fat, resulting in a person having a weight for a given height that is greater than some accepted standard but is not considered obese. A BMI of 25 to 29.9 is considered overweight.

- Obesity is defined as having excess body fat that adversely affects health, resulting in a person having a weight for a given height that is substantially greater than some accepted standard. A BMI of 30 to 39.9 is considered obese. Morbid obesity occurs when a person's body weight exceeds 100% of normal, which puts him or her at very high risk for serious health consequences. A BMI of 40 or above is considered morbidly obese.

- The waist-to-hip ratio and waist circumference are used to determine patterns of fat storage. People with large waists (as compared to the hips) have an apple-shaped fat pattern. People with large hips (as compared to the waist) have a pear-shaped fat pattern. Having an apple-shaped pattern increases your risk for heart disease, type 2 diabetes, and other chronic diseases.

- We lose or gain weight based on changes in our energy intake, the food we eat, and our energy expenditure (both at rest and when physically active).

- Basal metabolic rate (BMR) is the energy needed to maintain the body's resting functions. BMR accounts for 60% to 75% of our total daily energy needs.

- The thermic effect of food is the energy we expend to process the food we eat. It accounts for 5% to 10% of the energy content of a meal and is higher for processing proteins and carbohydrates than for fats.

- The energy cost of physical activity represents energy that we expend for physical movement or work we do above basal levels. It accounts for 15% to 35% of our total daily energy output.

- Our genetic heritage influences our body weight, and factors such as possessing a thrifty gene (or genes) and maintaining a weight set point may affect a person's risk for obesity.

- Eating a diet proportionally higher in fat may increase the risk for obesity, as dietary fat is stored more easily as adipose tissue than is dietary carbohydrate or protein.

- Metabolic factors, such as low BMR, low spontaneous physical activity, low sympathetic nervous system activity, and low fat oxidation, influence weight loss and gain.

- Physiologic factors that influence body weight include alterations in various hormones that influence hunger and satiety, including leptin, ghrelin, peptide YY, uncoupling proteins, beta-endorphins, serotonin, and cholecystokinin.

- Cultural and social factors, such as easy access to large portions of inexpensive and high-fat foods and excessive use of electronic devices for entertainment, also contribute to obesity. Mood and emotional state also affect appetite.

- Fad diets are weight-loss programs that enjoy short-term popularity and are sold based on a marketing gimmick that appeals to the public's desires and fears. They typically promise rapid weight loss, often without increased physical activity or long-term behavioral modification, and they rarely result in long-term maintenance of weight loss.

- Diet plans that restrict intake of certain macronutrients can help many people lose weight, but some have unhealthful side effects.

- A sound weight-loss plan involves gradually reducing energy intake, incorporating physical activity into each day, and practicing changes in behavior that can assist in meeting realistic weight-change goals.

- Being underweight can be detrimental to one's health. Most of the products marketed for weight gain have been shown to be ineffective. Healthful weight gain involves consuming more energy than expended by selecting ample servings of nutritious, high-energy foods and exercising regularly by including resistance training and aerobic exercise.

- Overweight is not as detrimental to health as obesity, but it is associated with an increased risk for high blood pressure, heart disease, type 2 diabetes, sleep disorders, osteoarthritis, gallstones, and gynecological abnormalities.

- Obesity and morbid obesity are associated with significantly increased risks for many diseases and for premature death. Obesity can be treated with low-energy diets and regular physical activity, prescription medications, and surgery when necessary.

MasteringNutrition™

To further your understanding, go online and apply what you've learned to real-life case studies that will help you master the content!

Review Questions

1. The ratio of a person's body weight to height is represented as his or her
   a. body composition.
   b. basal metabolic rate.
   c. bioelectrical impedance.
   d. body mass index.

2. The body's total daily energy expenditure includes
   a. basal metabolic rate, thermal effect of food, and effect of physical activity.
   b. basal metabolic rate, movement, standing, and sleeping.
   c. effect of physical activity, standing, and sleeping.
   d. body mass index, thermal effect of food, and effect of physical activity.

3. All people gain weight when they
   a. eat a high-fat diet (>35% fat).
   b. take in more energy than they expend.
   c. fail to exercise.
   d. take in less energy than they expend.

4. The set-point theory proposes that
   a. obese people have a gene not found in slender people that regulates their weight so that it always hovers near a given set point.
   b. obese people have a gene that causes them to be energetically thrifty.
   c. all people have a genetic set point for their body weight.
   d. all people have a hormone that regulates their weight so that it always hovers near a given set point.

5. A body protein that increases appetite is
   a. leptin.
   b. ghrelin.
   c. PYY.
   d. orlistat.

6. **True or false?** Pear-shaped fat patterning is known to increase a person's risk for many chronic diseases, including diabetes and heart disease.

7. **True or false?** One pound of fat is equal to about 3,500 kcal.

8. **True or false?** Weight-loss medications are typically prescribed for people who have a body mass index greater than or equal to 18.5 kg/m².

9. **True or false?** Recommendations for weight gain include avoiding both aerobic and resistance exercise for the duration of the weight-gain program.

10. **True or false?** More than half of American adults are currently either overweight or obese.

11. Identify at least four characteristics of a healthful weight.

12. Describe a sound weight-loss program, including recommendations for diet, physical activity, and behavioral modifications.

13. Can you increase your basal metabolic rate? Is it wise to try? Defend your answer.

14. Identify at least four societal factors that may have influenced the rise in obesity rates in the United States since 1963.

Math Review

15. Your friend Misty joins you for lunch and confesses that she is discouraged about her weight. She says that she has been trying "really hard" for 3 months to lose weight but that, no matter what she does, she cannot drop below 148 lb. Based on her height of 5'8", calculate Misty's BMI. Is she overweight?

You know Misty exercises regularly. What questions would you suggest she think about? How would you advise her?

16. Misty's level of physical activity would classify her as moderately active. Approximately how many kcal does she need each day to maintain her current body weight?

Answers to Review Questions and Math Review can be found online in the MasteringNutrition Study Area.

Web Links

www.ftc.gov
Federal Trade Commission
Click on "For Consumers" and then "Diet, Health and Fitness" to find how to avoid false weight-loss claims.

www.consumer.gov/weightloss
Partnership for Healthy Weight Management
Visit this site to learn about successful strategies for achieving and maintaining a healthy weight.

www.eatright.org
Academy of Nutrition and Dietetics
Go to this site to learn more about fad diets and nutrition facts.

www.niddk.nih.gov/health/nutrit/nutrit.htm
National Institute of Diabetes and Digestive and Kidney Diseases
Find out more about healthy weight loss and how it pertains to diabetes and digestive and kidney diseases.

www.sne.org
Society for Nutrition Education
Click on "Resources and Relationships" and then "Weight Realities Resources" for additional resources related to positive attitudes about body image and healthful alternatives to dieting.

www.oa.org
Overeaters Anonymous
Visit this site to learn about ways to reduce compulsive overeating.

References

1. 60 Minutes Overtime Staff. (2012, February 12). Adele Talks About Her Body Image and Weight. *CBS News.* www.cbsnews.com/8301-504803_162-57376080-10391709/adele-talks-about-her-body-image-and-weight/. (Accessed February 2012.)

2. Manore, M. M., N. L. Meyer, and J. L. Thompson. 2009. *Sport Nutrition for Health and Performance,* 2nd edn. Champaign, IL: Human Kinetics.

3. Wang, Y. 2004. Epidemiology of childhood obesity—methodological aspects and guidelines: what is new? *Int. J. Obes.* 23:S21–S28.

4. Shai, I., R. Jiang, J. E. Manson, M. J. Stampfer, W. C. Willett, G. A. Colditz, and F. B. Hu. 2006. Ethnicity, obesity, and risk of type 2 diabetes in women. *Diab. Care.* 29:1585–1590.

5. Galgani, J., and E. Ravussin. 2008. Energy metabolism, fuel selection and body weight regulation. *Int. J. Obes.* 32:S109–S119.

6. Stunkard, A. J., T. I. A. Sørensen, C. Hanis, T. W. Teasdale, R. Chakraborty, W. J. Schull, and F. Schulsinger. 1986. An adoption study of human obesity. *N. Engl. J. Med.* 314:193–198.

7. Bouchard, C. 2010. Defining the genetic architecture of the predisposition to obesity: a challenging but not insurmountable task. *Am. J. Clin. Nutr.* 91:5–6.

8. Bloss, C. S., N. J. Stork, and E. J. Topol. 2011. Effect of direct-to-consumer genomewide profiling to assess disease risk. *N. Engl. J. Med.* 364(6):524–534.

9. Razquin, C., A. Marti, and J. A. Martinez. 2011. Evidences on three relevant obesogenes: MC4R, FTO, and PPARR. *Mol. Nutr. Food Res.* 55(1):136–149.

10. Kilpeläinen, T. O., L. Qi, S. Brage, S. J. Sharp, E. Sonestedt, E. Demerath, T. Ahmad, et al. 2011. Physical activity attenuates the influence of FTO variants on obesity risk: a meta-analysis of 218,166 adults and 19,268 children. *PLoS Med.* 8(11)e1001116, Epub 2011 Nov 1.

11. Bouchard, C., A. Tremblay, J. P. Després, A. Nadeau, P. J. Lupien, G. Thériault, J. Dussault, S. Moorjani, S. Pinault, and G. Fournier. 1990. The response to long-term overfeeding in identical twins. *N. Engl. J. Med.* 322:1477–1482.

12. Sumithran, P., L. A. Prendergast, E. Delbridge, K. Purcell, A. Shulkes, A. Kriketos, and J. Proietto. 2011. Long-term persistence of hormonal adaptations to weight loss. *N. Engl. J. Med.* 365:1597–1604.

13. Druce, M. R., A. M. Wren, A. J. Park, J. E. Milton, M. Patterson, G. Frost, M. A. Ghatei, C. Small, and S. R. Bloom. 2005. Ghrelin increases food intake in obese as well as lean subjects. *Int. J. Obes.* 29:1130–1136.

14. Suzuki, K., C. N. Jayasena, and S. R. Bloom. 2011. The gut hormones in appetite regulation. *J. Obes.* DOI: 10.1155/2011/528401. www.hindawi.com/journals/jobes/2011/528401/. (Accessed February 2012.)

15. Virtanen, K. A., M. E. Lidell, J. Orava, M. Heglind, R. Westergren, T. Niemi, M. Taittonen, J. Laine, N.-J. Savito, S. Enerbäck, and P. Nuutila. 2009. Functional brown adipose tissue in healthy adults. *N. Engl. J. Med.* 360(15):1518–1525.

16. Cypess, A. M., S. Lehman, G. Williams, I. Tal, D. Rodman, A. B. Goldfine, F. C. Kuo, E. L. Palmer, Y.-H. Tseng, A. Doria, G. M. Kolodny, and C. R. Kahn. 2009. Identification and importance of brown adipose tissue in adult humans. *N. Engl. J. Med.* 360(15):1509–1517.

17. Eyler, A. E., D. Matson-Koffman, D. Rohm-Young, S. Wilcox, J. Wilbur, J. L. Thompson, B. Sanderson, and K. R. Evenson. 2003. Quantitative study of correlates of physical activity in women from diverse racial/ethnic groups: The Women's Cardiovascular Health Network Project. *Am. J. Prev. Med.* 25(3Si):93–103.

18. Eyler, A. E., D. Matson-Koffman, J. R. Vest, K. R. Evenson, B. Sanderson, J. L. Thompson, J. Wilbur, S. Wilcox, and D. Rohm-Young. 2002. Environmental, policy, and cultural factors related to physical activity in a diverse sample of women: The Women's Cardiovascular Health Network Project—summary and discussion. *Women and Health* 36:123–134.

19. Black, J. L., and J. MacinkoJ. 2008. Neighborhoods and obesity. *Nutr. Rev.* 66(1):2–20.

20. Ding, D., T. Sugiyama, and N. Owen. 2012. Habitual active transport, TV viewing and weight gain: a four-year follow-up study. *Prev. Med.* 54:201–204.

21. Lumeng, J. C., P. Forrest, D. P. Appugliese, N. Kaciroti, R. F. Corwyn, and R. H. Bradley. 2010. Weight status as a predictor of being bullied in third through sixth grades. *Pediatrics* 125(6):1301–1307.

22. Academy of Nutrition and Dietetics. 2012. Tip of the Day. Say No to the Dangers of Fad Diets. www.eatright.org/Public/content.aspx?id=6442465356&terms=fad+diets. (Accessed February 2012.)

23. Prentice, R. L., B. Caan, R. T. Chlebowski, et al. 2006. Low-fat dietary pattern and risk of invasive breast cancer: the Women's Health Initiative Randomized Controlled Dietary Modification Trial. *JAMA* 295:629–642.

24. Beresford, S. A., K. C. Johnson, C. Ritenbaugh, et al. 2006. Low-fat dietary pattern and risk of colorectal cancer: the Women's Health Initiative Randomized Controlled Dietary Modification Trial. *JAMA* 295:643–654.

25. Howard, B. V., L. Van Horn, J. Hsia, et al. 2006. Low-fat dietary pattern and risk of cardiovascular disease: the Women's Health Initiative Randomized Controlled Dietary Modification Trial. *JAMA* 295:655–666.

26. Howard, B. V., J. E. Manson, M. L. Stefanick, et al. 2006. Low-fat dietary pattern and weight change over 7 years: the Women's Health Initiative Dietary Modification Trial. *JAMA* 295:39–49.

27. Hession, M., C. Rolland, U. Kulkarni, A. Wise, and J. Broom. 2009. Systematic review of randomized controlled trials of low-carbohydrate vs. low-fat/low-calorie diets in the management of obesity and its co-morbidities. *Obes. Rev.* 10(1):36–50.

28. Ello-Martin, J. A., J. H. Ledikwe, and B. J. Rolls. 2005. The influence of food portion size and energy density on energy intake: implications for weight management. *Am. J. Clin. Nutr.* 82(suppl.):236S–241S.

29. Flood, J. E., L. S. Roe, and B. J. Rolls. 2006. The effect of increased beverage portion size on energy intake at a meal. *J. Am. Diet. Assoc.* 106:1984–1990.

30. Ello-Martin, J.A., L. S. Roe, J. H. Ledikwe, A. M. Beach, and B. J. Rolls. 2007. Dietary energy density in the treatment of obesity: a year-long trial comparing 2 weight-loss diets. *Am. J. Clin. Nutr.* 85(6):1465–1477.

31. Rolls, B. J., L. S. Roe, and J. S. Meengs. 2006. Reductions in portion size and energy density of foods are additive and lead to sustained decreases in energy intake. *Am. J. Clin. Nutr.* 83(1):11–17.

32. Wing, R. R., and S. Phelan. 2005. Long-term weight loss maintenance. *Am. J. Clin. Nutr.* 82(suppl):222S–225S.

33. American College of Sports Medicine, American Dietetic Association, and Dietitians of Canada. 2009. Nutrition and athletic performance. Joint Position Stand. *Med. Sci. Sports Exerc.* 41(3):709–731.

34. Ogden, C. L., M. D. Carroll, B. K. Kitt, and K. M. Flegal. 2012. Prevalence of obesity in the United States, 2009–10. NCHS data brief no 82. www.cdc.gov/nchs/data/databriefs/db82.pdf. (Accessed February 2012.)

35. Grundy, S. M., B. Hansen, S. C. Smith, J. I. Cleeman, and R. A. Kahn. 2004. Clinical management of metabolic syndrome: report of the American Heart Association/National Heart, Lung, and Blood Institute/American Diabetes Association Conference on Scientific Issues Related to Management. *Circulation* 109:551–556.

36. MyHealthyWaist.org. 2011. The Concept of CMR. www.myhealthywaist.org/the-concept-of-cmr/index.html. (Accessed February 2012.)

37. Agency for Healthcare Research and Quality, National Guideline Clearinghouse. 2011. Cardiometabolic risk management in primary care. www.guideline.gov/content.aspx?id=34113&search=cardiometabolic+risk+management+in+primary+care. (Accessed February 2012.)

38. Ervin, R. B. 2009. Prevalence of metabolic syndrome among adults 20 years of age and over, by sex, age, race and ethnicity, and body mass index: United States, 2003–2006. *Nat. Health Stat. Rep.* 13:1–4. http://www.cdc.gov/nchs/data/nhsr/nhsr013.pdf. (Accessed February 2012.)

39. National Institute of Diabetes and Digestive and Kidney Diseases. Weight-control Information Network. 2008. Understanding Adult Obesity. NIH Publication No. 06-3680. www.win.niddk.nih.gov/publications/understanding.htm. (Accessed February 2012.)

40. Bibbins-Domingo, K., P. Coxson, M. J. Pletcher, J. Lightwood, and L. Goldman. 2007. Adolescent overweight and future adult coronary heart disease. *N. Engl. J. Med.* 357:2371–2379.

41. Christakis, N. A., and J. H. Fowler. 2007. The spread of obesity in a large social network over 32 years. *N. Engl. J. Med.* 357(4):370–379.

42. Institute of Medicine, Food and Nutrition Board. 2002. *Dietary Reference Intakes for Energy, Carbohydrate, Fiber, Fat, Fatty Acids, Cholesterol, Protein, and Amino Acids (Macronutrients).* Washington, DC: National Academies Press.

43. Bérubé-Parent, S., D. Prud'homme, S. St-Pierre, E. Doucet, and A. Tremblay. 2001. Obesity treatment with a progressive clinical tri-therapy combining sibutramine and a supervised diet-exercise intervention. *Int. J. Obes.* 25:1144–1153.

44. Chanoine, J.-P., S. Hampl, C. Jensen, M. Boldrin, and J. Hauptman. 2005. Effect of orlistat on weight and body composition in obese adolescents. A randomized controlled trial. *JAMA* 293(23):2873–2883.

45. Hutton, B., and D. Fergusson. 2004. Changes in body weight and serum lipid profile in obese patients treated with orlistat in addition to a hypocaloric diet: a systemic review of randomized clinical trials. *Am. J. Clin. Nutr.* 80:1461–1468.

46. Saper, R. B., D. M. Eisenberg, and R. S. Phillips. 2004. Common dietary supplements for weight loss. *Am. Fam. Phys.* 70(9):1731–1738.

47. Allison, D. B., K. R. Fontaine, S. Heshka, J. L. Mentore, and S. B. Heymsfield. 2001. Alternative treatments for weight loss: a critical review. *Crit. Rev. Food Sci. Nutr.* 41(1):1–28.

48. Sjöström, L., A.-K. Lindroos, M. Peltonen, J. Torgerson, C. Bouchard, B. Carlsson, S. Dahlgren, B. Larsson, K. Narbro, C. D. Sjöström, M. Sullivan, and H. Wedel. 2004. Lifestyle, diabetes, and cardiovascular risk factors 10 years after bariatric surgery. *N. Engl. J. Med.* 351(26):2683–2693.

Nutrition DEBATE

High-Carbohydrate, Moderate-Fat Diets—Have They Been Oversold?

For the past 30 years, dietary fat has been demonized and touted as the cause of obesity, cardiovascular disease, type 2 diabetes, and many types of cancers. As a result, researchers and health professionals have emphasized the health benefits of eating a moderate-fat, high-carbohydrate diet (one in which approximately 20–30% of energy comes from fat and 55–60% of energy comes from carbohydrate), with national dietary guidelines being developed and promoted around this message. Recently published results from the Women's Health Initiative Randomized Controlled Dietary Modification Trial have shaken the nutrition and health world and caused experts to seriously question the existing beliefs that moderate-fat diets are the key to reducing our risks for many chronic diseases.

The Women's Health Initiative Randomized Controlled Dietary Modification Trial involved 48,835 ethnically diverse postmenopausal women aged 50 to 79 years.[1] Women were randomized into either a control group that received a copy of the Dietary Guidelines for Americans and other health materials or an intervention group. Women randomized to the intervention group received an intensive behavioral modification program involving eighteen group sessions in the first year of the study, followed by quarterly maintenance sessions. The intervention promoted dietary changes to achieve a goal of 20% of energy intake from fat (7% of energy intake from saturated fat), an increase in fruit and vegetable intake to at least 5 servings per day, and an increase in whole grains to at least 6 servings per day. However, the diet was not intended to reduce energy intake or induce weight loss. The average length of time to follow up participants was 8 years.

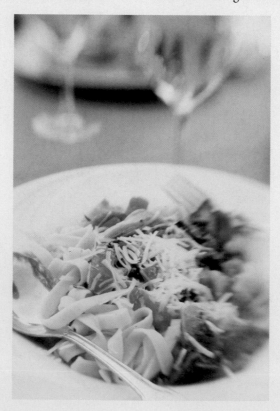

The results from this study, which is the most expensive study of diet ever conducted, surprised many experts. At the end of the follow-up period, there was no significant health benefit in the intervention group—there was no reduction in risk for cardiovascular disease, breast cancer, or colorectal cancer.[1–3] One benefit that was observed was that women in the intervention group lost weight during the first year (a loss of approximate 4.8 pounds), and they maintained a lower weight than women in the control group over 7.5 years.[4] Some women in the control group also lost weight, and the greatest amount of weight lost in both groups occurred in those who decreased their percentage of energy intake from fat.

What do these results mean? Should we no longer be concerned about the risks of dietary fat? Should we eat however we choose? The study had a number of limitations that need to be recognized, and an editorial published by the Harvard School of Public Health has helped put these findings into perspective.[5] Although participants in the intervention reduced their fat intake from 38% to 29% of total energy intake, they did not reach the target goal of consuming no more than 20% of energy intake from fat. Thus, it has been suggested that a lower-fat diet might be more effective in reducing the risk for chronic diseases. In addition, the participants were postmenopausal women, and it might be that intervening at this age is too late to prevent the development of cardiovascular disease and various cancers. Because dietary intake was self-reported, it might also be possible that the women over-reported the actual dietary changes they made, meaning that they did not improve their diet as reported and thus no health changes would result. Another issue is that it may take longer than 8 years to see the health benefits of this type of diet, and thus a much longer study would be needed to detect health benefits.

However there is now a growing body of evidence that the key to reducing chronic disease risks is focusing on changing the *type* of dietary fat consumed, not the total amount.[5] The challenge with reducing dietary fat is that many people choose to substitute low-fiber, highly refined carbohydrate foods in place of fat. This substitution leads to negative changes in blood lipids and blood glucose. Reducing our intake of saturated and *trans* fats, and increasing our intake of plant oils and food sources high in poly- and mono-unsaturated fats, appears to be the healthiest approach. In fact, the current Dietary Guidelines for Americans support the consumption of these foods. Lowering total fat intake may not be critically important unless a person is trying to reduce total energy intake. Even under these circumstances, people should be encouraged to optimize their intake of healthy fats and avoid replacing fat with refined carbohydrates.

Another take-home message is that too many Calories from any source will lead to weight gain. As noted in this chapter, both overweight and obesity are associated with an increased risk for heart disease and other chronic diseases.

CRITICAL THINKING QUESTIONS

- Should you adopt a high-carb, moderate-fat diet?

- Is this type of diet compatible with your personal needs, preferences, health risks, and lifestyle?

- Do you think that other diets are better or worse alternatives to higher-carbohydrate, lower-fat diets? Why or why not?

- What diet do you think would work best to help you maintain a healthful weight and muscle mass and provide enough energy and nutrients to maintain your lifestyle and your long-term health?

REFERENCES

1. Howard, B.V., L. Van Horn, J. Hsia, J. E. Manson, M. L. Stefanick, S. Wassertheil-Smoller, M. D. Kuller, et al. 2006. Low-fat dietary pattern and risk of cardiovascular disease. The Women's Health Initiative Randomized Controlled Dietary Modification Trial. *JAMA* 295(6):655–666.

2. Prentice, R. L., B. Caan, R. T. Chlebowski, R. Patterson, L. H. Kuller, J. K. Ockene, K. L. Margolis, et al. 2006. Low-fat dietary pattern and risk of invasive breast cancer. The Women's Health Initiative Randomized Controlled Dietary Modification Trial. *JAMA* 295(6):629–642.

3. Beresford, S. A. A., K. C. Johnson, C. Ritenbaugh, N. L. Lasser, L. G. Snetselaar, H. R. Black, G. L. Anderson, et al. 2006. Low-fat dietary pattern and risk of colorectal cancer. The Women's Health Initiative Randomized Controlled Dietary Modification Trial. *JAMA* 295(6):643–654.

4. Howard, B. V., J. E. Manson, M. L. Stefanick, S. A. Beresford, G. Frank, B. Jones, R. J. Rodabough, et al. 2006. Low-fat dietary pattern and weight change over 7 years. The Women's Health Initiative Randomized Controlled Dietary Modification Trial. *JAMA* 295(6):39–49.

5. Harvard School of Public Health. 2012. Low-Fat Diet Not a Cure-All. *The Nutrition Source.* www.hsph.harvard.edu/nutritionsource/nutrition-news/low-fat/. (Accessed February 2012.)

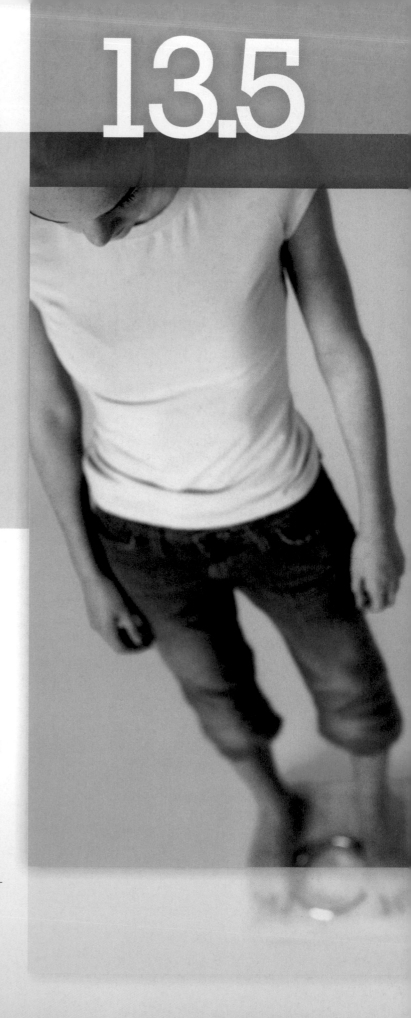

Disordered Eating

Want to find out . . .

- what is the leading cause of death in females age 15 through 24?
- whether men experience disordered eating?
- what keeps some overweight people up all night?

READ ON.

On August 2, 2006, Uruguayan fashion model Luisel Ramos collapsed during a fashion show. Just 22 years old, she was pronounced dead of heart failure brought on by anorexia nervosa, a condition of self-imposed starvation. Family members say that, in the months prior to her death, she had adopted a diet of lettuce leaves and diet cola, and at 5'9" tall, her weight had dropped to just 98 pounds. The following month, Madrid's "Fashion Week" responded to Ramos' death by banning from its runway fashion models who could not meet a minimum BMI of 18.0. The Milan fashion show quickly responded by imposing a minimum of 18.5. In addition, several modeling agencies began to require prospective models to present medical records attesting to their health. Although promising, such measures alone were clearly inadequate, as at least four more fashion models had died from self-starvation by the end of 2010. Early in 2012, the Council of Fashion Designers of America (CFDA) released new guidelines for the hiring of runway models, including measures such as educating staff to recognize the warning signs of an eating disorder. The CFDA imposed no sanctions, however, for noncompliance. Then, in March of 2012, Israel took a major step forward in the fight against eating disorders. The government passed a law banning the use of underweight models in advertisements. The new law states that models with a BMI under 18.5 cannot be hired unless a doctor explicitly confirms that they are not underweight.

Do only fashion models develop eating disorders, or can they occur in people like you? When does normal dieting cross the line into disordered eating? What early warning signs might tip you off that a friend was crossing that line? If you noticed the signs in a friend or family member, would you confront him or her? If so, what would you say? In the following pages, we explore *In Depth* some answers to these important questions.

Eating Behaviors Occur on a Continuum

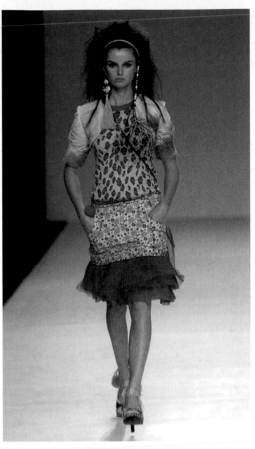

A string of models have died as a result of eating disorders.

Disordered eating is a general term used to describe a variety of atypical eating behaviors that people use to achieve or maintain a lower body weight. These behaviors may be as simple as going on and off diets or as extreme as refusing to eat any fat. Such behaviors don't usually continue for long enough to make the person seriously ill, nor do they significantly disrupt the person's normal routine.

In contrast, some people restrict their eating so much or for so long that they become dangerously underweight. These people have an **eating disorder,** a psychiatric condition that involves extreme body dissatisfaction and long-term eating patterns that negatively affect body functioning. The two more commonly diagnosed eating disorders are anorexia nervosa and bulimia nervosa. **Anorexia nervosa** is a potentially life-threatening eating disorder that is characterized by self-starvation, which eventually leads to a severe nutrient deficiency. In contrast, **bulimia nervosa** is characterized by recurrent episodes of extreme overeating and compensatory behaviors to prevent weight gain, such as self-induced vomiting, misuse of laxatives, fasting, or excessive exercise. Both disorders will be discussed in more detail shortly.

When does normal dieting cross the line into disordered eating? Eating behaviors occur on a *continuum*, a spectrum

that can't be divided neatly into parts. An example is a rainbow—where exactly does the red end and the orange begin? Thinking about eating behaviors as a continuum makes it easier to understand how a person can progress from relatively normal eating behaviors to a pattern that is disordered. For instance, let's say that for several years you've skipped breakfast in favor of a mid-morning snack, but now you find yourself avoiding the cafeteria until early afternoon. Is this normal? To answer that question, you'd need to consider your feelings about food and your **body image**—the way you perceive your body.

Take a moment to study the Eating Issues and Body Image Continuum (**Figure 1**). Which of the five columns best describes your feelings about food and your body? If you find yourself identifying with the statements on the left side of the continuum, you probably have few issues with food or body image. Most likely you accept your body size and view food as a normal part of maintaining your health and fueling your daily physical activity. As you progress to the right side of the continuum, food and body image become bigger issues, with food restriction becoming the norm. If you identify with the statements on the far right, you are probably afraid of eating and dislike your body. If so, what can you do to begin to move toward the left side of the continuum? How can you begin to develop a more healthful approach to food selection and to

---

disordered eating   A general term used to describe a variety of abnormal or atypical eating behaviors that are used to keep or maintain a lower body weight.

eating disorder   A clinically diagnosed psychiatric disorder characterized by severe disturbances in body image and eating behaviors.

anorexia nervosa   A serious, potentially life-threatening eating disorder that is characterized by self-starvation, which eventually leads to a deficiency in the energy and essential nutrients required by the body to function normally.

bulimia nervosa   A serious eating disorder characterized by recurrent episodes of binge eating and recurrent inappropriate compensatory behaviors in order to prevent weight gain, such as self-induced vomiting, fasting, excessive exercise, or misuse of laxatives, diuretics, enemas, or other medications.

body image   A person's perception of his or her body's appearance and functioning.

549

• I am not concerned about what others think regarding what and how much I eat. • When I am upset or depressed I eat whatever I am hungry for without any guilt or shame. • I feel no guilt or shame no matter how much I eat or what I eat. • Food is an important part of my life but only occupies a small part of my time. • I trust my body to tell me what and how much to eat.	• I pay attention to what I eat in order to maintain a healthy body. • I may weigh more than what I like, but I enjoy eating and balance my pleasure with eating with my concern for a healthy body. • I am moderate and flexible in goals for eating well. • I try to follow Dietary Guidelines for healthy eating.	• I think about food a lot. • I feel I don't eat well most of the time. • It's hard for me to enjoy eating with others. • I feel ashamed when I eat more than others or more than what I feel I should be eating. • I am afraid of getting fat. • I wish I could change how much I want to eat and what I am hungry for.	• I have tried diet pills, laxatives, vomiting, or extra time exercising in order to lose or maintain my weight. • I have fasted or avoided eating for long periods of time in order to lose or maintain my weight. • I feel strong when I can restrict how much I eat. • Eating more than I wanted to makes me feel out of control.	• I regularly stuff myself and then exercise, vomit, or use diet pills or laxatives to get rid of the food or Calories. • My friends/family tell me I am too thin. • I am terrified of eating fat. • When I let myself eat, I have a hard time controlling the amount of food I eat. • I am afraid to eat in front of others.
FOOD IS NOT AN ISSUE	**CONCERNED/WELL**	**FOOD PREOCCUPIED/OBSESSED**	**DISRUPTIVE EATING PATTERNS**	**EATING DISORDERED**
BODY OWNERSHIP	**BODY ACCEPTANCE**	**BODY PREOCCUPIED/OBSESSED**	**DISTORTED BODY IMAGE**	**BODY HATE/DISASSOCIATION**
• Body image is not an issue for me. • My body is beautiful to me. • My feelings about my body are not influenced by society's concept of an ideal body shape. • I know that the significant others in my life will always find me attractive. • I trust my body to find the weight it needs to be at so I can move and feel confident about my physical body.	• I base my body image equally on social norms and my own self-concept. • I pay attention to my body and my appearance because it is important to me, but it only occupies a small part of my day. • I nourish my body so it has the strength and energy to achieve my physical goals. • I am able to assert myself and maintain a healthy body without losing my self-esteem.	• I spend a significant amount time viewing my body in the mirror. • I spend a significant amount of time comparing my body to others. • I have days when I feel fat. • I am preoccupied with my body. • I accept society's ideal body shape and size as the best body shape and size. • I believe that I'd be more attractive if I were thinner, more muscular, etc.	• I spend a significant amount of time exercising and dieting to change my body. • My body shape and size keep me from dating or finding someone who will treat me the way I want to be treated. • I have considered changing or have changed my body shape and size through surgical means so I can accept myself. • I wish I could change the way I look in the mirror.	• I often feel separated and distant from my body—as if it belongs to someone else. • I hate my body and I often isolate myself from others. • I don't see anything positive or even neutral about my body shape and size. • I don't believe others when they tell me I look OK. • I hate the way I look in the mirror.

FIGURE 1 The Eating Issues and Body Image Continuum. The progression from normal eating (far left) to disordered eating (far right) occurs on a continuum. (*Source:* Data from Smiley, L., L. King, and H. Avery. University of Arizona Campus Health Service. Original Continuum, C. Shlaalak. Preventive Medicine and Public Health. Copyright © 1997 Arizona Board of Regents.)

view your body in a more positive light? Before you can begin to find solutions, you need to understand the many complex factors that contribute to eating disorders and disordered eating and the differences between these terms.

Many Factors Contribute to Disordered Eating Behaviors

The factors that contribute to the development of disordered eating in any particular individual are very complex.

Influence of Genetic Factors

Overall, the diagnosis of anorexia nervosa and bulimia nervosa is several times more common in siblings and other blood relatives who also have the diagnosis than in the general population.[1, 2] Data from twin studies estimate that genetic factors account for 50–83% of the variance in eating disorders.[2] These observations might imply the existence of an "eating disorder gene"; however, it is difficult to separate the contribution of genetic and environmental factors within families.

Influence of Family

Research suggests that family conditioning, structure, and patterns of interaction can influence the development and maintenance of an eating disorder. Based on observational studies, compared to families without a member with an eating disorder, there are three traits that run within families of people with eating disorders:[3]

- *Anxiety.* Within families, anxiety can be contagious and can maintain or even exacerbate a pattern of disordered eating. For example, parents may display a high level of anxiety in response to a child's disordered eating behaviors. The child senses this anxiety and responds by more intensive food avoidance.
- *Compulsivity.* The families of individuals with eating disorders are characterized by inflexibility, rigidity, and the need for order. Thus, when the family experiences an unpredictable event, the individual with an eating disorder may turn to compulsive behaviors—such as refusing food or obsessively exercising—to adapt.
- *Abnormal eating behavior in one family member.* A pattern of disordered eating may already be present within the family, leading other family members to view this behavior as normal or acceptable.

Influence of Media

As media saturation has increased over the last century, so has the incidence of eating disorders among white women.[4] Every day, we are confronted with advertisements in which computer-enhanced images of very lean, beautiful women promote everything from beer to cars (**Figure 2**). Most adult men and women understand that these images are unrealistic, but adolescents, who are still developing a sense of their identity and body image, lack the same ability to distance themselves from what they see.[5] Because body image influences eating behaviors, it is likely that the barrage of media models may be contributing to the increase in eating disorders. However, scientific evidence demonstrating that the media are *causing* increased eating disorders is difficult to obtain.

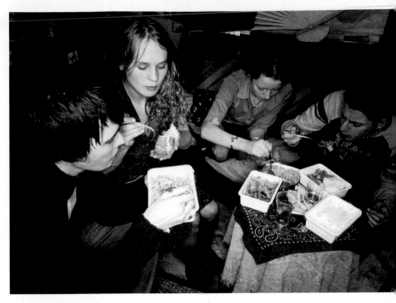

Hectic schedules often induce busy people to grab a quick meal "on the go."

Influence of Social and Cultural Values

Eating disorders are significantly more common in white females in Western societies than in other women worldwide.[6] This may be due in part to the white Western culture's association of slenderness with attractiveness, wealth, and high fashion. In contrast, until recently, the prevailing view in developing societies has been that excess body fat is desirable as a sign of health and material abundance.

The members of society with whom we most often interact—our family members, friends, classmates, and co-workers—also influence the way we see ourselves. Their comments related to our body weight or shape can be particularly hurtful—enough so to cause some people to start down the path of disordered eating. For example, individuals with bulimia nervosa report that they perceived greater pressure from

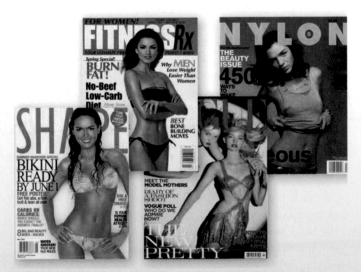

FIGURE 2 Photos of models and celebrities are routinely airbrushed or altered to "enhance" physical appearance. Unfortunately, many young people believe these portrayals are accurate and strive to meet unrealistic physical goals.

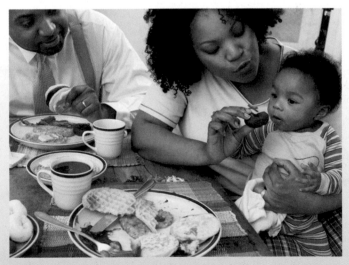

Family environment influences when, what, and how much we eat.

their peers to be thin than controls, while research shows that peer teasing about weight increases body dissatisfaction and eating disturbances.[7] Thus, our comments to others regarding their weight do count. Peer relationships also appear to be highly influential in the development of anorexia. A 2011 study from the London School of Economics concluded that anorexia is primarily socially induced. The higher the BMI of one's peers, the lower the risk of developing anorexia.[8]

Influence of Personality

A number of studies suggest that people with anorexia nervosa exhibit increased rates of obsessive-compulsive behaviors and perfectionism. They also tend to be socially inhibited, compliant, and emotionally restrained.[9] Unfortunately, many studies observe these behaviors only in individuals who are very ill and in a state of starvation, which may affect personality. Thus, it is difficult to determine if personality is the cause or effect of the disorder.

In contrast to people with anorexia nervosa, people with bulimia nervosa tend to be more impulsive, have low self-esteem, and demonstrate an extroverted, erratic personality style that seeks attention and admiration. In these people, negative moods are more likely to cause overeating than food restriction.[9]

Anorexia Nervosa Is a Potentially Deadly Eating Disorder

According to the American Psychiatric Association, 90% to 95% of individuals with anorexia nervosa are young girls or women.[1] Approximately 0.5% to 3.7% of American females develop anorexia, and 20% of these women will die prematurely from complications related to their disorder, including suicide and heart problems.[10] These statistics make anorexia nervosa the most common and most deadly psychiatric disorder diagnosed in women and the leading cause of death in females

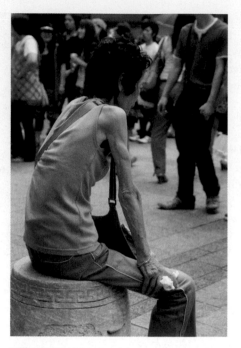

FIGURE 3 People with anorexia nervosa experience an extreme drive for thinness, resulting in potentially fatal weight loss.

between the ages of 15 and 24 years.[10, 11] As the statistics indicate, anorexia nervosa also occurs in males, but the prevalence is much lower than in females.

Signs and Symptoms of Anorexia Nervosa

The classic sign of anorexia nervosa is an extremely restrictive eating pattern that leads to self-starvation (**Figure 3**). These individuals may fast completely, restrict energy intake to only a few kilocalories per day, or eliminate all but one or two food groups from their diet. They also have an intense fear of weight gain, and even small amounts (for example, 1–2 lb) trigger high stress and anxiety.

In females, **amenorrhea** (the condition of having no menstrual periods for at least 3 continuous months) is a common feature of anorexia nervosa. It occurs when a young woman consumes insufficient energy to maintain normal body functions.

The American Psychiatric Association identifies the following conditions of anorexia nervosa (reprinted with permission from the *Diagnostic and Statistical Manual of Mental Disorders, Text Revision,* © 2000 American Psychiatric Association):

- Refusal to maintain body weight at or above a minimally normal weight for age and height
- Intense fear of gaining weight or becoming fat, even though considered underweight by all medical criteria
- Disturbance in the way in which one's body weight or shape is experienced, undue influence of body weight or shape on self-evaluation, or denial of the seriousness of the current low body weight
- Amenorrhea in females who are past puberty. Amenorrhea is defined as the absence of at least three consecutive menstrual cycles. A woman is considered to have amenorrhea if her periods occur only when given hormones, such as estrogen or oral contraceptives.

The signs of an eating disorder such as anorexia nervosa may be somewhat different in males. Females say they feel fat even though they typically are normal weight or even underweight before they develop the disorder. In contrast, males are more likely to have actually been overweight or even obese.[12, 13] Thus, the male's fear of "getting fat again" is based on reality. In addition, males with disordered eating are less concerned with actual body weight (scale weight) than females but are more concerned with body composition (percentage of muscle mass compared to fat mass).

---

amenorrhea The absence of menstruation. In females who had previously been menstruating, it is defined as the absence of menstrual periods for 3 or more continuous months.

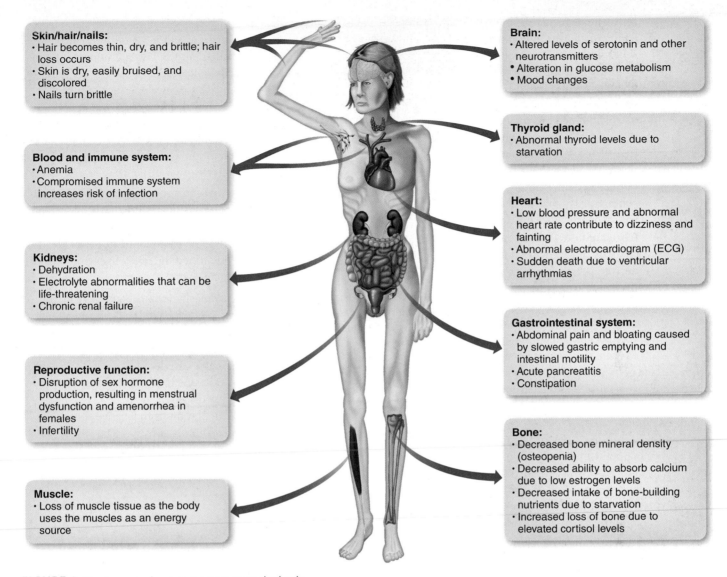

Skin/hair/nails:
- Hair becomes thin, dry, and brittle; hair loss occurs
- Skin is dry, easily bruised, and discolored
- Nails turn brittle

Blood and immune system:
- Anemia
- Compromised immune system increases risk of infection

Kidneys:
- Dehydration
- Electrolyte abnormalities that can be life-threatening
- Chronic renal failure

Reproductive function:
- Disruption of sex hormone production, resulting in menstrual dysfunction and amenorrhea in females
- Infertility

Muscle:
- Loss of muscle tissue as the body uses the muscles as an energy source

Brain:
- Altered levels of serotonin and other neurotransmitters
- Alteration in glucose metabolism
- Mood changes

Thyroid gland:
- Abnormal thyroid levels due to starvation

Heart:
- Low blood pressure and abnormal heart rate contribute to dizziness and fainting
- Abnormal electrocardiogram (ECG)
- Sudden death due to ventricular arrhythmias

Gastrointestinal system:
- Abdominal pain and bloating caused by slowed gastric emptying and intestinal motility
- Acute pancreatitis
- Constipation

Bone:
- Decreased bone mineral density (osteopenia)
- Decreased ability to absorb calcium due to low estrogen levels
- Decreased intake of bone-building nutrients due to starvation
- Increased loss of bone due to elevated cortisol levels

FIGURE 4 The impact of anorexia nervosa on the body.

The methods that men and women use to achieve weight loss also appear to differ. Males are more likely to use excessive exercise as a means of weight control, whereas females tend to use severe energy restriction, vomiting, and laxative abuse. These weight-control differences may stem from sociocultural biases; that is, dieting is considered to be more acceptable for women, whereas the overwhelming sociocultural belief is that "real mean don't diet."[13] For more information on eating disorders in men, see the nearby **Highlight** box.

Health Risks of Anorexia Nervosa

Left untreated, anorexia nervosa eventually leads to a deficiency in energy and other nutrients that are required by the body to function normally. The body will then use stored fat and lean tissue (for example, organ and muscle tissue) as an energy source to maintain brain tissue and vital body functions. The body will also shut down or reduce nonvital body functions to conserve energy. Electrolyte imbalances can lead to heart failure and death. **Figure 4** highlights

many of the health problems that occur in people (specifically, women and girls) with anorexia nervosa. The best chance for recovery is when an individual receives intensive treatment early.

Bulimia Nervosa Is Characterized by Binge Eating and Purging

Bulimia nervosa is an eating disorder characterized by repeated episodes of **binge eating** followed by some form of **purging.** While binge eating, the person feels a loss of

---

binge eating   Consumption of a large amount of food in a short period of time, usually accompanied by a feeling of loss of self-control.

purging   An attempt to rid the body of unwanted food by vomiting or other compensatory means, such as excessive exercise, fasting, or laxative abuse.

self-control, including an inability to end the binge once it has started.[14] At the same time, the person feels a sense of euphoria not unlike a drug-induced high. A binge is usually defined as a quantity of food that is large for the person and for the amount of time in which it is eaten (**Figure 5**). For example, a person may eat a dozen brownies with 2 quarts of ice cream in a period of just 30 minutes.

The prevalence of bulimia nervosa is higher than anorexia nervosa and is estimated to affect 1% to 4% of women.[10] Like anorexia nervosa, bulimia nervosa is found predominantly in women: six to ten females are diagnosed for every one male. The mortality rate for bulimia nervosa is estimated at approximately 4%.[10]

Although the prevalence of bulimia nervosa is much higher in women, rates for men are significant in some predominantly "thin-build" sports in which participants are encouraged to maintain a low body weight (for example, horse racing, wrestling, crew, and gymnastics). Individuals in these sports typically do not have all the characteristics of bulimia nervosa, however, and the purging behaviors they practice typically stop once the sport is discontinued.

An individual with bulimia nervosa typically purges after most episodes, but not necessarily on every occasion, and weight gain as a result of binge eating can be significant. Methods of purging include vomiting, laxative or diuretic abuse, enemas, fasting, and excessive exercise. For example, after a binge, a runner may increase her daily mileage to equal the "calculated" energy content of the binge.

Symptoms of Bulimia Nervosa

As with anorexia nervosa, the American Psychiatric Association has identified conditions of bulimia nervosa (reprinted with permission from the Diagnostic and Statistical Manual of Mental Disorders, Text Revision, © 2000 American Psychiatric Association):

- Recurrent episodes of binge eating (for example, eating a large amount of food in a short period of time, such as within 2 hours)
- Recurrent inappropriate compensatory behavior in order to prevent weight gain, such as self-induced vomiting; misuse of laxatives, diuretics, enemas, or other medications; fasting; or excessive exercise

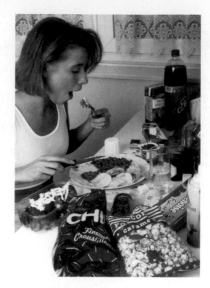

FIGURE 5 People with bulimia nervosa often consume large amounts of food in relatively brief periods of time.

- Binge eating occurs on average at least twice a week for 3 months
- Body shape and weight unduly influence self-evaluation
- The disturbance does not occur exclusively during episodes of anorexia nervosa. Some individuals will have periods of binge eating and then periods of starvation, which makes classification of their disorder difficult.

How can you tell if someone has bulimia nervosa? In addition to the recurrent and frequent binge eating and purging episodes, the National Institutes of Health[15] have identified the following symptoms of bulimia nervosa:

- Chronically inflamed and sore throat
- Swollen glands in the neck and below the jaw
- Worn tooth enamel and increasingly sensitive and decaying teeth as a result of exposure to stomach acids
- Gastroesophageal reflux disorder
- Intestinal distress and irritation from laxative abuse
- Kidney problems from diuretic abuse
- Severe dehydration from purging of fluids

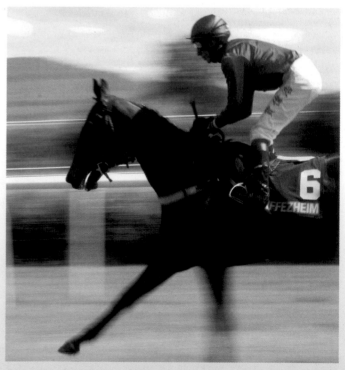

Men who participate in "thin-build" sports, such as jockeys, have a higher risk for bulimia nervosa than men who do not.

Muscle Dysmorphia: The Male Eating Disorder?

Is there a reverse form of anorexia nervosa unique to men? For decades, bodybuilders have recognized that some men view themselves as "puny" even when they are normal size or even very muscular; work out obsessively; and adhere to an extremely restrictive diet. Recognizing the syndrome they observed as a sort of "reverse anorexia," they coined the name "bigorexia."[1]

Recently, many psychiatric researchers and clinicians have confirmed that this disorder exists. They call it *muscle dysmorphia* (in medicine, a *dysmorphia* is an abnormality of structure). Some classify the disorder as a subtype of *body dysmorphic disorder*, a psychiatric illness in which the person is preoccupied with a physical flaw that is either extremely minor or doesn't actually exist. Others classify it as an eating disorder, pointing out that the patients' pathological pursuit of weight gain causes them to engage in highly disordered eating behaviors quite similar to those of patients with anorexia. They also note that the risk factors for muscle dysmorphia and anorexia nervosa and the approaches found to be successful in treating the two disorders are similar.[2]

No matter how the disorder is classified, the fundamental characteristic, as with anorexia nervosa, is a body image distortion. Men with muscle dysmorphia perceive themselves as small and frail even though they may actually be quite large and muscular. As a result, they are pathologically preoccupied with muscularity, spend long hours lifting weights, and follow a meticulous diet, often consisting of excessive high-protein foods and dietary supplements, such as protein powders. But no matter how "buff" they become, their reflection in the mirror does not match their idealized body size and shape. That said, studies suggest that as many as half of men with muscle dysmorphia do recognize at least to a "fair" extent that their perceptions about their physique are flawed.[2]

Men with muscle dysmorphia also share other characteristics with men and women with anorexia. For instance, they also report "feeling fat" and express significant discomfort with the idea of having to expose their body to others (for example, take off their clothes in the locker room). They also have increased rates of other psychiatric illnesses, including anxiety and depression.[3]

There are some outward indications that someone may be struggling with muscle dysmorphia. Not all of them apply to all men with the disorder. If you notice any of these behaviors in a friend or relative, talk about it with him and let him know that help is available.

- Rigid and excessive schedule of weight training
- Strict adherence to a high-protein, muscle-enhancing diet
- Use of anabolic steroids, protein powders, or other muscle-enhancing drugs or supplements
- Poor attendance at work, school, or sports activities because of interference with a rigid weight-training schedule
- Avoidance of social engagements in which the person will not be able to follow his strict diet
- Avoidance of situations in which the person would have to expose his body to others
- Frequent and critical self-evaluation of body composition

Like anorexia nervosa, muscle dysmorphia can cause significant distress and despair, and can even be life-threatening. Men with the disorder are more likely to report substance abuse—including the use of anabolic steroids—and are more likely to have attempted suicide. In one study, half of the men diagnosed with muscle dysmorphia had attempted suicide.[1] Therapy—especially participation in an all-male support group—can help.

References

1. Pope, C. G., H. G. Pope, W. Menard, C. Fay, R. Olivardia, and K. A. Phillips. 2005. Clinical features of muscle dysmorphia among males with body dysmorphic disorder. *Body Image* 2(4):395–400.
2. Murray, S. B., E. Rieger, S. W. Touyz, and Y. de la Garza Garcia. 2010. Muscle dysmorphia and the DSM-V conundrum: where does it belong? *International Journal of Eating Disorders* 43(6):483–491. http://onlinelibrary.wiley.com/doi/10.1002/eat.20828/pdf. (Accessed March 2012.)
3. Weltzin, T. E. 2012. A Silent Problem: Males with Eating Disorders in the Workplace. National Association of Anorexia Nervosa and Associated Disorders. www.anad.org/get-information/males-eating-disorders/medical-director-on-males-with-eds-in-the-workplace/. (Accessed March 2012.)

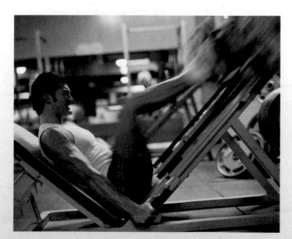

Men are more likely than women to exercise excessively in an effort to control their weight.

Health Risks of Bulimia Nervosa

The destructive behaviors of bulimia nervosa can lead to illness and even death. The most common health consequences associated with bulimia nervosa are

- Electrolyte imbalance typically caused by dehydration and the loss of potassium and sodium from the body with frequent vomiting. This can lead to irregular heartbeat and even heart failure and death.
- Gastrointestinal problems: inflammation, ulceration, and possible rupture of the esophagus and stomach from frequent bingeing and vomiting. Chronic irregular bowel movements and constipation may result in people with bulimia who chronically abuse laxatives.
- Dental problems: tooth decay and staining from stomach acids released during frequent vomiting

As with anorexia nervosa, the chance of recovery from bulimia nervosa increases, and the negative effects on health decrease, if the disorder is detected at an early stage. Familiarity with the warning signs of bulimia nervosa can help you identify friends and family members who might be at risk.

Binge-Eating Disorder Can Cause Significant Weight Gain

When was the last time a friend or relative confessed to you about "going on an eating binge"? Most likely, he or she explained that the behavior followed some sort of stressful event, such as a problem at work, the breakup of a relationship, or a poor grade on an exam. Many people have one or two binge episodes every year or so, in response to stress. But in people with **binge-eating disorder,** the behavior occurs an average of twice a week or more and is not usually followed by purging. This lack of compensation for the binge distinguishes binge-eating disorder from bulimia nervosa and explains why the person tends to gain a lot of weight.

The prevalence of binge-eating disorder is estimated to be 2% to 5% of the adult female population[10] and 8% of the obese population.[16] In contrast to anorexia and bulimia, binge-eating disorder is also common in men. Our current food environment, which offers an abundance of good-tasting, cheap food any time of the day, makes it difficult for people with binge-eating disorder to avoid food triggers.

As you would expect, the increased energy intake associated with binge eating significantly increases a person's risk of being overweight or obese. In addition, the types of foods individuals typically consume during a binge episode are high in fat and sugar, which can increase blood lipids. Finally, the stress associated with binge eating can have psychological consequences, such as low self-esteem, avoidance of social contact, depression, and negative thoughts related to body size.

Night-Eating Syndrome Can Lead to Obesity

Night-eating syndrome was first described in a group of patients who were not hungry in the morning but spent the evening and night eating and reported insomnia. Like binge-eating disorder, it is associated with obesity because, although night eaters don't binge, they do consume significant energy in their frequent snacks, and they don't compensate for the excess energy intake.

The distinguishing characteristic of night-eating syndrome is the time during which most of the day's energy intake occurs. Night eaters eat relatively little during the day, consuming the majority of their energy between 8:00 PM and 6:00 AM. They even get up in the night to eat. Night eating is also characterized by a depressed mood and by insomnia. In short, night eaters appear to have a unique combination of three disorders: an eating disorder, a sleep disorder, and a mood disorder.[17]

Night-eating syndrome is important clinically because of its association with obesity, which increases the risk for several chronic diseases, including heart disease, high blood pressure, stroke, type 2 diabetes, and arthritis. Obesity also increases the risk for sleep apnea, which can further disrupt the night eater's already abnormal sleeping pattern.

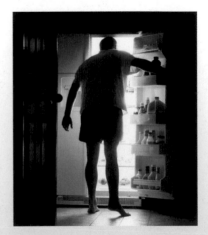

People with night-eating syndrome consume most of their daily energy between 8 PM and 6 AM.

---

binge-eating disorder A disorder characterized by binge eating an average of twice a week or more, typically without compensatory purging.

night-eating syndrome Disorder characterized by intake of the majority of the day's energy between 8:00 PM and 6:00 AM. Individuals with this disorder also experience mood and sleep disorders.

The Female Athlete Triad Consists of Three Disorders

The *female athlete triad* is a serious syndrome that consists of three clinical conditions in some physically active females:[18]

- Low energy availability (such as inadequate energy intake to maintain menstrual function or to cover energy expended in exercise) with or without eating disorders
- Menstrual dysfunction, such as amenorrhea (the absence of menstruation for 3 months or more)
- Low bone density (**Figure 6**)

Certain sports that strongly emphasize leanness or a thin body build may place a young girl or a woman at risk for the female athlete triad. These sports typically include figure skating, gymnastics, and diving; classical ballet dancers are also at increased risk for the disorder.

Active women experience the general social and cultural demands placed on women to be thin, as well as pressure from their coach, teammates, judges, and/or spectators to meet weight standards or body-size expectations for their sport. Failure to meet these standards can result in severe consequences,

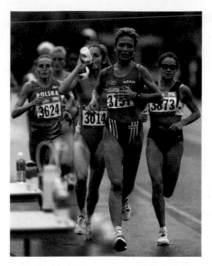

Sports that emphasize leanness or require athletes to wear body-contouring clothing increase the risk for female athlete triad.

such as being cut from the team, losing an athletic scholarship, or decreased participation with the team.

As the pressure to be thin mounts, active women may restrict their energy intake, typically by engaging in disordered eating behaviors. Energy restriction combined with high levels of physical activity can disrupt the menstrual cycle and result in amenorrhea. Menstrual dysfunction can also occur in active women who are not dieting and don't have an eating disorder. These women are just not eating enough to cover the energy costs of their exercise training and all the other energy demands of the body and daily living. Female athletes with menstrual dysfunction, regardless of the cause, typically have reduced levels of the reproductive hormones estrogen and progesterone. When estrogen levels in the body are low, it is difficult for bone to retain calcium, and gradual loss of bone mass occurs. Thus, many female athletes develop premature bone loss (osteoporosis) and are at increased risk for fractures.

Recognition of an athlete with one or more of the components of the female athlete triad can be difficult, especially if the athlete is reluctant to be honest when questioned about the symptoms. For this reason, familiarity with the early warning signs is critical. These include excessive dieting and/or weight loss, excessive exercise, stress fractures, and self-esteem that appears to be dictated by body weight and shape. (See Chapter 11, pages 460–461, for additional information on this topic.)

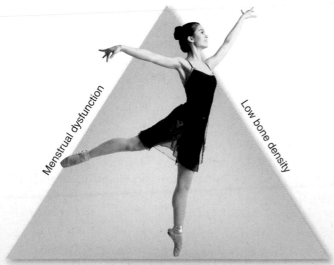

Menstrual dysfunction

Low bone density

Low energy availability

FIGURE 6 The female athlete triad is a syndrome composed of three coexisting disorders: low energy availability (with or without eating disorders), menstrual dysfunction (such as amenorrhea), and low bone density (such as osteoporosis). Energy availability is defined as dietary energy intake minus exercise energy expenditure.

Treatment for Disordered Eating Requires a Multidisciplinary Approach

As with any health problem, prevention is the best treatment for disordered eating. People having trouble with eating and body image issues need help to deal with these issues before they develop into something more serious.

Treating anyone with disordered eating requires a multidisciplinary approach. In addition to a physician and psychologist, a nutritionist, the person's coach and trainer (if an athlete), and family members and friends all must work together. Patients who are severely underweight, display signs of malnutrition, are medically unstable, or are suicidal may require immediate hospitalization. Conversely, patients who are underweight but are still medically stable may enter an outpatient program designed to meet their specific needs.

Some outpatient programs are extremely intensive, requiring patients to come in each day for treatment, whereas others are less rigorous, requiring only weekly visits for meetings with a psychiatrist or eating disorder specialist.

Nutritional Therapies Are Used in Treating Anorexia Nervosa

The goals of nutritional therapies are to restore the individual to a healthy body weight and resolve the nutrition-related eating issues. For hospitalized patients, the expected weight gain per week ranges from 1 to 3 pounds. For outpatient settings, the expected weight gain is much lower (0.5 to 1 pound/week). During the weight-gain phase of a treatment program, energy intake goals may be set at 1,000 to 1,600 kcal/day, depending on body size, severity of the disease, and achievable levels of intake.

Patients frequently try a variety of methods to avoid consuming the food presented to them. They may discard the food, vomit, exercise excessively, or engage in a high level of non-exercise motor activity to eliminate the calories they have just consumed. For this reason, patients are carefully watched by hospital staff or parents to make sure they swallow all their food. In addition to increasing amounts of food, patients may be given vitamin and mineral supplements to ensure that adequate micronutrients are consumed.

Nutrition counseling is an important aspect of the treatment to deal with the body image issues that occur as weight is regained. Once the patient reaches an acceptable body weight, nutrition counseling will address issues such as the acceptability of certain foods; dealing with food situations, such as family gatherings and eating out; and learning to put together a healthful food plan for weight maintenance.

Nutrition Counseling Is Important in Treating Bulimia Nervosa

Most individuals with bulimia nervosa are of normal weight or overweight, so restoring body weight is generally not the focus of treatment as it is with anorexia nervosa. Instead, nutrition counseling generally focuses on identifying and dealing with events and feelings that trigger binge eating, reducing purging, and establishing eating behaviors that can maintain a healthful body weight. In addition, nutrition counseling will address negative feelings about foods and the fear associated with uncontrolled binge eating.

Talking About Disordered Eating

Discussing a friend's eating behaviors can be difficult. It is important to choose an appropriate time and place to raise your concerns and to listen closely and with great sensitivity to your friend's feelings. Here, we outline an approach you might use.

Before approaching a friend or family member you suspect of having an eating disorder, learn as much as you possibly can about the eating disorder. Make sure you know the difference between the facts and myths about eating disorders. Locate a health professional specializing in eating disorders to whom you can refer your friend, and be ready to go with your friend if he or she does not want to go alone. If you are at a university or college, check with your local health center to see if it has an eating disorder team or can recommend someone to you. Set the stage for your discussion by finding a relaxed and private setting.[19]

The National Eating Disorders Association recommends the following steps to take during your discussion:[19]

- Schedule a time to talk. Set aside a time and place for a private discussion in which you can share your concerns openly and honestly in a caring and supportive way. Make sure the setting is quiet and away from other distractions.
- Communicate your concerns. Share your memories of specific times when you felt concerned about your friend's eating or exercise behaviors. Explain that you think these things may indicate that there is a problem that needs professional attention.

Nutri-Case | Liz

"I used to dance with a really cool modern company, where everybody looked sort of healthy and 'real.' No waifs! When they folded after Christmas, I was really bummed, but this spring, I'm planning to audition for the City Ballet. My best friend dances with them, and she told me that they won't even look at anybody over 100 pounds. So I've just put myself on a strict diet. Most days, I come in under 1,200 Calories, though some days I cheat and then I feel so out of control. Last week, my dance teacher stopped me after class and asked me whether or not I was menstruating. I thought that was a pretty weird question, so I just said sure, but then when I thought about it, I realized that I've been so focused and stressed out lately that I really don't know! The audition is only a week away, so I'm going on a juice fast this weekend. I've just got to make it into the City Ballet!"

What factors increase Liz's risk for the female athlete triad? What, if anything, do you think Liz's dance teacher should do? Is intervention even necessary, since the audition is only a week away?

- Ask your friend to explore these concerns with a counselor, doctor, nutritionist, or other health professional who is knowledgeable about eating issues. If you feel comfortable doing so, offer to help your friend make an appointment or accompany your friend on the first visit.
- Avoid conflicts or a "battle of the wills" with your friend. If your friend refuses to acknowledge that there is a problem, or any reason for you to be concerned, restate your feelings and the reasons for them and leave yourself open and available as a supportive listener.
- Avoid placing shame, blame, or guilt on your friend regarding his or her actions or attitudes. Do not use accusatory "you" statements, such as "You just need to eat" or "You are acting irresponsibly." Instead, use "I" statements—for example, "I'm concerned about you because I never see you in the cafeteria anymore" or "It makes me afraid when I hear you vomit."
- Avoid giving simple solutions—for example, "If you would just stop, everything would be fine."
- Express your continued support. Remind your friend that you care and want your friend to be healthy and happy.

 # Web Links

www.harriscentermgh.org

Harris Center for Education and Advocacy in Eating Disorders, Massachusetts General Hospital
This site provides information about current eating disorder research, as well as sections on understanding eating disorders and resources for those with eating disorders.

www.nimh.nih.gov

National Institute of Mental Health (NIMH) Office of Communications and Public Liaison
Search this site for "disordered eating" or "eating disorders" to find numerous articles on the subject.

www.anad.org

National Association of Anorexia Nervosa and Associated Disorders
Visit this site for information and resources about eating disorders.

www.nationaleatingdisorders.org

National Eating Disorders Association
This site is dedicated to expanding public understanding of eating disorders and promoting access to treatment for those affected and support for their families.

 # References

1. American Psychiatric Association. 1994. *Diagnostic and Statistical Manual of Mental Disorders (DSM-IV),* 4th edn. Washington, DC: Author.

2. Grave, R. D. 2011. Eating disorders: Progress and challenges. *Europ. J. Internal. Med.* 22:153–160.

3. Treasure, J. A., R. Sepulved, P. MacDonald, W. Whitaker, C. Lopez, M. Zabala, O. Kyracou, and G. Todd. 2008. The assessment of the family of people with eating disorders. *Europ. Eating Disorder Review.* 16:247–255.

4. Striegel-Moore, R. H., and L. Smolak. 2002. Gender, ethnicity, and eating disorders. In: Fairburn, D. G., and K. D. Brownell, eds. *Eating Disorders and Obesity: A Comprehensive Handbook,* 2nd edn. New York: Guilford Press, pp. 251–255.

5. Steinberg, L. 2002. *Adolescence,* 6th edn. New York: McGraw-Hill.

6. Treasure, J. A., M. Claudino, and N. Zucker. 2010. Eating disorders. *Lancet* 375:583–593.

7. Stice, E. 2002. Sociocultural influences on body image and eating disturbances. In: Fairburn, D. G., and K. D. Brownell, eds. *Eating Disorders and Obesity: A Comprehensive Handbook,* 2nd edn. New York: Guilford Press, pp. 103–107.

8. Costa-Font, J., and M. Jofre-Bonet. (2011, November). Anorexia, Body Image, and Peer Effects: Evidence from a Sample of European Women. *Centre for Economic Performance*: CEP discussion paper No. 1098. http://cep.lse.ac.uk/pubs/download/dp1098.pdf. (Accessed March 2012.)

9. Wonderlich, S. A. 2002. Personality and eating disorders. In: Fairburn, D. G., and K. D. Brownell, eds. *Eating Disorders and Obesity: A Comprehensive Handbook,* 2nd edn. New York: Guilford Press, pp. 204–209.

10. National Association of Anorexia Nervosa and Associated Disorders. 2012. Eating Disorder Statistics. www.anad.org/get-information/about-eating-disorders/eating-disorders-statistics/. (Accessed March 2012.)

11. Patrick, L. 2002. Eating disorders: a review of the literature with emphasis on medical complication and clinical nutrition. *Altern. Med. Rev.* 7(3):184–202.

12. Robb, A. S., and M. J. Dadson. 2002. Eating disorders in males. *Child Adolesc. Psychiatric. Clin. N. Am.* 11:399–418.

13. Beals, K. A. 2004. *Disordered Eating in Athletes: A Comprehensive Guide for Health Professionals.* Champaign, IL: Human Kinetics.

14. Garfinkel, P. E. 2002. Classification and diagnosis of eating disorders. In: Fairburn, D. G., and K. D. Brownell, eds. *Eating Disorders and Obesity: A Comprehensive Handbook,* 2nd edn. New York: Guilford Press, pp. 155–161.

15. National Institutes of Health. 2011. Eating Disorders. www.nimh.nih.gov/health/publications/eating-disorders/eating-disorders.pdf. (Accessed March 2012.)

16. Grilo, C. M. 2002. Binge eating disorder. In: Fairburn, D. G., and K. D. Brownell, eds. *Eating Disorders and Obesity: A Comprehensive Handbook,* 2nd edn. New York: Guilford Press, pp.178–182.

17. Stunkard, A. J. 2002. Night eating syndrome. In: Fairburn, D. G., and K. D. Brownell, eds. *Eating Disorders and Obesity: A Comprehensive Handbook,* 2nd edn. New York: Guilford Press, pp. 183–187.

18. Nattiv A., A. B. Loucks, M. M. Manore, C. F. Sanborn, J. Sundgot-Borgen, and M. P. Warren. 2007. The female athlete triad. *Med. and Sci. in Sport and Exer.* 39(10):1867–1882.

19. National Eating Disorders Association. 2005. What Should I Say? Tips for Talking to a Friend Who May Be Struggling with an Eating Disorder. www.nationaleatingdisorders.org/p.asp?WebPage_ID5322&Profile_ID541174. (Accessed March 2012.)

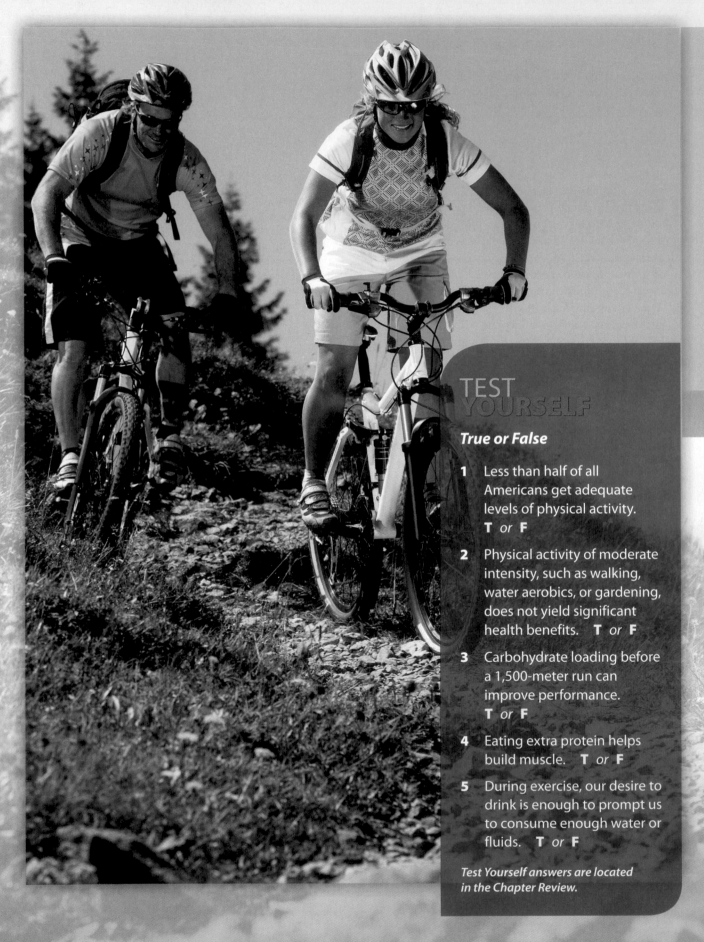

TEST YOURSELF

True or False

1 Less than half of all Americans get adequate levels of physical activity. **T** *or* **F**

2 Physical activity of moderate intensity, such as walking, water aerobics, or gardening, does not yield significant health benefits. **T** *or* **F**

3 Carbohydrate loading before a 1,500-meter run can improve performance. **T** *or* **F**

4 Eating extra protein helps build muscle. **T** *or* **F**

5 During exercise, our desire to drink is enough to prompt us to consume enough water or fluids. **T** *or* **F**

Test Yourself answers are located in the Chapter Review.

14

Nutrition and Physical Activity: Keys to Good Health

Learning Objectives

After studying this chapter, you should be able to:

1. Compare and contrast the concepts of physical activity, leisure-time physical activity, exercise, and physical fitness, *p. 562.*

2. Define the four components of fitness, *pp. 562–563.*

3. List at least four health benefits of being physically active on a regular basis, *pp. 562–563.*

4. Describe the main components of a sound fitness program, *pp. 565–569.*

5. Describe the FITT principle, and calculate your maximal and training heart rate range, *pp. 567–570.*

6. List and describe at least three processes we use to break down fuels to support physical activity, *pp. 571–576.*

7. Discuss at least three changes in nutrient needs that can occur in response to an increase in physical activity or vigorous exercise training, *pp. 577–583.*

8. Describe the concept of carbohydrate loading, and discuss situations in which this practice may be beneficial to athletic performance, *pp. 581–582.*

9. Define the heat illnesses, including heat syncope, heat cramps, heat exhaustion, and heat stroke, *pp. 584–585.*

10. Define the term *ergogenic aids,* and discuss the potential benefits and risks of at least four ergogenic aids that are currently on the market, *pp. 592–594.*

MasteringNutrition™

Go online for chapter quizzes, pre-tests, Interactive Activities, and more!

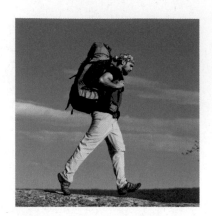

Hiking is a leisure-time physical activity that can contribute to your physical fitness.

In June 2011, Dottie Gray of Missouri won four gold medals in track and field at the National Senior Games. In the 800-meter dash, she clocked 5:33.71 to break the American record in her age class. If her record-breaking time doesn't impress you, perhaps it will when you consider her age: at the time she gave these winning performances, Dottie Gray was 86 years old! How does she stay so fit? Gray reports that she does her best to run a 5K every weekend.[1]

There's no doubt about it: regular physical activity dramatically improves a person's strength, stamina, health, and longevity. But what qualifies as "regular physical activity"? In other words, how much does a person need to do to reap the benefits? And if people do become more active, do their diets have to change too?

You may be asking yourself why a nutrition textbook includes a chapter on physical activity. One reason is that a healthful diet and regular physical activity are like two sides of the same coin, interacting in a variety of ways to improve strength and stamina and to increase resistance to many chronic diseases and acute illnesses. Physical activity affects how we store and metabolize various nutrients, and our nutritional status impacts our ability to perform physical activity. Additionally, the nutrition and physical activity recommendations for reducing the risks for heart disease also reduce the risks for various nutrition-related chronic diseases, including high blood pressure, type 2 diabetes, obesity, and some forms of cancer! In this chapter, we define physical activity, identify its many benefits, and discuss the nutrients needed to maintain an active life.

Why Engage in Physical Activity?

The term **physical activity** describes any movement produced by muscles that increases energy expenditure. Different categories of physical activity include occupational, household, leisure-time, and transportation.[2] **Leisure-time physical activity** is any activity not related to a person's occupation that includes competitive sports, planned exercise training, and recreational activities, such as hiking, walking, and bicycling. **Exercise** is therefore considered a subcategory of leisure-time physical activity and is activity that is purposeful, planned, and structured.[3]

Physical Activity Increases Our Fitness

A lot of people are looking for a "magic pill" that will help them maintain weight loss, reduce their risk for diseases, make them feel better, and improve their quality of sleep. Although they may not be aware of it, regular physical activity is this "magic pill." That's because it promotes **physical fitness**: the ability to carry out daily tasks with vigor and alertness, without undue fatigue, and with ample energy to enjoy leisure-time pursuits and meet unforeseen emergencies.[2]

The four components of physical fitness are cardiorespiratory fitness, which is the ability of the heart, lungs, and blood vessels to supply working muscles; musculoskeletal fitness, which is fitness of the muscles and bones; flexibility; and body composition (**Table 14.1**).[4] These are achieved through three types of exercise:

- **Aerobic exercise** involves the repetitive movement of large muscle groups, which increases the body's use of oxygen and promotes cardiovascular health. In your daily life, you get aerobic exercise when you walk to school, work, or a bus stop or take the stairs to a third-floor classroom.
- **Resistance training** is a form of exercise in which our muscles work against resistance, such as against handheld weights. Carrying grocery bags or books and moving heavy objects are everyday activities that make our muscles work against resistance.
- **Stretching** exercises are those that increase flexibility, as they involve lengthening muscles using slow, controlled movements. You can perform stretching exercises even while you're sitting in a classroom by flexing, extending, and rotating your neck, limbs, and extremities.

physical activity Any movement produced by muscles that increases energy expenditure; includes occupational, household, leisure-time, and transportation activities.

leisure-time physical activity Any activity not related to a person's occupation; includes competitive sports, recreational activities, and planned exercise training.

exercise A subcategory of leisure-time physical activity; any activity that is purposeful, planned, and structured.

physical fitness The ability to carry out daily tasks with vigor and alertness, without undue fatigue, and with ample energy to enjoy leisure-time pursuits and meet unforeseen emergencies.

aerobic exercise Exercise that involves the repetitive movement of large muscle groups, increasing the body's use of oxygen and promoting cardiovascular health.

resistance training Exercise in which our muscles act against resistance.

stretching Exercise in which muscles are gently lengthened using slow, controlled movements.

TABLE 14.1 The Components of Fitness

Fitness Component	Examples of Activities One Can Do to Achieve Fitness in Each Component
Cardiorespiratory	Aerobic-type activities, such as walking, running, swimming, cross-country skiing
Musculoskeletal fitness	Resistance training, weight lifting, calisthenics, sit-ups, push-ups
Muscular strength	Weight lifting or related activities using heavier weights with few repetitions
Muscular endurance	Weight lifting or related activities using lighter weights with more repetitions
Flexibility	Stretching exercises, yoga
Body composition	Aerobic exercise, resistance training

Physical Activity Reduces Our Risk for Chronic Diseases

In addition to contributing to our fitness, physical activity can reduce our risk for certain diseases. Specifically, the following are some of the health benefits of physical activity:

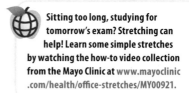

Sitting too long, studying for tomorrow's exam? Stretching can help! Learn some simple stretches by watching the how-to video collection from the Mayo Clinic at www.mayoclinic.com/health/office-stretches/MY00921.

- *Reduces our risk for, and complications of, heart disease, stroke, and high blood pressure.* Regular physical activity increases high-density lipoprotein (HDL) cholesterol and lowers triglycerides in the blood, improves the strength of the heart, helps maintain healthy blood pressure, and limits the progression of atherosclerosis.
- *Reduces our risk for obesity.* Regular physical activity maintains lean body mass and promotes more healthful levels of body fat, may help in appetite control, and increases energy expenditure and the use of fat as an energy source.
- *Reduces our risk for type 2 diabetes.* Regular physical activity enhances the action of insulin, which improves the cells' uptake of glucose from the blood, and it can improve blood glucose control in people with diabetes, which in turn reduces the risk for, or delays the onset of, diabetes-related complications.
- *May reduce our risk for colon cancer.* Although the exact role that physical activity may play in reducing colon cancer risk is still unknown, we do know that regular physical activity enhances gastric motility, which reduces the transit time of potential cancer-causing agents through the gut.
- *Reduces our risk for osteoporosis.* Regular physical activity, especially weight-bearing exercise, increases bone density and enhances muscular strength and flexibility, thereby reducing the likelihood of falls and the incidence of fractures and other injuries when falls occur.

Regular physical activity is also known to improve our sleep patterns, reduce our risk for upper respiratory infections by improving immune function, and reduce anxiety and mental stress. It also can be effective in treating mild and moderate depression.

Most Americans Are Inactive

For most of our history, humans were very physically active. This was not by choice but because their survival depended on it. Prior to the industrial age, humans expended a considerable amount of energy

Nutrition
MILESTONE

Although the benefits of exercise have been touted throughout history, it wasn't until **1953** that a significant link between physical health and exercise was confirmed. After returning from military service in World War II, Dr. Jeremiah "Jerry" Morris and other public health researchers in the United Kingdom became aware of the growing modern epidemic of coronary heart disease. Some evidence suggested that a person's occupation may play a key role in their risk of having a heart attack. Dr. Morris was able to prove his hypothesis in a landmark paper, published in *The Lancet*, which discussed his research on London transport employees.

This study showed that the heart attack rates of the bus drivers (who sat most of the day) were more than twice as high as those of conductors (who ran up and down the stairs of double-decker buses all day). He documented the waist circumferences of the bus employees via their pant waistband sizes, which indicated that the physically active conductors had a significantly lower risk for heart attack, no matter what the size of their waist! Dr. Morris is recognized as the father of physical activity epidemiology, and he continued to be an avid exerciser and active public health researcher until his death in 2009 at the age of 99.

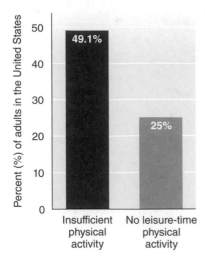

FIGURE 14.1 Rates of physical inactivity in the United States. Almost 50% of the U.S. population does not do enough physical activity to meet national health recommendations, and 25% report doing no leisure-time physical activity. (*Sources*: Data from National Center for Health Statistics. 2012. Health, United States, 2011: With Special Feature on Socioeconomic Status and Health. Hyattsville, MD. www.cdc.gov/nchs/data/hus/hus11.pdf#073; and Centers for Disease Control and Prevention. 2008. 1988–2007 No Leisure-Time Physical Activity Trend Chart. www.cdc.gov/nccdphp/dnpa/physical/stats/leisure_time.htm.)

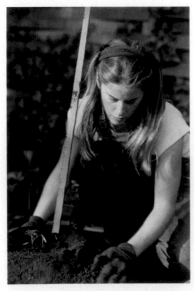

Moderate physical activity, such as gardening, helps maintain overall health.

each day foraging and hunting for food, planting and harvesting food, preparing food once it was acquired, and securing shelter. In addition, their diet was composed primarily of small amounts of lean meats and naturally grown vegetables and fruits. This lifestyle pattern contrasts considerably with today's, which is characterized by sedentary jobs, easy access to an overabundance of energy-dense foods, and few opportunities for or little interest in expending energy through occupational or recreational activities.

Given these changes, it isn't surprising that most people find the "magic pill" of physical activity hard to swallow. The Centers for Disease Control and Prevention reports that almost 50% of adults in the United States do not do enough physical activity to meet national health recommendations, and 25% admit to doing no leisure-time physical activity at all (**Figure 14.1**).[5,6] These statistics mirror the reported increases in obesity, heart disease, and type 2 diabetes in industrialized countries.

This trend toward inadequate physical activity levels is also occurring in young people. Among high school students, only 18.5% of girls and 38.3% of boys are meeting the recommended 60 minutes per day on 5 or more days per week.[7] Although physical education (PE) is part of the mandated curriculum in most states, only 27.2% of girls and 34.6% of boys participate in daily PE. Since our habits related to eating and physical activity are formed early in life, it is imperative that we provide opportunities for children and adolescents to engage in regular, enjoyable physical activity. An active lifestyle during childhood increases the likelihood of an active, healthier life as an adult.

How Much Physical Activity Is Enough?

As you've just read, most Americans do not engage in enough regular physical activity to meet current national recommendations. But what are the current recommendations, and what must a person do to achieve them?

In 1996, a report of the Surgeon General recommended that Americans engage in at least 30 minutes of physical activity on most days of the week.[2] Then, in 2002, the Institute of Medicine (IOM), which is part of the National Academy of Sciences, released a recommendation that Americans be active 60 minutes per day to optimize health.[8] As this amount and frequency of physical was significantly higher than the Surgeon General's recommendation, it caused a great deal of confusion and controversy. What was the basis for this more challenging recommendation?

The IOM recommendation was derived from metabolic studies specifically examining the energy expenditure associated with maintaining a healthful body weight (defined as a BMI of 18.5 to 25 kg/m^2). After reviewing a large number of studies that assessed energy expenditure and BMI, the IOM concluded that participating in about 60 minutes of moderately intense physical activity per day will move people to an active lifestyle and will allow them to maintain a healthful body weight.

The IOM recommendation was not based on evidence supporting the wider range of health benefits that result when a person moves from doing no physical activity to at least some level of physical activity. The growing body of evidence regarding the health benefits of physical activity clearly indicates that doing at least some physical activity is better than doing none, and doing more physical activity is better than doing less.

In 2008, the United States Department of Health and Human Services released the Physical Activity Guidelines for Americans.[9] These include guidelines for children and adolescents, adults, and older adults, with additional information for women who are pregnant; people with disabilities, type 2 diabetes, or osteoarthritis; and people who are cancer survivors. These guidelines build upon the Surgeon General's recommendation of 30 minutes per day on most, if not all, days of the week. Specifically, the 2008 guidelines for adults state the following:

■ Inactivity should be avoided. Participating in any amount of physical activity will provide some health benefits.

- To gain substantial health benefits, adults should do a minimum of 150 minutes per week of moderate-intensity activity, or 75 minutes per week of vigorous intensity activity, or an equivalent combination of these two intensities of activity. The activities should be aerobic in nature and performed in episodes of at least 10 minutes' duration, spread throughout the week.
- To gain additional and more extensive health benefits, adults should increase their aerobic activity level to 300 minutes per week of moderate-intensity activity, or 150 minutes per week of vigorous-intensity activity, or an equivalent combination of these two intensities.
- Adults should also participate in muscle-strengthening activities that are moderate or vigorous in intensity and involve all major muscle groups on at least 2 days per week.

Thus, the 2008 Physical Activity Guidelines for Americans incorporate the range of available evidence and promote a *minimum* of 150 minutes per week of moderate-intensity aerobic physical activity, with additional encouragement to increase both the intensity and the duration of activity throughout the week to gain even more health benefits.

RECAP

Physical activity is any movement produced by muscles that increases energy expenditure. Physical fitness is the ability to carry out daily tasks with vigor and alertness, without undue fatigue, and with ample energy to enjoy leisure-time pursuits and meet unforeseen emergencies. Physical activity provides a multitude of health benefits, including reducing our risk for obesity and other chronic diseases and relieving anxiety and stress. Most people in the United States, including many children, are insufficiently active. The 2008 Physical Activity Guidelines for Americans suggest that adults do a minimum of 150 minutes of moderate-intensity aerobic activity per week or 75 minutes of vigorous-intensity aerobic activity per week, or an equivalent combination of the two. It is also recommended that adults engage in moderate- or vigorous-intensity muscle strengthening exercises at least 2 days per week. ■

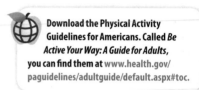

Download the Physical Activity Guidelines for Americans. Called *Be Active Your Way: A Guide for Adults*, you can find them at www.health.gov/paguidelines/adultguide/default.aspx#toc.

What Is a Sound Fitness Program?

Several widely recognized qualities of a sound fitness program, as well as guidelines to help people design one that is right for them, are explored in this section. Keep in mind that people with heart disease, high blood pressure, diabetes, obesity, asthma, osteoporosis, or arthritis should get approval to exercise from their healthcare practitioner prior to starting a fitness program. In addition, a medical evaluation should be conducted before starting an exercise program for an apparently healthy but currently inactive man 40 years or older or woman 50 years or older.

A Sound Fitness Program Meets Your Personal Goals

A fitness program that may be ideal for you is not necessarily right for everyone. Before designing or evaluating any program, it is important that each person define his or her personal fitness goals. Do you want to prevent osteoporosis, diabetes, or another chronic disease that runs in your family? Do you simply want to increase energy and stamina? Or do you intend to compete in athletic events? Each of these scenarios requires a unique fitness program. This concept is referred to as the specificity principle: specific actions yield specific results.

Training is generally defined as activity leading to skilled behavior. Training is very specific to any activity or goal. For example, if you want to train for athletic competition, a traditional approach that includes planned, purposive exercise sessions under the guidance of a trainer or coach would be beneficial. If you wanted to achieve cardiorespiratory fitness, you might be advised to participate in an aerobics class at least three times per week or jog for at least 20 minutes three times per week.

In contrast, if your goal is to transition from doing no regular physical activity to doing enough physical activity to maintain your overall health, you could follow the minimum recommendations put forth in the 2008 Physical Activity Guidelines for Americans.[9] To gain significant health benefits, including reducing the risk for chronic diseases, you can participate in at least 30 minutes per day of moderate-intensity aerobic physical activity (such as gardening, brisk walking, or basketball). The activity need not be completed in one session. You can divide the amount of physical activity into two or more shorter sessions throughout the day, as long as the total cumulative time is achieved (for example, brisk walking for 10 minutes three times per day). Although these minimum guidelines are appropriate for achieving health benefits, performing physical activities at a higher intensity and for longer duration will confer even greater health benefits and more significant improvements in physical fitness.

A Sound Fitness Program Is Varied, Consistent, and Fun!

A number of factors motivate us to be active. Some are *intrinsic* factors, which are those done for the satisfaction a person gains from engaging in the activity. Others are *extrinsic*, which are those done to obtain rewards or outcomes that are separate from the behavior itself.[10] Examples of intrinsic factors that motivate us to engage in physical activity include the desire to gain competence, the desire to be challenged by the activity and enhance our skills, and enjoyment. Some of the most common extrinsic factors are desires to improve appearance and to increase fitness. Recently, some employers have been offering financial incentives to log in time at the company's fitness center, another example of an extrinsic factor.

Whether we are more motivated by intrinsic or extrinsic factors is related to the type of activity in which we engage and whether we're a regular or infrequent exerciser. People who are regularly active tend to be more motivated by intrinsic factors, whereas extrinsic factors appear to be more important to people who are not regularly active or are trying to engage in activity for the first time.[11]

Thus, an important motivator in maintaining regular physical activity is enjoyment—or fun! People who enjoy being active find it easy to maintain their physical fitness. What activities do you consider fun? If you enjoy the outdoors, hiking, camping, fishing, and rock climbing are potential activities for you. If you would rather exercise with friends between classes, walking, climbing stairs, jogging, roller-blading, or bicycle riding may be more appropriate. Or you may prefer to use the programs and equipment at your campus or community fitness center or purchase your own treadmill and free weights.

Variety is also important to maintaining your fitness and your interest in being regularly active. Although some people enjoy doing similar activities day after day, many get bored with the same fitness routine. Incorporating a variety of activities into your fitness program will help maintain your interest and increase your enjoyment while promoting the various types of fitness identified in Table 14.1. Variety can be achieved in the following ways:

- Combining aerobic exercise, resistance training, and stretching
- Combining indoor and outdoor activities throughout the week
- Taking different routes when you walk or jog each day
- Watching a movie, reading a book, or listening to music while you ride a stationary bicycle or walk on a treadmill
- Participating in different activities each week, such as walking, dancing, bicycling, yoga, weight lifting, swimming, hiking, and gardening

This "smorgasbord" of activities can increase your fitness without leading to monotony and boredom.

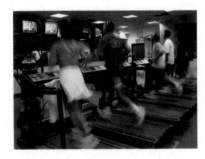

Watching television or listening to music can provide variety while running on a treadmill.

Are you ready to get fit? Take the adult fitness test from the President's Council on Fitness, Sports, and Nutrition at www.adultfitnesstest.org.

A Sound Fitness Program Appropriately Overloads the Body

In order to improve fitness, an extra physical demand must be placed on the body. This is referred to as the **overload principle.** A word of caution is in order here: *the overload principle does not advocate subjecting the body to inappropriately high stress,* because this can lead to exhaustion and injuries. In contrast, an appropriate overload on various body systems will result in healthy improvements in fitness. For example, a gain in muscle strength and size that results from repeated work that overloads the muscle is referred to as **hypertrophy.** When muscles are not worked adequately, they **atrophy,** or decrease in size and strength.

To achieve an appropriate overload, four factors should be considered, collectively known as the **FITT principle:** *f*requency, *i*ntensity, *t*ime, and *t*ype of activity. The FITT principle can be used to design either a general physical fitness program or a performance-based exercise program. **Figure 14.2** shows how the FITT principle can be applied to a cardiorespiratory and muscular fitness program.

Let's consider each of the FITT principle's four factors in more detail.

Frequency

Frequency refers to the number of activity sessions per week. Depending on the goals for fitness, the frequency of activities will vary. The Physical Activity Guidelines for Americans recommend engaging in aerobic (cardiorespiratory) activities for at least 150 minutes a week. To achieve cardiorespiratory fitness, training should be at least 3 to 5 days per week. On the other hand, training more than 6 days per week does not cause significant gains

overload principle   Placing an extra physical demand on your body in order to improve your fitness level.

hypertrophy   The increase in strength and size that results from repeated work to a specific muscle or muscle group.

atrophy   A decrease in the size and strength of muscles that occurs when they are not worked adequately.

FITT principle   The principle used to achieve an appropriate overload for physical training; FITT stands for *f*requency, *i*ntensity, *t*ime, and *t*ype of activity.

frequency   Refers to the number of activity sessions per week you perform.

	Frequency	Intensity	Time
Cardiorespiratory fitness 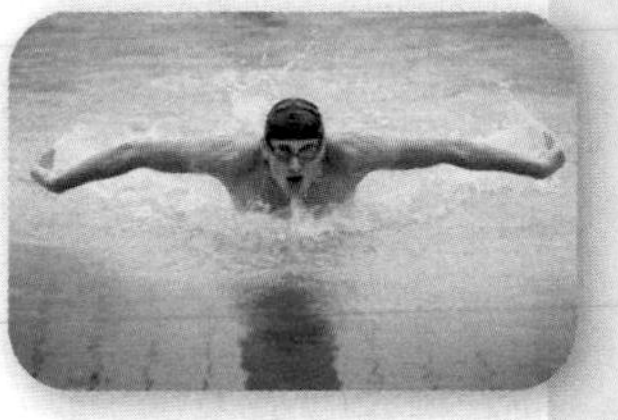	Most days of the week	50–70% maximal heart rate for moderate intensity; 70–85% maximal heart rate for vigorous intensity	At least 30 consecutive minutes
Muscular fitness 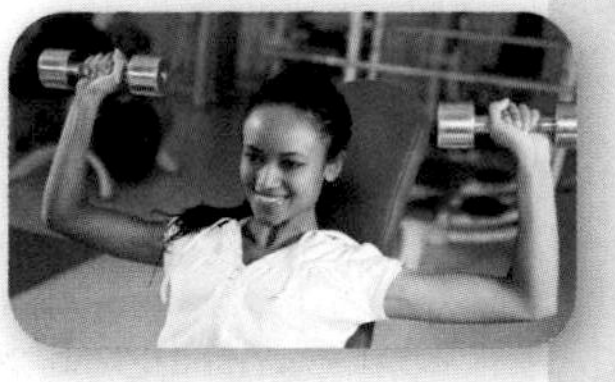	2–3 days per week	70–85% maximal weight you can lift	1–3 sets of 8–12 lifts* for each set *A minimum of 8–10 exercises involving the major muscle groups such as arms, shoulders, chest, abdomen, back, hips, and legs, is recommended.
Flexibility 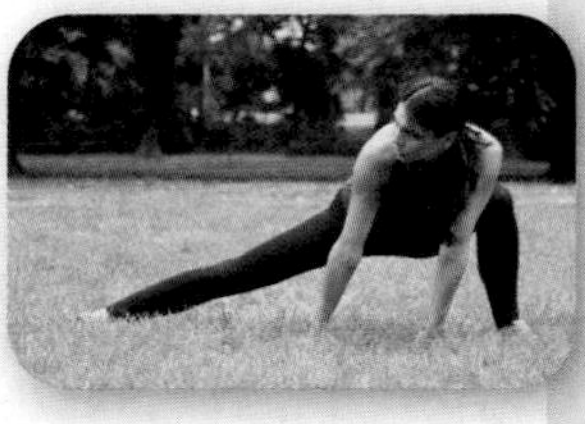	2–4 days per week	Stretching through full range of motion	2–4 repetitions per stretch* *Hold each stretch for 15–30 seconds.

FIGURE 14.2 Using the FITT principle to achieve cardiorespiratory and musculoskeletal fitness and flexibility. The recommendations in this figure follow the 2008 Physical Activity Guidelines for Americans (still in effect today).

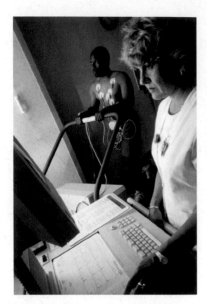

Testing in a fitness lab is the most accurate way to determine maximal heart rate.

in fitness but can substantially increase the risks for injury. Training 3 to 6 days per week appears optimal to achieve and maintain cardiorespiratory fitness. In contrast, only 2 to 3 days of training are needed to achieve muscular fitness.

Intensity

Intensity refers to the amount of effort expended, or to how difficult the activity is to perform. We can describe the intensity of activity as low, moderate, or vigorous:

- **Low-intensity activities** are those that cause very mild increases in breathing, sweating, and heart rate. Examples include walking at a leisurely pace, fishing, and light house-cleaning.
- **Moderate-intensity activities** cause moderate increases in breathing, sweating, and heart rate. For instance, you can carry on a conversation, but not continuously. Examples include brisk walking, water aerobics, doubles tennis, ballroom dancing, and bicycling slower than 10 miles per hour.
- **Vigorous-intensity activities** produce significant increases in breathing, sweating, and heart rate, so that talking is difficult when exercising. Examples include jogging, running, racewalking, singles tennis, aerobics, bicycling 10 miles per hour or faster, jumping rope, and hiking uphill with a heavy backpack.

Traditionally, heart rate has been used to indicate level of intensity during aerobic activities. You can calculate the range of exercise intensity that is appropriate for you by estimating your **maximal heart rate,** which is the rate at which your heart beats during maximal-intensity exercise. Maximal heart rate is estimated by subtracting your age from 220.

Figure 14.3 shows an example of a heart rate training chart, which you can use to estimate the intensity of your own workout. The Centers for Disease Control and Prevention makes the following recommendations:[12]

- To achieve moderate-intensity physical activity, your target heart rate should be 50–70% of your estimated maximal heart rate. Older adults and anyone who has been inactive for a long time may want to exercise at the lower end of the moderate-intensity range.

intensity The amount of effort expended during an activity, or how difficult the activity is to perform.

low-intensity activities Activities that cause very mild increases in breathing, sweating, and heart rate.

moderate-intensity activities Activities that cause moderate increases in breathing, sweating, and heart rate.

vigorous-intensity activities Activities that produce significant increases in breathing, sweating, and heart rate; talking is difficult when exercising at a vigorous intensity.

maximal heart rate The rate at which the heart beats during maximal-intensity exercise.

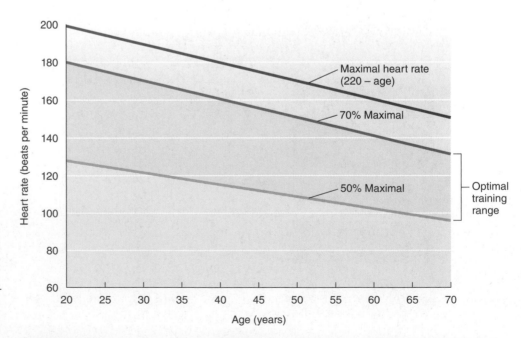

FIGURE 14.3 This heart rate training chart can be used to estimate aerobic exercise intensity. The top line indicates the predicted maximal heart rate value for a person's age (220 – age). The shaded area represents the heart rate values that fall between 50% and 70% of maximal heart rate, which is the range generally recommended to achieve aerobic fitness.

- To achieve vigorous-intensity physical activity, your target heart rate should be 70–85% of your estimated heart rate. Those who are physically fit or are striving for a more rapid improvement in fitness may want to exercise at the higher end of the vigorous-intensity range.
- Competitive athletes generally train at a higher intensity, around 80–95% of their maximal heart rate.

Although the calculation of *220 minus age* has been used extensively for years to predict maximal heart rate, it was never intended to accurately represent everyone's true maximal heart rate or to be used as the standard of aerobic training intensity. The most accurate way to determine your own maximal heart rate is to complete a maximal exercise test in a fitness laboratory; however, this test is not commonly conducted with the general public and can be very expensive. Although not completely accurate, the estimated maximal heart rate method can still be used to give you a general idea of your aerobic training range.

So what is your maximal heart rate and training range? To find out, try the easy calculation in the **You Do the Math** box (page 570).

Time of Activity

Time of activity refers to how long each session lasts. To achieve general health, a person can do multiple, short bouts of activity that add up to 30 minutes each day. However, to achieve higher levels of fitness, it is important that the activities be done for at least 20 to 30 consecutive minutes.

For example, let's say you want to compete in triathlons. To be successful during the running segment of the triathlon, you will need to be able to run quickly for at least 5 miles. Thus, it is appropriate for you to train so that you can complete 5 miles during one session and still have enough energy to swim and bicycle during the race. You will need to train consistently at a distance of 5 miles; you will also benefit from running longer distances.

Type of Activity

Type of activity refers to the range of physical activities a person can engage in to promote health and physical fitness. Many of the types of physical activities one can engage in are shown in Table 14.1 (page 563) and Figure 14.2 (page 567). The types of activity you choose to engage in will depend on your goals for health and physical fitness, your personal preferences, and the range of activities available to you.

A Sound Fitness Plan Includes a Warm-Up and a Cool-Down Period

To properly prepare for and recover from an exercise session, warm-up and cool-down activities should be performed. **Warm-up,** also called preliminary exercise, includes general activities, such as gentle aerobics, calisthenics, and then stretching followed by specific activities that prepare a person for the actual activity, such as jogging or swinging a golf club. The warm-up should be brief (5 to 10 minutes), gradual, and sufficient to increase muscle and body temperature. It should not cause fatigue or deplete energy stores.

Warming up prior to exercise is important, as it properly prepares your muscles for exertion by increasing blood flow and body temperature. It enhances the body's flexibility and may also help prepare you psychologically for the exercise session or athletic event.

Cool-down activities are done after the exercise session. The cool-down should be gradual and allow the body to recover slowly. The cool-down should include some of the same activities performed during the exercise session, but at a low intensity, and should allow ample time for stretching. Cooling down after exercise assists in the prevention of injury and may help reduce muscle soreness.

Tips for Increasing Your Physical Activity

Now that you know the benefits of regular physical activity and the characteristics of a sound fitness plan, how do you get started? If you have not been active until now, it's

Want to learn more about the various tools used to measure physical activity levels? Go to the University of Pittsburgh Physical Activity Resource Center for Public Health at www.parcph.org/assess.aspx to find out more.

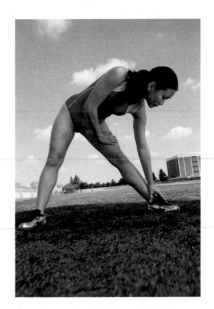

Stretching should be included in the warm-up and the cool-down for exercise.

time of activity   How long each exercise session lasts.

type of activity   The range of physical activities a person can engage in to promote health and physical fitness.

warm-up   Also called preliminary exercise; includes activities that prepare you for an exercise bout, including stretching, calisthenics, and movements specific to the exercise bout.

cool-down   Activities done after an exercise session is completed; should be gradual and allow your body to slowly recover from exercise.

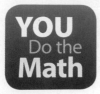

Calculating Your Maximal and Training Heart Rate Range

Judy was recently diagnosed with type 2 diabetes, and her healthcare provider has recommended she begin an exercise program. She is considered obese, according to her body mass index, and she has not been regularly active since she was a teenager. Judy's goals are to improve her cardiorespiratory fitness and achieve and maintain a more healthful weight. Fortunately, Valley Hospital, where she works as a nurse's aide, recently opened a small fitness center for its employees. Judy plans to begin by either walking on the treadmill or riding the stationary bicycle at the fitness center during her lunch break.

Judy needs to exercise at an intensity that will help her improve her cardiorespiratory fitness and lose weight. She is 38 years of age, is obese, has type 2 diabetes, and has been approved to do moderate-intensity activity by her healthcare provider. Even though she does a lot of walking and lifting in her work as a nurse's aide, her doctor has recommended that she set her exercise intensity range to begin at a heart rate at the low end of the currently recommended moderate intensity, or 50% to 70% of estimated maximal heart rate.

Let's calculate Judy's maximal heart rate values:

- Maximal heart rate: 220 − age = 220 − 38 = 182 beats per minute (bpm)
- Lower end of intensity range: 50% of 182 bpm = 0.50 × 182 bpm = 91 bpm
- Higher end of intensity range: 70% of 182 bpm = 0.70 × 182 bpm = 127 bpm

Because Judy is a trained nurse's aide, she is skilled at measuring a heart rate, or pulse. To measure your own pulse, take the following steps:

- Place your second (index) and third (middle) fingers on the inside of your wrist, just below the wrist crease and near the thumb. Press lightly to feel your pulse. Don't press too hard, or you will occlude the artery and be unable to feel its pulsation.
- If you can't feel your pulse at your wrist, try the carotid artery at the neck. This is located below your ear, on the side of your neck directly below your jaw. Press lightly against your neck under the jaw bone to find your pulse.
- Begin counting your pulse with the count of "zero"; then count each beat for 15 seconds.
- Multiply that value by 4 to estimate heart rate over 1 minute.
- Do not take your pulse with your thumb, as it has its own pulse, which would prevent you from getting an accurate estimate of your heart rate.

As you can see from these calculations, when Judy walks on the treadmill or rides the bicycle, her heart rate should be between 91 and 127 bpm; this will put her in her aerobic training zone and allow her to achieve cardiorespiratory fitness. It will also help her lose weight, assuming she consumes less energy than she expends each day.

Now you do the math. Sam is a recreational runner who is 70 years old and wishes to train to compete in track and field events at the National Senior Games. His doctor has approved him for competition and has advised that Sam train at 75% to 80% of his maximal heart rate. (A) Calculate Sam's maximal heart rate. (B) What is Sam's heart rate training range in bpm?

Answers are located online in the MasteringNutrition Study Area.

---

important to set realistic goals you can achieve in a short period of time—for instance, "I want to perform at least 10 minutes of physical activity each day on at least 5 days next week." Here are some tips for how you incorporate more regular physical activity into your daily life and, as a result, improve your health:

For a quick estimate of your training heart rate range, go to www.mayoclinic.com/health/target-heart-rate/SM00083.

- Walk as often and as far as possible: Park your car farther away from your dorm, a lecture hall, or shops. Walk to school or work. Go for a brisk walk between classes. Get on or off the bus one stop away from your destination. And don't be in such a rush to reach your destination—take the long way and burn a few more Calories.
- At every opportunity, take the stairs instead of the escalator or elevator.
- When working on the computer for long periods of time, take a 3- to 5-minute break every hour to stretch, walk to another room, or make a cup of tea.
- Exercise while watching television—for example by doing sit-ups, stretching, or using a treadmill or stationary bike.
- While talking on your cell phone, memorizing vocabulary terms, or practicing your choral part, don't stand still—pace!
- Turn on some music and dance!

- Get an exercise partner: join a friend for walks, hikes, cycling, skating, tennis, or a fitness class.
- Take up a group sport.
- Register for a class from the physical education department in an activity you've never tried before, maybe yoga or fencing.
- Register for a dance class, such as jazz, tap, or ballroom.
- Use the pool, rock-climbing wall, or other facilities at your campus fitness center, or join a health club, gym, or YMCA/YWCA in your community.
- Join an activity-based club, such as a skating, tennis, or hiking club.
- Play golf without using a golf cart—choose to walk and carry your clubs instead.
- Choose a physically active vacation that provides daily activities combined with exploring new surroundings.

RECAP

A sound fitness program must meet your personal fitness goals. It should be fun and include variety and consistency to help you maintain interest and achieve fitness in all components. It must also place an extra physical demand, or an overload, on your body. To achieve appropriate overload, follow the FITT principle: *Frequency* refers to the number of activity sessions per week. *Intensity* refers to how difficult the activity is to perform. *Time* refers to how long each activity session lasts. *Type* refers to the range of physical activities one can engage in. Warm-up exercises prepare the muscles for exertion by increasing blood flow and temperature. Cool-down activities help prevent injury and may help reduce muscle soreness. ■

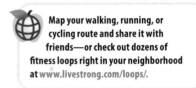

Map your walking, running, or cycling route and share it with friends—or check out dozens of fitness loops right in your neighborhood at www.livestrong.com/loops/.

What Fuels Our Activities?

In order to perform exercise, or muscular work, we must be able to generate energy. **Figure 14.4** (page 572) provides an overview of all of the metabolic pathways that result in the generation of energy to support exercise. As this figure shows, the body can use carbohydrates, fats, and even relatively small amounts of proteins to fuel physical activity.

The common currency of energy for virtually all cells in the body is adenosine triphosphate, or ATP (see Chapter 7, Figure 7.2). Remember that, when one of the three phosphates in ATP is cleaved, energy is released. The products remaining after this reaction are adenosine diphosphate (ADP) and an independent inorganic phosphate group (Pi). In a mirror image of this reaction, the body regenerates ATP by adding a phosphate group back to ADP. In this way, energy is continually provided to the cells both at rest and during exercise.

The amount of ATP stored in a muscle cell is very limited; it can keep the muscle active for only about 1 to 3 seconds. Thus, we need to generate ATP from other sources to fuel activities for longer periods of time. Fortunately, we are able to generate ATP from the breakdown of carbohydrate, fat, and protein, providing the cells with a variety of sources from which to receive energy. The primary energy systems that provide energy for physical activities are the adenosine triphosphate–creatine phosphate (ATP–CP) energy system and the anaerobic and aerobic breakdown of carbohydrates. Our bodies also generate energy from the breakdown of fats. As you will see, the type, intensity, and duration of the activities performed determine the amount of ATP needed and therefore the energy system that is used.

The ATP–CP Energy System Uses Creatine Phosphate to Regenerate ATP

As previously mentioned, muscle cells store only enough ATP to maintain activity for 1 to 3 seconds. When more energy is needed, a high-energy compound called **creatine phosphate (CP)** (also called phosphocreatine, or PCr) can be broken down to support the regeneration of ATP (**Figure 14.5**, page 572). Because this reaction can occur in the absence of oxygen, it is referred to as an anaerobic reaction (meaning "without oxygen").

creatine phosphate (CP) A high-energy compound that can be broken down for energy and used to regenerate ATP.

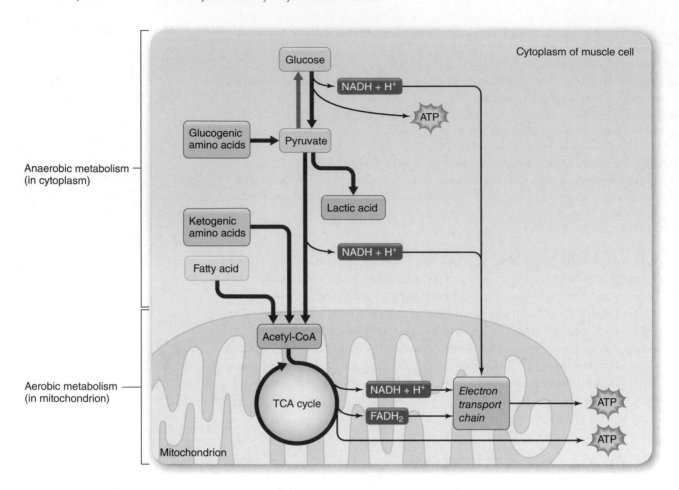

FIGURE 14.4 An overview of the metabolic pathways that result in ATP production during exercise. Carbohydrate, in the form of glucose, and proteins, in the form of amino acids, can be metabolized via anaerobic and aerobic pathways, whereas fatty acids are predominantly metabolized via aerobic pathways.

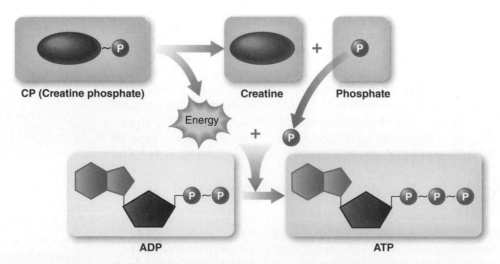

FIGURE 14.5 When the compound creatine phosphate (CP) is broken down into a molecule of creatine and an independent phosphate molecule, energy is released. This energy, along with the independent phosphate molecule, can then be used to regenerate ATP.

Muscle tissue contains about four to six times as much CP as ATP, but there is still not enough CP available to fuel long-term activity. CP is used the most during very intense, short bouts of activity, such as lifting, jumping, and sprinting (**Figure 14.6**). Together, the stores of ATP and CP can only support a *maximal* physical effort for about 3 to 15 seconds. The body must rely on other energy sources, such as carbohydrate and fat, to support activities of longer duration.

The Breakdown of Carbohydrates Provides Energy for Both Brief and Long-Term Exercise

During activities lasting about 30 seconds to 3 minutes, the body needs an energy source that can be used quickly to produce ATP. The breakdown of carbohydrates, specifically glucose, provides this quick energy through glycolysis. The most common source of glucose during exercise comes from glycogen stored in the muscles and glucose found in the blood. For every glucose molecule that goes through glycolysis, two ATP molecules are produced (see Chapter 7, Figure 7.7). The primary end product of glycolysis is pyruvate, which is converted to lactic acid (lactate) when oxygen availability is limited in the cell.

For years it was assumed that lactic acid was a useless, even potentially toxic, by-product of high-intensity exercise. We now know that lactic acid is an important intermediate of glucose breakdown and that it plays a critical role in supplying fuel for working muscles, the heart, and resting tissues. But does lactic acid buildup cause muscle fatigue and soreness? See the **Nutrition Myth or Fact?** box (page 574) for the answer. Any excess lactic acid that is not used by the muscles is transported in the blood back to the liver, where it is converted back into glucose via the Cori cycle (**Figure 14.7**, page 574). The glucose produced in the liver via the Cori cycle can recirculate to the muscles and provide energy as needed.

The major advantage of glycolysis is that it is the fastest way to generate ATP for exercise, other than the ATP–CP system. However, this high rate of ATP production can be sustained only for a brief period of time, generally less than 3 minutes. To perform exercise that lasts longer than 3 minutes, the body relies on the aerobic energy system.

In the aerobic energy system, pyruvate goes through the additional metabolic pathways of the TCA cycle and the electron transport chain in the presence of oxygen (see Chapter 7, Figure 7.12). Although this process is slower than glycolysis occurring under anaerobic conditions, the breakdown of one glucose molecule going through aerobic metabolism yields thirty-six to thirty-eight ATP molecules for energy, whereas the anaerobic process yields only two ATP molecules. Thus, this aerobic process supplies eighteen times more energy! Another advantage of the aerobic process is that it does not result in the significant production of acids and other compounds that contribute to muscle fatigue, which means that a low-intensity activity can be performed for hours. Aerobic metabolism of glucose is the primary source of fuel for our muscles during activities lasting from 3 minutes to 4 hours.

The body can store only a limited amount of glycogen. An average, well-nourished man who weighs about 154 lb (70 kg) can store about 200 to 500 g of muscle glycogen, which is equal to 800 to 2,000 kcal of energy. Although trained athletes can store more muscle glycogen than the average person, even their bodies do not have enough stored glycogen to provide an unlimited energy supply for long-term activities.

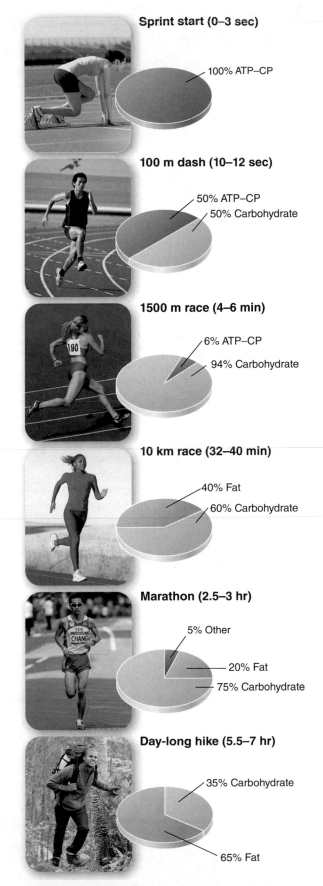

Sprint start (0–3 sec)
100% ATP–CP

100 m dash (10–12 sec)
50% ATP–CP
50% Carbohydrate

1500 m race (4–6 min)
6% ATP–CP
94% Carbohydrate

10 km race (32–40 min)
40% Fat
60% Carbohydrate

Marathon (2.5–3 hr)
5% Other
20% Fat
75% Carbohydrate

Day-long hike (5.5–7 hr)
35% Carbohydrate
65% Fat

FIGURE 14.6 The relative contributions of ATP–CP, carbohydrate, and fat to activities of various durations and intensities.

Nutrition
Myth OR **Fact?**

Does Lactic Acid Cause Muscle Fatigue and Soreness?

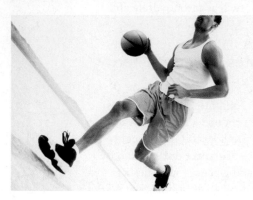

Theo and his teammates won their basketball game last night, but just barely. With two of the players sick, Theo got more court time than usual, and when he got back to the dorm, he could hardly get his legs to carry him up the stairs. This morning, Theo's muscles ache all over, and he wonders if a buildup of lactic acid is to blame.

Lactic acid is a by-product of glycolysis. For many years, both scientists and athletes believed that lactic acid causes muscle fatigue and soreness. Does recent scientific evidence support this belief?

The exact causes of muscle fatigue are not known, and there appear to be many contributing factors. Recent evidence suggests that fatigue may be due not only to the accumulation of many acids and other metabolic by-products, such as inorganic phosphate,[1] but also to the depletion of creatine phosphate and changes in calcium in the cells that affect muscle contraction. Depletion of muscle glycogen, liver glycogen, and blood glucose, as well as psychological factors, can all contribute to fatigue.[2] Thus, it appears that lactic acid only contributes to fatigue and does not cause it independently.

So what factors cause muscle soreness? As with fatigue, there are probably many factors. It is hypothesized that soreness usually results from microscopic tears in the muscle fibers as a result of strenuous exercise. This damage triggers an inflammatory reaction, which causes an influx of fluid and various chemicals to the damaged tissue area. These substances work to remove damaged tissue and initiate tissue repair, but they may also stimulate pain. However, it appears highly unlikely that lactic acid is an independent cause of muscle soreness.

Recent studies indicate that lactic acid is produced even under aerobic conditions! This means it is produced at rest as well as during exercise at any intensity. The reasons for this constant production of lactic acid are still being studied. What we do know is that lactic acid is an important fuel for resting tissues, for working cardiac and skeletal muscles, and even for the brain both at rest and during exercise.[3,4] We also know that endurance training improves the muscle's ability to use lactic acid for energy. Thus, contrary to being a waste product of glucose metabolism, lactic acid is actually an important energy source for muscle cells during rest and exercise.

References

1. Westerblad, H., D. G. Allen, and J. Lännergren. 2002. Muscle fatigue: lactic acid or inorganic phosphate the major cause? *News Physiol. Sci.* 17(1):17–21.
2. Brooks, G., T. Fahey, and K. Baldwin. 2005. *Exercise Physiology: Human Bioenergetics and Its Applications*. New York: McGraw-Hill.
3. Brooks, G. A. 2009. Cell–cell and intracellular lactate shuttles. *J. Physiol.* 587(23):5591–5600.
4. Van Hall, G., M. Stromstad, P. Rasmussen, O. Jans, M. Zaar, C. Gam, B. Quistorff, N. H. Secher, and H. B. Nielsen. 2009. Blood lactate is an important energy source for the human brain. *J. Cerebral Blood Flow & Metab.* 29(6):1121–1129.

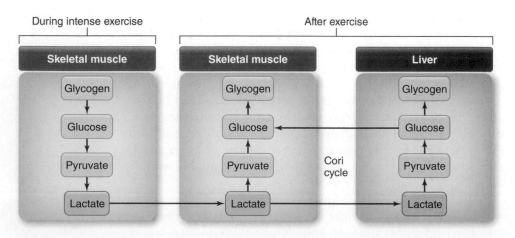

FIGURE 14.7 The Cori cycle is the metabolic pathway by which excess lactic acid can be converted into glucose in the liver.

Thus, we also need a fuel source that is abundant and can be broken down under aerobic conditions, so that it can support activities of lower intensity and longer duration. This fuel source is fat.

Aerobic Breakdown of Fats Supports Exercise of Low Intensity and Long Duration

When we refer to fat as a fuel source, we mean stored triglycerides. Their fatty acid chains provide much of the energy needed to support long-term activity. The longer the fatty acid, the more ATP that can be generated from its breakdown. For instance, palmitic acid is a fatty acid with 16 carbons. If palmitic acid is broken down completely, it yields 129 ATP molecules! Obviously, far more energy is produced from this 1 fatty acid molecule than from the aerobic breakdown of a glucose molecule.

There are two major advantages of using fat as a fuel. First, fat is an abundant energy source, even in lean people. For example, a man who weighs 154 lb (70 kg) who has a body fat level of 10% has approximately 15 lb of body fat, which is equivalent to more than 50,000 kcal of energy! This is significantly more energy than can be provided by his stored muscle glycogen (800 to 2,000 kcal). Second, fat provides 9 kcal of energy per gram, more than twice as much energy per gram as carbohydrate. The primary disadvantage of using fat as a fuel is that the breakdown process is relatively slow; thus, fat is used predominantly as a fuel source during activities of lower intensity and longer duration. Fat is also our primary energy source during rest, sitting, and standing in place.

What specific activities are fueled by fat? Walking long distances uses fat stores, as does hiking, long-distance cycling, and other low- to moderate-intensity forms of exercise. Fat is also an important fuel source during endurance events such as marathons (26.2 miles) and ultra-marathon races (49.9 miles). Endurance exercise training improves our ability to use fat for energy, which may be one reason that people who exercise regularly tend to have lower body fat levels than people who do not exercise.

It is important to remember that we are almost always using some combination of carbohydrate and fat for energy. At rest, very little carbohydrate is used, and the body relies mostly on fat. During maximal exercise (at 100% effort), the body uses mostly carbohydrate and very little fat. However, most activities done each day involve some use of both fuels (**Figure 14.8**).

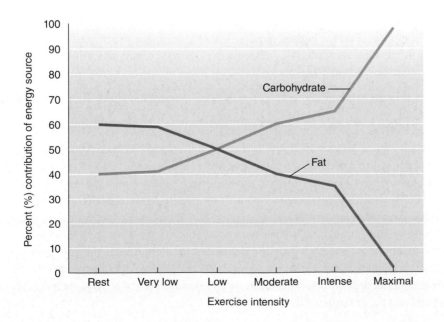

FIGURE 14.8 For most daily activities, including exercise, we use a mixture of carbohydrate and fat for energy. At lower exercise intensities, we rely more on fat as a fuel source. As exercise intensity increases, we rely more on carbohydrate for energy. (*Source*: Data adapted from Brooks, G. A., and J. Mercier. 1994. Balance of carbohydrate and lipid utilization during exercise: the "crossover" concept. *J. Appl. Physiol.* 76[6]:2253–2261.)

If you want to decrease body fat, is it better to do low-intensity exercise or moderate- and high-intensity exercises? The answer to this question depends on how long you are able to engage in an activity. Even though fat is the primary fuel source during low-intensity activities, such as sitting and standing, to decrease body fat you would obviously want to do activities of higher intensity to expend additional energy and decrease body fat stores. If you have a low fitness level and can walk for 20 minutes but can jog for only 2 minutes, then the overall amount of fat used and energy expended for walking is higher than for jogging, and walking is the better choice to decrease body fat in this case. Recent evidence suggests that engaging in high-intensity interval training (HIT) is a time-efficient strategy to optimize aerobic fitness and the use of fat as a fuel to support exercise.[13] Beneficial changes have been observed with only about 15 minutes of very intense exercise; however the potential of applying this type of training to people who are highly unfit or with disease is not known.

When it comes to eating properly to support regular physical activity or exercise training, the nutrient to focus on is carbohydrate. This is because most people store more than enough fat to support exercise, whereas our storage of carbohydrate is limited. It is especially important that adequate stores of glycogen are maintained for moderate to intense exercise. Dietary recommendations for fat, carbohydrate, and protein are reviewed shortly.

Amino Acids Are Not Major Sources of Fuel During Exercise

Proteins—more specifically, amino acids—are not major energy sources during exercise. Although they can be used directly for energy if necessary, they are more often used to make glucose to maintain blood glucose levels during exercise. The carbon skeletons of amino acids can be converted into pyruvate or acetyl-CoA, or they can feed directly into the TCA cycle to provide energy during exercise if necessary. (See Chapter 7, Figure 7.19.) Amino acids also help build and repair tissues after exercise. Depending on the intensity and duration of the activity, amino acids may contribute about 3% to 6% of the energy needed.[14]

Given this, why is it that so many active people are concerned about their protein intakes? As you've learned (in Chapter 6), muscles are not stimulated to grow by exclusively consuming extra dietary protein. Only appropriate physical training combined with an adequate intake of dietary protein can stimulate muscles to grow and strengthen. Thus, while adequate dietary protein is needed to support activity and recovery, consuming very high amounts does not necessarily provide an added benefit. The protein needs of athletes are somewhat higher than the needs of non-athletes, but most people eat more than enough protein to support even the highest requirements for competitive athletes! Thus, there is generally no need for recreationally active people or even competitive athletes to consume protein or amino acid supplements.

RECAP

The amount of ATP stored in a muscle cell is limited and can keep a muscle active for only about 1 to 3 seconds. For intense activities lasting about 3 to 15 seconds, creatine phosphate can be broken down to provide energy and support the regeneration of ATP. To support activities that last from 30 seconds to 2 minutes, energy is produced from glycolysis. Fatty acids can be broken down aerobically to support activities of low intensity and longer duration. The two major advantages of using fat as a fuel are that it is an abundant energy source and it provides more than twice the energy per gram as carbohydrate. Amino acids may contribute from 3% to 6% of the energy needed during exercise, depending on the intensity and duration of the activity. Amino acids help build and repair tissues after exercise. ■

What Kind of Diet Supports Physical Activity?

Lots of people wonder "Do my nutrient needs change if I become more physically active?" The answer to this question depends on the type, intensity, and duration of the chosen activities. It is not necessarily true that our requirement for every nutrient is greater if we are physically active.

People who are performing moderate-intensity, daily activities for health can follow the general guidelines put forth in the USDA Food Patterns. For smaller or less active people, the lower end of the range of recommendations for each food group may be appropriate. For larger or more active people, the higher end of the range is suggested. Modifications may be necessary for people who exercise vigorously every day, and particularly for athletes training for competition. **Table 14.2** provides an overview of the nutrients that can be affected by regular, vigorous exercise training. Each of these nutrients is described in more detail in the following section.

Vigorous Exercise Increases Energy Needs

Athletes generally have higher energy needs than moderately active or sedentary people. The amount of extra energy needed to support regular training is determined by the type, intensity, and duration of the activity. In addition, the energy needs of male athletes are higher than those of female athletes, because male athletes weigh more, have more muscle mass, and expend more energy during activity. This is relative, of course: a large woman

TABLE 14.2 Suggested Intakes of Nutrients to Support Vigorous Exercise

Nutrient	Functions	Suggested Intake
Energy	Supports exercise, activities of daily living, and basic body functions	Depends on body size and the type, intensity, and duration of activity. For many female athletes: 1,800 to 3,500 kcal/day For many male athletes: 2,500 to 7,500 kcal/day
Carbohydrate	Provides energy, maintains adequate muscle glycogen and blood glucose; high complex carbohydrate foods provide vitamins and minerals	45–65% of total energy intake Depending on sport and gender, should consume 6–10 g of carbohydrate per kg body weight per day
Fat	Provides energy, fat-soluble vitamins, and essential fatty acids; supports production of hormones and transport of nutrients	20–35% of total energy intake
Protein	Helps build and maintain muscle; provides building material for glucose; is an energy source during endurance exercise; aids recovery from exercise	10–35% of total energy intake Endurance athletes: 1.2–1.5 g per kg body weight Strength athletes: 1.3–1.8 g per kg body weight
Water	Maintains temperature regulation (adequate cooling); maintains blood volume and blood pressure; supports all cell functions	Consume fluid before, during, and after exercise Consume enough to maintain body weight Consume at least 8 cups (64 fl. oz) of water daily to maintain regular health and activity Athletes may need up to 10 liters (170 fl. oz) every day; more is required if exercising in a hot environment
B-vitamins	Critical for energy production from carbohydrate, fat, and protein	May need slightly more (1–2 times the RDA) for thiamin, riboflavin, and vitamin B_6
Calcium	Builds and maintains bone mass; assists with nervous system function, muscle contraction, hormone function, and transport of nutrients across cell membrane	Meet the current RDA: 14–18 yr: 1,300 mg/day 19–50 yr: 1,000 mg/day 51–70 yr: 1,000 mg/day (men); 1,200 mg/day (women) 71 yr and older: 1,200 mg/day
Iron	Primarily responsible for the transport of oxygen in blood to cells; assists with energy production	Consume at least the RDA: Males: 14–18 yr: 11 mg/day 19 and older: 8 mg/day Females: 14–18 yr: 15 mg/day 19–50 yr: 18 mg/day 51 and older: 8 mg/day

who trains 3 to 5 hours each day will probably need more energy than a small man who trains 1 hour each day. The energy needs of athletes can range from only 1,500 to 1,800 kcal per day for a small female gymnast to more than 7,500 kcal per day for a male cyclist competing in the Tour de France cross-country cycling race.

Figure 14.9 shows an example of 1 day's meals and snacks, totalling about 1,800 kcal and 4,000 kcal, with the carbohydrate content of these foods meeting more than 60% of total energy intake. As you can see, athletes who need more than 4,000 kcal per day need to

Eating for Athletes: Meeting High Energy Demands

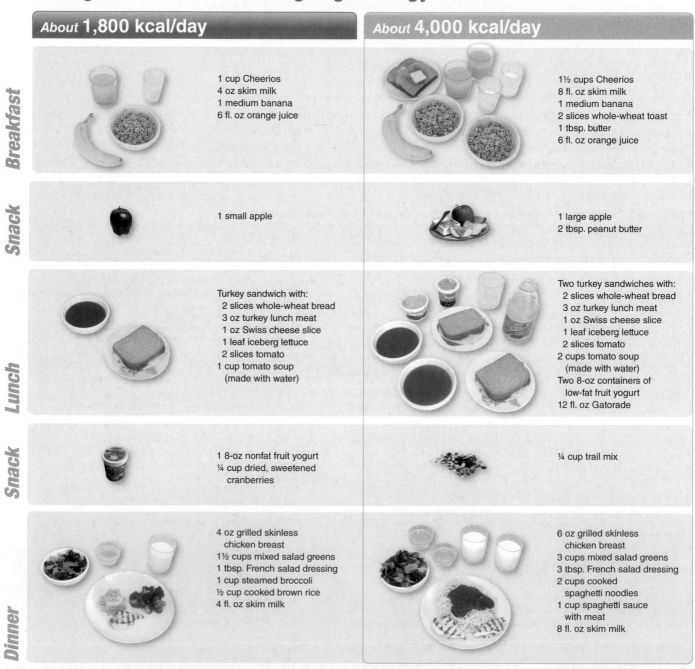

FIGURE 14.9 High-carbohydrate (approximately 60% of total energy) meals and snacks that contain approximately 1,800 kcal per day (left) and 4,000 kcal per day (right). Athletes must plan their diets carefully to meet energy demands, particularly those with very high energy needs.

consume very large quantities of food. However, the heavy demands of daily physical training, work, school, and family responsibilities often leave these athletes with little time to eat adequately. Thus, many athletes meet their energy demands by planning regular meals and snacks and **grazing** (eating small meals throughout the day) consistently. They may also take advantage of the energy-dense snack foods and meal replacements specifically designed for athletes participating in vigorous training. These steps help athletes maintain their blood glucose levels and energy stores.

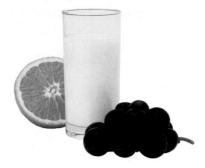

Small, healthful snacks can help you meet daily energy demands.

If an athlete is losing body weight, his or her energy intake is inadequate. Conversely, weight gain may indicate that energy intake is too high. Weight maintenance is generally recommended to maximize performance. If weight loss is warranted, food intake should be lowered no more than 200 to 500 kcal per day, and athletes should try to lose weight prior to the competitive season, if at all possible. Weight gain may be necessary for some athletes and can usually be accomplished by consuming 500 to 700 kcal per day more than needed for weight maintenance. The extra energy should come from a healthy balance of carbohydrate (45% to 65% of total energy intake), fat (20% to 35% of total energy intake), and protein (10% to 35% of total energy intake).

Many athletes are concerned about their weight. Jockeys, boxers, wrestlers, judo athletes, and others are required to "make weight"—to meet a predefined weight category. Others, such as distance runners, gymnasts, figure skaters, and dancers, are required to maintain a very lean figure for performance and aesthetic reasons. These athletes tend to eat less energy than they need to support vigorous training, which puts them at risk for inadequate intakes of all nutrients. These athletes are also at a higher risk of suffering from health consequences resulting from poor energy and nutrient intake, including eating disorders, osteoporosis, menstrual disturbances (in women), dehydration, heat and physical injuries, and even death. It is also important to understand that athletes should not adopt low-carbohydrate diets in an attempt to lose weight. As we discuss next, carbohydrates are a critical energy source for maintaining exercise performance.

Carbohydrate Needs Increase for Many Active People

Carbohydrate (in the form of glucose) is one of the primary sources of energy for a body in training. Both endurance athletes and strength athletes require adequate carbohydrate to maintain their glycogen stores and provide quick energy.

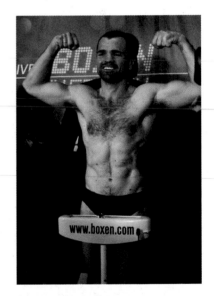

Some athletes diet to meet a predefined weight category.

How Much of an Athlete's Diet Should Be Composed of Carbohydrate?

Recall (from Chapter 4) that the AMDR for carbohydrate is 45% to 65% of total energy intake. Athletes should consume carbohydrate intakes within this recommended range. Although high-carbohydrate diets (greater than 60% of total energy intake) have been recommended in the past, this percentage value may not be appropriate for all athletes.

To illustrate the importance of carbohydrate intake for athletes, let's see what happens to Theo when he participates in a study designed to determine how carbohydrate intake affects glycogen stores during a period of heavy training. Theo was asked to go to the exercise laboratory at the university and ride a stationary bicycle for 2 hours a day for 3 consecutive days at 75% of his maximal heart rate. Before and after each ride, samples of muscle tissue were taken from his thighs to determine the amount of glycogen stored in the working muscles. Theo performed these rides under two different experimental conditions—once when he had eaten a high-carbohydrate diet (80% of total energy intake) and again when he had eaten a moderate-carbohydrate diet (40% of total energy intake). As you can see in **Figure 14.10** (page 580), Theo's muscle glycogen levels decreased dramatically after each training session. More important, his muscle glycogen levels did not recover to baseline levels over the 3 days when Theo ate the lower-carbohydrate diet. He was able to maintain his muscle glycogen levels only when he was eating the higher-carbohydrate diet. Theo also told the researchers that completing the 2-hour rides was much more difficult when he had eaten the moderate-carbohydrate diet as compared to when he was eating the diet that was higher in carbohydrate.

grazing Consistently eating small meals throughout the day; done by many athletes to meet their high energy demands.

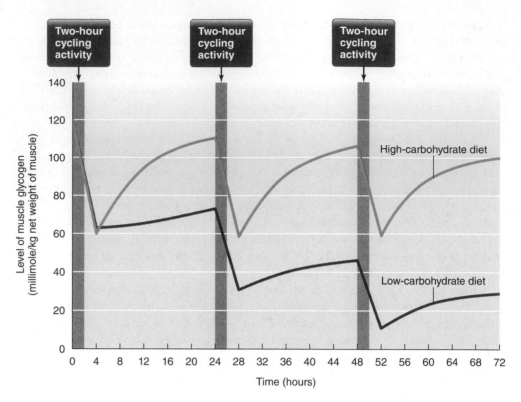

FIGURE 14.10 The effects of a low-carbohydrate diet on muscle glycogen stores. When a low-carbohydrate diet is consumed, glycogen stores cannot be restored during a period of regular, vigorous training. (*Source:* Data adapted from Costill, D. L., and J. M. Miller. 1980. Nutrition for endurance sport: CHO and fluid balance. *Int. J. Sports Med.* 1:2–14. Copyright © 1980 Georg Thieme Verlag. Used with permission.)

When Should Carbohydrates Be Consumed?

It is important for athletes not only to consume enough carbohydrate to maintain glycogen stores but also to time their intake optimally. The body stores glycogen very rapidly during the first 24 hours of recovery from exercise, with the highest storage rates occurring during the first few hours.[15] Higher carbohydrate intakes during the first 24 hours of recovery from exercise are associated with higher amounts of glucose being stored as muscle glycogen. It is recommended that athletes consume a daily carbohydrate intake of approximately 6 to 10 g of carbohydrate per kg body weight to optimize muscle glycogen stores. However, the need may be much greater in athletes who are training heavily daily, as they have less time to recover and require more carbohydrate to support both training and storage needs.

If an athlete has to perform or participate in training bouts that are scheduled less than 8 hours apart, then he or she should try to consume enough carbohydrate in the few hours after training to allow for ample glycogen storage. However, with a longer recovery time (generally 12 hours or more), the athlete can eat when he or she chooses, and glycogen levels should be restored as long as the total carbohydrate eaten is sufficient.

Interestingly, studies have shown that muscle glycogen can be restored to adequate levels in the muscle whether the food is eaten in small, multiple snacks or in larger meals,[15] although some studies show enhanced muscle glycogen storage during the first 4 to 6 hours of recovery when athletes are fed large amounts of carbohydrate every 15 to 30 minutes.[16,17] There is also evidence that consuming high glycemic index foods during the immediate postrecovery period results in higher glycogen storage than is achieved as a result of eating low glycemic index foods. This may be due to a greater malabsorption of the

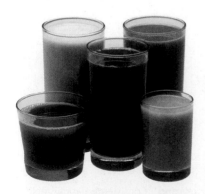

Fruit and vegetable juices can be a good source of carbohydrates.

carbohydrates in low glycemic index foods, as these foods contain more indigestible forms of carbohydrate.[15]

What Food Sources of Carbohydrates Are Good for Athletes?

What are good carbohydrate sources to support vigorous training? In general, fiber-rich, less processed carbohydrate foods, such as whole grains and cereals, fruits, vegetables, and juices, are excellent sources that also supply fiber, vitamins, and minerals. Guidelines recommend that intake of simple sugars be less than 10% of total energy intake, but some athletes who need very large energy intakes to support training may need to consume more. In addition, as previously mentioned, glycogen storage can be enhanced by consuming foods with a high glycemic index immediately postrecovery. Thus, there are advantages to consuming a wide variety of carbohydrate sources.

As a result of time constraints, many athletes have difficulties consuming enough food to meet carbohydrate demands. Sports drinks and energy bars have been designed to help athletes increase their carbohydrate intake. **Table 14.3** identifies some energy bars and other simple, inexpensive snacks and meals that provide 50 to 100 g of carbohydrate.

When Does Carbohydrate Loading Make Sense?

As you know, carbohydrate is a critical energy source to support exercise —particularly endurance-type activities—yet we have a limited capacity to store it. So it's not surprising that discovering ways to maximize carbohydrate storage has been at the forefront of sports nutrition research for many years. The practice of **carbohydrate loading**, also called *glycogen loading,* involves altering both exercise duration and carbohydrate intake to maximize the amount of muscle glycogen. **Table 14.4** (page 582) provides a schedule for carbohydrate loading for an endurance athlete.

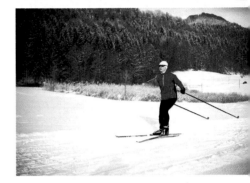

Carbohydrate loading may benefit endurance athletes, such as cross-country skiers.

TABLE 14.3 Carbohydrate and Total Energy in Various Foods

Food	Amount	Carbohydrate (g)	Energy from Carbohydrate (%)	Total Energy (kcal)
Sweetened applesauce	1 cup	50	97	207
Large apple with Saltine crackers	1 each 8 each	50	82	248
Whole-wheat bread with jelly and skim milk	1 oz slice 4 tsp 12 fl. oz	50	71	282
Spaghetti (cooked) with tomato sauce	1 cup ¼ cup	50	75	268
Brown rice (cooked) with mixed vegetables and apple juice	1 cup ½ cup 12 fl. oz	100	88	450
Grape-Nuts cereal with raisins and skim milk	½ cup ³/₈ cup 8 fl. oz	100	84	473
Clif Bar (chocolate chip)	2.4 oz	43	75	230
Meta-Rx (fudge brownie)	100 g	41	41	400
Power Bar (chocolate)	1 bar	45	75	240
PR Bar Ironman	50 g	22	44	200

Source: Data adapted from Manore, M. M., N. L. Meyer, and J. L. Thompson. 2009. *Sport Nutrition for Health and Performance.* 2nd edn. Champaign, IL: Human Kinetics.

carbohydrate loading A process that involves altering training and carbohydrate intake so that muscle glycogen storage is maximized; also known as *glycogen loading.*

TABLE 14.4 Recommended Carbohydrate Loading Guidelines for Endurance Athletes

Days Prior to Event	Exercise Duration (in minutes)	Carbohydrate Content of Diet (g per kg body weight)
6	90 (at 70% max effort)	5 (moderate)
5	40 (at 70% max effort)	5 (moderate)
4	40 (at 70% max effort)	5 (moderate)
3	20 (light training)	10 (high)
2	20 (light training)	10 (high)
1	Rest	10 (high)
Day of race	Competition	Precompetition food and fluid

Source: Data adapted from *Current Trends in Performance Nutrition*, by Marie Dunford. Copyright © 2005 by Human Kinetics, Champaign IL. Reprinted with permission.

Athletes who may benefit from carbohydrate loading are those competing in marathons, ultra-marathons, long-distance swimming, cross-country skiing, and triathlons. Athletes who compete in baseball, American football, 10-kilometer runs, walking, hiking, weight lifting, and most swimming events will not gain any performance benefits from this practice, nor will people who regularly participate in moderately intense physical activities to maintain fitness.

It is important to emphasize that, even in endurance events, carbohydrate loading does not always improve performance. There are many adverse side effects of this practice, including extreme gastrointestinal distress, particularly diarrhea. We store water along with the extra glycogen in the muscles, which leaves many athletes feeling heavy and sluggish. Athletes who want to try carbohydrate loading should experiment prior to competition to determine whether it is an acceptable and beneficial approach for them.

Nutri-Case

Theo

"Ever since I did that cycling test in the fitness lab, I've been watching my carbohydrates. Lately, I've been topping 500 grams of carbs a day. But now I'm beginning to wonder, am I getting enough protein? I'm starting to feel really wiped out, especially after games. We've won four out of the last five games, and I'm giving it everything I've got, but today I was really dragging myself through practice. I'm eating about 180 grams of protein a day, but I think I'm going to try one of those protein powders they sell at my gym. I guess I just feel like, when I'm competing, I need some added insurance."

Theo's weight averages about 200 lb. Given what you've learned about the role of the energy nutrients in vigorous physical activity, what do you think might be causing Theo to feel "wiped out"? Would you recommend that Theo try the protein supplement? What other strategies might be helpful for him to consider?

Moderate Fat Consumption Is Enough to Support Most Activities

Fat is an important energy source for both moderate physical activity and vigorous endurance training. When athletes reach a physically trained state, they are able to use more fat for energy; in other words, they become better "fat burners." This can also occur in people who are not athletes but who regularly participate in aerobic-type fitness activities. This training effect occurs for a number of reasons, including an increase in the number and activity of various enzymes involved in fat metabolism, an improved ability of the muscles to store fat, and an improved ability to extract fat from the blood for use during exercise. By using fat as a fuel, athletes can spare carbohydrate, so they can use it during prolonged, intense training or competition.

Many athletes concerned with body weight and physical appearance believe they should eat less than 15% of their total energy intake as fat, but this is inadequate for vigorous activity. Instead, a fat intake of 20% to 35% of total energy intake is generally recommended for most athletes, with less than 10% of total energy intake as saturated fat. The same recommendations are put forth for non-athletes. Fat provides not only energy but also the fat-soluble vitamins and essential fatty acids that are critical to maintaining general health. If fat consumption is too low, inadequate levels of these can eventually prove detrimental to training and performance. Athletes who have chronic disease risk factors, such as high blood lipids, high blood pressure, or unhealthful blood glucose levels, should work with their physician to adjust their intake of fat and carbohydrate according to their health risks.

Many Athletes Have Increased Protein Needs

The protein intakes suggested for active people range from 1.0 to 1.8 grams per kg body weight. At the lower end of this range are people who exercise four to five times a week for 30 minutes or less. At the upper end are athletes who train five to seven times a week for more than an hour a day. Protein intakes as high as 1.8 to 2.0 grams per kg per day may help prevent loss of lean body mass during periods when an athlete is restricting energy to promote fat loss.[18]

Most inactive people and many athletes in the United States consume more than enough protein to support their needs.[19] However, some athletes do not consume enough protein, including those with very low energy intakes, vegetarians or vegans who do not consume high-protein food sources, and young athletes who are growing and are not aware of their higher protein needs.

In 1995, Dr. Barry Sears published *The Zone: A Dietary Road Map,* a book that claims numerous benefits of a high-protein, low-carbohydrate diet for athletes.[20] Since that time, Sears has published more than a dozen spin-offs, all of which recommend the consumption of a 40–30–30 diet, or one composed of 40% carbohydrate, 30% fat, and 30% protein. Dr. Sears claims that high-carbohydrate diets impair athletic performance because of the unhealthful effects of insulin. These claims have not been supported by research, and, in fact, many of Dr. Sears' claims are not consistent with human physiology. The primary problem with the Zone Diet for athletes is that it is too low in both energy and carbohydrate to support training and performance.

High-quality protein sources include lean meats, poultry, fish, eggs, low-fat dairy products, legumes, and soy products. By following their personalized MyPlate food patterns, people of all fitness levels can consume more than enough protein without the use of supplements or specially formulated foods. Many athletes use protein shakes and other products in an attempt to build muscle mass and strength; some even use *ergogenic aids* to try to enhance performance. To learn more about ergogenic aids, and whether they are effective and safe, refer to the **Nutrition Debate** at the end of this chapter.

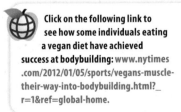

Click on the following link to see how some individuals eating a vegan diet have achieved success at bodybuilding: www.nytimes.com/2012/01/05/sports/vegans-muscle-their-way-into-bodybuilding.html?_r=1&ref=global-home.

RECAP

The type, intensity, and duration of activities a person participates in determine his or her nutrient needs. Carbohydrate needs may increase for some active people. In general, athletes should consume 45% to 65% of their total energy as carbohydrate. Carbohydrate loading involves altering physical training and the diet such that the storage of muscle glycogen is maximized. Active people use more fat than carbohydrates for energy, because they experience an increase in the number and activity of the enzymes involved in fat metabolism, and they have an improved ability to store fat and extract it from the blood for use during exercise. A dietary fat intake of 20% to 35% is recommended for athletes, with less than 10% of total energy intake as saturated fat. Although protein needs can be higher for athletes, most people in the United States already consume more than twice their daily needs for protein. ■

Water is essential for maintaining fluid balance and preventing dehydration.

Regular Exercise Increases Our Need for Fluids

In this section we review some of the basic functions of water and its role during exercise. (For a detailed discussion of fluid and electrolyte balance, see Chapter 9.)

Functions of Water

Water serves many important functions in the body. It is all of the following:

- A lubricant that bathes the tissues and cells
- A transport medium for nutrients, hormones, and waste products
- An important component of many chemical reactions, particularly those related to energy production
- A structural part of body tissues such as proteins and glycogen
- A vital component in temperature regulation; without adequate water, the body cannot cool properly through sweating, which can result in severe heat illness and even death

Cooling Mechanisms

Heat production can increase by fifteen to twenty times during heavy exercise! The primary way in which this heat is dissipated is through sweating, which is also called **evaporative cooling.** When body temperature rises, more blood (which contains water) flows to the surface of the skin. In this way, heat is carried from the core of the body to the surface of the skin. By sweating, the water (and body heat) leaves our bodies, and the air around us picks up the evaporating water from our skin, cooling our bodies.

Dehydration and Heat-Related Illnesses

Heat illnesses occur because, when we exercise in the heat, our muscles and skin constantly compete for blood flow. When there is no longer enough blood flow to simultaneously provide adequate blood to our muscles and our skin, muscle blood flow takes priority and evaporative cooling is inhibited. Exercising in heat plus humidity is especially dangerous; whereas the heat dramatically raises body temperature, the high humidity inhibits evaporative cooling—that is, the environmental air is already so saturated with water that it is unable to absorb the water in sweat. Body temperature becomes dangerously high, and heat illness is likely.

Dehydration significantly increases our risk for heat illnesses. **Figure 14.11** identifies the symptoms of dehydration during heavy exercise.

Heat illnesses include heat syncope, heat cramps, heat exhaustion, and heat stroke:

- **Heat syncope** is dizziness that occurs when people stand for too long in the heat and the blood pools in their lower extremities. It can also occur when people stop suddenly after a race or stand rapidly from a lying position.

evaporative cooling   Sweating, which is the primary way in which the body dissipates heat.

heat syncope   Dizziness that results from blood pooling in the lower extremities; often results from standing too long in hot weather, standing rapidly from a lying position, or stopping suddenly after physical exertion.

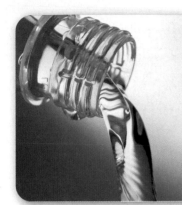

Symptoms of Dehydration During Heavy Exercise:
- Decreased exercise performance
- Increased level in perceived exertion
- Dark yellow or brown urine color
- Increased heart rate at a given exercise intensity
- Decreased appetite
- Decreased ability to concentrate
- Decreased urine output
- Fatigue and weakness
- Headache and dizziness

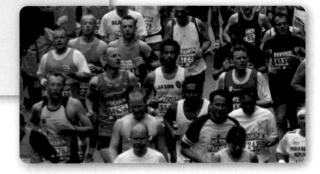

FIGURE 14.11 Symptoms of dehydration during heavy exercise.

- **Heat cramps** are muscle spasms that occur during exercise or several hours after strenuous exercise or manual labor. They are most commonly felt in the legs, arms, or abdomen after a person cools down. They occur when sweat losses and fluid intakes are high, urine volume is low, and sodium intake is inadequate to replace these losses.
- **Heat exhaustion** and **heat stroke** occur on a continuum, with unchecked heat exhaustion leading to heat stroke. Early signs of heat exhaustion include excessive sweating, cold and clammy skin, rapid but weak pulse, weakness, nausea, dizziness, headache, and difficulty concentrating. As this condition progresses, consciousness becomes impaired. Signs that a person is progressing to heat stroke are hot, dry skin; rapid and strong pulse; vomiting; diarrhea; a body temperature greater than or equal to 104°F; hallucinations; and coma. Prompt medical care is essential to save the person's life.

Guidelines for Proper Fluid Replacement

How can we prevent dehydration and heat illnesses? Obviously, adequate fluid intake is critical before, during, and after exercise. Unfortunately, our thirst mechanism cannot be relied upon to signal when we need to drink. If we rely on our feelings of thirst, we will not consume enough fluid to support exercise.

General fluid replacement recommendations are based on maintaining body weight. Athletes who are training and competing in hot environments should weigh themselves before and after the training session or event and should regain the weight lost over the subsequent 24-hour period. They should avoid losing more than 2% to 3% of body weight during exercise, as performance can be impaired with fluid losses as small as 1% of body weight.

Table 14.5 (page 586) reviews guidelines for proper fluid replacement. For activities lasting less than 1 hour, plain water is generally adequate to replace fluid losses. However, for training and competition lasting longer than 1 hour in any weather, sports beverages containing carbohydrates and electrolytes are recommended. These beverages are also recommended for people who will not drink enough water because they don't like the taste. If drinking these beverages will guarantee adequate hydration, they are appropriate to use. (For more specific information about sports beverages, see Chapter 9, pages 384–385.)

Inadequate Intakes of Some Vitamins and Minerals Can Diminish Health and Performance

When people train vigorously for athletic events, their requirements for certain vitamins and minerals may be altered. Many highly active people do not eat enough food or a variety

heat cramps Muscle spasms that occur several hours after strenuous exercise; most often occur when sweat losses and fluid intakes are high, urine volume is low, and sodium intake is inadequate.

heat exhaustion A heat illness characterized by excessive sweating, weakness, nausea, dizziness, headache, and difficulty concentrating. Unchecked, heat exhaustion can lead to heat stroke.

heat stroke A potentially fatal heat illness characterized by hot, dry skin; rapid heart rate; vomiting; diarrhea; elevated body temperature; hallucinations; and coma.

TABLE 14.5 Guidelines for Fluid Replacement

Activity Level	Environment	Fluid Requirements (liters per day)
Sedentary	Cool	2–3
Active	Cool	3–6
Sedentary	Warm	3–5
Active	Warm	5–10

Before Exercise or Competition

- Drink adequate fluids during the 24 hours before event; should be able to maintain body weight.
- Slowly drink about 0.17 to 0.24 fl. oz per kg body weight of water or a sports drink at least 4 hours prior to exercise or event to allow time for excretion of excess fluid prior to event.
- Slowly drink another 0.10 to 0.17 fl. oz per kg body weight about 2 hours before the event.
- Consuming beverages with sodium and/or small amounts of salted snacks at a meal will help stimulate thirst and retain fluids consumed.

During Exercise or Competition

- Drink early and regularly throughout the event to sufficiently replace all water lost through sweating.
- Amount and rate of fluid replacement depend on individual sweating rate, exercise duration, weather conditions, and opportunities to drink.
- Fluids should be cooler than the environmental temperature and flavored to enhance taste and promote fluid replacement.

During Exercise or Competition That Lasts More Than 1 Hour

- Fluid replacement beverage should contain 5–10% carbohydrate to maintain blood glucose levels; sodium and other electrolytes should be included in the beverage in amounts of 0.5–0.7 g of sodium per liter of water to replace the sodium lost by sweating.

Following Exercise or Competition

- Consume about 3 cups of fluid for each pound of body weight lost.
- Fluids after exercise should contain water to restore hydration status, carbohydrates to replenish glycogen stores, and electrolytes (for example, sodium and potassium) to speed rehydration.
- Consume enough fluid to permit regular urination and to ensure the urine color is very light or light yellow in color; drinking about 125–150% of fluid loss is usually sufficient to ensure complete rehydration.

In General

- Products that contain fructose should be limited, as these may cause gastrointestinal distress.
- Caffeine and alcohol should be avoided, as these products increase urine output and reduce fluid retention.
- Carbonated beverages should be avoided, as they reduce the desire for fluid intake due to stomach fullness.

Sources: Data adapted from Murray, R. 1997. Drink more! Advice from a world class expert. *ACSM's Health and Fitness Journal* 1:19–23; American College of Sports Medicine Position Stand. 2007. Exercise and fluid replacement. *Med. Sci. Sports Exerc.* 39(2):377–390; and Casa, D. J., L. E. Armstrong, S. K. Hillman, S. J. Montain, R. V. Reiff, B. S. E. Rich, W. O. Roberts, and J. A. Stone. 2000. National Athletic Trainers' Association position statement: fluid replacement for athletes. *J. Athlet. Train.* 35:212–224.

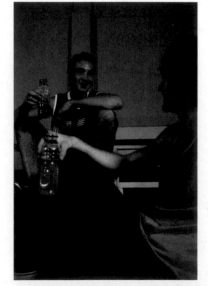

Drinking sports beverages during training or competition lasting more than 1 hour replaces fluid, carbohydrates, and electrolytes.

of foods that allows them to consume enough of these nutrients, yet it is imperative that active people do their very best to eat an adequate, varied, and balanced diet to try to meet their increased needs.

B-Vitamins

The B-vitamins are directly involved in energy metabolism (see Chapter 8 for full treatment of the nutrients involved in energy metabolism). There is reliable evidence that—as a population—active people may require slightly more thiamin, riboflavin, and vitamin B_6 than the current RDA because of increased production of energy and inadequate dietary intake in some active people.[19] However, these increased needs are easily met by consuming adequate energy and plenty of fiber-rich carbohydrates. Active people at risk for poor B-vitamin status are those who consume inadequate energy or who consume mostly refined-carbohydrate foods, such as soda pop and sugary snacks. Vegan athletes and active individuals may be at risk for inadequate intake of vitamin B_{12}; food sources enriched with this nutrient include soy and cereal products.

Calcium

Calcium supports proper muscle contraction and ensures bone health. Calcium intakes are inadequate for most women in the United States, including both sedentary and active women. This is most likely due to a failure to consume foods that are high in calcium, particularly dairy products. Although vigorous training does not appear to directly increase our need for calcium, we need to consume enough calcium to support bone health. If we do not, stress fractures and severe loss of bone can result.

Some female athletes suffer from a syndrome known as the *female athlete triad* (see Chapter 13.5, page 557). In the female athlete triad, nutritional inadequacies cause irregularities in the menstrual cycle and hormonal disturbances that can lead to a significant loss of bone mass. Thus, for female athletes, consuming the recommended amounts of calcium is critical. For female athletes who are physically small and consume lower energy intakes, calcium supplementation may be needed to meet current recommendations.

Iron

Iron, a part of the hemoglobin molecule, is critical for the transport of oxygen in the blood to the cells and working muscles. Iron is also involved in energy production. Active individuals lose more iron in their sweat, feces, and urine than do inactive people, and endurance runners lose iron when their red blood cells break down in their feet as a result of the impact of running. Female athletes and non-athletes lose more iron than male athletes because of menstrual blood losses, and females in general tend to eat less iron in their diets. Vegetarian athletes and active people may also consume less iron. Thus, many athletes and active people are at higher risk for iron deficiency. Depending on its severity, poor iron status can impair athletic performance and the ability to maintain regular physical activity.

A phenomenon known as *sports anemia* was identified in the 1960s. Sports anemia is not true anemia but a transient decrease in iron stores that occurs at the start of an exercise program for some people, as well as in some athletes who increase their training intensity. Exercise training increases the amount of water in the blood (called *plasma volume*); however, the amount of hemoglobin does not increase until later into the training period. Thus, the iron content in the blood appears to be low but instead is falsely depressed due to increases in plasma volume. Sports anemia, since it is not true anemia, does not affect performance.

In general, it appears that physically active females are at relatively high risk of suffering from the first stage of iron depletion, in which iron stores are low.[21] Because of this, it is suggested that blood tests of iron stores and monitoring of dietary iron intakes be part of routine healthcare for active people.[21] In some cases, iron needs cannot be met through the diet and supplementation is necessary. Iron supplementation should be done with a physician's approval and proper medical supervision.

RECAP

Regular exercise increases fluid needs. Fluid is critical to cool internal body temperature and prevent heat illnesses. Dehydration is a serious threat during exercise in extreme heat and high humidity. Heat illnesses include heat syncope, heat cramps, heat exhaustion, and heat stroke. Active people may need more thiamin, riboflavin, and vitamin B_6 than inactive people. Exercise itself does not increase calcium needs, but most women, including active women, do not consume enough calcium. Some female athletes suffer from the female athlete triad, a condition that involves the interaction of low energy availability, osteoporosis, and amenorrhea. Many active individuals require more iron, particularly female athletes and vegetarian athletes. ■

Chapter Review

TEST YOURSELF | *ANSWERS*

1. **T** Almost 50% of Americans do not get enough physical activity, and 25% report doing no leisure-time physical activity at all.

2. **F** Walking, water aerobics, heavy gardening, and other forms of moderate physical activity do yield significant health benefits if you engage in these activities for approximately 30 minutes a day most days of the week.

3. **F** Carbohydrate loading may help improve performance for endurance events, such as marathons and triathlons, but does not improve performance in nonendurance types of athletic events, such as a 1,500-meter run.

4. **F** Our muscles are not stimulated to grow when we eat extra protein, whether as food or supplements. Weight-bearing exercise appropriately stresses the body and produces increased muscle mass and strength.

5. **F** Unfortunately, our thirst mechanism cannot be relied upon to signal when we need to drink. If we rely solely on our feelings of thirst, we will not consume enough fluid to support exercise.

Summary

- Physical activity is any movement produced by muscles that increases energy expenditure.

- Leisure-time physical activity is any activity not related to a person's occupation and includes competitive sports and recreational activities. Exercise is a subcategory of leisure-time physical activity and is purposeful, planned, and structured.

- Physical fitness has many components and is defined as the ability to carry out daily tasks with vigor and alertness, without undue fatigue, and with ample energy to enjoy leisure-time pursuits and meet unforeseen emergencies.

- Physical activity provides a multitude of health benefits, including reducing our risks for heart disease, stroke, high blood pressure, obesity, type 2 diabetes, and osteoporosis. Despite these benefits, most Americans are inactive.

- The components of fitness include cardiorespiratory fitness, musculoskeletal fitness (which includes muscular strength and muscular endurance), flexibility, and body composition. Physical fitness is specific to each one of these components.

- A sound fitness program is one that meets your personal goals; is varied, consistent, and enjoyable; appropriately overloads the body; and includes a warm-up and a cool-down period.

- To achieve the appropriate overload for fitness, the FITT principle should be followed. *Frequency* refers to the number of activity sessions per week. *Intensity* refers to how difficult the activity is to perform. *Time* refers to how long each activity session lasts. *Type* refers to the range of physical activities a person can engage in to promote health and physical fitness.

- Warm-up exercises prepare the muscles for exertion by increasing blood flow and temperature. Cool-down activities assist in the prevention of injury and may help reduce muscle soreness.

- The amount of ATP stored in a muscle cell is limited and can keep a muscle active for only about 1 to 3 seconds.

- For activities lasting about 3 to 15 seconds, creatine phosphate can be broken down in an anaerobic reaction to provide energy and support the regeneration of ATP.

- To support activities that last from 30 seconds to 2 minutes, energy is produced from glycolysis. Glycolysis produces two ATP molecules for every glucose molecule broken down. Pyruvate is the final end product of glycolysis.

- The further metabolism of pyruvate in the presence of adequate oxygen provides energy for activities that last from 3 minutes to 4 hours. During this aerobic process, each molecule of glucose can yield thirty-six to thirty-eight ATP molecules.

- Fat can be broken down aerobically to support activities of low intensity and long duration.

- Amino acids can be used to make glucose to maintain our blood glucose levels during exercise and can contribute from 3% to 6% of the energy needed during exercise. Amino acids also help build and repair tissues after exercise.

- Vigorous-intensity exercise requires extra energy, and male athletes typically need more energy than female athletes because of their higher muscle mass and larger body weight. Athletes who are concerned with making a competitive weight or with the aesthetic demands of their sport may be at risk for insufficient energy and nutrient intakes.

- It is generally recommended that athletes consume 45% to 65% of their total energy as carbohydrate.

- Carbohydrate loading involves altering physical training and the diet such that the storage of muscle glycogen is maximized in an attempt to enhance endurance performance.

- A dietary fat intake of 20% to 35% is generally recommended for athletes, with less than 10% of total energy intake as saturated fat.

- Protein needs can be higher for athletes and regularly active people, but most people in the United States already consume more than twice their daily needs for protein.

- Regular exercise increases our fluid needs to help cool our internal body temperature and prevent heat illnesses. Heat illnesses include heat syncope, heat cramps, heat exhaustion, and heat stroke. Adequate fluid intake before, during, and after exercise will help prevent heat illnesses.

- Active people may need more thiamin, riboflavin, and vitamin B_6 than inactive people. Most women, including active women, do not consume enough calcium. Many active individuals also require more iron, particularly female athletes and vegetarian athletes.

MasteringNutrition™

To further your understanding, go online and apply what you've learned to real-life case studies that will help you master the content!

Review Questions

1. For achieving and maintaining cardiorespiratory fitness, the intensity range typically recommended is
   a. 25% to 50% of your estimated maximal heart rate.
   b. 35% to 75% of your estimated maximal heart rate.
   c. 50% to 70% of your estimated maximal heart rate.
   d. 75% to 95% of your estimated maximal heart rate.

2. The amount of ATP stored in a muscle cell can keep a muscle active for about
   a. 1 to 3 seconds.
   b. 10 to 30 seconds.
   c. 1 to 3 minutes.
   d. 1 to 3 hours.

3. To support a long afternoon of gardening, the body predominantly uses which nutrient for energy?
   a. carbohydrate
   b. fat
   c. amino acids
   d. lactic acid

4. Creatine
   a. enhances performance in aerobic-type events.
   b. increases an individual's risk for bladder cancer.
   c. can increase strength gained in resistance exercise.
   d. is stored in the liver.

5. Which of the following statements about carbohydrate loading is true?
   a. It supports activities across a wide range of intensities, including baseball and marathon running.
   b. It is recommended only for athletes at risk for type 2 diabetes.
   c. It involves altering both exercise duration and carbohydrate intake to maximize the amount of muscle glycogen.
   d. It is consistently shown to improve endurance performance.

6. **True or false?** A sound fitness program overloads the body.

7. **True or false?** A dietary fat intake of 15% to 25% is generally recommended for athletes.

8. **True or false?** If heat exhaustion goes unchecked, it can lead to heat stroke.

9. **True or false?** Sports anemia is a chronic decrease in iron stores that occurs in some athletes who have been training intensely for several months to years.

10. **True or false?** FITT stands for frequency, intensity, time, and type of activity.

11. You decide to start training for your school's annual marathon. After studying this chapter, which of the following preparation strategies would you pursue, and why?
    - Use of B-vitamin supplements
    - Use of creatine supplements
    - Use of sports beverages
    - Carbohydrate loading

12. Given what you have learned about Gustavo in the Nutri-Cases in previous chapters, would you advise him to begin a planned exercise program of low to moderate intensity? Why or why not? If so, what steps should he take before starting an exercise program?

13. Marisa and Conrad are students at the same city college. Marisa walks to and from school each morning from her home seven blocks away. Conrad lives in a suburb 12 miles away and drives to school. Marisa, an early childhood education major, covers the lunch shift, 2 hours a day, at the college's day care center, cleaning up the lunchroom and supervising the children on the playground. Conrad, an accounting major, works in his department office 2 hours a day, entering data into computer spreadsheets. On weekends, Marisa and her sister walk downtown and go shopping. Conrad goes to the movies with his friends. Neither Marisa nor Conrad participates in sports or scheduled exercise sessions. Marisa has maintained a normal, healthful weight throughout the school year, but in the same period of time, Conrad has gained several pounds. Identify at least two factors that might play a role in Marisa's and Conrad's current weights.

14. Write a plan for a weekly activity/exercise routine that does the following:
    - Meets your personal fitness goals
    - Is fun for you to do
    - Includes variety and consistency
    - Uses all components of the FITT principle
    - Includes a warm-up and cool-down period

Math Review

15. Liz is a dance major. She participates in two 90-minute dance classes each day on five days a week, plus does a 60-minute strength-training workout during her lunch break twice a week. She is a vegetarian, and her current energy intake is 1,800 kcal per day. She weighs 105 lb. After referring to Table 6.2 (Chapter 6, page 238) Liz estimates her protein intake should be 1.5 g per kg body weight, and she wants to keep her fat intake relatively low at 20% of her total daily energy intake. Based on this information, calculate how many grams of protein, fat, and carbohydrate Liz needs to consume daily to support this activity program. Does Liz's carbohydrate intake fall within the AMDR, which is 45% to 65% of total energy intake?

Answers to Review Questions and Math Review can be found online in the MasteringNutrition Study Area.

Web Links

www.heart.org/HEARTORG
American Heart Association
The "Getting Healthy" part of this site has sections on health tools, exercise and fitness, healthy diet, lifestyle management, and more.

www.acsm.org
American College of Sports Medicine
Click on "Access Public Information" under the "Brochures and Fact Sheets" section for guidelines on healthy aerobic activity and calculating your exercise heart rate range, as well as under the "Newsletters" section to access the ACSM's Fit Society Page newsletter.

www.choosemyplate.gov
USDA ChooseMyPlate.gov
Visit this site to learn more about physical activity and how to find ways to incorporate more physical activity into your daily life.

www.webmd.com
WebMD
Visit this site to learn about a variety of lifestyle topics, including fitness and exercise.

www.hhs.gov
US Department of Health and Human Services
Review this site for multiple statistics on health, exercise, and weight, as well as information on supplements, wellness, and more.

www.win.niddk.nih.gov/publications/physical.htm
Weight-Control Information Network
Find out more about healthy fitness programs.

www.ods.od.nih.gov
NIH Office of Dietary Supplements
Look on this National Institutes of Health site to learn more about the health effects of specific nutritional supplements.

www.fnic.nal.usda.gov/dietary-supplements
USDA National Agricultural Library Food and Nutrition Information Center
Visit this page for links to detailed information about ergogenic aids.

References

1. Miner, D. 2011. 32nd St. Louis Senior Olympics Kick Off in Creve Coeur. *Creve Coeur Patch.* http://crevecoeur.patch.com/articles/32nd-st-louis-senior-olympics-kick-off-in-creve-coeur.

2. US Department of Health and Human Services. 1996. *Physical Activity and Health: A Report of the Surgeon General.* Atlanta: US Department of Health and Human Services, Centers for Disease Control and Prevention, National Centers for Chronic Disease Prevention and Health Promotion.

3. Caspersen, C. J., K. E. Powell, and G. M. Christensen. 1985. Physical activity, exercise, and physical fitness: definitions and distinctions for health-related research. *Public Health Rep.* 100:126–131.

4. Heyward, V. H. 2010. *Advanced Fitness Assessment and Exercise Prescription.* 6th edn. Champaign, IL: Human Kinetics.

5. National Center for Health Statistics. 2012. Health, United States, 2011: With Special Feature on Socioeconomic Status and Health. www.cdc.gov/nchs/data/hus/hus11.pdf#073.

6. Centers for Disease Control and Prevention. 2008. 1988–2007 No Leisure-Time Physical Activity Trend Chart. www.cdc.gov/nccdphp/dnpa/physical/stats/leisure_time.htm.

7. Centers for Disease Control and Prevention. 2012. Youth risk behavior surveillance—United States, 2011. *Morbid. Mortal.Weekly Rev.* 61:SS-4. www.cdc.gov/healthyyouth/physicalactivity/facts.htm.

8. Institute of Medicine, Food and Nutrition Board. 2002. *Dietary Reference Intakes for Energy, Carbohydrates, Fiber, Fat, Protein and Amino Acids (Macronutrients).* Washington, DC: National Academy of Sciences.

9. US Department of Health and Human Services. 2009. 2008 Physical Activity Guidelines for Americans. http://health.gov/paguidelines/guidelines/default.aspx#toc.

10. Ryan, R. M., C. M. Frederick, D. Lepes, N. Rubio, and K. M. Sheldon. 1997. Intrinsic motivation and exercise adherence. *Int. J. Sport Psychol.* 28:335–354.

11. Buckworth, J., R. E. Lee, G. Regan, L. K. Schneider, and C. C. DeClemente. 2007. Decomposing intrinsic and extrinsic motivation for exercise: application to stages of motivational readiness. *Psychol. Sport Exerc.* 8(4):441–461.

12. Centers for Disease Control and Prevention. 2011. Physical Activity for Everyone. Target Heart Rate and Estimated Maximum Heart Rate. www.cdc.gov/physicalactivity/everyone/measuring/heartrate.html.

13. Gibala, M. J., and S. L. McGee. 2008. Metabolic adaptations to short-term high-intensity interval training: a little pain for a lot of gain? *Exerc. Sport Sci. Rev.* 36(2):58–63.

14. American College of Sports Medicine, American Dietetic Association, and Dietitians of Canada. 2009. Nutrition and athletic performance. Joint position statement. *Med. Sci. Sports Exerc.* 41:709–731.

15. Burke, L. 2010. Nutrition for recovery after competition and training. In: Burke, L., and V. Deakin, eds. *Clinical Sports Nutrition.* 4th edn. New York: McGraw-Hill, pp. 358–392.

16. van Hall, G., S. M. Shirreffs, and J. A. L. Calbert. 2000. Muscle glycogen resynthesis during recovery from cycle exercise: no effect of additional protein ingestion. *J. Appl. Physiol.* 88:1631–1636.

17. Jentjens, R. L., L. J. C. van Loon, C. H. Mann, A. J. M. Wagenmakers, and A. E. Jeukendrup. 2001. Addition of protein and amino acids to carbohydrates does not enhance postexercise muscle glycogen synthesis. *J. Appl. Physiol.* 91:839–846.

18. Phillips, S. M., and L. J. C van Loon. 2011. Dietary protein for athletes: from requirements to optimum adaptation. *J. Sports Sci.* 29(S1):S29–S38.

19. Manore, M. M, N. L. Meyer, and J. L. Thompson. 2009. *Sports Nutrition for Health and Performance.* 2nd edn. Champaign, IL: Human Kinetics.

20. Sears, B. 1995. *The Zone: A Dietary Road Map.* New York: HarperCollins.

21. Sinclair, L. M., and P. S. Hinton. 2005. Prevalence of iron deficiency with and without anemia in recreationally active men and women. *J. Am. Diet. Assoc.* 105(6):975–978.

Are Ergogenic Aids Necessary for Active People?

Many competitive athletes and even some recreationally active people continually search for that something extra that will enhance their performance. **Ergogenic aids** are substances used to improve exercise and athletic performance. For example, nutrition supplements can be classified as ergogenic aids, as can anabolic steroids and other pharmaceuticals. Interestingly, people report using ergogenic aids not only to enhance athletic performance but also to improve their physical appearance, prevent or treat injuries and diseases, and help them cope with stress. Some people even report using them because of peer pressure!

As you have learned in this chapter, adequate nutrition is critical to athletic performance and to regular physical activity, and products such as sports bars and beverages can help athletes maintain their competitive edge. However, as we will explore shortly, many ergogenic aids are not effective, some are dangerous, and most are very expensive. For the average consumer, it is virtually impossible to track the latest research findings for these products. In addition, many have not been adequately studied, and unsubstantiated claims surrounding them are rampant. How can you become a more educated consumer?

Previously (in Chapter 1) we included a discussion of how to determine if a website is reliable and how to evaluate research and claims made by companies promoting their products, some of which include companies promoting ergogenic aids (pages 28–29). A recent review of the evidence underpinning sports performance products, which includes drinks, supplements, clothing, and footwear, found that there was inadequate information available to perform a critical appraisal of approximately half of the products.[1] In addition, when studies were conducted to assess a product's effectiveness, only 2.7% of the studies were judged to be of high quality and at low risk of bias. Thus, the authors of this review concluded that the currently available evidence is not of sufficient quality to inform the public about the benefits and risks of various sports products.

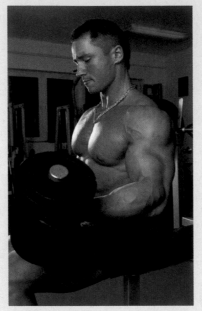

Anabolic substances are often marketed to people striving to increase muscle size, but many cause harmful side effects.

New ergogenic aids are available virtually every month. It is therefore not possible to discuss every available product in this debate. However, a brief review of a number of currently popular ergogenic aids is provided.

Anabolic Products Are Touted as Muscle and Strength Enhancers

Many ergogenic aids are said to be **anabolic,** meaning that they build muscle and increase strength. Most anabolic substances promise to increase testosterone, which is the hormone associated with male sex characteristics and that increases muscle size and strength. Although some anabolic substances are effective, they are generally associated with harmful side effects.

Anabolic Steroids

Anabolic steroids are testosterone-based drugs that have been known to be effective in increasing muscle size, strength, power, and speed. They have been used extensively by strength and power athletes; however, these products are illegal in the United States, and their use is banned by all major collegiate and professional sports organizations, in addition to both the U.S. and the International Olympic Committees. Proven long-term and irreversible effects of steroid use include infertility; early closure of the plates of the long bones, resulting in permanently shortened stature; shriveled testicles, enlarged breast tissue (that can be removed only surgically), and other signs of "feminization" in men; enlarged clitoris, facial hair growth, and other signs of "masculinization" in women; increased risk for certain forms of cancer; liver damage; unhealthful changes in blood lipids; hypertension; severe acne; hair thinning or baldness; and depression, delusions, sleep disturbances, and extreme anger (so-called roid rage).

---

ergogenic aids Substances used to improve exercise and athletic performance.

anabolic The characteristic of a substance that builds muscle and increases strength.

Androstenedione and Dehydroepiandrosterone

Androstenedione ("andro") and dehydroepiandrosterone (DHEA) are precursors of testosterone. Manufacturers of these products claim that taking them will increase testosterone levels and muscle strength. Androstenedione became very popular after baseball player Mark McGwire claimed he used it during the time he was breaking home run records. A national survey found that, in 2002, about one of every forty high school seniors had used "andro" in the past year.[2] Contrary to popular claims, recent studies have found that neither androstenedione nor DHEA increases testosterone levels, and androstenedione has been shown to increase the risk for heart disease in men aged 35 to 65 years.[3] There are no studies that support the products' claims of improving strength and increasing muscle mass.

Gamma-Hydroxybutyric Acid

Gamma-hydroxybutyric acid, or GHB, is a central nervous system depressant. It was once promoted as an alternative to anabolic steroids for building muscle. The production and sale of GHB were never approved in the United States; however, it was illegally produced and sold on the black market as a dietary supplement. For many users, GHB caused only dizziness, tremors, or vomiting, but others experienced severe side effects, including seizures, respiratory depression, sedation, and coma. Many people were hospitalized, and some died.

In 2001, the federal government placed GHB on the controlled substances list, making its manufacture, sale, and possession illegal. A form of GHB is available by prescription for the treatment of narcolepsy, a rare sleep disorder, but extra paperwork is required by the prescribing physician, and prescriptions are closely monitored. After the ban, a similar product (gamma-butyrolactone, or GBL) was marketed in its place. This product was also found to be dangerous and was removed from the market by the FDA. Recently, another replacement product called BD (also known as 1,4-butanediol) was banned by the FDA because it has caused at least seventy-one deaths, with forty more under investigation. BD is an industrial solvent and is listed on ingredient labels as tetramethylene glycol, butylene glycol, or sucol-B. Side effects include wild, aggressive behavior; nausea; incontinence; and sudden loss of consciousness.

Creatine

Creatine is a supplement that has become wildly popular with strength and power athletes. Creatine, or creatine phosphate, is found in meat and fish and stored in our muscles. As described earlier, our bodies use creatine phosphate (CP) to regenerate ATP. It is theorized that creatine supplements make more CP available to replenish ATP, which prolongs a person's ability to train and perform in short-term, explosive activities, such as weight lifting and sprinting. Between 1994 and 2012, more than 1,700 research articles related to creatine and exercise in humans were published. Creatine does not seem to enhance performance in aerobic-type events but has been shown to increase the work performed and amount of strength gained during resistance exercise and to enhance sprint performance in swimming, running, and cycling.[4]

In January 2001, the *New York Times* reported that the French government had claimed that creatine use could lead to cancer.[5] The news spread quickly across national and international news organizations and over the Internet. Subsequently, these claims were found to be false, as there are no studies in humans that suggest an increased risk for cancer with creatine use. In fact, numerous studies show an anti-cancer effect.[6,7] Although side effects such as dehydration, muscle cramps, and gastrointestinal disturbances have been reported with creatine use, there is very little information on how long-term use impacts health. Further research is needed to determine the effectiveness and safety of creatine use over prolonged periods of time.

Protein and Amino Acid Supplements

Protein and amino acid supplements have long been popular and are widely available in health food stores and on the Internet. Examples of these products include various protein powders and individual amino acids, such as glutamine and arginine. Although manufacturers claim that these products build muscle mass and enhance strength, research indicates that they do not.[8-10]

Some Products Are Said to Optimize Fuel Use During Exercise

Certain ergogenic aids are touted as increasing energy levels and improving athletic performance by optimizing the use of fat, carbohydrate, and protein. The products reviewed here are caffeine, ephedrine, carnitine, chromium, and ribose.

Caffeine

Caffeine is a stimulant that makes us feel more alert and energetic, decreasing feelings of fatigue during exercise. In addition, caffeine has been shown to increase the use of fat as a fuel during endurance exercise, which spares muscle glycogen and improves performance.[11,12] Energy drinks that contain high amounts of caffeine, such as Red Bull, have become popular with athletes and many college students. These drinks should be avoided during exercise, however, as severe dehydration can result due to the combination of fluid loss from exercise and caffeine consumption. Research also indicates that energy drinks are associated with serious side effects in children, adolescents, and young adults with conditions such as seizures, diabetes, and mood behavior disorders.[13] It should be recognized that caffeine is a controlled or restricted drug in the athletic world, and athletes can be banned from Olympic competition if their urine levels are too high. However, the amount of caffeine that is banned is quite high, and athletes would need to consume caffeine in pill form to reach this level. Side effects of caffeine use include increased blood pressure, increased heart rate, dizziness, insomnia, headache, and gastrointestinal distress.

Ephedrine is made from the herb *Ephedra sinica* (Chinese ephedra).

Ephedrine

Ephedrine, also known as ephedra, Chinese ephedra, and *ma huang*, is a strong stimulant marketed as a weight-loss supplement and energy enhancer. In reality, many products sold as Chinese ephedra (or herbal ephedra) contain ephedrine synthesized in a laboratory and other stimulants, such as caffeine. The use of ephedra does not appear to enhance performance, but supplements containing both caffeine and ephedra have been shown to prolong the amount of exercise that can be done until exhaustion is reached.[14] Ephedra is known to reduce body weight and body fat in sedentary women, but its impact on weight loss and body fat levels in athletes is unknown. Side effects of ephedra use include headaches, nausea, nervousness, anxiety, irregular heart rate, and high blood pressure; and at least seventeen deaths have been attributed to its use. It is currently illegal to sell ephedra-containing supplements in the United States.

Carnitine

Carnitine is a compound made from amino acids and is found in the membranes of mitochondria in our cells. Carnitine helps shuttle fatty acids into the mitochondria, so that they can be used for energy. It has been proposed that exercise training depletes our cells of carnitine and that supplementation should restore carnitine levels, thereby enabling us to improve our use of fat as a fuel source. Thus, carnitine is marketed not only as a performance-enhancing substance but also as a "fat burner." Research studies of carnitine supplementation do not support these claims, as neither the transport of fatty acids nor their oxidation appears to be enhanced with supplementation.[15] The use of carnitine supplements has not been associated with significant side effects.

Chromium

Chromium is a trace mineral that enhances insulin's action of increasing the transport of amino acids into the cell. It is found in whole-grain foods, cheese, nuts, mushrooms, and asparagus. It is theorized that many people are chromium deficient and that supplementation will enhance the uptake of amino acids into muscle cells, which will increase muscle growth and strength. Like carnitine, chromium is marketed as a fat burner, as it is speculated that its effect on insulin stimulates the brain to decrease food intake. Chromium supplements are available as chromium picolinate and chromium nicotinate. Early studies of chromium supplementation showed promise, but more recent, better-designed studies do not support any benefit of chromium supplementation on muscle mass, muscle strength, body fat, or exercise performance.[16]

Ribose

Ribose is a five-carbon sugar that is critical to the production of ATP. Ribose supplementation is claimed to improve athletic performance by increasing work output and by promoting a faster recovery time from vigorous training. While ribose has been shown to improve exercise tolerance in patients with heart disease, several studies have reported that ribose supplementation has no impact on athletic performance.[17–20]

CRITICAL THINKING QUESTIONS

- After reading this debate, do you think there are any ergogenic aids that you would try? If so, why?

- Under what circumstances do you believe it is acceptable to use ergogenic aids?

- Do you feel there should be more strict regulations on the promotion and sales of ergogenic aids? Why or why not?

REFERENCES

1. Heneghan, C., J. Howick, B. O'Neill, P. J. Gill, D. S. Lasserson, D. Cohen, R. Davis, A. Ward, A. Smith, G. Jones, and M. Thompson. 2012. The evidence underpinning sports performance products: a systematic assessment. *BMJ Open* 2:e001702. DOI:10.1136/bmjopen-2012-001702.

2. US Department of Health and Human Services (HHS). 2004. News release. HHS Launches Crackdown on Products Containing Andro. www.hhs.gov/news/press/2004pres/20040311.html.

3. Broeder, C. E., J. Quindry, K. Brittingham, L. Panton, J. Thomson, S. Appakondu, K. Breuel, R. Byrd, J. Douglas, C. Earnest, C. Mitchell, M. Olson, T. Roy, and C. Yarlagadda. 2000. The Andro Project: physiological and hormonal influences of androstenedione supplementation in men 35 to 65 years old participating in a high-intensity resistance training program. *Arch. Intern. Med.* 160:3093–3104.

4. Tarnopolsky, M. A. 2010. Caffeine and creatine use in sport. *Ann. Nutr. Metab.* 57(suppl 2):1–8.

5. Reuters. 2001. Creatine use could lead to cancer, French government reports. *New York Times,* January 25. www.nytimes.com.

6. Jeong, K. S., S. J. Park, C. S. Lee, T. W. Kim, S. H. Kim, S. Y. Ryu, B. H. Williams, R. L. Veech, and Y. S. Lee. 2000. Effects of cyclocreatine in rat hepatocarcinogenesis model. *Anticancer Res.* 20(3A):1627–1633.

7. Ara, G., L. M. Gravelin, R. Kaddurah-Daouk, and B. A. Teicher. 1998. Antitumor activity of creatine analogs produced by alterations in pancreatic hormones and glucose metabolism. *In Vivo* 12:223–231.

8. Manore, M. M., N. L. Meyer, and J. L. Thompson. 2009. *Sports Nutrition for Health and Performance.* 2nd edn. Champaign, IL: Human Kinetics.

9. Finn, K. J., R. Lund, and M. Rosene-Treadwell. 2003. Glutamine supplementation did not benefit athletes during short-term weight reduction. *J. Sports Sci. Med.* 2:163–168.

10. Campbell, B. I., P. M. La Bounty, and M. Roberts. 2004. The ergogenic potential of arginine. *J. Int. Soc. Sports Nutr.* 1(2):35–38.

11. Anderson, M. E., C. R. Bruce, S. F. Fraser, N. K. Stepto, R. Klein, W. G. Hopkins, and J. A. Hawley. 2000. Improved 2000-meter rowing performance in competitive oarswomen after caffeine ingestion. *Int. J. Sport Nutr. Exerc. Metab.* 10:464–475.

12. Spriet, L. L., and R. A. Howlett. 2000. Caffeine. In: Maughan, R. J., ed. *Nutrition in Sport.* Oxford: Blackwell Science, pp. 379–392.

13. Seifert, S. M., J. L. Schaechter, E. R. Hershorin, and S. E. Lipshultz. 2011. Health effects of energy drinks on children, adolescents, and young adults. *Pediatrics* 127(3):511–528.

14. Bucci, L. 2000. Selected herbals and human exercise performance. *Am. J. Clin. Nutr.* 72:624S–636S.

15. Hawley, J. A. 2002. Effect of increased fat availability on metabolism and exercise capacity. *Med. Sci. Sports Exerc.* 34(9):1485–1491.

16. Vincent, J. B. 2003. The potential value and toxicity of chromium picolinate as a nutritional supplement, weight loss agent and muscle development agent. *Sports Med.* 33(3):213–230.

17. Pliml, W., T. von Arnim, A. Stablein, H. Hofmann, H. G. Zimmer, and E. Erdmann. 1992. Effects of ribose on exercise-induced ischaemia in stable coronary artery disease. *Lancet* 340(8818):507–510.

18. Earnest, C. P., G. M. Morss, F. Wyatt, A. N. Jordan, S. Colson, T. S. Church, Y. Fitzgerald, L. Autrey, R. Jurca, and A. Lucia. 2004. Effects of a commercial herbal-based formula on exercise performance in cyclists. *Med. Sci. Sports Exerc.* 36(3):504–509.

19. Hellsten, Y., L. Skadhauge, and J. Bangsbo. 2004. Effect of ribose supplementation on resynthesis of adenine nucleotides after intense intermittent training in humans. *Am. J. Physiol. Regul. Integr. Comp. Physiol.* 286:R182–R188.

20. Kreider, R. B., C. Melton, M. Greenwood, C. Rasmussen, J. Lundberg, C. Earnest, and A. Almada. 2003. Effects of oral D-ribose supplementation on anaerobic capacity and selected metabolic markers in healthy males. *Int. J. Sport Nutr. Exerc. Metab.* 13(1):76–86.

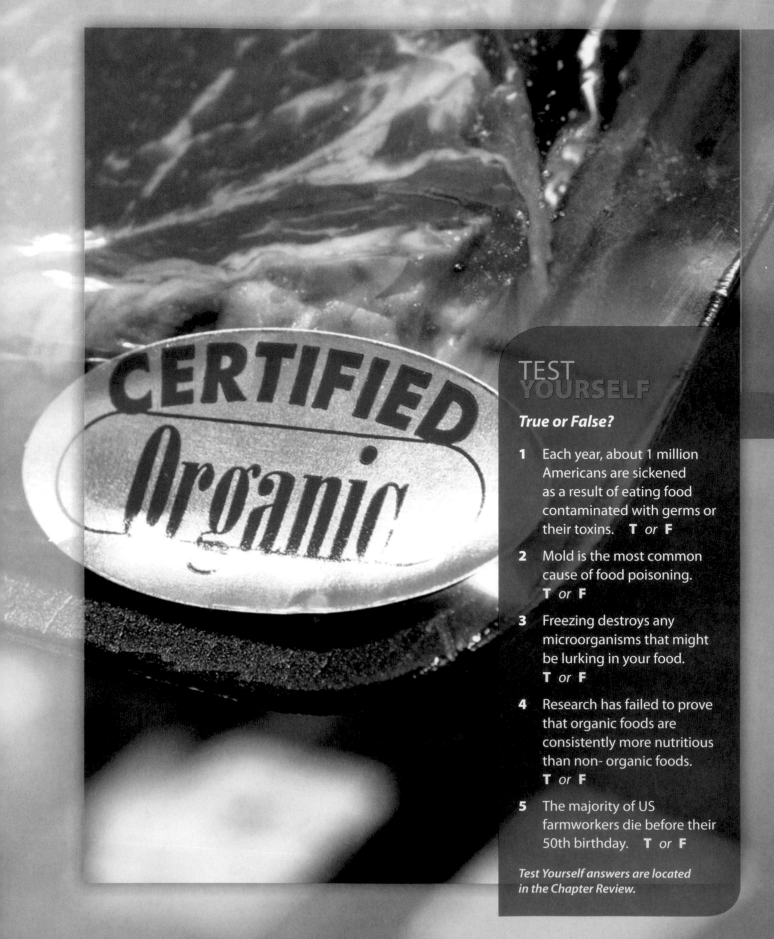

True or False?

1   Each year, about 1 million Americans are sickened as a result of eating food contaminated with germs or their toxins.   **T** *or* **F**

2   Mold is the most common cause of food poisoning. **T** *or* **F**

3   Freezing destroys any microorganisms that might be lurking in your food. **T** *or* **F**

4   Research has failed to prove that organic foods are consistently more nutritious than non- organic foods. **T** *or* **F**

5   The majority of US farmworkers die before their 50th birthday.   **T** *or* **F**

Test Yourself answers are located in the Chapter Review.

15

Consumer Issues: Food Safety, Production, and Impact on the Environment

Learning Objectives

After studying this chapter, you should be able to:

1. Describe what foodborne illness is and why it is of concern, *pp. 598–599.*

2. Identify the causes of most foodborne illness and how the body responds to contaminants, *pp. 601–607.*

3. Describe strategies for preventing foodborne illness at home, while eating out, and when traveling to other countries, *pp. 607–612.*

4. Compare and contrast the various methods manufacturers use to preserve foods, *pp. 613–614.*

5. Debate the safety of food additives, including the role of the GRAS list, *pp. 614–616.*

6. Describe the process of genetic modification and discuss the potential risks and benefits associated with genetically modified organisms, *pp. 616–617.*

7. Describe the process by which persistent organic pollutants accumulate in foods, *pp. 618–619.*

8. Identify the relative benefits and drawbacks of foods grown with and without conventional pesticides, *pp. 619–620.*

9. Describe the roles that growth hormones and anitbiotics in anmials, and chemical residues from packaging, play in food safety, *pp. 620–621.*

10. Discuss the primary tenets of the burgeoning "food movement," and the role that personal choices can play in helping to promote food equity, *pp. 622–626.*

MasteringNutrition™

Go online for chapter quizzes, pre-tests, Interactive Activities, and more!

The winter of 2012 was not a good season for produce. By mid-January, sixty-eight people had been sickened, and twenty-one hospitalized, following infection with a species of bacterium called *Salmonella enteritidis*, contracted at the same restaurant chain. The culprits were thought to be contaminated lettuce and/or tomatoes.[1] A few weeks later, twenty-nine people in eleven states became ill—seven of them requiring hospitalization—after consuming raw sprouts contaminated with a different bacterium, this time *E. coli* O26.[2] But crops are not the only source of contamination in our food supply. For example, *Salmonella* bacteria are routinely found in raw poultry and eggs, and in 2011 it showed up in ground turkey and ground beef.[1] And *E. coli* is a common resident of raw and undercooked meats: in recent years, *E. coli*–contaminated beef has caused several outbreaks of severe illness, including kidney failure and death.[2] What's worse, *Salmonella* and *E. coli* are just two of the many bacteria and other contaminants that cause foodborne illness.

How do disease-causing agents enter our food and water supplies, and how can we protect ourselves from them? What makes foods spoil, and what techniques help keep foods fresh longer? How do practices in the U.S. food industry protect consumers, and how are consumers responding to practices that put us—and our environment—at risk? We explore these and other questions in this chapter.

Why Is Foodborne Illness a Critical Concern?

Foodborne illness is a term used to encompass any symptom or disorder that arises from ingesting food or water contaminated with disease-causing (pathogenic) microscopic organisms (called microorganisms), their toxic secretions, or chemicals (such as mercury or **pesticides**). You probably refer to foodborne illness more commonly as *food poisoning*.

Foodborne Illness Affects Millions of Americans Annually

According to the Centers for Disease Control and Prevention (CDC), approximately 48 million Americans—1 out of every 6—report experiencing foodborne illness each year. Of these, 128,000 are hospitalized and 3,000 die.[3] The following people are most at risk for serious foodborne illness:

- Developing fetuses, infants, and young children, as their immune system is immature
- People who are very old or have a chronic illness, as their immune system may be compromised
- People with acquired immunodeficiency syndrome (AIDS)
- People who are receiving immune system–suppressing drugs, such as transplant recipients and cancer patients

Although the statistics may seem frightening, most experts consider our food supply safe. That's partly because not all cases of food contamination make all people sick; in fact, even virulent strains cause illness in only a small percentage of people who consume the tainted food. Moreover, modern technology has given us a wide array of techniques to preserve foods. We discuss these later in this chapter.

Finally, food safety in the United States is monitored by several government agencies. In addition to the CDC, mentioned earlier, the United States Department of Agriculture (USDA), Food and Drug Administration (FDA), and Environmental Protection Agency (EPA) monitor and regulate food production and preservation. Information about these agencies and how to access them appears in **Table 15.1**.

foodborne illness An illness transmitted by food or water contaminated by a pathogenic microorganism, its toxic secretions, or a toxic chemical.

pesticides Chemicals used either in the field or in storage to decrease destruction by predators or disease.

TABLE 15.1 Government Agencies That Regulate Food Safety

Name of Agency	Year Established	Role in Food Regulations	Website
US Department of Agriculture (USDA)	1785	Oversees safety of meat, poultry, and eggs sold across state lines; also regulates which drugs can be used to treat sick cattle and poultry	www.usda.gov
US Food and Drug Administration (FDA)	1862	Regulates food standards of food products (except meat, poultry, and eggs) and bottled water; regulates food labeling and enforces pesticide use as established by EPA	www.fda.gov
Centers for Disease Control and Prevention (CDC)	1946	Works with public health officials to promote and educate the public about health and safety; is able to track information needed in identifying foodborne illness outbreaks	www.cdc.gov
Environmental Protection Agency (EPA)	1970	Regulates use of pesticides and which crops they can be applied to; establishes standards for water quality	www.epa.gov

Food Production Is Increasingly Complex

Despite safeguards, foodborne illness has emerged as a major public health threat in recent years. One reason is that more foods are mass-produced than ever before, with a combination of ingredients from a much greater number of sources, including fields, feedlots, and processing facilities all over the world. These various sources can remain hidden not only to consumers but even to food companies using the ingredients. Contamination can occur at any point from farm to table (**Figure 15.1**, page 600), and when it does, it can be difficult to trace.

At the same time, federal oversight of food-production facilities decreased in the last decades of the 20th century. Thirty-five years ago, the FDA inspected about half of the nation's food-processing facilities annually. By 2008, the inspection rate had dropped below 5%. Not surprisingly, in 2009, the CDC warned that, after decades of steady progress, the safety of the nation's food supply was no longer improving. The same year, President Barack Obama announced the creation of the Food Safety Working Group to sponsor changes in food-safety laws. The U.S. Congress responded by crafting a new food-safety bill, the Food Safety Modernization Act, which was passed into law in January 2011. Among its provisions are the following:[4]

- New requirements for actions that food processors must take to prevent contamination
- New requirements for food importers to verify the safety of food from their suppliers
- New FDA enforcement tools, including mandatory recall authority
- A new, more rigorous inspection schedule

It's too soon to judge the effectiveness of these provisions; however, in May 2012, the CDC published data showing that in 2010 the overall rate of foodborne infections again began to decline.[5]

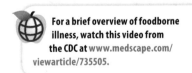

For a brief overview of foodborne illness, watch this video from the CDC at www.medscape.com/viewarticle/735505.

RECAP

Foodborne illness affects 48 million Americans a year. Contamination can occur at any point from farm to table. The Centers for Disease Control and Prevention, the Food and Drug Administration, the United States Department of Agriculture, and the Environmental Protection Agency monitor and regulate food production and preservation. The Food Safety Modernization Act of 2011 increased the oversight of food production by federal agencies and authorized the FDA to swiftly recall contaminated foods from the market. ■

FIGURE 15.1 Food is at risk for contamination at any of the five stages from farm to table, but following food-safety guidelines can reduce the risks.

Farms

Animals raised for meat can harbor harmful microorganisms, and crops can be contaminated with pollutants from irrigation, runoff from streams, microorganisms or toxins in soil, or pesticides. Contamination can also occur during animal slaughter or from harvesting, sorting, washing, packing, and/or storage of crops.

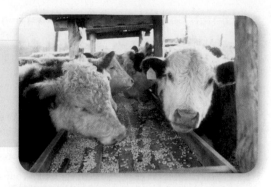

Processing

Some foods, such as produce, may go from the farm directly to the market, but most foods are processed. Processed foods may go through several steps at different facilities. At each site, people, equipment, or environments may contaminate foods. Federal safeguards, such as cleaning protocols, testing, and training, can help prevent contamination.

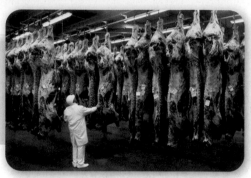

Transportation

Foods must be transported in clean, refrigerated vehicles and containers to prevent multiplication of microorganisms and microbial toxins.

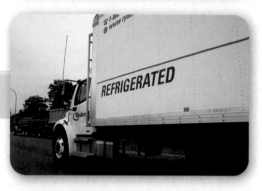

Retail

Employees of food markets and restaurants may contaminate food during storage, preparation, or service. Conditions such as inadequate refrigeration or heating may promote multiplication of microorganisms or microbial toxins. Establishments must follow FDA guidelines for food safety and pass local health inspections.

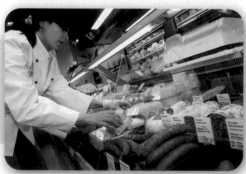

Table

Consumers may contaminate foods with unclean hands, utensils, or surfaces. They can allow the multiplication of microorganisms and microbial toxins by failing to follow the food-safety guidelines for storing, preparing, cooking, and serving foods discussed in this chapter.

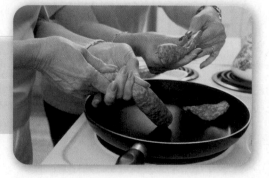

What Causes Most Foodborne Illness?

The consumption of food containing pathogenic microorganisms—those capable of causing disease—results in food infections. Food intoxications result from consuming food in which microorganisms have secreted harmful substances called toxins. Naturally occurring plant and marine toxins also contaminate food. Finally, chemical residues in foods, such as pesticides and pollutants in soil or water, can cause illness. Residues are discussed later in this chapter.

Several Types of Microorganisms Contaminate Foods

The microorganisms that most commonly cause food infections are bacteria and viruses; however, other tiny organisms and nonliving particles can also contaminate foods.

Bacteria are microorganisms that lack a true cell nucleus and reproduce either by division or by spore formation. Many thrive in the intestines of birds and mammals, including poultry, pigs, and cattle, so foodborne infection often results from consuming undercooked or raw foods or fluids contaminated with infected animal feces. Bacteria cause about 39% of all foodborne illnesses.[6] A few of the most common culprits are identified in **Table 15.2** (pages 602–603). Of these, the bacterium responsible for the most illnesses, hospitalizations, and deaths is *Salmonella* (**Figure 15.2**).[3]

Viruses are much smaller than bacteria, and they can't survive apart from living cells. Just one type, called *norovirus*, causes nearly all foodborne viral illness in the United States, and more foodborne illnesses than all other microorganisms put together (**Figure 15.3**).[7] Norovirus is so common and contagious that it's commonly referred to simply as "the stomach flu." Norovirus illness typically comes on suddenly as *gastroenteritis*, inflammation of the lining of the stomach and intestines, and results in stomach cramps, vomiting, and diarrhea. In healthy people, the symptoms typically resolve spontaneously within a day or two. Raw foods can harbor norovirus, and it can spread from person to person and commonly from infected food-service workers who handle foods with unclean hands. College campuses commonly report outbreaks of norovirus. In 2012, for instance, outbreaks occurred on several campuses in New Jersey and Washington, DC, sending hundreds of students to their campus health center or to the hospital. Hepatitis A and hepatitis E viruses can also contaminate foods and water supplies. They can cause a range of responses from mild, self-limiting illness to acute liver damage and even death.

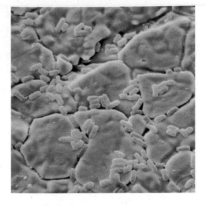

FIGURE 15.2 *Salmonella* is the leading cause of bacterial foodborne illness; it can cause fever, diarrhea, and abdominal cramps, and cells of some strains can perforate the intestines and invade the blood, causing systemic infection and death.

bacteria Microorganisms that lack a true nucleus and reproduce by division or by spore formation.

viruses A group of infectious agents that are much smaller than bacteria, lack independent metabolism, and are incapable of growth or reproduction outside of living cells.

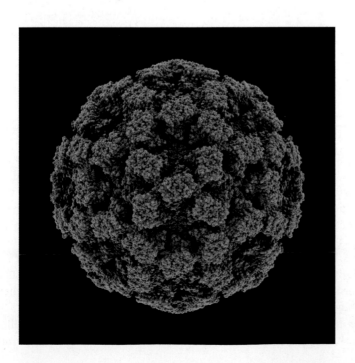

FIGURE 15.3 Norovirus is the leading cause of foodborne infection in the United States. It is responsible for more foodborne illness than all other viruses, bacteria, and parasites combined.

TABLE 15.2 Common Bacterial Causes of Foodborne Illness

Bacterium	Incubation Period	Duration	Symptoms	Foods Most Commonly Affected
Salmonella (more than 2,300 types)	12–24 hours	4–7 days	Diarrhea Abdominal pain Chills Fever Vomiting Dehydration	Raw or undercooked eggs, poultry, and meat Raw milk and dairy products Seafood Fruits and vegetables
Clostridium perfringens	6–24 hours	1 day	Abdominal cramps Diarrhea	Beef Poultry Gravies Dried foods Cooked foods prepared in large quantities Leftovers
Campylobacter jejuni	1–7 days	7–10 days	Fever Headache and muscle pain followed by diarrhea (sometimes bloody) Nausea Abdominal cramps	Raw and undercooked meat, poultry, or shellfish Raw eggs Cake icing Untreated water Unpasteurized milk
Escherichia coli (O157:H7 and other strains that can cause human illness)	2–4 days	5–10 days	Diarrhea (may be bloody) Abdominal cramps Nausea Can lead to kidney and blood complications	Contaminated water Raw milk Raw or rare ground beef, sausages Unpasteurized apple juice or cider Uncooked fruits and vegetables
Staphylococcus aureus	1–6 hours	2–3 days	Severe nausea and vomiting Abdominal cramps Diarrhea	Custard- or cream-filled baked goods Ham Poultry Dressings, sauces, and gravies Eggs Mayonnaise-based salads
Listeria monocytogenes	2 days–3 weeks	None reported	Fever Muscle aches Nausea Diarrhea Headache, stiff neck, confusion, loss of balance, or convulsions if infection spreads to nervous system Infections during pregnancy can lead to miscarriage or stillbirth	Uncooked meats and vegetables Soft cheeses Lunch meats and hot dogs Unpasteurized milk

(Table continued on next page)

Parasites are microorganisms that simultaneously derive benefit from and harm their host. They are responsible for only about 2% of foodborne illnesses. The most common culprits are the following:

- **Helminths** are multicellular worms, such as tapeworms (**Figure 15.4**), flukes, and roundworms. They reproduce by releasing their eggs into vegetation or water. Animals, including fish, then consume the contaminated matter. The eggs hatch inside their host, and larvae develop in the host's tissue. The larvae can survive in the flesh long after the host is killed for food. Thoroughly cooking beef, pork, or fish destroys the larvae. In contrast, people who eat contaminated foods either raw or undercooked consume living larvae, which then mature into adult worms in their small intestine. Some worms cause mild symptoms, such as nausea and diarrhea, but others can grow large enough to cause intestinal obstruction or even death.

- **Protozoa** are single-celled organisms that commonly cause waterborne illness. One of the most common culprits worldwide is *Giardia*, various species of which cause a

parasite A microorganism that simultaneously derives benefit from and harms its host.

helminth A multicellular microscopic worm.

protozoa Single-celled, mobile microorganisms.

fungi Plantlike, spore-forming organisms that can grow as either single cells or multicellular colonies.

TABLE 15.2 continued

Bacterium	Usual Sources of Contamination	Steps for Prevention
Salmonella (more than 2,300 types)	Intestinal tract and feces of poultry *Salmonella enteritidis* in raw shell eggs	Cook foods thoroughly. Avoid cross-contamination. Use sanitary practices.
Clostridium perfringens	Widely found in environment and in intestinal tracts of animals and humans Can survive in little or no oxygen	Cook foods thoroughly. Serve hot. Refrigerate leftovers promptly. Reheat leftovers thoroughly before serving.
Campylobacter jejuni	Intestinal tracts of animals and birds Raw milk Untreated water and sewage sludge	Drink only pasteurized milk. Cook foods properly. Avoid cross-contamination.
Escherichia coli (O157:H7 and other strains that can cause human illness)	Intestinal tracts of cattle Raw milk Unchlorinated water	Thoroughly cook meat. Avoid cross-contamination.
Staphylococcus aureus	Human skin Infected cuts Pimples Noses and throats	Refrigerate foods. Use sanitary practices.
Listeria monocytogenes	Intestinal tract and feces of animals Soil and manure used as fertilizer Raw milk	Thoroughly cook all meats. Heat hot dogs until they are steaming hot. Wash produce before eating. Avoid cross-contamination. Wash hands after handling hot dogs, lunch meats, and other meats. Avoid unpasteurized milk and foods made with unpasteurized milk. People at high risk should avoid eating refrigerated smoked seafood unless it is cooked.

Sources: Data from Iowa State University Extension, Food Safety and Quality Project. 2000. Safe Food: It's Your Job Too! www.extension.iastate.edu/foodsafety/Lesson/L1.html; US Food and Drug Administration (FDA). How Can I Prevent Foodborne Illness? www.cfsan.fda.gov/~dms/qa-fdb1.html; and Centers for Disease Control and Prevention (CDC). 2011. 2011 Estimates of Foodborne Illness in the United States. www.cdc.gov/Features/dsFoodborneEstimates/.

diarrheal illness called *giardiasis*.[8] *Giardia* lives in the intestines of infected animals and humans and is passed into the environment from their stools. People typically consume *Giardia* by swallowing contaminated water (in lakes, streams, rivers, swimming pools, and so on) or by eating contaminated food. Symptoms include diarrhea, stomach cramps, and upset stomach, usually beginning within 1 to 2 weeks of being infected and generally lasting 2 to 6 weeks.

■ **Fungi** are plantlike, spore-forming organisms that can grow as either single cells or multicellular colonies. Three common types are yeasts, which are globular; molds, which are long and thin; and the familiar mushrooms. Fewer than 1% of foodborne illnesses are caused by fungi.[3] This is due in part to the fact that very few species of fungi cause serious disease in people with healthy immune systems, and those that do cause disease in humans are not typically foodborne. In addition, unlike bacterial growth, which is invisible and often tasteless, fungal growth typically makes food look and taste so unappealing that we immediately discard it (**Figure 15.5**, page 604).

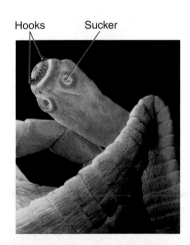

Hooks   Sucker

FIGURE 15.4 Tapeworms have long bodies with hooks and suckers they use to attach to a host's tissue.

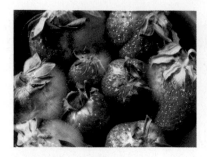

FIGURE 15.5 Molds rarely cause foodborne illness, in part because they look so unappealing that we throw the food away.

A foodborne illness in beef cattle that has had front-page exposure in recent years is mad cow disease, or *bovine spongiform encephalopathy (BSE)*. This neurologic disorder is caused by a **prion,** a proteinaceous infectious particle that is self-replicating. Prions are normal proteins of animal tissues that can misfold and become infectious. When they do, they can transform other normal proteins into abnormally shaped prions until they eventually cause illness.

The human form of BSE can develop in people who consume contaminated meat or tissue. If you eat beef, are you at risk? See the **Nutrition Myth or Fact?** box (page 605) to find out.

Some Foodborne Illness Is Due to Toxins

The microorganisms just discussed cause illness by directly infecting and destroying body cells. In contrast, other bacteria and fungi secrete chemicals, called **toxins,** that are responsible for serious and even life-threatening illnesses. These toxins bind to body cells and can cause a variety of symptoms, such as diarrhea, vomiting, organ damage, convulsions, and paralysis. Toxins can be categorized depending on the type of cell they bind to; the two primary types of toxins associated with foodborne illness are neurotoxins, which damage the nervous system and can cause paralysis, and enterotoxins, which target the gastrointestinal system and generally cause severe diarrhea and vomiting.

Bacterial Toxins

One of the most common and deadly neurotoxins is produced by the bacterium *Clostridium botulinum*. This botulism toxin blocks nerve transmission to muscle cells and causes paralysis, including of the muscles required for breathing. A common source of contamination is food in a damaged (split, pierced, or bulging) can. If you spot damaged canned goods while shopping, notify the store manager. If you inadvertently purchase food in a damaged can, or find that the container spurts liquid when you open it, throw it out immediately. Never taste the food, as even a microscopic amount of botulism toxin can be deadly.[9] Other common sources of *C. botulinum* are foods improperly canned at home and raw honey.

Some strains of *E. coli*, including those involved in the outbreaks mentioned at the beginning of this chapter, are particularly dangerous because they produce a toxin called *Shiga toxin*. These types are referred to as *Shiga toxin-producing* E. coli, or STEC. The most common STEC is *E. coli* O157. STECs are particularly dangerous because, in the vulnerable populations mentioned earlier, infection can result in kidney failure and, in some cases, death.

Eating spoiled fish—commonly tuna or mackerel—is unwise because the bacteria responsible for the spoilage release toxins into the fish. The result is *scombrotoxic fish poisoning*, which causes headache, vomiting, a rash, sweating, and flushing within a few minutes to 2 hours after consumption. Symptoms are usually mild and resolve within a few hours in healthy people.[10]

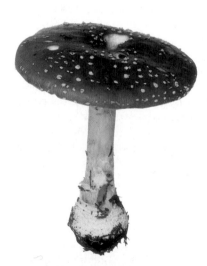

FIGURE 15.6 Some mushrooms, such as this fly agaric, contain fungal toxins that can cause illness or even death.

Fungal Toxins

Some fungi produce poisonous chemicals called *mycotoxins*. (The prefix *myco-* means "fungus.") These toxins are typically found in grains stored in moist environments. In some instances, moist conditions in the field encourage fungi to reproduce and release their toxins on the surface of growing crops. Long-term consumption of mycotoxins can cause organ damage or cancer.

A highly visible fungus that causes food intoxication is the poisonous mushroom. Most mushrooms are not toxic, but a few, such as the deathcap mushroom (*Amanita phalloides*), can be fatal. Some poisonous mushrooms are quite colorful (**Figure 15.6**), a fact that helps explain why the victims of mushroom poisoning are often children.[11]

prion A protein that misfolds and becomes infectious; prions are not living cellular organisms or viruses.

toxin Any harmful substance; in microbiology, a chemical produced by a microorganism that harms tissues or causes harmful immune responses.

Nutrition Myth OR Fact?

Mad Cow Disease: Is It Safe to Eat Beef?

Mad cow disease is a fatal brain disorder in cattle caused by a prion, which is an abnormally folded, infectious protein. Prions influence other proteins to take on their abnormal shape, and these abnormal proteins cause brain damage. Mad cow disease is also called *bovine spongiform* (spongelike) *encephalopathy (BSE)*. The disease eats away at a cow's brain, leaving it full of holes. Eventually, the brain can no longer control vital life functions and the cow literally "goes mad." Unfortunately, people who eat meat from infected cattle will also be infected. Symptoms may take years to appear, but eventually the person may develop the human form of mad cow disease, called *variant Creutzfeldt-Jakob disease (vCJD)*. As of June 2012, this disease had killed 176 people in Great Britain, as well as 25 people in France and several in other nations.[1]

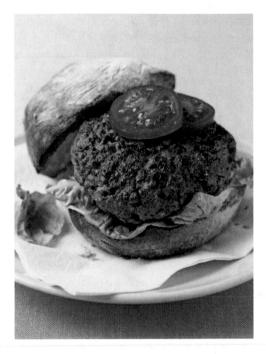

Scientists are not certain how the prions are introduced to cattle. They think that cattle become infected by eating feed containing tissue from the brains and spinal cords of other infected cattle. Decades ago in Great Britain and Europe, it was common practice to feed livestock with meal made from other animals. This practice has ceased, however, and the number of deaths attributed to vCJD declined from its peak of 28 in the year 2000 to just 5 in 2011.[1]

For many years, experts in North America believed BSE to be a problem limited to Europe. But then, eight cases of BSE were found in cows in Canada from 2003 to 2006. And in December 2003, the first case of mad cow disease was reported in the United States. Since then, three additional cases have been confirmed, the most recent in April of 2012.[2] So if you eat beef, are you at risk?

To date, only one case of vCJD has been confirmed in Canada and one in the United States, and these individuals are thought to have acquired the disease while in the United Kingdom. Although the precise etiology of vCJD anywhere in the world is not known, the low incidence in North America may reflect longstanding preventive practices. For instance, the United States has a system of three interlocking safeguards against BSE. The first and most important of these is the practice of removing, prior to slaughter, the parts of an animal that would contain BSE, should an animal have the disease. The second is rigorous control of the quality of animal feed. The third safeguard—which led to the April 2012 detection in a cow culled for lameness—is an ongoing BSE surveillance program in which carcasses are routinely sampled for BSE.[2]

So is it safe for Americans to eat beef? The US Department of Agriculture, the FDA, the National Institutes of Health, and the Centers for Disease Control and Prevention are working together to eliminate the use of unapproved animal feed and to improve technologies and procedures to detect BSE before an animal is approved for meat consumption. The US beef industry is highly motivated to comply with safety regulations, since reduced beef intake translates into millions of dollars in lost income. Although it may not be possible to absolutely guarantee the safety of U.S. beef, adherence to these strict safety standards does minimize the risk of an outbreak of vCJD.

References

1. International Society for Infectious Diseases. 2012, June 12. Prion Disease Update. www.promedmail.org/direct.php?id=20120612.1164648.
2. US Department of Agriculture Animal and Plant Health Inspection Service. 2012, April 24. Update from APHIS Regarding a Detection of Bovine Spongiform Encephalopathy (BSE) in the United States. www.aphis.usda.gov/newsroom/2012/05/bse_update_050212.shtml.

Toxic Algae

In April 2012, scientists predicted that a "red tide" could cause the closure of shellfish beds along as much as 250 miles of the northern New England coastline. Shellfish beds are closed to protect the public from a foodborne illness called *paralytic shellfish poisoning (PSP)*

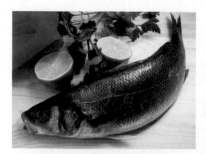

Sea bass may look appealing, but like several other large predatory tropical fish, it can be contaminated with a high concentration of marine toxins.

in anyone consuming mussels or clams harvested during a red tide.[12] Red tides are caused by the excessive production of certain species of toxic algae, whose bloom turns ocean waters purple, pink, or red. The blooms occur most commonly along the Gulf of Maine and on the Gulf Coast of Florida, but they also appear in U.S. West Coast waters. Humans don't consume these marine toxins directly; rather, mussels, clams, and other seafoods consume the toxic algae. When people consume the affected seafood—which typically looks, smells, and tastes normal—PSP results.[12] Finfish can also be contaminated with toxic algae. *Ciguatoxins* are marine toxins commonly found in fresh fish caught off the coasts of Hawaii, Puerto Rico, the Virgin Islands, and other tropical regions. They are produced by algae called *dinoflagellates*, which are consumed by small fish. The toxins become progressively more concentrated as larger fish eat these small fish, and high concentrations can be present in fish such as grouper, sea bass, snapper, and a number of other large fish from tropical regions. Symptoms of ciguatoxin poisoning include nausea, vomiting, diarrhea, headache, itching, a "pins-and-needles" feeling, and even nightmares or hallucinations, but the illness is rarely fatal and typically resolves within a few weeks.[10]

Plant Toxins

A variety of plants contain toxins that, if consumed, can cause illness. As humans evolved, we learned to avoid such plants. However, one plant toxin is still commonly found in kitchens. Potatoes that have turned green contain the toxin *solanine*, which forms during the greening process. The green color is actually due to chlorophyll, a harmless pigment that forms when the potatoes are exposed to light. Although the production of solanine occurs simultaneously with the production of chlorophyll, the two processes are separate and unrelated. Solanine is very toxic even in small amounts, and potatoes that appear green beneath the skin should be thrown away. Toxicity causes vomiting, diarrhea, fever, headache, and other symptoms and can progress to shock. Rarely, the poisoning can be fatal.[13] You can avoid the greening of potatoes by storing them for only short periods in a dark cupboard or brown paper bag in a cool area. Wash the potato to expose its color, and throw it away if it has turned green.

The Body Responds to Contaminants with Acute Illness

Many contaminants are killed in the mouth by antimicrobial enzymes in saliva or in the stomach by hydrochloric acid. Any that survive these chemical assaults usually trigger vomiting and/or diarrhea as the gastrointestinal tract attempts to expel them. Simultaneously, the white blood cells of the immune system are activated, and a generalized inflammatory response causes the person to experience nausea, fatigue, fever, and muscle aches. Depending on the state of one's health, the precise microorganism or toxin involved, and the "dose" ingested, symptoms can range from mild to severe.

To diagnose a foodborne illness, a specimen—usually blood or stool—must be analyzed. Treatment usually involves keeping the person hydrated and comfortable, as most foodborne illness tends to be self-limiting; that is, the person's vomiting and diarrhea, though unpleasant, rid the body of the offending agent. In more severe cases, hospitalization may be necessary.

In the United States, all confirmed cases of foodborne illness must be reported to the state health department, which in turn reports these illnesses to the CDC in Atlanta, Georgia. The CDC monitors its reports for indications of epidemics of foodborne illness and assists local and state agencies in controlling such outbreaks.

Certain Conditions Help Microorganisms Multiply in Foods

Given the correct environmental conditions, microorganisms can thrive in many types of food. Four factors affect the survival and reproduction of food microorganisms:

- *Temperature.* Many microorganisms capable of causing human illness thrive at warm temperatures, from about 40°F to 140°F (4°C to 60°C). You can think of this range of temperatures as the **danger zone** (**Figure 15.7**). These microorganisms can be destroyed by thoroughly heating or cooking foods, and their reproduction can be slowed by refrigeration and freezing. Safe cooking and food-storage temperatures are identified later in this chapter.
- *Humidity.* Many microorganisms require a high level of moisture; thus, foods such as boxed dried pasta do not make suitable microbial homes, although cooked pasta left at room temperature would prove hospitable.
- *Acidity.* Most microorganisms have a preferred pH range in which they thrive. For instance, *Clostridium botulinum* thrives in alkaline environments. It cannot grow or produce its toxin in acidic environments, so the risk for botulism is decreased in citrus fruits, pickles, and tomato-based foods. In contrast, alkaline foods, such as fish and most vegetables, are a magnet for *C. botulinum*.
- *Oxygen content.* Many microorganisms require oxygen to function; thus, food-preservation techniques that remove oxygen, such as industrial canning and bottling, keep foods safe for consumption. In contrast, *C. botulinum* thrives in an oxygen-free environment. For this reason, the canning process heats foods to an extremely high temperature to destroy this organism. In March 2011, a food producer voluntarily recalled thousands of cases of canned beets because of concerns that the food had not been heated high enough to destroy *C. botulinum*.

In addition, microorganisms need an entryway into a food. Just as our skin protects our bodies from microbial invasion, the peels, rinds, and shells of many foods seal off access to the nutrients within. Eggshells are a good example of a natural food barrier. Once such a barrier is removed, however, the food loses its primary defense against contamination.

RECAP

Food infections result from the consumption of food containing living microorganisms, such as bacteria, whereas food intoxications result from consuming food containing toxins. The body has several defense mechanisms that help rid us of offending microorganisms or their toxins. In order to reproduce in foods, microorganisms require a precise range of temperature, humidity, acidity, and oxygen content. ■

How Can You Prevent Foodborne Illness?

The United States Department of Agriculture's Fight BAC! logo identifies four basic rules for food safety (**Figure 15.8**, page 608).

Clean: Wash Your Hands and Kitchen Surfaces Often

One of the easiest and most effective ways to prevent foodborne illness is to consistently wash your hands before and after handling food. Remove any rings or bracelets before you begin, because jewelry can harbor bacteria. Scrub for at least 20 seconds with a mild soap, being sure to wash underneath your fingernails and between your fingers. Rinse under warm, running water. Although you should wash dishes in hot water, it's too harsh for hand washing: it causes the surface layer of the skin to break down, increasing the risk that microorganisms will be able to penetrate your skin. Dry your hands on a clean towel or fresh paper towel.

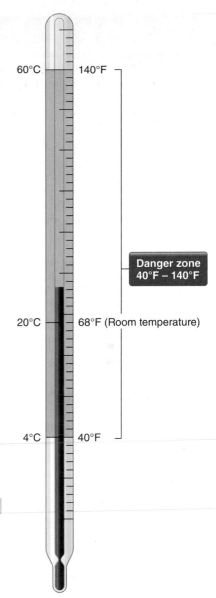

FIGURE 15.7 The danger zone is a temperature range within which many pathogenic microorganisms thrive. Notice that "room temperature" (about 68°F) is within the danger zone!

danger zone The range of temperature (about 40°F to 140°F, or 4°C to 60°C) at which many microorganisms capable of causing human disease thrive.

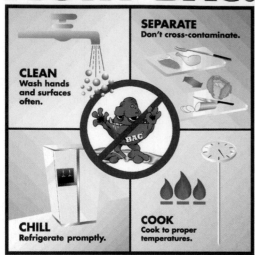

FIGHT BAC!

CLEAN Wash hands and surfaces often.

SEPARATE Don't cross-contaminate.

CHILL Refrigerate promptly.

COOK Cook to proper temperatures.

Keep Food Safe From Bacteria

FIGURE 15.8 Fight BAC! is the food-safety logo of the United States Department of Agriculture.

Thoroughly wash utensils, containers, cutting boards, and countertops with soap and hot water. Rinse. You can sanitize them with a solution of 1 tablespoon of chlorine bleach to 1 gallon of water. Flood the surface with the bleach solution and allow it to air dry. Wash fruits and vegetables thoroughly under running water just before eating, cutting, or cooking them. Washing fruits and vegetables with soap or detergent, or using commercial produce washes, is not recommended.[14]

Separate: Don't Cross-Contaminate

Cross-contamination is the spread of microorganisms from one food to another. This commonly occurs when raw foods, such as chicken and vegetables, are cut using the same knife, prepared on the same cutting board, or stored on the same plate. Keep raw meat, poultry, eggs, and seafood and their juices away from ready-to-eat food. Use separate cutting boards, utensils, and plates. When preparing meals with a marinade, reserve some of the fresh marinade in a clean container; then add the raw ingredients to the remainder. In this way, some uncontaminated marinade will be available if needed later in the cooking process. When marinating raw food, you should always keep it in the refrigerator.[14]

Beware of cross-contamination while food shopping. For example, the displaying of food products such as cooked shrimp on the same bed of ice as raw seafood is not safe, nor is slicing cold cuts with the same knife used to trim raw meat. Report such practices to your local health authorities.

Chill: Store Foods in the Refrigerator or Freezer

The third rule for keeping food safe from bacteria is to promptly refrigerate or freeze it. Remember the danger zone: microorganisms that cause foodborne illness can reproduce in temperatures above 40°F. To keep them from multiplying in your food, keep it cold. Refrigeration (at or below 40°F) and freezing (at or below 0°F)[15] do not kill all microorganisms, but cold temperatures diminish their ability to reproduce in quantities large enough to cause illness. Also, many naturally occurring enzymes that cause food spoilage are deactivated at cold temperatures.

Shopping for Perishable Foods

When shopping for food, purchase refrigerated and frozen foods last. Put packaged meat, poultry, or fish into a plastic bag before placing it in your shopping cart. This prevents drippings from those foods from coming into contact with others in your cart.

When choosing perishable foods, check the "sell by" or "best used by" date on the label. The "sell by" date indicates the last day a product can be sold and still maintain its quality during normal home storage and consumption. The "best used by" date tells you how long a product will maintain optimum quality before eating.[16] If the stamped date has passed, don't purchase the item and notify the store manager. These foods should be promptly removed from the shelves.

After you purchase perishable foods, get them home and into the refrigerator or freezer within 1 hour. If your trip home will be longer than an hour, take along a cooler to transport them in.

Refrigerating Foods at Home

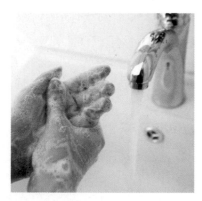

One of the most effective strategies for preventing foodborne illness is simply to wash your hands thoroughly.

As soon as you get home from shopping, put meats, eggs, cheeses, milk, and any other perishable foods in the refrigerator. Store meat, poultry, and seafood in the back of the refrigerator away from the door, so that they stay cold, and on the lowest shelf, so that their juices do not drip onto any other foods. If you are not going to use raw poultry, fish,

cross-contamination Contamination of one food by another via the unintended transfer of microorganisms through physical contact.

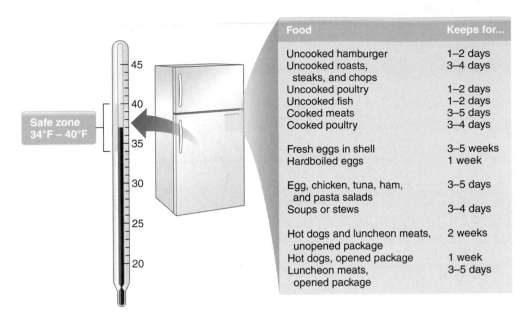

Food	Keeps for...
Uncooked hamburger	1–2 days
Uncooked roasts, steaks, and chops	3–4 days
Uncooked poultry	1–2 days
Uncooked fish	1–2 days
Cooked meats	3–5 days
Cooked poultry	3–4 days
Fresh eggs in shell	3–5 weeks
Hardboiled eggs	1 week
Egg, chicken, tuna, ham, and pasta salads	3–5 days
Soups or stews	3–4 days
Hot dogs and luncheon meats, unopened package	2 weeks
Hot dogs, opened package	1 week
Luncheon meats, opened package	3–5 days

Safe zone 34°F – 40°F

FIGURE 15.9 While it's important to keep a well-stocked refrigerator, it's also important to know how long foods will keep. (*Source:* Data from US Department of Agriculture, Food Safety and Inspection Service. May 11, 2010. Fact Sheets. Safe Food Handling. Refrigeration and Food Safety.)

or ground beef within 2 days of purchase, store it in the freezer. A guide for refrigerating foods is provided in **Figure 15.9**.

After a meal, refrigerate leftovers promptly—even if still hot—to discourage microbial growth. The standard rule is to refrigerate leftovers within 2 hours of serving. If the ambient temperature is 90°F or higher, such as at a picnic, foods should be refrigerated within 1 hour.[1] A larger quantity of food takes longer to cool, so divide and conquer: separate leftovers into shallow containers for quicker cooling.[16] Finally, avoid keeping leftovers for more than a few days (Figure 15.9). If you don't plan to finish a dish within the recommended time frame, freeze it.

Freezing and Thawing Foods

The temperature in your freezer should be set at 0°F. Use a thermometer and check it periodically. If your electricity goes out, avoid opening the freezer until the power is restored. When the power does come back on, check the temperature on the top shelf. If it is at or below 40°F, the food should still be safe to eat, or refreeze.

As with refrigeration, smaller packages will freeze more quickly. Rather than attempting to freeze an entire casserole, divide the food into multiple, small portions in freezer-safe containers; then freeze.

Sufficient thawing will ensure adequate cooking throughout, which is essential to preventing foodborne illness. Thaw poultry on the bottom shelf of the refrigerator, in a large bowl to catch its juices. **Table 15.3** (page 610) shows recommended poultry thawing times based on weight. Never thaw frozen meat, poultry, or seafood on a kitchen counter or in a basin of warm water. Room temperatures allow the growth of bacteria on the surface of food. You can also thaw foods in your microwave, following the manufacturer's instructions.

Dealing with Molds in Refrigerated Foods

Some molds like cool temperatures. Mold spores are common in the atmosphere, and they randomly land on food in open containers. If the temperature and acidity of the food are hospitable, they will grow.

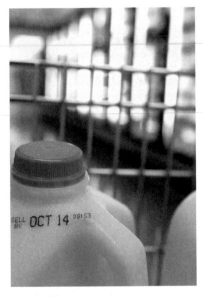

The "sell by" date tells the store how long to display the product for sale.

Thinking about drinking raw milk? The CDC advises you to think again. Watch three Americans tell their stories of foodborne illness following raw milk consumption at www.cdc.gov/foodsafety/rawmilk/raw-milk-videos.html.

TABLE 15.3 A Guide to Thawing Poultry

Method Needed	Size of Poultry	Approximate Length of Time
Refrigerator	1–3 pounds, small chickens, pieces 3–6 pounds, large chickens, ducks, small turkeys 6–12 pounds, large turkeys 12–16 pounds, whole turkey 16–20 pounds, whole turkey	1 day 2 days 3 days 3–4 days 4–5 days
Microwave (read instructions)	1–3 pounds, small chickens, pieces 3–6 pounds, large chickens, ducks, small turkeys	8–15 minutes* (standing time 10 minutes) 15–30 minutes* (standing time 20 minutes)

*Approximate;, read microwave's instructions.
Note: Turkeys purchased stuffed and frozen with the USDA or state mark of inspection on the packaging are safe because they have been processed under controlled conditions. These turkeys should not be thawed before cooking. Follow package directions for safe handling.
Sources: Data from Lacey, R. W. 1994. *Hard to Swallow: A Brief History of Food.* Cambridge: Cambridge University Press, pp. 85–187; and US Department of Agriculture, Food Safety and Inspection Service. 2000. *Turkey Basics: Safe Thawing.* www.fsis.usda.gov/Fact_Sheets/Poultry_Preparation_Fact_Sheets/index.asp.

If the surface of a small portion of a solid food, such as hard cheese, becomes moldy, it is generally safe to cut off that section down to about an inch and eat the unspoiled portion. However, if soft cheese, sour cream, tomato sauce, or another soft or fluid product becomes moldy, discard it.

Cook: Heat Foods Thoroughly

> The safe minimum cooking temperatures for the doneness of meat, poultry, seafood, eggs, and leftovers are identified in a table at www.foodsafety.gov/keep/charts/mintemp.html.

Thoroughly cooking food is a sure way to kill the intestinal worms discussed earlier and many other microorganisms. Color and texture are unreliable indicators of safety. Use a food thermometer to ensure that you have cooked food to a safe minimum internal temperature to destroy any harmful bacteria. Place the thermometer in the thickest part of the food, away from bone, fat, or gristle. See the **Highlight** box for tips about grilling and barbequing foods.[14]

Microwave cooking is convenient, but you need to be sure your food is thoroughly and evenly cooked and that there are no cold spots in the food where bacteria can thrive. For best results, cover food, stir often, and rotate for even cooking. Raw and semi-raw (such as marinated or partly cooked) fish delicacies, including sushi and sashimi, may be tempting, but their safety cannot be guaranteed. Always cook fish thoroughly. When done, fish should be opaque and flake easily with a fork. If you're wondering how sushi restaurants can guarantee the safety of their food, the short answer is they can't. All fish to be used for sushi must be flash frozen in a process that effectively kills any parasites that are in the fish, but it does not necessarily kill bacteria or viruses. In April 2012, 316 people in twenty-six states experienced foodborne illness after consuming sushi made with tuna contaminated with *Salmonella* bacteria.[17] Thus, eating raw seafood remains risky. For this reason, pregnant women and others at increased risk for foodborne illness are advised to avoid it.[18]

You may have fond memories of licking cake or brownie batter off a spoon when you were a kid, but such practices are no longer considered safe. That's because most cake batter contains raw eggs, one of the most common sources of *Salmonella*. The USDA recommends that you cook eggs until they are firm.

Protect Yourself from Toxins in Foods

Killing microorganisms with heat is an important step in keeping food safe, but it won't protect you against their toxins. That's because many toxins are unaffected by heat and are capable of causing severe illness even when the microorganisms that produced them have been destroyed.

For example, let's say you prepare a casserole for a team picnic. Too bad you forget to wash your hands before serving it to your teammates, because you contaminate the

Food-Safety Tips for Your Next Barbecue

HIGHLIGHT

It's the end of the term and you and your friends are planning a lakeside barbecue to celebrate! Here are some tips from the Center for Food Safety and Applied Nutrition at the US Food and Drug Administration for preventing foodborne illness at any outdoor gathering.

- **Wash your hands, utensils, and food-preparation surfaces.** Even in outdoor settings, food safety begins with hand washing. Take along a water jug, some soap, and paper towels or a box of moist, disposable towelettes. Keep all utensils and platters clean when preparing foods.

- **Keep foods cold during transport.** Use coolers with ice or frozen gel packs to keep food at or below 40°F. It's easier to maintain a cold temperature in small coolers. Consider packing three: put beverages in one cooler, washed fruits and vegetables and containers of potato salad in another, and wrapped, frozen meat, poultry, and seafood in another. Keep coolers in the

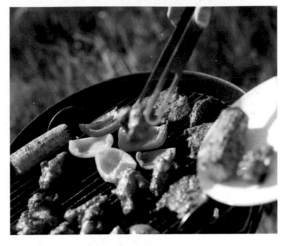

At a barbecue, it's essential to heat foods to the proper temperature.

air-conditioned passenger compartment of your car, rather than in a hot trunk.

- **Grill foods thoroughly.** Use a food thermometer to be sure the food has reached an adequate internal temperature before serving.

- **Avoid cross-contamination.** When taking food from the grill to the table, never use the same platter or utensils that previously held raw meat or seafood!

- **Keep hot foods hot.** Keep grilled food hot until it is served by moving it to the side of the grill, just away from the coals, so that it stays at or above 140°F. If grilled food isn't going to be eaten right away, wrap it well and place it in an insulated container.

- **Keep cold foods cold.** Cold foods, such as chicken salad, should be kept in a bowl of ice during your barbecue. Drain off water as the ice melts and replace the ice frequently. Don't let any perishable food sit out longer than 2 hours. In temperatures above 90°F, don't let food sit out for more than 1 hour.

Source: Data from US Food and Drug Administration. 2012, May 9. Food Facts. Eating Outdoors. Handling Food Safely. www.fda.gov/Food/ResourcesForYou/Consumers/ucm109899.htm.

casserole with the bacterium *Staphylococcus aureus*, which is commonly found on skin. You and your friends go off and play soccer, leaving the food in the sun, and a few hours later you take the rest of the casserole home. At supper, you heat the leftovers thoroughly, thinking that this will kill any bacteria that multiplied while it was left out. That night you experience nausea, severe vomiting, and abdominal pain. What happened? While your food was left out, *Staphylococcus* multiplied in the casserole and produced a toxin (**Figure 15.10**). When you reheated the food, you killed the microorganisms, but their toxin was unaffected by the heat. When you then ate the food, the toxin made you sick.

Be Choosy When Eating Out—Close to Home or Far Away

When choosing a place to eat out, avoid restaurants that don't look clean. Grimy tabletops and dirty restrooms indicate indifference to hygiene. On the other hand, the cleanliness of areas used by the public doesn't guarantee that the kitchen is clean. That is why health inspections are important. Public health inspectors randomly visit and inspect the food-preparation areas of all businesses that serve food, whether eaten in or taken out. When in doubt, check the inspection results posted in the restaurant.

Another way to protect yourself when dining out is by ordering foods to be cooked thoroughly. If you order a hamburger and it arrives pink in the middle, or scrambled eggs and they arrive runny, send the food back to be cooked thoroughly.

To listen to any of dozens of podcasts on food safety at home, go to www.fsis.usda.gov/News_&_Events/Food_Safety_at_Home_Podcasts/index.asp?src_location=content&src_page=FSEd.

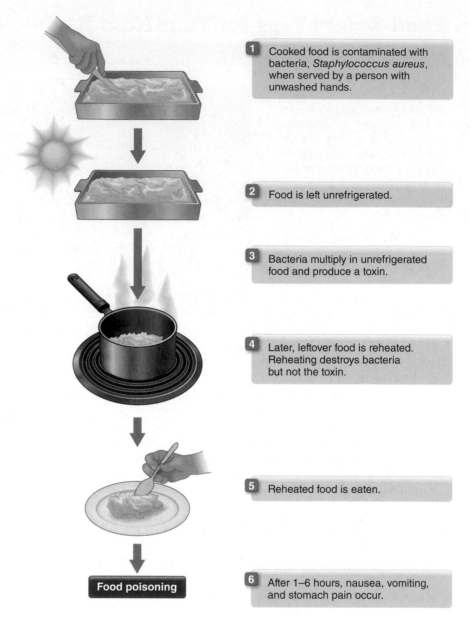

1 Cooked food is contaminated with bacteria, *Staphylococcus aureus*, when served by a person with unwashed hands.

2 Food is left unrefrigerated.

3 Bacteria multiply in unrefrigerated food and produce a toxin.

4 Later, leftover food is reheated. Reheating destroys bacteria but not the toxin.

5 Reheated food is eaten.

Food poisoning

6 After 1–6 hours, nausea, vomiting, and stomach pain occur.

FIGURE 15.10 Food contamination can occur long after the microorganism itself has been destroyed.

Find more information about how to ensure food and water safety when traveling by visiting the CDC's website: wwwnc.cdc.gov/travel/content/safe-food-water.aspx.

processed foods Foods that are manipulated mechanically or chemically.

pasteurization A form of sterilization using high temperatures for short periods of time.

irradiation A sterilization process in which food is exposed to gamma rays or high-energy electron beams to kill microorganisms. Irradiation does not impart any radiation to the food being treated.

When planning a trip, tell your physician your travel plans and ask about vaccinations you need or any medications you should take along in case you get sick. Pack a waterless antibacterial hand cleanser and use it frequently. When dining, select foods and beverages carefully (see Chapter 3). All raw food has the potential for contamination.

RECAP

Foodborne illness can be prevented at home by following four tips: (1) Clean: wash your hands and kitchen surfaces often. (2) Separate: isolate foods to prevent cross-contamination. (3) Chill: store foods in the refrigerator or freezer. (4) Cook: heat foods long enough and at the correct temperatures to ensure proper cooking. When eating out, avoid restaurants that don't look clean, and ask that all food be cooked thoroughly. ■

How Is Food Spoilage Prevented?

Any food that has been harvested and that people aren't ready to eat must be preserved in some way or, before long, it will degrade enzymatically and become home to a variety of microorganisms. Even **processed foods**—foods that are manipulated mechanically or chemically—have the potential to spoil.

The most ancient methods of preserving foods are salting, sugaring, drying, and smoking, all of which draw the water out of plant or animal cells. By dehydrating the food, these methods make it inhospitable to microorganisms and dramatically slow the action of enzymes that would otherwise degrade the food. We still use many of these methods today to preserve and prepare foods and meats, such as the salted Italian Parma ham.

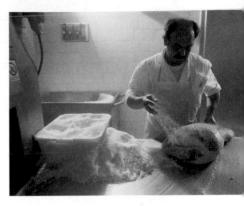

A worker salting a Parma ham.

Natural methods of cooling have also been used for centuries, including storing foods in underground cellars, caves, running streams, and even "cold pantries"—north-facing rooms of the house that were kept dark and unheated, often stocked with ice. The forerunner of the modern refrigerator—the miniature icehouse, or icebox—was developed in the early 1800s, and in cities and towns a local iceman would make rounds delivering ice to homes.

More recently, technological advances have helped food producers preserve the integrity of their products for months and even years between harvesting and consumption:

- *Canning.* Developed in the late 1700s, canning involves washing and blanching food, placing it in cans, siphoning out the air, sealing the cans, and then heating them to a very high temperature. Canned food has an average shelf life of at least 2 years from the date of purchase.
- *Pasteurization.* The technique called **pasteurization** exposes a beverage or other food to heat high enough to destroy microorganisms, but for a short enough period of time that the taste and quality of the food are not affected. For example, in flash pasteurization, milk or other liquids are heated to 162°F (72°C) for 15 seconds.
- *Irradiation.* The **irradiation** process exposes foods to gamma rays from radioactive metals. Energy from the rays penetrates food and its packaging, killing or disabling microorganisms in the food. The process does not cause foods to become radioactive! A few nutrients, including thiamin and vitamins A, E, and K, are lost, but these losses are also incurred in conventional processing and preparation. Although irradiated food has been shown to be safe, the FDA requires that all irradiated foods be labeled with a "radura" symbol and a caution against irradiating the food again (**Figure 15.11**).

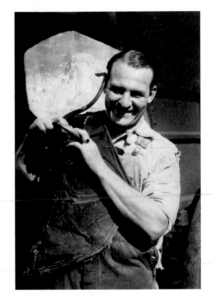

Before the modern refrigerator, an "iceman" would deliver ice to homes and businesses.

FIGURE 15.11 The US Food and Drug Administration requires the radura—the international symbol of irradiated food—to be displayed on all irradiated food sold in the United States.

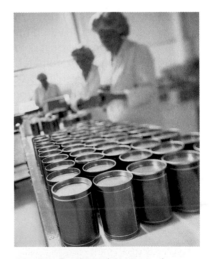

Canning food involves several steps to ensure all microorganisms in the food are killed.

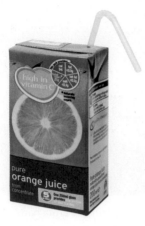

Aseptic packaging allows foods to be stored unrefrigerated for several months without spoilage.

- *Aseptic packaging.* You probably know aseptic packaging best as "juice boxes." Food and beverages are first heated, then cooled, then placed in sterile containers. The process uses less energy and materials than traditional canning, and the average shelf life is about 6 months.
- *Modified atmosphere packaging.* In this process, the oxygen in a package of food is replaced with an inert gas, such as nitrogen or carbon dioxide. This prevents a number of chemical reactions that spoil food, and it slows the growth of bacteria that require oxygen. The process can be used with a variety of foods, including meats, fish, vegetables, and fruits.
- *High-pressure processing.* In this technique, the food to be preserved is subjected to an extremely high pressure, which inactivates most bacteria while retaining the food's quality and freshness.

RECAP

Salting, sugaring, drying, smoking, and cooling have been used for centuries to preserve food. Canning, pasteurization, irradiation, and several packaging techniques are used to preserve a variety of foods during shipping, as well as on grocer and consumer shelves. ■

What Are Food Additives, and Are They Safe?

Have you ever picked up a loaf of bread and started reading its ingredients? You'd expect to see flour, yeast, water, and some sugar, but what are all those other items? They are collectively called *food additives*, and they are in almost every processed food. **Food additives** are not foods in themselves but, rather, natural or synthetic chemicals added to foods to enhance them in some way. More than 3,000 different food additives are currently used in the United States. **Table 15.4** identifies only a few of the most common.

Food Additives Include Nutrients and Preservatives

Vitamins and minerals are added to foods as nutrients and as preservatives. Vitamin E is usually added to fat-based products to keep them from going rancid, and vitamin C is used as an antioxidant in many foods. Iodine is added to table salt to help decrease the incidence of goiter, a condition that causes the thyroid gland to enlarge. Vitamin D is added to milk, and calcium is added to soy milk, rice milk, almond milk, and some juices to help prevent osteoporosis. Folate is added to cereals, breads, and other foods to help prevent certain types of birth defects.

The following two preservatives have raised health concerns:

- *Sulfites.* A small segment of the population is sensitive to sulfites, preservatives used in many beers and wines and some other processed foods. These people can experience asthma, headaches, or other symptoms after eating food containing the offending preservatives.
- *Nitrites.* Commonly used to preserve processed meats, nitrites can be converted to nitrosamines during the cooking process. Nitrosamines have been found to be carcinogenic in animals, so the FDA has required all foods with nitrites to contain additional antioxidants to decrease the formation of nitrosamines.

Nutrition MILESTONE

In **1859**, French chemist and microbiologist Louis Pasteur boiled a meat broth in a flask that had a long, slender, curved neck that allowed air, but not dust, access to the broth. The flask remained free of contamination by microorganisms. However, when the neck of the flask was changed so that dust could enter, the broth quickly became contaminated. This experiment disproved a belief held for 2,000 years that life could arise spontaneously from inanimate matter. Just 3 years later, in 1862, Pasteur showed that the growth of microorganisms is responsible for spoiling beverages such as beer, wine, and milk. He heated milk to a very high temperature, theorizing that the heat would kill any microorganisms present. The experiment was a success, and the technique, called pasteurization, bears his name.

food additive A substance or mixture of substances intentionally put into food to enhance its appearance, safety, palatability, and quality.

Other Food Additives Include Flavorings, Colorings, and Other Agents

Flavoring agents are used to replace the natural flavors lost during food processing. In contrast, *flavor enhancers* have little or no flavor of their own but accentuate the natural flavor

TABLE 15.4 Examples of Common Food Additives

Food Additive	Foods Found In
Coloring Agents	
Beet extract	Beverages, candies, ice cream
Beta-carotene	Beverages, sauces, soups, baked goods, candies, macaroni and cheese mixes
Caramel	Beverages, sauces, soups, baked goods
Tartrazine	Beverages, cakes and cookies, ice cream
Preservatives	
Alpha-tocopherol (vitamin E)	Vegetable oils
Ascorbic acid (vitamin C)	Breakfast cereals, cured meats, fruit drinks
BHA	Breakfast cereals, chewing gum, oils, potato chips
BHT	Breakfast cereals, chewing gum, oils, potato chips
Calcium proprionate/sodium proprionate	Bread, cakes, pies, rolls
EDTA	Beverages, canned shellfish, margarine, mayonnaise, processed fruits and vegetables, sandwich spreads
Propyl gallate	Mayonnaise, chewing gum, chicken soup base, vegetable oils, meat products, potato products, fruits, ice cream
Sodium benzoate	Carbonated beverages, fruit juice, pickles, preserves
Sodium chloride (salt)	Most processed foods
Sodium nitrate/sodium nitrite	Bacon, corned beef, lunch meats, smoked fish
Sorbic acid/potassium sorbate	Cakes, cheese, dried fruits, jellies, syrups, wine
Sulfites (sodium bisulfite, sulfur dioxide)	Dried fruits, processed potatoes, wine
Texturizers, Emulsifiers, and Stabilizers	
Calcium chloride	Canned fruits and vegetables
Carageenan/pectin	Ice cream, chocolate milk, soy milk, frostings, jams, jellies, cheese, salad dressings, sour cream, puddings, syrups
Cellulose gum/guar gum/gum arabic/locust gum/xanthan gum	Soups and sauces, gravies, sour cream, ricotta cheese, ice cream, syrups
Gelatin	Desserts, canned meats
Lecithin	Mayonnaise, ice cream
Humectants	
Glycerin	Chewing gum, marshmallows, shredded coconut
Propylene glycol	Chewing gum, gummy candies

of foods. One of the most common flavor enhancers is monosodium glutamate (MSG). In some people, MSG causes symptoms such as headaches, difficulty breathing, and heart palpitations.

Common food *colorings* include beet juice, which imparts a red color; beta-carotene, which gives a yellow color; and caramel, which adds brown color. The coloring tartrazine (FD&C Yellow #5) causes an allergic reaction in some people, and its use must be indicated on the product packaging.

Texturizers are added to foods to improve their texture. *Emulsifiers* help keep fats evenly dispersed within foods. *Stabilizers* give foods "body" and help them maintain a desired texture or color. *Humectants* keep foods such as marshmallows, chewing gum, and shredded coconut moist and stretchy. *Desiccants* prevent the absorption of moisture from the air; for example, they are used to prevent table salt from forming clumps.[19]

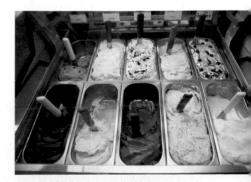

Many foods, such as ice cream, contain colorings.

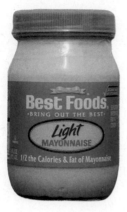

Mayonnaise contains emulsifiers to prevent separation of fats.

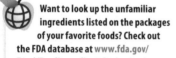

Want to look up the unfamiliar ingredients listed on the packages of your favorite foods? Check out the FDA database at www.fda.gov/Food/FoodIngredientsPackaging/GenerallyRecognizedasSafeGRAS/GRASSubstancesSCOGSDatabase/default.htm.

Generally Recognized as Safe (GRAS) A list established by Congress to identify substances used in foods that are generally recognized as safe based on a history of long-term use or on the consensus of qualified research experts.

genetic modification The process of changing an organism by manipulating its genetic material.

recombinant DNA technology A type of genetic modification in which scientists combine DNA from different sources to produce a transgenic organism that expresses a desired trait.

Are Food Additives Safe?

Federal legislation was passed in 1958 to regulate food additives. The Delaney Clause, also enacted in 1958, states, "No additive may be permitted in any amount if tests show that it produces cancer when fed to man or animals or by other appropriate tests." Before a new additive can be used in food, the producer of the additive must demonstrate its safety to the FDA by submitting data on its reasonable safety. The FDA determines the additive's safety based on these data.

Also in 1958, the U.S. Congress recognized that many substances added to foods would not require this type of formal review by the FDA prior to marketing and use, as their safety had already been established through long-term use or because their safety had been recognized by qualified experts through scientific studies. These substances are exempt from the more stringent testing criteria for new food additives and are referred to as substances that are **Generally Recognized as Safe (GRAS).** The GRAS list identifies substances that either have been tested and determined by the FDA to be safe and approved for use in the food industry or are deemed safe as a result of consensus among experts qualified by scientific training and experience.

In 1985, the FDA established the Adverse Reaction Monitoring System (ARMS). Under this system, the FDA investigates complaints from consumers, physicians, and food companies about food additives.

RECAP

Food additives are chemicals intentionally added to foods to enhance their color, flavor, texture, nutrient density, moisture level, or shelf life. Although there is continuing controversy over food additives in the United States, the FDA regulates additives used in our food supply and considers safe those it approves. ■

How Is Genetic Modification Used in Food Production?

In **genetic modification,** also referred to as *genetic engineering*, the genetic material, or DNA, of an organism is altered to bring about specific changes in its seeds or offspring. Selective breeding is one example of genetic modification; for example, Brahman cattle, which have poor-quality meat but high resistance to heat and humidity, are bred with English shorthorn cattle, which have good meat but low resistance to heat and humidity. The outcome of this selective breeding process is Santa Gertrudis cattle, which have the desired characteristics of higher-quality meat and resistance to heat and humidity. Although selective breeding is effective and has helped increase crop yields and improve the quality and quantity of our food supply, it is a relatively slow and imprecise process, as a great deal of trial and error typically occurs before the desired characteristics are achieved.

Recently, advances in biotechnology have moved genetic modification beyond selective breeding. These advances include the manipulation of the DNA of living cells of one organism to produce the desired characteristics of a different organism. Called **recombinant DNA technology,** the process commonly begins when scientists isolate from an animal, a plant, or a microbial cell a particular segment of DNA—one or more genes—that codes for a protein conferring a desirable trait, such as salt tolerance in tomato plants (**Figure 15.12**). Scientists then splice the DNA into a "host cell," usually a microorganism. The cell is cultured to produce many copies, a *gene library,* of the beneficial gene. Then, many scientists can readily obtain the gene to modify other organisms that lack the desired trait—for example, traditional tomato plants. The modified DNA causes the plant's cells to build the protein of interest, and the plant expresses the desired trait. The term *genetically modified organism (GMO)* refers to any organism in which the DNA has been altered using recombinant DNA technology.

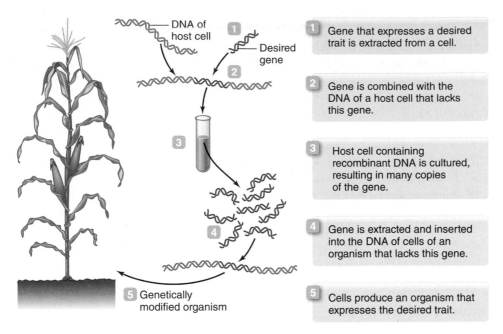

1. Gene that expresses a desired trait is extracted from a cell.

2. Gene is combined with the DNA of a host cell that lacks this gene.

3. Host cell containing recombinant DNA is cultured, resulting in many copies of the gene.

4. Gene is extracted and inserted into the DNA of cells of an organism that lacks this gene.

5. Cells produce an organism that expresses the desired trait.

FIGURE 15.12 Recombinant DNA technology involves producing plants and other organisms that contain modified DNA, which enables them to express desirable traits that are not present in the original organism.

In agriculture, GMOs are used to induce resistance to herbicides and pesticides. For example, genetically modified corn crops can be sprayed with chemicals that kill weeds without harming the corn. Genetic modification can also increase resistance to insects or viruses that cause disease in plants. Scientists can also insert a gene to make crops more tolerant of environmental conditions, such as drought or poor soil. Another use is to increase the nutritional value of a crop. For instance, researchers have modified soybeans and canola to increase their content of monounsaturated fatty acids.

Since 1996, many crops have been genetically modified and incorporated into our current food market. The most common GMO food crops are corn and soybeans. The US Department of Agriculture reports that, in 2011, 88% of all corn crops and 94% of all soybean crops grown in the United States were genetically engineered varieties, chosen for their greater tolerance of pesticides and resistance to insects.[20]

The relative benefits and harm of genetic modification have been debated worldwide. For more information, see the **Nutrition Debate** at the end of this chapter.

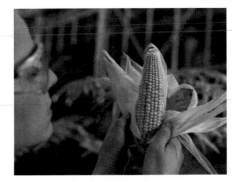

Corn is one of the most widely cultivated genetically modified crops.

RECAP

In genetic modification, the genetic material, or DNA, of an organism is altered to enhance certain qualities. In agriculture, genetic modification is often used to improve crop protection or to increase nutrients in the resulting food. Genetic modification is also used in animals and microorganisms. ■

How Do Residues Harm Our Food Supply?

Food **residues** are chemicals that remain in foods despite cleaning and processing. Four types of residues of global concern are persistent organic pollutants, pesticides, hormones and antibiotics used in animals, and packaging residues. Although residues can cause nerve damage, skin rashes, and other health problems, the most common concern related to residues is an increased risk for cancer.

residues Chemicals that remain in foods despite cleaning and processing.

Persistent Organic Pollutants Can Cause Illness

Many different chemicals are released into the atmosphere as a result of industry, agriculture, automobile emissions, and improper waste disposal. These chemicals, collectively referred to as **persistent organic pollutants (POPs),** can travel thousands of miles in gases or as airborne particles, in rain, snow, rivers, and oceans, eventually entering the food supply through the soil or water.[21] If a pollutant gets into the soil, a plant can absorb the chemical into its structure and pass it on as part of the food chain. Animals can also absorb the pollutant into their tissues or consume it when feeding on plants growing in the polluted soil. Fat-soluble pollutants are especially problematic, as they tend to accumulate in the animal's body tissues in ever greater concentrations as they move up the food chain. This process is called **biomagnification.** The POPs are then absorbed by humans when the animal is used as a food source (**Figure 15.13**).

POP residues have been found in virtually all categories of foods, including baked goods, fruit, vegetables, meat, poultry, fish, and dairy products. Significant levels have been detected all over the Earth, even in pristine regions of the Arctic thousands of miles from any known source.[21]

Mercury and Lead Are Nerve Toxins

Mercury, a naturally occurring element, is found in soil, rocks, and water. It is also released into the air by pulp and paper processing and the burning of garbage and fossil fuels. As mercury falls from the air, it finds its way to streams, rivers, lakes, and the ocean, where it accumulates. Fish absorb mercury as they feed on aquatic organisms, and this mercury is

persistent organic pollutants (POPs) Chemicals released into the environment as a result of industry, agriculture, or improper waste disposal; automobile emissions also are considered POPs.

biomagnification The process by which persistent organic pollutants become more concentrated in animal tissues as they move from one creature to another through the food chain.

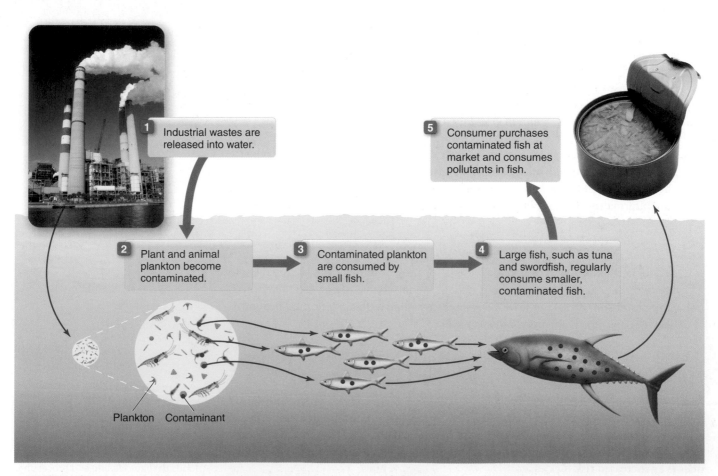

1 Industrial wastes are released into water.

5 Consumer purchases contaminated fish at market and consumes pollutants in fish.

2 Plant and animal plankton become contaminated.

3 Contaminated plankton are consumed by small fish.

4 Large fish, such as tuna and swordfish, regularly consume smaller, contaminated fish.

Plankton Contaminant

FIGURE 15.13 Biomagnification of persistent organic pollutants in the food supply.

passed on to us when we consume the fish. As mercury accumulates in the body, it has a toxic effect on the nervous system.

Large predatory fish, such as swordfish, shark, king mackerel, and tilefish, tend to contain the highest levels of mercury.[22] Because mercury is especially toxic to the developing nervous system of fetuses and growing children, pregnant and breastfeeding women and young children are advised to avoid eating these types of fish. Canned tuna, salmon, cod, pollock, sole, shrimp, mussels, and scallops do not contain high levels of mercury and are safe to consume; however, the FDA recommends that pregnant women and young children eat no more than two servings (12 oz) per week of any type of fish.[22]

Lead is another POP of concern. It can be found naturally in the soil, water, and air, but it also occurs as industrial waste from leaded gasoline, lead-based paints, and lead-soldered cans, now outlawed but decomposing in landfills. Some ceramic mugs, containers, and dishes are fired with lead-based glaze; thus, residues can build up in foods exposed to them. Excessive lead exposure can cause learning and behavioral impediments in children and cardiovascular and kidney disease in adults.

Dioxins Are Carcinogens

Dioxins are industrial pollutants typically formed as a result of combustion processes, such as waste incineration or the burning of wood, coal, or oil. Dioxins enter the soil and can persist in the environment for many years. Thus, even though dioxin levels have been declining for the last 30 years, largely as a result of increased regulation, some of the dioxins emitted decades ago will still be in the environment years from now.

There is concern that long-term exposure to dioxins can result in an increased risk for cancer and other disorders.[23] Because dioxins easily accumulate in the fatty tissues of animals, most dioxin exposure in humans occurs through the dietary intake of animal fats.[24] Whereas the EPA has been working to reduce dioxin emissions into the environment, the USDA and the FDA have been collaborating on efforts to monitor the dioxin levels in the U.S. food supply and to reduce the levels of all types of dioxins. If a particular food is shown to have high dioxin levels and the source can be determined, the agencies work to eliminate that source. To reduce your personal exposure to dioxins, eat meat less frequently, trim the fat from the meats you consume, and avoid fatty meats. Choose nonfat milk and yogurt, and low-fat cheeses, and replace butter with plant oils.

Pesticides Protect Against Crop Losses

Pesticides are a family of chemicals used in both fields and farm storage areas to decrease the destruction and crop losses caused by weeds, animals, insects, and fungi. Pesticides also help reduce the potential spread of disease by decreasing the level of microorganisms on crops. They increase overall crop yield and allow for greater crop diversity. The following are the three most common types of pesticides used in food production:

- *Herbicides*, which are used to control weeds and other unwanted plant growth
- *Insecticides*, which are used to control insects that can infest crops
- *Fungicides*, which are used to control plant-destroying fungal growth

Some pesticides used today are naturally derived and/or have a low impact on the environment. These include **biopesticides,** which are species-specific and work to suppress a pest's population, not eliminate it. For example, pheromones are a biopesticide that disrupts insect mating by attracting males into traps. Biopesticides also do not leave residues on crops—most degrade rapidly and are easily washed away with water.

In contrast, pesticides made from petroleum-based products can leave residues on foods. The liver is responsible for detoxifying these chemicals. But if the liver is immature, as in a fetus, an infant, or a child, or if the liver is stressed by disease or other toxins, such as excessive alcohol, then it cannot effectively remove pesticide residues. These residues have the potential to accumulate and cause nerve damage, cancer, birth defects, and other problems. It is therefore essential to wash all produce carefully.

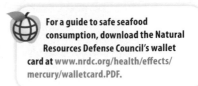

For a guide to safe seafood consumption, download the Natural Resources Defense Council's wallet card at www.nrdc.org/health/effects/mercury/walletcard.PDF.

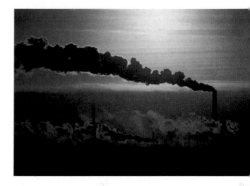

One of the ways mercury is released into the environment is by burning fossil fuels.

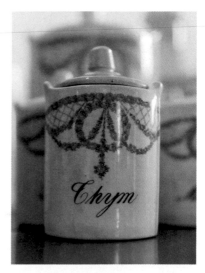

Antique porcelain is often coated with lead-based glaze.

biopesticides Primarily insecticides, these chemicals use natural methods to reduce damage to crops.

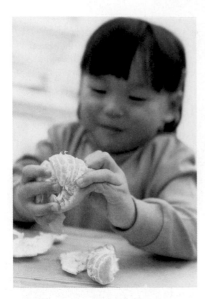

Peels protect foods against contamination; however, you should still wash the fruit before peeling.

The EPA is responsible for regulating the labeling, sale, distribution, use, and disposal of all pesticides in the United States. Before the EPA can accept a pesticide for use, it must be determined that it performs its intended function with minimal impact to the environment. Once the EPA has certified a pesticide, states can set their own regulations for its use. The following are some tips from the EPA for reducing your level of exposure to pesticides:[25]

- Wash and scrub all fresh fruits and vegetables thoroughly under running water.
- Peel fruits and vegetables whenever possible, and discard the outer leaves of leafy vegetables, such as cabbage and lettuce. Trim the excess fat from meat and remove the skin from poultry and fish, because some pesticide residues collect in the fat.
- Eat a variety of foods from various sources, as this can reduce the risk of exposure to a single pesticide.
- Consume more organically grown foods. **Table 15.5** identifies the twelve foods most likely to contain high levels of pesticide residue and the fifteen foods lowest in pesticide residues. If your food budget is limited, spend your money on the organically grown versions of the "dirty dozen."
- If you garden, avoid using fertilizers and pesticides to keep these chemicals out of your groundwater, as well as your foods.
- Filter your tap water, whether it comes from a municipal water system or a well, to reduce your exposure to pesticides, fertilizers, and other contaminants.

Growth Hormones and Antibiotics Are Used in Animals

Introduced into the U.S. food supply in 1994, **recombinant bovine growth hormone (rBGH)** is a genetically engineered growth hormone. It is used in beef herds to induce animals to grow more muscle tissue and less fat. It is also injected into a third of U.S. dairy cows to increase milk output. Although the FDA has allowed the use of rBGH in the United States, both Canada and the European Union have banned it for two reasons:

- The available evidence shows an increased risk for mastitis (inflamed udders) in dairy cows injected with rBGH.[26] Farmers treat mastitis with antibiotics, promoting the development of strains of pathogenic bacteria that are resistant to antibiotics.

recombinant bovine growth hormone (rBGH) A genetically engineered hormone injected into dairy cows to enhance their milk output.

TABLE 15.5 Shopper's Guide to Pesticides in Produce

The "Dirty Dozen": Buy These Organic	The "Clean Fifteen": Lowest in Pesticides
1. Peaches	1. Onions
2. Apples	2. Avocados
3. Bell peppers	3. Sweet corn
4. Celery	4. Pineapples
5. Nectarines	5. Mangoes
6. Strawberries	6. Asparagus
7. Cherries	7. Sweet peas
8. Kale	8. Kiwi
9. Lettuce	9. Cabbage
10. Grapes (imported)	10. Eggplant
11. Carrots	11. Papayas
12. Pears	12. Watermelon
	13. Broccoli
	14. Tomatoes
	15. Sweet potatoes

- The milk of cows receiving rBGH has higher levels of a hormone called insulin-like growth factor (IGF-1). This hormone can pass into the bloodstream of humans who drink milk from cows that receive rBGH, and some studies have shown that an elevated level of IGF-1 in humans may increase the risk for certain cancers. However, the evidence from these studies is inconclusive.[26]

The American Cancer Society suggests that more research is needed to help better appraise these health risks. In the meantime, consumer concerns about rBGH have caused a significant decline in the sales of milk from cows treated with rBGH.[26]

Antibiotics are used not only in dairy cows but also in other animals raised for food. For example, they are routinely added to the feed of swine to reduce the number of disease outbreaks in overcrowded pork-production facilities. Many researchers are concerned that cows, pigs, and other animals treated with antibiotics are becoming significant reservoirs for the development of a particularly virulent antibiotic-resistant strain of bacteria known as *methicillin-resistant Staphylococcus aureus (MRSA)*.[27] This type of *Staphylococcus aureus* cannot be effectively treated with methicillin or other beta-lactam antibiotics, including penicillin and amoxicillin. Infection with MRSA can cause symptoms ranging from a mild skin rash to a "flesh-eating" destruction of tissues to death: each year, MRSA is responsible for thousands of deaths in the United States.[28] In a study conducted on hog farms in Illinois and Iowa, 100% of the swine aged 9 and 12 weeks tested positive for MRSA, and the prevalence among their workers was 64%.[27]

You can reduce your exposure to antibiotics, growth hormones, and toxic runoff from livestock feedlots by choosing organic eggs, milk, yogurt, and cheeses and by eating free-range meat from animals raised without the use of these chemicals. You can also reduce your risk by eating vegetarian and vegan meals more often.

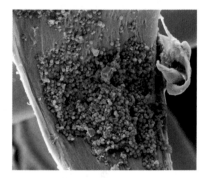

The resistant strain of bacteria responsible for methicillin-resistant *Staphylococcus aureus* (MRSA).

Residues Can Also Persist in Packaging

In December 2009, *Consumer Reports* magazine published the results of a study that shocked food-safety experts nationwide. It had found a chemical called bisphenol A, or BPA, in nearly all of the canned foods it had tested, from soups to infant formula. Why the concern about BPA? Although the effects of this chemical on humans are unknown, it's a form of synthetic estrogen, a female reproductive hormone, and both the National Toxicology Program of the National Institutes of Health and the FDA have some concern about its potential effects on the brain, behavior, and prostate gland of fetuses, infants, and young children.[29] Some studies have linked BPA to genital abnormalities and breast cancer in both males and females, prostate cancer, miscarriage, reduced sperm count, and even heart disease and diabetes.

In 2010, the FDA announced that it was conducting research into BPA and supporting industry efforts to remove it from all packaging. In addition to cans, BPA is found in beverage containers (including baby bottles), plastic dinnerware, auto parts, toys, dental sealants, and other products. So it's no wonder that scientists at the CDC have found measurable levels of BPA in the urine of nearly all the people it has tested.[30]

What to do? Although you can't control the level of BPA in canned foods you eat, you can control your use of plastics. Avoid carrying, storing, or microwave-heating foods or liquids in bottles with the recycling code 3 or 7. Although number 2, 4, 5, and 6 plastics are generally considered to be BPA-free and safe for carrying or storing food, water, and other beverages, always use glass or ceramics when heating foods and fluids in the microwave.[29]

RECAP

Persistent organic pollutants (POPs) of concern include mercury, lead, and dioxins. Pesticides are used to prevent or reduce food crop losses but are potential toxins; therefore, it is essential to wash all produce carefully. The use of recombinant bovine growth hormone (rBGH) and antibiotics raises concerns about bovine and human health. BPA in packaging leaves a residue in foods that may be responsible for neurologic and other abnormalities, especially in infants and children. ∎

What's Behind the Rising "Food Movement"?

In 1993, four children in Washington State died after eating fast-food hamburgers contaminated with *E. coli*. Although certainly not the first food-safety incident to capture public attention, it marked a turning point, after which Americans increasingly questioned the assumption that all of our food is always entirely safe to eat. A national debate about food safety and food politics began; a series of investigative news articles, books, and films explored not only the health risks but also the environmental and social costs of contemporary methods of food production. Advocates for public health, animal welfare, farmland preservation, the rights of farmworkers, and environmental quality all came together in a common cause. The food movement was born. Although a comprehensive discussion of the food movement isn't possible here, let's take a brief look at some of its most recognizable concerns.

Organic Agriculture Reduces the Use of Pesticides

In the population boom that followed the end of World War II, the demand for food increased dramatically. The American chemical industry helped increase agricultural production by providing a variety of new fertilizers and pesticides, including an insecticide called DDT, which began poisoning not just insects but also fish and birds from the time it was first released for agricultural use in 1945. Then, in 1962, marine biologist Rachel Carson published *Silent Spring*, a book in which she described the harmful effects of DDT and other synthetic pesticides. The book's title referred to the effect of pesticides on songbirds, whose extinction would someday lead to a "silent spring." Scientists found Carson's research convincing, and readers flocked to her cause, creating a small but ever-growing demand for organic food.

The term *organic* describes foods that are grown without the use of toxic and persistent fertilizers and pesticides, genetic engineering, or irradiation. A recent national survey indicates that approximately 4% of all food products sold in the United States are now organic. Between 1990 and 2008, sales of organic products in the United States skyrocketed from $1 billion to over $28 billion.[31]

To Be Labeled Organic, Foods Must Meet Federal Standards

In 2002, the National Organic Program (NOP) of the USDA established organic standards that provide uniform definitions for all organic products. Any product claiming to be organic must comply with the following definitions:

- *100% organic:* products containing only organically produced ingredients, excluding water and salt
- *Organic:* products containing 95% organically produced ingredients by weight, excluding water and salt, with the remaining ingredients consisting of those products not commercially available in organic form
- *Made with organic ingredients:* a product containing more than 70% organic ingredients

If a processed product contains less than 70% organically produced ingredients, those products cannot use the term *organic* in the principal display panel, but ingredients that are organically produced can be specified on the ingredients statement on the information panel. Products that are "100% organic" and "organic" may display the USDA organic seal (**Figure 15.14**).

Farms certified as organic must pass an inspection by a government-approved certifier, who verifies that the farmer is following all USDA organic standards.[32] Organic farming methods are strict and require farmers to find natural alternatives to many common problems, such as weeds and insects. Contrary to common belief, organic farmers can use pesticides as a final option for pest control when all other methods have failed or are known to be ineffective, but they are restricted to a limited number that have been approved for use. Organic farmers emphasize the use of renewable resources and the conservation of soil and water. Once a crop is harvested, a winter crop (usually a legume) is planted to help fix nitrogen in the soil and decrease erosion, which also lessens the need for fertilizers.

Organic meat, poultry, eggs, and dairy products come from animals fed only organic feed, and if the animals become ill, they are removed from the others until well again. None of these animals are given growth hormones to increase their size or ability to produce milk.

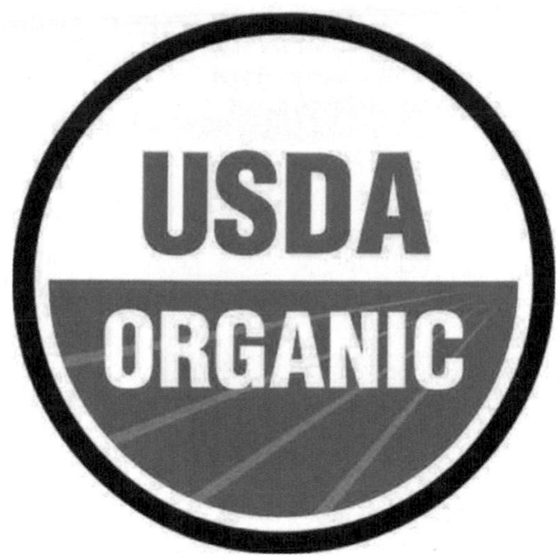

Research Data Supporting a Nutritional Advantage of Organically Grown Foods Are Inconclusive

Over the past decade, many studies have found that some organically grown fruits and vegetables, from strawberries to corn, are higher in certain vitamins and antioxidant phytochemicals than their non-organic counterparts.[33-36] However, a 2009 systematic review of 162 studies published from 1958 through 2008 found no nutritional superiority of organically produced foods over foods conventionally produced. The study's lead author concluded that there is no evidence to support the selection of organic foods for nutritional superiority.[37] Still, many people choose organic produce because of concerns about their exposure to pesticides.

FIGURE 15.14 The USDA organic seal identifies foods that are at least 95% organic.

Sustainable Agriculture Preserves the Environment and Promotes Food Diversity

Another issue at the heart of the food movement is sustainability. The EPA defines **sustainability** as the ability to meet, or satisfy, basic economic, social, and security needs now and in the future without undermining the natural resource base and environmental quality on which life depends.[38] Whereas some people view sustainability as a lofty but impractical ideal, others point out that it's a necessary condition of human survival. That's because sustainable practices can reduce the pollution of our soil and water and help reverse America's declining food diversity. To achieve both of these goals, experts argue that we must reduce our dependence on corporate farming. To understand the impact of corporate farming, let's review some history.

Beginning in the 1960s, revisions of the federal Agricultural Adjustment Act, commonly called the *farm bill*, provided financial incentives for America's farmers to "get big or get out."[39] The number of small farms dwindled, and the remaining industrial operations focused on increasing their production of the few subsidized crops, such as corn. To do so, industrial farming relied on pesticides, fertilizers, and antibiotics on feedlots, practices that prompted a sharp increase in soil and water pollution. In the Salinas and lower San Joaquin valleys of California, for example, pollution from chemical fertilizers and manure has contaminated the groundwater, making it undrinkable for at least the next 30 years.[39]

How have corporate farms reduced food diversity? When the farm bill began to subsidize target crops, those crops—especially corn—began to monopolize the food supply. As a result, the average American diet lost its variety, which is a key component of a healthful diet. As food expert Michael Pollan writes, if you are what you eat, most Americans are "corn": meat and poultry are corn-fed, french fries are cooked in corn oil, soft drinks are sweetened with high-fructose corn syrup, and fillers, binders, and dozens of other additives in processed foods are derived from corn.[40] Since no subsidies were paid for the production of fresh fruits and vegetables, their availability and variety plummeted, and they became more expensive. Americans soon discovered that they could enjoy an entire meal of corn-based foods for less than the cost of a pint of fresh raspberries.

Recently, various efforts within the food movement have begun to challenge the monopolization of our food supply. The following are a few examples of the many ways

sustainability The ability to meet, or satisfy, basic economic, social, and security needs now and in the future without undermining the natural resource base and environmental quality on which life depends.

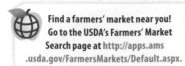

Find a farmers' market near you!
Go to the USDA's Farmers' Market
Search page at http://apps.ams
.usda.gov/FarmersMarkets/Default.aspx.

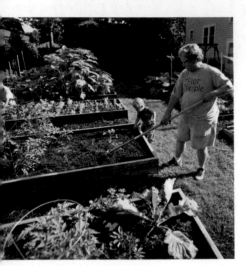

Modified farming techniques, such as using raised beds, enable urban and suburban residents to grow their own fruits and vegetables.

that individuals, communities, and corporations are promoting sustainability and food diversity:

■ *Family farms.* For the first time in decades, the number of farms in the United States has been increasing. The USDA's most recent Census of Agriculture showed a 4% increase in the number of farms between 2002 and 2007—a net increase of more than 75,000 farms.[41] And many of the new farmers are young adults taking advantage of programs offering land, financial support, and mentoring. Moreover, many are dedicated to organic farming, crop diversity, and other practices of sustainable agriculture.

■ *Community supported agriculture (CSA).* In CSA programs, a farmer sells a certain number of "shares" to the public. Shares typically consist of a box of produce from the farm on a regular basis, such as once weekly throughout the growing season. Farmers get cash early on, as well as guaranteed buyers. Consumers get fresh, locally grown food. Together, farmers and consumers develop ongoing relationships as they share the bounty in a good year, as well as the losses when weather extremes or blight reduces yield. Although there is no national database on CSA programs, the organization LocalHarvest lists over 4,000.[42] For more information on CSA programs, including a map locating programs in the United States, go to www.localharvest.org/csa/.

■ *Farmers' markets.* There are now more than 7,000 farmers' markets in the United States, more than four times the number when the USDA began compiling these data in 1994.[43] Along with CSAs, farmers' markets represent a growing trend toward the consumption of "local food"—that is, food grown within a few hundred miles of the consumer. Supporters claim that consuming local food limits energy use and greenhouse gas emissions from transportation (so-called food miles) and that these foods are fresher and nutritionally superior. Although researchers agree that the lowest environmental impact is associated with consuming foods harvested in-season from a local farm, this is not possible year-round in the many regions of the world with short growing seasons. In such cases, the resource costs of both greenhouse cultivation and long-term storage of foods may exceed the energy costs of transported foods.[44]

■ *Urban agriculture.* Urban agriculture is on the rise. From Pittsburgh to San Francisco, city governments are changing zoning codes to encourage the cultivation of vegetable gardens on rooftops, in abandoned parking lots, and even as part of the landscaping on municipal properties.[45]

Nutri-Case

Theo

"I got really sick yesterday after eating lunch in the cafeteria. I had a turkey sandwich, potato salad, and a cola. A few hours later, in the middle of basketball practice, I started to shake and sweat. I felt really nauseated and barely made it to the bathroom before vomiting. Then I went back to my dorm room and crawled into bed. This morning I still feel a little sick to my stomach, and sort of weak. I asked a couple of my friends who ate in the cafeteria yesterday if they got sick, and neither of them did, but I still think it was the food. I'm going off-campus for lunch from now on!"

Do you think that Theo's illness was foodborne? If so, what food(s) do you most suspect? What do you think of his plan to go off-campus for lunch from now on?

- *School gardens.* The School Garden Association of America was founded in 1910, and in 1914 the federal government created the Office of School and Home Gardening within the US Bureau of Education.[46] During World Wars I and II, school gardening became part of the war effort; however, in the postwar decades, the number of school gardens dwindled. Recently, growing concerns about childhood obesity, the poor quality of children's diets, and their reduced opportunities for physical activity has renewed interest in school gardens. In partnership with the AmeriCorps Service Network, a new effort called FoodCorps was launched in 2009 to increase school garden programs across the United States. In addition to promoting student acceptance of fruits and vegetables, school garden programs teach valuable lessons in nutrition, agriculture, and even cooking. In many schools, cafeterias incorporate the foods into the school lunch menu. In the 2011–2012 school year, FoodCorps served nearly 50,000 children.[47]

- *Corporate involvement.* Whereas many smaller natural-food companies have long made sustainable agriculture part of their company identity, only recently has the food movement moved into corporate America. In 2010, the world's largest retailer, Walmart, unveiled a set of global sustainable agriculture goals the company intends to reach by the year 2015. Those goals include selling $1 billion in foods from small and mid-size local farms and providing training in sustainable farming practices to 1 million farmers.[48] In early 2011, McDonald's Corporation announced its own new sustainable agriculture commitment, and other retailers and restaurant chains are expected to follow suit.

Public health experts point out that these efforts to promote sustainability also have the potential to reduce the number of so-called **food deserts**—areas such as some inner-city neighborhoods and isolated rural regions where people lack access to affordable, nutritious food. For example, Philadelphia has the highest obesity rate and the greatest percentage of people in poverty of any large American city. As part of a new national initiative called Healthy Corner Stores, Philadelphia in 2012 invested $900,000 in 600 of the city's corner stores to increase city residents' access to healthy foods, such as fresh produce.[49]

Personal Choices Can Help Promote Food Equity

You might think of the food movement as affluent Americans shopping at a farmers' market. However, the introduction of corporate farming has displaced small-scale farmers and reduced food diversity in developing as well as developed nations. Currently, just four companies control 75% of the international grain trade.[50] Monopoly control of genetically modified, nonrenewable seed has had tragic consequences. By one estimate, a quarter million farmers have taken their lives because of debt induced by the high cost of nonrenewable seed.[51]

Corporate farming has also monopolized agricultural labor, forcing farmworkers to accept poverty-level wages, and substandard and even dangerous living conditions for their labor. In the past decade, for example, the owners of seven Florida farms have been convicted of beating, chaining, and stealing from laborers in what a Florida district attorney described as "slavery." While performing backbreaking labor, America's 6 million farmworkers are continually exposed to UV radiation, pesticides, and crop dusts and pests, and they often lack basic sanitation, access to shade and water, and healthcare.[39] Not surprisingly, the life expectancy of U.S. farmworkers is just 49 years.[50]

In a climate in which power over food is ever more tightly controlled, the food movement is providing ordinary citizens a means to promote change. Across national boundaries, people just like you are making simple choices—such as purchasing only **fair trade** goods or supporting local farms—that are making a difference.

food desert A community in which residents lack access to affordable fresh fruits and vegetables and other healthful foods.

fair trade A trading partnership promoting equity in international trading relations, and contributing to sustainable development by securing the rights of marginalized producers and workers.

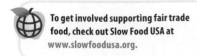

To get involved supporting fair trade food, check out Slow Food USA at www.slowfoodusa.org.

As Francis Moore Lappé, author of the groundbreaking book *Diet for a Small Planet*, explains, the food movement encourages us to think with an "eco-mind," refusing to accept scarcity and oppression for some in the name of production for many. By promoting the values of fairness, connection, and abundance, involvement in the movement encourages us to make choices in ways that can change our world.[50]

RECAP

The food movement promotes individual and collective action to preserve the environment, increase food diversity, and promote equity. The USDA regulates organic farming standards and inspects and certifies farms that follow all USDA organic standards. The USDA organic seal identifies foods that are at least 95% organic. The goal of sustainable agriculture initiatives, such as community supported agriculture and farmers' markets, is to produce an abundance of diverse foods without depleting natural resources or environmental quality. The value of equity requires us to make choices that reject exploitation and promote fair trade. ■

Chapter Review

TEST YOURSELF | ANSWERS

1 **F** Foodborne illness actually sickens about 48 million Americans each year, and about 3,000 die.

2 **F** Most cases of foodborne illness are caused by just one species of virus, called norovirus. Bacteria also commonly cause foodborne illness.

3 **F** Freezing destroys some microorganisms but only inhibits the ability of other microorganisms to reproduce. When the food is thawed, these cold-tolerant microorganisms resume reproduction.

4 **T** Although some studies have found higher levels of certain vitamins and antioxidant phytochemicals in organic foods, there are not enough studies published on this topic to state with confidence that organic foods are consistently more nutritious than nonorganic foods.

5 **T** Poverty, harsh labor, inadequate healthcare, exposure to pesticides, reduced access to safe drinking water, and many other factors reduce the life expectancy of U.S. farmworkers by nearly 30 years as compared to that of other Americans.

Summary

- Approximately 48 million Americans experience foodborne illness each year, and approximately 3,000 die as a result.

- Foodborne illness results from the consumption of food containing living microorganisms or their toxins.

- The majority of foodborne illnesses are due to a species of virus called norovirus. *Salmonella* is the most common bacterium involved in foodborne illness.

- Common food toxins include those produced by bacteria and fungi, toxic algae in fish and shellfish, and plant toxins.

- The body has several defense mechanisms, such as saliva, stomach acid, vomiting, diarrhea, and the inflammatory response, that help rid us of offending microorganisms and toxins.

- In order to reproduce in foods, microbes require a precise range of temperature, humidity, acidity, and oxygen content.

- You can prevent foodborne illness at home by following these tips: Clean: wash your hands and kitchen surfaces often. Separate: isolate foods to prevent cross-contamination. Chill: refrigerate or freeze perishable foods. Cook: heat foods long enough and at the required temperature to ensure proper cooking.

- Common food preservation techniques include canning, pasteurization, special packaging, the addition of preservatives, and irradiation.

- Food additives are natural or synthetic ingredients added to foods during processing to enhance them in some way. They include flavorings, colorings, nutrients, texturizers, and other additives.

- The GRAS list identifies several hundred substances that have either been tested and found to be safe and approved for use in the food industry or are deemed safe as a result of consensus among experts qualified by scientific training and experience.

- In genetic modification, the DNA of an organism is manipulated to enhance certain qualities, such as herbicide resistance or nutrient concentration.

- Persistent organic pollutants (POPs) are chemicals released into the atmosphere as a result of industry, agriculture, automobile emissions, and improper waste disposal. Plants, animals, and fish absorb the chemicals from contaminated soil or water and pass them on as part of the food chain.

- Large predatory fish, such as swordfish, shark, king mackerel, and tilefish, tend to contain high levels of mercury, which is toxic to the nervous system.

- Although pesticides prevent or reduce crop losses, they are potential toxins; thus, the EPA regulates their use.

- Recombinant bovine growth hormone (rBGH) is injected into beef and dairy cows to increase their yield.

- Cows and pigs administered antibiotics have become significant reservoirs for the development of MRSA, an antibiotic-resistant strain of bacteria.

- Organic Standards in 2002 established uniform definitions for all organic products sold in the United States.

- The food movement encompasses a variety of initiatives intended to promote sustainability, preserve natural resources, increase access to a variety of nutritious foods, and reduce the exploitation of farmers and consumers throughout the world.

MasteringNutrition™

To further your understanding, go online and apply what you've learned to real-life case studies that will help you master the content!

Review Questions

1. The temperature in your refrigerator should be at or below
   a. 0°F.
   b. 20°F.
   c. 40°F.
   d. 60°F.

2. Leftovers from a meal should be refrigerated
   a. immediately after serving.
   b. within 30 minutes of serving.
   c. within 2 hours of serving.
   d. within 3 hours of serving.

3. Yeasts are
   a. a type of mold used in baked goods as a stabilizer.
   b. a type of bacterium that can cause food intoxication.
   c. a type of fungus used to ferment foods.
   d. a type of mold inhibitor used as a food preservative.

4. The potential spread of MRSA is a public health concern because
   a. MRSA is a strain of bacterium resistant to conventional antibiotics.
   b. MRSA readily spreads from animal populations to humans.
   c. MRSA can be fatal.
   d. all of the above.

5. Foods that are labeled 100% organic
   a. contain only organically produced ingredients, excluding water and salt.
   b. may display the EPA's organic seal.
   c. were produced without the use of pesticides.
   d. contain foods from plant sources only.

6. **True or false?** You prepare a potato, egg, and red onion salad with mayonnaise at 10:00 AM for a 2:00 PM barbecue. It is safe to leave the salad at room temperature until the barbecue.

7. **True or false?** Recombinant bovine growth hormone (rBGH) is used to increase the amount and quality of meat in beef herds and milk production in dairy cows.

8. **True or false?** In the United States, farms certified as organic are allowed to use pesticides under certain conditions.

9. **True or false?** Irradiation makes foods radioactive.

10. **True or false?** BPA is a persistent organic pollutant.

11. A box of macaroni and cheese has the words *Certified Organic* on the front and the following ingredients listed on the side: organic durum semolina pasta (organic durum semolina, water), organic cheddar cheese (organic cultured pasteurized milk, salt, enzymes), whey, salt. Is this food 100% organic? Why or why not? Does it contain any food additives? If so, identify them.

12. Steven and Dante go to a convenience store after a tennis match, looking for something to quench their thirst. Steven chooses a national brand of pasteurized orange juice, and Dante chooses a bottle of locally produced, organic, unpasteurized apple juice. Steven points out to Dante that his juice is not pasteurized, but Dante shrugs and says, "I'm more afraid of the pesticides they used on the oranges in your juice than I am of microorganisms in mine!" Which juice would you choose, and why?

13. Pickling is a food-preservation technique that involves soaking foods, such as cucumbers, in a solution containing vinegar (acetic acid). Why is pickling effective in preventing food spoilage?

14. In the 1950s and 1960s in Minamata, Japan, more than 100 cases of a similar illness were recorded: patients, many of whom were infants or young children, suffered irreversible damage to the nervous system. A total of forty-six people died. Adults with the disease and mothers of afflicted young children had one thing in common: they had frequently eaten fish caught in Minamata Bay. What do you think might have been the cause of this illness? Using key words from this description, research the event on the Internet and identify the culprit(s).

15. Your sister Joy, who attends a culinary arts school, is visiting you for dinner. You want to impress her, so you've decided to make chicken marsala. You begin that afternoon by removing two chicken breasts from the freezer and putting them in a bowl in the refrigerator to thaw. Then you go shopping for fresh salad ingredients. When you get home from the market, you take the chicken breasts from the refrigerator and set them on a clean cutting board. You then take the lettuce, red pepper, and scallions you just bought, put them in a colander, and rinse them. Next, you slice them with a clean knife on your marble countertop and toss them together in a salad. You put the chicken breasts in a frying pan and cook them until they lose their pink color. In a separate pan, you prepare the sauce. Finally, using a clean knife, you slice some freshly baked bread on the countertop. You then wash the knives and the cutting board you used for the chicken. Joy arrives and admires your skill in cooking. Later that night, you both wake up vomiting. Identify at least two aspects of your food preparation that might have contributed to your illness.

Answers to Review Questions can be found online in the MasteringNutrition Study Area.

Web Links

www.foodsafety.gov
Foodsafety.gov
Use this website as a gateway to a range of government food safety information; it contains updates, safety reports, help with reporting illnesses and product complaints, news on foodborne pathogens, and more.

www.cdc.gov/foodsafety/index.html
CDC Food Safety Homepage
This section of the larger CDC website focuses on issues specifically related to food safety, with a range of informational resources.

www.fightbac.org
Partnership for Food Safety Education
The website of the Partnership for Food Safety Education (PFSE), features the Fight BAC! food safety initiative, designed to educate consumers about food safety issues.

www.epa.gov/pesticides
US Environmental Protection Agency: Pesticides
This site provides information on agricultural and home-use pesticides, pesticide-related health and safety issues, environmental effetcs, and government regulation of pesticide types and uses.

www.ams.usda.gov
USDA National Organic Program
Click on "National Organic Program" to get to the web page describing the NOP's standards and labeling program, consumer information, and publications.

www.ota.com
Organic Trade Association
This website provides lots of detailed information in support of the OTA's mission to promote and protect organic trade to benefit the environment, farmers, the public, and the economy.

www.fsis.usda.gov/food_safety_education/index.asp
The Food Safety and Inspection Service area of the larger USDA website is designed to educate the public about safe food handling practices, and reduce the risks from foodborne illnesses through a variety of tools, resources, and links to related topic areas.

References

1. US Centers for Disease Control and Prevention (CDC). 2012, May 30. Salmonella Outbreaks. www.cdc.gov/salmonella/outbreaks.html.
2. US Centers for Disease Control and Prevention (CDC). 2012, June 10. E. coli Outbreak Investigations. www.cdc.gov/ecoli/outbreaks.html.
3. US Centers for Disease Control and Prevention (CDC). 2012, June 11. Estimates of Foodborne Illness in the United States. www.cdc.gov/foodborneburden/index.html.
4. Hamburg, M. A. 2011, January 3. Food Safety Modernization Act: Putting the Focus on Prevention. www.whitehouse.gov/blog/2011/01/03/food-safety-modernization-act-putting-focus-prevention.
5. US Centers for Disease Control and Prevention (CDC). 2012, May 22. Trends in Foodborne Illness in the United States, 1996–2010. www.cdc.gov/foodborneburden/trends-in-foodborne-illness.html.
6. Scallan, E., R. M. Hockstra, F. J. Angulo, R. V. Tauxe, M. A. Widdowso, S. L. Roy, et al. 2011. Foodborne illness acquired in the United States—major pathogens. Emerg. Infect. Dis. DOI: 10.3201/eid1701.P11101.
7. Hall, A. J. 2011, March 22. Norovirus in the News. www.foodsafety.gov/blog/norovirus.html.
8. US Centers for Disease Control and Prevention (CDC). 2011, March 8. Parasites—Giardia. www.cdc.gov/parasites/giardia/.
9. US Department of Agriculture Food Safety and Inspection Service. 2011, March 17. Common Questions: Food Safety. www.fsis.usda.gov/help/faqs_hotline_preparation/index.asp#10.
10. US Centers for Disease Control and Prevention (CDC). (2010, July 20). Marine Toxins. www.cdc.gov/nczved/divisions/dfbmd/diseases/marine_toxins.
11. Habal, R. 2011, July 27. Mushroom Toxicity. Medscape Reference. http://emedicine.medscape.com/article/167398-overview 10.
12. Woods Hole Oceanographic Institution. 2012, April 4. Researchers Report Potential for a "Moderate" New England "Red Tide" in 2012. www.whoi.edu/main/news-releases?tid=3622&cid=133929.
13. National Institutes of Health. 2011, December 15. Potato Plant Poisoning: Green Tubers and Sprouts. MedlinePlus. www.nlm.nih.gov/medlineplus/ency/article/002875.htm.
14. US Department of Agriculture Food Safety and Inspection Service. 2011, June 28. Be Food Safe. www.fsis.usda.gov/Be%5FFoodSafe/.
15. US Department of Agriculture Food Safety and Inspection Service. 2010. Fight Bac FactSheet: Chill. www.fightbac.org/storage/documents/flyers/chill_%20fightbac_factsheet_2010_color.pdf.
16. US Department of Agriculture Food Safety and Inspection Service. 2011, September 16. Food Product Dating. Fact Sheets: Food Labeling. www.fsis.usda.gov/Factsheets/Food_Product_Dating/.

17. US Centers for Disease Control and Prevention (CDC). 2012, May 17. Multistate Outbreak of *Salmonella* Bareilly and *Salmonella* Nchanga Infections Associated with a Raw Scraped Ground Tuna Product. www.cdc.gov/salmonella/bareilly-04-12/index.html.

18. FoodSafety.gov. (n.d.). Checklist of Foods to Avoid During Pregnancy. www.foodsafety.gov/poisoning/risk/pregnant/chklist_pregnancy.html.

19. Center for Science in the Public Interest (CSPI). 2012. Chemical Cuisine. Learn About Food Additives. www.cspinet.org/reports/chemcuisine.htm.

20. US Department of Agriculture Economic Research Service. 2011, July 1. Data Sets: Adoption of Genetically Engineered Crops in the US. www.ers.usda.gov/Data/BiotechCrops.

21. US Environmental Protection Agency (EPA). 2012, April 19. Persistent Organic Pollutants: A Global Issue, a Global Response. www.epa.gov/international/toxics/pop.html.

22. Food and Drug Administration (FDA). 2011, October 25. What You Need to Know About Mercury in Fish and Shellfish. www.fda.gov/Food/ResourcesForYou/Consumers/ucm110591.htm.

23. US Environmental Protection Agency (EPA). 2012, February 17. EPA's Reanalysis of Key Issues Related to Dixoin Toxicity and Response to NAS Comments, Volume 1. EPA 600/R-10/038F. www.epa.gov/iris/supdocs/dioxinv1sup.pdf.

24. US Food and Drug Administration (FDA). 2012, February. Questions and Answers About Dioxins and Food Safety. www.fda.gov/Food/FoodSafety/FoodContaminantsAdulteration/ChemicalContaminants/DioxinsPCBs/ucm077524.htm?utm_campaign=Google2&utm_source=fdaSearch&utm_medium=website&utm_term=questions%20and%20answers%20about%20dioxins&utm_content=1.

25. US Environmental Protection Agency (EPA). 2012, May 9. Pesticides and Food: Healthy, Sensible Food Practices. www.epa.gov/pesticides/food/tips.htm.

26. American Cancer Society. 2011, February 18. Recombinant Bovine Growth Hormone. www.cancer.org/cancer/cancercauses/othercarcinogens/athome/recombinant-bovine-growth-hormone.

27. Smith, T. C., et al. 2009. Methicillin-Resistant *Staphylococcus aureus* (MRSA) Strain ST398 Is Present in Midwestern U.S. Swine and Swine Workers. *PLoS ONE* 4(1):e4258. Doi: 10.1371/journal.pone.0004258.

28. US Centers for Disease Control and Prevention (CDC). 2011, April 15. Methicillin-Resistant *Staphylococcus aureus* (MRSA) Infections. www.cdc.gov/mrsa/.

29. US Food and Drug Administration (FDA). 2012, March 30. Bisphenol A (BPA): Use in Food Contact Application. www.fda.gov/NewsEvents/PublicHealthFocus/ucm064437.htm.

30. US Centers for Disease Control and Prevention (CDC). 2010, February 11. Fact Sheet: Bisphenol A (BPA). www.cdc.gov/exposurereport/BisphenolA_FactSheet.html.

31. Organic Trade Association. 2011. OTA's 2011 Organic Industry Survey. www.ota.com/pics/documents/2011OrganicIndustrySurvey.pdf.

32. US Department of Agriculture Agricultural Marketing Service. National Organic Program. Understanding Organic. 2010, February 5. www.ams.usda.gov/AMSv1.0/ams.fetchTemplateData.do?template=TemplateA&leftNav=NationalOrganicProgram&page=NOPUnderstandingOrganic&description=Understanding%20Organic&acct=nopgeninfo.

33. Reganold, J. P., P. K. Andrews, J. R. Reeve, L. Carpenter-Boggs, C. W. Schadt, J. R. Alldredge, C. F. Ross, N. M. Davies, and J. Zhou. 2010. Fruit and soil quality of organic and conventional strawberry agroecosystems. *Plos ONE* 5(9):e123456.

34. Asami, D. K., Y. J. Hong, D. M. Barrett, and A. E. Mitchell. 2003. Comparison of the total phenolic and ascorbic acid content of freeze-dried and air-dried marionberry, strawberry, and corn grown using conventional, organic, and sustainable agricultural practices. *J. Agric. Food Chem.* 51(5):1237–1241.

35. Carbonaro, M., M. Mattera, S. Nicoli, P. Bergamo, and M. Cappelloni. 2002. Modulation of antioxidant compounds in organic vs conventional fruit (peach, *Prunus persica* L., and pear, *Pyrus communis* L.). *J. Agric. Food Chem.* 50(19):5458–5462.

36. Grinder-Pedersen, L., S. E. Rasmussen, S. Bügel, L. O. Jørgensen, D. Vagn Gundersen, and B. Sandström. 2003. Effect of diets based on foods from conventional versus organic production on intake and excretion of flavonoids and markers of antioxidative defense in humans. *Agric. Food Chem.* 51(19):5671–5676.

37. Dangour, A. D., S. K. Dodhia, A. Hayter, E. Allen, K. Lock, and R. Uauy. 2009. Nutritional quality of organic foods: a systematic review. *Amer. J. of Clin. Nut.* DOI:10.3945/ajcn.2009.28041. www.ajcn.org/cgi/content/abstract/ajcn.2009.28041v1.

38. US Environmental Protection Agency (EPA). 2011, March 2. What Is Sustainability? www.epa.gov/sustainability/basicinfo.htm.

39. Imhoff, D., and M. Dimock. 2012, June 8. America needs a farm bill that works. *Los Angeles Times.* www.latimes.com/news/opinion/commentary/la-oe-imhoff-farm-bill-20120608,0,7923048.story.

40. Pollan, M. 2006. *The Omnivore's Dilemma: A Natural History of Four Meals.* New York: Penguin.

41. US Department of Agriculture. 2008. 2007 Census of Agriculture. www.agcensus.usda.gov/Publications/2007/Online_Highlights/Fact_Sheets/farm_numbers.pdf.

42. LocalHarvest. 2011. Community Supported Agriculture. www.localharvest.org/csa/.

43. US Department of Agriculture Agricultural Marketing Service. 2011, August 8. Farmers Market Growth: 1994–2011. www.ams.usda.gov/AMSv1.0/ams.fetchTemplateData.do?template=TemplateS&navID=WholesaleandFarmersMarkets&leftNav=WholesaleandFarmersMarkets&page=WFMFarmersMarketGrowth&description=Farmers%20Market%20Growth&acct=frmrdirmkt.

44. Edwards-Jones, G. 2010. Does eating local food reduce the environmental impact of food production and enhance consumer health? *Proceedings of the Nutrition Society* 69:582–591.

45. Bittman, M. 2011. Food: six things to feel good about. *The New York Times,* March 22. http://opinionator.blogs.nytimes.com/2011/03/22/food-six-things-to-feel-good-about/?emc=eta1.

46. Library of Congress. 2010, July 20. School Gardens with Constance Carter. Journeys and Crossings. www.loc.gov/rr/program/journey/schoolgardens-transcript.html.

47. Eschmeyer, D. 2012, June 19. FoodCorps is one of several efforts to give children healthy foods. *Washington Post*. www.washingtonpost.com/postlive/foodcorps-is-one-of-several-efforts-to-give-children-healthy-foods/2012/06/18/gJQAepNLoV_story.html.

48. Walmart. 2010, October 14. Walmart Sustainable Agriculture: Fact Sheet. http://graphics8.nytimes.com/packages/pdf/opinion/Fact_Sheet_Walmart_Sustainable.pdf.

49. Healthy Corner Stores Network. 2012, June 20. Food Deserts. www.healthycornerstores.org/tag/food-deserts.

50. Moore Lappé, F. 2011, September 14. The Food Movement: Its Power and Possibilities. The Nation. www.thenation.com/article/163403/food-movement-its-power-and-possibilities.

51. Shiva, V. 2011, September 14. Resisting the Corporate Theft of Seeds. The Nation. www.thenation.com/article/163401/resisting-corporate-theft-seeds.

Nutrition DEBATE

Genetically Modified Organisms: A Blessing or a Curse?

Current advances in biotechnology have opened the door to one of the most controversial topics in food science: genetically modified organisms (GMOs). GMOs are organisms created through *genetic engineering*, the standard U.S. term for a process in which foreign genes are spliced into a nonrelated species, creating an entirely new (*transgenic*) organism. *Biotech foods, gene foods, bioengineered food, gene-altered foods,* and *transgenic foods* are other terms used to describe foods that have been created through genetic engineering.

Developing GMOs is a lengthy, tedious, and costly process requiring years of research and testing. After carefully selecting and cultivating cells from an organism with a desired trait, the DNA is removed and scientists identify, isolate, and extract individual genes that code for the desired functions. Using bacteria to transfer these genes, scientists incorporate them into new cells, where the introduced genes trigger the synthesis of proteins that accomplish the chosen functions. By using bacteria as the selected medium, DNA can be easily and efficiently produced and incorporated into any cell. Any plant, animal, or microorganism (such as bacteria or yeast) that has had its DNA altered in a laboratory to enhance or change certain characteristics is considered genetically engineered. For example, *Bacillus thuringiensis* (Bt) is a genetically engineered bacterium that is used as a pesticide.

Since 1996, hundreds of genetically modified foods have been incorporated into our food market. In addition, several important medical therapeutics have been developed using genetic engineering, including human insulin, human growth factor, and factor VIII (a protein needed for blood clotting in people with hemophilia). Many scientists are working on *gene therapy*—that is, replacing defective genes in patients with genetic diseases such as sickle cell anemia with genes from people without the disease. Currently, research labs around the world are devoted to expanding the capabilities and applications of genetic engineering.

Many people envision an ever-expanding role for genetic engineering in food production. They base their support on the numerous potential benefits resulting from the application of this technology:

- Enhanced taste and nutritional quality of food
- Crops that grow faster, have higher yields, can be grown in inhospitable soils, and have increased resistance to pests, disease, herbicides, and spoilage
- Increased production of high-quality meat, eggs, and milk
- Improved animal health due to increased disease resistance and overall hardiness

- Environmentally responsible outcomes, such as a 9.1% reduction in pesticide use between 1996 and 2010, the use of less harmful herbicides and insecticides, conservation of water due largely to the development of drought-tolerant species of corn, reduced use of energy and emission of greenhouse gases because of reduced need for ploughing and pesticide spraying, and soil conservation due to higher productivity on arable land[1]
- Increased food security for countries struggling with food insecurity and starvation by increasing the income of small farmers, improving crop yields, and producing food crops with greater resistance to drought[1]

Despite these benefits, there is significant opposition to genetic engineering. Detractors cite a wide range of concerns related to environmental hazards, human health risks, and economic instability:

- Gene transfer from GM foods to cells of the body or to bacteria in the gastrointestinal tract, which could adversely affect human health; for example, if antibiotic-resistant genes were transferred, susceptibility to infectious disease could increase[2]
- Unintentional transfer of genes to nontarget species through cross-pollination, which could result in undesirable plants, such as superweeds that are tolerant to conventional herbicides or a food tainted with non-food-grade ingredients; the risk of such transfer is real, as was shown when traces of a type of maize that was approved for use only in animal feed appeared in maize products for human consumption in the United States[2]
- Loss of biodiversity of plants and animals
- Increased risk of either creating a new allergen or causing allergic reactions in susceptible individuals
- Development of new diseases that can attack plants, animals, and humans
- Production of bacteria that are resistant to all antibiotics
- Potential for only a few food companies and countries to control the majority of world food production; for example, the seed industry has become increasingly concentrated as large bioengineering firms have bought up smaller seed companies, then increased seed prices for crops such as corn and soybeans[3]
- Inadequate or nonexistent labeling laws that prevent consumers from knowing if they are consuming foods that are genetically modified
- Creation of biological weapons and increased risk of bioterrorism

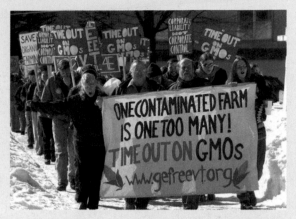

Many people oppose the genetic engineering of foods for environmental, health, or economic reasons.

Some who oppose genetic engineering believe that it is unnatural and unethical to alter the genes of any organism. Most opponents base their concern on the fact that the potential long-term risks and dangers are unknown and may far outweigh the potential short-term benefits. Many argue that, at the very least, all GM foods should be labeled, so that consumers know what they are purchasing. As of 2012, the US Food and Drug Administration did not require that all genetically engineered foods be identified as such; however, in March 2012, fifty-five members of Congress signed a letter to the FDA requesting support of a petition to require mandatory labeling of all GM foods.[4]

Genetically modified crops are grown in twenty-nine countries; however, the top two producers—the United States (43% of global total) and Brazil (19% of global total)—produce more GM crops than the other twenty-seven countries combined.[4] The primary crops in the United States are corn, soybeans, cotton, canola, sugarbeets, alfalfa, papaya, and squash. Brazil's GM crops are limited to soybeans, corn, and cotton. Even though the United States and Canada are among the top five, regions within these countries have succeeded in banning the production of GMOs. These include several counties in California, including Mendocino, Trinity, and Marin, and the Canadian province of Prince Edward Island.

The European Union (EU) has strict regulations regarding GMOs, including having mechanisms in place to track GMO products through production and distribution chains and to monitor any effect of GMOs on the environment. All foods produced for human consumption and all animal feed products that contain GMOs must be clearly labeled. In addition, any foods that are produced from GMO ingredients must be clearly labeled, even if the final food product does not contain the DNA or protein of the original GMO. Currently, only two biotech crops—corn and potatoes—are approved for cultivation in the EU,[1,5] and only fifteen genetically modified foods are marketed in the EU. Companies that wish to market GMOs and genetically modified foods in the EU must submit an application that includes a full environmental risk assessment and a safety assessment. This report is then reviewed by the designated government agencies and a decision is made regarding the application. Recently, scientific opinion in the EU appears to have shifted toward greater support of GM foods: in October 2011, a large group of Swedish and UK scientists publicly urged the revision of current European legislation to allow society to benefit from the production of GM crops.[1]

As GMOs and genetically modified foods have been available for only a few years, it will take more time to understand their impact on the world.

CRITICAL THINKING QUESTIONS

- What's your view of the controversy around the genetic engineering of food?
- Based on your current knowledge of GMOs and genetically modified foods, do you support their use and mass distribution both within the United States and around the world?
- Do you think that genetically modified foods should be clearly labeled for consumers?
- Do you have any reservations about buying and consuming genetically modified foods? If so, what are they?

REFERENCES

1. International Service for the Acquisition of Agri-Biotech Applications (ISAAA). 2012. *Global Status of Commercialized Biotech/GM Crops: 2011.* ISAAA Brief No. 43-2011: Executive summary. Ithaca, NY: ISAAA. www.isaaa.org/resources/publications/briefs/43/executivesummary/default.asp.
2. World Health organization (WHO). 2010. Twenty Questions on Genetically Modified (GM) Foods. www.who.int/foodsafety/publications/biotech/20questions/en/.
3. Neuman, W. 2010. Justice Dept. Tells Farmers It Will Press Agriculture Industry on Antitrust. *The New York Times,* March 12. www.nytimes.com/2010/03/13/business/13seed.html.
4. Congress of the United States. 2012, March 12. Letter to Margaret Hamburg, Commissioner of the Food and Drug Administration. www.centerforfoodsafety.org/wp-content/uploads/2012/03/Final-Signed-GE-Labeling-Letter.pdf.
5. Kanter, J. 2010. E.U. Clears Biotech Potato for Cultivation. *The New York Times,* March 3. www.nytimes.com/2010/03/03/business/global/03potato.html.

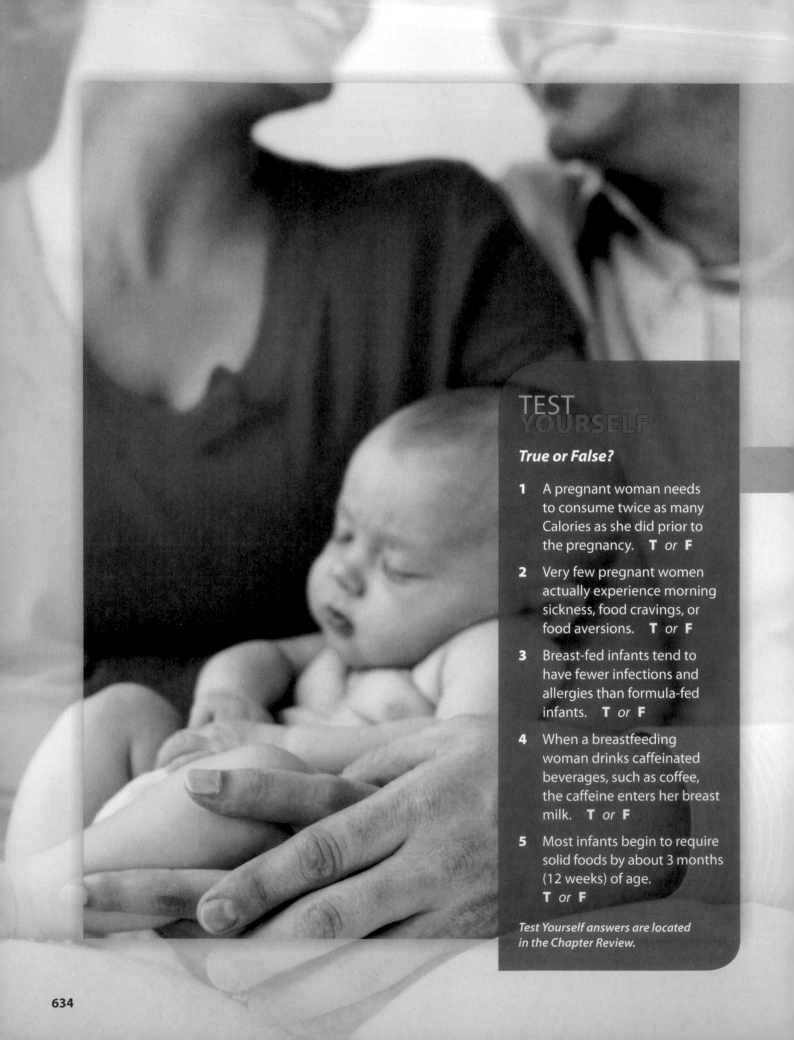

True or False?

1   A pregnant woman needs to consume twice as many Calories as she did prior to the pregnancy.   **T** *or* **F**

2   Very few pregnant women actually experience morning sickness, food cravings, or food aversions.   **T** *or* **F**

3   Breast-fed infants tend to have fewer infections and allergies than formula-fed infants.   **T** *or* **F**

4   When a breastfeeding woman drinks caffeinated beverages, such as coffee, the caffeine enters her breast milk.   **T** *or* **F**

5   Most infants begin to require solid foods by about 3 months (12 weeks) of age.   **T** *or* **F**

Test Yourself answers are located in the Chapter Review.

16

Nutrition Through the Life Cycle: Pregnancy and the First Year of Life

Learning Objectives

After studying this chapter, you should be able to:

1. List four reasons that maintaining a nutritious diet is important for a woman of childbearing age even prior to conception, *pp. 636–637.*

2. Explore the relationship among fetal development, physiologic changes in the pregnant woman, and increasing nutrient requirements during the course of a pregnancy, *pp. 637–641.*

3. Identify the ranges of optimal weight gain for pregnant women, and the implications of too little or too much weight gain during pregnancy for both the mother and the developing baby, *pp. 641–643.*

4. Identify the macronutrient and micronutrient needs of pregnant women, including for supplements and fluids, *pp. 644–649.*

5. Discuss the key nutrient-related disorders commonly experienced by women during pregnancy, *pp. 649–653.*

6. Describe the key nutritional issues for pregnant adolescents and vegetarians, and exercise recommendations for most pregnant women, *pp. 653–655.*

7. Describe the physiologic aspects of lactation, and identify the key nutrient recommendations for and needs of breastfeeding women, *pp. 658–666.*

8. Review the perspectives surrounding the advantages and disadvantages of breastfeeding, including the role of fathers and siblings in infant bonding, *pp. 661–666.*

9. Identify the nutrient needs and growth patterns of developing infants, including their needs for supplements and fluids, *pp. 665–670.*

10. Identify the pros and cons of using formula, the challenges surrounding introducing solid foods, and the key areas of nutrient-related concerns for infants, *pp. 670–677.*

MasteringNutrition™

Go online for chapter quizzes, pre-tests, Interactive Activities, and more!

635

An active, curious 2-year-old, Tomas brings joy and laughter to his parents and family. That wasn't always the case, however. Tomas weighed just over 3 lb 5 oz at birth—about half of what an average full-term newborn weighs. Even today, Tomas is still small for his age and continues to struggle with his coordination and speech. Although the United States has an extensive and expensive healthcare system, the rate of low-birth-weight babies remains above 8%.[1] Moreover, our infant mortality rate—the number of deaths of infants before their first birthday—is now higher than that of over forty other developed, and under-developed, countries: in 2011, the United States recorded 6.1 infant deaths for every 1,000 live births, as compared to just 1.8 for Monaco, 2.2 for Japan, 2.3 for Singapore, and 2.7 for Sweden.[2]

What contributes to these troubling statistics? What are the short- and long-term effects of low birth weight on developing children? And what role does prenatal diet play in determining the future health and well-being of a child? In this chapter, we discuss how adequate nutrition supports fetal development, maintains a pregnant woman's health, and contributes to lactation. We then explore the nutrient needs of breastfeeding and formula-feeding infants.

Starting Out Right: Healthful Nutrition in Pregnancy

At no stage of life is nutrition more crucial than during fetal development and infancy. From conception through the end of the first year of life, adequate nutrition is essential for tissue formation, neurologic development, and bone growth, modeling, and remodeling. The ability to reach peak physical and intellectual potential in adult life is partly determined by the nutrition received during fetal development and the first year of life. Public health officials view pregnancy-related nutrition as so important to the health of the nation that several *Healthy People 2020* objectives are specific to prenatal and postnatal nutrition.[3] These objectives will be identified throughout this chapter.

Is Nutrition Important Before Conception?

Several factors make adequate nutrition important even before **conception,** the point at which a woman's ovum (egg) is fertilized with a man's sperm. First, some problems related to nutrient deficiency develop extremely early in the pregnancy, typically before the mother even realizes she is pregnant. An adequate and varied preconception diet reduces the risk for such problems, providing "insurance" during those first few weeks of pregnancy.

For example, failure of the spinal cord to close results in *neural tube defects;* these defects are closely related to inadequate folate status during the first few weeks after conception. For this reason, all women capable of becoming pregnant are encouraged to consume 400 µg of folic acid from fortified foods such as cereals or supplements daily, in addition to natural sources of folate from a varied, healthful diet. This recommendation should be followed by all women of childbearing age whether or not they plan to become pregnant.

Second, adopting a healthful diet and lifestyle prior to conception requires women to avoid alcohol, illegal drugs, tobacco, and other known *teratogens* (substances that cause birth defects). Women should also consult their healthcare provider about their consumption of caffeine, medications, herbs, and supplements; and if they smoke, they should attempt to quit.

Third, a healthful diet and appropriate levels of physical activity can help women achieve and maintain an optimal body weight prior to pregnancy. Women with a pre-pregnancy body mass index (BMI) between 19.8 and 26.0 have the best chance of an uncomplicated pregnancy and delivery, with low risk for negative outcomes, such as prolonged labor and cesarean section. As we will discuss in greater detail shortly, women with a BMI below or above this range prior to conception are at greater risk for pregnancy-related complications.

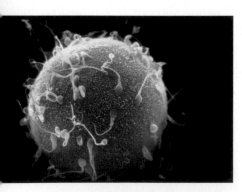

During conception, a sperm fertilizes an egg, creating a zygote.

conception The uniting of an ovum (egg) and sperm to create a fertilized egg, or zygote; also called *fertilization.*

Finally, maintaining a balanced and nourishing diet before conception reduces a woman's risk of developing a nutrition-related disorder during her pregnancy. These disorders, which we discuss later in the chapter, include gestational diabetes and hypertensive disorders. Although genetic and metabolic abnormalities are beyond the woman's control, following a healthful diet prior to conception is something a woman can do to help her fetus develop into a healthy baby.

A man's nutrition and lifestyle prior to conception is important as well. Malnutrition, such as severe zinc deficiency, contributes to abnormalities in sperm. Both sperm number and *motility* (ability to move) are reduced by alcohol consumption, as well as the use of certain prescription and illegal drugs. Moreover, smoking is known to damage sperm and reduce male fertility. Additionally, infections accompanied by a high fever can destroy sperm; so, to the extent that adequate nutrition keeps the immune system strong, it also promotes a man's fertility.

Why Is Nutrition Important During Pregnancy?

A balanced, nourishing diet throughout pregnancy provides the nutrients needed to support fetal growth and development without depriving the mother of nutrients she needs to maintain her own health. It also minimizes the risks of excess energy intake. A full-term pregnancy, also called the period of **gestation**, lasts 38 to 42 weeks and is divided into three **trimesters,** with each trimester lasting about 13 to 14 weeks.

The First Trimester

About once each month, a nonpregnant woman of childbearing age experiences *ovulation*, the release of an ovum (egg cell) from an ovary. The ovum is then drawn into the uterine (fallopian) tube. The first trimester (approximately weeks 1 through 13) begins when the ovum and sperm unite to form a single, fertilized cell called a **zygote.** As the zygote travels through the uterine tube, it further divides into a ball of twelve to sixteen cells, which at about day 4, arrives in the uterus (**Figure 16.1**). By day 10, the inner portion of the zygote,

gestation The period of intrauterine development from conception to birth.

trimester Any one of three stages of pregnancy, each lasting approximately 13 to 14 weeks.

zygote A fertilized egg (ovum) consisting of a single cell.

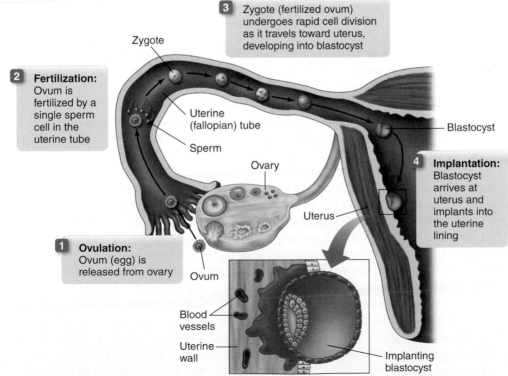

FIGURE 16.1 Ovulation, conception, and implantation.

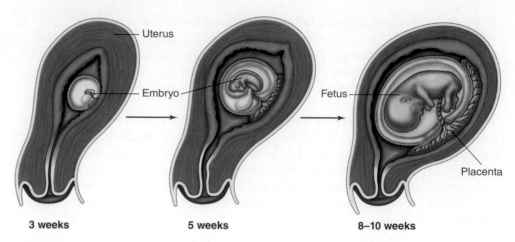

FIGURE 16.2 Human embryonic development during the first 10 weeks. Organ systems are most vulnerable to teratogens during this time, when cells are dividing and differentiating.

called the *blastocyst,* implants into the uterine lining. The outer portion becomes part of the placenta, which is discussed shortly.

Further cell growth, multiplication, and differentiation occur, resulting in the formation of an **embryo.** Over the next 6 weeks, embryonic tissues fold into a primitive, tubelike structure with limb buds, organs, and facial features recognizable as human (**Figure 16.2**). It isn't surprising, then, that the embryo is most vulnerable to teratogens during this time. Not only alcohol and illegal drugs but also prescription and over-the-counter medications, megadoses of supplements such as vitamin A, certain herbs, viruses, cigarette smoking, and radiation can interfere with embryonic development and cause birth defects.[3] In some cases, the damage is so severe that the pregnancy is naturally terminated in a **spontaneous abortion** (*miscarriage*), which occurs most often in the first trimester.

During the first weeks of pregnancy, the embryo obtains its nutrients from cells lining the uterus. But by the fourth week, a primitive **placenta** has formed in the uterus from both embryonic and maternal tissue. Within a few more weeks, the placenta will be a fully functioning organ through which the mother will provide nutrients and remove fetal wastes (**Figure 16.3**).

By the end of the embryonic stage, about 8 weeks postconception, the embryo's tissues and organs have differentiated dramatically. A primitive skeleton, including fingers and toes, has formed. Muscles have begun to develop in the trunk and limbs, and some movement is now possible. A primitive heart has also formed and begun to beat, and the digestive system is differentiating into distinct organs (stomach, liver, and so forth). The brain and cranial nerves have differentiated, and the head has a mouth, eyespots with eyelids, and primitive ears.

The third month of pregnancy marks the transition from embryo to **fetus.** The fetus requires abundant nutrients from the mother's body to support its dramatic growth during this period. The placenta is now a mature organ and can provide these nutrients. It is connected to the fetal circulatory system via the **umbilical cord,** an extension of fetal blood vessels emerging from the fetus's navel (called the *umbilicus*). Blood rich in oxygen and nutrients flows through the placenta and into the umbilical vein (see Figure 16.3). Once inside the fetus's body, the blood travels to the fetal liver and heart. Wastes are excreted in blood returning from the fetus to the placenta via the umbilical arteries. Although many people think there is a mixing of blood from the fetus and the mother, the two blood supplies remain separate; the placenta is the "go-between" that allows the transfer of nutrients and wastes.

Because the formation of body limbs, eyes and ears, and organs occurs during the first trimester, nutrient deficiencies during this time can lead to irreversible structural or functional damage. At the same time, nutrient toxicities as well as exposure to drugs, alcohol,

embryo The human growth and developmental stage lasting from the third week to the end of the eighth week after fertilization.

spontaneous abortion The natural termination of a pregnancy and expulsion of pregnancy tissues because of a genetic, developmental, or physiologic abnormality that is so severe that the pregnancy cannot be maintained; also called *miscarriage.*

placenta A pregnancy-specific organ formed from both maternal and embryonic tissues. It is responsible for oxygen, nutrient, and waste exchange between mother and fetus.

fetus The human growth and developmental stage lasting from the beginning of the ninth week after conception to birth.

umbilical cord The cord containing arteries and veins that connects the baby (from the navel) to the mother via the placenta.

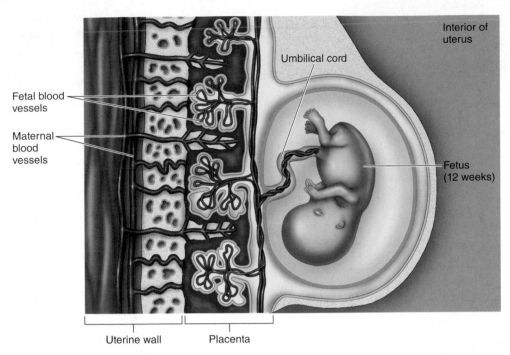

Interior of uterus

Umbilical cord

Fetal blood vessels

Maternal blood vessels

Fetus (12 weeks)

Uterine wall   Placenta

FIGURE 16.3 Placental development. The placenta is formed from both embryonic and maternal tissues. When the placenta is fully functional, fetal blood vessels and maternal blood vessels are intimately intertwined, allowing the exchange of nutrients and wastes between the two. The mother transfers nutrients and oxygen to the fetus, and the fetus transfers wastes to the mother for disposal.

certain medications, or microbes during this trimester can also result in fetal malformation. The consequences of specific nutrient deficiencies and toxicities are discussed shortly.

The Second Trimester

During the second trimester (approximately weeks 14 through 27 of pregnancy), the fetus continues to grow and mature (**Figure 16.4**, page 640). The fetus can suck its thumb, its ears begin to hear, and its eyes can open and close and react to light. The placenta is now fully functional. At the beginning of the second trimester, the fetus is about 3 inches long and weighs about 1.5 lb. By the end of the second trimester, the fetus is generally more than a foot long and weighs more than 2 lb. Some babies born prematurely in the last weeks of the second trimester survive with intensive **neonatal** care.

The Third Trimester

The third trimester (approximately week 28 to birth) is a time of remarkable growth for the fetus. During 3 short months, the fetus gains nearly half its body length and three-quarters of its body weight! At the time of birth, an average baby is approximately 18 to 22 inches long and about 7.5 lb in weight (see Figure 16.4). Brain growth (which continues to be rapid for the first 2 years of life) is also quite remarkable, and the lungs become fully mature. Because of the intense growth and maturation of the fetus during the third trimester, it continues to be critical that the mother eat an adequate and balanced diet.

Impact of Nutrition on Newborn Maturity and Birth Weight

An adequate, nourishing diet is one of the most important modifiable variables increasing the chances for birth of a mature newborn. Proper nutrition also increases the likelihood that the newborn's weight will be appropriate for his or her gestational age. Generally, a birth weight of at least 5.5 lb is considered a marker of a successful pregnancy.

neonatal Referring to a newborn.

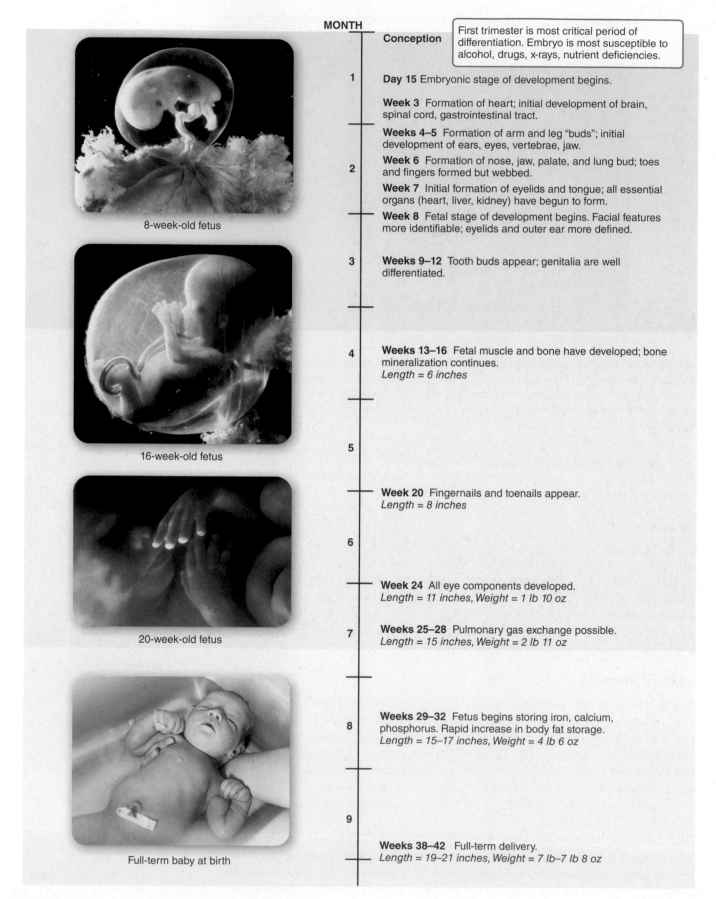

MONTH

Conception

First trimester is most critical period of differentiation. Embryo is most susceptible to alcohol, drugs, x-rays, nutrient deficiencies.

1

Day 15 Embryonic stage of development begins.

Week 3 Formation of heart; initial development of brain, spinal cord, gastrointestinal tract.

Weeks 4–5 Formation of arm and leg "buds"; initial development of ears, eyes, vertebrae, jaw.

Week 6 Formation of nose, jaw, palate, and lung bud; toes and fingers formed but webbed.

2

Week 7 Initial formation of eyelids and tongue; all essential organs (heart, liver, kidney) have begun to form.

Week 8 Fetal stage of development begins. Facial features more identifiable; eyelids and outer ear more defined.

8-week-old fetus

3

Weeks 9–12 Tooth buds appear; genitalia are well differentiated.

4

Weeks 13–16 Fetal muscle and bone have developed; bone mineralization continues.
Length = 6 inches

16-week-old fetus

5

Week 20 Fingernails and toenails appear.
Length = 8 inches

6

Week 24 All eye components developed.
Length = 11 inches, Weight = 1 lb 10 oz

20-week-old fetus

7

Weeks 25–28 Pulmonary gas exchange possible.
Length = 15 inches, Weight = 2 lb 11 oz

8

Weeks 29–32 Fetus begins storing iron, calcium, phosphorus. Rapid increase in body fat storage.
Length = 15–17 inches, Weight = 4 lb 6 oz

Full-term baby at birth

9

Weeks 38–42 Full-term delivery.
Length = 19–21 inches, Weight = 7 lb–7 lb 8 oz

FIGURE 16.4 A timeline of embryonic and fetal development.

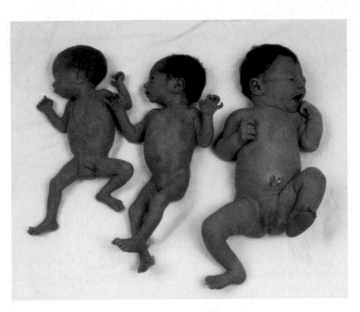

FIGURE 16.5 A healthy 2-day-old infant (right) compared to two low-birth-weight infants.

An undernourished mother is likely to give birth to a **low-birth-weight** infant who is at increased risk for infection, learning disabilities, impaired physical development, and death in the first year of life (**Figure 16.5**).[4] Many low-birth-weight infants are born **preterm**— that is, before 38 weeks of gestation. Others are born at term but weigh less than would be expected for their gestational age; this condition is called **small for gestational age (SGA).** Although nutrition is not the only factor contributing to maturity and birth weight, its role cannot be overstated.

RECAP

A full-term pregnancy lasts from 38 to 42 weeks and is traditionally divided into trimesters lasting 13 to 14 weeks. During the first trimester, cells differentiate and divide rapidly to form the various tissues of the human body. The fetus is especially susceptible to nutrient deficiencies, toxicities, and teratogens during this time. The second and third trimesters are characterized by continued growth and maturation. Nutrition is important before and throughout pregnancy to support fetal development without depleting the mother's reserves. An adequate, nourishing diet increases the chance that a baby will be born after 37 weeks and will weigh at least 5.5 lb. ■

How Much Weight Should a Pregnant Woman Gain?

Recommendations for weight gain vary according to a woman's weight *before* she became pregnant and whether the pregnancy is singleton (one fetus) or multiple (two or more fetuses). As you can see in **Table 16.1** (page 642), the average recommended weight gain for women of normal pre-pregnancy weight is 25 to 35 lb; underweight women should gain a little more than this amount, and overweight and obese women should gain somewhat less.[5] Adolescents should follow the same recommendations as those for adults. Women of normal pre-pregnancy weight who are pregnant with twins are advised to gain 37 to 54 lb.[5]

Women who have a low pre-pregnancy BMI (<18.5) or gain too little weight during their pregnancy increase their risk of having a preterm or low-birth-weight baby and of dangerously depleting their own nutrient reserves. Gaining *too much* weight during pregnancy or being overweight (BMI >25) or obese (BMI >30) prior to conception is also

low birth weight An infant weight of less than 5.5 lb at birth.

preterm The birth of a baby prior to 38 weeks of gestation.

small for gestational age (SGA) A condition in which infants whose birth weight for gestational age falls below the 10th percentile.

TABLE 16.1 Recommended Weight Gain for Women During Pregnancy

Pre-Pregnancy Weight Status	Body Mass Index (kg/m²)	Recommended Total Weight Gain (lb)
Normal	18.5–24.9	25–35
Underweight	<18.5	28–40
Overweight	25.0–29.9	15–25
Obese	>30.0	11–20

Source: Rasmussen, K.M., and A.L. Yaktine, eds. 2009. *Weight Gain During Pregnancy: Reexamining the Guidelines.* Institute of Medicine; National Research Council. Washington, DC: National Acaedemy Press.

risky—and much more common. Excessive pre-pregnancy weight or prenatal weight gain increases the risk that the fetus will be large for his or her gestational age, and large babies have an increased risk for trauma during vaginal delivery and for cesarean birth. Also, children born to overweight or obese mothers have higher rates of childhood obesity[6] and childhood metabolic syndrome.[7] A high birth weight has also been linked to increased risk for adolescent obesity. In addition, the more weight gained during pregnancy, the more difficult it is for the mother to return to her pre-pregnancy weight and the more likely it is that her weight gain will be permanent. This weight retention can become especially problematic if the woman has two or more children; the extra weight also increases her long-term risk for type 2 diabetes and high blood pressure. One goal of *Healthy People 2020* is to increase the proportion of mothers who achieve a recommended weight gain during their pregnancies, thus avoiding excessive and inadequate weight gains.[3]

In addition to the amount of weight, the *pattern* of weight gain is important. During the first trimester, a woman of normal weight should gain no more than 3 to 5 lb. During the second and third trimesters, an average of about 1 lb a week is considered healthful for normal-weight women. For overweight women, a gain of 0.6 lb/week is considered appropriate, and obese women are advised to gain no more than 0.5 lb/week.[5] Many healthcare providers feel the guidelines for overweight and obese women are too generous, especially when you consider that 60% of overweight and 25% of obese women exceed the guidelines.[8] In fact, some healthcare practitioners are starting to encourage otherwise healthy overweight or obese women not to gain any weight during pregnancy and, if carefully supervised, actually to lose a few pounds. If weight gain is excessive within a single week, month, or trimester, the woman should attempt to slow the rate of weight gain. On the other hand, if a woman has not gained sufficient weight in the early months of her pregnancy, she should gradually increase her energy and nutrient intake. The newborns of women who lose weight during the first trimester—due to severe nausea and vomiting, for example—are likely to be of lower birth weight than newborns of women with appropriate weight gain. In short, weight gain throughout pregnancy should be slow and steady.

In a society obsessed with thinness, it is easy for pregnant women to worry about weight gain. Focusing on the quality of food consumed, rather than the quantity, can help women feel more in control. In addition, following a physician-approved exercise program helps pregnant women maintain a positive body image and prevent excessive weight gain. The 2010 Dietary Guidelines for Americans advises pregnant women to ensure an appropriate weight gain as specified by the 2009 Institute of Medicine Guidelines.[9]

A pregnant woman may also feel less anxious about her weight gain if she understands how that weight is distributed. Of the total weight gained in pregnancy, 10 to 12 lb are accounted for by the fetus itself, the amniotic fluid, and the placenta (**Figure 16.6**). Another 3 to 4 lb represents an increase of 40% to 50% in maternal blood volume. A woman can expect to be about 10 to 12 lb lighter immediately after giving birth and,

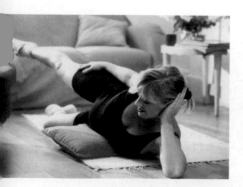

Following a physician-approved exercise program helps pregnant women maintain a positive body image and prevent excess weight gain.

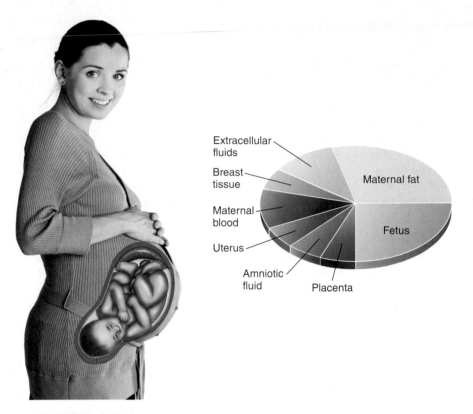

FIGURE 16.6 The weight gained during pregnancy is distributed between the mother's own tissues and the pregnancy-specific tissues.

within about 2 weeks, another 5 to 8 lb lighter because of fluid loss (from plasma and interstitial fluid).

After the first 2 weeks following giving birth, losing the remainder of pregnancy weight requires that more energy be expended than is taken in. Appropriate physical activity can help women lose those extra pounds. Also, because production of breast milk requires significant energy, breastfeeding helps many new mothers lose some of the remaining weight. Moderate weight reduction is safe while breastfeeding and will not compromise the weight gain of the nursing infant.

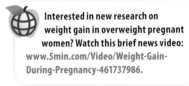

Interested in new research on weight gain in overweight pregnant women? Watch this brief news video: www.5min.com/Video/Weight-Gain-During-Pregnancy-461737986.

RECAP

Sufficient Calories should be consumed so that a pregnant woman gains an appropriate amount of weight, typically 25 to 35 lb, to ensure adequate growth of the fetus. The Calories consumed during pregnancy should be nutrient-dense, so that both the mother and the fetus obtain the nutrients they need from food. ■

What Are a Pregnant Woman's Nutrient Needs?

The requirements for nearly all nutrients increase during pregnancy to accommodate the growth and development of the fetus without depriving the mother of the nutrients she needs to maintain her own health. With the exception of iron, most women can meet these increased needs by carefully selecting foods high in nutrient density. The Choose MyPlate .gov website provides a useful tool that reinforces the concepts of adequacy, balance, and variety in food choices; it also suggests food patterns for pregnant women. See the Web Links at the end of this chapter.

Macronutrient Needs of Pregnant Women

In pregnancy, macronutrients provide necessary energy for building tissue. They are also the very building blocks for the fetus, as well as for the mother's pregnancy-associated tissues.

Energy   Given what you've learned about pregnancy weight gain, you've probably figured out that energy requirements increase only modestly during pregnancy. In fact, during the first trimester, a woman should consume approximately the same number of Calories daily as during her nonpregnant days. Instead of eating more, she should attempt to maximize the nutrient density of what she eats. For example, drinking low-fat milk or calcium-fortified soy milk is preferable to drinking soft drinks. Low-fat milk and fortified soy milk provide valuable protein, vitamins, and minerals to feed the fetus's rapidly dividing cells, whereas soft drinks provide nutritionally empty Calories.

During the last two trimesters of pregnancy, energy needs increase by about 350 to 450 kcal/day. For a woman normally consuming 2,000 kcal/day, an extra 400 kcal represents only a 20% increase in energy intake, a goal that can be met more easily than many pregnant women realize. For example, 1 cup of low-fat yogurt and a graham cracker with jam is about 400 kcal. At the same time, some vitamin and mineral needs increase by as much as 50%—so again, the key for getting adequate micronutrients while not consuming too many extra Calories is choosing nutrient-dense foods.

Protein   During pregnancy, protein needs increase to about 1.1 grams per day per kilogram body weight over the entire 9-month period.[10] This is an increase of 25 g of protein per day. One half of a turkey (2 oz) and cheese (1 oz) sandwich would provide the extra 25 g of protein. For a pregnant woman weighing approximately 142 lb, the total recommended intake would average 71 g per day. Keep in mind that many women already eat this much protein each day, especially in the United States. Dairy products, meats, fish, poultry, eggs, and soy products are all rich sources of protein, as are legumes, nuts, and seeds. Still, it can be challenging for vegetarian and vegan women to meet their increased protein needs. To try designing a protein-rich snack for a vegetarian mother-to-be, see the **You Do the Math** box (page 645).

Carbohydrate   Pregnant women are advised to aim for a carbohydrate intake of at least 175 g per day.[10] All pregnant women should be counseled on the potential hazards of very-low-carbohydrate diets. Glucose is the primary metabolic fuel of the developing fetus; thus, pregnant women need to consume healthful sources of carbohydrate throughout the day. The recommended intake will also prevent ketosis (discussed in detail in Chapter 4, page 132) and help maintain normal blood glucose levels. Additional carbohydrate may be needed to support daily physical activity.

The recommendation of 175 g is easily met by consuming a balanced diet. The majority of carbohydrate intake should come from whole foods, such as whole-grain breads and cereals, brown rice, fruits, vegetables, and legumes. Not only are these carbohydrate-rich foods good sources of micronutrients, such as the B-vitamins, but they also contain a lot of fiber, which can help prevent constipation. Fiber-rich foods contribute to one's sense of fullness and can be an advantage to women who need to be careful not to gain too much weight.

Fat   The guideline for the percentage of daily Calories that comes from fat does not change during pregnancy.[10] Pregnant women should be aware that, because new tissues and cells are being built, adequate consumption of dietary fat is even more important than in the nonpregnant state. In addition, during the third trimester, the fetus stores most of its own body fat, which is a critical source of fuel in the newborn period. Without adequate fat stores, newborns cannot effectively regulate their body temperature.

Consumption of the right kinds of fats is important. Like anyone else, pregnant women should limit their intakes of saturated and *trans* fats because of their negative impact on cardiovascular health (as discussed in Chapter 5). Poly- and monounsaturated fats should be chosen whenever possible. The omega-3 polyunsaturated fatty acid

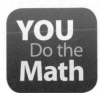

Planning a Protein-Packed Snack

Earlier in this chapter we pointed out that, during the last two trimesters of pregnancy, a woman's energy needs increase by about 350 to 450 kcal/day. At the same time, a pregnant woman's need for protein increases by 25 g per day. To help you appreciate how important it is for pregnant women to choose nutrient-dense foods, here's a two-part challenge:

Part 1. Annabelle is 6 months pregnant with her first child. She is an ovo-lacto vegetarian. Before she was pregnant, she never ate a mid-afternoon snack at work. Now, she eats a snack consisting of one slice of whole-wheat bread topped with 2 tablespoons of peanut butter, along with an 8-ounce carton of calcium-fortified orange juice. Let's see if this snack fulfills her need for extra Calories, as well as her increased protein needs.

1. List each food item, the kcal, and the g protein provided:

One slice whole-wheat bread:	110 kcal	5 g protein
2 tablespoons peanut butter:	190 kcal	8 g protein
8 ounces orange juice:	110 kcal	2 g protein

2. Calculate the total kcal in this snack: 110 + 190 + 110 = 410.

3. Does the snack meet her increased energy needs? Yes

4. Calculate the total g protein in this snack: 5 + 8 + 2 = 15.

5. Does the snack meet her increased protein needs? No. This snack meets 60% of Annabelle's increased protein needs: 15/25 = .60. She could increase the protein content of her snack by choosing a different beverage, such as milk or soy milk. Alternatively, she could decide to increase the amount of protein in other meals she eats during the day.

Part 2. Now it's your turn. Design a mid-afternoon snack for Annabelle that would meet but not exceed her needs for both increased Calories and increased protein.

Answers will vary according to individual inputs.

---

docosahexaenoic acid (DHA) has been found to be uniquely critical for both neurologic and eye development. Because the fetal brain grows dramatically during the third trimester, DHA is especially important in the maternal diet. Good sources of DHA are oily fish, such as anchovies, mackerel, salmon, and sardines. It is also found in lower amounts in tuna, chicken, and eggs (some eggs are DHA-enhanced by feeding hens a DHA-rich diet).

Pregnant women who eat fish should be aware of the potential for mercury contamination, as even a limited intake of mercury during pregnancy can impair a fetus's developing nervous system. Pregnant women should avoid large fish, such as swordfish, shark, tilefish, and king mackerel, and should limit their intake of white (albacore) tuna to 6 ounces per week.[9] Other than these specific limitations, however, pregnant women can safely consume up to 12 oz of most other types of fish per week, as long as it is appropriately cooked.[9]

> Interested in learning more about the pros and cons of consuming fish during pregnancy? A short video from the March of Dimes explains which foods to choose and which to avoid when you are pregnant: go to www.marchofdimes.com/pregnancy/nutrition_risks.html.

Micronutrient Needs of Pregnant Women

The need for micronutrients increases during pregnancy because of the expansion of the mother's blood supply and growth of the uterus, placenta, breasts, body fat, and the fetus itself. In addition, the increased need for energy during pregnancy correlates with an increased need for micronutrients involved in the metabolism of macronutrients and ATP production. Discussions about the micronutrients most critical during pregnancy follow. Refer to **Table 16.2** (page 646) for an overview of the changes in micronutrient needs with pregnancy.

Folate   Because folate is necessary for cell division, it follows that, during a time when both maternal and fetal cells are dividing rapidly, the requirement for this vitamin would be increased. Adequate folate is especially critical during the first 28 days after conception, when it is required for the formation and closure of the **neural tube**, an embryonic structure that eventually becomes the brain and spinal cord. Folate deficiency is associated

neural tube Embryonic tissue that forms a tube, which eventually becomes the brain and spinal cord.

TABLE 16.2 Changes in Nutrient Recommendations with Pregnancy for Adult Women

Micronutrient	Pre-Pregnancy	Pregnancy	% Increase
Folate	400 µg/day	600 µg/day	50
Vitamin B$_{12}$	2.4 µg/day	2.6 µg/day	8
Vitamin C	75 mg/day	85 mg/day	13
Vitamin A	700 µg/day	770 µg/day	10
Vitamin D	5 µg/day	5 µg/day	0
Calcium	1,000 mg/day	1,000 mg/day	0
Iron	18 mg/day	27 mg/day	50
Zinc	8 mg/day	11 mg/day	38
Sodium	1,500 mg/day	1,500 mg/day	0
Iodine	150 µg/day	220 µg/day	47

spina bifida An embryonic neural tube defect that occurs when the spinal vertebrae fail to completely enclose the spinal cord, allowing it to protrude.

anencephaly A fatal neural tube defect in which there is partial absence of brain tissue, most likely caused by failure of the neural tube to close.

with neural tube defects, such as **spina bifida** (**Figure 16.7**) and **anencephaly,** a fatal defect in which there is partial absence of brain tissue. Adequate folate intake does not guarantee normal neural tube development, as the precise cause of neural tube defects is unknown, and in some cases there is a genetic component. It is estimated, however, that up to 70% of all neural tube defects could be prevented by simply improving maternal intake of folic acid or folate.[11] One goal of *Healthy People 2020* is to reduce the occurrence of spina bifida and other neural tube defects by increasing the dose for women in their childbearing years to an intake of at least 400 µg of folic acid from fortified foods or dietary supplements.[3]

So, to reduce the risk for neural tube defects, all women capable of becoming pregnant are encouraged to consume 400 µg of folic acid per day from supplements, fortified foods, or both in addition to a variety of foods naturally high in folates. The emphasis on obtaining folic acid from supplements and fortified foods is due to the higher bioavailability of these sources. Of course, folate remains very important even after the neural tube has closed. The RDA for folate for pregnant women is therefore 600 µg/day, a full 50% increase over the RDA for a nonpregnant female.[12] A deficiency of folate during pregnancy

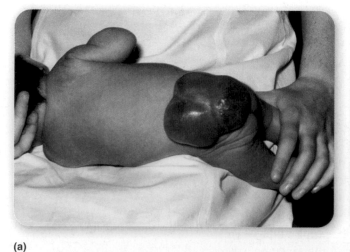

(a)

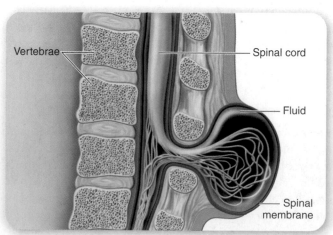

Vertebrae — Spinal cord

Fluid

Spinal membrane

(b)

FIGURE 16.7 Spina bifida, a common neural tube defect. **(a)** An external view of an infant with spina bifida. **(b)** An internal view of the protruding spinal membrane and fluid-filled sac.

can result in macrocytic anemia (a condition in which blood cells do not mature properly) and has been associated with low birth weight, preterm delivery, and failure of the fetus to grow properly. Sources of food folate include orange juice; green, leafy vegetables (such as spinach and broccoli); and lentils. For more than two decades, the Food and Drug Administration (FDA) has mandated that all enriched grain products, such as cereals, breads, and pastas, be fortified with folic acid; thus, including these foods, ideally as whole grains, in the daily diet can further increase folate intake.

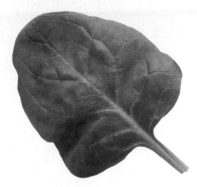

Spinach is an excellent source of folate.

Vitamin B$_{12}$ Vitamin B$_{12}$ (cobalamin) is vital during pregnancy, because it regenerates the active form of folate. Not surprisingly, deficiencies of vitamin B$_{12}$ can also result in macrocytic anemia, yet the RDA for vitamin B$_{12}$ for pregnant women is only 2.6 µg/day, a mere 8% increase over the RDA of 2.4 µg/day for nonpregnant women.[12] How can this be? One reason is that, during pregnancy, absorption of vitamin B$_{12}$ is more efficient. The required amount of vitamin B$_{12}$ can easily be obtained from animal food sources, such as meats, dairy products, and eggs. However, deficiencies have been observed in women who have followed a vegan diet for several years; these deficiencies have also been observed in the infants of some mothers who follow a vegan diet. Fortified foods or supplementation provides these women with the needed amounts of vitamin B$_{12}$.

Vitamin C Because blood plasma volume increases during pregnancy, and because vitamin C is being transferred to the fetus, the concentration of vitamin C in maternal blood decreases. Vitamin C deficiency during pregnancy has been associated with an increased risk for premature birth and other complications. The RDA for vitamin C during pregnancy is increased by a little more than 10% over the RDA for nonpregnant women (from 75 mg to 85 mg per day for adult pregnant women, 80 mg per day for pregnant adolescents). Women who smoke during pregnancy should consume even higher levels of vitamin C, because smoking lowers both serum and amniotic fluid levels. Many foods are rich sources of vitamin C, such as citrus fruits and juices, peppers, and numerous other fruits and vegetables.

Vitamin A Vitamin A needs increase during pregnancy by about 10%, to 770 µg per day for adult pregnant women and 750 µg per day for pregnant adolescents.[13] Vitamin A deficiency during pregnancy has been linked to an increased risk for low birth weight, growth problems, and preterm delivery. However, excess preformed vitamin A exerts teratogenic effects. Consumption of excessive preformed vitamin A, particularly during the first trimester, increases the risk for birth of an infant with craniofacial malformations, including cleft lip or palate; heart defects; and abnormalities of the central nervous system.[13] A well-balanced diet supplies sufficient vitamin A, so supplementation during pregnancy is not recommended. Note that provitamin A, in the form of beta-carotene (which is converted to vitamin A in the body), has not been associated with birth defects.

Vitamin D Despite the role of vitamin D in calcium absorption, the RDA for this nutrient does not increase during pregnancy. According to the Institute of Medicine, the amount of vitamin D transferred from the mother to the fetus is relatively small and does not appear to affect overall maternal vitamin D status.[14] Pregnant women who receive adequate exposure to sunlight do not need vitamin D supplements. However, pregnant women with darkly pigmented skin and/or limited sun exposure who do not regularly drink milk will benefit from vitamin D supplementation. It has been estimated that almost 30% of dark-skinned pregnant women living in the northeastern United States are in a state of vitamin D deficiency, which may result in impaired fetal growth, preeclampsia, placental infections, preterm birth, and increased risk for type 1 diabetes later in the offspring's life.[15] Most prenatal vitamin supplements contain 10 µg/day of vitamin D, which is considered safe and acceptable, although some researchers view that level as inadequate for maintaining normal serum levels of vitamin D.[14] Because vitamin D is fat soluble, pregnant women should avoid consuming excessive vitamin D from supplements, as toxicity can cause developmental disability in the newborn.

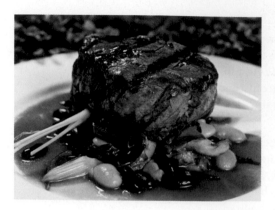

Meats provide complete protein, which is essential for building and maintaining both maternal and fetal tissues.

Calcium Growth of the fetal skeleton requires as much as 30 g of calcium, most during the last trimester. However, the RDA for calcium does not change during pregnancy; it remains at 1,300 mg/day for pregnant adolescents (14–18 y) and 1,000 mg/day for adult pregnant women (19–50 y).[14] Why is there no increase? First, pregnant women absorb dietary calcium more efficiently than do nonpregnant women, assuming adequate vitamin D status. Second, the extra demand for calcium has not been found to cause permanent demineralization of the mother's bones or to increase fracture risk; thus, there is no justification for recommending higher intakes. Sources of calcium include milk, calcium-fortified soy milk and other milk substitutes, calcium-fortified juices, yogurt and cheese, fortified breakfast cereals, tofu, and a variety of green, leafy vegetables.

Iron Recall (from Chapter 12) the importance of iron in the formation of red blood cells, which transport oxygen throughout the body so that cells can produce ATP. During pregnancy, the demand for red blood cells increases to accommodate the needs of the expanded maternal blood volume, growing uterus, placenta, and fetus itself. Thus, more iron is needed. Fetal demand for iron increases even further during the last trimester, when the fetus stores iron in the liver for use during the first few months of life. This iron storage is protective, because breast milk is low in iron. While recognizing that iron supplements are routinely prescribed to pregnant women, the 2010 Dietary Guidelines for Americans specifically advises women capable of becoming pregnant to eat foods high in heme iron, such as meat, fish, and poultry, and/or to consume iron-rich plant foods, such as legumes, or iron-fortified foods with vitamin C–rich foods.[9]

Severely inadequate iron intake certainly has the potential to harm the fetus, resulting in an increased rate of low birth weight, preterm birth, stillbirth, and death of the newborn in the first weeks after birth. However, in most cases, the iron-deprived fetus builds adequate stores by "robbing" maternal iron, resulting in iron-deficiency anemia in the mother. During pregnancy, maternal iron deficiency causes extreme paleness and exhaustion, but at birth it endangers the mother's life: anemic women are more likely to die during or shortly after childbirth, because they are less able to tolerate blood loss and fight infection. One goal of *Healthy People 2020* is to reduce iron deficiency among pregnant females.[3]

The RDA for iron during pregnancy is 27 mg per day, compared to 18 mg per day for nonpregnant women and 15 mg per day for nonpregnant adolescents.[13] This represents a 50% to 80% increase, despite the fact that iron loss is minimized during pregnancy because menstruation ceases. Typically, women of childbearing age have poor iron stores, and the demands of pregnancy are likely to produce a deficiency. To ensure adequate iron stores during pregnancy, an iron supplement (as part of, or separate from, a total prenatal supplement) is routinely prescribed during the last two trimesters. Vitamin C enhances iron absorption, as do dietary sources of heme iron; however, substances in coffee, tea, milk, bran, and oxalate-rich foods decrease absorption. Therefore, many healthcare providers recommend taking iron supplements with foods high in vitamin C and/or heme iron.

Zinc The RDA for zinc for adult pregnant women increases by about 38% over the RDA for nonpregnant adult women, from 8 mg per day to 11 mg per day, and the RDA increases from 9 mg per day to 12 mg per day for pregnant adolescents.[13] Because zinc has critical roles in DNA, RNA, and protein synthesis, it is extremely important that adequate zinc status be maintained during pregnancy to ensure proper growth and development of both maternal and fetal tissues. Inadequate zinc can lead to fetal malformations, premature birth, decreased birth size, and extended labor. The absorption of zinc from supplements is inhibited by high intakes of non-heme iron, such as those found in iron supplements, when these two minerals are taken with water.[16] However, when food sources of iron and zinc are consumed together in a meal, absorption of zinc is not affected, largely because the amount of iron in the meal is not high enough to block zinc uptake. Good dietary sources of zinc include red meats, shellfish, and fortified cereals.

Sodium and Iodine   During pregnancy, the AI for sodium is the same as for a nonpregnant adult woman, or 1,500 mg (1.5 g) per day.[17] Although too much sodium is associated with fluid retention and bloating, as well as high blood pressure, increased body fluids are a normal and necessary part of pregnancy, so some sodium is needed to maintain fluid balance.

Iodine needs increase significantly during pregnancy, but the RDA of 220 μg per day is easy to achieve by using a modest amount of iodized salt (sodium chloride) during cooking. Sprinkling salt onto food at the table is unnecessary; a balanced, healthful diet will provide all the iodine needed during pregnancy.

Do Pregnant Women Need Supplements?

Prenatal multivitamin and mineral supplements are not strictly necessary during pregnancy, but most healthcare providers recommend them. Meeting all the nutrient needs would otherwise take careful and somewhat complex dietary planning. Prenatal supplements are especially good insurance for vegans, adolescents, and others whose diets might normally be low in one or more micronutrients. It is important that pregnant women understand, however, that supplements are to be taken *in addition to,* not as a substitute for, a nutrient-rich diet.

Fluid Needs of Pregnant Women

Fluid plays many vital roles during pregnancy. It allows for the necessary increase in the mother's blood volume, acts as a lubricant, aids in regulating body temperature, and is necessary for many metabolic reactions. Fluid that the mother consumes also helps maintain the **amniotic fluid** that surrounds, cushions, and protects the fetus in the uterus. The AI for total fluid intake, which includes drinking water, beverages, and food, is 3 liters per day (about 12.7 cups). This recommendation includes approximately 2.3 liters (10 cups) of fluid as total beverages, including drinking water.[17]

Drinking adequate fluid helps combat two common discomforts of pregnancy: fluid retention and, possibly, constipation. Drinking lots of fluids (and going to the bathroom as soon as the need is felt) will also help prevent **urinary tract infections,** which are common in pregnancy. Fluids also combat dehydration, which can develop if a woman with morning sickness has frequent bouts of vomiting. For these women, fluids such as soups, juices, and sports beverages are usually well tolerated and can help prevent dehydration.

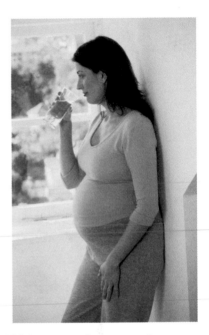

It's important that pregnant women drink about 10 cups of fluid a day.

RECAP

Protein, carbohydrates, and fats provide the building blocks for fetal growth. Folate deficiency has been associated with neural tube defects. Most healthcare providers recommend prenatal supplements for pregnant women to ensure that sufficient micronutrients, such as iron, are consumed. Fluid provides for increased maternal blood volume and amniotic fluid. ■

Nutrition-Related Concerns for Pregnant Women

Pregnancy-related conditions involving a particular nutrient, such as iron-deficiency anemia, have already been discussed. The following sections describe some of the most common discomforts and disorders of pregnant women that are related to their general nutrition.

Morning Sickness

Morning sickness, or *nausea and vomiting of pregnancy* (NVP), is extremely common and almost always appears during the first trimester.[18] It can vary from occasional, mild queasiness to constant nausea with bouts of vomiting. In truth, "morning sickness" is not an

amniotic fluid   The watery fluid within the innermost membrane of the sac containing the fetus. It cushions and protects the growing fetus.

urinary tract infection   A bacterial infection of the urethra, the tube leading from the bladder to the body exterior.

morning sickness   A condition characterized by varying degrees of nausea and vomiting associated with pregnancy, most commonly in the first trimester.

appropriate name because the nausea and vomiting can begin at any time of the day and may last all day. NVP usually resolves by week 12 to 16 and the mother and fetus do not suffer lasting harm. However, some women experience such frequent vomiting that it becomes a serious medical condition, requiring hospitalization or in-home intravenous (IV) therapy. There is no cure for morning sickness. However, here are some practical tips for reducing the severity:

- Eat small, frequent meals and snacks throughout the day. An empty stomach can trigger nausea.
- Consume most of the day's fluids between meals. Frozen ice pops, watermelon, gelatin desserts, and mild broths are often well-tolerated sources of fluid.
- Keep snacks such as crackers at the bedside to ease nighttime queasiness or to eat before rising.
- Take prenatal supplements at a time of day when vomiting is least likely.
- Avoid sights, sounds, smells, and tastes that bring on or worsen queasiness. Cold or room-temperature foods are often better tolerated than hot foods.
- For some women, alternative therapies, such as acupuncture, acupressure wrist bands, biofeedback, meditation, and hypnosis, help. Always check with your healthcare provider to ensure that the therapy you are using is safe and does not interact with other medications or supplements.

Cravings and Aversions

It seems as if nothing is more stereotypical about pregnancy than the image of a frazzled husband getting up in the middle of the night to run to the convenience store to get his pregnant wife some pickles and ice cream. This image, although humorous, is far from reality. Although some women have specific cravings, most crave a particular type of food (such as "something sweet" or "something salty") rather than a particular food.

Why do pregnant women crave certain tastes? Does a desire for salty foods mean that the woman is experiencing a sodium deficit? Although there may be some truth to the assertion that we crave what we need, scientific evidence for this claim is lacking.

Most cravings are, of course, for edible substances. But a surprising number of pregnant women crave nonfoods, such as laundry starch, chalk, and clay. This craving, called **pica,** may result in nutritional or health problems for the mother and fetus and is the subject of the **Highlight** box (page 651).

Food aversions are also common during pregnancy and may originate from social, cultural, or religious beliefs. In some cultures, for example, women traditionally avoid shellfish ("it causes allergies") or duck ("child will be born with webbed feet"). Such aversions and taboos are often strongly woven into the family's belief system.

Gastroesophageal Reflux

Gastroesophageal reflux, also termed *heartburn*, is common during pregnancy. Pregnancy-related hormones relax lower esophageal smooth muscle, increasing the incidence of heartburn. During the last two trimesters, the enlarging uterus pushes up on the stomach, compounding the problem. Practical tips for minimizing heartburn during pregnancy include the following:

- Avoid excessive weight gain.
- Eat small, frequent meals and chew food slowly.
- Don't wear tight clothing.
- Wait for at least 1 hour after eating before lying down.
- Sleep with your head elevated.
- Ask your healthcare provider to recommend an antacid that is safe for use during pregnancy.

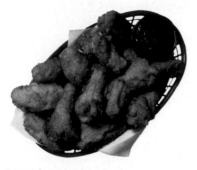

Deep-fried foods are often unappealing to pregnant women.

pica An abnormal craving to eat various nonfood substances, such as clay, chalk, or soap.

The Danger of Nonfood Cravings

HIGHLIGHT

A few weeks after she learned she was pregnant, Darlene started feeling "funny." She experienced bouts of nausea lasting several hours every day, and her appetite seemed to disappear. At the grocery store, she wandered through the aisles with an empty cart, confused about what foods she should be eating and unable to find anything that appealed to her. Eventually, she'd return home with a few small items—and a large bag of ice. At the assembly plant where she worked, she took cupfuls of ice from the soda machine and ate it throughout the day. Each weekend, she went through more than a boxful of popsicles to "settle her stomach."

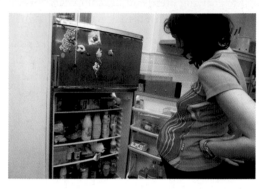

Pica is the condition of craving nonfood substances, such as dirt, chalk, pebbles, or soap.

At Darlene's next checkup, her nurse became concerned because she had lost weight. Darlene was too embarrassed to admit to that the only thing she wanted to eat was ice.

Some people believe that pregnant women with unusual cravings are intuitively seeking out nutrients their bodies need. Arguing against this theory is the phenomenon of *pica*—the craving and persistent consumption of nonfood material— which can occur during pregnancy. Pica is not the same as the common cravings for out-of-the-ordinary foods that many women experience while pregnant. A woman with pica may crave ice, clay, dirt, chalk, coffee grounds, baking soda, laundry starch, hair, burnt matches, stones, charcoal, mothballs, toothpaste, soap, rocks, and many other nonfood items, including even feces.[1] The cause of these cravings for nonfood substances of little or no nutritional value is not known; however, it is more common among children, and people with developmental disabilities are also at increased risk.[2] Underlying biochemical disorders, lower socioeconomic status, and family stress have been implicated as possible causes, as have cultural factors. For example, in the United States, pica is more common among pregnant African American women than women from other racial or ethnic groups; among recent immigrants vs. non-immigrants; and among lower-socioeconomic groups compared to higher ones.[3,4] Nutrient deficiencies have also been associated with pica, although it is not at all clear that nutrient deficiencies cause it. In fact, inhibition of nutrient absorption caused by the ingestion of clay and other substances can produce nutrient deficiencies.

Whatever the cause, pica is often dangerous. Excessive consumption of ice can lead to inadequate weight gain in pregnancy if the ice substitutes for food. Ingestion of clay, starch, and other materials can not only inhibit absorption of nutrients but may also cause constipation, intestinal blockage, and even excessive weight gain. Women with pica are at greater risk for high exposure to lead, as well as to other toxic substances, which can impair the neurodevelopment of the fetus and increase the risk for pregnancy-related complications.[4] In addition, ingestion of certain substances, such as talcum powder, can lead to severe weight loss and lung disease.[5]

Some pregnant women with pica are able to find foods they can substitute for the craved nonfood items—for instance, peanut butter instead of clay, or nonfat powdered milk instead of starch. If a woman experiences pica, she should talk with her healthcare provider immediately to identify strategies to avoid eating dangerous substances and instead consume healthful foods that will support optimal growth and development of her fetus. In addition, women consuming dirt, clay, or paint should be tested for blood lead levels to minimize risk for fetal lead exposure.[4] Pica should not be viewed as "weird" or "awful"—it is a potentially dangerous condition that should be addressed in a sensitive and caring manner. In this way, pregnant women with pica will be more likely to be open and honest with their healthcare providers about their cravings, opening the door for appropriate support.

References

1. Uher, R., and M. Rutter. 2012. Classification of feeding and eating disorders: review of evidence and proposals for ICD-11. *World Psychiatry* 11:80–92.
2. Matson, J. L., B. Belava, M. A. Hattier, and M. L. Matson. 2011. Pica in persons with developmental disabilities: characteristics, diagnosis, and assessment. *Res. Autism Spectrum Disorders.* 5:1459–1464.
3. Gavrelis, N., A. Sertkaya, L. Bertelsen, B. Cuthbertson, L. Phillips, and J. Moya. 2011. An analysis of the proportion of the U.S. population that ingests soil or other non-food substances. *Human Ecological Risk Assessment: An International Journal* 17:996–1012.
4. Thihalolipavan, S., B. M Candalla, and J. Ehrlich. 2012. Examining pica in NYC pregnant women with elevated blood lead levels. *Matern. Child Health J.* DOI:10.1007/s10995-012-0947-5.
5. Devasahayam, J., U. Pillai, and A. Lacasse. 2011. Talcum powder pica as the cause of interstitial lung disease. *Q. J. Med.* DOI:10.1093/qjmed/hcr106.

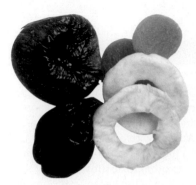

Consuming foods high in fiber, such as dried fruits, may reduce the chances of constipation.

Constipation

Hormone production during pregnancy causes the smooth muscles to relax, including the muscles of the large intestine, slowing colonic movement of food residue. Pressure exerted by the growing uterus on the colon can slow movement even further, making elimination difficult. Practical hints that may help a woman avoid constipation include the following:

- Include 25 to 35 g of fiber in the daily diet, concentrating on fresh fruits and vegetables, dried fruits, legumes, and whole grains.
- Keep fluid intake high as fiber intake increases. Drink plenty of water and eat water-rich fruits and vegetables, such as melons, citrus, and lettuce.
- Keep physically active, as exercise is one of many factors that help increase motility of the large intestine.

Pregnant women should use over-the-counter fiber supplements only as a last resort and should not use any laxative product without first discussing it with their healthcare provider.

Gestational Diabetes

Gestational diabetes, diagnosed in up to 10% of all U.S. pregnancies, is usually a temporary condition in which a pregnant woman is unable to produce sufficient insulin or becomes insulin resistant, and thus develops elevated levels of blood glucose. Fortunately, gestational diabetes has no ill effects on either the mother or the fetus if blood glucose levels are strictly controlled through diet, physical activity, and/or medication. Screening for gestational diabetes is routine for almost all healthcare practitioners and is necessary because several of the symptoms, which include frequent urination, fatigue, and an increase in thirst and appetite, mimic what is seen in a normal pregnancy. If poorly controlled or untreated, gestational diabetes can result in a baby who is too large as a result of receiving too much glucose across the placenta during fetal life. Infants who are overly large are at risk for early birth and trauma during vaginal birth, and often need to be born by cesarean section. There is also evidence that exposing a fetus to maternal diabetes significantly increases the risk for overweight and metabolic disorders later in life.[19,20]

Women who are obese, who are age 35 years or older, who have a family history of diabetes, and who are of Native American, African American, or Hispanic origin have a greater risk of developing gestational diabetes, as do women who previously delivered a large-for-gestational-age infant. Almost 20% of woman with gestational diabetes develop type 2 diabetes within the next 9 years.[21] As with any type of diabetes, attention to diet, weight control, and physical activity reduces the risk for gestational diabetes.

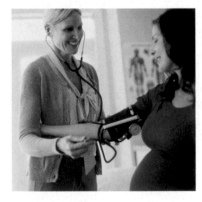

Pregnant women should have their blood pressure measured to screen for pregnancy-related hypertension.

Hypertensive Disorders in Pregnancy

About 7% to 8% of U.S. pregnancies are complicated by some form of hypertension, or high blood pressure, yet it accounts for almost 16% of pregnancy-related deaths in industrialized nations, such as the United States.[22] The term *hypertensive disorders in pregnancy* encompasses several different conditions. A woman who develops high blood pressure, with no other symptoms, during the pregnancy is said to have *gestational hypertension.* **Preeclampsia** is characterized by a sudden increase in maternal blood pressure during pregnancy with the presence of swelling, excessive and rapid weight gain unrelated to food intake, and protein in the urine. If left untreated, it can progress to eclampsia, a condition characterized by seizures and kidney failure and, if untreated, fetal and/or maternal death.

No one knows exactly what causes the various hypertensive disorders in pregnancy, but women who are pregnant for the first time, either adolescents or over the age of 35 to 40 years, African American, diabetic, smokers, obese, or from a low-income background, as well as those who have a family or personal history of eclampsia, are at greater risk.[22] Management of preeclampsia focuses mainly on blood pressure control. Typical treatment includes bed rest and medical oversight. Ultimately, the only thing that will cure the condition is childbirth. Today, with good prenatal care, gestational hypertension is nearly always

gestational diabetes Insufficient insulin production or insulin resistance that results in consistently high blood glucose levels, specifically during pregnancy; the condition typically resolves after birth occurs.

preeclampsia High blood pressure that is pregnancy-specific and accompanied by protein in the urine, edema, and unexpected weight gain.

detected early and can be appropriately managed, and prospects for both mother and fetus are usually very good. In nearly all women without prior chronic high blood pressure, blood pressure returns to normal within about a day or so after the birth, although recent studies suggest that women with preeclampsia are at greater risk for cardiovascular disease later in life.[23]

Adolescent Pregnancy

Throughout the adolescent years, girls' bodies are still changing and growing. Peak bone mass has not yet been reached, and full physical stature may not have been attained; thus, pregnant adolescents have higher needs for bone-related nutrients, such as calcium, phosphorus, and magnesium. Teens also commonly begin pregnancy in an iron-deficient state and, so, have an increased iron need.[24] Teens are also more likely to be underweight than are young adult women, and they are more likely to fail to gain adequate weight during pregnancy. In addition, many adolescents have not established healthful nutritional patterns. Thus, adhering to a diet that provides the appropriate level of energy to meet the adolescent's own needs as well as those of her fetus can be a challenge. At the same time, higher rates of prenatal alcohol use, smoking, and drug use also contribute to higher rates of preterm births, low-birth-weight babies, and other complications.

Many pregnant adolescents delay or fail to seek prenatal care. This is especially unfortunate because, in the adolescent age group, prenatal care is the most significant factor in pregnancy outcome. With regular prenatal care and close attention to proper nutrition and other healthful behaviors, the likelihood of a positive outcome for both the adolescent mother and the infant is similar to that for older mothers and their infants.[24]

In 2010, the adolescent birthrate dropped to 34.3 births for every 1,000 U.S. women aged 15–19. Although this is the lowest teen birth-rate since the 1940s, it is also among the highest of all industrialized nations. One of the goals of *Healthy People 2020* is to reduce pregnancies among adolescent females.[3]

> If you'd like to get involved reducing teen pregnancy, visit the website of the National Campaign to Prevent Teen and Unplanned Pregnancy at www.thenationalcampaign.org.

Vegetarianism

With the possible exception of iron and zinc, vegetarian women who consume dairy products and eggs (lacto-ovo-vegetarians) have no nutritional challenges beyond those encountered by every pregnant woman. In contrast, women who are totally vegetarian (vegan) need to be more vigilant than usual about their intake of nutrients that are derived primarily or wholly from animal products. These include vitamin D (unless regularly exposed to sunlight throughout the pregnancy), vitamin B_6, vitamin B_{12}, calcium, iron, and zinc. Supplements containing these nutrients are usually necessary. A regular prenatal supplement will fully meet the vitamin, iron, and zinc needs of a vegan woman but does not fulfill calcium needs, so a separate calcium supplement, or consumption of calcium-fortified soy milk or orange juice, is usually required.

Exercise

Physical activity during pregnancy is recommended for all women experiencing normal pregnancies. Women who rarely, if ever, exercised before becoming pregnant and overweight and obese women can benefit greatly from increased activity but should begin slowly and progress gradually under the guidance of their healthcare provider. Women should avoid exercising outdoors when it is hot and humid and should always maintain appropriate fluid intake. Exercise during pregnancy benefits both mother and fetus in the following ways:

- Reduces risk for gestational diabetes and preeclampsia
- Helps prevent excessive prenatal weight and body fat gain
- Improves mood, energy level, and sleep patterns
- Enhances posture and balance
- Improves muscle tone, strength, and endurance

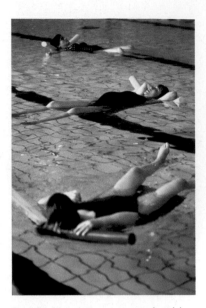

During pregnancy, women should adjust their physical activity to comfortable, low-impact exercise.

- Reduces lower back pain and shortens the duration of active labor
- Lowers the risk for preterm birth and large-for-gestational age infants

Recent guidelines suggest exercises that engage large muscle groups in a continuous manner, including a combination of moderate-intensity aerobic activity (brisk walking, leisurely swimming, dancing), vigorous-intensity aerobic activity (very brisk walking, swimming at a moderate-to-hard pace, cycling on a stationary bike, indoor rowing), and muscle-strengthening activities.[25] The terms *moderate* and *vigorous* are relative, since each woman enters and moves through her pregnancy at an individual level of fitness. Moderate activity is often described as one during which it is still possible to carry on a normal conversation; vigorous activity produces sweating, noticeable increases in breathing rate and depth, and an inability to converse normally. The more vigorous the activity, the less total time is needed to reap its benefits: 6.5 hours/week of brisk walking vs. fewer than 3 hours/week of stationary cycling.

Recommendations for muscle-strengthening exercise during pregnancy are straightforward:[24]

- Choose lighter weights and more repetitions.
- Opt for resistance bands over free weights, which might accidentally hit or fall on the abdomen.
- Don't lift weights while lying on your back, which might compress a major blood vessel and restrict blood flow to the fetus.
- Avoid moves that require sudden movements or might place you off balance, such as lunges or twists.
- Pay attention to your body's signals!

What about yoga and Pilates? Both offer classes tailored to pregnant women, adapting certain exercises to accommodate the body's changing center of gravity and increased joint flexibility. Activities that strengthen body core, abdominals, and pelvic floor or Kegel muscles make for an easier pregnancy and delivery. See **Table 16.3** for a sample program of physical activity for a pregnant woman.

Pregnant women should avoid activities such as horseback riding, scuba diving, water or snow skiing, hockey, gymnastics, and soccer. They need to stay hydrated, especially in

TABLE 16.3 Exercise Plan for Pregnant Women

Day of the Week	Warm-Up	Aerobic Activity	Muscle Strengthening	Cool-Down
Monday	5–10 min	30–45 min, moderate-intensity activity (leisurely lap swimming)		5 min
Tuesday	5–10 min		30 min light weights, high repetitions; upper and lower body	5 min
Wednesday	5–10 min	30 min vigorous activity (indoor cycling or rowing)		5 min
Thursday	5–10 min		45 min yoga, Pilates, or other core exercises	5 min
Friday	5–10 min	30–45 min moderate-intensity activity (outdoor hike, flat or gentle slope)		5 min
Saturday	5–10 min		30 minutes light weights, high repetitions; upper and lower body	5 min

Note: Women with established pre-pregnancy exercise routines should aim for the higher duration; women who rarely/never exercised before pregnancy should start with short durations of low-intensity activity and gradually build endurance.

hot and humid weather, and dress comfortably. If symptoms of stress, such as dizziness, shortness of breath, chest pain, vaginal bleeding or leakage, or uterine contractions, occur, all physical activity should stop and a healthcare provider contacted immediately.[26]

Want more details on maintaining fitness while pregnant? Watch this slideshow on exercise during and after pregnancy: www.webmd.com/baby/ss/slideshow-pregnancy-fitness-moves.

Caffeine Consumption

Caffeine, a stimulant found in coffee, tea, soft drinks, and some foods, crosses the placenta and thus reaches the fetus, whose ability to metabolize caffeine is limited. Current thinking holds that pregnant women who consume less than about 200–300 mg of caffeine per day (the equivalent of one to two cups of coffee) are very likely doing no harm to the fetus.[27,28] Evidence suggests that consuming higher daily doses of caffeine (the higher the dose, the more compelling the evidence) may slightly increase the risk for miscarriage and stillbirth and impair fetal growth.[29] It is sensible, then, for pregnant women to limit their daily caffeine intake to no more than the equivalent of two cups of coffee. See **Table 16.4** for a list of common sources of caffeine.

Another reason for avoiding coffee and caffeinated soft drinks during pregnancy is that they can make one feel full and, if sweetened, provide considerable Calories. If a pregnant woman retains a very strong desire for coffee, she might try a low- or nonfat decaf café latte, known to Latinas as *café con leche,* which offers a healthier nutrient profile than just coffee alone.

Alcohol Consumption

Alcohol is a known teratogen that readily crosses the placenta and accumulates in the fetal bloodstream. The immature fetal liver cannot readily metabolize alcohol, and its presence in fetal blood and tissues is associated with a variety of birth defects. These effects are dose dependent: the more the mother drinks, the greater the potential harm to the fetus. The term *fetal alcohol spectrum disorders (FASD)* encompasses a range of complications that can develop when a pregnant woman consumes alcohol.[30]

Excessive drinking (greater than three to four drinks per day) during pregnancy can result in the birth of a baby with *fetal alcohol syndrome (FAS)*, the most severe form of

TABLE 16.4 Caffeine Content of Common Foods and Beverages

Food/Beverage Name	Portion Size	Caffeine (mg) per Portion
Brewed coffee	16 fl. oz	200–325
Decaffeinated coffee	16 fl. oz	5–25
Espresso	2 fl. oz	150
Brewed tea	16 fl. oz	100–250
Iced green tea	16 fl. oz	15
Mountain Dew	12 fl. oz	54
Dr Pepper	12 fl. oz	43
Pepsi	12 fl. oz	38
7-Up, Sprite, Sierra Mist	12 fl. oz	0
Fresca, Fanta, Mug Root Beer	12 fl. oz	0
Monster Energy, Full Throttle, Red Bull, Amp	16 fl. oz	145–160
Coffee ice cream	8 fl. oz	50–70
Coffee yogurt	6 oz	36
Hershey's Special Dark Chocolate Bar	1.45 oz	30
Baking chocolate	1 oz	23
Hershey's Kisses	5 pieces	5

FASD. (For details on FAS and FASD, see Chapter 4.5, In Depth: Alcohol, page 165.) These infants have a high mortality rate, and those who do survive suffer from malformations of the face, limbs, heart, and nervous system and typically face lifelong emotional, behavioral, social, and learning problems. Another form of FASD, *alcohol-related neurodevelopmental disorder (ARND)*, is a more subtle set of alcohol-related abnormalities. These include developmental and behavioral problems (for example, hyperactivity, attention deficit disorder, and impaired cognition).[31]

In addition to FASD, frequent drinking (more than seven drinks per week) or occasional binge drinking (more than four to five drinks on one occasion) during pregnancy can increase the risk for miscarriage, complications during delivery, low birth weight, neonatal asphyxia, and intrauterine growth retardation.[32]

Although some pregnant women do have the occasional alcoholic drink with no apparent ill effects, there is no amount of alcohol that is known to be safe. The best advice regarding alcohol during pregnancy is to abstain, if not from before conception then as soon as pregnancy is suspected. As with other critical national health concerns, *Healthy People 2020* directly addresses this issue with the stated goals of increasing abstinence from alcohol among pregnant women and reducing the incidence of FAS.[3]

Smoking

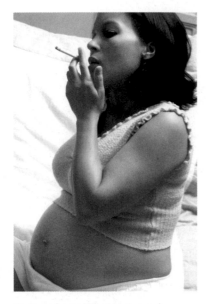

Maternal smoking is extremely harmful to the developing fetus.

Despite the well-known consequences of cigarette smoking and the growing social stigma associated with smoking during pregnancy, more than 13% of pregnant women smoked during their last trimester of pregnancy, and the rate was even higher among adolescents.[33,34]

Maternal smoking exposes the fetus to toxins such as lead, cadmium, cyanide, nicotine, and carbon monoxide. Fetal blood flow is reduced, which limits the delivery of oxygen and nutrients, resulting in impaired fetal growth and development. Maternal smoking greatly increases risk for miscarriage, stillbirth, placental abnormalities, intrauterine growth retardation, preterm delivery, and low birth weight. Rates of sudden infant death syndrome, overall neonatal mortality (within the first 28 days of life), respiratory illnesses, risk for cleft lip or cleft palate, and allergies are higher in the infants and children of smokers compared to nonsmokers.

Healthy People 2020 has the goal of increasing the number of women who stop smoking during their first trimester and stay off cigarettes for the duration of their pregnancy.[3] It has been estimated that the potential exists to save almost $40,000 in healthcare expenses for preventing just one smoking-related low-birth-weight baby.[35]

Illegal Drugs

Despite the fact that illegal drug use during pregnancy is unquestionably harmful to the fetus, nearly 5% of U.S. pregnant women between the ages of 15 and 44 years report having used illicit drugs. Over 16% of pregnant adolescents (15–17 years) used illicit drugs, as did 7% of young adult pregnant women (18–25 years).[36] Most drugs pass through the placenta into the fetal blood, where they accumulate in fetal tissues and organs, including the liver and brain.

Drugs such as marijuana, cocaine, heroin, ecstasy, and amphetamines all pose similar risks: impaired placental blood flow (thus, reduced transfer of oxygen and nutrients to the fetus) and higher rates of low birth weight, premature delivery, placental defects, and miscarriage. Newborns suffer signs of withdrawal, including tremors, excessive crying, sleeplessness, and poor feeding.[37] Even after several years, children born to women who used illicit drugs during pregnancy are at greater risk for developmental delays, impaired learning, and behavioral problems. Recently, inappropriate use of certain prescription medications, including prescription narcotics, have created additional problems for pregnant women and their infants.

All women are strongly advised to stop taking illegal and inappropriate prescription drugs *before* becoming pregnant. There is no safe level of use for illegal drugs during pregnancy.

Food Safety

The US Departments of Health and Human Services and of Agriculture recommend that pregnant women avoid unpasteurized milk, raw or partially cooked eggs, raw or undercooked meat/fish/poultry, unpasteurized juices, and raw sprouts.[38] Women who are or could become pregnant, as well as breastfeeding mothers, are advised to avoid eating large fish, such as shark, swordfish, and king mackerel, and to limit their intake of canned albacore tuna because of their high mercury content. Pregnant women should consult their state or county health department for information on the safety of locally caught fish.

Fish, shellfish, and a variety of meats may be contaminated with dioxins, persistent organic pollutants associated with a variety of health problems. The effect of dioxins may be most significant on the developing fetal organs, including the nervous system, and on birth weight.[39] As with mercury, state or country health departments can provide information about dioxin levels in the local food supply.

Soft cheeses, such as brie, feta, Camembert, and Mexican-style cheeses (called *queso blanco* or *queso fresco*), should be avoided unless the label specifically states the product is made with pasteurized milk. Unpasteurized milk and cheeses may be contaminated with the bacterium *Listeria monocytogenes*, which triggers miscarriage, premature birth, or fetal infection when consumed during pregnancy. Pregnant women should follow safe food-handling practices to ensure a healthy pregnancy outcome (see Chapter 15).

RECAP

About half of all pregnant women experience morning sickness, and many crave or feel aversions to specific types of foods. Gastroesophageal reflux and constipation in pregnancy are related to hormonal relaxation of smooth muscle. Gestational diabetes and hypertensive disorders can seriously affect maternal and fetal well-being. The nutrient needs of pregnant adolescents are so high that adequate nourishment becomes difficult. Women who follow a vegan diet usually need to consume multivitamin and mineral supplements, plus supplemental calcium, during pregnancy. Exercise (provided the mother has no contraindications) can enhance the health of a pregnant woman. Caffeine intake should be limited; and use of alcohol, cigarettes, and illegal drugs should be completely avoided during pregnancy. Safe food-handling practices are especially important during pregnancy. ■

*Nutri-*Case

Judy

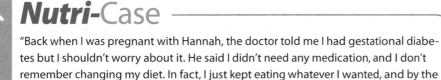

"Back when I was pregnant with Hannah, the doctor told me I had gestational diabetes but I shouldn't worry about it. He said I didn't need any medication, and I don't remember changing my diet. In fact, I just kept eating whatever I wanted, and by the time Hannah was born, I had gained almost 60 pounds. I never did lose all that extra weight."

Judy has recently been diagnosed with type 2 diabetes. If Judy were pregnant today, what information would her healthcare provider probably share with her? Is it common that women with gestational diabetes develop type 2 diabetes years later? What are some things Judy could have done to lower her risk for type 2 diabetes?

Lactation: Nutrition for Breastfeeding Mothers

Throughout most of human history, infants have thrived on only one food: breast milk. As early as 1867, however, synthetic milk substitutes became available. During the first half of the 20th century, commercially prepared infant formulas slowly began to replace breast milk as many women's preferred feeding method. Aggressive marketing campaigns promoting formula as more nutritious than breast milk convinced many families, even in developing nations, to switch. Soon formula-feeding became a status symbol, proof of a family's wealth and modern thinking.

In the 1970s, this trend began to reverse with a renewed appreciation for the natural simplicity of breastfeeding. At the same time, several international organizations, including the World Health Organization, UNICEF, and La Leche League, began to promote the nutritional, immunologic, financial, and emotional advantages of breastfeeding and developed programs to encourage and support breastfeeding worldwide.

These efforts have paid off. In 2010, almost 75% of new U.S. mothers initiated breastfeeding in the hospital, an all-time high, and more than 44% of mothers were still breastfeeding their babies at 6 months of age.[40] Worldwide, slightly more than half of all women breastfeed *exclusively* for at least 6 months; however, this value is significantly lower in the United States, where only 15% of children are breast-fed exclusively at 6 months of age.[40]

One goal of *Healthy People 2020* is to increase early postpartum breastfeeding to 82% of U.S. mothers, with 60% of women still breastfeeding at 6 months and 34% at 12 months postpartum.[3] Although U.S. mothers have nearly achieved the early postpartum goal, they still fall well below the 6- and 12-month goals.

How Does Lactation Occur?

Lactation, the production of breast milk, is a process that is set in motion during pregnancy in response to several hormones. Once established, lactation can be sustained as long as the mammary glands continue to receive the proper stimuli.

The Body Prepares During Pregnancy

Throughout pregnancy, the placenta produces the hormones estrogen and progesterone. In addition to performing various functions to maintain the pregnancy, these hormones physically prepare the breasts for lactation. The breasts increase in size, and milk-producing glands (alveoli) and milk ducts are formed (**Figure 16.8**). Toward the end of pregnancy, the hormone *prolactin* increases. Prolactin is released by the anterior pituitary gland and is responsible for milk synthesis. However, estrogen and progesterone suppress the effects of prolactin during pregnancy.

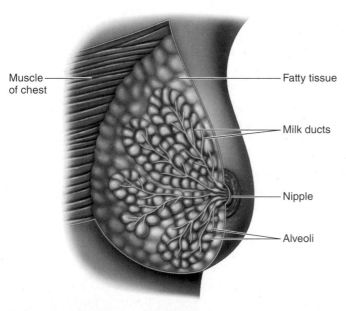

Muscle of chest — Fatty tissue — Milk ducts — Nipple — Alveoli

FIGURE 16.8 Anatomy of the breast. During pregnancy, estrogen and progesterone secreted by the placenta foster the preparation of breast tissue for lactation. This process includes breast enlargement and development of the milk-producing glands, or alveoli.

lactation The production of breast milk.

colostrum The first fluid made and secreted by the breasts from late in pregnancy to about a week after birth. It is rich in immune factors and protein.

What Happens After Childbirth

By the time a pregnancy has come to full term, the level of prolactin is about ten times higher than it was at the beginning of pregnancy. At birth, the suppressive effect of estrogen and progesterone ends, and prolactin is free to stimulate milk production. The first substance to be released from the breasts for intake by the newborn is **colostrum,** sometimes called premilk or first milk. It is thick, yellowish in color, and rich in protein, and it includes antibodies that help protect the newborn from infection. It is also relatively high in vitamins and minerals. Colostrum also contains a factor that fosters the growth of "friendly" bacteria in the infant's GI tract. These bacteria in turn prevent the growth of other, potentially harmful bacteria. Finally, colostrum has a laxative effect in infants, helping the infant to expel *meconium,* the sticky "first stool." Within 2 to 4 days, colostrum is fully replaced by mature milk. Mature breast milk contains protein, fat, and carbohydrate (as the sugar lactose).

Mother–Infant Interaction Maintains Milk Production

Continued, sustained breast milk production depends entirely on infant suckling (or a similar stimulus, such as a mechanical pump). Infant suckling stimulates the continued production of prolactin, which in turn stimulates more milk production. The longer and more vigorous the feeding, the more milk will be produced. Thus, even twins and triplets can be successfully breastfed.

Prolactin allows for milk to be produced, but that milk has to move through the milk ducts to the nipple in order to reach the baby's mouth. The hormone responsible for this "let-down" of milk is *oxytocin.* Like prolactin, oxytocin is produced by the pituitary gland, and its production is dependent on the suckling stimulus at the beginning of a feeding (**Figure 16.9**). This response usually occurs within 10 to 30 seconds but can be inhibited by stress. Finding a relaxed environment in which to breastfeed is therefore important. Many women experience let-down in response to other cues, such as hearing a baby cry or even thinking about their infant.

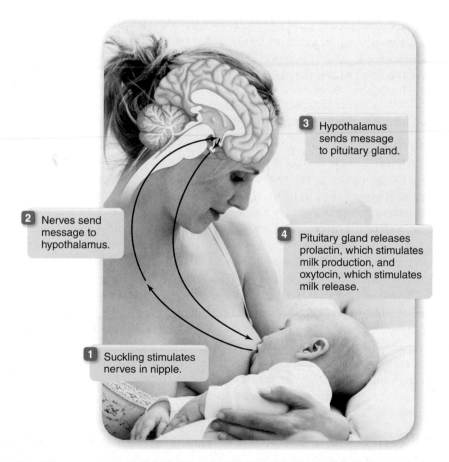

3 Hypothalamus sends message to pituitary gland.

2 Nerves send message to hypothalamus.

4 Pituitary gland releases prolactin, which stimulates milk production, and oxytocin, which stimulates milk release.

1 Suckling stimulates nerves in nipple.

FIGURE 16.9 Sustained milk production depends on the mother–child interaction during breastfeeding, specifically the suckling of the infant. Suckling stimulates the continued production of prolactin, which is responsible for milk production, and oxytocin, which is responsible for the let-down response.

What Are a Breastfeeding Woman's Nutrient Needs?

You might be surprised to learn that breastfeeding requires even more energy and nutrients than pregnancy! This is because breast milk has to supply an adequate amount of all the nutrients an infant needs to grow and develop.

Energy and Macronutrient Recommendations for Breastfeeding Women

It is estimated that milk production requires about 700 to 800 kcal/day. It is generally recommended that lactating women aged 19 years and above consume 330 kcal/day above their pre-pregnancy energy needs during the first 6 months of breastfeeding and 400 additional kcal/day during the second 6 months.[10] This additional energy is sufficient to support adequate milk production. At the same time, the remaining energy deficit will assist in the gradual loss of excess body weight gained during pregnancy. It is critical that lactating women avoid severe energy restriction, as this practice can result in decreased milk production.

The weight loss that occurs during breastfeeding should be gradual, approximately 1 to 4 lb per month. Participating in regular physical activity can assist with weight loss and prevent excess weight gain up to 10 years later.[41] Moderate aerobic exercise (45 min/day, 5 days/week) does not affect breast milk volume or composition, nor does it reduce infant growth. There are, however, some very active women who may lose too much weight during breastfeeding and must either increase their energy intake or reduce their activity level to maintain health and milk production.

A lactating woman's needs for carbohydrate and protein increase over pregnancy requirements. Increases of 15 to 20 g of protein per day and 80 g of carbohydrate per day above pre-pregnancy requirements are recommended.[10] Women who breastfeed also need good dietary sources of DHA to support the rapid brain growth that occurs during the first 3 months of life. The DHA in the mother's diet is incorporated into the breast milk, to the benefit of the infant.

Micronutrient Recommendations for Breastfeeding Women

Micronutrient requirements for several vitamins and minerals increase over the requirements of pregnancy. These include vitamins A, C, E, riboflavin, vitamin B_{12}, biotin, and choline and the minerals copper, chromium, manganese, iodine, selenium, and zinc. The requirement for folate during lactation is 500 µg/day, which is decreased from the 600 µg/day required during pregnancy but is higher than pre-pregnancy needs (400 µg/day).[12]

Requirements for iron decrease significantly during lactation, to a mere 9 mg/day. This is because iron is not a significant component of breast milk, and breastfeeding usually suppresses menstruation for at least a few months, minimizing iron losses.[13]

Calcium is a significant component of breast milk; however, as in pregnancy, calcium absorption is enhanced during lactation, and urinary loss of calcium is decreased. In addition, some calcium appears to come from the demineralization of the mother's bones, and increased dietary calcium does not prevent this. Thus, the recommended intake for calcium for a lactating woman 19 years or older is unchanged from pregnancy and nonpregnant guidelines: 1,000 mg/day. Because of their own continuing growth, however, teen mothers (14–18 years) who are breastfeeding should continue to consume 1,300 mg/day.[14] Typically, if calcium intake is adequate, a woman's bone density returns to normal shortly after lactation ends.

Do Breastfeeding Women Need Supplements?

If a breastfeeding woman appropriately increases her energy intake, and does so with nutrient-dense foods, her nutrient needs can usually be met without supplements. The USDA's ChooseMyPlate.gov website provides recommendations for food choices for women who are breastfeeding their infants (see Web Links at the end of this chapter). However, there is nothing wrong with taking a basic multivitamin, as long as it is not considered a substitute for proper nutrition. Lactating women should consume omega-3 fatty acids either in fish or in supplements to increase breast milk levels of DHA. Women who do not consume dairy products should monitor their calcium intake carefully and may need supplements.

Fluid Recommendations for Breastfeeding Women

Because extra fluid is expended with every feeding, lactating women need to consume about an extra quart (about 1 liter) of fluid per day. The AI for total water is 3.8 liters per day for breastfeeding women, including about 13 cups of beverages.[17] This extra fluid enhances milk production and reduces the risk for dehydration. Many women report that, within a minute or two of beginning to nurse their baby, they become intensely thirsty. To prevent this thirst and achieve the recommended fluid intake, women are encouraged to drink a nutritious beverage (water, juice, milk, and so forth) each time they nurse their baby. However, women should avoid drinking hot beverages while nursing, because accidental spills could burn the infant.

RECAP

Lactation is the result of the coordinated effort of several hormones. Breasts are prepared for lactation during pregnancy, and infant suckling provides the stimulus that sustains the production of prolactin and oxytocin needed to maintain the milk supply. It is recommended that lactating women consume extra energy above pre-pregnancy guidelines, including increased protein, certain vitamins and minerals, and fluids. The requirements for folate and iron decrease from pregnancy levels, while the requirement for calcium remains the same. If nutrient intake is inadequate, milk production will decline and the woman will produce a smaller volume of breast milk. ■

Getting Real About Breastfeeding: Advantages and Challenges

Breastfeeding is recognized as the preferred method of infant feeding because of the nutritional value and health benefits of human milk.[42] However, the technique does require patience and practice, and teaching from an experienced mother or a certified lactation consultant is important. La Leche League International is an advocacy group for breastfeeding: its website (included at the back of this chapter under Web Links), publications, and local meetings are all valuable resources for breastfeeding mothers and their families. Many HMOs offer lactation classes for their members, and some U.S. hospitals, designated as "Baby Friendly," have adopted policies that enhance lactation success.[43]

Advantages of Breastfeeding

As adept as formula manufacturers have been at simulating components of breast milk, an exact replica has never been produced. In addition, there are other benefits that mother and baby can access only through breastfeeding.

Nutritional Superiority of Breast Milk   The amount and types of proteins in breast milk are ideally suited to the human infant. The main protein in breast milk, lactalbumin, is easily digested in infants' immature GI tracts, reducing the risk for gastric distress. Other proteins in breast milk bind iron and prevent the growth of harmful bacteria that require iron. Antibodies from the mother are additional proteins that help prevent infection while the infant's immune system is still immature. Certain proteins in human milk improve the absorption of iron; this is important because breast milk is low in iron. Cow's milk contains too much protein for infants, and the types of protein in cow's milk are harder for the infant to digest.

The primary carbohydrate in breast milk is lactose; its galactose component is important in nervous system development. Lactose provides energy and prevents ketosis in the infant, promotes the growth of beneficial bacteria, and increases the absorption of calcium. Breast milk has more lactose than cow's milk.

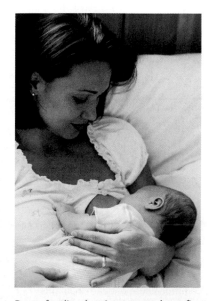

Breastfeeding has important benefits for both the mother and the infant.

The amounts and types of fat in breast milk are ideally suited to the human infant. DHA and arachidonic acid (ARA) are fatty acids that have been shown to be essential for the growth and development of the infant's nervous system and for development of the retina of the eyes. Until 2002, these fatty acids were omitted from commercial infant formulas in the United States, although they were available in formulas in other parts of the world. Interestingly, the concentration of DHA in breast milk varies considerably, is sensitive to maternal diet, and is highest in women who consume large quantities of fish during pregnancy and/or lactation.[44]

The fat content of breast milk, which is higher than that of whole cow's milk, changes according to the gestational age of the infant and during the course of every feeding: the milk that is initially released (called *foremilk*) is watery and low in fat, somewhat like skim milk. This milk is thought to satisfy the infant's initial thirst. As the feeding progresses, the milk acquires more fat and becomes more like whole milk. Finally, the very last 5% or so of the milk produced during a feeding (called the *hindmilk*) is very high in fat, similar to cream. This milk is thought to satiate the infant. It is important to let infants suckle for at least 20 minutes at each feeding, so that they get this hindmilk. Breast milk is also relatively high in cholesterol, which supports the rapid growth and development of the brain and nervous system.

Another important aspect of breastfeeding (or any type of feeding) is the fluid it provides the infant. Because of their small size, infants are at risk for dehydration, which is one reason feedings must be consistent and frequent. This topic will be discussed at greater length in the section on infant nutrition.

In terms of micronutrients, breast milk is a good source of readily absorbed calcium and magnesium. It is low in iron, but the iron it does contain is easily absorbed. Because healthy full-term infants store iron in preparation for the first few months of life, most experts agree that their iron needs can be met by breast milk alone for the first 6 months, after which iron-rich foods are needed. Although breast milk has some vitamin D, the American Academy of Pediatrics recommends that all breast-fed infants be provided with a vitamin D supplement.[45]

Breast milk composition continues to change as the infant grows and develops. Because of this ability to change as the baby changes, breast milk alone is entirely sufficient to sustain infant growth for the first 6 months of life. Throughout the next 6 months of infancy, as solid foods are gradually introduced, breast milk remains the baby's primary source of superior-quality nutrition. The American Academy of Pediatrics encourages exclusive breastfeeding (no food or other source of sustenance) for the first 6 months of life, continuing breastfeeding for at least the first year of life and, if acceptable within the family unit, into the second year of life.[46]

Protection from Infections, Allergies, and Residues Immune factors from the mother, including antibodies and immune cells, are passed directly from the mother to the newborn through breast milk. These factors provide important disease protection for the infant while its immune system is still immature. It has been shown that breast-fed infants have a lower incidence of respiratory tract, gastrointestinal tract, and ear infections than formula-fed infants.[46] Even a few weeks of breastfeeding is beneficial, but the longer a child is breastfed, the greater the level of passive immunity from the mother. In the United States, exclusive breastfeeding for 6 months has the potential to lower healthcare costs by as much as $13 billion per year, in large part due to a reduction in infant mortality rates related to **sudden infant death syndrome (SIDS)** and necrotizing enterocolitis (a disorder that causes tissue death in the intestine) in breast-fed infants.[47]

In addition, breast milk is nonallergenic, and breastfeeding is associated with a reduced risk for allergies during childhood and adulthood. Breast-fed babies also have a decreased chance of developing diabetes, overweight and obesity, hypercholesterolemia, and chronic digestive disorders.[46]

sudden infant death syndrome (SIDS) The sudden death of an otherwise healthy infant; the most common cause of death in infants older than 1 month of age.

Exclusively breast-fed infants are also protected from exposure to known and unknown contaminants and residues that may be found in baby bottles and cans of infant formulas. Recent concerns have centered on bisphenol A (BPA), a toxic chemical that has been found in a few brands of reusable bottles and formulas. As of 2009, the major U.S. manufacturers of baby bottles and infant feeding cups, which account for 90% of U.S. sales, discontinued the sale of products using BPA for the U.S. market.[48]

Physiologic Benefits for Mother Breastfeeding causes uterine contractions that quicken the return of the uterus to pre-pregnancy size and reduce bleeding. Many women also find that breastfeeding helps them lose the weight they gained during pregnancy, particularly if it continues for more than 6 months. In addition, breastfeeding appears to be associated with a decreased risk for breast cancer.[49] The relationship between breastfeeding and osteoporosis is still unclear, and more research on this topic is needed.[50]

Breastfeeding also suppresses ovulation, lengthening the time between pregnancies and giving a mother's body the chance to recover before she conceives again. This benefit can be life-saving for malnourished women living in countries that discourage or outlaw the use of contraceptives. Ovulation may not cease completely, however, so it is still possible to become pregnant while breastfeeding. Healthcare providers typically recommend the use of additional birth control methods while breastfeeding to avoid another conception too soon to allow a mother's body to recover from the earlier pregnancy.

Mother–Infant Bonding Breastfeeding is among the most intimate of human interactions. Ideally, it is a quiet time away from distractions when mother and baby begin to develop an enduring bond of affection known as *attachment*. Breastfeeding enhances attachment by providing the opportunity for frequent, direct skin-to-skin contact, which stimulates the baby's sense of touch and is a primary means of communication.[25] The cuddling and intense watching that occur during breastfeeding begin to teach the mother and baby about the other's behavioral cues. Breastfeeding also reassures the mother that she is providing the best possible nutrition for her baby. Healthcare providers recommend that hospitals permit continuous rooming-in of breast-fed infants throughout the day and night to enhance the initiation and continuation of breastfeeding.[43]

Undoubtedly, bottle-feeding does not preclude parent–infant attachment! As long as attention is paid to closeness, cuddling, and skin contact, bottle-feeding can foster bonding as well.

Convenience and Cost Breast milk is always ready, clean, at the right temperature, and available on demand, whenever and wherever it's needed. In the middle of the night, when the baby wakes up hungry, a breastfeeding mother can respond almost instantaneously, and both are soon back to sleep. In contrast, formula-feeding is a time-consuming process: parents have to continually wash and sterilize bottles, and each batch of formula must be mixed and heated to the proper temperature.

In addition, breastfeeding costs nothing other than the price of a modest amount of additional food for the mother. In contrast, formula can be relatively expensive, and there are the additional costs of bottles and other supplies, as well as the cost of energy used for washing and sterilization. A hidden cost of formula-feeding is its effect on the environment—the energy used and waste produced during formula manufacturing, marketing, shipping and distribution, preparation, and disposal of used packaging. In contrast, breastfeeding is environmentally responsible, using no external energy and producing no external wastes.

Challenges Associated with Breastfeeding

For some women and infants, breastfeeding is easy from the very first day. Others experience some initial difficulty, but with support from an experienced nurse, lactation consultant, or volunteer mother from La Leche League, the experience becomes successful and pleasurable. Some families, however, encounter difficulties that make formula-feeding their best choice, temporarily or permanently.

Effects of Drugs and Other Substances on Breast Milk   Many substances, including prescription and over-the-counter medications, pass into breast milk. Breastfeeding mothers should inform their physician that they are breastfeeding. If a safe and effective form of the necessary medication cannot be found, the mother will have to avoid breastfeeding while she is taking the drug. During this time, she can pump and discard her breast milk, so that her milk supply will be adequate when she resumes breastfeeding.

Caffeine, alcohol, nicotine, and illicit drugs also enter breast milk. Caffeine, nicotine, and other stimulant drugs can make the baby agitated and fussy and can disturb infant sleep patterns. Breastfeeding women should reduce their caffeine intake to no more than two or three cups of coffee per day (or the equivalent of other caffeine-containing beverages and foods) and avoid caffeine intake within 2 hours prior to nursing their infant. They should also quit smoking and avoid the use of illicit drugs. Alcohol can make the baby sleepy, depress the central nervous system, and slow motor development, in addition to inhibiting the mother's milk supply. Breastfeeding women should abstain from alcohol in the early stages of lactation, since it easily passes into the breast milk and infants 0–3 months of age metabolize alcohol at a rate half that of adults. It takes about 2 to 3 hours for the alcohol from a single serving of beer or wine to be eliminated from the body, so it is possible for breastfeeding women to plan ahead and coordinate moderate alcohol intake with their breastfeeding schedule.

Environmental contaminants, including pesticides, industrial solvents, and heavy metals such as lead and mercury, can pass into breast milk when breastfeeding mothers are exposed to these chemicals.[51,52] Mothers can limit their infants' exposure to these harmful substances by controlling their environment. Fresh fruits and vegetables should be thoroughly washed and peeled to minimize exposure to pesticides and fertilizer residues. Exposure to solvents, paints, gasoline fumes, furniture strippers, and similar products should also be limited. Even with some exposure to these environmental contaminants, U.S. and international health agencies all agree that the benefits of breastfeeding almost always outweigh potential concerns.

Food components that pass into the breast milk may seem innocuous; however, some substances, such as those found in garlic, onions, peppers, broccoli, and cabbage, are distasteful enough to the infant to prevent proper feeding. Some babies have allergic reactions to foods the mother has eaten, such as wheat, cow's milk, eggs, or citrus, and suffer gastrointestinal upset, diaper rash, or another reaction. The offending foods must then be identified and avoided.

Maternal HIV Infection and Other Diseases   HIV, the virus that causes AIDS, can be transmitted from mother to baby through breast milk. Thus, HIV-positive women in the United States and Canada are encouraged to feed their infants formula. This recommendation does not apply to all women worldwide, however, because the low cost and sanitary nature of breast milk, as compared to the high cost and potential for waterborne diseases with formula-feeding, often make exclusive breastfeeding the best choice for women in developing countries.[53] The United Nations recently published new guidelines on infant feeding for HIV-infected women.[54]

Conflict Between Breastfeeding and the Mother's Employment   Breast milk is absorbed more readily than formula, making more frequent feedings necessary. Newborns commonly require breastfeeding every 1 to 3 hours versus every 2 to 4 hours for formula-feeding. Mothers who are exclusively breastfeeding and return to work within the first 6 months after the baby's birth must leave several bottles of pumped breast milk for others to feed the baby in their absence each day. This means that working women have to pump their breasts to express the breast milk during the work day. This can be a challenge in companies that do not provide the time, space, and privacy required, a scenario most often seen in low-paying jobs.

Work-related travel is also a concern: if the mother needs to be away from home for longer than 24 to 48 hours, she can typically pump and freeze enough breast milk for others to give the baby in her absence. Understandably, many women cite returning to work as the reason they switch to formula-feeding.[55]

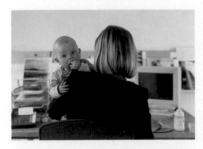

Working moms can be discouraged from—or supported in—breastfeeding in a variety of ways.

Some working women successfully combine breastfeeding with formula-feeding. For example, a woman might breastfeed in the morning before she leaves for work, as soon as she returns home, and again at bedtime. Other feedings are formula given by the infant's father or a childcare provider. Women who choose this approach usually find that their bodies adapt quickly and produce ample milk for the remaining breastfeedings.

Social Concerns   In North America, women have at times been insulted or otherwise harassed for breastfeeding in public. Over the past decade, however, both social customs and state laws have become more accommodating and supportive of nursing mothers. Some states have passed legislation preserving a woman's right to breastfeed in public. Advocacy groups and greater social and cultural awareness have also contributed to a more forgiving climate for women to breastfeed. When women feel free (and legally protected) to do so, the baby's feeding schedule becomes much less confining. For more information on the work of La Leche League and other organizations that provide support for breastfeeding mothers, see the **Highlight** box (page 666).

What About Bonding for Fathers and Siblings?

With all the attention given to attachment between a breastfeeding mother and an infant, it is easy for fathers and siblings to feel left out. One option that allows other family members to participate in infant feeding is to supplement breastfeeding with bottle-feedings of stored breast milk or formula as soon as breastfeeding has become well established. That way, the mother's milk supply will be established, and the infant will not be confused by the artificial nipple. Fathers and other family members can also bond with the infant when bathing and/or dressing them, as well as through everyday cuddling and play.

Although breastfeeding in public is a much more common practice today than in the past, some people still consider it inappropriate.

RECAP

Breastfeeding provides many benefits to both mother and newborn, including superior nutrition, heightened immunity, mother–infant bonding, convenience, and cost. However, breastfeeding may not be the best option for every family. A mother may need to use a medication that enters the breast milk and makes it unsafe for consumption. A mother's job may interfere with the baby's requirement for frequent feedings. The infant's father and siblings can participate in feedings using a bottle filled with either pumped breast milk or formula. ■

Infant Nutrition: From Birth to 1 Year

Most first-time parents are amazed at how rapidly their infant grows and develops. Optimal nutrition is extremely important during the first year, as the baby's organs and nervous system continue to develop and mature and as the baby grows physically and acquires new skills.

During the first year of an infant's life, breast milk remains the food of choice; however, iron-fortified formula is an acceptable substitute for those families who have decided that breastfeeding is not an option. After approximately 6 months, most infants are ready for *complementary* foods, such as baby cereals and strained meats, which provide key nutrients and introduce the infant to new tastes and textures. An infant who is lovingly and consistently fed when hungry will feel secure and well cared for. A relaxed, consistent feeding relationship between parent and child fosters a positive and healthy outlook toward food. In many ways, an infant's diet during his or her first year of life "sets the stage" for future health and development.

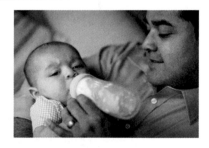

Fathers and siblings can bond with infants through bottle-feeding.

Typical Infant Growth and Activity Patterns

In the first year of life, an infant generally grows about 10 inches in length and triples in weight—a growth rate more rapid than will ever occur again. To support this phenomenal growth, energy needs per unit body weight are also the highest they will ever be,

Finding Support for Breastfeeding Moms

Although one of life's most natural processes, the "art of breastfeeding" for many women requires a certain amount of education, support, and practice. Fortunately, women today have more opportunities to learn about and practice breastfeeding than ever before.

Prenatal classes (classes held before the birth) are one such opportunity. Typically taught by certified nurse practitioners, midwives, or other childbirth specialists, these classes provide essential information—including information about breastfeeding—to parents-to-be. In many communities, special breastfeeding classes are offered by certified lactation consultants or other maternity healthcare providers, to help women who plan to breastfeed for the first time or who want to improve upon a previous breastfeeding experience.

Many hospitals and birthing centers also now provide breastfeeding support. Hospitals can seek the designation "Baby Friendly" based on the World Health Organization/UNICEF Baby-Friendly Hospital Initiative, meaning their facilities have shown that they have adopted certain practices to support successful breastfeeding. The following are some of those practices:[1]

- Having a written breastfeeding policy that is communicated to all healthcare staff

- Informing all pregnant women about the benefits and management of breastfeeding

- Helping mothers initiate breastfeeding within a half-hour of birth and helping them maintain lactation

- Giving newborn infants no food or drink other than breast milk, unless medically indicated

- Practicing rooming-in to encourage breastfeeding on demand

- Fostering the establishment of breastfeeding support groups and referring mothers to them on discharge from the hospital or clinic

Unfortunately, as of May 2012, there were only 143 Baby Friendly hospitals and clinics in the United States, a discouragingly low number.[2] A current list can be found at www.babyfriendlyusa.org. Even without this designation, however, many hospitals and clinics are becoming more actively supportive of breastfeeding than in years past.

La Leche League International is a worldwide organization dedicated to supporting breastfeeding mothers. La Leche League offers local meetings and conferences, as well as books, CDs, podcasts, online forums, and other materials, to help pregnant women and new moms succeed in breastfeeding. However, its most significant contribution may be the free in-home visits offered by experienced members to help women establish or maintain breastfeeding and troubleshoot problems. La Leche League also offers resources for moms of multiples (twins, triplets, and so on), premature infants, or special-healthcare-need babies, as well as materials for working mothers and those who want to provide their infants with breast milk even though they themselves can't nurse. Resources are now available in dozens of languages, providing education and support to millions of women in the United States and across the globe. Other grassroots organizations provide additional assistance to breastfeeding women and their babies.

To help families identify qualified lactation consultants, groups such as the International Board of Lactation Consultant Examiners develop and administer certification examinations. When searching for a qualified lactation consultant, parents-to-be can thus confirm a candidate's professional qualifications.

In some communities, local mothers serve as *doulas*—knowledgeable, experienced lay companions who stay with the new mom and family through labor, birth, and beyond, often supporting the breastfeeding process. While these women may not have academic or professional credentials, they are typically well known and respected within the local community.

References

1. Goodman, K., and E. DiFrisco. 2012. Achieving baby-friendly designation; step-by-step. *MCN Am. J. Matern. Child Nurs.* 37:146–152.
2. Baby Friendly Hospitals, USA. 2012. U.S. Baby-Friendly Birth Facilities. www.babyfriendlyusa.org/eng/03.html. (Accessed July 2012.)

approximately triple that of adults. Energy needs are also very high, because the basal metabolic rates of babies are high (**Figure 16.10**). This is in part because the body surface area of a baby is large compared to its body size, increasing its loss of body heat. Still, the limited physical activity of a baby keeps total energy expenditure relatively low.

For the first few months of life, an infant's activities consist mainly of eating and sleeping. As the first year progresses, the range of activities gradually expands to include rolling over, sitting up, crawling, standing, and finally taking the first few wobbly steps. As shown in Figure 16.10, the relative need for energy to support growth slows during the second 6 months of life, just as activity begins to increase.

Growth charts—one set for girls and one set for boys—are routinely used by healthcare providers and parents to track growth. They are available from the Centers for Disease Control and Prevention (CDC) free of charge. An example is provided in **Figure 16.11**. Charts for children birth to 36 months assess length-for-age, weight-for-age, and weight-for-length, all expressed as percentiles. If an infant is in the 90th percentile for length, he or she is longer than 89% of U.S. infants of that age and gender and thus is considered very long. If an infant is in the 10th percentile for weight, only 10% of U.S. infants of the same age and gender weigh less than he or she does, so that baby can be viewed as relatively underweight compared to other infants. Although every infant is unique, in general, healthcare providers look for a close correlation between length and weight rankings. In other words, an infant who is in the 60th percentile for length is usually in about the 50th to 70th percentile for weight. A child in the 50th percentile for length but the 5th percentile for weight may be malnourished. Consistency over time is also a consideration: for example, an infant who suddenly drops well below his or her established profile for weight might be underfed or ill. The CDC has also developed BMI-for-age charts for children over 24 months of age.

Although growth charts are effective tools for assessing an infant's nutrition status, there are some limitations. For example, it is important to consider the physical stature of the baby's parents. If both parents are tall, you would expect the infant to remain close to the upper percentiles for length. Exclusively breast-fed infants often track at a lower percentile weight-for-age compared to formula-fed infants, although no differences in length-for-age or head circumference are noted. Families need to know that this slower rate of weight gain has not been associated with any negative outcomes. Indeed, many healthcare providers believe that the slower growth rate of breast-fed infants should be considered the norm, not the exception, because formula-feeding is a relatively recent cultural phenomenon.

The growth of the brain is more rapid during the first year than at any other time, and infants' heads are typically large in proportion to the rest of their bodies, approximately one-fourth of their total length. Pediatricians use head circumference as an additional tool for the assessment of growth and nutritional status; CDC growth charts for head-circumference-for-age are available for infants and toddlers birth to 36 months of age. After around 18 months of age, the rate of brain growth slows, and gradually the body "catches up" to head size, resulting in body proportions that are closer to those of a child.

As infants grow and develop, their proportions of muscle, fat, and bone evolve. Body fat, as a percentage of total body weight, increases after birth and peaks around 9 months of age. Muscle tissue increases slowly but steadily, and body calcium, a marker for skeletal growth, more than doubles during the first year of life.[14] Body water, as a percentage of total body weight, is highest in newborns and gradually decreases through and beyond early childhood.[17]

Nutrient Needs of Infants

Three characteristics of infants combine to make their nutritional needs unique. These are (1) their high energy needs per unit body weight to support rapid growth, (2) their immature digestive tracts and kidneys, and (3) their small size.

Macronutrient Needs of Infants

An infant needs to consume about 40 to 50 kcal/lb of body weight per day, with newborns at the higher end of the range and infants 6 to 12 months old at the lower end. This amounts to about 600 (girls) to 650 (boys) kcal/day at around 6 months of age.[10] Given the immature digestive tracts and kidneys of infants, as well as their high fluid needs, providing this much energy may seem difficult. Fortunately, breast milk and commercial formulas are energy dense, providing about 650 kcal/L of fluid.[10] When complementary (solid) foods are introduced, they provide even more energy in addition to the breast milk or formula.

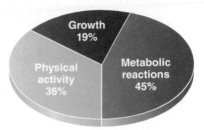

0–6 months

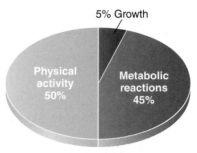

6–12 months

FIGURE 16.10 Energy expenditure during infancy. During the first 6 months of life, infants expend more energy to support growth and less energy on physical activity than in the second 6 months of life.

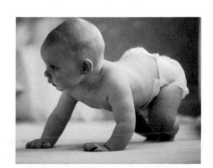

The proportions of muscle, fat, and bone in the bodies of infants change as they grow and become more active.

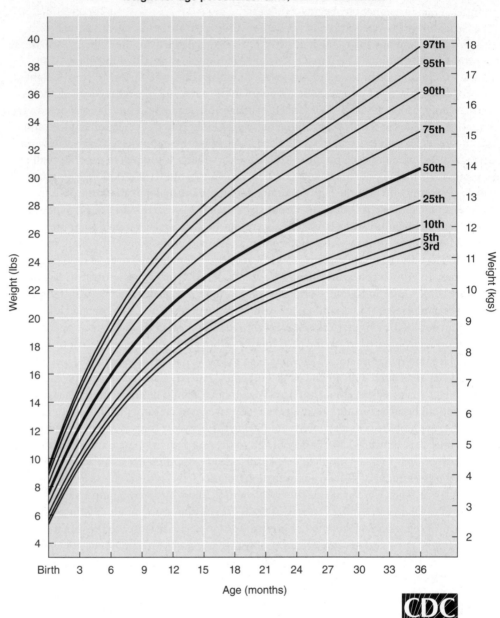

FIGURE 16.11 This weight-for-age growth chart is a much smaller version of charts used by healthcare practitioners to monitor and assess the growth of an infant/toddler from birth to 36 months. This example shows the growth curves of girls over time, each at different percentiles. (*Source:* Data from The National Center for Health Statistics in collaboration with the National Center for Chronic Disease Prevention and Health Promotion, 2000.)

Infants are not small versions of adults; they are growing rapidly compared to the typically stable adult phase of life. The proportions of macronutrients they require differ from adult proportions, as do the types of food they can tolerate. It is generally agreed that about 40% to 50% of an infant's diet should come from fat during the first year of life (30–31 g/day) and that fat intakes below this level can be harmful before the age of 2 years. Given the high energy needs of infants, it makes sense to take advantage of the energy density of fat (9 kcal/g). Breast milk and commercial formulas are both high in fat (about 50% of total energy).

Specific fatty acids are essential for the rapid brain growth, maturation of the retina of the eye, and nervous system development that happen in the first 1 to 2 years of life. The Adequate Intake (AI) fatty acid guidelines for infants are based on the composition of breast milk, which is always the standard for infant nutrient guidelines. For infants 7 to 12 months of age, the contributions of complementary foods are considered. The infant AI for omega-6 fatty acids is 4.4 to 4.6 g/day, about 6% to 8% of total Calories, whereas the infant AI for omega-3 fatty acids is 0.5 g/day, approximately 1% of total Calories.[10] Breast milk is an excellent source of the fatty acids arachidonic acid (AA) and docosahexaenoic acid (DHA), although levels of DHA vary widely with the mother's diet. Both of these fats have been associated with short-term improvements in visual function and, possibly, cognitive development. Many formula manufacturers are now adding AA and DHA to their products.

The recommended carbohydrate intake for infants 0 to 6 months of age is based on the lactose content of human milk.[10] The AI for infants 0 to 6 months of age is 60 g/day of carbohydrate. The carbohydrate AI for older infants 7 to 12 months of age reflects the intake of human milk and complementary foods and is set at 95 g/day.

The recommended intake of protein for infants 0 to 6 months of age is 9.1 g/day, or about 1.5 g/kg body weight per day.[10] Again, this value is based on the protein content of human milk. Formula-fed infants typically consume higher amounts of protein compared to breast-fed infants; however, the proteins in commercial formulas are less efficiently digested and absorbed. The protein guideline for infants 7 to 12 months of age is 9.9 g/day, or 1.1 g/kg body weight per day.[10] Recall (from Chapter 6) that the adult RDA for protein is 0.8 g/day. The relatively higher intake for infants is to accommodate their rapid growth. However, no more than 20% of an infant's daily energy requirement should come from protein. Immature infant kidneys are not able to process and excrete the excess amine groups from higher-protein diets. Breast milk and commercial formulas both provide adequate total protein and appropriate essential amino acids to support growth and development.

Micronutrient Needs of Infants

An infant's micronutrient needs are also high to accommodate rapid growth and development. Micronutrients of particular note include iron, vitamin D, zinc, fluoride, and, for infants of breastfeeding vegans, vitamin B_{12}. Fortunately, breast milk and commercial formulas provide most of the micronutrients needed for infant growth and development, with some special considerations, discussed later in this chapter.

In addition, all infants are routinely given an injection of vitamin K shortly after birth. This provides vitamin K until the infant's intestine can develop its own healthful bacteria, which provide vitamin K thereafter.

Do Infants Need Supplements?

Breast milk and commercial formulas provide most of the vitamins and minerals infants need. However, breast milk is low in vitamin D, and deficiencies of this nutrient have been detected in breast-fed infants with dark skin and in those with limited sunlight exposure.[56] Breast-fed infants and those consuming less than 1 L of vitamin D–fortified formula should be prescribed a supplement containing vitamin D.[57]

Breast-fed infants also require additional iron beginning no later than 6 months of age, because the infant's iron stores become depleted and breast milk is a poor source of iron. Iron is extremely important for cognitive development and prevention of iron-deficiency anemia. Puréed meats and infant rice cereal fortified with iron can serve as additional iron sources and are excellent choices when introducing solid food.

Fluoride is important for strong tooth development, but fluoride supplementation is not recommended during the first 6 months of life. Depending on the fluoride content of the household water supply, breast-fed infants over the age of 6 months may need a fluoride supplement. Most brands of bottled water have low levels of fluoride, and many home water treatment systems remove fluoride. On the other hand, fluoride toxicity may be a risk for infants simultaneously exposed to fluoridated toothpaste and rinses, fluoridated water, and fluoride supplements.

There are special conditions in which additional supplements may be needed for breast-fed infants. For example, if a woman is a vegan, her breast milk may be low in vitamin B_{12}, and a supplement of this vitamin should be given to the baby.

For formula-fed infants, the need for supplementation depends on the formula composition and other factors. Many formulas are already fortified with iron, for example; thus, no additional iron supplement is necessary. If the baby is getting adequate vitamin D through either the ingestion of at least 1 liter of vitamin D–fortified formula or via regular sun exposure, an extra supplement may not be necessary.

If a supplement is given, careful consideration should be given to dose. The supplement should be formulated specifically for infants, and the recommended daily dose should not be exceeded. High doses of micronutrients can be dangerous. For example, too much iron can be fatal, and too much fluoride can cause mottling, pitting, and staining of the teeth. Excessive vitamin D can cause abnormally high levels of serum calcium and calcification of soft tissues, such as the kidney.

Fluid Recommendations for Infants

Fluid is critical for everyone, but for infants the balance is more delicate for two reasons. First, they proportionally lose more water through evaporation from the skin surface area than adults. Second, their kidneys are immature and unable to concentrate urine. Hence, they are at even greater risk for dehydration. An infant needs about 2 oz of fluid per pound of body weight, and either breast milk or formula is almost always adequate in providing this amount. Experts recently confirmed that "infants exclusively fed human milk do not require supplemental water."[18] This is true for infants living in hot and humid climates as well as more moderate environments. Parents can be reassured that their infant's fluid intake is appropriate if the infant produces six to eight wet diapers per day.

Certain conditions, such as diarrhea, vomiting, fever, or extreme hot weather, can accelerate fluid loss. In these instances, supplemental fluid, ideally as water, may be needed. Because too much fluid can be dangerous for an infant, supplemental fluids (whether water or an infant electrolyte formula) should be given only under the advice of a physician. Generally, it is advised that supplemental fluids not exceed 4 oz per day. Parents should avoid giving breast-fed or formula-fed infants sugar water, fruit juices, or sweetened beverages in a bottle, especially at bedtime, as the practice can cause decay of developing teeth.

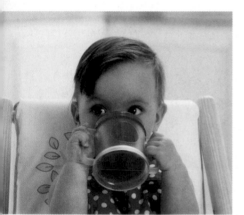

Infants are at high risk for dehydration and should be offered water and other nutritious beverages on a regular basis.

RECAP

Infancy is characterized by the most rapid rate of growth a human being will ever experience, and an infant's energy needs are correspondingly high. Assessment of the infant's growth pattern can provide important clues to his or her nutritional state.

Breast milk is the ideal infant food for the first 6 months of life; iron-fortified formula also provides the necessary nutrients for young infants. Vitamin D supplements are recommended for exclusively breast-fed infants; iron and fluoride supplements may be prescribed for infants older than 6 months of age. ∎

What Types of Formula Are Available?

We discussed the advantages of breastfeeding earlier in this chapter, and indeed both national and international healthcare organizations consider breastfeeding the best choice for infant nutrition, when possible. However, if breastfeeding is not feasible, several types of commercial formulas provide nutritious alternatives. In the United States, as many as 80% to 85% of infants are fed commercial formula by the age of 1 year. Formula manufacturers must comply with the Infant Formula Act of 1980 (since revised), which established minimum and maximum levels for twenty-nine nutrients. Although most formula manufacturers try to mimic the nutritional value of breast milk, these formulas still cannot completely duplicate the immune factors, enzymes, and other unique components of human milk.

Most formulas are based on cow's milk that is modified to make it more appropriate for human infants. The amount of total protein is reduced and levels of milk proteins are altered in order to mirror the types of proteins in breast milk. In addition, the product is heated to denature the proteins and make them more digestible. The naturally occurring lactose may be supplemented with sucrose to provide adequate carbohydrate. Vegetable oils and/or microbiologically produced fatty acids replace the naturally occurring butterfat. A range of vitamins and minerals, such as iron, is added to meet national standards. Recently, some manufacturers have added compounds such as taurine, carnitine, and the fatty acids AA and DHA to more closely mimic the nutrient profile of breast milk. This chapter's **Nutrition Label Activity** box (page 672) gives you the opportunity to review some of these ingredients.

Soy-based formulas are effective alternatives for infants who are lactose intolerant (although this is rare in infants). While soy formulas may also be used with infants who cannot tolerate the proteins in cow's milk–based formulas, many infants who are allergic to cow's milk protein are also allergic to soy protein. Soy formulas will satisfy the requirements of families who are strict vegans. However, soy-based formulas are not without controversy.[58] Because soy contains isoflavones, or plant forms of estrogens, there is some concern over the effects these compounds have on growing infants.[59] Currently, it is believed that soy formulas are safe, but they should only be used when breast milk or cow's milk–based formulas are contraindicated. Soy-based formulas are not the same as soy milk, which is not suitable for infant feeding.

Finally, there are specialized formulas for specific medical conditions. Some contain proteins that have been predigested, for example, or have nutrient compositions designed to accommodate certain genetic abnormalities. Others have been developed to meet the unique nutritional needs of preterm infants. Many of these specialized or medical formulas are available only through a physician.

Commercial formulas provide infants with a nutritious alternative to breast milk. Cow's milk, including fresh, evaporated, condensed, and dried milks, should not be introduced to infants until after 1 year of age. Cow's milk is too high in protein, the protein is difficult to digest, and the poor digestibility may contribute to gastrointestinal bleeding. In addition, cow's milk has too much sodium, too little iron, and a poor balance of other vitamins and minerals. Goat's milk is also inappropriate for infants and should not be used as a substitute for breast milk or formula.

When Do Infants Begin to Need Solid Foods?

As the result of declining nutrient stores, particularly iron, and continued growth, infants begin to need complementary, or solid, foods at around 6 months of age (**Table 16.5**, page 673). As previously noted, the American Academy of Pediatrics recommends exclusive breastfeeding for the first 6 months of life, but also recognizes that there is no evidence of significant harm if complementary foods are offered no earlier than 4 months of age.

Nutrition MILESTONE

The practice of "hand feeding" infants with animal milk and/or grain-based mixtures is documented going as far back as 2000 BC. These mixtures, however, were so incompatible with infant nutritional needs that as many as 90% or more of "formula-fed" infants died, up through the early 1800s. It wasn't until the nutrient differences between cow's and human milk were understood that successful infant formulas were developed. Justus von Liebig is credited with developing and marketing the

first commercial powdered infant formula in **1867**. Made from cow's milk, wheat, malt flour, and potassium bicarbonate, it quickly became a popular option for well-to-do families. By 1883, twenty-seven brands of this or similar infant formulas were available.

In the United States, the first federal regulations related to infant formulas were established in 1941. In 1951, concentrated liquid formulas were introduced, followed by the marketing of iron-fortified formulas in 1959. In the 1960s, manufacturers modified their protein sources to create whey-dominant formulas, and formulas made with highly digestible isolated soy protein became widely available. More recently, as the science of infant feeding has advanced, formula manufacturers have improved vitamin and mineral levels and have added components such as DHA and taurine. Infant formulas have also been enhanced through the addition of *probiotics*, which are certain types of live bacteria known to be beneficial to health. With these types of improvements, infants who are fed commercial formulas today can sustain growth and development that are nearly on par with breast-fed infants.

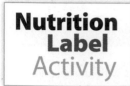

Reading Infant Food Labels

Imagine that you are a new parent shopping for infant formula. **Figure 16.12** shows the label from a typical can of formula. As you can see, the ingredients list is long and has many technical terms. Even well-informed parents would probably be stumped by many of them. Fortunately, with the information you learned in previous chapters, you can probably answer the following questions:

- The first ingredient listed is a modified form of *whey protein*. What common food is the source of *whey*?

- The fourth ingredient listed is *lactose*. Is lactose a form of protein, fat, or carbohydrate? Why is lactose important for infants?

- The front label states the formula has a blend of DHA (docosahexaenoic acid) and ARA (arachidonic acid). Are DHA and ARA forms of protein, fat, or carbohydrate? Why are these two nutrients thought to be important for infants?

The label also claims that this formula is "Our Closest Formula to Breast Milk." Can you think of some differences between breast milk and this formula that still exist? Look at the list of nutrients on the label. You'll notice that there is no "% Daily Value" column, which you see on most food labels. Next time you are at the grocery store, look at other baby food items, such as baby cereal or puréed fruits. Do their labels simply list the nutrient content, or is the "% Daily Value" column used? Why do you think infant formula has a different label format?

Let's say you are feeding a 6-month-old infant who needs about 500 kcal/day. Using the information from the nutrition section of the label, you can calculate the number of fluid ounces of formula the baby needs (this assumes that no cereal or other foods are eaten):

There are 100 kcal per 5 fl. oz:

100 kcal ÷ 5 fl. oz = 20 kcal/fl. oz

500 kcal ÷ 20 kcal/fl. oz = 25 fl. oz of formula per day to meet this baby's energy needs

A 6-month-old infant needs about 210 mg calcium per day. Based on an intake of 25 fl. oz of formula per day, as just calculated, you can use the label nutrition information to calculate the amount of calcium that is provided:

There are 78 mg calcium per 5 fl. oz serving of formula:

78 mg ÷ 5 fl. oz = 15.6 mg calcium per fl. oz

15.6 mg calcium per fl. oz X 25 fl. oz = 390 mg calcium per day

You can see that the infant's need for calcium is easily met by the formula alone.

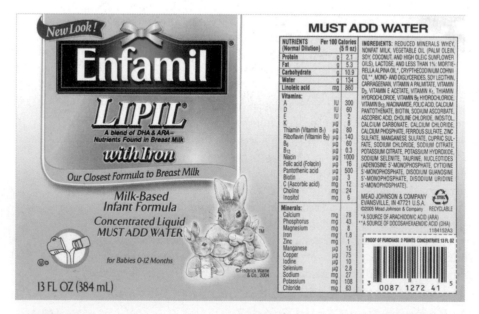

FIGURE 16.12 An infant formula label. Notice that there is a long list of ingredients and no % Daily Value.

TABLE 16.5 Guidelines for the Introduction of Foods to Infants

Guideline	Explanation
Introduce single-item foods, one at a time, at 3- to 5-day intervals. Avoid multigrain cereals and mixed dishes.	This makes it easier to identify possible food allergies.
Start with foods that provide key nutrients, such as iron-fortified infant cereals and puréed meats.	Iron and zinc are the most common nutrient deficiencies in infants. Meat provides both.
One hundred percent undiluted fruit juices should not be introduced until the infant is at least 6 months of age. When introduced, limit to 4 to 6 oz/day and vary the types of juice offered.	High juice intake displaces calcium- and protein-rich breast milk and formula. Many popular juices, such as apple juice, offer limited nutritional value.
Do not introduce cow's milk until the infant is at least 1 year old. When introduced, provide whole milk, not reduced-fat milk.	The nutrient profile of cow's milk is not optimal to meet the needs of the growing infant. Healthy 1-year-olds need the energy provided by whole milk.
Introduce a variety of foods by the age of 1 year.	Variety and diversity in foods improve nutrient intake; stimulate the senses of taste, odor, and touch; and positively influence future eating habits.

One factor limiting an infant's ability to take solid foods is the *extrusion reflex.* During infant feeding, the suckling response depends on a particular movement of the tongue that draws liquid out of the breast or bottle. But when solid foods are introduced with a spoon, this tongue movement (the extrusion reflex), causes the baby to push most of the food back out of the mouth. The extrusion reflex begins to lessen around 4 to 5 months of age.

Another factor is muscle development. To minimize the risk for choking, the infant must have gained muscular control of the head and neck and must be able to sit up (with or without support).

Still another part of being ready for solid foods is sufficient maturity of the digestive and kidney systems. Infants can digest and absorb lactose from birth; however, the ability to digest starch does not fully develop until the age of 3 to 4 months. If an infant is fed cereal, for example, before he or she can digest the starch, diarrhea and discomfort may develop. In addition, early introduction of solid foods can lead to improper absorption of intact, undigested proteins, setting the stage for allergies. Finally, the kidneys must have matured, so that they are better able to process nitrogen wastes from proteins and concentrate urine.

The need for solid foods is also related to nutrient needs. At about 6 months of age, infant iron stores become depleted; thus, puréed meats or iron-fortified infant cereals are often the first foods introduced. Rice cereal rarely provokes an allergic response and is easy to digest. If cereal is the iron source of choice and all goes well with the rice cereal, another single-grain cereal (other than wheat, which is highly allergenic) can be introduced. If meat is the first food introduced, the family may then gradually introduce single-item, vitamin C–rich strained vegetables or fruits.

Commercial baby foods are convenient and are typically made without added salt; some are made only with organic ingredients. Dessert items and dinner-type foods are not recommended, because they contain added sugars and starches. Parents can use an inexpensive food grinder to prepare homemade baby foods that are inexpensive and reflect the cultural diversity of the family.

Throughout the first year, solid foods should only be a supplement to, not a substitute for, breast milk or iron-fortified formula. Infants still need the nutrient density and energy that breast milk and formula provide.

What *Not* to Feed an Infant

The following foods should never be offered to an infant:

- *Foods that could cause choking.* Foods such as grapes, hot dogs, nuts, popcorn, raw carrots, raisins, and hard candies cannot be chewed adequately by infants and can cause choking.

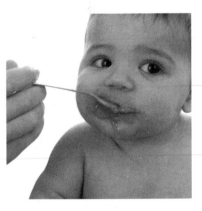

The extrusion reflex will push solid food out of an infant's mouth.

- *Corn syrup and honey.* These may contain spores of the bacterium *Clostridium botulinum.* These spores can germinate and grow into viable bacteria in the immature digestive tracts of infants, where they produce a potent toxin that can be fatal. Children older than 1 year can safely consume these substances, however, because their digestive tracts are mature enough to kill any *C. botulinum* bacteria.
- *Goat's milk.* Goat's milk is notoriously low in many nutrients that infants need, such as folate, vitamin C, vitamin D, and iron.
- *Cow's milk.* For children under 1 year, cow's milk is too concentrated in minerals and protein and contains too few carbohydrates to meet infant energy needs. Infants can begin to consume whole cow's milk after the age of 1 year. Infants and toddlers should not be given reduced-fat cow's milk before the age of 2 years, as it does not contain enough fat and is too high in mineral content for the kidneys to handle effectively. Infants should not be given evaporated milk or sweetened condensed milk.
- *Large quantities of fruit juices.* Fruit juices are poorly absorbed in the infant digestive tract, causing diarrhea if consumed in excess. Large quantities of fruit juice can make an infant feel full and reject breast milk or formula at feeding time, thus causing him or her to miss out on essential nutrients. Many fruit juices are also high in sugar. Plain water will also effectively quench an infant's thirst.
- *Too much salt and sugar.* Infant foods should not be seasoned with salt or other seasonings or sweetened. Cookies, cakes, and other excessively sweet, processed foods also should be avoided.
- *Too much breast milk or formula.* As nutritious as breast milk and formula are, once infants reach the age of 6 months, solid foods should be introduced gradually. Six months of age is a critical time, as that is when a baby's iron stores begin to be depleted. In addition, infants are physically and psychologically ready to incorporate solid foods at this time, and solid foods can help appease their increasing appetites. Between 6 months and the time of weaning (from breast or bottle), solid foods should gradually make up an increasing proportion of the infant's diet. Overreliance on breast milk or formula, to the exclusion or displacement of iron-rich foods, can result in a condition known as *milk anemia.*

RECAP

In the absence of breastfeeding, iron-fortified formulas provide adequate nutrition for infants. Solid foods can gradually be introduced into an infant's diet at 4 to 6 months of age, beginning with puréed meats or iron-fortified rice cereal (or other non-wheat cereals), then moving to single-item vegetables and fruits. Parents should carefully select and prepare the foods to be given to their infants, avoiding those that represent a choking hazard and limiting high-sugar foods and beverages. Solid foods expand the infant's exposure to tastes and textures and represent an important developmental milestone. ■

Nutrition-Related Concerns for Infants

Nutrition is one of the biggest concerns of new parents. Infants cannot speak, and their cries are sometimes indecipherable. Feeding time can be very frustrating for parents, especially if the child is not eating, is not growing appropriately, or has problems such as diarrhea, vomiting, or persistent skin rashes. Following are some nutrition-related concerns for infants.

Allergies

Many foods have the potential to stimulate an allergic reaction. Breastfeeding reduces the risk for allergy development, as does delaying the introduction of solid foods until the age of 6 months. One of the most common allergies in infants is to the proteins in cow's milk–based formulas. Egg whites, peanuts, soy, and wheat are other common triggers to allergic reactions. Every food should be introduced in isolation, so that any allergic reaction can be identified and the particular food avoided.

Symptoms of an allergic reaction vary but may include gastrointestinal distress such as diarrhea or vomiting, rashes or hives, runny nose or sneezing, or even difficulty breathing. Peanut allergy is the leading cause of fatal food reactions in a pediatric population.[60] While many infants who are allergic to cow's milk, wheat, soy, and eggs develop a tolerance for them, very few infants allergic to peanuts are able to outgrow the allergy.[61]

Colic

Perhaps nothing is more frustrating to new parents than the relentless crying spells of some infants, typically referred to as **colic.** In this condition, newborns and young infants who appear happy, healthy, and well nourished suddenly begin to cry or even shriek and continue no matter what their caregiver does to console them. The spells tend to occur at the same time of day, typically late in the afternoon or early in the evening, and often occur daily for a period of several weeks. Crying may last for hours at a time. Overstimulation of the nervous system, feeding too rapidly, swallowing of air, and intestinal gas pain are considered possible culprits, but the precise cause is unknown.

As with allergies, if a colicky infant is breastfed, breastfeeding should be continued, but the mother should try to determine whether eating certain foods seems to prompt crying and, if so, eliminate the offending food(s) from her diet. Avoidance of spicy or other strongly flavored foods may also help. Formula-fed infants may benefit from a change in type of formula. In the worst cases of colic, a physician may prescribe medication. Fortunately, most cases disappear spontaneously, possibly because of maturity of the GI tract, around 3 months of age.

Gastroesophageal Reflux

The regurgitation, or reflux, of stomach contents into the esophagus often results in the all too familiar "spitting up" of young infants. Particularly common in preterm infants, gastroesophageal reflux occurs in about 3% of newborns. Typically, as the gastrointestinal tract matures within the first 12 months of life, this condition resolves. Caretakers should avoid overfeeding the infant, keep the infant upright after each feeding, and watch for choking or gagging.

Failure to Thrive

At times, seemingly healthy infants reach an inappropriate plateau or decline in their growth. Pediatric healthcare providers describe **failure to thrive (FTT)** as a condition in which, in the absence of disease or physical abnormalities, the infant's weight or weight-for-height is below the 3rd percentile, or the infant has fallen more than two percentile lines on the NCHS growth charts after a previously stable pattern of growth. Acute malnutrition often results in *wasting*, or low weight-for-height, and chronic malnutrition typically produces growth *stunting*, in which the child has low height-for-age.

Psychosocial factors that increase the risk for FTT include poverty, inadequate knowledge, extreme nutritional beliefs, social isolation, domestic violence, and/or substance abuse. If not corrected in a timely manner, FTT may result in developmental, motor, and cognitive delays typically associated with infants in developing nations.

Feeding Challenges in Special Populations

Feeding problems are common among children born with physical abnormalities such as *cleft lip* or *cleft palate* (**Figure 16.13**, page 676), infants with genetic or inborn errors of metabolism, and those with developmental delays.[62] In many cases, occupational and speech therapists, registered dietitians, and other health professionals provide the family with the necessary skills and knowledge to ensure the nutritional health and well-being of their children.

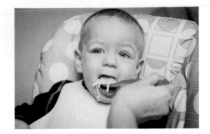

Early introduction of solid foods may play a role in the development of food allergies, especially if infants are introduced to highly allergenic foods early on.

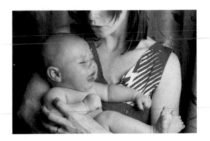

Colicky babies will cry for no apparent reason, even if they otherwise appear well nourished and happy.

colic   A condition of unconsolable infant crying of unknown origin that can last for hours at a time.

failure to thrive (FTT)   A condition in which an infant's weight gain and growth are far below typical levels for age and previous patterns of growth, for reasons that are unclear or unexplained.

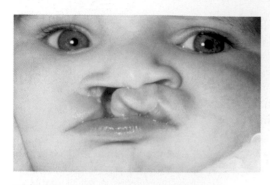

FIGURE 16.13 This baby has a condition known as unilateral cleft lip, also sometimes called *hare lip*. Cleft lip results from failure of the tissues of a fetus's face and mouth to fuse properly during the second and third months of pregnancy. Cleft lip is closely related to the condition of cleft palate, and the two often occur together.

While most infants born with cleft lip alone have few feeding problems, babies born with cleft palate can't create enough suction to withdraw milk from the breast or bottle. Specialized bottles and nipples are available that can provide the infant with formula or breast milk that has been expressed. While there is no firm consensus, many doctors consider the best age range to surgically repair cleft palate to be between approximately 5 and 15 months of age, or earlier. Cleft lip and cleft palate often occur together.

Infants with inborn errors of metabolism may have neuromuscular disorders that decrease their muscular strength, endurance, and coordination and contribute to a slow pace of feeding, difficulty swallowing and/or chewing, and poor head control. Some infants with developmental delays demonstrate poor lip closure, abnormal gag reflex, tongue thrust, or hypersensitivity to temperature or texture. Each infant requires careful evaluation by a pediatric dietitian and feeding team to develop an individualized feeding plan.

Anemia

As previously noted, full-term infants are born with sufficient iron stores to last for approximately the first 6 months of life. In older infants and toddlers, however, iron is the mineral most likely to be deficient. Iron-deficiency anemia causes pallor, lethargy, and impaired growth. Iron-fortified formula is a good source for formula-fed infants. Some pediatricians prescribe a supplement containing iron especially formulated for infants. Iron for older infants is typically supplied by iron-fortified rice cereal or puréed meats. Overconsumption of cow's milk remains a common cause of anemia among U.S. infants and children.

Dehydration

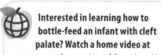

Interested in learning how to bottle-feed an infant with cleft palate? Watch a home video at www.youtube.com/watch?v=--luzt-j0wA.

Whether the cause is diarrhea, vomiting, prolonged fever, or inadequate fluid intake, dehydration is extremely dangerous to infants and if left untreated can quickly result in death. (The factors behind infants' increased risk for dehydration were discussed earlier in this chapter on page 670.) Treatment includes providing fluids, a task that is difficult if vomiting is occurring. In some cases, the physician may recommend that a pediatric electrolyte solution, readily available at most grocery and drug stores, be administered on a temporary basis. In more severe cases, hospitalization may be necessary. If possible, breastfeeding should continue throughout an illness. A physician or other healthcare provider should be consulted on decisions related to the use of formula and solid foods.

Nursing Bottle Syndrome

Infants should never be left alone with a bottle, whether lying down or sitting up. As infants manipulate the nipple of the bottle, the high-carbohydrate fluid (whether breast milk, formula, or fruit juice) drips out, coming into prolonged contact with the developing teeth. This high-carbohydrate fluid provides an optimal food source for the bacteria that are the underlying cause of dental caries (cavities). Severe tooth decay can result (**Figure 16.14**). Encouraging the use of a cup around the age of 8 months helps prevent nursing bottle syndrome, as does weaning the baby from a bottle entirely by the age of 15 to 18 months. In addition, infants' gum tissue and emerging teeth should be gently cleaned with a wash cloth to minimize bacterial growth and increase acceptance of a toothbrush use when introduced.

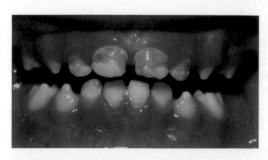

FIGURE 16.14 Leaving a baby alone with a bottle can result in the tooth decay of nursing bottle syndrome.

Lead Poisoning

Lead is especially toxic to infants and children, because their brains and central nervous systems are still developing. Lead poisoning can result in decreased mental capacity, behavioral problems, anemia, impaired growth, impaired

hearing, and other problems. Unfortunately, lead in old pipes and lead paint can still
be found in older homes and buildings. Measures to reduce lead exposure include the
following:

- Allowing tap water to run for a minute or so before use, to clear the pipes of any lead-contaminated water
- Using only cold tap water for drinking, cooking, and infant formula preparation, as hot tap water is more likely to leach lead
- Professionally removing lead-based paint or painting it over with latex paint

RECAP

Risk for food allergies can be reduced by delaying the introduction of solid foods until the infant is at least 6 months of age. Infants with colic or gastroesophageal reflux present special challenges, but both conditions generally improve over time. Infants who present with failure to thrive require close monitoring by healthcare providers, as do infants experiencing severe dehydration. Anemia is easily prevented through the use of iron-fortified formulas and cereals. Families need the support and guidance of healthcare professionals when feeding infants with birth defects, metabolic disorders, or developmental delays. Nursing bottle syndrome is characterized by dental caries in infants left lying down or sitting up with a bottle containing any carbohydrate-containing fluid. Lead poisoning can result in cognitive, behavioral, and other problems. ■

Chapter Review

TEST YOURSELF | ANSWERS

1 **F** Energy needs after the first trimester increase by only about 20% above a woman's pre-pregnant needs. This translates to an extra 350 to 450 additional Calories per day during the second and third trimesters, not a doubling of Calories.

2 **F** More than half of all pregnant women experience morning sickness, and food cravings or aversions are also common.

3 **T** Breast milk contains various immune factors (antibodies and immune system cells) from the mother that protect about the infant against infection. The nutrients in breast milk are structured to be easily digested by an infant, resulting in fewer symptoms of gastrointestinal distress and fewer allergies.

4 **T** Caffeine quickly passes into breast milk, as do alcohol and most prescription and over-the-counter medications.

5 **F** Most infants do not have a physiologic need for solid food until about 6 months of age.

Summary

- Nutrition is important before conception, because critical stages of cell division, tissue differentiation, and organ development occur in the early weeks of pregnancy, often before a woman even knows she is pregnant.

- A plentiful, nourishing diet is important throughout pregnancy to provide the nutrients needed to support fetal development without depriving the mother of nutrients she needs to maintain her own health.

- A normal pregnancy progresses over the course of 38 to 42 weeks. This time is divided into three trimesters of 13 to 14 weeks. Each trimester is associated with particular developmental phases of the embryo/fetus.

- Pregnant women of normal weight should consume adequate energy to gain 25 to 35 lb during pregnancy. Women who are underweight should gain slightly more, and women who are overweight or obese should gain less.

- Pregnant women need to be especially careful to consume adequate amounts of folate, vitamin B_{12}, vitamin C, vitamin D, calcium, iron, and zinc. A supplement is often prescribed to ensure adequate intake of these nutrients.

- Many pregnant women experience nausea and/or vomiting during pregnancy, and many crave or feel aversions to specific types of foods and nonfood substances.

- Gastroesophageal reflux and constipation in pregnancy are related to the relaxation of smooth muscle caused by certain pregnancy-related hormones.

- Gestational diabetes and gestational hypertension are nutrition-related disorders that can seriously affect maternal and fetal health.

- The bodies of adolescents are still growing and developing; thus, their nutrient needs during pregnancy are higher than those of older pregnant women.

- Alcohol is a teratogen and should not be consumed in any amount during pregnancy.

- Cigarette smoking reduces placental transfer of oxygen and nutrients, limiting fetal growth and development.

- Successful breastfeeding requires the coordination of several hormones, including estrogen, progesterone, prolactin, and oxytocin. These hormones govern the preparation of the breasts, as well as actual milk production and the let-down response.

- Breastfeeding women require more energy than they needed during pregnancy. Protein needs increase, and an overall nutritious diet with plentiful fluids is important in maintaining milk quality and quantity, as well as preserving the mother's health.

- The advantages of breastfeeding include the nutritional superiority of breast milk, protection from infections and allergies, promotion of attachment, convenience, and lower cost.

- Breastfeeding exclusively for the first 6 months of a baby's life is recommended by North American and international healthcare organizations.

- Challenges that might be encountered with breastfeeding include the effect of medications on breast milk, concerns related to transmission of HIV to a breastfeeding infant, scheduling conflicts for mothers who return to work, and social concerns.

- Infants are characterized by their extremely rapid growth and brain development.

- Physicians use length and weight measurements as the main tools for assessing an infant's nutritional status.

- Because infant stores of iron become depleted after about 6 months, an iron supplement is sometimes prescribed for breastfeeding infants.

- Breast milk or formula is entirely sufficient for the first 6 months of life. After that, solid foods can be introduced (for example, puréed meat or rice cereal fortified with iron) and expanded gradually, with breast milk or formula remaining very important throughout the first year.

- Infants need to be monitored carefully for appropriate growth and daily for appropriate number of wet diapers to assess nutrient intake and hydration.

- Nutrition-related concerns for infants include the potential for allergies, colic, gastroesophageal reflux, dehydration, failure to thrive, feeding challenges, anemia, nursing bottle syndrome, and ingestion of lead. Infants with special medical needs benefit from the support of a pediatric dietitian and other feeding professionals.

MasteringNutrition™

To further your understanding, go online and apply what you've learned to real-life case studies that will help you master the content!

Review Questions

1. Folate deficiency in the first weeks after conception has been linked with which of the following problems in the newborn?
   a. anemia
   b. neural tube defects
   c. low birth weight
   d. preterm birth

2. Which of the following hormones is responsible for the let-down response?
   a. progesterone
   b. estrogen
   c. oxytocin
   d. prolactin

3. Which of the following nutrients should be added to the diet of breast-fed infants when they are around 6 months of age?
   a. protein
   b. fat
   c. iron
   d. vitamin A

4. A pregnancy weight gain of 28 to 40 lb is recommended for
   a. all women.
   b. women who begin their pregnancy underweight.
   c. women who begin their pregnancy overweight.
   d. women who begin their pregnancy at a normal weight.

5. One of the best solid foods to introduce first to infants is
   a. Cream of Wheat cereal.
   b. applesauce.
   c. teething biscuits.
   d. puréed meat.

6. **True or false?** Major developmental errors and birth defects are most likely to occur in the third trimester of pregnancy.

7. **True or false?** Infant suckling is a critical component of successful and continued lactation.

8. **True or false?** Growth is a key indicator of adequate infant nutrition.

9. **True or false?** Alcohol easily passes from the mother's bloodstream into fetal blood and, in breastfeeding women, into the breast milk.

10. **True or false?** If gestational diabetes is not well controlled, the fetus may not receive enough glucose and is at high risk for low birth weight.

11. Identify five advantages and five disadvantages of breastfeeding. Can you think of others?

12. You are a registered dietitian in a public health clinic. A pregnant 15-year-old is referred to you for nutrition-related counseling and services. Identify at least three topics that you would discuss with this client.

13. Your cousin, who is pregnant with her first child, tells you that her physician prescribed supplemental iron tablets for her but that she decided not to take them. "You know me," she says, "I'm a natural food nut! I'm absolutely certain that my careful diet is providing all the nutrients my baby needs!" Is it possible that your cousin is partly right and partly wrong? Explain.

14. You visit your neighbors one afternoon to congratulate them on the birth of their new daughter, Katie. While you are there, 2-week-old Katie suddenly starts crying as if she is in terrible pain. "Oh, no," Katie's dad says to his wife. "Here we go again!" He turns to you and explains, "She's been like this every afternoon for the past week, and it goes on until sunset. I just wish we could figure out what we're doing wrong." What would you say?

15. You are on a picnic with your sister at a park, who drapes a shawl over her shoulders and breastfeeds her 11-month-old son. A woman walking by stops and says, "Isn't that child getting too old for that?" What information could you share with the woman in response to her question?

Math Review

16. Mature breast milk averages about 700 kcal per liter, with 35 g of fat and 9 g of protein. Calculate the % of kcal from fat and protein. How do these values compare to those recommended for a healthy young adult? Why are the nutrient proportions of breast milk appropriate for infants?

Answers to Review Questions and Math Review can be found online in the MasteringNutrition Study Area.

Web Links

www.aap.org
American Academy of Pediatrics
Visit this website for information on infants' and children's health. Clinical information as well as guidelines for parents and caregivers can be found. Searches can be performed for topics such as "neural tube defects" and "infant formulas."

www.choosemyplate.gov/pregnancy-breastfeeding
ChooseMyPlate Plans for Pregnant and Breastfeeding Women
This website is designed for pregnant and breastfeeding women and provides meal plans that can be personalized to address the needs of women who are pregnant or breastfeeding.

www.fnic.nal.usda.gov
Food and Nutrition Information Center of the USDA
Click on "Lifecycle Nutrition." This page provides links to topics on pregnancy, breastfeeding, and infant nutrition.

www.emedicine.com/ped
eMedicine: Pediatrics
This site provides references for numerous infant health and nutrition issues. Select "Toxicology" and then "Toxicity, Iron" to learn about accidental iron poisoning and its signs in children and infants.

www.marchofdimes.com
March of Dimes
Click on "Pregnancy & Newborn" to find links on nutrition during pregnancy, breastfeeding, and baby care.

www.llli.org
La Leche League
This site provides information about breastfeeding; search or browse to find multiple articles on the health effects of breastfeeding for mother and infant.

www.nofas.org
National Organization on Fetal Alcohol Syndrome
This site provides news and information relating to fetal alcohol syndrome.

www.helppregnantsmokersquit.org
National Partnership to Help Pregnant Smokers Quit
This is a site created to educate healthcare providers and smokers about the dangers of smoking while pregnant and to provide tools to help pregnant smokers quit.

References

1. Martin, J. A., B. E. Hamilton, S. J. Ventura, M. J. Osterman, S. Kirmeyer, T. J. Mathews, and E. C. Wilson. 2011. Births: final data for 2009. *Natl. Vital Stat. Rep.* 60:1–70.

2. Kaiser Family Foundation. 2011. Infant Mortality Rate (Total Deaths per 1,000 Live Births) 2011. www.globalhealthfacts.org/data/topic/map.aspx?ind=91. (Accessed June 2012.)

3. US Department of Health and Human Services. *Healthy People 2020* Objectives and Topics. www.healthypeople.gov/2020/topicsobjectives2020/default.aspx. (Accessed June 2012.)

4. Han, Z., S. Mulla, J. Beyene, G. Liao, and S. D. McDonald on behalf of the Knowledge Synthesis Group. 2011. Maternal underweight and the risk of preterm birth and low birth weight: a systematic review and meta-analyses. *Int. J. Epidemiology.* 40:65–101.

5. Rasmussen, K. M., and A. L. Yaktine, eds. 2009. *Weight Gain During Pregnancy: Reexamining the Guidelines.* Washington, DC: National Academy Press.

6. Margerison-Zilko, B. P. Shrimali, B. Eskenazi, M. Lahiff, A. R. Lindquist, and B. F. Abrams. 2011. Trimester of maternal gestational weight gain and offspring body weight at birth and age five. *Matern. Child Health J.* DOI:10.1007/s10995-011-0846-1.

7. Fraser, A., K. Tilling, C. Macdonald-Wallis, N. Sattar, S. M. Nelson, and D. A. Lawlor. 2010. Association of maternal weight gain in pregnancy with offspring obesity and metabolic and vascular traits in childhood. *Circulation* 121:2557–2564.

8. Barbour, L. A. 2012. Weight gain in pregnancy: is less truly more for mother and infant? *Obstetric Medicine* 5:58–64.

9. US Department of Agriculture and US Department of Health and Human Services. December 2010. *Dietary Guidelines for Americans 2010.* 7th edn. Washington, DC: US Government Printing Office. www.cnpp.usda.gov/dietaryguidelines.htm.

10. Institute of Medicine, Food and Nutrition Board. 2002. *Dietary Reference Intakes for Energy, Carbohydrate, Fiber, Fat, Fatty Acids, Cholesterol, Protein, and Amino Acids.* Washington, DC: National Academy Press.

11. Spina Bifida Association. Folic Acid. www.spinabifidaassociation.org/site/c.liKWL7PLLrF/b.2700277/k.2112/Folic_Acid.htm.

12. Institute of Medicine, Food and Nutrition Board. 1998. *Dietary Reference Intakes for Thiamin, Riboflavin, Niacin, Vitamin B_6, Folate, Vitamin B_{12}, Pantothenic Acid, Biotin, and Choline.* Washington, DC: National Academy Press.

13. Institute of Medicine, Food and Nutrition Board. 2001. *Dietary Reference Intakes for Vitamin A, Vitamin K, Arsenic, Boron, Chromium, Copper, Iodine, Iron, Manganese, Molybdenum, Nickel, Silicon, Vanadium, and Zinc.* Washington, DC: National Academy Press.

14. Institute of Medicine, Food and Nutrition Board. 2011. *Dietary Reference Intakes for Calcium and Vitamin D.* Washington, DC: National Academy Press.

15. Rosen, C. J., J. S. Adams, D. D. Bikle, D. M. Black, M. B. Demay, J. E. Manson, M. H. Murad, and C. S. Kovacs. 2012. The non-skeletal effects of vitamin D: an endocrine society scientific statement. *Endocrine Rev.* 33:456–492.

16. Olivares, M., F. Pizarro, M. Ruz, and D. Lópex de Romaňa. 2012. Acute inhibition of iron bioavailability by zinc: studies in humans. *Biometals* 25:657–664.

17. Institute of Medicine, Food and Nutrition Board. 2004. *Dietary Reference Intakes for Water, Potassium, Sodium, Chloride, and Sulfate*. Washington, DC: National Academy Press.

18. Chan, R. L., A. F. Olshan, D. A. Savitz, A. H. Herring, J. L. Daniels, H. B. Peterson, and S. L. Martin. 2011. Maternal influences on nausea and vomiting in early pregnancy. *Matern. Child Health.* 15:122–127.

19. Malcolm, J. 2012. Preventing diabetes in women with gestational diabetes. Through the looking glass: gestational diabetes as a predictor of maternal and offspring long-term health. *Diab/Metab. Res. Rev.* 28:307–311.

20. Baptiste-Roberts, K., W. K. Nicholson, N. Wang, and F. L. Brancati. 2012. Gestational diabetes and subsequent growth patterns of offspring: the National Collaborative Perinatal Project. *Matern. Child Health J.* 16:125–132.

21. Shah, B. R., L. L. Lipscombe, D. S. Feig, and J. M. Lowe. 2011. Missed opportunities for type 2 diabetes testing following gestational diabetes: a population-based cohort study. *Brit. J. Obstet. Gynec.* 118:1484–1490.

22. Jutcheon, J. A., S. Lisonkova, and K. S. Joseph. 2011. Epidemiology of pre-eclampsia and the other hypertensive disorders of pregnancy. *Best Practice & Research Clinical Obstetrics and Gynaecology* 25:391–403.

23. Mongraw-Chaffin, M. L., P. M. Cirillo, and B. A. Cohn. 2010. Preeclampsia and cardiovascular disease death. Prospective evidence from the Child Health and Development Studies cohort. *Hypertension* 56:166–171.

24. Davidson, M., M. London, and P. Ladewig. 2012. *Maternal-Newborn Nursing and Women's Health*. 9th edn. Upper Saddle River, NJ: Pearson.

25. Zavorsky, G. S., and L. D. Longo. 2011. Exercise guidelines in pregnancy: New perspectives. *Sports Med.* 41:345–360.

26. American College of Obstetricians and Gynecologists. 2011. Frequently Asked Questions: Exercise during Pregnancy. www.acog.org. (Accessed July 2012.)

27. March of Dimes. 2010. Caffeine in Pregnancy. www.marchofdimes.com/pregnancy/nutrition_caffeine.html.

28. Jarosz, M., R. Wierzejska, and M. Siuba. 2012. Maternal caffeine intake and its effect on pregnancy outcomes. *Europ. J. Obstet. Gynecol. Reproductive Biol.* 160:156–160.

29. Stefanidou, E. M., L. Caramellino, A. Patriarca, and G. Menato. 2011. Maternal caffeine consumption and *sine causa* recurrent miscarriage. *Europ. J. Obstet. Gynecol. Reproductive Biol.* 158:220–224.

30. Riley, E. P., M. A. Infante, and K. R. Warren. 2011. Fetal alcohol spectrum disorders: an overview. *Neuropsychol. Rev.* 21:73–80.

31. Jully-Martens, K., K. Denys, S. Treit, S. Tamana, and C. Rasmussen. 2012. A review of social skills deficits in individuals with fetal alcohol spectrum disorders and prenatal alcohol exposure: Profiles, mechanisms, and interventions. *Alcoholism: Clin. Exper. Res.* 36:568–576.

32. Meyer-Leu, Y., S. Lemola, J. Daeppen, O. Deriaz, and S. Gerber. 2011. Association of moderate alcohol use and binge drinking during pregnancy with neonatal health. *Alcoholism: Clin. Exper. Res* 35:1669–1677.

33. Centers for Disease Control and Prevention. 2012. Tobacco Use and Pregnancy. www.cdc.gov/reproductivehealth/tobaccousepregnancy/. (Accessed July 2012.)

34. Committee on Health Care for Underserved Women and Committee on Obstetric Practice of the American College of Obstetricians and Gynecologists. 2010. Committee opinion: Smoking cessation during pregnancy. *Obstet. Gynecol.* 116:1241–1244.

35. Campaign for Tobacco-Free Kids. 2008. Smoking and Pregnancy: The Harms of Continued Smoking and the Benefits of Quitting. www.cdc.gov/reproductivehealth/tobaccousepregnancy/. (Accessed July 2012.)

36. Substance Abuse and Mental Health Services Administration. 2011. Results from the 2010 National Survey on Drug Use and Health: Summary of National Findings, NSDUH Series H-41, HHS Publication No. (SMA) 11-4658. Rockville, MD: Substance Abuse and Mental Health Services Administration.

37. National Institute on Drug Abuse. 2011. Topics in Brief: Prenatal Exposure to Drugs of Abuse—May 2011. www.drugabuse.gov/publications/topics-in-brief/prenatal-exposure-to-drugs-abuse. (Accessed July 2012.)

38. US Food & Drug Administration. 2011. *Food Safety for Moms-to-Be.* www.fda.gov/food/resourcesforyou/healtheducators/ucm081819.htm. (Accessed July 2012.)

39. Tsukimori, K., H. Uchi, C. Mitoma, F. Yasukawa, T. Chiba, T. Todaka, J. Kajiwara, T. Yoshimura, T. Hirata, K. Fukushima, N. Wake, and M. Furue. 2012. Maternal exposure to high levels of dioxins in relation to birth weight in women affected by Yusho disease. *Environ. Int.* 38:79–86.

40. Centers for Disease Control and Prevention. Breastfeeding Report Card—United States—2011. www.cdc.gov/breastfeeding/pdf/2011BreastfeedingReportCard.pdf. (Accessed July 2012.)

41. Lovelady, C. 2011. Symposium on "nutrition: getting the balance right in 2010. Session 1: balancing intake and output: food v. exercise. Balancing exercise and food intake with lactation to promote post-partum weight loss. *Proc. Nutr. Soc.* 70:181–184.

42. US Department of Health and Human Services. 2011. *The Surgeon General's Call to Action to Support Breastfeeding.* Washington, DC: US Department of Health and Human Services, Office of the Surgeon General.

43. Goodman, K., and E. DiFrisco. 2012. Achieving baby-friendly designation; step-by-step. *MCN Am. J. Matern. Child Nurs.* 37:146–152.

44. Urwin, H. J., E. A. Miles, P. S. Noakes, L. Kremmyda, M. Vlachava, N. D. Diaper, F. J. Pérez-Cano, K. M. Godfrey, P. C. Calder, and P. Yaqoob. 2012. Salmon consumption during pregnancy alters fatty acid composition and secretory IgA concentration in breast milk. *J. Nutr.* DOI:10.3945/jn.112.160804.

45. Perrine, C. G., A. J. Sharma, M. E. D. Jefferds, M. K. Serdula, and K. S. Scanlon. 2010. Adherence to vitamin D recommendations among US infants. *Pediatrics* 125:627–632.

46. American Academy of Pediatrics, Section on Breastfeeding. 2012. Breastfeeding and the use of human milk policy statement. *Pediatrics* 129:e827–841.

47. Bartick, M., and A. Reinhold. 2010. The burden of suboptimal breastfeeding in the United States: a pediatric cost analysis. *Pediatrics* 125:e1048–1056.

48. US Department of Health & Human Services. Bisphenol A (BPA) Information for Parents. www.hhs.gov/safety/bpa/. (Accessed July 2012.)

49. Kotsopoulos, J., J. Lubinshi, L. Salmena, H. T. Lynch, C. Kim-Sing, W. D. Foulkes, P. Ghadirian, S. L. Neuhausen, R. Demsky, N. Tung, P. Ainsworth, L. Senter, A. Eisen, C. Eng, C. Singer, O. Ginsburg, J. Blum, T. Huzarski, A. Poll, P. Sun, and S. A. Narod for the Hereditary Breast Cancer Clinical Study Group. 2012. Breastfeeding and the risk of breast cancer in *BRAC1* and *BRAC2* mutation carriers. *Breast Cancer Research* 14:R42.

50. Bjørnerem, L., A. Ahmed, L. Jørgensen, J. Størmer, and R. M. Joakimsen. 2011. Breastfeeding protects against hip fracture in postmenopausal women: the Tromsø study. *J. Bone Mineral Research.* 26:2843–2850.

51. Borjan, M., S. Marcella, B. Blount, M. Greenberg, J. Zhang, E. Murphy, L. Valentin-Blasini, and M. Robson. 2011. Perchlorate exposure in lactating women in an urban community in New Jersey. *Science of the Total Environment* 409:460–464.

52. Park, J., J. She, A. Holden, M. Sharp, R. Gephart, G. Souders-Mason, V. Zhang, J. Chow, B. Leslie, and K. Hooper. 2011. High postnatal exposure to polybrominated diphenyl ethers (PBDEs) and polychlorinated biphenyls (PCBs) via breast milk in California: does BDE-209 transfer to breast milk? *Environmental Science & Technology* 45:4579–4585.

53. Kindra, G., A. Coutsoudis, F. Exposito, and T. Esterhuizen. 2012. Breastfeeding in HIV exposed infants significantly improves child health: a prospective study. *Matern. Child Health J.* 16:632–640.

54. World Health Organization. 2010. Antiretroviral Drugs for Treating Pregnant Women and Preventing HIV Infection in Infants: Recommendations for a Public Health Approach. 2010 Version. Geneva, Switzerland: WHO Press.

55. Adams, C., R. Berger, P. Conning, L. Cruikshank, and K. Dore. 2001. Breastfeeding trends at a community breastfeeding center; an evaluation survey. *J. Obstet. Gynecol. Neonatal Nurs.* 30(4): 392–400.

56. Holick, M. F., N. C. Binkley, H. A. Bischoff-Ferrari, C. M. Gordon, D. A. Hanley, R. P. Heaney, M. H. Murad, and C. M. Weaver. 2011. Evaluation, treatment, and prevention of vitamin D deficiency: an Endocrine Society clinical practice guideline. *J. Clin. Endocrinol. Metab.* 96:1911–1930.

57. Merewood, A., S. D. Mehta, X. Grossman, T. C. Chen, J. Mathieu, M. F. Holick, and H. Bauchner. 2012. Vitamin D status among 4-month-old infants in New England: a prospective cohort study. *J. Human Lactation.* 28:159–166.

58. Vandenplas, Y., E. De Greef, T. Devreker, and B. Hauser. 2011. Soy infant formula: is it that bad? *Acta Pædiatrica* 100:162–166.

59. Adgent, M. A., J. L. Daniels, L. J. Edwards, A. M. Siega-Riz, and W. J. Rogan. 2011. Early-life soy exposure and gender-role play behavior in children. *Environmental Health Perspectives* 119:1811–1816.

60. Sicherer, S. H. 2011. Epidemiology of food allergy. *J. Allergy Clin. Immunology.* 127:594–602.

61. McWilliams, L., T. Mousallem, and W. Burks. 2012. Future therapies for food allergy. *Human Vaccines & Immunotherapeutics* 8:etext prior to publication. www.landesbioscience.com/journals/vaccines/article/20868/?show_full_text=true&.

62. Cloud, H. 2012. Developmental disabilities. In: Samour, P. Q., and K. King, eds. *Pediatric Nutrition.* 4th edn. Sudbury, MA: Jones & Bartlett Learning.

The Fetal Environment: Does It Leave a Lasting Impression?

Would you be surprised to learn that your risk of developing obesity and certain chronic diseases as an adult can be influenced by what happened even before you were born? Research suggests that the fetal environment, including the mother's nutritional status, influences the risks for obesity and chronic diseases later in life. This relationship is described as the "fetal origins theory" or the theory of "developmental origins of adult health and disease."

Exposure to Famine

Some of the earliest research into the fetal origins theory investigated the health of adults born during or shortly after a famine in the Netherlands from 1944 to 1945. During World War II, the Dutch population had been relatively well nourished until October 1944, when the Germans placed an embargo on all food transport into the western Netherlands. At the same time, an unusually early and harsh winter set in. As a result, a severe famine hit the western Netherlands. For several months, food intake was limited and energy intakes were as low as 500 kcal/day. In May 1945, with the liberation of the country, food supplies were restored and dietary intake rapidly normalized. Luckily for scientists, the Dutch maintained an excellent system of healthcare records, providing important information about not only pregnancy outcomes but also the health of the offspring over the next 60 years. Not surprisingly, maternal weight gain and infant birth weight were much lower than normal. What was surprising, however, was the long-term impact of the famine as these "embargo babies" progressed through adulthood.[1,2]

Exposure to famine during the first trimester of pregnancy resulted in a much higher risk among the offspring for obesity, abdominal obesity, coronary heart disease, abnormal serum lipid profile, and metabolic syndrome during adulthood. If the pregnancy had progressed to the third trimester by the time the famine began, there was a higher rate of glucose intolerance and type 2 diabetes in adulthood along with an increased risk for schizophrenia and, oddly, a greater preference for fatty foods among the embargo babies.[1]

Why, you might wonder, would low pregnancy weight gain and low birth weight lead to an increased risk for obesity and a variety of other diseases some 50 years later? While there are many theories, most relate to a process known as **fetal adaptation**.[3,4] This occurs when a fetus who is exposed to a harmful environment, such as maternal starvation or malnutrition, goes into survival mode. The

body's production of hormones shifts in favor of those that promote energy storage, the activity of certain enzymes may change, and the size and functioning of body organs such as the liver, kidney, and pancreas are impacted. There may even be changes in the activation—and thus the expression—of certain genes. Although these adaptations are beneficial to the fetus, allowing it to survive the harmful prenatal environment, the same hormonal, enzymatic, organ, and genetic changes may contribute to the development of chronic diseases over the life span.

The results of other "natural experiments" suggest that the effects of the prenatal environment on adult health depend heavily on the precise circumstances in each situation. For example, Leningrad (now St. Petersburg) was under siege by the Germans during World War II for over 2½ years, and as a result the population experienced starvation—over a million people died. And yet, adults who were born during this period did not have the same increased disease risks as found in those exposed, *in utero*, to the Dutch famine.[5,6] How could this be, since the Leningrad babies were exposed to conditions far worse than those experienced by the Dutch babies? Researchers theorize that the impact of fetal exposure to malnutrition is actually worsened if followed by high nutrient intakes shortly after birth.[6] This was a key difference between the Netherlands and Leningrad famines: once the Dutch embargo was lifted, the population returned to a nourishing, adequate diet. This allowed the underweight infants to experience rapid weight gain and catch-up growth during their first year of life. In contrast, the Leningrad infants who survived into adulthood may have continued to suffer from malnutrition throughout infancy and even into toddlerhood, remaining underweight and underfed. Catch-up growth in the postnatal period is associated with a more severe increase in blood pressure and other chronic diseases during adulthood.

More recently, people born during weather- and war-related famines in Africa and other parts of the world have

---

fetal adaptation Physiologic adaptations comprising a "survival mode" that occur when a fetus is exposed to harmful prenatal environment, such as maternal starvation or malnutrition. Hormone production shifts toward promoting energy storage, and the activity of certain enzymes may change. There may also be changes in the size and functioning of body organ, as well as in the expression of some genes. These adaptations, while enabling a fetus to survive, may also contribute to the development of chronic diseases over the life span.

provided researchers with additional information on the impact of the fetal environment on adult health/disease outcomes. For instance, some recent studies confirm the association between low birth weight and high blood pressure and other forms of cardiovascular disease.[7]

Exposure to Specific Nutrient Deficiencies

By definition, a famine is a widespread lack or severe reduction in all food. Thus, research on the long-term health effects of famines cannot identify or describe the impact of *in utero* deficiencies of specific nutrients. Other studies, however, have been able to look at the impact of specific food patterns or nutrient deficiencies. For example, evidence suggests that poor maternal intake of calcium increases risk for hypertension in adult offspring. Moreover, poor maternal folate status has been linked not only to neural tube defects in the newborn but also to early signs of atherosclerosis in adult offspring.[4,8,9] Thus, fetal stressors that influence adult health include not only starvation and inadequate energy but also specific micronutrient deficiencies.

Exposure to Dietary Excesses

Strong evidence also links maternal dietary excesses to poor health outcomes in adult offspring. Maternal obesity has been linked not only to an increased risk for childhood[10] and adult[11] obesity but also to changes in the "programming" of the fetal brain, resulting in altered feeding behaviors.[12] Maternal obesity is also linked to a higher risk for birth defects, many of which have lifelong implications for health.[13] Population studies have also reported an association between high birth weight, common in infants born to obese women, and an increased risk for breast cancer in adulthood.

Maternal diabetes and its high-glucose environment has been shown to greatly increase the risk for type 2 diabetes, overweight, excess adiposity, and metabolic syndrome in adult offspring.[14,15,16] The children of diabetic women are up to eight times more likely to develop type 2 diabetes or pre-diabetes as adults compared to the general population.[15] High blood levels of triglycerides, increased waist circumference, and increased blood pressure are other measures of adult-onset diseases associated with maternal diabetes.

Prenatal exposure to excessive levels of individual nutrients also has lifelong implications. A high maternal intake of vitamin A as retinol (but not as its precursor, beta-carotene)

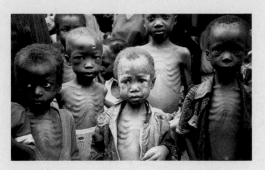

The consequences of fetal exposure to malnutrition, and childhood starvation, are often lifelong.

is associated with an increased risk for congenital heart defects,[16] skull abnormalities, and other defects.[17] Scientists continue to investigate the possible lifelong effects of other nutrient excesses, including the impact of high maternal intake of sodium on risk for hypertension in their adult offspring and the effect of high maternal saturated fat intake on risk for congenital defects.

In short, research suggests that there are lifelong consequences to any type of nutrient imbalance during pregnancy, whether the imbalance is a total energy deficit, a single nutrient deficiency, or an energy or nutrient excess.

Exposure to Alcohol, Tobacco, and Other Toxic Agents

You've already learned of the lifelong impact of fetal alcohol syndrome, resulting from exposure to high maternal blood alcohol levels. In addition, maternal smoking has been shown to negatively impact the long-term health of the offspring. Not only are the offspring of women who smoked during pregnancy at high risk for preterm delivery and low birth weight, but they are also at higher risk for childhood allergies and respiratory diseases, adult-onset high blood pressure, childhood behavioral problems,[4] and cleft lip and palate.[18] New evidence also confirms a link between maternal smoking and increased risk for adult-onset diabetes among offspring, as well as a lifelong higher risk for obesity.[19]

Not surprisingly, maternal exposure to lead increases the risk for developmental delays, behavioral and learning problems, and hearing loss.[20] Maternal exposure to mercury can result in irreversible damage to the baby's nervous system and subsequent learning disabilities. In each of these examples, the mother's dietary intake and her immediate environment can lead to harmful effects that persist into and throughout adulthood.

Individual Health Implications

If your mother experienced some type of nutritional, metabolic, or environmental stress during pregnancy, you certainly are not doomed to suffer from one or more of the health problems mentioned here. That's because the research described reported on large groups of people, not individuals. Moreover, it calculated increases in risk for—or susceptibility to—certain conditions, but it did not and cannot condemn anyone to any particular disease.

Any type of fetal programming or genetic influence that develops as a result of the fetal environment is just one factor in your wellness. A much more significant influence is your own lifestyle, especially your personal food choices, dietary patterns, activity habits, alcohol intake, and smoking.

CRITICAL THINKING QUESTIONS

■ In most states, pregnant women can be arrested for child abuse if, at the time of their delivery, they are found to have cocaine, heroin, or other illegal drugs in their system. Do you think similar laws should be enacted for pregnant women with alcohol or nicotine in their blood? Why or why not?

■ If you were a member of a women's health care team, would you advise an obese client to avoid known pregnancy risks by deferring pregnancy until she was able to bring her weight and blood glucose level down to a recommended range? Why or why not? If you went forward with the advice, how would you present it?

REFERENCES

1. Lussana, F., R. C. Painter, M. C. Ocke, H. R. Buller, P. M. Bossuyt, and T. J. Roseboom. 2008. Prenatal exposure to the Dutch famine is associated with a preference for fatty foods and a more atherogenic lipid profile. *Am. J. Clin. Nutr.* 88:1648–1652.

2. Lumey, L. H., A. D. Stein, H. S. Kahn, and J. A. Romijn. 2009. Lipid profiles in middle-aged men and women after famine exposure during gestation: the Dutch Hunger Winter Families Study. *Am. J. Clin. Nutr.* 90:1737–1743.

3. Kaijser, M., A. K. E. Bonamy, O. Akre, S. Cnattingius, F. Granath, M. Norman, and A. Ekbom. 2009. Perinatal risk factors for diabetes in later life. *Diabetes* 58:523–526.

4. Jaddoe, V. W. V. 2008. Fetal nutritional origins of adult diseases: challenges for epidemiological research. *Eur. J. Epidemiol.* 23:767–771.

5. Stanner, S. A., K. Bulmer, C. Andres, O. E. Lantseva, V. Borodina, V. V. Poteen, and J. S. Yudkin. 1997. Does malnutrition in utero determine diabetes and coronary heart disease in adulthood? Results from the Leningrad siege study, a cross sectional study. *Brit. Med. J.* 315:1342–1348.

6. Stanner, S. A., and J. S. Yudkin. 2001. Fetal programming and the Leningrad siege study. *Twin Research* 4:287–292.

7. Juonala, M., C. G. Magnussen, G. S. Berenson, A. Venn, T. L. Burns, M. A. Sabin, S. R. Srinivasan, S. R. Daniels, P H. Davis, W. Chen, C. Sun, M. Cheung, J. S. Viikari, T. Dwyer, and O. T. Raitakari. 2011. Childhood adiposity, adult adiposity, and cardiovascular risk factors. *N. Engl. J. Med.* 365:1876–1885.

8. Miranda, J. J., S. Kinra, J. P. Casas, G. Davey Smith, and S. Ebrahim. 2008. Non-communicable diseases in low- and middle-income countries: context, determinants and health policy. *Trop. Med. Int. Health.* 13:1225–1234.

9. Maret, W., and H. H. Sandstead. 2008. Possible roles of zinc nutriture in the fetal origins of disease. *Experimental Gerontology* 43:378–381.

10. Catalano, P. M., K. Farrell, A. Thomas, L. Huston-Presley, P. Mencin, S. Hauguel de Mouson, and S. B. Amini. 2009. Perinatal risk factors for childhood obesity and metabolic dysregulation. *Am. J. Clin. Nutr.* 90:1303–1313.

11. Stuebe, A. M., M. R. Forman, and K. B. Michels. 2009. Maternal-recalled gestational weight gain, pre-pregnancy body mass index, and obesity in the daughter. *Intl. J. Obesity.* 33:743–752.

12. Bouret, S .G. 2010. Role of early hormonal and nutritional experiences in shaping feeding behavior and hypothalamic development. *J. Nutr.* 140:653–657.

13. Stothard, K. J., P. W. G. Tennant, R. Bell, and J. Rankin. 2009. Maternal overweight and obesity and the risk of congenital anomalies: a systematic review and meta-analysis. *JAMA.* 301:636–650.

14. Garcia-Vargas, L., S. S. Addison, R. Nistala, D. Kurukula-suriya, and J. R. Sowers. 2012 Gestational diabetes and the offspring: implications in the development of the cardio-renal metabolic syndrome in offspring. *Cardiorenal Med.* 2:134–142.

15. Clausen, T. D., E. R. Mathiesen, T. Hansen, O. Pedersen, D. M. Jensen, J. Lauenborg, L. Schmidt, and P. Damm. 2009. Overweight and the metabolic syndrome in adult offspring of women with diet-treated gestational diabetes mellitus or type 1 diabetes. *J. Clin. Endocrinology Metab.* 94:2464–2470.

16. Nielsen, G. L., C. Dethlefsen, S. Lundbye-Christensen, J. F. Pedersen, L. Mølsted-Pedersen, and M. W. Gillman. 2012. Adiposity in 277 young adult male offspring of women with diabetes compared with controls: a Danish population-based cohort study. *Acta Obstetricia et Gynecologica Scandinavica* 91:838–843.

17. Cetin, I., C. Berti, and S. Calabrese. 2009. Role of micronutrients in the periconceptual period. *Hum. Reproduction Update.* 16:80–95.

18. Dixon, M. J., M. L. Marazita, T. H. Beaty, and J. C. Murray. 2011. Cleft lip and palate: understanding genetic and environmental influences. *Nature Reviews: Genetics.* 12:167–178.

19. Zucker, M. 2002. Smoking during pregnancy: even worse than you think. *Pulmonary* Reviews.com 7(3). www.pulmonaryreviews.com/march02/smoking.html. (Accessed March 2010.)

20. March of Dimes. 2007. Quick Reference Fact Sheets: Environmental Risks and Pregnancy. www.marchofdimes.com/professionals/14332_9146.asp. (Accessed March 2010.)

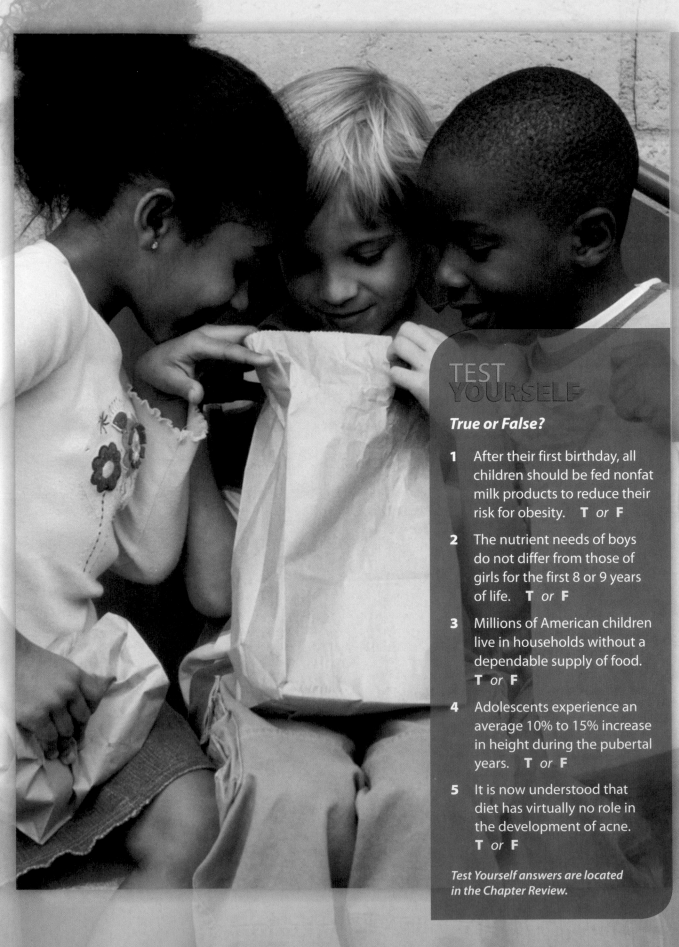

True or False?

1 After their first birthday, all children should be fed nonfat milk products to reduce their risk for obesity. **T** *or* **F**

2 The nutrient needs of boys do not differ from those of girls for the first 8 or 9 years of life. **T** *or* **F**

3 Millions of American children live in households without a dependable supply of food. **T** *or* **F**

4 Adolescents experience an average 10% to 15% increase in height during the pubertal years. **T** *or* **F**

5 It is now understood that diet has virtually no role in the development of acne. **T** *or* **F**

Test Yourself answers are located in the Chapter Review.

17

Nutrition Through the Life Cycle: Childhood and Adolescence

Learning Objectives

After studying this chapter, you should be able to:

1. Describe the key nutrient needs for toddlers, including for energy, macronutrients, micronutrients, fluids, and supplements (if any), *pp. 688–691.*

2. Describe the issues involved in encouraging toddlers to eat nutritious foods, and ways in food choices for adults and children differ, *pp. 691–694.*

3. Identify and describe the areas of toddler-specific nutritional concerns, *pp. 694–695.*

4. Identify the nutrition-related issues of preschool and school-age children, taking into account their growth and activity patterns and specific nutrient needs, *pp. 695–699.*

5. Discuss the nutritional issues surrounding vegan diets, encouraging nutritious food choices, and school attendance and lunch programs for young children, *pp. 699–701.*

6. Identify and describe the areas of nutritional concern for children, *pp. 701–703.*

7. Describe the nutritional issues for adolescents, taking into account their psychosocial development, growth and activity patterns, and nutrient needs, *pp. 703–707.*

8. Identify and discuss the main areas of nutrition-related concern for adolescents, *pp. 707–709.*

9. Describe the central issues underlying the concerns over pediatric obesity, and identify the "seeds" of the problem, *p. 710.*

10. Discuss the dietary and lifestyle options for preventing childhood obesity, including the roles of the family and school, *pp. 711–715.*

MasteringNutrition™

Go online for chapter quizzes, pre-tests, Interactive Activities, and more!

C
hristina is a happy 7-year-old who loves school, her kitten, and TV. According to her mother, Christina never "grew out" of her baby fat and, because she is often teased by other children, rarely goes outside to play. Her school's 30-minute physical education classes twice a week provide the only real exercise Christina gets. Six weeks ago, at the start of the school year, the school nurse sent home a note explaining that Christina's weight and height ratio indicated she is obese. Following up on the nurse's advice, Christina and her mom visited a local clinic specializing in pediatrics and found out that Christina has hypertension, high triglycerides, high total and LDL cholesterol, low HDL cholesterol, and type 2 diabetes. "How can my baby have diabetes?" asked her mom. "My dad didn't get it until he was almost 60 years old and I didn't get it until I was 42 years old." Unfortunately, Christina is one of a growing number of children under the age of 10 who are diagnosed with what used to be regarded as adult diseases. Why are more and more children developing these diseases at such young ages? How can families, healthcare providers, school personnel, and society as a whole work together to improve the health of America's children?

This chapter will help answer these and related questions. Although most topics are discussed within specific age groupings (toddlers, children, and adolescents), the chapter closes with an in-depth review of pediatric obesity, which affects children of all ages.

Nutrition for Toddlers

When babies celebrate their first birthday, they transition out of infancy and into the active world of toddlers. Personality and behavioral changes introduce potential conflict into mealtimes, and parents who have been accustomed to making all decisions about their child's diet must now begin to consider the child's preferences. In addition, toddlers attending day care may be exposed to foods that are more or less nutritious than the foods served at home. These and other circumstances add new challenges to the feeding process.

Toddler Growth and Activity Patterns

The rapid growth rate of infancy begins to slow during toddlerhood, the second and third years of life. A toddler will grow a total of about 5.5 to 7.5 inches and gain an average of 9 to 11 pounds. Toddlers expend more energy in order to fuel their increasing levels of activity as they explore their expanding world and develop new skills. They progress from taking a few wobbly steps to running, jumping, and climbing with confidence, and they begin to dress, feed, and toilet themselves. Thus, their diet should provide an appropriate quantity and quality of nutrients to fuel their growth and activity.

What Are a Toddler's Nutrient Needs?

Nutrient needs increase as a child progresses from infancy to toddlerhood. Refer to **Table 17.1** (page 689) for a review of specific nutrient recommendations.

Energy and Macronutrient Recommendations for Toddlers

Although the energy requirement per kilogram of body weight for toddlers is just slightly less than for infants, total energy requirements are higher because toddlers are larger and much more active than infants. The *estimated energy requirement (EER)*, or the total energy needed per day, varies according to a toddler's age, body weight, and level of activity.

Although there is currently insufficient evidence available to set a DRI for fat for toddlers, healthy toddlers of appropriate body weight need to consume 30% to 40% of their

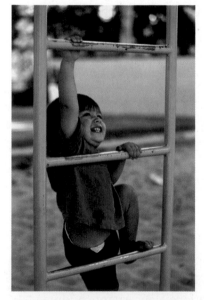

Toddlers expend significant amounts of energy actively exploring their world.

TABLE 17.1 Nutrient Recommendations for Children and Adolescents

Nutrient	Children Age 1–3 Years	Children Age 4–8 Years	Children Age 9–13 Years	Adolescents Age 14–18 Years
Fat	No DRI	No DRI	No DRI	No DRI
Protein	1.10 g/kg body weight per day	0.95 g/kg body weight per day	0.95 g/kg body weight per day	0.85 g/kg body weight per day
Carbohydrate	130 g/day	130 g/day	130 g/day	130 g/day
Vitamin A	300 µg/day	400 µg/day	600 µg/day	Boys = 900 µg/day Girls = 700 µg/day
Vitamin C	15 mg/day	25 mg/day	45 mg/day	Boys = 75 mg/day Girls = 65 mg/day
Vitamin E	6 mg/day	7 mg/day	11 mg/day	15 mg/day
Calcium	500 mg/day	800 mg/day	1,300 mg/day	1,300 mg/day
Iron	7 mg/day	10 mg/day	8 mg/day	Boys = 11 mg/day Girls = 15 mg/day
Zinc	3 mg/day	5 mg/day	8 mg/day	Boys = 11 mg/day Girls = 9 mg/day
Fluid	1.3 L/day	1.7 L/day	Boys = 2.4 L/day Girls = 2.1 L/day	Boys = 3.3 L/day Girls = 2.3 L/day

total daily energy intake as fat.[1] That's because fat provides a concentrated source of energy in a relatively small amount of food, and this is important for toddlers, especially those who are fussy eaters or have little appetite. Fat is also necessary during the toddler years to support the continuously developing nervous system.

Toddlers' protein needs increase modestly, because they weigh more than infants and are still growing rapidly. The RDA for protein for toddlers is 1.1 g/kg body weight per day, or approximately 13 g of protein daily.[1] Recall that 2 cups of milk alone provide 16 g of protein; thus, most toddlers have little trouble meeting their protein needs.

The RDA for carbohydrate for toddlers is 130 g/day, and carbohydrate intake should be about 45% to 65% of total energy intake.[1] As is the case for older children and adults, most of the carbohydrates eaten should be complex, and refined carbohydrates from high-fat/high-energy foods, such as cookies and candy, should be kept to a minimum. Fruits and 100% fruit juices are nutritious sources of simple carbohydrates that can also be included in a toddler's diet. Keep in mind, however, that too much fruit juice can displace other foods and nutrients and can cause diarrhea. If consumed at bedtime or between meals, the sugars in fruit juice may also contribute to tooth decay. The American Academy of Pediatrics (AAP) recommends that the intake of fruit juice be limited to 4 to 6 fl. oz per day for children 1 to 6 years of age.[2]

Adequate fiber is important for toddlers to maintain regularity. The AI is 14 g of fiber per 1,000 kcal of energy, or, based on the average energy intake of this age group, 19 g/day.[1] Unfortunately, dietary fiber intake is inadequate in most U.S. children.[3] Whole-grain cereals, fresh fruits and vegetables, and whole-grain breads are healthful choices for toddlers' meals and snacks. Too much fiber, however, can inhibit the absorption of several nutrients, such as iron and zinc; harm toddlers' small digestive tracts; and cause them to feel too full to consume adequate nutrients.

Determining the macronutrient requirements of toddlers can be challenging. See the **You Do the Math** box (page 690) for analysis of the macronutrient levels in one toddler's daily diet.

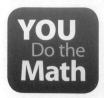

Is This Menu Good for a Toddler?

A dedicated mother and father want to provide the best nutrition for their young son, Ethan, who is now 1 ½ years old and has just been completely weaned from breast milk. Ethan weighs about 26 lb (11.8 kg). Following is a typical day's menu for Ethan. Grams of protein, fat, and carbohydrate are given for each food. The day's total energy intake is 1,168 kcal. Calculate the percentage of Ethan's calories that come from protein, fat, and carbohydrate (numbers may not add up to exactly 100% because of rounding). Where are Ethan's parents doing well, and where could they use some advice for improvement?

Note: This activity focuses on the macronutrients. It does not ask you to consider Ethan's intake of micronutrients or fluids.

There is a total of 47.5 g protein in Ethan's menu:

$$47.5 \text{ g} \times 4 \text{ kcal/g} = 190 \text{ kcal}$$

$$190 \text{ kcal protein}/1{,}168 \text{ total kcal} \times 100 = 16\% \text{ protein}$$

There is a total of 25.75 g fat in Ethan's menu:

$$25.75 \text{ g} \times 9 \text{ kcal/g } 5 \text{ 232 kcal}$$

$$232 \text{ kcal fat}/1{,}168 \text{ total kcal} \times 100 = 20\% \text{ fat}$$

There is a total of 186.5 g carbohydrate in Ethan's menu:

$$186.5 \text{ g} \times 4 \text{ cal/g} = 746 \text{ kcal}$$

$$746 \text{ kcal carbohydrate}/1{,}168 \text{ total kcal} \times 100$$

$$= 64\% \text{ carbohydrate}$$

Ethan's parents are doing very well at offering a wide range of foods from various food groups; they are especially doing well with fruits and vegetables. Also, according to his EER, Ethan requires about 970 kcal/day, and he is consuming 1,168 kcal/day, thus meeting his energy needs.

Ethan's total carbohydrate intake for the day is 186.5 g, which is higher than the RDA of 130 g per day; however, this value falls within the recommended 45% to 65% of total energy intake that should come from carbohydrates. Thus, high carbohydrate intake is adequate to meet his energy needs.

However, Ethan is being offered far more than enough protein. The DRI for protein for toddlers is about 13 g per day, and Ethan is being offered more than three times that much!

It is also readily apparent that Ethan is being offered too little fat for his age. Toddlers need at least 30% to 40% of their total energy intake from fat, and Ethan is only consuming about 20% of his calories from fat. He should be drinking whole milk, not 1% milk. He should occasionally be offered higher-fat foods, such as cheese for his snacks or macaroni and cheese for a meal. Yogurt is fine, but it shouldn't be nonfat at Ethan's age.

In conclusion, Ethan's parents should be commended for offering a variety of nutritious foods but should be counseled that a little more fat is critical for toddlers' growth and development. Some of the energy currently being consumed as protein and carbohydrate should be shifted to fat.

Meal	Foods	Protein (g)	Fat (g)	Carbo-hydrate (g)
Breakfast	Oatmeal (½ cup, cooked)	2.5	1.5	13.5
	Brown sugar (1 tsp.)	0	0	4
	Milk (1%, 4 fl. oz)	4	1.25	5.5
	Grape juice (4 fl. oz)	0	0	20
Mid-morning Snack	Banana slices (1 small banana)	0	0	16
	Yogurt (nonfat fruit-flavored, 3 fl. oz)	5.5	0	15.5
	Orange juice (4 fl. oz)	1	0	13
Lunch	Whole-wheat bread (1 slice)	1.5	0.5	10
	Peanut butter (1 tbsp.)	4	8	3.5
	Strawberry jam (1 tbsp.)	0	0	13
	Carrots (cooked, ⅛ cup)	0	0	2
	Applesauce (sweetened, ¼ cup)	0	0	12
	Milk (1%, 4 fl. oz)	4	1.25	5.5
Afternoon Snack	Bagel (½)	3	1	20
	American cheese product (1 slice)	3	5	1
	Water	0	0	0
Dinner	Scrambled egg (1)	11	5	1
	Baby food spinach (3 oz)	2	0.5	5.5
	Whole-wheat toast (1 slice)	1.5	0.5	10
	Mandarin orange slices (¼ cup)	0.5	0	10
	Milk (1%, 4 fl. oz)	4	1.25	5.5

Micronutrient Recommendations for Toddlers

As toddlers grow, their micronutrient needs increase. Of particular concern with toddlers are adequate intakes of the micronutrients associated with fruits and vegetables. In addition, vitamin D, calcium, and iron have been identified as "priority nutrients" for children aged 2 to 4 years.

Vitamin D intake often decreases in toddlers is closely linked to milk consumption. The American Academy of Pediatrics recommends vitamin D supplements for all children who consume less than 1 liter of vitamin D–fortified dairy products each day—a group that includes the majority of U.S. children.[4] Vitamin D–fortified soy milk and other milk alternatives, in adequate amounts, are also acceptable.

Calcium is necessary to promote optimal bone mass through early adulthood. For toddlers 1 to 3 years, the RDA for calcium is 700 mg/day.[5] Dairy products are excellent sources of calcium. When a child reaches the age of 1 year, whole cow's milk can be given; however, reduced-fat milk (2% or less) should *not* be given until age 2. If dairy products are not feasible, calcium-fortified orange juice and milk alternatives can supply calcium, or children's calcium supplements can be given. Toddlers generally cannot consume enough food to be able to depend on alternate calcium sources, such as dark-green vegetables.

Iron-deficiency anemia is the most common nutrient deficiency in young children in the United States and around the world. Iron-deficiency anemia can affect a child's energy level, attention span, and ability to learn. The RDA for iron for toddlers is 7 mg/day.[6] Good sources of well-absorbed heme iron include lean meats, fish, and poultry; non-heme iron is provided by egg yolks, legumes, greens, and fortified foods such as breakfast cereals. When toddlers consume non-heme sources of iron, such as beans or greens, a rich source of vitamin C at the same meal will enhance the absorption of iron from these sources.

Fluid Recommendations for Toddlers

Toddlers lose less fluid from evaporation than infants, and their more mature kidneys are able to concentrate urine, conserving the body's fluid. However, as toddlers become active, they start to lose significant fluid through sweat, especially in hot weather. Parents need to make sure an active toddler is drinking adequately. The recommended fluid intake for toddlers is listed in Table 17.1 and includes about 4 cups as beverages, including water.[7] Suggested beverages include plain water, milk, calcium-fortified beverages, and foods high in water content, such as vegetables and fruits.

Do Toddlers Need Nutritional Supplements?

Toddlers can be well nourished by consuming a balanced, varied diet. But given their typically erratic eating habits, the child's physician may recommend a multivitamin/multimineral supplement as a precaution against deficiencies. The toddler's physician or dentist may also prescribe a fluoride supplement if the community water supply is not fluoridated. Supplements should also be considered for children in vegan families, children from families who cannot afford adequate amounts of nourishing foods, children with certain medical conditions or dietary restrictions, and very picky or erratic eaters.

As many as 30% of U.S. children between the ages of 2 and 5 years use nutrient supplements, although many take them on an irregular basis.[4] As always, if a supplement is given, it should be formulated especially for toddlers and the recommended dose should not be exceeded. A supplement should not contain more than 100% of the Daily Value of any nutrient per dose.

Many parents choose special cereals, snack foods, and packaged dinners for their young children. How do the nutrient values of these foods compare to those of similar versions for adults? See the **Nutrition Label Activity** box (page 692) to find out.

Encouraging Nutritious Food Choices with Toddlers

Parents and pediatricians have long known that toddlers tend to be choosy about what they eat. Some avoid entire foods groups, such as all meats or vegetables. Others refuse all but one or two favorite foods (such as peanut butter on crackers) for several days or longer. Still others eat in extremely small amounts, seemingly satisfied by a single slice of apple or

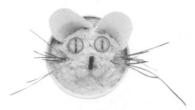

Most toddlers are delighted by food prepared in a "fun" way.

two bites of toast. These behaviors frustrate and worry many parents, but in fact, as long as a variety of healthful food is available, most normal-weight toddlers are able to match their food intake with their needs. A toddler will most likely make up for one day's nutrient or energy deficiency later in the week. Food should never be "forced" on a child, as doing so sets the stage for eating and control issues later in life.

Toddlers' stomachs are still very small, and they cannot consume all of the energy they need in three meals. They need small meals, interspersed with nutritious snacks, every 2 to 3 hours. A successful technique is to create a snack tray filled with small portions of nutritious food choices, such as one-third of a banana, two pieces of cheese, and two whole-grain crackers, and leave it within reach of the child's play area. The child can then "graze" on these healthful foods while he or she plays. Limiting their food alternatives can also be effective in helping toddlers eat nutritiously. For example, parents can say, "It's snack time! Would you like apples and cheese, or bananas and yogurt?"

Foods prepared for toddlers should be developmentally appropriate. Nuts, carrots, grapes, raisins, and cherry tomatoes are difficult for a toddler to chew and pose a choking hazard. Foods should be soft and sliced into strips or wedges that are easy for children to grasp. As a child develops more teeth and becomes more coordinated, the foods offered can become more varied. Though certainly not necessary, several food companies now market "toddler foods" geared specifically to their developmental stage. The **Nutrition Label Activity** box provides the opportunity to compare labeling practices for toddler and adult foods.

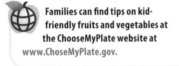

Families can find tips on kid-friendly fruits and vegetables at the ChooseMyPlate website at www.ChoseMyPlate.gov.

Foods prepared for toddlers should also be fun. Parents can use cookie cutters to turn a peanut-butter sandwich into a pumpkin face, or arrange cooked peas or carrot slices to create a smiling face on top of mashed potatoes. Juice and yogurt can be frozen into "popsicles" or blended into "milkshakes."

Nutrition Label Activity

Comparing Foods for Children and Adults

Parents who purchase foods such as "junior dinners" for their toddlers often check the Nutrition Facts Panel for information on the ingredients and nutrient value of the products. Many of these parents may not realize that the FDA and USDA have specific label requirements for products aimed at children less than 2 years old and for those who are 2 to 4 years old. Food products designed for children under 2 years of age cannot list the amount of saturated, polyunsaturated, or monounsaturated fat; the amount of cholesterol; or the calories from fat on the label. This is to avoid the impression that fat is bad for young children; recall that dietary fat should not be restricted in children under the age of 2 years.

Compare the labels of the infant chicken noodle dinner" (**Figure 17.1a**) and the adult chicken noodle dinner (Figure 17.1b). What other differences in the Nutrition Facts Panel do you see? Compare the ingredient list for the two products. What is the most prevalent ingredient in the toddler food? Does the toddler food contain all or any of the food additives listed in the adult product? Why do you believe there is a difference?

Foods for children under 2 years of age cannot be labeled with nutrient claims ("low-fat") or health claims that often appear on food labels. Labels of foods for children under the age

of 2 years are, however, allowed to make statements such as "Provides 100% of the Daily Value for vitamin C." They can also describe the product as *unsweetened* or *unsalted,* because those terms describe taste features more than nutrient value. Terms such as *no sugar added* and *sugar free* cannot be used on foods for children 2 years and under, although they are permitted on dietary supplements for children.

The small size of children 4 years and under means they have lower nutrient needs than adults. Nutrition Facts information for products marketed to young children is therefore based on smaller serving sizes and age-appropriate Daily Values. Some products, such as infant cereal, have nutrient information both for infants up to 1 year and for children 1 to 4 years (Figure 17.1c). This approach provides families with nutrient guidelines for all young children. Because there are no Daily Values (DVs) for fat (total or saturated), cholesterol, sodium, or fiber for children under the age of 4 years, there are also no %DV figures for those nutrients on the labels of foods aimed at these children. Use the baby cereal label (Figure 17.1c) to identify the one nutrient for which the DV is actually *higher* for infants than for children 1 to 4 years of age. (*Hint:* It is a mineral.)

(a)

Chicken Noodle Dinner

INSPECTED FOR U.S. DEPARTMENT OF AGRICULTURE

NET WT 4 OZ (113g)

Nutrition Facts

Serv Size: 1 jar
Calories 80

Amount Per Serving			
Total Fat	3g	Total Carb	11g
Trans Fat	1g	Fiber	2g
Sodium	40mg	Sugars	4g ★
Potassium	200mg	Protein	3g

% Daily Value	• Protein 16%	• Vitamin A 270%
Vitamin C 0%	• Calcium 2%	• Iron 4% • Zinc 10%

★ CONTAINS NATURAL VEGETABLE SUGARS ONLY

INGREDIENTS: WATER, CARROTS, FINELY GROUND CHICKEN, GREEN SPLIT PEAS, ENRICHED EGG NOODLES (DURUM WHEAT FLOUR, EGG SOLIDS, NIACIN, FERROUS SULFATE, THIAMIN MONONITRATE, RIBOFLAVIN, FOLIC ACID), RICE FLOUR, CHICKEN FAT, ONION POWDER, SOYBEAN OIL AND EXTRACTIVES OF CELERY.

• Unsalted
• No artificial flavors, colors or preservatives

(b)

Nutrition Facts

Serving Size 2/3 cup mix (60g) Makes 1 cup prepared
Servings Per Container 2

Amount Per Serving	Mix	Prepared as Directed
Calories	220	260
Calories from Fat	30	80

	% Daily Value**	
Total Fat 3.5g*	**5%**	**13%**
Saturated Fat 1g	**4%**	**10%**
Trans Fat 0g		
Cholesterol 50mg	**17%**	**17%**
Sodium 860mg	**36%**	**38%**
Total Carbohydrate 40mg	**13%**	**13%**
Dietary Fiber 2g	**6%**	**6%**
Sugars 2g		
Protein 8g		
Vitamin A	6%	10%
Vitamin C	10%	10%
Calcium	2%	2%
Iron	10%	10%
Thiamin	30%	30%
Riboflavin	15%	15%
Niacin	15%	15%
Folate	25%	25%

*Amount in Mix. 1/2 tbsp. of margarine add 40 calories, 5g fat (1g saturated), and 50mg sodium.

**Percent Daily Values are based on a 2,000 calorie diet. Your daily values may be higher or lower depending on your calorie needs.

	Calories:	2,000	2,500
Total Fat	Less than	65g	80g
Sat. Fat	Less than	20g	25g
Cholesterol	Less than	300mg	300mg
Sodium	Less than	2,400mg	2,400mg
Total Carbohydrate		300g	375g
Dietary Fiber		25g	30g

INGREDIENTS: ENRICHED EGG NOODLES (WHEAT FLOUR, EGGS, NIACIN, FERROUS SULFATE, THIAMIN MONONITRATE, RIBOFLAVIN, FOLIC ACID), CORN STARCH, SALT, CORN SYRUP*, ONION*, MALTODEXTRIN, CHICKEN FAT*, CHICKEN BROTH*, NATURAL FLAVORS, HYDROLYZED PROTEIN (SOY, CORN), AUTOLYZED YEAST EXTRACT, BELL PEPPER*, GARLIC*, PARTIALLY HYDROGENATED SOYBEAN OIL, PARSLEY*, SPICES (INCLUDING PAPRIKA), XANTHAN AND GUAR GUMS, GUM ARABIC, WHEY, SODIUM CASEINATE, DISODIUM PHOSPHATE, DISODIUM INOSINATE, DISODIUM GUANYLATE, ANNATTO AND OLEORESIN TURMERIC (FOR COLOR).
*DEHYDRATED
CONTAINS: EGG, WHEAT, SOY, MILK

(c)

Oatmeal
CEREAL FOR BABY

Nutrition Facts

Serving Size 1/4 cup (15g)
Servings Per Container About 15

Amount Per Serving

Calories 60

Total Fat	1g
Trans Fat	0g
Sodium	0mg
Potassium	50mg
Total Carbohydrate	10g
Fiber	1g
Sugars	2g
Protein	2g

% Daily Value	Infants 0–1	Children 1–4
Protein	10%	9%
Vitamin A	0%	0%
Vitamin C	0%	0%
Calcium	15%	10%
Iron	45%	60%
Vitamin E	15%	8%
Thiamin	25%	15%
Riboflavin	25%	20%
Niacin	25%	20%
Vitamin B$_6$	25%	10%
Folate	25%	10%
Vitamin B$_{12}$	25%	15%
Phosphorus	15%	10%
Zinc	20%	10%

INGREDIENTS: OAT FLOUR, TRI- AND DICALCIUM PHOSPHATE, SOY OIL-LECITHIN, TOCOPHEROLS (VITAMIN E), ELECTROLYTIC IRON, ZINC SULFATE, NIACINAMIDE (A B VITAMIN), RIBOFLAVIN (VITAMIN B-2), PYRIDOXINE HYDROCHLORIDE (VITAMIN B-6), THIAMIN (VITAMIN B-1), FOLIC ACID (A B VITAMIN) AND VITAMIN B-12 (CYANOCOBALAMIN).

FIGURE 17.1 Label guidelines for foods targeting infants and children under the age of 2 years differ from the labeling regulations for other foods. **(a)** Label from infant chicken noodle dinner. **(b)** Label from an adult chicken noodle meal. Note the listing of *trans* and saturated fat contents, among other differences. **(c)** Label from oatmeal cereal for infants and young children. (*Source:* United States Food and Drug Administration.)

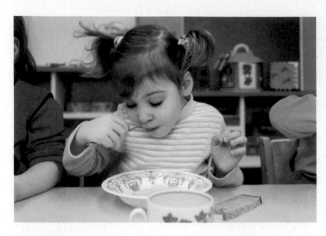

FIGURE 17.2 Portion sizes for toddlers and preschoolers are much smaller than for older children. Use the following guideline: 1 tablespoon of the food for each year of age equals 1 serving. For example, the meal shown here—2 tablespoons of rice, 2 tablespoons of black beans, and 2 tablespoons of chopped tomatoes—is appropriate for a 2-year-old toddler.

A positive environment helps toddlers develop good mealtime habits as well. Parents should consistently seat the toddler in the same place at the table and make sure that the child is served first. Television and other distractions should be turned off, and pleasant conversation should include the toddler, even if the toddler hasn't begun to speak. Toddlers should not be forced to sit still until they finish every bite, as they still have short attention spans.

Even at mealtime, portion sizes should be small. One tablespoon of a food for each year of age constitutes a serving throughout the toddler and preschool years (**Figure 17.2**). Realistic portion sizes can give toddlers a sense of accomplishment when they "eat it all up" and reduce parents' fears that their child is not eating enough.

New foods should be introduced gradually. Most toddlers are leery of new foods, spicy foods, hot (temperature) foods, mixed foods such as casseroles, and foods with strange textures. A helpful rule is to encourage the child to eat at least one bite of a new food: if the child does not want the rest, nothing negative should be said, and the child should be praised just for the willingness to try. The same food should be reintroduced a few weeks later. Eventually, after several tries, the child might accept the food. Some foods, however, won't be accepted until well into adulthood as tastes expand and develop. Parents should never bribe with food—for example, promising dessert if the child finishes her squash. Bribing teaches children that food can be used to reward and manipulate. Instead, parents should try to positively reinforce good behaviors—for example, "Wow! You ate every bite of your squash! That's going to help you grow big and strong!"

Role modeling is important because toddlers mimic older children and adults: if they see their parents eating a variety of healthful foods, toddlers will be likely to do so as well. Adults have a significant impact on the nutrient intakes and diet quality of their children's choices.[7] Finally, toddlers are more likely to eat food they help prepare: encourage them to assist in the preparation of simple foods, such as helping pour a bowl of cereal or helping arrange raw vegetables on a plate.

Nutrition-Related Concerns for Toddlers

Just as toddlers have their own specific nutrient needs, they also have toddler-specific nutrition concerns.

Continued Allergy Watch

As during infancy, wheat, peanuts, cow's milk, soy, citrus, egg whites, and seafood remain common food allergens. New foods should be presented one at a time, and the toddler should be monitored for allergic reactions for a week before additional new foods are introduced. To prevent the development of food allergies, even foods that are established in the diet should be rotated rather than served every day.

Vegetarian Families

For toddlers, an ovo-lacto-vegetarian diet in which eggs and dairy foods are included can be as wholesome as a diet including meats and fish.[8] However, because meat, fish, and poultry are important sources of zinc and heme iron, the most bioavailable form of iron, vegetarian families must be careful to include enough zinc and iron from other sources in their child's diet.

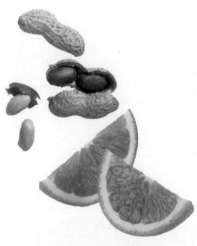

Foods that may cause allergies, such as peanuts and citrus fruits, should be introduced to toddlers one at a time.

In contrast, a vegan diet, in which no foods of animal origin are consumed, poses several potential nutritional risks for toddlers:

- *Protein:* Vegan diets can be too low in protein for toddlers, who need protein for growth and increasing activity. Few toddlers can consume enough legumes and whole grains to provide sufficient protein. The high-fiber content of these foods quickly produces a sense of fullness for the toddler, decreasing total food intake.
- *Calcium, iron, and zinc:* Calcium is a concern because of the avoidance in a vegan diet of milk, yogurt, and cheese. As with protein, few toddlers can consume enough calcium from plant sources to meet their daily requirement, and supplementation is advised. Iron and zinc are also commonly low in vegan diets due to the absence of meat, fish, and poultry. They need to be provided by fortified cereals, legumes, and possibly supplements.
- *Vitamins D and B$_{12}$:* Both vitamins are typically lower in vegan diets. Some cereals and soy milks are now fortified with vitamin D; however, some toddlers may still need a vitamin D–containing supplement if they consume less than 1 liter of fortified soy milk daily. Vitamin B$_{12}$, though found in many fortified breakfast cereals, is not naturally available in any amount from plant foods and must be supplemented.
- *Fiber:* Vegan diets often contain a higher amount of fiber than is recommended for toddlers, resulting in lowered absorption of iron and zinc, as well as a premature sense of fullness or satiety at mealtimes.

The practice of feeding a vegan diet to infants and young children is highly controversial. See **Nutrition Myth or Fact? Are Vegan Diets Inappropriate for Young Children?** (page 696) for more information about this controversy.

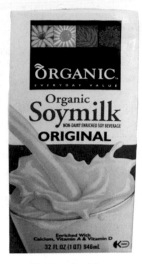

Enriched and fortified foods, such as fortified soy milk, provide important nutrient supplementation that should be included in vegan diets given to toddlers.

RECAP

Growth during toddlerhood is slower than during infancy; however, toddlers are highly active, and thus total energy, fat, and protein requirements are higher than for infants. Toddlers require small, frequent, nutritious meals and snacks. Until age 2, toddlers should drink whole milk rather than reduced-fat (2% or lower) milk. Iron deficiency is a concern and can be avoided by feeding toddlers lean meats, fish, poultry, eggs, and iron-fortified foods. Toddlers need to drink about 4 cups of beverages, including water. Role modeling by parents and access to ample healthful foods can help toddlers make nutritious choices. Feeding vegan diets to toddlers is controversial and poses a risk for potential deficiencies of calcium, iron, zinc, vitamin D, and vitamin B$_{12}$. ■

Nutrition for Preschool and School-Age Children

Children develop increased language fluency, improved decision-making skills, and greater physical coordination and dexterity as they progress through the preschool and school-age years. The nutrient requirements and nutrition issues of importance to children are discussed in this section.

Childhood Growth and Activity Patterns

Children at this stage of development experience a slow and steady rate of growth, averaging 2 to 4 inches per year, until the rapid growth of adolescence begins. Activity levels among children vary dramatically—some love sports and physical activity, whereas others prefer quieter activities, such as reading and drawing. Television, computer use, and electronic games often tempt children into a sedentary lifestyle. All children can be encouraged to have fun using their muscles in various ways that suit their interests (**Figure 17.3,** page 698).

Nutrition Myth OR Fact?

Are Vegan Diets Inappropriate for Young Children?

The health benefits to adults consuming vegan diets are well known.[1] In contrast, the practice of feeding a vegan diet to infants or young children is a subject of heated controversy. Many who support veganism feel that consumption of any type of animal product is immoral, that feeding animal products to children fosters a lifetime of obesity and chronic disease, and that consumption of animal products wastes natural resources and contributes to environmental damage. In contrast, opponents emphasize that feeding a vegan diet to young children deprives them of a healthful level of essential nutrients that can only be obtained if the child consumes animal products. Some people even suggest that veganism for young children is, in essence, a form of child abuse.

As with many controversies, there are valid concerns on both sides. For example, there have been documented cases of children failing to thrive, and even dying, on extreme vegan diets.[2] Cases have been cited of vitamin B_{12}, calcium, zinc, iron, and vitamin D deficiencies in vegan children. Inadequate intakes of omega-3 fatty acids, iodine, and riboflavin have also been reported. These nutrients are found primarily or almost exclusively in animal products, and deficiencies can have serious and lifelong consequences. For example, not all of the neurologic impairments caused by vitamin B_{12} deficiency can be reversed by timely B_{12} supplement intervention.[3] In addition, inadequate zinc, calcium, and vitamin D can result in impaired bone growth and strength, increased susceptibility to fracture,[4] and failure to reach peak bone mass.

However, most examples of nutrition-related illness or death in vegan children stem from lack of education, fanaticism, and/or extremism. A 6-week-old infant, weighing only 3.5 pounds (half the birth weight of a healthy, full-term newborn), died after being fed a vegan diet of mainly soy milk and apple juice.[2] Another example is discussed in a video news feature found at www.newsy.com/videos/mother-s-vegan-diet-blamed-for-baby-s-death/. Informed parents following responsible vegan diets are rarely involved in cases of child neglect, death, or malnutrition. Families must recognize that veganism is not a lifestyle one can safely undertake without a thorough education. Parents need to know the need for supplementation of those nutrients not provided in adequate amounts on a plant-based diet, including calcium, zinc, and vitamins B_{12} and D. They also must recognize how difficult it is for a young child to maintain normal iron status without including sources of heme iron, which are totally absent in a vegan diet. Parents also need to understand that typical vegan diets are high in fiber and low in fat and that this combination can lead to inappropriately low weight gain and impaired growth in very young

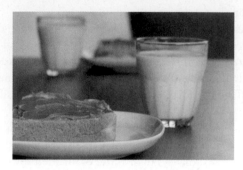

Most nutrition experts recommend a more moderate diet—one that includes fish, dairy products, and eggs—rather than a vegan diet for young children. This snack of peanut butter sandwiches and milk is a healthful choice.

children. Moreover, certain staples of the vegan diet, such as wheat, soy, and nuts, commonly provoke allergic reactions in children; when this happens, finding a plant-based substitute that contains adequate nutrients can be challenging.

On the other hand, both the American Dietetic Association and the American Academy of Pediatrics have stated that a vegan diet can promote normal growth and development—*provided* that adequate supplements and/or fortified foods are consumed to account for the nutrients that are normally found in animal products. However, most healthcare organizations stop short of outright endorsement of a vegan diet for young children. Instead, many advocate a more moderate approach during the early childhood years. Reasons for this level of caution include several factors:

- Some vegan parents are not adequately educated on the planning of meals and the inclusion of supplements to ensure adequate levels of all nutrients.

- Most young children are picky eaters and are hesitant to eat certain food groups, particularly vegetables.

- The high fiber content of vegan diets may not be appropriate for very young children.

- Young children have small stomachs and are often not able to consume enough plant-based foods to ensure adequate intakes of all nutrients and energy.

Because of these concerns, most nutrition experts advise parents to take a more moderate dietary approach, one that emphasizes plant foods but also includes some animal-based foods, such as fish, dairy, and/or eggs. Once children reach school age, the benefits of a well-planned vegan diet (low fat, abundant fiber, antioxidant rich) will promote good health as they progress into adulthood.

References

1. Craig, W. J. 2009. Health effects of vegan diets. *Am. J. Clin. Nutr.* 89(suppl.):1627S–1633S.
2. Planck, N. 2007. Death by veganism. *The New York Times,* May 21. www.nytimes.com/2007/05/21/opinion/21planck.html?pagewanted. (Accessed July 2012.)
3. Benton, D. 2012. Vitamins and cognitive development and performance—vitamins and neural and cognitive development outcomes in children. *Proc. Nutr. Soc.* 71:14–26.
4. Bachmann, M., M. S. Gaston, and F. Hefti. 2011. Supracondylar stress fracture of the femur in a child. *J. Pediatric Orthopaedics B.* 20:70–73.

Activity-based interactive DVD games can be an excellent option for children who must remain indoors for extended periods of time.

What Are a Child's Nutrient Needs?

Three-year-olds have the same set of nutrient recommendations that apply to toddlers (see Table 17.1). From age 4 through 8, the values for most nutrients increase. Until age 9, the nutrient needs of young boys do not differ significantly from those of girls; because of this, the DRI values for macronutrients, fiber, and micronutrients are grouped together for boys and girls aged 4 to 8 years. The onset of sexual maturation, however, has a dramatic effect on the nutrient needs of children. Boys' and girls' bodies develop differently in response to gender-specific hormones. Because the process of sexual maturation begins subtly between the ages of 8 and 9, the DRI values are separately defined for boys and girls beginning at age 9[1,5–7] (see Table 17.1).

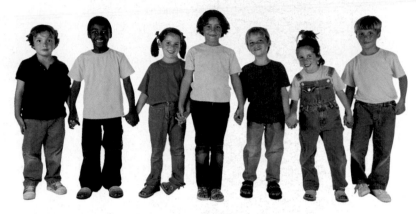

School-age children grow an average of 2 to 3 inches per year.

Energy and Macronutrient Recommendations for Children

Total energy requirements continue to increase throughout childhood because of increasing body size and, for some children, higher levels of physical activity. The EER varies according to a child's age, body weight, and level of activity.[1] Parents should provide diets that support normal growth and appropriate physical activity while minimizing risk for excess weight gain.

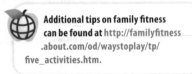

Additional tips on family fitness can be found at http://familyfitness .about.com/od/waystoplay/tp/ five_activities.htm.

Fat   Although dietary fat remains a key macronutrient in the preschool years, as a child ages, total fat should gradually be reduced to a level closer to that of an adult, around 25% to 35% of total energy.[1] One easy way to start reducing dietary fat is to limit intake of fried foods, high-fat protein sources such as hot dogs, baked goods, and high-fat snacks. This is also a good time to transition to lower-fat dairy products, such as 2% or 1% milk, low-fat yogurt, and low-fat mozzarella cheese sticks. A diet providing fewer than 25% of Calories from fat is not recommended for children, as they are still growing, developing, and maturing. In fact, unless a child is overweight or has specific health concerns, parents should avoid putting too much emphasis on fat restriction during this age span. Impressionable and peer-influenced children may be prone to categorizing foods as "good" or "bad." This may lead to skewed views of food and inappropriate dietary restrictions.

Carbohydrate   The RDA for carbohydrate for children is 130 g/day, which is about 45% to 65% of total daily energy intake.[1] Complex carbohydrates from whole grains, fruits, vegetables, and legumes should be emphasized. Simple sugars should come from fruits and 100% fruit juices, with foods high in refined sugars, such as such as cakes, cookies, and candies, saved for occasional indulgences. The AI for fiber for children is 14 g/1,000 kcal, which can be met by the consumption of fresh fruits, vegetables, legumes, and whole grains.[1] As is the case with toddlers, too much fiber can be detrimental, because it can make a child feel full and can interfere with adequate food intake and lower the absorption of certain nutrients, such as iron and zinc.

Protein   Total need for protein (shown in Table 17.1) increases for children because of their larger size, even though their growth rate has slowed. The RDA for protein is 0.95 g/kg body weight per day.[1] This protein requirement is easily met by portions such as one chicken drumstick and two glasses of milk or ½ cup of pinto beans, 1 oz of cheese, and half a peanut butter sandwich. Lean meats, fish, poultry, lower-fat dairy products, soy-based foods, and legumes are nutritious sources of protein that can be provided to children of all ages.

Children who follow a vegetarian diet can meet their protein needs by following dietary guidelines such as those illustrated by the Power Plate graphic, which can be found at http:// pcrm.org/health/diets/pplate/ power-sources.

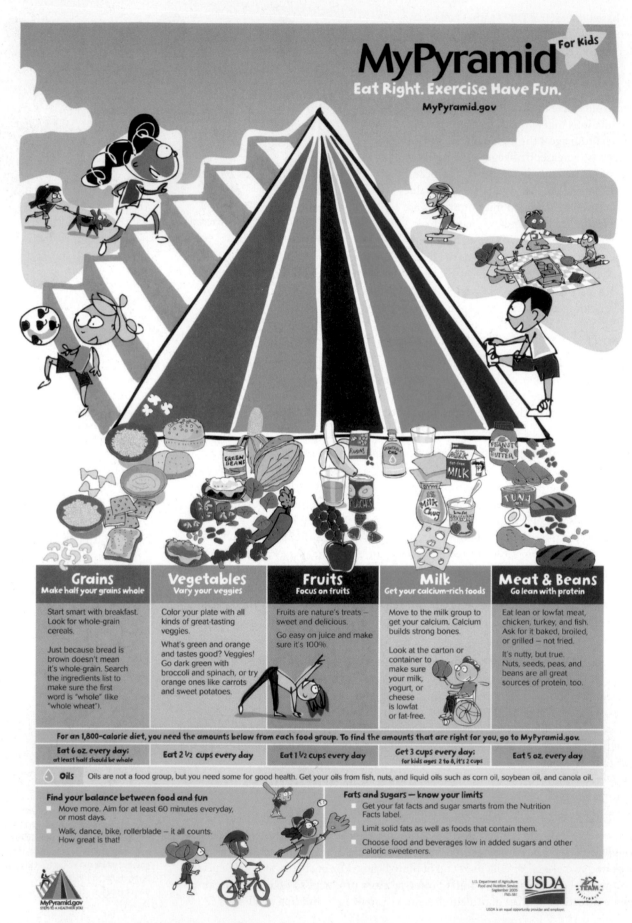

FIGURE 17.3 MyPyramid for Kids. This graphic tool depicts the nutrition needs for children and encourages them to "Eat Right. Exercise. Have Fun." (*Source*: Figure from the United States Department of Agriculture.)

Micronutrient Recommendations for Children

The need for most micronutrients increases slightly for children up to age 8 because of their increasing size. A sharper increase occurs during the transition years approaching adolescence; this increase is due to the impending adolescent growth spurt and the early phases of sexual maturation. Children who fail to consume the recommended amount of fruits and vegetables each day may become deficient in vitamins A, C, and E. Offering fruits and fresh vegetables as snacks as well as during mealtimes can increase intakes of these vitamins as well as fiber and potassium, two priority nutrients found lacking in the diets of low-income children.

The RDA for calcium is 1,000 mg/day for children aged 4 to 8 years and 1,300 mg/day for children aged 9 to 13 years.[5] Because peak bone mass is achieved in the late teens or early twenties, childhood and adolescence are critical times to ensure adequate deposition of bone tissue. Inadequate calcium intake during childhood and adolescence leads to poor bone health and potentially osteoporosis in later years. Milk, yogurt, cheese, fortified milk alternatives, and fortified fruit juices are child-friendly and convenient sources of calcium. The problem of "milk displacement," when children stop drinking milk in favor of soda, punch, energy drinks, and fruit drinks, is a recognized factor in low calcium intake.[9] Diets that are low in calcium also tend to be low in other nutrients, such as protein vitamin D and magnesium, so attention to calcium intake can help ensure a more healthful overall diet for children.

The RDAs for children aged 4 to 8 years for iron and zinc increase slightly to 10 mg/day and 5 mg/day, respectively.[6] The RDA for iron drops to 8 mg/day for boys and girls aged 9 to 13 years. These recommendations are based on the assumption that most girls do not begin menstruation until after age 13.[6] Mild-flavored, tender cuts of meat and poultry are readily accepted by most children, and legumes offer a fiber-rich, fat-free alternative that will also add iron and zinc to the diet. Refer again to Table 17.1 for a review of the micronutrient needs of children.

If there is any concern that a child's nutrient needs are not being met for any reason, such as missed meals or inadequate family resources, vitamin and mineral supplements may help correct any deficit. If used, the supplement should be age-specific, and the recommended dose (not more than 100% DV) should not be exceeded.[4]

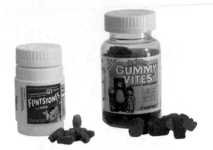

Children's multivitamins often appear in shapes or bright colors.

Fluid Recommendations for Children

The fluid recommendations for children are summarized in Table 17.1 and average about 5 to 8 cups of beverages per day, including water.[7] The exact amount of fluid needed varies according to the child's level of physical activity and weather conditions. At this point in their lives, children are mostly in control of their own fluid intake. However, as they become more active during school, in sports, and while playing, young children in particular may need reminders to drink in order to stay properly hydrated, especially if the weather is hot. Most, if not all, of the beverages offered should be free of caffeine and added sugars.

Encouraging Nutritious Food Choices in Children

Peer pressure can be extremely difficult for both parents and their children to deal with during this stage of life. Most children want to feel that they "belong" and will mirror the actions of children they view as popular. Some children have their own spending money, and most are very susceptible to TV and other messages encouraging unhealthful food choices. Children also spend more time visiting friends and eating more meals and snacks without their parents' supervision. The impact of this increasing autonomy on the health of children can be profound, yet parents remain important role models.[10]

Parents and children can work together to find compromises by planning and talking about healthful foods. Families who plan, prepare, and eat meals together are more

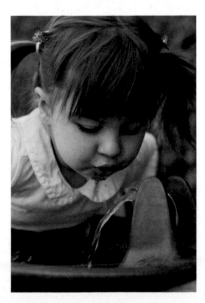

Fluid intake is important for young children, who may become so involved in their play that they ignore the sensation of thirst.

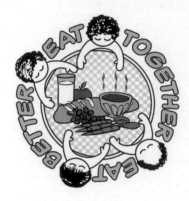

FIGURE 17.4 "Eat Better, Eat Together" promotes family mealtimes as a way to improve children's diets. (*Source*: Figure from Washington State University Extension.)

successful at promoting good food choices. The "Eat Better, Eat Together" nutrition education program promotes family mealtime (**Figure 17.4**). Parents should continue to demonstrate healthy eating and physical activity patterns to maintain a consistent message to their children.

What Is the Effect of School Attendance on Nutrition?

School attendance can affect a child's nutrition in several ways. First, hectic schedules and long bus or car rides cause many children to minimize or skip breakfast completely. School-age children who don't eat breakfast may not get a chance to eat until lunch. If the entire morning is spent in a state of hunger, children are more likely to do poorly on schoolwork, have decreased attention spans, and have more behavioral problems than their peers who do eat breakfast. For this reason, many schools offer low/no-cost school breakfasts, and many offer "in-class breakfast," which is free to all students, removing any stigma previously associated with cafeteria-based breakfast programs. These breakfasts help children optimize their nutrient intake, avoid the behavioral and learning problems associated with hunger in the classroom, and have the potential to improve math and reading achievement, particularly among low-performing students.[11]

Another consequence of attending school is that, with no one monitoring what they eat, children do not always consume adequate amounts of food. If they buy a school lunch, they might not like the foods being served, or their peers might influence them to skip certain foods. Even nutritious homemade lunches may be left uneaten or traded for less nutritious fare. Many children rush through lunch in order to spend more time on the playground; as a result, some schools send students to the playground first, allowing the children time to burn off their pent-up energy as well as build their hunger and thirst.

Finally, some schools continue to accept revenues from food companies in exchange for the right to advertise and sell their products to children. Although increasing numbers of states and school districts are strictly limiting sales of foods low in nutrient value during the school day, some schools still provide vending machines filled with snacks that are high in empty Calories.

Do School Lunches Improve Child Health and Nutrition?

The impact of the National School Lunch Program (NSLP) on children's diets is enormous: 99% of public schools participate, serving over 32 million children.[12] On the surface, it would appear that school lunches are expected to improve children's diets, because they must meet the nutritional standards of the newly implemented Healthy, Hunger-Free Kids Act:

- Students must be offered both fruits and vegetables every day.
- Milk must be fat-free or low-fat.
- Offerings of whole-grain-rich foods must be substantially increased and, by July 2014, all grains must be whole-grain-rich.
- Calories, averaged over a week, and portion sizes must be appropriate for the age of the children being served.
- Sodium, saturated fats, and *trans* fats must be reduced to specified levels.[13]

These guidelines also apply to the School Breakfast Program. In addition, vending machines and other sources of food on school campuses must meet specific nutrient guidelines. Finally, those schools that are able to improve their meals get additional federal funding.

While these new regulations represent the first major enhancement of nutritional standards in over 15 years, some caution remains. The actual amount of nutrients a student *gets* depends on what the student actually *eats*. So a child might eat a slice of whole-wheat

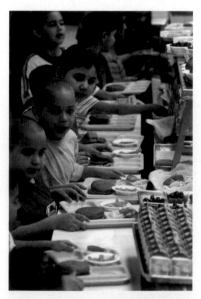

School-age children may receive a standard school lunch, but many choose less healthful foods when given the opportunity.

cheese pizza and low-fat milk but skip an apple and carrot sticks. Keep in mind also that children can still bring high-fat and high-sugar snacks and beverages from home or trade with classmates who bring them.

The good news is that many schools are working to ensure a more healthful food environment. Most states have adopted policies that restrict the types of competitive (non-NSLP) foods and beverages that can be sold on school campuses. School districts are required to develop wellness policies that address nutrition. Increased attention to nutrition has resulted in the offering of healthful options such as salad bars, fresh fruit bowls, baked potato bars, and soup stations to entice students into more healthful choices. Many schools now cultivate a garden on school grounds or even on the school rooftop where children help grow the vegetables that will be used in their lunches. The US Department of Agriculture has developed several programs to encourage children to adopt healthy lifestyles, for example by providing children with less common fruits and vegetables they might not otherwise have had the chance to try.

As nutritionists, school foodservice directors, educators, and parents continue to work together to improve the school meal programs, efforts will focus on increasing the use and consumption of fruits, vegetables, and whole grains in order to meet the nutrient needs of the children while minimizing risk for hunger and obesity.[14]

Nutrition MILESTONE

In **1853**, the Children's Aid Society of New York began serving meals to students attending its vocational school. It took another 50 years, however, for the idea to gain acceptance with other charitable groups. In 1894, *penny lunches* were begun in one Philadelphia school and the practice quickly spread to eight others. By 1910, Boston, Cleveland, St. Louis, Cincinnati, Chicago, and Milwaukee were offering meals to elementary and high school students. By the 1920s, many boards of education had recognized their responsibility to feed children, "train them in sane habits of eating, and teach them to choose wisely what food they buy." During the Great Depression in the 1930s, the number of hungry and malnourished children exploded, and many school lunch programs were funded by state and city governments.

It wasn't until 1946 that President Harry Truman initiated the National School Lunch Program, prompted in part by the large numbers of young men reporting for World War II military duty in a malnourished state. The federal legislation served multiple purposes: to ensure national security, to safeguard the health and well-being of the nation's children, and to encourage the domestic consumption of nutritious agricultural commodities and other food. In 1966, President Lyndon Johnson expanded the initiative by including more options for school breakfast programs, followed in 1968 by a further expansion into a Summer Meals Program. From its modest beginnings as a community-based charitable effort, the Federal School Lunch and Breakfast Program currently serves 32 million meals per year, two-thirds of which are free or reduced-price.

Nutrition-Related Concerns During Childhood

In addition to potential nutrient deficiencies that have already been discussed, new concerns arise during childhood. The issue of childhood obesity is discussed in more detail at the end of this chapter.

Iron-Deficiency Anemia

Despite the best efforts of public health nutritionists and other healthcare providers, iron-deficiency anemia remains a significant problem for many children. Rates of iron-deficiency anemia are higher among children from Mexican American and low-income families, emphasizing the need to evaluate each child in light of his or her family's unique risk factors. Meat, fish, and poultry provide well-absorbed sources of heme iron, and child-friendly foods such as iron-fortified cereals, dried fruits, and legumes can provide additional iron. Children who have very poor appetites or erratic eating habits may need to use an iron-containing supplement, although parents must provide careful supervision because of iron's high potential for childhood toxicity.

If left untreated, iron deficiency with or without anemia can lead to behavioral, cognitive, and motor deficits, developmental delays, and impaired immune response. In those children exposed to lead, iron deficiency increases the rate of lead absorption and severity of lead toxicity.[2] Iron-deficiency anemia reduces a child's energy level and contributes to passivity and lethargy. The cognitive and behavioral consequences of iron deficiency in

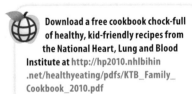

Download a free cookbook chock-full of healthy, kid-friendly recipes from the National Heart, Lung and Blood Institute at http://hp2010.nhlbihin .net/healthyeating/pdfs/KTB_Family_ Cookbook_2010.pdf

young children can be long-standing, making prevention a critical goal. Early detection through dietary assessments and simple blood tests, followed by effective treatment, ensures all children will enter school healthy and ready to learn.

Dental Caries

Dental caries, or cavities, occur when bacteria in the mouth feed on carbohydrates deposited on teeth. As a result of metabolizing the carbohydrates, the bacteria secrete acid that begins to erode tooth enamel, leading to tooth decay. The occurrence of dental caries can be minimized by limiting between-meal sweets, especially jelly beans, caramels, and others that stick to teeth. Frequent brushing helps eliminate the sugars on teeth, as well as the bacteria that feed on them.

Fluoride, either through a municipal water supply or through supplements, will also help deter the development of dental caries. Because "baby teeth" make room for and guide the permanent teeth into position, preschoolers need regular dental care as much as older children do. Children should start having regular dental visits at the age of 3 years.

Body-Image Concerns

As children approach puberty, appearance and body image play increasingly important roles in food choices by both girls and boys. These concerns are not necessarily detrimental to health, particularly if they result in children making more healthful food choices, such as eating more whole grains, fruits, and vegetables. However, it is important for children to understand that being thin does not guarantee health, popularity, or happiness and that a healthy body image includes accepting our own individual body type and recognizing that we can be physically fit and healthy at a variety of weights, shapes, and sizes (**Figure 17.5**). Excessive concern with thinness can lead children to experiment with fad diets, food restriction, and other behaviors that can result in under nutrition and perhaps even trigger a clinical eating disorder.

Childhood Food Insecurity

Although most children in the United States grow up with an abundant and healthful supply of food, millions of American children are faced with food insecurity and hunger. Food insecurity occurs when a household is not able to ensure a consistent, dependable supply of safe and nutritious food.[15] Approximately 21% of U.S. households with children can be classified as food insecure, with much higher rates among low-income households with children (47%), low-income female-headed households (50%), and those with "complex living arrangements" (53%). These statistics are definitely at odds with America's image as "the land of plenty."

The effects of food insecurity and hunger can be very harmful to children.[15] Without an adequate breakfast, they will not be able to concentrate or pay attention to their parents, teachers, or other caretakers. Impaired nutrient status can blunt children's immune responses, making them more susceptible to common childhood illnesses. Increased rates of hospitalizations have been linked to food insecurity. Children's psychosocial health is also impacted by food insecurity: rates of anxiety and suicide are associated with food insecurity. Finally, maternal depression is more common within food-insecure households, creating an environment that often leads to poor mental health outcomes in the child.

Options for families facing food insecurity include a number of government and privately funded programs, including school breakfast and lunch programs and the Supplementary Nutrition Assistance Program (previously termed the Food Stamp program). Families who face economic difficulties should be referred to public health or social service agencies and encouraged to apply for available nutrition benefits. Private and faith-based food pantries and kitchens can provide a narrow range of foods for a limited period of time but cannot be relied on to meet the nutritional needs of children and their families over an extended period of time.

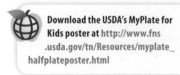

Download the USDA's MyPlate for Kids poster at http://www.fns .usda.gov/tn/Resources/myplate_ halfplateposter.html

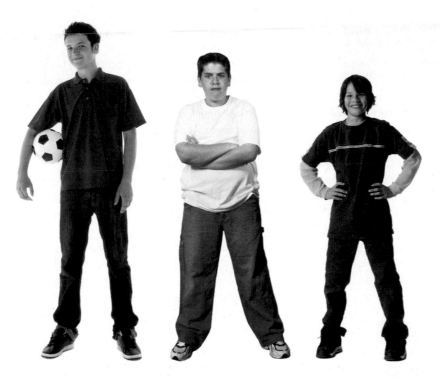

FIGURE 17.5 Normal, healthy school-age children come in a variety of shapes and sizes.

RECAP

Children have a slower growth rate than toddlers, yet their larger body size and greater level of physical activity increase their total energy and nutrient needs. Children need a lower percentage of energy from fat than toddlers but slightly more than adults. Among highly active children, fluid intake should be monitored and encouraged.

Peer pressure has a strong influence on nutritional choices in school-age children, but parents can encourage healthful eating and act as role models. Calcium needs increase as children mature but intake often declines. Iron deficiency is a common problem and can lead to severe behavioral, learning, and motor deficits. School lunch programs are designed to improve children's nutrient intake, but not all children take full advantage of the programs. Body-image concerns arise in both boys and girls as they approach the adolescent years. Families facing economic challenges can be assisted by a number of government and privately funded programs. ■

Nutrition for Adolescents

The adolescent years are typically defined as beginning with the onset of **puberty,** the period in life in which secondary sexual characteristics develop and there is the capacity for reproducing. Adolescence continues through age 18.

Adolescent Psychosocial Development

Adolescence is a period when emotions and behaviors often seem unpredictable and confusing. It is characterized by increasing independence as the adolescent establishes a personal sense of identity and works toward greater self-reliance. Adolescents may, for example, decide to follow a vegetarian or vegan diet as a means of setting themselves apart

puberty The period in life in which secondary sexual characteristics develop and the body becomes biologically capable of reproduction.

Hannah

Nutri-Case

"When I was a kid, I always dreaded gym class, especially games with teams. Three of us who were overweight always got picked last for every sport. What made it even worse was hearing my teammates complain about having me on their team. The summer before I started middle school, I wanted to lose weight so bad that I just plain stopped eating. My mom had to leave early to work at the hospital and didn't get home until evening, so I'd tell her I'd been eating all day and wasn't hungry for dinner. But one rainy Saturday morning my mom went out to run some errands and I was home alone with nothing to do, and without even thinking about it, I opened the fridge and saw half of a pizza from the night before. I ate a slice. It tasted so good! Then I ate another slice, and another, until it was gone, and then I started in on some cookies. I would have finished those, too, if my mom hadn't come home. She was pretty upset about me eating all the leftover pizza, so I told her how hungry I was because I'd been fasting all week, and she started to cry. She said she'd gone through the same teasing when she was a kid. After that we both tried to eat better for a while, but it didn't last. So I'm glad I'm taking a nutrition course, because now I know how to make better choices to get down to a weight that's right for me. And maybe I can use what I've learned to help my mom!"

Given what you know about Hannah and her mother, why do you think their initial attempts "to eat better" didn't last? What advice would you give her about talking with her mom about nutrition? Have you shared anything you've learned in this course with family members? If so, how did they respond to the information?

from the family unit. Whereas younger adolescents tend to be self-centered, living for the present, older teens typically focus on defining their role in life. All teens deal with their emerging sexuality, and many experiment with risky lifestyle choices—such as drugs, alcohol, or cigarettes—that lie outside their traditional cultural or social boundaries. During this developmental phase, they may be unresponsive to parental guidance and ignore attempts to improve their diet and activity patterns. Most adolescents, however, successfully navigate the many challenges of this life stage and mature into emotionally stable, self-reliant, productive adults.

Adolescent Growth and Activity Patterns

Growth during adolescence is primarily driven by hormonal changes, including increased levels of testosterone for boys and estrogen for girls. Both boys and girls experience growth spurts, or periods of accelerated growth, during later childhood and adolescence. Growth spurts for girls tend to begin around 10 to 11 years of age, and growth spurts for boys begin around 12 to 13 years of age. These growth periods last about 2 years.

Adolescents experience an average 20% to 25% increase in height during the pubertal years. During an average 1-year spurt, girls tend to grow 3.5 inches and boys tend to grow 4 inches. The average girl reaches almost full height by the onset of menstruation (called **menarche**). Boys typically experience continual growth throughout adolescence, and some even grow slightly taller during early adulthood.

Skeletal growth ceases once closure of the *epiphyseal plates* occurs (**Figure 17.6**). The **epiphyseal plates** are plates of cartilage located toward the end of the long bones (that is,

menarche The onset of menstruation, or the menstrual period.

epiphyseal plates Plates of cartilage located toward the end of long bones that provide for growth in the length of long bones.

the bones of the arms and legs) that provide for growth in length. In some circumstances, such as malnutrition or use of anabolic steroids, the epiphyseal plates can close early in adolescents and result in a failure to reach full stature.

Weight and body composition also change dramatically during adolescence. Weight gain is extremely variable during this time and reflects the adolescent's energy intake, physical activity level, and genetics. The average weight gained by girls and boys during these years is 35 and 45 lb, respectively. The weight gained by girls and boys is dramatically different in terms of its composition. Girls tend to gain significantly more body fat than boys, with this fat accumulating around the buttocks, hips, breasts, thighs, and upper arms. Although many girls are uncomfortable or embarrassed by these changes, they are a natural result of maturation. Boys gain significantly more muscle mass than girls, and they experience an increase in muscle definition. Other changes that occur with sexual maturation include a deepening of the voice in boys and the growth of pubic hair in both boys and girls.

The physical activity levels of adolescents are highly variable. Many are physically active in sports, dance, or other organized activities, whereas others become more interested in intellectual or artistic pursuits. This variability in activity levels of adolescents results in highly individual energy needs. Although the rapid growth and sexual maturation that occur during puberty require a significant amount of energy, adolescence is often a time in which overweight begins.

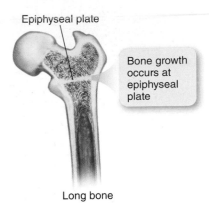

Epiphyseal plate

Bone growth occurs at epiphyseal plate

Long bone

FIGURE 17.6 Skeletal growth ceases once closure of the epiphyseal plates occurs.

What Are an Adolescent's Nutrient Needs?

The nutrient needs of adolescents are influenced by rapid growth, weight gain, and sexual maturation, in addition to the demands of physical activity.

Energy and Macronutrient Recommendations for Adolescents

Adequate energy intake is necessary to maintain adolescents' health, support their dramatic growth and maturation, and fuel their physical activity. Because of these competing demands, the energy needs of adolescents can be quite high. To calculate the EER for this life stage, you must know the person's age, physical activity level, weight, and height.[1]

As with the younger age groups, there is no DRI for fat for adolescents.[1] However, adolescents are at risk for the same chronic diseases as adults, including type 2 diabetes, obesity, coronary heart disease, and various cancers. Thus, it is prudent for adolescents to consume 25% to 35% of total energy from fat and to consume no more than 10% of total energy from saturated fat sources.

The RDA for carbohydrate for adolescents is 130 g/day.[1] As with adults, this amount of carbohydrate covers what is needed to supply adequate glucose to the brain, but it does not cover the amount of carbohydrate needed to support daily activities. Thus, it is recommended that adolescents consume more than the RDA, or about 45% to 65% of their total energy as carbohydrate, and most carbohydrate should come from complex carbohydrate sources. The AI for fiber for adolescent girls is 26 g/day and for adolescent boys is 38 g/day. These levels are virtually the same as for adult women and men.

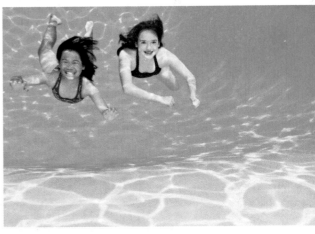

Because of rapid growth and the active lifestyle of many adolescents, their energy needs can be quite high.

The RDA for protein for adolescents, at 0.85 g protein per kilogram of body weight per day, is similar to that of adults, which is 0.80 g per kilogram body weight.[1] This amount is assumed to be sufficient to support health and to cover the additional needs of growth and development during the adolescent stage. As with adults, most U.S. adolescents consume protein in amounts that far exceed the RDA.

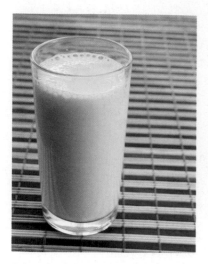

Adequate calcium intake during adolescence is necessary to achieve peak bone mass, in addition to other critical body and cell functions.

Micronutrient Recommendations for Adolescents

Micronutrients of particular concern for adolescents include calcium, iron, and vitamin A. Adequate calcium intake is critical to achieve peak bone density, and the RDA for calcium for adolescents 14–18 years of age is 1,300 mg/day.[4] This amount of calcium can be difficult for many adolescents to consume, because the quality of foods they select is often less than optimal to meet their nutrient needs. To achieve this level of calcium intake, adolescents need to eat at least 4 servings of dairy foods or calcium-fortified products daily. Green, leafy vegetables and legumes also provide calcium, although the per-serving amount and bioavailability may be lower than in dairy and calcium-fortified foods.

The iron needs of adolescents are relatively high; this is because iron is needed to replace the blood lost during menstruation in girls and to support the growth of muscle mass in boys. The RDA for iron for boys is 11 mg/day, and the RDA for girls is 15 mg/day.[5] If energy intake is adequate and adolescents consume heme-iron food sources, such as animal products, each day, they should be able to meet the RDA for iron. However, some young people adopt a vegetarian lifestyle during this life stage, or they consume foods that have limited nutrient density. Both of these situations can prevent adolescents from meeting the RDA for iron.

Vitamin A is critical to support the rapid growth and development that occurs during adolescence. The RDA for vitamin A is 900 µg per day for boys and 700 µg per day for girls,[5] which can be met by consuming 5 to 9 servings of fruits and vegetables each day. As with iron and calcium, meeting the RDA for vitamin A can be a challenging goal in this age group due to their potential to make less healthful food choices.

If an adolescent is unable or unwilling to eat adequate amounts of nutrient-dense foods, then a multivitamin and mineral supplement that provides no more than 100% of the Daily Value for the micronutrients can be beneficial as a safety net. As with younger children and adults, a supplement should not be considered a substitute for a balanced, healthful diet.

Fluid Recommendations for Adolescents

The fluid needs of adolescents are higher than those for children because of their higher physical activity levels and the extensive growth and development that occurs during this phase of life. The recommended daily fluid intakes for adolescents are summarized in Table 17.1 and average about 11 cups of beverages, including water, for boys and 10 cups for girls.[6] Boys are generally more active than girls and have more lean tissue; thus, they require a higher fluid intake to maintain fluid balance. Very active adolescents who are exercising in the heat may have higher fluid needs than the AI, and these individuals should be encouraged to drink often to quench their thirst and avoid dehydration.

Encouraging Nutritious Food Choices with Adolescents

Adolescents make many of their own food choices and buy a significant amount of the foods they consume. Although parents can still be effective role models, adolescents are generally strongly influenced by their peers, mass media, personal preferences, and their own developing sense of what foods make up an adequate diet.

Areas of particular concern in the adolescent diet are the lack of vegetables, fruits, and whole grains. Many teens eat on the run, skip meals, and select fast foods and convenience foods, because they are inexpensive and accessible, and taste good. Parents, caretakers, and school foodservice programs can capitalize on adolescents' preferences for pizza, burgers, spaghetti, and sandwiches by providing more healthful meat and cheese alternatives, whole-grain breads, and plenty of appealing vegetable-based side-dishes. In addition, keeping healthful snacks, such as fruits and vegetables, that are already cleaned and prepared in

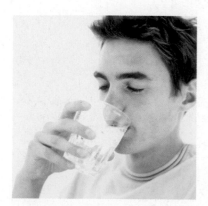

Adolescents have higher fluid needs than younger children.

easy-to-eat pieces may encourage adolescents to consume more of these foods as between-meal snacks. Teens should also be encouraged to consume adequate milk and other calcium-enriched beverages.

Many teens move out of their family home when they attend college or get their first full-time job. The **Highlight** feature box **On Your Own: Stocking Your First Kitchen** (page 708) identifies staples to keep on hand for healthful snacks and meals.

Nutrition-Related Concerns for Adolescents

Nutrition-related concerns for adolescents include bone density and body-image issues, as well as the health of their skin and hair. Additional concerns include cigarette smoking and the use of alcohol and illegal drugs.

Bone Density Watch

Early adolescence, 13 to 15 years of age, is a crucial time for ensuring adequate dietary calcium in order to maximize bone calcium uptake and bone mineral density over the next several years.[5] Achieving and maintaining optimal bone density during adolescence and into young adulthood is critical for delaying or preventing the onset of osteoporosis.

As previously noted, meeting the adolescent RDA for calcium (1,300 mg/day) is challenging.[16] Historically, one of the most reliable sources of calcium in the US diet has been dairy foods, yet by age 18, average fluid milk consumption has fallen by more than 25% compared to intake at age 8 years, whereas soda intake has tripled. Although not the only factor, milk consumption during adolescence is strongly linked to higher bone mineral content and lower risk for adult bone fractures.[16] A national "Milk Matters" campaign, coordinated by the National Institute of Child Health and Human Development in conjunction with the US Department of Health and Human Services, distributes teen-friendly materials to encourage greater intakes of milk and other dairy foods (**Figure 17.7**). Campaign materials are available free of charge from its website (see the Web Links at the end of this chapter).

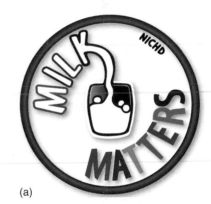

(a)

Disordered Eating and Eating Disorders

An initially healthful concern about body image and weight can turn into a dangerous obsession during this emotionally challenging life stage. Clinical eating disorders frequently begin during adolescence and can occur in boys as well as girls. Warning signs include rapid and excessive weight loss, a preoccupation with weight and body image, habitual bathroom visits after meals, and signs of frequent vomiting or laxative use. (Disordered eating is discussed In Depth on pages 548–559.)

Adolescent Acne and Diet

Acne flare-ups plague many adolescents. Acne is an inflammation of the sebaceous (oil) glands associated with hair follicles. These glands produce an oily secretion, called *sebum*, that normally flows out onto the skin surface, keeping skin soft and moist and repelling microbes. In acne, excessive sebum collects in and plugs up hair follicles. "Blackheads" occur when follicles are exposed to air, and the top layer of sebum oxidizes. They are not caused by dirt! "Whiteheads" are collections of sebum in follicles not exposed to air.

The hormonal changes that occur during puberty are largely responsible for the sudden appearance of acne in many adolescents. Emotional stress, genetic factors, and personal hygiene are most likely secondary contributors. But what about foods? For decades, chocolate, fried foods, fatty foods, sweets, and other foods have been wrongfully linked to acne; it is now believed that individual foods play virtually no role in its development. On

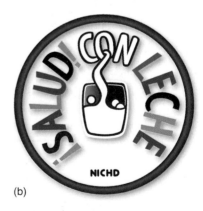

(b)

FIGURE 17.7 Milk Matters/Salud con Leche. These logos are part of a new government program to encourage milk consumption in children and adolescents. They are provided **(a)** in English and **(b)** in Spanish. (*Source:* "Milk Matters" and "Salud Con Leche" from National Institute of Child Health and Human Development website.)

On Your Own: Stocking Your First Kitchen

HIGHLIGHT

Many teens move out of the house around age 18 or 19 and settle into apartments, college or university housing, or shared housing. One question teens often have is how to stock their first kitchen. What basic foods—or staples—do they need to always have on hand, so that they can quickly and easily assemble healthful meals and snacks? The following checklist includes the foods that many Americans consider staples. It can be modified to include items that are staples in non-Western cultures and to address vegetarian, vegan, low-fat, low-sodium, and other diets. By stocking healthful foods like the ones listed here, you'll be much more likely to make healthful food choices every day!

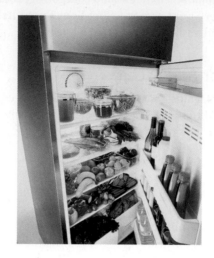

Keep your refrigerator stocked with the following:

Low-fat or skim milk and/or soy milk
Calcium-enriched orange juice
Hard cheeses
Eggs
Lean deli meats
Tofu
Hummus, peanut butter, low-fat cream cheese, and/or other perishable spreads
Two- to 3-day supply of dark-green lettuce and other salad fixings or ready-to-eat salads
Two- to 3-day supply of other veggies
Two- to 3-day supply of fresh fruits
Low-fat salad dressings, mustards, salsas, and so forth
Whole-grain breads, rolls, bagels, pizza crusts
Tortillas: corn, whole-wheat flour; whole-wheat pita bread

Stock your freezer with the following:

Individual portions of chicken breast, extra-lean ground beef, pork loin chops, fish fillets, veggie (black bean) "burgers" or soy alternatives

Lower-fat frozen entrées ("boost" with salad, whole-grain roll, and extra veggies)
Frozen veggies (no sauce)
Frozen cheese or veggie pizza ("boost" with added mushrooms, green peppers, and so forth)
Low-fat ice cream, sherbet, or sorbet

Stock your kitchen cupboards with the following:

Potatoes, sweet potatoes, onions, garlic, and so forth, as desired
Canned or vacuum-packed tuna, salmon, crab (in water, not oil)
Canned low/no-sodium veggies: corn, tomatoes, mushrooms, and so forth
Canned low/no-sodium legumes: black beans, refried beans, pinto/kidney beans, garbanzo beans
Canned soups that are low in sodium and fat and high in fiber—read the Nutrition Facts Panels
Dried beans and/or lentils, if desired
Pasta and rice, preferably whole-grain; barley, couscous, tabouli
Bottled tomato-based pasta sauces
Canned fruit in juice
Dried fruits, including golden raisins, dried cranberries, apricots, cherries, plums (prunes)
Nuts, including peanuts, almonds, walnuts, and so forth
Whole-grain ready-to-eat cereals for breakfast and snacking; whole-grain cooked cereals, such as oatmeal
Whole-grain, lower-fat crackers
Pretzels, low-fat tortilla/corn chips, low/no-fat microwave popcorn
Salt, pepper, balsamic vinegar, soy sauce, other condiments and spices as desired
Olive oil, canola oil, and so forth, as desired

the other hand, a healthful diet, rich in fruits, vegetables, whole grains, and lean meats, can provide vitamin A, vitamin C, zinc, and other nutrients to optimize skin health and maintain an effective immune system. In addition, this dietary pattern can be described as having a low glycemic load, which has been linked to a reduced occurrence and severity of adolescent acne.[17]

Prescription medications, including the vitamin A derivative 13-*cis*-retinoic acid (Accutane), effectively control severe forms of acne. Neither Accutane nor any other prescription vitamin A derivative should be used by women who are pregnant, are planning a pregnancy, or may become pregnant. Accutane is a known *teratogen*, causing severe fetal malformations. The teratogenic effect is so severe that the FDA now requires all women of childbearing age who use Accutane to register in a risk management program, iPLEDGE, to ensure that pregnancies do not occur while under treatment. Incidentally, vitamin A taken in supplement form is not effective in acne treatment and, due to its own risk for toxicity, should not be used in amounts that exceed 100% of the Daily Value.

Use of Tobacco, Alcohol, and Illegal Drugs

Adolescents are naturally curious, and many are open to experimenting with tobacco, alcohol, and illegal drugs. Cigarette smoking diminishes appetite and can interfere with nutrient metabolism. In fact, it is often used by adolescent girls to achieve or maintain a low body weight.[18] Other effects of smoking on young people include the following:

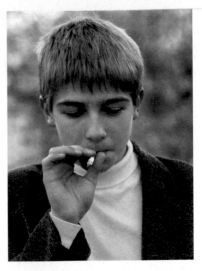

Cigarette smoking can interfere with nutrient metabolism.

- Addiction to nicotine and continuation as adult smoker
- Reduced rate of lung growth
- Impaired athletic performance and endurance
- Shortness of breath
- Early signs of heart disease and stroke
- Increased risk for lung cancer and other smoking-related cancers as adults

Among adolescents, smoking is also associated with an increased incidence of participation in other risky behaviors, such as abuse of alcohol and other drugs, fighting, and having unprotected sex. There is also a link between pediatric/adolescent smoking and early onset of depression and anxiety disorders.[19]

Alcohol and drug use can start at early ages, even in school-age children. The primary cause of death among high school–age youth is a motor vehicle accident; alcohol is a factor in 14% of deaths in motor vehicle accidents.[20] Alcohol can also interfere with proper nutrient absorption and metabolism, and it can take the place of foods in an adolescent's diet; these adverse effects of alcohol put adolescents at risk for various nutrient deficiencies. Alcohol consumption and use of many illegal drugs are also associated with "the munchies," a feeling of food craving that usually results in the intake of large quantities of high-fat, high-sugar, nutrient-poor foods. This behavior can result in overweight or obesity, and it increases the risk for nutrient imbalance. Teens who use drugs and alcohol are typically in poor physical condition, are either underweight or overweight, have poor appetites, and perform poorly in school.

RECAP

Adolescents experience rapid increases in height, weight, and lean body mass and fat mass. Adequate energy is needed to support growth, maturation, and physical activity. Fat intake should be 25% to 35% of total energy, and carbohydrate intake should be 45% to 65% of total energy intake. Calcium is needed to optimize bone growth and to achieve peak bone density, and iron needs are increased due to increased muscle mass in boys and to menstruation in girls. Adolescents' food choices are influenced by peer pressure and personal preferences. They may select fast foods and high-fat/high-energy snack foods in place of whole grains, fruits, and vegetables. Adolescents with lower levels of physical activity may therefore experience overweight for the first time during this period. Suboptimal bone density, disordered eating behaviors, acne, cigarette smoking, and use of alcohol and illegal drugs are also concerns for this age group. ■

Pediatric Obesity Watch: A Concern for Children and Adolescents

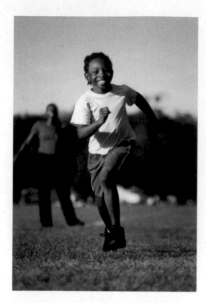

Active, healthy-weight children are less likely to become overweight adults.

Although the prevalence of obesity has stabilized for U.S. children and adolescents since 2007, rates remain unacceptably high.[21] Currently, about 12% of preschoolers are obese. Among older children the rate is even higher, with 18% of youth age 6 to 19 classified as obese. Using the Centers for Disease Control and Prevention (CDC) classification system, children are considered to be obese if their BMI is at or above the 95th percentile; that is, when when their BMI is higher than that of 95% of U.S. children of the same age and gender who made up the reference group at the time these charts were developed.[21]

We may feel shocked at the sight of an obese preschooler, but children's health experts point out that we should be more concerned by what we don't see. Even in early childhood, significant overweight can exacerbate asthma, cause sleep apnea, impair a child's mobility, and lead to intense teasing, low self-esteem, depression, and social isolation. Fatty liver is diagnosed in one-third of obese children, and increasing numbers of obese children are experiencing high blood lipids, high blood pressure, metabolic syndrome, skeletal disorders, and other medical problems.[21] Also, it's been estimated that about 70% of obese children maintain their higher weight as adults, making prevention of childhood overweight all the more important for long-term health and well-being.[22,23] Reversal of the epidemic of pediatric obesity can be accomplished only through an aggressive, comprehensive, nationwide health campaign.

The Seeds of Pediatric Obesity

The relatively recent surge in pediatric obesity results from a complex interaction among genetic, environmental, and sociocultural factors. A child's weight or BMI is closely related to parental weight or BMI: children with one overweight or obese parent are twice as likely to be overweight as those with no overweight or obese parent, while children in families where both those parents are overweight or obese are nearly four times as likely to be overweight. Some research suggests that, among boys, risk for overweight is more influenced by their father's weight status than their mother's.[24] Genetic risk factors, however, can be overcome: young adults who are physically active have a lower BMI than would be predicted by their genetic background.[25]

Lower parental education and income are associated with increased risk for pediatric obesity, as are environmental factors such as access to playgrounds, safe bicycle/walking paths, and grocery stores with a full range of healthful foods.[23] Cultural influences, particularly among recent immigrant families, may also exert a strong influence on risk for childhood obesity.

Believe it or not, overweight and obesity can occur as early as the toddler years, as can early signs of risk. Toddlers should not be denied nutritious food; however, parents and caretakers should not aggressively feed them or feed them out of habit. Nor should toddlers be encouraged to eat when they say or take actions that indicate they are full. In the toddler years, a child who is above the 80th percentile for weight should be monitored.

The preschool years are also an important time for parents to be watchful of actual or potential overweight and obesity. Preschoolers should be encouraged and supported in increasing their physical activity, and as for all children, foods with low nutrient density, such as sodas, cookies, and candies, should be limited. Parents should not be offended if the child's pediatrician, school nurse, or other healthcare provider expresses concern over the child's weight status; early intervention and the promotion of a healthy lifestyle are often the most effective measures against lifelong obesity. Not only are healthcare providers closely monitoring the weight status of children, but the National Heart, Lung, and Blood Institute recommends that *all* children undergo cholesterol screening between the ages of 9 and 11 years, with additional follow-up in late adolescence.[26]

Pediatric Obesity: Prevention Through a Healthful Diet

Nutrition and healthcare experts agree that the main contributors to childhood obesity are similar to those involved in adult obesity: eating and drinking too many Calories and moving around too little. Parental overweight, parental consumption of sugar-sweetened beverages, and other "obesogenic" behaviors certainly influence childhood obesity.[27] The introduction and retention of healthful eating habits are key interventions in the fight against pediatric obesity.

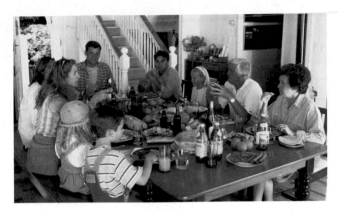

Parents should ensure that families take part in shared meals regularly.

The Role of the Family in Healthful Eating

Children typically mimic their parents, especially at the younger ages, so rather than singling out overweight children and placing them on restrictive diets, experts encourage family wide improvements in food choices, mealtime habits, and other behaviors.[28] Parents should encourage children to eat a healthful breakfast every morning, and sit down to a shared family meal each evening, as regularly as possible.

Parents should strive to provide consistently nutritious snacks, and retain control over the purchasing and preparation of foods until older children and teens are responsible and knowledgeable enough to make healthful decisions. Parents can keep a selection of fruits, vegetables, whole-grain products, and low-fat dairy foods readily available as healthful alternatives to high-fat, high-sugar snacks (positive parenting). For active children who frequently eat on the run, parents can keep a supply of nonperishable snacks, such as granola bars, dried fruits, and nuts, along with kid-friendly fruits, such as apples, bananas, and oranges, to grab as everyone dashes out the door. Mealtimes, especially dinner, should offer a colorful variety of foods, with the emphasis on green, yellow, orange, and red vegetables and deep-brown grains. If available foods are healthful, children can be free to choose among them and will gain confidence in their ability to make good food choices (self-efficacy).

Whenever possible, parents should minimize the number of meals eaten in restaurants, especially fast-food franchises. When families do eat out, parents should share large portion sizes and order grilled, broiled, or baked foods instead of fried foods and encourage other family members to do the same.

Many children and adolescents resent parental oversight and involvement in their weight-control program. Parents should not allow the dinner table or kitchen to turn into a war zone; instead, they should model healthful eating behaviors, provide a diverse array of healthful foods, and encourage healthful lifestyle choices, including physical activity. Even if a child's weight stabilizes rather than declines, parents should praise the absence of additional weight gain as a positive step.

The Role of the School in Healthful Eating

As previously noted, the National School Lunch Program is designed to limit the amount of fat, sugar, and sodium served to students. Several states now ban vending machines at elementary and middle schools; efforts at high schools have generally been less successful. Consistent and repeated school-based messages on good nutrition can reinforce the efforts of parents and healthcare providers.

Many schools have embraced "garden-based learning," an educational strategy aimed at improving student's learning and social skills, as well as their intakes of fresh produce.[29] Children are encouraged to apply what they have learned in math, science, health, geography, and other subjects. Several states have developed grade-specific curricula offering pre-planned lessons and activities designed to meet state education

Many schools take advantage of nutrition education programs offered through agencies such as state or county health departments, local Dairy Councils, and the Produce for Better Health Foundation, at www .fruitsandveggiesmorematters.org.

standards. Research has shown that children who are actively involved in growing fruits and vegetables are more likely to accept unfamiliar foods, increase their total fruit and vegetable consumption, and understand the links between dietary choices and health.[30]

Pediatric Obesity: Prevention Through an Active Lifestyle

Increased energy expenditure through increased physical activity is essential for successful weight management among children. The Institute of Medicine recommends that children participate in physical activity and exercise for at least an hour each day;[1] the 2008 Physical Activity Guidelines for Americans also advise bone- and muscle-strengthening activities at least 3 days each week.[31] For younger children, this can be divided into two or three shorter sessions, allowing them to regroup, recoup, and refocus between activity sessions. Older children should be able to be active for an hour without stopping. Obese children are more likely to engage in physical activities that are noncompetitive, fun, and structured in a way that allows them to proceed at their own pace. Children should be exposed to a variety of activities, so that they move different muscles, play at various intensities, avoid boredom, and find out what they like and don't like to do (**Table 17.2**).

TABLE 17.2 Examples of Physical Activities for Children and Adolescents

Type of Physical Activity	Age Group: Children	Age Group: Adolescents
Moderate-intensity aerobic	■ Active recreation, such as hiking, skateboarding, rollerblading ■ Bicycle riding ■ Brisk walking	■ Active recreation, such as canoeing, hiking, skateboarding, rollerblading ■ Brisk walking ■ Bicycle riding (stationary or road bike) ■ Housework and yard work, such as sweeping or pushing a lawn mower ■ Games that require catching and throwing, such as baseball and softball
Vigorous-intensity aerobic	■ Active games involving running and chasing, such as tag ■ Bicycle riding ■ Jumping rope ■ Martial arts, such as karate ■ Running ■ Sports such as soccer, ice or field hockey, basketball, swimming, tennis ■ Cross-country skiing	■ Active games involving running and chasing, such as flag football ■ Bicycle riding ■ Jumping rope ■ Martial arts, such as karate ■ Running ■ Sports such as soccer, ice or field hockey, basketball, swimming, tennis ■ Vigorous dancing ■ Cross-country skiing
Muscle-strengthening	■ Games such as tug-of-war ■ Modified push-ups (with knees on the floor) ■ Resistance exercises using body weight or resistance bands ■ Rope or tree climbing ■ Sit-ups (curl-ups or crunches) ■ Swinging on playground equipment/bars	■ Games such as tug-of-war ■ Push-ups and pull-ups ■ Resistance exercises with exercise bands, weight machines, hand-held weights ■ Climbing wall ■ Sit-ups (curl-ups or crunches)
Bone-strengthening	■ Games such as hopscotch ■ Hopping, skipping, jumping ■ Jumping rope ■ Running ■ Sports such as gymnastics, basketball, volleyball, tennis	■ Hopping, skipping, jumping ■ Jumping rope ■ Running ■ Sports such as gymnastics, basketball, volleyball, tennis

Note: Some activities, such as bicycling, can be moderate or vigorous intensity, depending upon level of effort.

Source: 2008 Physical Activity Guidelines for Americans, from U.S. Department of Health and Human Services.

Nutrition Myth OR Fact?

Is Breakfast the Most Important Meal of the Day?

What did you eat for breakfast this morning? Whole-grain cereal with low-fat milk? A strawberry Pop-Tart? Or nothing at all? Why does it matter, anyway? Sure, you've heard the saying that breakfast is the most important meal of the day, but that's just a myth—isn't it? As long as you eat a nutritious lunch and dinner, why should skipping breakfast matter?

Actually, decades-long research has clearly confirmed the importance of a healthful breakfast.[1,2] Most studies highlight one or more of three key health benefits: First, breakfast improves overall nutritional status. Second, it enhances academic performance and mental functioning. Third, it helps maintain a healthful weight. Let's examine the evidence for each of these claims.

The word *breakfast* was initially used as a verb meaning "to break the fast"—that is, to end the hours of fasting that naturally occur while we sleep. When we fast, our bodies break down stored nutrients to provide energy to fuel the resting body. First, cells break down glycogen stores in the liver and muscle tissues, using the newly released glucose for energy. These stores last about 12 hours. But people who skip breakfast typically go without food for much longer than that: if they finish dinner around 7:00 PM and don't eat again until noon the next day, they are fasting (going without fuel) for 17 hours! Long before this point, essentially all stored glycogen is used up, and the body has turned to fatty acids and amino acids as fuel sources.

If you're like most people, when your blood glucose is low, not only are you hungry but you also may feel weak, shaky, and irritable and have poor concentration. So it's not surprising that children and teens who skip breakfast don't function as well as their breakfast-eating peers: their physical, academic, and behavioral performances are all negatively affected. Recent research confirms the following conclusions:[1,2]

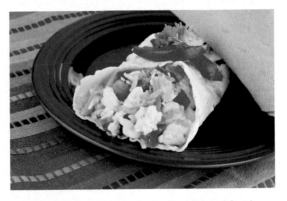

Breakfast doesn't have to be boring! A breakfast burrito with scrambled eggs, low-fat cheese, and vegetables wrapped in a whole-grain tortilla provides energy and nutrients to start your day off right.

- Skipping breakfast often leads to lower daily intakes of most vitamins and minerals and a higher consumption of fat. Nutrients such as calcium, fiber, vitamin D, protein, and iron that are not consumed during breakfast are not replaced at later meals.

- Missing breakfast and experiencing hunger impair students' ability to learn and overall cognitive performance. Exam scores are lower, memory recall is impaired, and reading, vocabulary, and math performance lags.

- Students who skip breakfast demonstrate reduced attention span, with more behavioral problems, than students who arrive at school in a well-nourished state.

- Breakfast decreases tardiness and improves school attendance.

- Consumption of a protein-rich or low glycemic index breakfast decreases subsequent caloric intake at lunch. Many studies report an association between breakfast consumption and lower body fat and/or body weight.[3]

It is clear that the importance of breakfast in optimizing physical and mental functioning is no myth!

References

1. Imberman, S. A., and A. D. Kugler. 2012. The effect of providing breakfast on student performance: evidence from an in-class breakfast program. National Bureau of Economic Research, NBER Working Paper No. 17720.
2. Hasz, L. A., and M. A. Lamport. 2012. Breakfast and adolescent academic performance: an analytical review of recent research. *Europ. J. Bus. Soc. Sci.* 1:61–79.
3. Kral, T. V. E., L. M. Whiteford, M. Heo, and M. S. Faith. 2011. Effects of eating breakfast compared with skipping breakfast on ratings of appetite and intake at subsequent meals in 8- to 10-year-old children. *Am. J. Clin. Nutr.* 93:284–291.

The Role of the Family in Physical Activity

As with healthful eating, parental and adult role models are vital in any effort to increase the physical activity level of children and adolescents. When parents and children are active together, healthful activity patterns are established early. To encourage activity throughout the day, parents should encourage shared activities, such as ball games, bicycle rides, hikes, and skating outings. In addition, community organizations, such as the YMCA and municipal recreational centers have supervised youth-oriented weight-training programs, climbing walls, skateboard parks, and other nontraditional activity options that are typically open to the whole family.

In the past, children played freely outdoors and even kept active indoors in times of bad weather. In recent years, however, multiple factors have prompted childhood activities to become increasingly sedentary. One factor is the availability and attraction of sedentary entertainment technologies, including television, video games, computer games, and smart phones. The American Academy of Pediatrics recommends no media use for children younger than 2 years[32] and no more than 2 hours per day of TV viewing for preschoolers.[33] Children who watch more TV and have higher total screen time are at increased risk for obesity.[34] Too much television and screen time can interfere with the acquisition of physical skills and can hinder children's use of their own imaginations, dampening creativity. Moreover, most television commercials airing during children's programs advertise foods such as sweetened breakfast cereals made with refined grains, candies, pastries, and high-fat snacks.[35] Even parents who limit television watching should sit with their younger children during several commercials and explain to them, in age-appropriate language, that these foods are made to look appealing to kids but are not healthful choices.

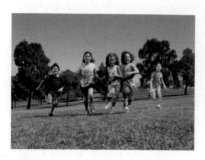

Encouraging physical play with friends is a good way to combat childhood obesity.

Another factor contributing to low levels of physical activity among America's youth is the high number of households in which no adult is home after school, either because of single-parent families or because both parents must work to support the family. Safety concerns may cause working parents to forbid their children, when they are home alone after school, to venture out of the house. If this is the case, the family may consider investing in electronic game systems that offer virtual tennis, step aerobics, dancing, and other active simulations.

By increasing their physical activity, many obese children are able to "catch up" to their weight as they grow taller without restricting their food (and thus nutrient) intake. Increased activity also helps children acquire motor skills and muscle strength, establish good sleep patterns, and develop self-esteem as they feel themselves becoming faster, stronger, and more skilled. Regular physical activity also optimizes bone mass, strengthens muscles, enhances cardiovascular and respiratory function, and lowers emotional stress in obese children.

The Role of the School in Physical Activity

As academic standards increase across the country, many schools are reducing or eliminating physical education classes and, in elementary schools, recess periods. Budget cuts have also led to the reduction or elimination of physical activity programs, including high school sports programs. Unfortunately, these decisions are short-sighted, because daily physical activity not only helps regulate body weight but also improves academic performance. Researchers have noted that, when children have the opportunity to take part in recess, classroom behavior improves, children are more attentive to their teachers, and students are more focused on assigned tasks.[36] In addition, children classified as physically fit have higher levels of academic achievement than unfit children.[37]

Parents, healthcare providers, and other community members can join forces to work with local school boards to optimize opportunities for physical activity in the schools. A program called We Can! (Ways to Enhance Children's Activity & Nutrition), a collaboration of several national health and government agencies, provides resources for parents, healthcare providers, schools, and communities, so that they can develop their own local physical activity and nutrition programs. We Can! is just one of many programs schools can use in developing their own action plans. Daily physical education in schools, continued funding for team and individual sports, and noncompetitive physical activity options outside of schools can help reduce the prevalence of obesity among

U.S. children and adolescents, slowly reversing what has been an alarming health trend for the past 30 years.

RECAP

Obesity is an important concern for children of all ages, their families, and their communities. Parents should model healthy eating and activity behaviors. Schools play an important role in providing nutritious breakfasts and lunches, and varied opportunities for daily physical activity. ■

Chapter Review

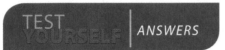

1 **F** Until they reach their second birthday, toddlers have a higher need for fat than do older children or adults, so they should consume foods that are higher in fat, including full-fat milk.

2 **T** The DRI guidelines do not differentiate between girls and boys until the age of 9 years.

3 **T** In 2010, 8.5 million children experienced food insecurity, as members of households that lacked dependable access to enough food for all members.

4 **F** Adolescents experience an average 20% to 25% increase in height during the pubertal years.

5 **T** Hormonal changes, emotional stress, genetic factors, and personal hygiene are the most likely contributors to adolescent acne.

Summary

- Toddlers grow more slowly than infants but are far more active. They require small, frequent, nutritious snacks and meals, and food should be cut in small pieces, so that it is easy to handle and swallow.

- For toddlers and young children, a serving of food equals 1 tablespoon for each year of age. For example, 4 tablespoons of yogurt is a full serving for a 4-year-old child.

- Energy, fat, and protein requirements are higher for toddlers than for infants. Many toddlers will not eat vegetables, so micronutrients of concern include vitamins A, C, and E.

- Until age 2, toddlers should drink whole milk rather than reduced-fat milk to meet calcium requirements. Iron deficiency is a concern in the toddler years and can be minimized by the consumption of foods naturally high in iron and iron-fortified foods.

- Feeding vegan diets to toddlers is controversial and poses potential deficiencies for protein, iron, calcium, zinc, vitamin D, and vitamin B_{12}.

- School-age children are more independent and can make more of their own food choices. Physical activity levels can vary dramatically.

- School-age children should eat 25% to 35% of their total energy as fat and 45% to 65% of their total energy as carbohydrate.

- Calcium needs increase as children mature. Consuming adequate calcium to support the development of peak bone mass is a primary concern for school-age children.

- Although iron needs decrease slightly in childhood, iron-deficiency anemia occurs in some children. Healthful food choices and, if appropriate, use of an iron supplement can prevent the fatigue, illness, and impaired learning that often accompany childhood iron deficiency.

■ Many school-age children skip breakfast and do not choose healthful foods during school lunch. Peer pressure and popularity are strong influences on food choices. School lunches are nutritious and meet federal guidelines, but the foods that children choose to eat at school, both during and outside the lunch break, can be high in fat, sugar, and energy and low in nutrients.

■ Families experiencing food insecurity should be referred to appropriate government and social service agencies; short-term solutions such as utilizing food pantries must be supported with long-term, multidimensional support.

■ Puberty is the period in life in which secondary sexual characteristics develop and the physical capability to reproduce begins. Puberty results in rapid increases in height, weight, lean body mass, and fat mass.

■ Energy needs for adolescents are variable and can be quite high, and adequate energy is needed to support growth, maturation, and physical activity. Fat intake should be 25% to 35% of total energy, and carbohydrate intake should be 45% to 65% of total energy intake.

■ Many adolescents replace whole grains, fruits, and vegetables with fast foods and high-fat/high-energy snack foods, placing themselves at risk for deficiencies of calcium, iron, and vitamin A. Calcium is needed to optimize bone growth and to achieve peak bone density, and iron needs are greater because of increased muscle mass in boys and menstruation in girls.

■ Disordered eating behaviors, eating disorders, personal appearance, cigarette smoking, and use of alcohol and illegal drugs are concerns for adolescents.

■ Obesity can begin to develop at any time from toddlerhood through adolescence if energy intake exceeds energy spent in physical activity. Both families and schools can play important roles in encouraging smart food choices and increased physical activity.

MasteringNutrition™

To further your understanding, go online and apply what you've learned to real-life case studies that will help you master the content!

Review Questions

1. The RDA for calcium for adolescents is
   a. less than that for young children.
   b. less than that for adults.
   c. less than that for pregnant adults.
   d. greater than that for young children, adults, and pregnant adults.

2. Carbohydrate should make up what percentage of total energy for school-age children?
   a. 25% to 40%
   b. 35% to 50%
   c. 45% to 65%
   d. 45% to 70%

3. Which of the following is a common nutrition-related concern for school-age children?
   a. inappropriately low fat intake
   b. skipping breakfast
   c. botulism
   d. protein deficiency

4. Which of the following breakfasts would be most appropriate to serve a 22-month-old child?
   a. 1 cup of iron-fortified cooked oat cereal, 2 tablespoons of mashed pineapple, and 1 cup of skim milk
   b. 2 tablespoons of plain yogurt, 2 tablespoons of applesauce, 2 tablespoons of fortified whole-grain oat cereal, and ½ cup of calcium-fortified orange juice
   c. ½ cup of iron-fortified cooked oat cereal, ½ cup of cubed pineapple, and 1 cup of low-fat milk
   d. two small link sausages cut in 1-inch pieces, two scrambled eggs, one slice of whole-wheat toast, four cherry tomatoes, ½ cup of applesauce, and 1 cup of whole milk

5. Which of the following statements about cigarette smoking is true?
   a. Cigarette smoking can interfere with the metabolism of nutrients.
   b. Cigarette smoking commonly causes food cravings, such as "getting the munchies."
   c. iPLEDGE is a program from the National Institutes of Health that encourages adolescents to stop smoking.
   d. All of these statements are true.

6. **True or false?** Toddlers need 30% to 40% of their total energy intake as fat.

7. **True or false?** Children are too young to understand and be influenced by the examples of their parents.

8. **True or false?** Among both males and females, the need for calcium decreases after the age of 16 due to the completion of bone growth.

9. **True or false?** National guidelines advise that all children and adolescents get 30 minutes of exercise 3 to 4 days each week.

10. **True or false?** Weight gain during adolescence is expected and healthful.

11. Identify some advantages and disadvantages of modern technology (such as television and computers) in terms of its impact on lifestyle and nutrition.

12. Explain why a toddler in a vegan family might be at risk for protein deficiency.

13. Imagine that you are taking care of four 5-year-old children for an afternoon. Design a menu for the children's lunch that is nutritious and that will be fun for them to eat.

14. Imagine that you plan meals for a high school cafeteria. Design a menu with three lunch choices that are nutritious and that are likely to be popular with teens.

15. Your classmate Lydia is a bit eccentric. An engineering major, she spends an average of 6 hours a day at her computer, drinking diet colas and eating pretzels. She is unusually slender, even though she admits to getting no regular exercise. Your university is in upstate New York, and Lydia is from Vermont. If you were a registered dietitian (RD) and Lydia were your client, what nutrition-related health concern(s) might you discuss with her? Identify *at least* three elements in Lydia's story that are known risk factors for the health problem(s) you identify.

Math Review

16. Your 16-year-old sister is following a vegan diet. Her RDA for calcium is 1,300 mg/day. If she ate a salad with 2 cups of raw spinach (115 mg calcium/cup), 2 ounces of firm tofu cubes (50 mg/oz), and ¾ cup of calcium-fortified orange juice (300 mg/cup), would she meet one-third of her calcium RDA?

Answers to Review Questions and Math Review can be found online in the MasteringNutrition Study Area.

Web Links

www.wecan.nhlbi.nih.gov
We Can!
We Can! (Ways to Enhance Children's Activity & Nutrition) provides materials for families, schools, and healthcare providers to use to help children increase their physical activity, make healthy food choices, and achieve healthy weights.

www.keepkidshealthy.com
Keep Kids Healthy.com
Find information about nutrition and health for toddlers, children, and adolescents on this website.

www.cdc.gov
Centers for Disease Control and Prevention (CDC)
Click on "Health Promotion"; then select topics such as "Adolescent Health" or "Project VERB™," plus many others.

www.vrg.org
Vegetarian Resource Group
Visit this website to learn more about vegetarianism for all ages. Included on the site are special sections for teens and kids, as well as recipes and guides for vegetarian and vegan eating in all kinds of situations.

www.health.gov/dietaryguidelines
Dietary Guidelines for Americans
Visit this site to read the 2005 Dietary Guidelines for Americans and to learn about their development.

www.fns.usda.gov
USDA Food & Nutrition Services
Read about government programs to provide food to all ages, including school meal programs, the Child and Adult Care Food Program, and the Women, Infants, and Children program.

www.eatright.org
American Dietetic Association
Visit this website to learn about healthy eating habits for all stages of life.

www.nichd.nih.gov/milk
Milk Matters
Need ideas on how to increase milk and other dairy foods intakes? This website provides practical tips and menus for children and adolescents.

References

1. Institute of Medicine, Food and Nutrition Board. 2002. *Dietary Reference Intakes for Energy, Carbohydrates, Fiber, Fat, Protein and Amino Acids (Macronutrients).* Washington, DC: The National Academy of Sciences.

2. Kleinman, R. E., ed. 2009. *Pediatric Nutrition Handbook.* 6th edn. Elk Grove Village, IL: American Academy of Pediatrics.

3. Kranz, S., M. Brauchla, J. L. Slavin, and K. B. Miller. 2012. What do we know about dietary fiber intake in children and health? The effects of fiber intake on constipation, obesity, and diabetes in children. *Adv. Nutr.* 3:47–53.

4. Vernacchio, L., J. P. Kelly, D. W. Kaufman, and A. A. Mitchell. 2011. Vitamin, fluoride, and iron use among U.S. children younger than 12 years of age: results from the Slone survey 1998–2007. *J. Amer. Dietetic Assoc.* 111:285–289.

5. Ross, A. C., C. L. Taylor, A. L. Yaktine, and H. B. Del Valle, eds. 2011. *Dietary Reference Intakes for Calcium and Vitamin D.* Washington, DC: National Academy Press.

6. Institute of Medicine, Food and Nutrition Board. 2001. *Dietary Reference Intakes for Vitamin A, Vitamin K, Arsenic, Boron, Chromium, Copper, Iodine, Iron, Manganese, Molybdenum, Nickel, Silicon, Vanadium, and Zinc.* Washington, DC: National Academy Press.

7. Institute of Medicine, Food and Nutrition Board. 2004. *Dietary Reference Intakes for Water, Potassium, Sodium, Chloride, and Sulfate.* Washington, DC: National Academy Press.

8. McEvoy, C. T., N. Temple, and J. V. Woodside. 2012. Vegetarian diets, low-meat diets and health: a review. *Public Health Nutrition* DOI:10.1017/S1368980012000936.

9. Fiorito, L. M., M. Marini, D. C. Mitchell, H. Smiciklas-Wright, and L. L. Birch. 2010. Girls' early sweetened carbonated beverage intake predicts different patterns of beverage and nutrient intake across childhood and adolescence. *J. Am. Diet. Assoc.* 110:543–550.

10. Zuercher, J. L., D. A. Wagstaff, and S. Kranz. 2011. Associations of food group and nutrient intake, diet quality, and meal sizes between adults and children in the same household: a cross-sectional analysis of U.S. households. *Nutr. J.* 10:131. DOI:10.1186/1475-2891-10-131.

11. Imberman, S. A., and A. D. Kugler. 2012. *The Effect of Providing Breakfast on Student Performance: Evidence from an In-Class Breakfast Program.* NBER Working Paper No.17720. Cambridge, MA: National Bureau of Economic Research.

12. Dillon, S. 2011. Lines grow long for free school meals, thanks to economy. *The New York Times,* November 29.

13. US Department of Agriculture, Food and Nutrition Service. 2012. USDA Unveils Historic Improvements to Meals Served in America's Schools. Release No. 0023.12. www.fns.usda.gov/cga/PressReleases/2012/0023.htm. (Accessed July 2012.)

14. Miller, C. H. 2009. A practice perspective on the third School Nutrition Dietary Assessment Study. *J. Am. Diet. Assoc.* 109:S14–S17.

15. Fiese, B. H., C. Gundersen, B. Koester, and L. Washington. 2011. Household food insecurity—serious concerns for child development. *Social Policy Report* 25:3–19.

16. Abrams, S. A. 2011. Calcium and vitamin D requirements for optimal bone mass during adolescence. *Current Opinion in Clinical Nutrition & Metabolic Care* 14:605–609.

17. Melnik, B. C. 2012. Diet in acne: further evidence for the role of nutrient signaling in acne pathogenesis. *Acta Derm.Venereol.* 92:228–231.

18. Hong, T., J. Rice, and C. Johnson. 2011. Social environmental and individual factors associated with smoking among a panel of adolescent girls. *Women & Health* 51:187–203.

19. Jamal, M., A. J. W. Van der Does, B. W. J. H. Penninx, and P. Cuijpers. 2011. Age at smoking onset and the onset of depression and anxiety disorders. *Nicotine & Tobacco Research* 13:809–819.

20. National Institute on Alcohol Abuse and Alcoholism. 2010. *Rethinking drinking: Alcohol and your health.* Available at http://rethinkingdrinking.niaaa.nih.gov/WhatsTheHarm/WhatAreTheRisks.asp.

21. Ogden, C. L., M. D. Carroll, B. K. Kit, and K. M. Flegal. 2012. Prevalence of obesity and trends in body mass index among U.S. children and adolescents, 1999–2010. *JAMA.* 307:483–490.

22. Bibbins-Domingo, K., P. Coxson, M.J. Pletcher, J. Lightwood, and L. Goldman. 2007. Adolescent overweight and future adult coronary heart disease. *N. Engl. J. Med.* 357:2371-2379.

23. Xu, L., L. Dubois, D. Burnier, M. Girard, and D. Prud'homme. 2011. Parental overweight/obesity, social factors, and child overweight/obesity at 7 years of age. *Pediatrics International* 53:826–831.

24. Silventoinen, K., A. L. Hasselbalch, T. Lallukka, L. Bogl, K. H. Pietiläinen, B. L. Heitmann, K. Schousboe, A. Rissanen, K. O. Kyvik, T. I. Sørensen, and J. Kaprio. 2009. Modification effects of physical activity and protein intake on heritability of body size and composition. *Am. J. Clin. Nutr.* 90:1096–1103.

25. Brennan, L., S. Castro, R. C. Brownson, J. Claus, and C. T. Orleans. 2011. *Ann. Rev. Public Health.* 32:199–223.

26. de Ferranti, S., and R. L. Washington. 2012. NHLBI guidelines on cholesterol in kids: what's new and how does this change practice? *AAP News* 33:1.

27. Sonneville, K. R., S. L. Rifas-Shiman, K. P. Kleinman, S. L. Gortmaker, M. W. Gillman, and E. M. Taveras. 2012. Associations of obesogenic behaviors in mothers and obese children participating in a randomized trial. *Obesity* 20:1449–1454.

28. Faith, M. S., L. Van Horn, L. J. Apel, L. E. Burke, J. A. S. Carson, H. A. Franch, J. M. Jakicic, T. V. E. Kral, A. Odoms-Young, B. Wansink, and J. Wylie-Rosett. 2012. *Circulation* 125:1186–1207.

29. U.C. Davis Center for Nutrition in Schools. 2012. *Garden-based learning.* Available at http://cns.ucdavis.edu/resources/garden/index.cfm.

30. California School Garden Network. 2012. *Why school gardens?* Available at http://www.csgn.org/why-school-gardens.

31. Physical Activity Guidelines Advisory Committee. 2008. *Physical Activity Guidelines Advisory Committee Report, 2008.* Washington, DC: US Department of Health and Human Services.

32. American Academy of Pediatrics Council on Communications and Media. 2011. Policy statement: media use by children younger than 2 years. *Pediatrics* 128:1040–1045.

33. American Academy of Pediatrics. 2010. Media education. *Pediatrics* 126:1–6.

34. de Jong, E., T. L. S. Visscher, R. A. HiraSing, M. W. Heymans, J. C. Seidell, and C. M. Renders. 2011. Association between TV viewing, computer use and overweight, determinants and competing activities of screen time in 4- to 13-year-old children. *Int. J. Obesity* DOI:10.1038/ijo.2011.244.

35. Boyland, E. J., J. A. Harrold, T. C. Kirkham, C. Corker, J. Cuddy, D. Evans, T. M. Dovey, C. L. Lawton, J. E. Blundell, and J. C. G. Halford. 2011. Food commercials increase preference for energy-dense foods, particularly in children who watch more television. *Pediatrics* 128:e93–e100.

36. Barros, R. M., E. J. Silver, and R. E. K. Stein. 2009. School recess and group classroom behavior. *Pediatrics* 123:431–436.

37. Chomitz, V. R., M. M. Slining, R. J. McGowan, S. E. Mitchell, G. F. Dawson, and K. A. Hacker. 2009. Is there a relationship between physical fitness and academic achievement? Positive results from public school children in the northeastern United States. *J. School Health.* 79:30–37.

Bariatric Surgery for Adolescents

Nearly 18% of U.S. adolescents are obese, with 1–2% classified as morbidly obese (BMI > 40 kg/m²).[1] While overall rates of pediatric obesity seem to be plateauing, rates of morbid obesity continue to increase. Adolescent morbid obesity is associated with an 80% chance of adult morbid obesity and high rates of medical comorbidities (type 2 diabetes, metabolic syndrome, hypertension, hyperlipidemia, sleep apnea) and psychosocial disorders (depression, anxiety, suicidal thoughts).[2,3] While prevention of obesity and morbid obesity is viewed as the best solution, effective prevention on a wide scale remains difficult to achieve. As a result, bariatric surgery is becoming a more common treatment approach.[4,5] Given the risks of any surgical procedure and the irreversible nature of some forms of bariatric surgery, is this intervention appropriate for adolescents as young as 13 years of age?

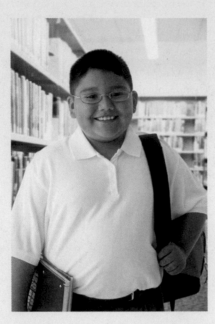

Bariatric surgery is becoming a more common treatment for seriously overweight adolescents.

While it is hard to accurately estimate how many adolescents undergo bariatric surgery each year, its frequency is increasing. There are two common bariatric surgical procedures for adolescents.[6] The *laparoscopic adjustable gastric banding (LAGB),* which restricts food intake, is reversible and does not interfere with normal digestion and absorption, however the weight loss results are more modest than achieved via other methods and it does not resolve the metabolic abnormalities associated with morbid obesity. The *Roux-en-Y gastric bypass (RYGBP)* is more invasive, drastically alters GI structure and absorptive functions, requires lifelong vitamin and mineral supplementation, and has a higher rate of complications. However, it also results in much greater weight loss, is FDA approved for adolescents, and effectively improves or fully resolves many of the metabolic abnormalities associated with morbid obesity.[2]

National and international organizations have established guidelines and best practices on the appropriate use of bariatric surgery in adolescents. Eligibility requirements for adolescents commonly include the following:[1,4]

- *Minimum age.* Eighteen years is the most common minimum age, although patient ages as young as 11, 13, and 15 years are cited in at least one set of guidelines. Some criteria are based on developmental (Tanner) stage, rather than chronological age.
- *Minimum BMI.* The minimum is >40 kg/m² or >35 kg/m²; the presence of comorbidities is often included.
- *History of 6 or more months of targeted weight loss efforts.* Previous lifestyle and behavioral efforts must have been proven ineffective in achieving significant weight loss before embarking on this course of action.
- *Demonstrated commitment to and understanding of all pre- and postoperative requirements.* Candidates must agree to regular follow-up for at least 1 year, adhere to nutritional guidelines, and, if female, avoid pregnancy for at least 1 year following the procedure.
- *Supportive family environment.* A supportive and involved family is a key aspect contributing to successful bariatric surgery for adolescents.

Adolescents who are pregnant or breastfeeding, abuse alcohol or drugs, have an eating disorder, or are diagnosed with certain medical conditions are not considered appropriate candidates for bariatric surgery.[4]

Long-term outcomes for bariatric surgery in adolescents are limited. One study followed adolescents up to 10 years after their RYGBP procedure.[2] While complications were reported, there were no deaths. Most, if not all, reported resolution of previous medical conditions, including diabetes, hyperlipidemia, hypertension, sleep apnea, gastroesophageal reflux, and arthritic symptoms. Quality of life often greatly improves following bariatric surgery, and psychological disorders are often improved or resolved. From a purely financial perspective, there is not enough data to evaluate the cost-effectiveness of adolescent bariatric surgery.[6,7]

CRITICAL THINKING QUESTIONS

There is no doubt that pediatric morbid obesity results in significant and often long-lasting medical, psychological, and social impairments. Lifestyle interventions, including nutrition, physical activity, and behavioral components, are inexpensive and low/no risk. Bariatric surgery is expensive and often irreversible, complications occur on a regular basis, and adolescents may not have the maturity to make an informed decision.

■ What is your opinion of a 15-year-old boy's request to "go under the knife" because he is tired of trying to diet and hates to exercise? How much effort is "enough" when looking at failure through lifestyle interventions for morbid obesity?

■ For our society, is adolescent bariatric surgery a good investment in terms of the health of the nation? What kind of information would you need in order to make a strong argument one way or the other?

REFERENCES

1. Michalsky, M., R. E. Kramer, M. A. Fullmer, M. Polfuss, R. Porter, W. Ward-Begnoche, E. A. Getzoff, M. Dreyer, S. Stolzman, and K. W. Reichard. 2011. Developing criteria for pediatric/adolescent bariatric surgery programs. *Pediatrics* 128:S65–S70.

2. Nijhawan, S., T. Martinez, and A. C. Wittgrove. 2012. Laparoscopic gastric bypass for the adolescent patient: long-term results. *Obes. Surg.* DOI: 10.1007/s11695-012-0670-8.

3. Kassira, N., V. A. Marks, and N. de la Cruz-Muñez. 2012. Bariatric surgery to reverse metabolic syndrome in adolescents. In: Lipshultz, S. E., et al., eds. *Pediatric Metabolic Syndrome*. London: Springer-Verlag.

4. Aikenhead, A., T. Lobstein, and C. Knai. 2011. Review of current guidelines on adolescent bariatric surgery. *Clinical Obesity* 1:3–11.

5. Fullmer, M. A., S. H. Abrams, K. Hrovat, L. Mooney, A. O. Scheimann, J. B. Hillman, and D. L. Suskind. 2012. Nutritional strategy for adolescents undergoing bariatric surgery: report of a working group of the Nutrition Committee of NASPGHAN/NACHRI. *J. Pediatric Gastroenterology & Nutrition* 54:125–135.

6. Aikenhead, A., C. Knai, and T. Lobstein. 2011. Effectiveness and cost-effectiveness of paediatric bariatric surgery: a systematic review. *Clinical Obesity* 1:12–25.

7. Woolford, S. J., S. J. Clark, B. J. Sallinen, J. D. Geiger, and G. L. Freed. 2012. Bariatric surgery decision making challenges: the stability of teens' decisions and the treatment failure paradox. *Pediatr. Surg. Int.* 28:455–460.

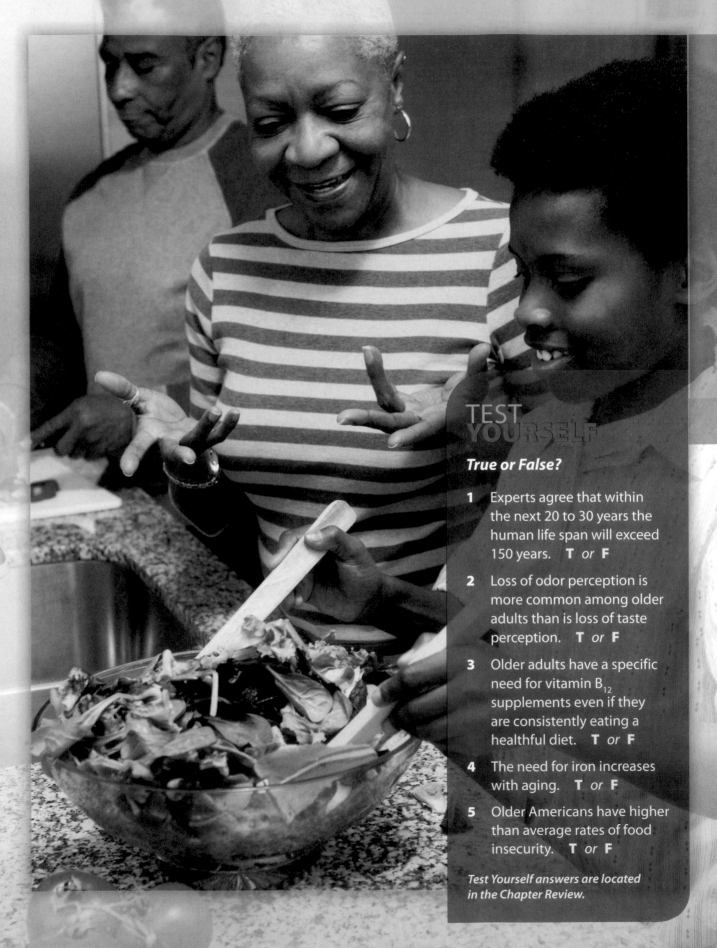

True or False?

1 Experts agree that within the next 20 to 30 years the human life span will exceed 150 years. **T** *or* **F**

2 Loss of odor perception is more common among older adults than is loss of taste perception. **T** *or* **F**

3 Older adults have a specific need for vitamin B_{12} supplements even if they are consistently eating a healthful diet. **T** *or* **F**

4 The need for iron increases with aging. **T** *or* **F**

5 Older Americans have higher than average rates of food insecurity. **T** *or* **F**

Test Yourself answers are located in the Chapter Review.

18

Nutrition Through the Life Cycle: The Later Years

Learning Objectives

After studying this chapter, you should be able to:

1. Describe the demographic changes related to the aging of America, *pp. 724–725.*

2. Identify current theories of human aging and how each relates to nutrient intake and/or status of older adults, *pp. 725–726.*

3. Describe the most common physiologic changes that occur as we age, *pp. 726–731.*

4. Explain how lifestyle choices can influence the rate at which we age, *p. 731.*

5. Compare and contrast the nutrient requirements of older adults to those of younger or middle-aged adults, including for energy, macronutrients, micronutrients, and fluids, *pp. 732–736.*

6. Identify and describe the range of nutrition-related concerns that pose health threats for older adults, *pp. 736–743.*

7. Discuss the issues surrounding the use of nutritional supplements by older adults, *p. 737.*

8. Identify the social and environmental factors that can affect the nutrition of older adults, *pp. 743–744.*

9. Discuss the various community services and nutrition programs available to U.S. elderly, including for those from varied ethnic or racial groups, *pp. 744–745.*

10. Evaluate the options for "end-of-life care" related to diet and nutritional support, *pp. 745–746.*

MasteringNutrition™

Go online for chapter quizzes, pre-tests, Interactive Activities, and more!

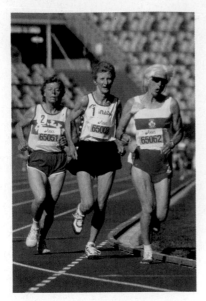

With the help of a nutritious diet and regular activity, many aging adults can remain highly active in their later years.

When Loretta finally retired from her job as a public school teacher at age 68, she looked forward to taking things a little easier. Then her daughter, Tina, a captain in the U.S. Army, was deployed to Afghanistan, leaving Tina's son, Chase, in his grandparents' care. Shortly after he moved in, Chase showed a budding interest in learning how to cook, so Loretta decided to enroll in a basic nutrition course at her local community college as a way to support Chase's new interest. When she arrived on campus, she was delighted to find that some of her fellow students were older than she was! Across the United States, colleges and universities are reporting a surge in the enrollment of older adults, some in their eighties and nineties. Many of these older students are fulfilling a lifelong dream of obtaining a college degree, whereas others, like Loretta, are taking classes for personal enrichment.

As our population continues to age, and seniors benefit from improvements in lifestyle and healthcare, life as an older adult now offers as many opportunities as challenges. Decades of research confirms the importance of a nutritious diet and regular physical activity in helping prevent chronic disease, enhance productivity, and improve quality of life as we age. What are the unique nutritional needs and concerns of older adults? How can diet and lifestyle affect the aging process? These and other questions will be addressed in this chapter.

What Are the Demographics of Aging?

Before we can discuss the nutrient needs and concerns of older adults, it's essential that we understand who makes up the older adult population in America—both their numbers and their characteristics.

The American Population Is Aging

The U.S. population is getting older each year. In 2010, over 40 million people aged 65 and older lived in the United States, representing about 13% of the population. Of these, 23 million were women, and 17 million were men.[1] It is estimated that by the year 2020 the elderly will account for about 16% of Americans, or more than 55 million adults.

By most measures, the quality of life of older Americans is improving. Older Americans are now healthier, more socially and physically active, and less likely to be confined to bed or have functional limitations than older adults living several decades ago. Many are choosing to work well beyond traditional retirement age, and increasing numbers are using the same technologies as their children and grandchildren. Ideally, this trend will continue for future generations of elderly as well.

The racial and ethnic profile of U.S. elderly continues to reflect the demographics of the country as a whole. Currently, about 20% of Americans over age 65 are minorities.[1] The proportion of non-Hispanic whites will sharply decline over the next several decades, whereas the older Hispanic population will grow at the fastest rate. The percentage of older Native Americans and African Americans will grow to a lesser extent. As we discuss later in this chapter, the growing diversity of the elderly population and its unique cultural needs will present a significant challenge to the medical and social service communities.

Those 85 years and over, known as the "very elderly" or "oldest of the old," currently represent the fastest-growing U.S. population subgroup, projected to increase 20%, from 5.5 million in 2010 to more than 6.6 million by the year 2020.[1] The number of *centenarians*, persons over the age of 100 years, and *super-centenarians*, over 110 years, continues to grow as well. In 2010, there were over 53,000 centenarians in the United States, a 50% increase from 1990!

Centenarians represent the future of U.S. elderly.

life expectancy The expected number of years remaining in one's life; typically stated from the time of birth. Children born in the United States in 2003 can expect to live, on average, 77.6 years.

Life Span Differs from Life Expectancy

Celebrating one's 60th birthday is common today. Yet when George Washington turned 60 years old in 1792, he had outlived most of his peers by about 15 years. U.S. **life expectancy,** about 47 years in the year 1900, has increased dramatically during the past century due largely to medical advances, better nutrition, and improved sanitation.

In 2010, the average U.S. life expectancy reached 78.3 years. Women live longer on average than men, and racial disparities in life expectancy exist. Life expectancy for African American males is 6 years less than for white males and for African American females is 4 years less than for white females.[2] While average U.S. life expectancy has increased over the past several decades, the rate of improvement is less than that of other high-income countries.[3] For example, life expectancy in Canada and several European nations is over 81 years, and in Monaco, the country with the highest life expectancy, it is just short of 90.[3] It has been estimated that this gap might be due at least in part to the growing rate of obesity in the United States.

For most older adults, the goal is not to live as long as possible but to live a life free of disability and disease for as long as possible. This concept of healthy longevity is often referred to as *active life expectancy, successful aging,* or *compression of morbidity.*

Life span is the age to which the longest-living member of the species has lived. Though very difficult to authenticate, one international volunteer organization estimates that there are about 70 super-centenarians living around the world, over 90% of them female.[4] Madame Jeanne Calment, born in France in 1875, survived to the age of 122 and is generally viewed as achieving the oldest age in the world. Although some researchers have sought ways of extending human life span (see the **Nutrition Debate** on energy restricted diets at the end of this chapter), most agree that a life span beyond 125 to 130 years is unlikely.

Why and How Do We Age?

The process of aging is natural and inevitable, influenced by genetic and environmental factors. Researchers have made great progress toward understanding the aging of humans, but much remains unknown. Scientists can't even agree when the aging process begins: some believe it starts at birth, whereas others argue it begins after peak reproductive age. While the debate continues, however, gerontologists agree that humans can positively influence the aging process through specific lifestyle and environmental choices.

Many Mechanisms Are Thought to Contribute to Aging

Aging occurs at the molecular, cellular, and tissue levels. Some signs of aging, such as the graying of hair, do not impair function or health. Other age-related changes, however, contribute to declines in functionality, health, and well-being. Scientists use the term **senescence** to describe those age-related processes that increase risk for disability, disease, and death.

Theories attempting to explain the mechanisms of aging can be categorized into two lines of research (**Table 18.1**). First are the **programmed theories of aging,** proposing that aging follows a biologically driven time line, similar to that of adolescence. In programmed theories of aging, nutrition has little, if any, potential or practical impact on senescence. For example, there is no doubt that genes exert tremendous influence on the aging process. Siblings of centenarians are four times more likely to live into their nineties than others. Researchers have even found a genetic mutation dubbed the "I'm Not Dead Yet" gene, which prolongs the life span of certain laboratory animals. Although researchers may never develop a "fountain of youth," they are well on their way to understanding how genetics contributes to cell senescence and human aging.

The second category consists of the **error theories of aging,** which argue that senescence occurs as a result of cell and tissue damage caused largely by environmental insults. These mechanisms include the following:

- As cells age, cell membrane function declines, allowing waste products to accumulate within the cell and decreasing normal uptake of nutrients and oxygen.
- Gerontologists have also linked the aging process to a progressive accumulation of free radicals, which are known to damage DNA and various cell proteins.

Wonder what it would be like to be a college student at the age of 95? Listen to what one woman has to say! www.msnbc.msn.com/id/18338864/ns/us_news-wonderful_world/t/woman-set-be-oldest-college-graduate/.

life span The highest age reached by any member of a species; currently, the human life span is 122 years.

senescence The progressive deterioration of bodily functions over time, resulting in increased risk for disability, disease, and death.

programmed theories of aging Aging is biologically determined, following a predictable pattern of physiologic changes, although the timing may vary from one person to another.

error theories of aging Aging is a cumulative process determined largely by exposure to environmental insults; the fewer the environmental insults, the slower the aging process.

TABLE 18.1 Theories of Aging

Model	Description	Nutrition Interface
Programmed Theories of Aging	Aging follows a biologically driven time line, similar to that of adolescence.	None evident
Hayflick theory of aging	Cells have a limited reproductive life span; in essence, cells can divide only so many times before they are no longer able to proliferate.	None evident
Theory of programmed longevity	Aging occurs when certain genes are turned on or off; the activation or suppression of these genes then triggers age-related loss of function.	Indirectly, a diet rich in antioxidants, such as vitamins C and E, could lower free-radical damage to DNA.
Endocrine theory of aging	Senescence is due to hormonal changes, such as declines in growth hormone, DHEA, estrogen, and/or testosterone.	None directly evident
Immunologic theory of aging	Aging is linked to loss of immune system activity and/or an increase in autoimmune diseases.	Adequate protein, zinc, iron, and vitamins A, C, and E help preserve remaining immune function.
Error Theories of Aging	Senescence occurs as a result of cell and tissue damage caused largely by environmental insults.	Several theoretical benefits of nutrient adequacy or supplementation
Wear-and-tear theory	Over time, cells simply wear out and eventually die. The greater the exposure to toxins and stressors, the more rapid the rate of decline.	Protein, zinc, and vitamins A and C could theoretically delay the aging process by improving cellular repair and recovery.
Cross-linkage theory	Abnormal cross-linkages of proteins, such as collagen, damage cells and tissues, impairing the function of organs.	Glycosylation, the abnormal attachment of glucose to proteins, can be limited by controlling blood glucose levels. Adequate intakes of vitamin C, selenium, and copper may reduce other types of protein cross-linkages.
Free-radical theory	Senescence is due to the cumulative damage caused by various free radicals.	Diets and/or supplements rich in vitamins C and E, selenium, and antioxidant phytochemicals may limit the cellular accumulation of free radicals.
Rate-of-living theory	In general, the higher the species' average basal metabolic rate (BMR), the shorter its life span.	Theoretically, energy restriction would lower BMR and prolong life (see the **Nutrition Debate** on pages 751–753).

- Cellular aging has also been linked to a progressive failure in DNA repair. Throughout the life cycle, human DNA is subjected to various insults, including free radicals, toxins, and random coding errors. Normally, the cell detects and repairs damaged DNA. With aging, however, the repair process becomes less efficient, leading to abnormal protein synthesis, which then results in cell, tissue, and organ senescence.
- Tissue and organ senescence has been linked to the process of **glycosylation.** This abnormal attachment of glucose to proteins results in loss of protein structure and function. As a result, lung tissue, blood vessels, and tendons become rigid and inflexible.

Changes identified by the error theories of aging are directly or indirectly linked to nutrient or energy status. Thus, consumption of adequate levels of antioxidant nutrients could theoretically delay some of these changes.

In truth, the programmed and error theories of aging are not mutually exclusive: it is likely that aging stems from a complex interplay of the factors identified in Table 18.1.

Characteristic Physiologic Changes Accompany Aging

Older adulthood is a time in which growth is complete and body systems begin to slow and degenerate. If the following discussion of this degeneration seems disturbing or depressing, remember that the changes described are at least partly within an individual's control. For instance, some of the decrease seen in muscle mass, bone mass, and muscle strength is due to low physical activity levels. Older adults who regularly participate in strengthening exercises and aerobic-type activities reduce their risks for low bone mass and muscle atrophy and weakness, which in turn reduces their risk for falls.

glycosylation The addition of glucose to blood and tissue proteins; typically impairs protein structure and function.

Age-Related Changes in Sensory Perception

For most individuals, eating is a social and pleasurable process; the sights, sounds, odors, and textures associated with food are closely linked to appetite. Odor, taste, tactile, and visual perception all decline with age; as they do, an older adult's food intake and nutritional status can decline as well.

More than half of elderly adults experience significant loss of olfactory (odor) perception, a condition more common than loss of taste perception, although "successfully aged" older adults experience less of a decline.[5] The enjoyment of food relies heavily on the sense of smell: think of your own response to the smell of bread baking in the oven or the aroma of grilled meat or poultry. Older adults who cannot adequately appreciate the appealing aromas of food may be unable to fully enjoy the foods offered within the meal. Loss of olfaction also restricts the ability to detect spoiled food, increasing the risk for food poisoning. Although often a simple consequence of aging, loss of odor perception can also be caused by zinc deficiency or can occur as a side effect of medication. If this is the case, a zinc supplement or change of medication may be a simple solution.

With increasing age, taste perception dims as well, which is one reason older adults seem to add so much salt to their foods or complain about the blandness of their foods. The ability to perceive sweetness and sourness also declines, but to a lesser extent. Some elderly experience **dysgeusia,** or abnormal taste perception, which can be caused by disease or medication use.

Loss of visual acuity has unexpected consequences for the nutritional health of the elderly. Many older adults have difficulty reading food labels, including nutrient information. Driving skills decline, limiting the ability of some older Americans to acquire healthy, affordable foods. Older adults with vision loss may not be able to see the temperature knobs on stoves or the controls on microwave ovens and may therefore choose cold meals, such as sandwiches, rather than meals that require heating. The visual appeal of a colorful, attractively arranged plate of food is also lost to visually impaired elderly, further reducing their desire to eat healthful meals.

Friends and family members can help older adults adjust to these sensory losses by encouraging appropriate food selections and preparation techniques. Flavor enhancers such as herbs and spices, meat concentrates, and sauces can increase the desirability of otherwise bland foods. Visual enhancements such as brightly colored garnishes and an array of different shapes and textures on the plate can also compensate for diminished olfaction.

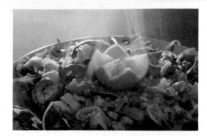

As people age, their ability to smell foods often declines.

Age-Related Changes in Gastrointestinal Function

Significant changes in the mouth and gastrointestinal tract occur with aging.[6] Some of these changes have the potential to increase the risk for nutrient deficiency.[7]

With increasing age, salivary production declines. In older adults with **xerostomia,** teeth are more susceptible to decay, chewing and swallowing become more difficult, and taste perception declines. Risk for fungal infections, such as candidiasis, increases. A diet rich in moist foods, including fruits and vegetables, sauces or gravies on meats, and high-fluid desserts such as puddings, is well tolerated by older adults with xerostomia. In the most severe cases, older adults can use an artificial saliva, which is sprayed into the mouth.

Some older adults, including those with Parkinson's disease, experience **dysphagia** (difficulty swallowing foods). Smooth, thick foods, such as cream soups or applesauce, are easy to swallow, but foods with mixed textures, such as gelatin with fruit pieces, should be avoided. Milkshakes, fruit nectars, and other thick or viscous beverages are better tolerated than thin liquids, such as water and coffee. Dysphagia requires professional assessment and treatment, drawing on the expertise of an occupational therapist, a physician, and a dietitian. If not accurately diagnosed and treated, dysphagia can lead to malnutrition, inappropriate weight loss, aspiration of food or fluid into the lungs, and pneumonia.

dysgeusia Abnormal taste perception.

xerostomia Dry mouth due to decreased saliva production.

dysphagia Abnormal swallowing.

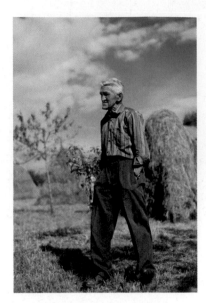

A variety of gastrointestinal and other physiologic changes can lead to weight loss in older adults.

Older adults are at risk for a reduced secretion of gastric acid, intrinsic factor, pepsin, and mucus.[6] **Achlorhydria,** a severe reduction in gastric hydrochloric acid production, limits the absorption of minerals, such as calcium, iron, and zinc, and food sources of folic acid and vitamin B_{12}. Lack of intrinsic factor, produced by the same cells that secrete gastric hydrochloric acid, reduces the absorption of vitamin B_{12} (see Chapter 8, page 326). These elderly, therefore, benefit from vitamin B_{12} supplements. Older adults may also experience a delay in gastric emptying, resulting in a prolonged sense of fullness and a reduced appetite. Although this may be viewed as a positive factor in people who are overweight or obese, it can lead to inappropriate weight loss.

There is increasing evidence that the gut microbiota of the elderly differs from that of younger adults, with important health implications.[8] Microbes in the gut digest fibers; produce short-chain fatty acids, which provide anti-inflammatory effects; and reduce the ability of pathogenic microorganisms to flourish. Age-related changes in dietary patterns, medication usage, and other lifestyle factors contribute to a reduction in the biodiversity of gut microbiota and an increase in pathogenic bacteria. The onset of the "aging gut" appears to be highly individualized and difficult to predict. The potential consequences, however, are clear: an increased inflammatory state, decreased immune functioning of the intestinal tract, and impaired functioning of the gut mucosal cells.

Recent research suggests that age-related changes in the release of appetite-regulating gut hormones may contribute to a condition known as "anorexia of aging."[9] Many elderly people report feeling less hunger and an increased sense of satiety, both of which contribute to inappropriately low food intake. Some studies suggest that the release of anorexigenic or satiety-inducing hormones (such as cholecystokinin (CCK)) is increased, and that of hunger-inducing ghrelin is decreased, in the elderly. These alterations would shift the regulation of appetite such that food intake would decline over the short and long term.

Compared to younger adults, the healthy elderly demonstrate no significant loss in digestive enzyme activity, the ability to absorb nutrients, or intestinal motility. Therefore, healthy elderly people generally digest and absorb protein, fat, and carbohydrate as efficiently as younger adults. The one exception is the digestion of lactose: only about 30% of older adults retain an "adequate" level of lactase enzyme activity. African American, Hispanic, Native American, and Asian elderly are at very high risk for lactose intolerance and may need to restrict their fluid milk intake to ½-cup servings, use lactose-reduced milk or lactase enzyme supplements, or eliminate milk from their diet entirely. Although tolerance for dairy foods may decrease with aging, the need for calcium does not. Older adults may need to turn to calcium-fortified soy, rice, or nut milks and fruit juices; fortified breakfast cereals; calcium-enriched tofu; leafy green vegetables; and other sources to ensure an adequate intake. Finally, although gastrointestinal function remains largely unaffected by aging, nutrient availability may be severely compromised if an older adult has a disease of the liver, pancreas, or GI tract that impairs digestion of food and absorption of nutrients.

Age-Related Changes in Body Composition

With aging, body fat increases and muscle mass declines. It has been estimated that women and men lose 20% to 25% of their lean body mass, respectively, as they age from 35 to 70 years. Decreased production of certain hormones, including testosterone and growth hormone, and chronic diseases contribute to this loss of muscle, as do poor diet and an inactive lifestyle. Older adults with **sarcopenia** (age-related, progressive loss of muscle mass, strength, and function) are often so weak that they are unable to rise from a seated position, climb stairs, or carry a bag of groceries. Along with adequate dietary intake, regular physical activity, including strength or resistance training, can help older

achlorhydria Lack of gastric acid secretion.

sarcopenia Age-related, progressive loss of muscle mass, muscle strength, and muscle function.

adults maintain their muscle mass and strength, delaying or preventing the need for institutionalization.

Body fat increases from young adulthood through middle age, peaking at approximately 55 to 65 years of age. Females experience a sharper increase in percent body fat compared to males. With aging, body fat shifts from subcutaneous stores, just below the skin, to internal or visceral fat stores, particularly in males. Increases in abdominal fat coincide with an increased risk for heart disease, diabetes, metabolic syndrome, functional impairments, and all-cause mortality.[10] Maintaining an appropriate energy intake and remaining physically active can help keep body fat to a healthful level.

An increasing number of elderly are at risk for **sarcopenic obesity,** which is strongly associated with metabolic dysfunction, frailty, disability, and inability to perform normal activities of daily living.[11] While total body weight and body fat are increased in these persons, their underlying muscle mass and strength are not adequate in amount or strength to support normal mobility and health. An intervention based on a higher protein intake (up to 1.6 g/kg/d or 45% of total Calories) and a regular program of resistance training could minimize or reverse this age-related loss of muscle mass while supporting moderate weight loss.

Bone mineral density declines with age and may eventually drop to the critical fracture zone. Among older women, the onset of menopause leads to a sudden and dramatic loss of bone due to the lack of estrogen (**Figure 18.1**). Although less dramatic, elderly males also experience loss of bone, due in part to decreasing levels of testosterone. (The nutrients recognized as essential to optimal bone health are identified in Chapter 11.) As noted in the **Highlight** box **Seniors on the Move,** bone health can be promoted through regular weight-bearing activity in adults well into their nineties and beyond.

Age-Related Changes in Organ Function

Aged organs are less adaptable to environmental or physiologic stressors. Young adults, for example, readily adapt to varying levels of fluid and sodium intakes because of the kidney's ability to maintain fluid balance. With increasing age, however, the kidneys lose their ability to concentrate waste products, leading to an increase in urine output and greater risk

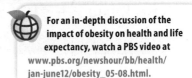

For an in-depth discussion of the impact of obesity on health and life expectancy, watch a PBS video at www.pbs.org/newshour/bb/health/jan-june12/obesity_05-08.html.

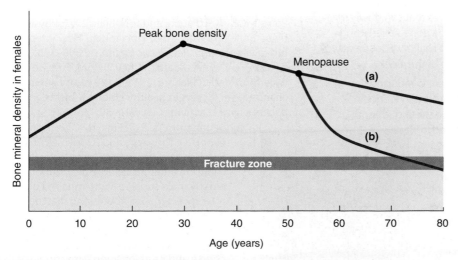

FIGURE 18.1 Bone mineral density in women tends to decline with aging. **(a)** A healthful lifestyle, an optimal diet, physical activity, and possible use of medication slow loss of bone. **(b)** The rapid loss of estrogen with menopause can cause a decrease in bone density and increased risk for bone fracture for women who do not adhere to a regimen of healthful lifestyle, diet, physical activity, and possibly medication.

sarcopenic obesity A condition in which increased body weight and body fat mass coexist with inappropriately low muscle mass and strength.

HIGHLIGHT

Seniors on the Move

Despite the proven benefits of an active lifestyle, relatively few older adults participate in regular leisure-time physical activity.

For a minor investment of time and energy, older adults reap benefits worth literally thousands of dollars in reduced healthcare costs. A regular program of physical activity lowers the risk for heart disease, hypertension, type 2 diabetes, obesity, macular degeneration, depression, and dementia.[1–4] The complications of arthritis can also be reduced with appropriate exercise, as can the risk for falls, bone fractures, and functional impairment.[5] The need for healthcare visits, diagnostics, medication, and other treatments to control blood glucose, serum cholesterol, blood pressure, and other factors in chronic illness can be reduced or eliminated with regular exercise.

Physically active elders live longer and enjoy better health while they live. Muscular strength and total daily energy expenditure are independently associated with lower risk for death among the elderly. The level of activity needed to improve health is not even that great: moderate- and even light-intensity activity greatly reduce risk for type 2 diabetes. Older adults should plan an activity program that includes four basic types of exercises:[1]

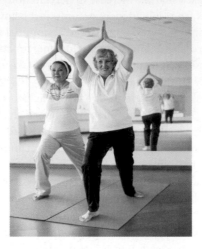

- **Flexibility exercises.** These activities set the stage for other forms of exercise by stretching the muscles and improving range of motion. Gentle arm swings, ankle circles, and torso twists are examples of moves that can slowly increase flexibility. Such exercises can be done while sitting in a chair, standing, or even while in a shallow pool. Ideally, older adults should stretch every day of the week.

- **Balance exercises.** Balance is important in reducing the risk for falls. Older adults should also have confidence in their ability to maintain balance before starting strength or endurance exercises. Toe raises, side leg raises, and rear leg swings are examples of balance activities; tai chi is another popular way to improve balance. Older adults to start balance exercises by holding a table or large chair with both hands, then progress to using one or no hands according to their abilities. Older adults should practice balance activities daily.

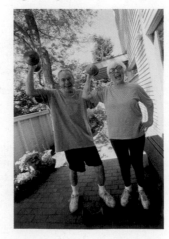

- **Strength or resistance training.** This type of activity can increase muscle mass and strength as well as enhance bone density, preserving the ability of older adults to maintain an independent lifestyle. Gains in muscle strength also improve balance and provide the foundation for endurance exercise. Ideally, older adults should engage in resistance training 2 to 3 days a week.

- **Endurance or aerobic exercise.** Activities such as brisk walking, bicycle riding, swimming, and dancing increase heart rate and improve cardiorespiratory function.

These activities should be low impact to minimize risk to aging bones, joints, and muscles. Older adults should aim for an intensity perceived as "fairly light" to "somewhat hard"—a level that is challenging but not exhausting. As with resistance training, older adults should check with their healthcare provider before starting on a program of endurance exercise. Once given approval, they aim for aerobic activities at least 3 days each week for 30 or more minutes a day.

Some seniors are vulnerable to exercise-related complications, such as dehydration, heat stress, fractures, or falls. Exercise rooms should offer appropriate temperature, ventilation and lighting, and supervised warm-up and cool-down periods should be incorporated into each activity. A thorough medical exam is advised prior to the start of programmed exercise.

The benefits of regular physical activity by older adults almost always far outweigh potential risks—the payoff is better health, more independence, less disability, and a longer, happier life!

References

1. Powell, K. E., A. E. Pauch, and S. N. Blair. 2011. Physical activity for health: what kind? How much? How intense? On top of what? *Annu. Rev. Public Health.* 32:349–365.
2. Genton, L., V. L. Karsegard, T. Chevalley, M. P. Kossovsky, P. Darmon, and C. Pichard. 2011. Body composition changes over 9 years in healthy elderly subjects and impact of physical activity. *Clin. Nutr.* 30:436–442.
3. Segerström, A. B., T. Elgzyri, K. Eriksson, L. Groop, O. Thorsson, and P. Wollmer. 2011. Exercise capacity in relation to body fat distribution and muscle fibre distribution in elderly male subjects with impaired glucose tolerance, type 2 diabetes and matched controls. *Diab. Res. Clin. Pract.* 94:57–63.
4. Middleton, L. E., D. E. Barnes, L. Lui, and K. Yaffe. 2010. Physical activity over the life course and its association with cognitive performance and impairment in old age. *J. Am. Geriatr. Soc.* 58:1322–1326.
5. Fahlman, M. M., N. McNevin, D. Boardley, A. Morgan, and R. Topp. 2011. Effects of resistance training on functional ability in elderly individuals. *Am. J. Health Promotion.* 25:237–243.

for dehydration. The aging liver is less efficient at breaking down drugs or alcohol, and the aging heart lacks the endurance to sustain a sudden increase in physical activity. The pancreas is less precise in regulating blood glucose levels, and bladder control may decline with aging. In most instances, older adults can adapt to these age-related changes through minor lifestyle adjustments, such as eating meals and snacks on a regular basis and ensuring an adequate fluid intake.

As a result of abnormal protein cross-linkages, connective tissues and blood vessels become increasingly stiff. Joint pain, elevated blood pressure, and impaired blood flow are typical consequences. The skin of older adults can become thin, dry, and fragile. Bruises and skin tears are very common and are slow to heal. The growth of nails slows and hair loss is common among elderly males and females. Although some of these consequences are simply cosmetic and represent no disease risk, the skin's tendency to bruise and tear may increase the risk for infection. A diet rich in vitamins C and A, zinc, copper, and protein may reduce the severity of bruising in some elderly.

The number of neurons in the brain decreases with age, impairing memory, reflexes, coordination, and learning ability. Whereas some believe that dementia is an inevitable part of the aging process, this is not true. As we discuss shortly, a healthful diet, regular physical activity, social interaction, intellectual stimulation, and other lifestyle choices can promote cognitive functioning.

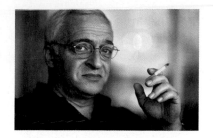

Older adults who smoke should remember that it's never too late to quit, and significant health improvements can manifest within weeks of quitting.

What Lifestyle Factors Accelerate Aging?

The way we live greatly influences the way we age. Whereas chronologic age is immovable, **biologic age** can be greatly influenced by personal choices and decisions. It is now possible to predict one's biologic age through a series of scored questions related to smoking habits, alcohol consumption, sun exposure, weight status, level of physical activity, and other factors. A similar approach is used to estimate potential longevity.

In addition to causing a variety of cancers, direct or secondhand exposure to cigarette and cigar smoke accelerates the aging process; inhalation of the thousands of toxins found in smoke impairs lung function, damages the cardiovascular system, increases the risk for osteoporosis, and impairs taste and odor perception. Smoking also causes premature facial wrinkling and impairs dental health. Older adults should be reminded that it is never too late to quit; improvements in taste perception, physical endurance, and lung function can be detected within weeks of smoking cessation.

Excessive consumption of alcohol also speeds up the aging process by interfering with nutrient intake and utilization, injuring the liver, increasing risk for osteoporosis, and contributing to accidental injuries and deaths (see the In Depth coverage of alcohol, pages 160–171). These effects are cumulative over the years, so the earlier the alcohol abuse begins, the greater the damage to body systems.

Sunlight exposure is the primary risk factor for age-related discoloration and thinning of the skin, as well as skin cancer. Most healthcare providers recommend that, after an initial 20 minutes of sun exposure to allow for skin production of vitamin D, people apply the application sunscreen in order to limit sun-induced skin damage.

Maintaining a normal weight is associated with healthy and successful aging. Excess body weight, at any age, speeds up the deterioration of joints, increasing the risk for osteoarthritis and numerous metabolic disorders, as well as contributing to functional limitations.[12] In addition, successful control of blood glucose—in part through weight management and physical activity—can delay the glycosylation of blood and tissue proteins. When people with diabetes fail to control their blood glucose levels, they experience chronic hyperglycemia and develop complications that seem to mimic the aging process. Obesity also accelerates age-related declines in cardiovascular health.

Lack of physical activity in older adults accelerates loss of muscle mass and bone density, increases risk for falls, is associated with depression and loss of cognitive function, and impairs the ability to perform simple activities of daily living.[13]

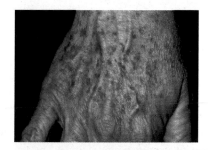

Lifelong exposure to sunlight can lead to discoloration and thinning of the skin in old age.

biologic age Physiologic age as determined by health and functional status; often estimated by scored questionnaires.

RECAP

The American population, as a whole, is aging. The very elderly—those 85 years of age and above—represent the fastest-growing segment of the U.S. population. Scientists are beginning to understand some of the basic cellular changes that contribute to aging and how diet and nutrition might influence the aging process. With aging, sensory perception declines, muscle mass is lost, fat mass increases, bone density decreases, and nutrient metabolism is impaired. Body organs can lose functional capacity and are less tolerant of stressors. These age-related changes influence the nutritional needs of older adults and their ability to consume a healthful diet. Tobacco use, alcohol abuse, excessive sun exposure, overweight, and inactivity accelerate the aging process. ■

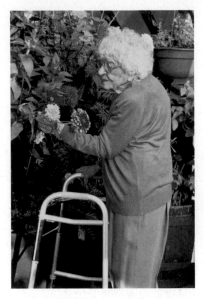

A less physically active lifestyle leads to lower total energy requirements in older adults.

What Are an Older Adult's Nutrient Needs?

The requirements for many nutrients are the same for older adults as for young and middle-aged adults. A few nutrient requirements increase, and a few are actually lower. **Table 18.2** identifies those recommendations that change with age, as well as the physiologic reason behind these changes.

Older Adults Have Lower Energy Needs

The energy needs of older adults are lower than those of younger adults, because loss of muscle mass and lean tissue results in a lower basal metabolic rate, and most older adults have a less physically active lifestyle. It is estimated that total daily energy expenditure decreases approximately 10 kcal each year for men and 7 kcal each year for women ages 19 and older. This means that a woman who needed 2,000 kcal at age 20 needs just 1,650 kcal at age 70. Some of this decrease in energy expenditure is in response to age-related decreases in muscle mass, but some of the decrease can be delayed or minimized by staying physically active.

TABLE 18.2 Nutrition Recommendations That Change with Increased Age

Changes in Nutrient Recommendations	Rationale for Changes
Increased need for vitamin D from 600 IU/day for adults up to age 70, to 800 IU/day for adults over 70	■ Decreased bone density ■ Decreased ability to synthesize vitamin D in the skin
Increased need for calcium from 1,000 mg/day for all adults up to age 51 and males 51–70 years of age to 1,200 mg/day for females 51 years of age and older and males over age 70 years	■ Decreased absorption of dietary calcium ■ Decreased bone density (earlier onset in women)
Decreased need for fiber from 38 g/day for males up to age 51 to 30 g/day for males 51 and older; decreases for females are from 25 g/day for females up to age 51 to 21 g/day for females 51 and older	■ Decreased energy intake
Increased need for vitamin B_6 in both males and females from 1.3 mg/day up to age 51 to 1.7 mg/day in males and 1.5 mg/day in females age 51 and older; need for vitamin B_{12} *from fortified foods or supplements*, as opposed to foods of animal origin	■ Increased need for these vitamins to maintain blood levels adequate to reduce homocysteine levels and to optimize immune function ■ Lower levels of stomach acid ■ Decreased absorption of food B_{12} from gastrointestinal tract
Decreased need for iron for females, from 18 mg/day up to age 51 to 8 mg/day for females 51 and older; no change in 8 mg/day iron recommendations for males	■ Cessation of menstruation in women; some loss of muscle and lean tissue in men and women

Because their total daily energy needs are lower, older adults need to pay particularly close attention to consuming a diet high in nutrient-dense foods but not too high in energy in order to avoid weight gain. The Human Nutrition Research Center at Tufts University has released a MyPlate for Older Adults, which is a helpful guide to food choices for this population (**Figure 18.2**).

Benjamin Franklin once noted, "To lengthen thy life, lessen thy meals." Refer to the **Nutrition Debate** at the end of this chapter to learn more about the theory of energy restriction, which proposes that Calorie-restricted diets may significantly prolong the human life span.

Macronutrient Recommendations Are Similar for Adults of All Ages

Because there is no evidence suggesting a minimal amount of dietary fat needed to maintain health, there is no DRI for total fat intake for older adults.[14] However, to reduce the risk for heart disease and other chronic diseases, it is recommended that total fat intake remain within 20% to 35% of total daily energy intake, with no more than 10% of total energy intake coming from saturated fat. Dietary sources of *trans* fatty acids should be kept to a minimum.

The RDA for carbohydrate for older adults is 130 g/day.[14] As with all other age groups, this level of carbohydrate is sufficient to support glucose utilization by the brain. There is no evidence to indicate what percentage of carbohydrate should come from sugars or starches. However, it is recommended that older individuals consume a diet that contains no more than 25% of total energy intake as sugars.[14]

The fiber recommendations are slightly lower for older adults than for younger adults, because older adults consume less energy. After age 50, 30 g of fiber per day for men and

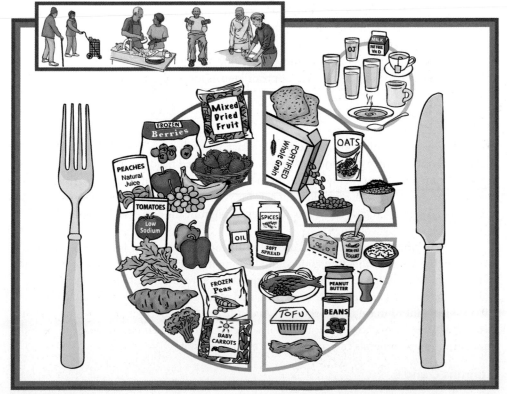

MyPlate for Older Adults

©2011 Tufts University   http://nutrition.tufts.edu/research/myplate-older-adults

FIGURE 18.2 The Tufts University MyPlate for Older Adults illustrates healthful food and fluid choices appropriate for older adults. (*Source:* Copyright 2011 Tufts University. For details about the MyPlate for Older Adults, please see http://nutrition.tufts.edu/research/myplate-older-adults.)

21 g per day for women is assumed sufficient to reduce the risks for constipation and diverticular disease, maintain healthful blood levels of glucose and lipids, and provide good sources of nutrient-dense, low-energy foods.

The DRI for protein is the same for adults of all ages: 0.8 g of protein per kilogram of body weight per day.[14] Although some researchers have argued for a higher protein allowance of 1.2 g/kg/day for older adults in order to optimize protein status, the benefits of a higher protein intake in the elderly remain unclear.[15] Protein is critical in helping reduce loss of muscle and lean tissue, maintaining immunity, enhancing wound healing and disease recovery, and helping prevent excessive loss of bone. Protein-rich foods are also important sources of vitamins and minerals that are typically low in the diets of older adults, including iron, zinc, and certain B-vitamins.

Some Micronutrient Recommendations Vary for Older Adults

The vitamins and minerals of particular concern for older adults are identified in Table 18.2.

Vitamin D and Calcium

Adequate vitamin D status is critical for preventing or minimizing the consequences of osteoporosis among older adults.[16] The requirement for vitamin D is higher than for younger adults because of an age-related reduction in the production of vitamin D in the skin. An increasing number of older adults are at risk for vitamin D deficiency because they are institutionalized and are not exposed to adequate amounts of sunlight. Others may limit intake of milk and dairy products due to lactose intolerance or perceived concerns over the fat content of these foods. Older adults living in the community are also at risk for vitamin D deficiency due to the widespread use of sunscreen; these creams and lotions are important to prevent skin cancer, but they block the sunlight needed for vitamin D synthesis in the skin. In addition to its role in bone health, vitamin D deficiency is associated with increased risk for cognitive impairment, falls, cardiovascular disease, diabetes, infectious diseases, and overall mortality.[17–19]

The RDA for calcium is higher for all adults over the age of 70 years and for women aged 51 to 70 years compared to younger adults. The calcium requirement increases at an earlier age for women compared to men due to the earlier onset of bone loss, typically at the onset of menopause.[16]

It is critical that older adults consume foods that are high in calcium and vitamin D and, when needed, use supplements in appropriate amounts and under the guidance of a healthcare provider.[20]

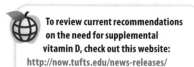

To review current recommendations on the need for supplemental vitamin D, check out this website:
http://now.tufts.edu/news-releases/ higher-not-lower-doses-vitamin-d-are- effectiv.

Iron and Zinc

Iron needs decrease with aging as a result of reduced muscle mass in both men and women and the cessation of menstruation in women. The decreased need for iron in older men is not significant enough to change the recommendations for iron intake in this group; thus, the RDA for iron is the same for older men as for younger, 8 mg/day. The RDA for iron in older women is also 8 mg/day, but this represents a significant decrease from the 18 mg/ day RDA for younger women.[21]

Although zinc recommendations are the same for all adults, zinc is especially critical for optimizing immune function and wound healing in older adults.[22] Intakes of both zinc and iron can be inadequate in older adults if they do not regularly eat red meats, poultry, and fish. These foods are relatively expensive, and older adults on a limited income may not be able to afford to eat them regularly. Also, the loss of teeth or use of dentures may increase the difficulty of chewing meats. Finally, age-related impairments in absorption and transport of these minerals can contribute to a deficient state.

Vitamins C and E

Although older adults are typically viewed as have increased levels of oxidative stress, the recommendations for vitamin C and vitamin E intakes are the same as for younger adults, because there is insufficient evidence that consuming amounts above the current RDA has any additional health benefits.[23–25] Researchers continue, however, to investigate the potential benefits of dietary or supplemental vitamin C and the roles it may play in lowering the risk for hypertension, impaired physical performance, and other age-related disorders.[23,24] Vitamin E also continues to be evaluated for its potential to reduce risk for cataracts, age-related macular degeneration, and other forms of oxidative stress.[26,27]

B-Vitamins

Older adults need to pay close attention to consuming adequate amounts of the B-vitamins, specifically vitamin B_6, vitamin B_{12}, and folate.[28] Inadequate intakes of these nutrients increases the level of the amino acid homocysteine in the blood, a state that has been linked to elevated risk for cardiovascular disease, age-related dementia (including Alzheimer's disease), and loss of cognitive function in the elderly.[29] Older adults with impaired vitamin B_6 and/or B_{12} status are at higher risk for depression and poor cognition.[30]

Vitamin B_6 recommendations are slightly higher for adults age 51 and older. The increased requirement is based on data indicating that more vitamin B_6 is required to maintain normal vitamin B_6 status as we age. These higher amounts appear necessary to reduce homocysteine levels and optimize attentiveness and cognition, as well as decrease risk for depression.[30]

The RDA for vitamin B_{12} is the same for younger and older adults; however, up to 30% of older adults experience atrophic gastritis and cannot absorb enough vitamin B_{12} from foods. It is therefore recommended that older adults consume foods that are fortified with vitamin B_{12} or take B_{12} supplements, because the vitamin B_{12} in these products is absorbed more readily.[31]

Vitamin A

Vitamin A requirements are the same for adults of all ages; however, older adults should be careful not to consume more than the RDA, as absorption of vitamin A is actually greater in older adults.[21] The consequences of vitamin A toxicity in the elderly can be significant: liver damage, neurologic problems, and increased risk for hip fracture.[32] Consuming foods high in beta-carotene or other carotenoids is safe and does not lead to vitamin A toxicity. In fact, increased intakes of lutein and zeaxanthin, two common carotenoids, reduce risk for late-onset age-related macular degeneration.[33]

Do Older Adults Need Micronutrient Supplements?

A variety of factors may limit an older adult's ability to eat healthfully.[34,35] Limited financial resources may prevent some older people from buying nutrient-dense foods on a regular basis; others may experience reduced appetite, social isolation, inability to prepare foods, or illnesses that limit nutrient absorption and metabolism. Thus, many older adults do benefit from taking a multivitamin and multimineral supplement that contains no more than the RDA for each nutrient. Healthcare providers typically encourage use of these supplements under the following conditions:

- When the amount and/or variety of food is so restricted that nutrient intake is probably deficient
- If the older adult eats fewer than two meals per day or limits food choices because of dental problems
- Whenever there are lifestyle or functional limitations that prevent adequate food intake
- If the older adult suffers from depression, dementia, social isolation, or extreme poverty
- If the older adult has a disease that impairs nutrient status or that could be relieved by nutrient supplementation
- If the older adult has osteoporosis, gastrointestinal diseases, or anemia

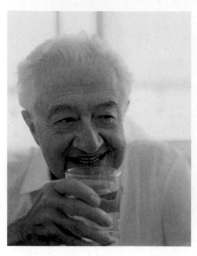

Older adults need the same amount of fluid as other adults.

Additional single-nutrient supplements, especially for vitamin B_{12}, may also be prescribed. In establishing the DRI for vitamin B_{12} for men and women over the age of 50 years, the Institute of Medicine stated, "It is advisable for most of this amount to be obtained by consuming foods fortified with B_{12} or a B_{12} containing supplement."[28] This is the first time that the IOM specifically acknowledged and supported the use of a nutrient supplement as an adjunct to a healthful diet. Many healthcare providers also recommend routine use of calcium and vitamin D supplements.

High-potency single-nutrient supplements can pose risks to the elderly. Older adults are more vulnerable to high-potency vitamin A supplements than younger adults, especially if they abuse alcohol. Vitamin D is also extremely toxic at high levels of intake, and megadoses of vitamin C can produce diarrhea and cramping. Inappropriate supplementation with iron leads to its accumulation in the liver, pancreas, and other soft tissues, particularly in middle-aged and older men. In short, older adults should avoid high-potency single-nutrient supplements unless they have been prescribed. The **Highlight** box, **Supplements for Seniors** (page 737), explains the formulation of commercial multivitamin-multimineral supplements designed specifically for older adults.

Fluid Recommendations Are the Same for All Adults

The AI for fluid is the same for all adults.[36] Men should consume 3.7 L (about 15.5 cups) of total water per day, which includes 3.0 L (about 13 cups) as total beverages, including drinking water. Women should consume 2.7 L (about 12.7 cups) of total water per day, which includes 2.2 L (about 9 cups) as total beverages, including drinking water.

In general, the elderly do not perceive thirst as effectively as do younger adults. Thus, they are at increased risk for chronic dehydration and hypernatremia (elevated blood sodium levels). Some older adults intentionally limit their beverage intake because they have urinary incontinence or do not want to be awakened for nighttime urination. This practice can endanger their health, so it is important for these individuals to seek treatment for the incontinence and continue to drink adequate amounts of fluids.

RECAP

Older adults have lower energy needs due to their loss of lean tissue and lower physical activity levels. They should consume 20% to 35% of total energy as fat and 45% to 65% as carbohydrate. Protein recommendations are currently the same as for younger adults, although some research suggests the need for slightly higher intakes. Micronutrients of concern for older adults include calcium, vitamin D, vitamin B_{12}, and others. Many older adults benefit from taking a multivitamin/multimineral supplement. Older adults are at risk for chronic dehydration and hypernatremia, so ample fluid intake should be encouraged. ∎

What Nutritional Concerns Threaten the Health of Older Adults?

In this section, we discuss several common nutrition-related concerns of older adults. As we explore each concern, we will attempt to answer two questions: (1) What, if any, nutrient concerns develop as a result of a specific medical disorder? (2) What, if any, effect does nutritional status have on the risk of developing that disorder?

Both Overweight and Underweight Are Serious Concerns

Not surprisingly, overweight and obesity are of concern for older adults.[37] In the United States, over 35% of adults over the age of 60 years are classified as obese, nearly 21 million elders. It is predicted that the rate of geriatric obesity will climb over the next few decades

HIGHLIGHT

Supplements for Seniors

Consumers have thousands of different options when shopping for nutritional supplements. Even if looking for a "simple" multivitamin/multimineral (MVMM) supplement, there are many available products, including those formulated specifically for seniors. How do these senior ("silver") products differ from other MVMM products? Are they actually better for seniors or just a marketing ploy? A close look at such products yields some interesting information.

Although every product line has its own formulation, a side-by-side comparison of the nutrients in one typical "adult" MVMM supplement with those in a "senior" MVMM product from the same manufacturer reveals very few differences. Of the thirty-three nutrients in the adult product, two (iron and tin) are omitted from the senior supplement, one (vitamin K) is provided at a lower dosage, three (calcium and vitamins E and B_6) are included at slightly higher levels, and one (vitamin B_{12}) is four times higher in the senior supplement. Although not all of these product modifications reflect age-specific DRI values (see the endpages of this book for DRI values), there are good reasons for most of these product adjustments. As you compare the product labels, remember that the US Food and Drug Administration (FDA) uses "% Daily Value" to describe nutrient levels, not the newer DRI recommendations.

Although the DRI for vitamin E does not change for males or females ages 19 to 70 years or above, there is good evidence that older adults are often in a state of "oxidative stress." Chronic inflammation, as occurs with arthritis and other conditions, is more common among older adults than younger populations and may increase the need for antioxidants, such as vitamin E. In addition, as previously discussed, there is preliminary, but inconsistent, research supporting the use of vitamin E in lowering the risk for age-associated eye disorders and dementia. Knowing that vitamin E has a relatively low risk for toxicity, the small increase provided in the senior supplement certainly poses no harm.

As with vitamin E, the DRI for vitamin K does not change with increased age. Why, then, does the senior supplement provide a lower dose? Persons on anticoagulant drugs, many of them elderly, are advised to tightly regulate vitamin K intake. By minimizing the amount of vitamin K in the senior supplement, there is less risk for a negative drug–nutrient interaction among seniors taking both the MVMM supplement and anticoagulant drugs. Some physicians might consider even 13% of the vitamin K Daily Value to be too much, so it would be important for each senior to

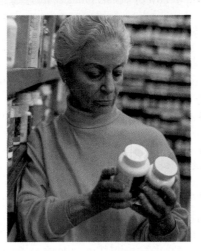

Many supplements are targeted for the elderly.

check with his or her doctor before using a MVMM with any vitamin K.

Although the senior supplement provides about 40 mg more calcium than the more general adult product, that amount does not go very far toward satisfying the DRI guideline of an additional 200 mg of calcium per day for adults 51 years and above. Calcium is too "bulky" for most MVMM supplements, so all adults, regardless of their stage of life, should choose a specific calcium supplement (possibly one with vitamin D and/or vitamin K) if their food choices do not provide adequate dietary calcium. The DRI for vitamin B_6 for adults 51 years and older is slightly higher than that for younger adults, and the senior supplement reflects that increase by providing 50% more vitamin B_6 than the MVMM product targeting the general adult population. This higher intake may provide additional protection against elevated serum homocysteine, a possible risk factor for heart disease.

As discussed earlier, many adults over the age of 50 years poorly absorb vitamin B_{12} from food sources. Older adults are advised to consume foods that are fortified with vitamin B_{12} or supplements, because the vitamin B_{12} in these sources is absorbed more readily than the vitamin B_{12} in food. Although the DRI recommends a change in the *source* of vitamin B_{12} rather than in the *amount,* the higher dosage in the senior supplement poses no harm.

What about the omission of iron from the senior supplement? Certainly, iron is a nutrient essential for good health; why would a manufacturer totally omit it from the product? A woman's need for iron decreases dramatically after menopause; most women can easily meet that need from food alone. In addition, risk for iron overload increases with age, particularly in older men; thus, eliminating iron from senior supplements actually lowers the risk for inappropriate iron loading. If an older adult has a specific need for supplemental iron—for example, following significant blood loss—his or her physician can recommend an iron-only supplement. Tin is the other mineral eliminated from the senior product; because tin has no Daily Value or DRI, there is no strong justification for including it in the senior supplement.

Each age-specific MVMM product line should be evaluated carefully to determine if the nutrient balance is appropriate for seniors. When consumed with a well-balanced diet, the small but important differences between supplements designed for seniors and supplements designed for middle-age adults can help seniors obtain the appropriate amounts of all the nutrients they need.

due to the higher rate of obesity in young and middle-aged adults and the earlier age of obesity onset. The elderly population as a whole has a high risk for heart disease, hypertension, type 2 diabetes, and cancer, and these diseases are more prevalent in older adults who are overweight or obese. Obesity increases the severity and consequences of osteoarthritis, limits the mobility of elderly adults, and is associated with functional declines in daily activities and cognition.

Although some healthcare providers may question the necessity or value of attempting weight loss at the age of 70 or 75 years, even moderate weight loss in obese elderly can improve metabolic and functional status. Weight loss should be encouraged in those elderly who are obese, as defined by measures of body composition, and who suffer from metabolic or functional complications. Older adults diagnosed with sarcopenic obesity need ongoing medical oversight if weight-loss efforts are undertaken. For all overweight or obese elderly, the goals are the same: clinically significant weight loss that minimizes muscle and bone loss.[37] The interventions for obese elderly are the same as for younger and middle-aged adults: lifestyle interventions, including the adoption of dietary modifications to achieve an energy deficit while retaining adequate nutrient intakes; gradual and medically appropriate initiation of physical activity to preserve lean body mass; and culturally appropriate behavior modification. In those cases where medications contribute to inappropriate weight gain, it may be possible to find an effective alternative medication that does not cause weight gain.

There are very few research studies on the effectiveness of anti-obesity drugs in the elderly. The benefit of bariatric (weight-loss) surgery for this population also is not clear. Obese elderly experience more complications, experience a smaller weight loss, and demonstrate less improvement in metabolic disorders following bariatric surgery compared to younger adults. However, with improvements in surgical techniques and postoperative care, there is general consensus that older adults should not be denied bariatric surgery only on the basis of their age.[37]

Recall that mortality rates are higher in adults who are underweight (BMI below 18.5) compared to people who are overweight (see Figure 13.2 on page 508). Significantly under weight older adults have fewer protein reserves to call upon during periods of catabolic stress, such as after surgery or after trauma, and are more susceptible to infection. Inappropriate weight loss suggests inadequate intake of both energy and nutrients. Chronic deficiencies of protein, vitamins, and minerals leave older adults at risk for poor wound healing and a depressed immune response.

Because underweight is so risky for elders, geriatric weight loss is an important healthcare concern. Gerontologists have identified nine "Ds" that account for most cases of geriatric weight loss (**Figure 18.3**). Several of these factors promote weight loss by reducing energy intake. They include drugs that decrease appetite, as well as eating impairments, such as dementia, poor dentition, dysgeusia, dysphagia, and dysfunction. Depression, which is common after the death of family members and friends or when adult children move out of the area, also contributes to reduced food intake. Treatment of inappropriate weight loss in the elderly is often a complex and lengthy process, relying on behavioral, medical, and psychological interventions.

In summary, any of the nine Ds can promote underweight, nutrient deficiencies, and frailty, significantly increasing the risk for serious illnesses, injuries, and death. A condition known as **geriatric failure-to-thrive,** also called "the dwindles," characterizes the complexity of age-related weight loss and related health factors.

Millions of Older Adults Have Osteoporosis

In the United States, about 10 million adults have osteoporosis; about 80% are female. Another 40 million are estimated to have low bone mass, a predictor of osteoporosis.[38] Among women, osteoporosis is typically diagnosed within a few years of menopause as estrogen levels sharply decline. Due in part to a higher peak bone density, the onset in males

geriatric failure-to-thrive Inappropriate, unexplained loss of body weight and muscle mass; usually results from a combination of environmental and health factors.

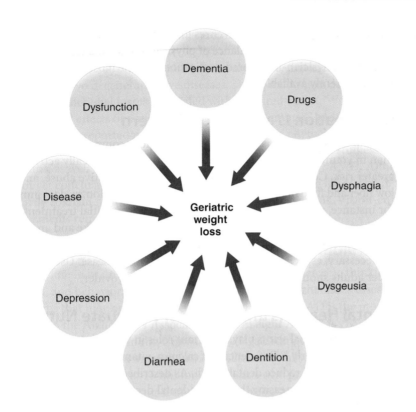

FIGURE 18.3 The nine Ds of geriatric weight loss: many factors contribute to inappropriate weight loss in the elderly.

is usually delayed until their seventies or eighties and is linked to declining testosterone levels, steroid therapy, and alcohol abuse. Men with osteoporosis are less likely to be diagnosed or treated for osteoporosis compared to women, although the medical community is now more aware of and responsive to the problem in men.

Many options are available for the treatment of osteoporosis, including a combination of dietary interventions, strength or resistance training, and medications. While calcium and vitamin D are typically associated with bone health, at least eight other minerals, four other vitamins, protein, and total energy are important in sustaining bone density and structure.[39] In addition, it is important to minimize an older adult's risk for a fall-induced fracture by assessing vision and balance, evaluating the need for a cane or walker, surveying the home environment for hazards, and reviewing medications.

Perhaps Half of Older Adults Experience Arthritis

Arthritis is one of the most prevalent chronic diseases among the elderly, affecting as many as half of all adults over the age of 65. It can affect one or multiple joints, cause pain on a daily or intermittent basis, and limit range of motion of one or more joints. The two most common forms of arthritis among the elderly are osteoarthritis and rheumatoid arthritis.

Osteoarthritis has been called a disease of "wear and tear." People with arthritis who are overweight or obese are strongly advised to lose weight and to participate in water exercise or other acceptable forms of physical activity. Pain medications and anti-inflammatory drugs may be prescribed. In extreme cases, hip or knee replacement surgery is required to reestablish normal mobility and function.

Rheumatoid arthritis (RA) typically strikes younger adults and is not associated with obesity or overuse syndromes. It often affects both hands, wrists, or knees. Because many people with RA are underweight, the nutritional goals focus on appropriate weight gain and a healthful, balanced intake of all nutrients. A wide range of medications is used to treat RA, but some of these interfere with nutrient utilization.

Arthritic adults may turn to nontraditional treatments. Glucosamine has shown some promise in relieving the symptoms of osteoarthritis; however, the majority of herbs, oils, and

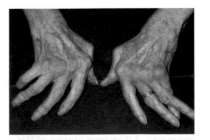

Rheumatoid arthritis often affects the hands.

TABLE 18.3 Examples of Common Drug–Nutrient Interactions

Category of Drug	Common Nutrient/Food Interactions
Antacids	May decrease the absorption of iron, calcium, folate, vitamin B_{12}
Antibiotics	May reduce the absorption of calcium, fat-soluble vitamins; reduce the production of vitamin K by gut bacteria
Anticonvulsants	Interfere with the activation of vitamin D
Anticoagulants ("blood thinners")	Oppose the clotting activity of vitamin K
Antidepressants	May cause weight gain as a result of increased appetite
Antiretroviral agents (treatment of HIV/AIDS)	Reduce the absorption of most nutrients
Aspirin	Decrease blood folate levels; increase loss of iron due to gastric bleeding
Diuretics	Some types may increase urinary loss of potassium, sodium, calcium, magnesium; others cause retention of potassium and other electrolytes
Laxatives	Increase fecal excretion of dietary fat, fat-soluble vitamins, calcium, other minerals

Numerous drugs are known to alter nutrient digestion and absorption. Long-term antibiotic therapy can lead to diarrhea and generalized malabsorption, as well as malabsorption of calcium specifically. Other drugs may block uptake of other micronutrients.

Many drugs negatively affect the activation or metabolism of nutrients such as vitamin D, folate, and vitamin B_6, contributing to secondary nutrient deficiencies even when nutrient intake is adequate. Several types of anti-epileptic drugs interfere with the activation of dietary vitamin D, leading to impaired bone health. Other medications increase the kidneys' excretion of nutrients.

Nutrition
MILESTONE

When nutritionists think of malnutrition, most immediately visualize an undernourished infant or child. It wasn't until the 1980s that geriatric malnutrition was recognized as a significant problem within the United States and across the globe.

In **1991**, researchers in France, Switzerland, and the United States began collaborating to develop a valid tool to assess the nutritional status of the elderly. The result was the Mini Nutritional Assessment (MNA), which today is considered the "gold standard." The MNA is composed of only eighteen questions but takes at least 10–15 minutes to complete, and it must be administered by a healthcare professional. In the 1990s, the American Dietetic Association, the American Academy of Family Physicians, and the National Council on Aging developed a shorter, self-administered nutrition questionnaire known by its acronym DETERMINE. Since then, other screening tools have been developed, each with its own strengths and disadvantages, but all with the potential to identify elderly, whether living in their own homes, in a care center, or in the hospital, who are at risk for malnutrition. The problem of geriatric malnutrition cannot be addressed unless it is first appropriately identified.

Effects of Nutritional Status or Intake on Medications

The activity of a specific drug is often impacted by nutritional status, including obesity, protein deficiency, and fluid imbalance. In other cases, micronutrient status or intake alters drug metabolism. For example, older adults taking the blood-thinning drug warfarin (Coumadin) should avoid consuming excess vitamin E, as vitamin E magnifies the effects of this drug. Both ibuprofen (Advil or Motrin) and acetaminophen (Tylenol) are commonly prescribed for muscle, joint, and headache pain, but taking these drugs with alcohol increases the risk for liver damage and bleeding, so alcohol should not be consumed with these medications. Consumption of iron supplements often reduces the absorption of certain antibiotics, and vitamin C deficiency prolongs the effect of pentobarbital.[49]

Some medications should be taken before or between meals, including those known to trigger gastrointestinal distress, whereas others are best absorbed and/or utilized when taken with meals. Foods as diverse as grapefruit juice, spinach, and

FIGURE 18.3 The nine Ds of geriatric weight loss: many factors contribute to inappropriate weight loss in the elderly.

Dementia

Dysfunction

Drugs

Disease

Dysphagia

Geriatric
weight
loss

Depression

Dysgeusia

Diarrhea

Dentition

is usually delayed until their seventies or eighties and is linked to declining testosterone levels, steroid therapy, and alcohol abuse. Men with osteoporosis are less likely to be diagnosed or treated for osteoporosis compared to women, although the medical community is now more aware of and responsive to the problem in men.

Many options are available for the treatment of osteoporosis, including a combination of dietary interventions, strength or resistance training, and medications. While calcium and vitamin D are typically associated with bone health, at least eight other minerals, four other vitamins, protein, and total energy are important in sustaining bone density and structure.[39] In addition, it is important to minimize an older adult's risk for a fall-induced fracture by assessing vision and balance, evaluating the need for a cane or walker, surveying the home environment for hazards, and reviewing medications.

Perhaps Half of Older Adults Experience Arthritis

Arthritis is one of the most prevalent chronic diseases among the elderly, affecting as many as half of all adults over the age of 65. It can affect one or multiple joints, cause pain on a daily or intermittent basis, and limit range of motion of one or more joints. The two most common forms of arthritis among the elderly are osteoarthritis and rheumatoid arthritis.

Osteoarthritis has been called a disease of "wear and tear." People with arthritis who are overweight or obese are strongly advised to lose weight and to participate in water exercise or other acceptable forms of physical activity. Pain medications and anti-inflammatory drugs may be prescribed. In extreme cases, hip or knee replacement surgery is required to reestablish normal mobility and function.

Rheumatoid arthritis (RA) typically strikes younger adults and is not associated with obesity or overuse syndromes. It often affects both hands, wrists, or knees. Because many people with RA are underweight, the nutritional goals focus on appropriate weight gain and a healthful, balanced intake of all nutrients. A wide range of medications is used to treat RA, but some of these interfere with nutrient utilization.

Arthritic adults may turn to nontraditional treatments. Glucosamine has shown some promise in relieving the symptoms of osteoarthritis; however, the majority of herbs, oils, and

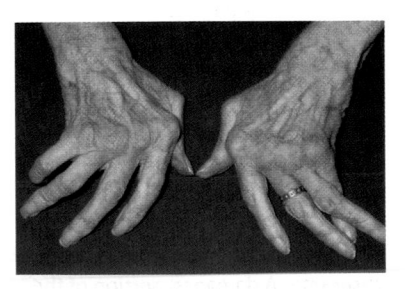

Rheumatoid arthritis often affects the hands.

supermarkets, may not be able to afford transportation to buy healthful food, and may fear leaving their homes to shop for groceries. Their homes may lack working refrigerators and/or stoves, limiting the types of foods that can be bought, stored, and prepared. Healthcare and social service providers should carefully probe for information on the ability of low-income elders to afford an adequate and healthful food supply.

Social Isolation Increases Health Risks

Older adults may become socially isolated for many reasons. Those who are restricted to bed or wheelchairs, have impaired walking, or are in poor health are prone to isolation even if they live in a household with others. The death of a spouse can precipitate isolation, especially among the very old who have also lost siblings and friends.

Lack of adequate transportation also increases the risk for isolation. Family members and friends may not always be able to offer rides, and even where public transportation is available, older adults may be concerned about cost and personal safety. Even if government-funded vans or buses are available for the elderly, transportation may be limited to weekdays and certain hours of the day.

Among minority elderly, particularly recent immigrants with language barriers, isolation can occur after the death of a bilingual spouse or as bilingual children move out of the household. These adults may lack the communication skills to navigate public transportation, shop, and secure social services. Ideally, communities with large immigrant populations can provide translators to help integrate these elderly into the community at large.

Social isolation increases the risk for alcohol and substance abuse, depression, and malnutrition. Personal healthcare habits decline, household maintenance is put off, and behavior becomes increasingly erratic. Isolated older adults are at high risk for victimization, such as telephone scams, and premature institutionalization. Religious, neighborhood, and social service agencies offer many programs to ensure that older adults are not forgotten within their homes.

Community Services Can Help Meet the Nutritional Needs of Older Adults

As the American population continues to age, greater demands are placed on social service agencies. This section identifies several programs available for older adults in need.

Community Nutrition Programs for Older Adults

The federal government has developed an extensive network of food and nutrition services for older Americans. Some are open to people of all ages, whereas others are restricted to people 60 years of age and up. Many are coordinated with state or local governments and community organizations. They include the following:

- *Supplemental Nutrition Assistance Program (SNAP):* This US Department of Agriculture (USDA) program, formerly known as the *Food Stamp Program,* provides food assistance for low-income households. Participants are provided with a monthly allotment, typically as a prepaid debit card. There are very few restrictions on the foods that can be purchased under this plan.
- *Senior Farmers' Market Nutrition Program:* This program is designed to provide fresh, unprocessed, locally grown fruits, vegetables, herbs, and honey from farmers' markets, Community Supported Agriculture (CSA) programs, and roadside stands. Low-income seniors are given coupons to be redeemed for eligible foods.
- *Child and Adult Care Program:* This program provides healthy meals and snacks to older and functionally impaired adults in qualified adult day-care settings.
- *Commodity Supplemental Food Program:* This program serves low-income pregnant women, infants and young children, and older adults. Income guidelines must be met. Specific commodity foods are distributed, including cereals, peanut butter, dry beans, rice or pasta, and canned juice, fruits, vegetables, meat, poultry, and tuna. Unlike SNAP, this program is not intended to provide a complete array of foods.

with surgery. As with macular degeneration, certain lifestyle habits, including dietary patterns, impact the risk for this disease.

Recent research suggests, but does not definitively prove, that dietary choices may slow the progress of these two degenerative eye diseases, saving millions of dollars and preventing or delaying the functional losses associated with impaired vision.[26,42,43] Several studies have shown beneficial effects of antioxidants, including vitamins C and E, on cataract formation, whereas others reported no significant benefit.[43] Two phytochemicals, lutein and zeaxanthin, have also been identified as protective by some, but not all, studies.[33,43] These four antioxidants, as well as zinc, may also provide protection against AMD. Although the research is not yet conclusive, older adults can benefit by consuming foods rich in these nutrients, primarily colorful fruits and vegetables, nuts, and whole grains. Vision-enhancing nutrient supplements remain an unproved therapy.

Age-Related Cognitive Impairment Is Not Inevitable

Dementia is a decline in brain functioning that typically affects memory, thinking, language, judgment, and behavior. An umbrella term, it includes Alzheimer's disease (AD) as well as other forms that may or may not be age-related; however, AD is the most common form. According to the Alzheimer's Association, one in eight Americans has AD, and it is the sixth leading cause of death in the United States. Healthcare costs for people with AD and other forms of dementia are more than $200 billion annually. This estimate does not include the labor of the more than 15 million Americans who provide unpaid care.[44]

Some research suggests that long-term intake of antioxidants, such as vitamin E, and certain unsaturated fatty acids, such as DHA, may lower the risk for dementia.[45] Elevated serum homocysteine, linked to deficiencies of folate and vitamins B_6 and B_{12}, has also been linked to Alzheimer's disease and dementia.[29,30]

Dementia is one of the "nine Ds" associated with geriatric weight loss. Many people with dementia and other forms of cognitive decline simply refuse to eat. Alzheimer's disease can trigger agitation and pacing, increasing energy expenditure.[46] As the disease progresses, the person loses the ability to manipulate utensils and eventually even to swallow. Helping people with dementia eat adequately can be challenging. Finger foods, such as cut-up fruit, cheese or meat cubes, vegetable slices, and small pieces of bread, can be eaten without utensils. Between-meal snacks and liquid nutritional supplements can also improve dietary intake. A multivitamin, multimineral supplement may also be necessary.

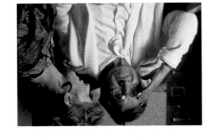

Many people with dementia have difficulty eating adequate portions of healthful food and require help to sustain sufficient energy intake.

Interactions Between Medications and Nutrition Can Be Harmful

Although the elderly account for less than 15% of the U.S. population, they take over 30% of all prescription medication.[47] A recent survey of U.S. community-dwelling older adults showed that a significant number of elderly people used more than five prescription medications at once, a condition termed **polypharmacy**.[48] Based on anecdotal reporting, it is expected that an unknown number of elderly people in the US likely use ten or more medications at once, a practice termed *excessive polypharmacy*. As life expectancy increases and medical management of chronic diseases improves, both of these conditions are likely to become more prevalent.

Effects of Medications on Nutrition

Prescription drugs interact not only with each other but also with nutrients (**Table 18.3**).[49] Some medications increase or decrease food intake, either directly or indirectly. For example, many medications impact neural or hormonal regulation of food intake, whereas others lead to nausea or vomiting or result in decreased production of saliva. The taste, aftertaste, and/or odor of oral medications may be so unpleasant that they reduce appetite. Some drugs cause visual impairment, lead to abnormal motor control, or alter cognition, all of which have the potential to interfere with food acquisition and preparation.

dementia A decline in brain function.

polypharmacy The concurrent use of five or more medications.

Want to learn more about the changes that take place in the brain of someone with AD? Watch this short video from the National Institute on Aging at www.nia.nih.gov/alzheimers/alzheimers-disease-video.

Nutrition

When nutritionists think of malnutrition, most immediately visualize an undernourished infant or child. It wasn't until the 1980s that geriatric malnutrition was recognized as a significant problem within the United States and across the globe.

In **1991**, researchers in France, Switzerland, and the United States began collaborating to develop a valid tool to assess the nutritional status of the elderly. The result was the Mini Nutritional Assessment (MNA), which today is considered the "gold standard". The MNA is composed of only eighteen questions but takes at least 10–15 minutes to complete, and it must be administered by a healthcare professional. In the 1990s, the American Dietetic Association, the American Academy of Family Physicians, and the National Council on Aging developed a shorter, self-administered nutrition questionnaire known by its acronym DETERMINE. Since then, other screening tools have been developed, each with its own strengths and disadvantages, but all with the potential to identify elderly, who are at risk for malnutrition. The problem of geriatric malnutrition cannot be addressed unless it is first appropriately identified.

the kidneys' excretion of nutrients.

Effects of Nutritional Status or Intake on Medications

The activity of a specific drug is often impacted by nutritional status, including obesity, protein deficiency, and fluid imbalance. In other cases, micronutrient status or intake alters drug metabolism. For example, older adults taking the blood-thinning drug warfarin (Coumadin) should avoid consuming excess vitamin E, as vitamin E magnifies the effects of this drug. Both ibuprofen (Advil or Motrin) and acetaminophen (Tylenol) are commonly prescribed for muscle, joint, and headache pain, but taking these drugs with alcohol increases the risk for liver damage and bleeding, so alcohol should not be consumed with these medications. Consumption of iron supplements often reduces the absorption of certain antibiotics, and vitamin C deficiency prolongs the effect of pentobarbital.[49]

Some medications should be taken before or between meals, including those known to trigger gastrointestinal distress, whereas others are best absorbed and/or utilized when taken with meals. Foods as diverse as grapefruit juice, spinach, and

Numerous drugs are known to alter nutrient digestion and absorption. Long-term antibiotic therapy can lead to diarrhea and generalized malabsorption, as well as malabsorption of calcium specifically. Other drugs may block uptake of other micronutrients. Many drugs negatively affect the activation or metabolism of nutrients such as vitamin D, folate, and vitamin B_6, contributing to secondary nutrient deficiencies even when nutrient intake is adequate. Several types of anti-epileptic drugs interfere with the activation of dietary vitamin D, leading to impaired bone health. Other medications increase

TABLE 18.3 Examples of Common Drug–Nutrient Interactions

Category of Drug	Common Nutrient/Food Interactions
Antacids	May decrease the absorption of iron, calcium, folate, vitamin B_{12}
Antibiotics	May reduce the absorption of calcium, fat-soluble vitamins; reduce the production of vitamin K by gut bacteria
Anticonvulsants	Interfere with the activation of vitamin D
Anticoagulants ("blood thinners")	Oppose the clotting activity of vitamin K
Antidepressants	May cause weight gain as a result of increased appetite
Antiretroviral agents (treatment of HIV/AIDS)	Reduce the absorption of most nutrients
Aspirin	Decrease blood folate levels; increase loss of iron due to gastric bleeding
Diuretics	Some types may increase urinary loss of potassium, sodium, calcium, magnesium; others cause retention of potassium and other electrolytes
Laxatives	Increase fecal excretion of dietary fat, fat-soluble vitamins, calcium, other minerals

aged cheese are known to react negatively with specific drugs.[50] Certain nutrient and herbal supplements have the ability to alter the activity of drug-metabolizing enzymes.

While the clinical implications of these interactions are not always clear, there is a potential for reduced or exaggerated drug effects.[49] Pharmacists and registered dietitians are able to provide information on such drug–food interactions and can give recommendations on dietary choices and the potential need for nutrient supplements. All older adults should be counseled on the potential for drug–food, drug–nutrient, and drug–supplement interactions.

RECAP

Osteoporosis, dental problems, arthritis, vision disorders, GI distress, and dementia are examples of "two-way streets" in which nutritional status influences an older adult's risk for the condition, while the condition itself has the potential to influence nutritional status. An older adult's nutritional status and intake can also influence the effectiveness of certain medications, and many of the drugs used by the elderly contribute to nutrient deficiencies. ■

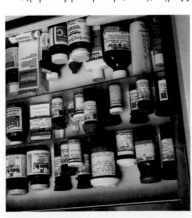

Medications taken by older adults can interact with nutrients.

What Social Concerns Affect the Nutrition of Older Adults?

We have explored the physical conditions that affect an older adult's nutritional status and needs, but social factors play a role as well. These include elder abuse and neglect, food insecurity, and social isolation.

Many Older Adults Experience Elder Abuse and Neglect

It has been estimated that up to one in ten U.S. elderly are abused by their spouses, children, neighbors, or paid caretakers each year.[51] Elder abuse can be physical, sexual, emotional, financial, neglectful, or unintentional. Denial of healthful food and adequate fluids falls within the scope of elder abuse and neglect. Although it can be difficult to detect, possible signs of such abuse include fear of the caregiver, anxiety, increased depression, and a desire for death. Home-bound elderly people may demonstrate new health problems, unexplained weight loss, dehydration and malnutrition, poor personal hygiene, and unexplained or suspicious physical injuries. Older adults without a trusted relative or friend may need to turn to a healthcare provider, court representative, or social service agency for protection and advice. Every state and local municipality has laws against elder abuse and can offer assistance if abuse or neglect is suspected. More information is available from the National Center on Elder Abuse (www.ncea.aoa.gov).

Food Insecurity Affects Nearly 4 Million Elderly

Food insecurity occurs when a family is not able to ensure a consistent, dependable supply of safe and nutritious food. "Very low food security" is a more severe economic state in which the family actually experiences reduced intake and disruption of normal eating patterns. In 2010, nearly 8% of households with elderly men and women in the United States were food insecure. This translates to nearly 4 million adults over the age of 60 years experiencing food insecurity. At greatest risk are African American, Hispanic, and other minorities; those living in the southern United States; and those living with one or more grandchildren.[52]

Older adults cope with food insecurity in several ways. Some make use of federal or local food assistance programs, such as the Supplemental Nutrition Assessment Program (formerly termed the *Food Stamp Program*), discussed shortly. A small number turn to food banks or food pantries for short-term assistance. Elderly adults can be embarrassed by their inability to provide for themselves and may resort to stealing food or going without adequate food. The most common cause of food insecurity and hunger among older adults is lack of income and poverty. Older adults in poverty often live in areas with few or no supermarkets, may not be able to afford transportation to buy healthful food, and may fear leaving their homes to shop for groceries. Their homes may lack working refrigerators and/or stoves, limiting the types of foods that can be bought, stored, and prepared. Healthcare and social service providers should carefully probe for information on the ability of low-income elders to afford an adequate and healthful food supply.

Social Isolation Increases Health Risks

Older adults may become socially isolated for many reasons. Those who are restricted to bed or wheelchairs, have impaired walking, or are in poor health are prone to isolation even if they live in a household with others. The death of a spouse can precipitate isolation, especially among the very old who have also lost siblings and friends.

Lack of adequate transportation also increases the risk for isolation. Family members and friends may not always be able to offer rides, and even where public transportation is available, older adults may be concerned about cost and personal safety. Even if government-funded vans or buses are available for the elderly, transportation may be limited to weekdays and certain hours of the day.

Among minority elderly, particularly recent immigrants with language barriers, isolation can occur after the death of a bilingual spouse or as bilingual children move out of the household. These adults may lack the communication skills to navigate public transporta-tion, shop, and secure social services. Ideally, communities with large immigrant popula-tions can provide translators to help integrate these elderly into the community at large. Social isolation increases the risk for alcohol and substance abuse, depression, and mal-nutrition. Personal healthcare habits decline, household maintenance is put off, and behavior becomes increasingly erratic. Isolated older adults are at high risk for victimization, such as tele-phone scams, and premature institutionalization. Religious, neighborhood, and social service agencies offer many programs to ensure that older adults are not forgotten within their homes.

Community Services Can Help Meet the Nutritional Needs of Older Adults

As the American population continues to age, greater demands are placed on social service agencies. This section identifies several programs available for older adults in need.

Community Nutrition Programs for Older Adults

The federal government has developed an extensive network of food and nutrition services for older Americans. Some are open to people of all ages, whereas others are restricted to people 60 years of age and up. Many are coordinated with state or local governments and community organizations. They include the following:

- *Supplemental Nutrition Assistance Program (SNAP):* This US Department of Agricul-ture (USDA) program, formerly known as the *Food Stamp Program,* provides food assistance for low-income households. Participants are provided with a monthly al-lotment, typically as a prepaid debit card. There are very few restrictions on the foods that can be purchased under this plan.
- *Senior Farmers' Market Nutrition Program:* This program is designed to provide fresh, unprocessed, locally grown fruits, vegetables, herbs, and honey from farmers' mar-kets, Community Supported Agriculture (CSA) programs, and roadside stands. Low-income seniors are given coupons to be redeemed for eligible foods.
- *Child and Adult Care Program:* This program provides healthy meals and snacks to older and functionally impaired adults in qualified adult day-care settings.
- *Commodity Supplemental Food Program:* This program serves low-income pregnant women, infants and young children, and older adults. Income guidelines must be met. Specific commodity foods are distributed, including cereals, peanut butter, dry beans, rice or pasta, and canned juice, fruits, vegetables, meat, poultry, and tuna. Unlike SNAP, this program is not intended to provide a complete array of foods.

■ *Nutrition Services Incentive Program:* The Administration on Aging provides cash and commodity foods to state agencies for meals for senior citizens. There is no income criteria; any person 60 years or above (plus his or her spouse, even if younger) can take part in this program. Although free, participants are encouraged to contribute what they can to cover meal costs. Lunch meals, designed to provide one-third of the RDA for key nutrients, are served at senior centers, churches, and other sites. Some provide "bag dinners" for evening meals, and others send home meals on Fridays for weekend use. Meals also can be delivered to the homes of qualified elders through the Meals on Wheels Association of America.

■ *The Emergency Food Assistance Program:* The USDA distributes commodity foods to state agencies for use by food banks, food pantries, and soup kitchens. Each state or agency establishes eligibility criteria, if any. The elderly are more likely to use the services of food banks and local food pantries, avoiding soup kitchens.

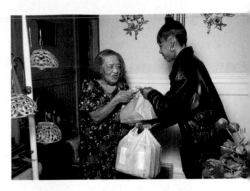

For home-bound disabled and older adults, community programs such as Meals on Wheels provide nourishing, balanced meals as well as vital social contact.

Participation in these community programs improves the dietary quality and nutrient intakes of older adults. Unfortunately, many programs have long waiting lists and are unable to meet current demands. As the number of elderly adults grows, the demand and need for these essential services will continue to increase.

Serving Minority Elderly

It is predicted that by 2020 nearly 25% of U.S. elderly will be classified as racial or ethnic minorities.[53] Hispanics have a life expectancy of almost 81 years, 2 years higher than that of whites and almost 8 years longer than African Americans.[54] The changing profile of the U.S. elderly population will require adaptations in current medical and social service interventions. For example, members of certain minority groups are at a greater risk for nutrition-related chronic diseases and their complications compared to non-Hispanic whites: Hispanics have higher rates of diabetes; African Americans experience greater rates of stroke, kidney failure, high blood pressure, colon cancer, and glaucoma; and Native Americans are at higher risk for diabetes, obesity, and alcohol abuse. Immigrants from around the world represent additional challenges for healthcare providers. Dietary counseling and other therapies can be used to lower the risk for such chronic diseases and their treatment. In order to meet the needs of minority elderly, nutrition professionals must develop an awareness of the cultures they serve, maintain flexibility in the foods/meals provided or prescribed, and work toward effective communication with their minority clients.

End-of-Life Care

Advances in medical care can prolong the lives of seriously ill persons, resulting in challenging legal and ethical issues. Healthcare providers must be well informed on end-of-life

Nutri-Case

Gustavo

"I don't believe in taking vitamins. If you eat good food, you get everything you need and it's the way nature intended it. My daughter kept nagging at my wife and me to start taking B-vitamins. She said when people get to be our age, they have problems with their nerves if they don't. I didn't fall for it, but my wife did, and then her doctor told her she needed calcium pills and vitamin D too. The kitchen counter is starting to look like a medicine chest! You know what I think? I think this whole vitamin thing is just a hoax to get you to empty your wallet."

Would you support Gustavo's decision to avoid taking a B-vitamin supplement? Given what you have learned in previous Nutri-Cases about Gustavo's wife, would you support or oppose her taking a B-vitamin, calcium, or vitamin D supplement? Explain your choices.

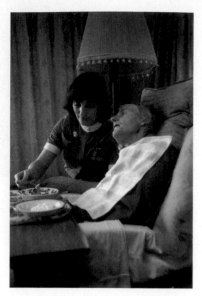

End-of-life care can be provided to elderly people who are terminally ill.

issues, including the provision of food and fluids, in order to help elderly clients and families make difficult decisions that honor the client's personal wishes. Ideally, an advance directive, such as a living will, is available to guide decision making.

The legalities surrounding end-of-life care are in continual flux as courts and legislative bodies enact, then modify, decisions on enteral nutrition (tube feeding), hydration, and other nutritional issues. Religious and cultural considerations often overlay legal issues, contributing to their complexity.

Healthcare providers, with agreement from the patient and/or appropriate legal authority, can provide **palliative care** to terminally ill individuals. With palliative care, no attempt is made to cure or treat the underlying condition; the care provided is designed primarily to minimize patient discomfort, offer social and spiritual support, and extend assistance to family and friends. Individuals who are facing imminent death rarely express hunger and have little or no thirst. If requested, specific foods or fluids are provided, even if they have no nutritional value, to comfort the patient. Hospice organizations are growing in number and availability and can provide palliative care to terminally ill individuals, either in their own homes or in a care facility.

palliative care Patient care aimed at reducing an individual's pain and discomfort without attempting to treat or cure.

RECAP

As many as 10% of older adults are estimated to experience abuse or neglect, including deprivation of nourishing food. Nearly 8% of U.S. elderly experience food insecurity. Disease, disability, death of a spouse, lack of transportation, and language barriers increase the risk for social isolation, which in turn increases the risk for malnutrition. Many social service agencies and programs exist to help older Americans with nutritional needs. Minority elderly may require help in overcoming language barriers and acquiring culturally appropriate foods. As older adults face end-of-life decisions, healthcare providers must be ready to assist them and their families with difficult decisions related to the provision of food and fluid. ■

Chapter Review

TEST YOURSELF | ANSWERS

1 **F** Experts agree it is unlikely that the human life span will increase much beyond 125 to 130 years.

2 **T** Older adults are more likely to lose their sense of smell than their sense of taste; however, loss of smell reduces the sense of taste.

3 **T** Because of an age-related decrease in gastric acid production, older adults are advised to get most of their vitamin B_{12} from supplements or fortified foods.

4 **F** Older men and women need less iron due to their loss of muscle mass, and older women require less iron due to the cessation of menstruation.

5 **F** In 2010, 7.9% of older Americans experienced food insecurity, whereas the national average was 14.5%.

Summary

- The U.S. population is aging at an unprecedented rate. Average life expectancy is now over 78 years. The very elderly, 85 and above, are the fastest-growing segment of the U.S. population; the numbers of centenarians and super-centenarians (over age 110) also continue to climb.

- The physiologic changes of aging include sensory declines, loss of muscle, increased fat mass, decreased bone density, and impaired ability to absorb and metabolize nutrients. Body organs lose functional capacity. These changes influence the nutritional needs of older adults and their ability to consume a healthful diet.

- Scientists are learning about various genetic and biochemical factors that contribute to senescence. Tobacco use, alcohol abuse, excessive sun exposure, overweight, and inactivity accelerate the aging process.

- Older adults need less energy, but some research suggests the need for slightly higher intakes of protein.

- Micronutrients of concern for older adults include calcium, vitamin D, and the B-vitamins. Iron needs decrease. Older adults also need slightly less fiber.

- Appropriate use of a multivitamin-multimineral supplement can enhance the nutritional status of older adults; however, certain high-dose, single-nutrient supplements can be dangerous unless prescribed. Calcium and vitamins B_{12} and D are single-nutrient supplements commonly prescribed for older adults.

- Older adults are at risk for chronic dehydration, so ample fluid intake should be encouraged.

- Nutritional status influences an older adult's risk for osteoporosis, dental problems, arthritis, vision problems, GI distress, and dementia; these conditions have the potential to influence nutritional status as well.

- An older adult's nutritional status and intake can alter the effectiveness of medications; many drugs used by the elderly contribute to nutrient deficiencies.

- Social issues affecting the nutrition of older adults include elder abuse and neglect, food insecurity, and social isolation.

- Demands on social service agencies increase as the population ages. As older adults face end-of-life decisions, healthcare providers must be ready to assist them and their families with difficult decisions related to the provision of food and fluid.

MasteringNutrition™

To further your understanding, go online and apply what you've learned to real-life case studies that will help you master the content!

Review Questions

1. Which of the following nutrients is needed in increased amounts in older adulthood?
   a. fiber
   b. vitamin D
   c. vitamin A
   d. iron

2. Abnormal taste perception is clinically known as
   a. dysgeusia.
   b. dysphagia.
   c. dysphasia.
   d. dysphonia.

3. Currently, the human life span is
   a. about 74 years.
   b. about 78 years.
   c. 114 years.
   d. 122 years.

4. Which of the following conditions results in defective protein cross-linkages and loss of tissue structure and function?
   a. xerostomia
   b. macular degeneration
   c. glycosylation
   d. achlorhydria

5. Providing cookies and lemonade to a terminally ill patient is an example of
   a. long-term care.
   b. geriatric care.
   c. palliative care.
   d. inappropriate care.

6. **True or false?** According to programmed theories of aging, nutrition has little, if any, potential or practical impact on disease, disability, or mortality.

7. **True or false?** Percentage of body fat typically continues to increase throughout an individual's life span.

8. **True or false?** Mortality rates are higher in underweight elderly than in overweight elderly.

9. **True or false?** The Institute of Medicine recommends that older adults obtain the DRI for vitamin B_{12} by consuming foods fortified with B_{12} or a B_{12}-containing supplement.

10. **True or false?** Older adults who regularly participate in strengthening and aerobic exercises have a reduced risk for fractures.

11. Identify four nutrient deficiencies that may arise from decreased production of gastric acid in older adults.

12. State two reasons a recent elderly immigrant from Southeast Asia may experience nutrient deficiencies after the death of her husband.

13. Identify several factors that increase the risk for dehydration in older adults.

14. Describe the nutritional counseling you would provide to a male client who is 86 years old and
    - eats only two meals per day: cold cereal with milk for breakfast and canned soup, crackers, and canned peaches or pears for dinner;
    - takes a daily antioxidant supplement containing levels of vitamins A, E, and C and selenium about five times higher than the DRI for these micronutrients; and
    - drinks three beers every night, so he can "sleep better."

15. Marta and her parents live in Dallas. A year ago, her maternal grandmother, who lives in Boston, stayed with them for several weeks after the death of Marta's grandfather. She seemed fit at the time, going for walks and cooking large meals for the family throughout her stay. Last night, Marta's mother received a phone call from a Boston hospital saying that her mother had been admitted after a hip fracture suffered in a fall at home and was battling significant dehydration and some cognitive impairment. Identify several factors that might have contributed to Marta's grandmother's condition.

Math Review

16. While helping her 72-year-old grandmother put away groceries, Kristina notices several new supplement bottles. One is a single-nutrient vitamin A supplement, which provides 3,333 µg/dose. Another is a special "Healthy Skin Formula," which also contains vitamin A, at 1,500 µg/dose. The third bottle is a multivitamin-multimineral supplement that provides 2,200 µg of vitamin A/dose. When Kristina asks about these new products, her grandmother explains that she read something online that said vitamin A made your skin look younger. So, her grandmother takes each of the three supplements every day to make her wrinkles go away faster! If Kristina's grandmother takes one dose of each of the three supplements per day, what percentage of the RDA does she consume? Of the UL? Do you see any potential problems with this level of intake?

Answers to Review Questions and Math Review can be found online in the MasteringNutrition Study Area.

Web Links

www.aarp.org
American Association of Retired Persons
A national advocacy group for the elderly; adults 50 years and above can join this organization of 35 million older Americans. The website has links to articles focusing on all aspects of health, finances, housing, and legal issues that are of importance to the elderly.

www.aoa.gov
Administration on Aging
Follow legislative updates on this website for information related to Congregate Meal and Meals on Wheels programs. Also provided are resources on Alzheimer's disease, elder rights and resources, housing, and elder nutrition.

www.cdc.gov
Centers for Disease Control and Prevention
Select "Health Promotion" and choose topics such as "Aging & Elderly Health" for accurate information on the health of America's seniors.

www.familydoctor.org
American Academy of Family Physicians
By selecting the "seniors" tab on the site's homepage, readers can find a thorough discussion of advance directives, living wills, and "do not resuscitate" orders.

www.fns.usda.gov/fns
Food & Nutrition Service, US Department of Agriculture
This site provides information on federal programs for low-income elderly, such as the Nutrition Services Incentive Program.

www.nia.nih.gov
National Institute on Aging
The National Institute on Aging provides information about how older adults can benefit from physical activity and good diet.

www.nihseniorhealth.gov
National Iinstitutes of Health: Senior Health
This web-based resource, displayed in large print, was developed specifically for older adults and offers up-to-date information on popular health topics for older Americans.

References

1. Administration on Aging. A Profile of Older Americans: 2011. www.aoa.gov/aoaroot/aging_statistics/Profile/2011/2.aspx. (Accessed July 2012.)
2. Murphy, S. L., J .Q. Xu, and K. D. Kochanek. 2012. Deaths: preliminary data for 2010. *National Vital Statistics Reports* 60(4).
3. Crimmins, E. M., S. H. Preston, and B. Cohen, eds. 2011. *Explaining Divergent Levels of Longevity in High Income Countries.* Washington, DC: National Academy Press.
4. Los Angeles Gerontology Research Group. 2012. Official Tables from the International Committee on Supercentenarians. www.grg.org/Adams/Tables.htm. (Accessed July 2012.)
5. Nordin, S., O. Almkvist, and B. Berglund. 2012. Is loss in odor sensitivity inevitable to the aging individual? A study of "successfully aged" elderly. *Chem. Percept.* 5:188–196.
6. Rughwani, N. 2011. Normal anatomic and physiologic changes with aging and related disease outcomes: a refresher. *Mt. Sinai J. Med.* 78:509–514.
7. Van Lancker, A., S. Verhaeghe, A. Van Hecke, K. Vanderwee, J. Goossens, and D. Beeckman. 2012. The association between malnutrition and oral health status in elderly in long-term care facilities: a systematic review. *International J. Nursing Studies.* doi.org/10.1016/j.injnurstu.2012.04.001.
8. Biagi, E., M. Candela, S. Fairweather-Tait, C. Franceschi, and P. Brigidi. 2012. Ageing of the human metaorganism: the microbial counterpart. *Age* 34:247–267.
9. Moss, C., W. S. Dhillo, G. Frost, and M. Hickson. 2011. Gastrointestinal hormones: the regulation of appetite and the anorexia of ageing. *J. Hum. Nutr. Diet.* 25:3–15.
10. Genton, L., V. L. Karsengard, T. Chevalley, M. P. Kossovsky, P. Darmon, and C. Pichard. 2011. Body compostion changes over 9 years in healthy elderly subjects and impact of physical activity. *Clin. Nutr.* 30:436–442.
11. Li, Z., and D. Heber. 2011. Sarcopenic obesity in the elderly and strategies for weight management. *Nutr. Rev.* 70:57–64.
12. Genton, L., V. L. Karsegard, T. Chevalley, M. P. Kossovsky, P. Darmon, and C. Pichard. 2011. Body composition changes over 9 years in healthy elderly subjects and impact of physical activity. *Clin. Nut.* 30:436–442.
13. Powell, K. E., A. E. Paluch, and S. N. Blair. 2011. Physical activity for health: what kind? How much? How intense? On top of what? *Annu. Rev. Public Health.* 32:349–365.
14. Institute of Medicine, Food and Nutrition Board. 2002. *Dietary Reference Intakes for Energy, Carbohydrates, Fiber, Fat, Protein and Amino Acids (Macronutrients).* Washington, DC: National Academy of Sciences.
15. Tieland, M., K. J. Borgonjen-Van den Berg, L. J. C. van Loon, L. C. P. G. M. de Groot. 2012. Dietary protein intake in community-dwelling, frail, and institutionalized elderly people: scope for improvement. *Eur. J. Nutr.* 51:173–179.
16. Institute of Medicine. 2011. *Dietary Reference Intakes for Calcium and Vitamin D.* Washington, DC: National Academy Press.
17. Virtanen, J. K., T. Nurmi, S. Voutilainen, J. Mursu, and T. Tuomainen. 2011. Association of serum 25-hydroxyvitamin D with the risk of death in a general older population in Finland. *Eur. J. Nutr.* 50:305–312.
18. Johansson, H., A. Odén, J. Kanis, E. McCloskey, M. Lorentzon, Ö. Ljunggren, M. K. Karlsson, P. M. Thorsby, Å. Tivesten, E. Barrett-Conner, C. Ohlsson, and D. Mellström. 2012. Low serum vitamin D is associated with increased mortality in elderly men: MrOS Sweden. *Osteoporosis Int.* 23:991–999.
19. Llewellyn, D. J., I. A. Lang, K. M. Langa, and D. Melzer. 2011. Vitamin D and cognitive impairment in the elderly U.S. population. *J. Gerontology: MEDICAL SCIENCES.* 66a:59–65.
20. Bolland, M .J., A. Grey, A. Avenell, G. D. Gamble, and I. R. Reid. 2011. Calcium supplements with or without vitamin D and risk of cardiovascular events: reanalysis of the Women's Health Initiative limited access dataset and meta-analysis. *BMJ.* DOI:10.1136/bmj.d2040.
21. Institute of Medicine, Food and Nutrition Board. 2001. *Dietary Reference Intakes for Vitamin A, Vitamin K, Arsenic, Boron, Chromium, Copper, Iodine, Iron, Manganese, Molybdenum, Nickel, Silicon, Vanadium, and Zinc.* Washington, DC: National Academy Press.
22. Mocchegiani, E., J. Romeo, M. Malavolta, L. Costarelli, R. Giacconi, L. Diaz, and A. Marcos. 2012. Zinc: dietary intake and impact of supplementation on immune function in elderly. *Age.* DOI: 10.1007/s11357-011-9377-3.
23. Saito, K., T. Yokoyama, H. Yoshida, H. Kim, H. Shimada, Y. Yoshida, H. Iwasa, Y. Shimizu, Y. Kondo, S. Handa, N. Maruyama, A. Ishigami, and T. Suzuki. 2011. A significant relationship between plasma vitamin C concentration and physical performance among Japanese elderly women. *J. Gerontol. A. Biol. Sci. Med. Sci.* DOI:10.1093/Gerona/glr174.
24. Juraschek, S. P., E. Guallar, L. J. Appel, and E. R. Miller III. 2012. Effects of vitamin C supplementation on blood pressure: a meta-analysis of randomized controlled trials. *Am. J. Clin. Nutr.* 95:1079–1088.
25. Institute of Medicine, Food and Nutrition Board. 2000. *Dietary Reference Intakes for Vitamin C, Vitamin E, Selenium, and Carotenoids.* Washington, DC: National Academy Press.
26. Klein, R., Ch. Chou, B. E. K. Klein, X. Zhang, S. M. Meuer, and J. B. Shaddine. 2011. Prevalence of age-related macular degeneration in the US population. *Arch. Opthalmol.* 129:75–80.
27. Sun, Y., A. Ma, Y. Li, X. Han, Q. Wang, and H. Liang. 2012. Vitamin E supplementation protects erythrocyte membranes from oxidative stress in healthy Chinese middle-aged and elderly people. *Nutr. Res.* 32:328–334.

28. Institute of Medicine, Food and Nutrition Board. 1998. *Dietary Reference Intakes for Thiamin, Riboflavin, Niacin, Vitamin B_6, Folate, Vitamin B_{12}, Pantothenic Acid, Biotin, and Choline.* Washington, DC: National Academy Press.

29. Hooshmand, B., A. Soloman, I. Kåreholt, M. Rusanen, T. Hänninen, J. Leiviskä, B. Winblad, T. Laatikainen, H. Soininen, and M. Kivipelto. 2012. Associations between serum homocysteine, holotranscolbalamin, folate and cognition in the elderly: a longitudinal study. *J. Int. Med.* 271:204–212.

30. Moorthyl, D., I. Peter, T. M. Scott, L. D. Parnell, C. Lai, J. W. Crott, J. M. Ordovás, J. Selhub, J. Griffith, I. H. Rosenberg, K. L. Tucker, and A. M. Troen. 2012. Status of vitamins B-12 and B-6 but not of folate, homocysteine, and the methylene-tetrahydrofolate reductase C677T polymorphism are associated with impaired cognition and depression in adults. *J. Nutr.* 142:1554–1560.

31. Wright, R. E., C. Hughes, and H. McNulty. 2011. The role of age on B_{12} biomarker response to dietary intakes of vitamin B_{12} and implications for dietary intake recommendations. *J. Hum. Nutr. Dietetics.* 24:309–310.

32. Ahmadieh, H., and A. Arabi. 2011. Vitamins and bone health: beyond calcium and vitamin D. *Nutr. Rev.* 69:584–598.

33. Ma, L., H. Dou, Y. Wu, Y. Huang, Y. Huang, X. Xu, Z. Zou, and X. Lin. 2011. Lutein and zeaxanthin intake and the risk of age-related macular degeneration: a systematic review and meta-analysis. *Brit. J. Nutr.* 107:350–359.

34. Troesch, B., M. Eggersdorfer, and P. Weber. 2012. 100 years of vitamins: adequate intake in the elderly is still a matter of concern. *J. Nutr.* 142:979–980.

35. Hankey, C. R., and W. Leslie. 2011. Nutritional issues and potential interventions in older people. *Rev. Clin. Gerontol.* 21:286–296.

36. Institute of Medicine, Food and Nutrition Board. 2004. *Dietary Reference Intakes for Water, Potassium, Sodium, Chloride, and Sulfate.* Washington, DC: National Academy Press.

37. Mathus-Vliegen, E. M. H., on behalf of the Obesity Management Task Force (OMTF) of the European Association for the Study of Obesity (EASO). 2012. Prevalence, pathophysiology, health consequences and treatment options of obesity in the elderly: a guideline. *Obesity Facts* 5:460–483.

38. National Osteoporosis Foundation. 2011. Prevalence Report. www.nof.org/print/219. (Accessed July 2012.)

39. Schulman, R.C., A. J. Weiss, and J. I Mechanick. 2011. Nutrition, bones, and aging: an integrative physiology approach. *Curr. Osteoporos Rep.* 9:184–195.

40. Van Lancker, A., S. Verhaeghe, A. Van Hecke, K. Vanderwee, J. Goossens, and D. Beeckman. 2012. The association between malnutrition and oral health status in elderly in long-term care facilities: a systematic review. *International J. Nursing Studies.* doi.org/10.1016/j.ijnurstu.2012.04.001.

41. Altenhoevel, A., K. Norman, C. Smoliner, and I. Peroz. 2012. The impact of self-perceived masticatory function on nutrition and gastrointestinal complaints in the elderly. *J. Nutr., Health, Aging.* 16:175–178.

42. Mares, J. A., R. P. Voland, S.A. Sondel, A. E. Millen, T. LaRowe, S. M. Moeller, M. L. Klein, B. A. Blodi, R. J. Chappell, L. Tinker, C. Ritenbaugh, K. M. Gehrs, G. E. Sarto, E. Johnson, D. M. Snodderly, and R. B. Wallace. 2011. Healthy lifestyles related to subsequent prevalence of age-related macular degeneration. *Arch. Ophthalmol.* 129:470–480.

43. Ho, L., R. van Leeuwen, J .C. M. Witteman, C. M. van Duijn, A. G. Uitterlinden, A. Hofman, P. T. V. M. de Jong, J. R. Vingerling, and C. C. W. Klaver. 2011. Reducing the genetic risk of age-related macular degeneration with dietary antioxidants, zinc, and ω-3 fatty acids. *Arch. Ophthalmol.* 129:758–766.

44. Alzheimer's Association. 2012. 2012 Alzheimer's disease facts and figures. *Alzheimer's & Dementia* 8(2):1–72.

45. Bazan, N. G., M. F. Molina, and W. C. Gordon. 2011. Docosahexaenoic acid signalolipidomics in nutrition: significance in aging, neuroinflammation, macular degeneration, Alzheimer's, and other neurodegenerative disease. *Ann. Rev. Nutr.* 31:321–351.

46. Middleton, L. E., T. M. Manini, E. M. Simonsick, T. B. Harris, D. E. Barnes, F. Tylavsky, J. S. Brach, J. E. Everhart, and K. Yaffe. 2011. Activity energy expenditure and incident cognitive impairment in older adults. *Arch. Intern. Med.* 171:1251–1257.

47. Mansur, N., A. Weiss, and Y. Beloosesky. 2012. Looking beyond polypharmacy: quantification of medication regimen complexity in the elderly. *Am. J. Geriatric Pharmacotherapy* doi.org/10.1016/j.amjopharm.2012.06.002.

48. Heuberger, R. A., and K. Caudell. 2011. Polypharmacy and nutritional status in older adults. *Drugs & Aging* 28:315–323.

49. Boullata, J. I., and L. M. Hudson. 2012. Drug-nutrient interactions: a broad view with implications for practice. *J. Acad. Nutr. Diet.* 112: 506–517.

50. Rodriguez-Fragoso, L., J. L. Martinez-Arismendi, D. Orozco-Bustos, J. Reyes-Esparza, E. Torres, and S. W. Burchiel. 2011. Potential risks resulting from fruit/vegetable-drug interactions: effects on drug-metabolizing enzymes and drug transporters. *J. Food Sci.* 76:R112–R124.

51. Dong, X., and M. A. Simon. 2011. Enhancing national policy and programs to address elder abuse. *JAMA.* 305:2460–2461.

52. Ziliak, J., and C. Gundersen. 2009. Senior hunger in the United States: differences across states and rural and urban areas. *University of Kentucky Center for Poverty Research Special Reports.* http://feedingamerica.org/hunger-in-america/hunger-facts/senior-hunger.aspx, (Accessed July 2012.)

53. Administration on Aging. 2011. Minority Aging. www.aoa.gov/aoaroot/aging_statistics/minority_aging/Index.aspx. (Accessed July 2012.)

54. Wright, D., and B. Blackburn. 2010. Why do Hispanics outlive white and black Americans? *ABC News.* http://abcnews.go.com/WN/us-hispanics-longer-life-expectancy-white-black-americans/story?id=11883156. (Accessed July 2012.)

Can We Live Longer by Eating a Low-Energy Diet?

How old do you want to live to be—80 years, 90, 100? Worldwide, throughout human history, legends have told of a "fountain of youth," which reverses decades of aging in anyone who drinks its waters. Of course, no one believes such tales any longer, but pick up a fashion or fitness magazine and you're likely to find modern equivalents: anti-aging diets, supplements, cosmetics, spa treatments, and other therapies. For instance, if you were to read that you could live to celebrate your 100th birthday in good health by eating about a quarter less than the average energy intake for your gender and height, would you do it? Or would you assume that this is just a fairy tale too? Believe it or not, a growing number of people are drastically cutting their Calorie intake in an effort to extend both their youthfulness and their longevity. Is this effective? What other actions can you take right now to live longer in good health? Let's find out.

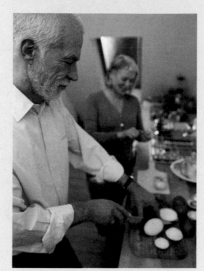

Maintaining a Calorically restricted diet that is also highly nutritious requires significant meal planning and preparation.

measures of health in humans and, thus, may be able to extend the human life span.[3]

How might CR prolong life span? The answer to this question is not fully understood, but it is thought that the reduction in metabolic rate that occurs with restricting energy intake results in a much lower production of free radicals, which in turn reduces oxidative damage to DNA, cell membranes, and other cell structures, possibly lowering chronic disease risk and prolonging life. Calorie restriction also causes marked improvements in insulin sensitivity and other hormonal changes that can lower the risk for chronic diseases, such as heart disease, stroke, and diabetes. There is also evidence that CR can alter gene expression in ways that reduce the effects of aging and lower the risk for cancer and other diseases. The following are some of the metabolic effects of CR reported in several, but not all, human studies:[1,3,4,5]

Does Calorie Restriction Increase Life Span?

A practice known as *Calorie restriction (CR)* has been getting a great deal of press lately. Although researchers haven't defined a precise number of Calories, or level of nutrients, that qualifies as a Calorie-restricted diet, the practice typically involves eating fewer Calories than your body needs to maintain your normal weight—while still getting enough vitamins and other nutrients to keep your body functioning in good health. In general—allowing for differences in how many Calories people are consuming prior to CR, as well as their gender, age, body composition, level of activity, and so forth—CR may call for a person to consume 20–30% fewer Calories than usual.[1]

Research has shown that CR can significantly extend the life span of rats, mice, fish, flies, and yeast cells, as well as nonhuman primates, such as monkeys.[2] But only in the past few years have researchers begun to design and conduct studies of CR in humans. The results of these preliminary studies suggest that CR can also improve metabolic

- Decreased fat mass and lean body mass
- Decreased blood glucose levels
- Decreased serum LDL- and total cholesterol; increased serum HDL-cholesterol
- Decreased core body temperature and blood pressure
- Decreased energy expenditure, beyond that expected for the weight loss that occurred, which suggests a generalized slowing of metabolic rate
- Decreased oxidative stress
- Reduced levels of DNA damage
- Lower levels of chronic inflammation
- Protective changes in various hormone levels

It is important to emphasize that species known to live longer with CR are fed highly nutritious diets. Situations such as starvation, anorexia nervosa, and extreme fad dieting, in which both energy and nutrient intakes are severely restricted, do not result in prolonged life, but are associated with an increased risk for premature death.

It's also essential to understand that the benefits of CR are thought to correlate to the age at which the program begins. The later in life the CR protocol is started, the lower the expected benefit. For example, if a person did not start CR until the age of 55 years, he or she would be expected to gain only 4 months of extended life![3]

What Are the Challenges of Calorie Restriction?

Although the benefits listed in the previous section appear promising, the research data supporting these benefits in humans are only preliminary. Research that can precisely study CR in humans might never be conducted because of logistical and ethical concerns. For instance, most people find it challenging to follow a Calorie-restricted diet for just a few months; compliance with this type of diet for a decades-long study could be almost impossible. There are also ethical concerns about the potential malnutrition that could occur.

In the absence of high-quality human studies, several CR groups, including the "CRONies" (Caloric Restriction with Optimal Nutrition), have provided researchers with some data. Most of the CRONies are males in their late thirties to mid-fifties. One report indicated that most CRONies had followed the CR diet for about 10 years and had reduced their Caloric intake by about 30%. Overall, members reported improved blood lipids and the other health benefits listed earlier. Still, researchers lack specific data on how well free-living adults actually follow the rigid and extensive demands of CR protocols.

You may be wondering how much less energy *you* would have to consume to meet the definition of Calorie restriction—and when you'd have to begin. It has been estimated that humans would need to restrict their typical energy intake by at least 20% for 40 years or more in order to gain an addition 4–5 years of healthy living. If you normally eat about 2,000 kcal/day, a 20% reduction would result in an energy intake of about 1,600 kcal per day. Although this might not seem excessive, it would be very difficult to maintain every day for a lifetime.

Also keep in mind that this diet must be of very high nutritional quality. This requirement presents a huge number of challenges, including meticulous planning of meals, limited options for eating meals outside of your home, and the challenge of working the demands of your special diet around the eating behaviors of family members and friends.

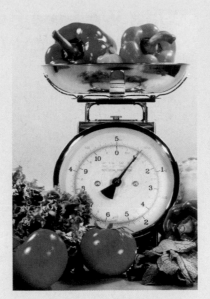

All foods must be carefully measured and weighed in a Calorie-restricted diet.

Also, those who follow the CR program report several side effects. The top three complaints are constant hunger, frequently feeling cold, and a loss of libido (sex drive).[3] Finally, the long-term effects of the diet are not known. There is concern that, if initiated in early adulthood, CR might reduce bone density or lead to inappropriate loss of muscle mass. And because the production of female reproductive hormones is linked to a certain level of body fat, CR could impair a woman's fertility. Interestingly, as noted earlier, most of the members of the CRONies are males.

Are There Alternatives to Calorie Restriction?

An interesting alternative to Caloric restriction is the practice of *intermittent fasting* (IF), also known as every-other-day-feeding (EODF) or alternate-day fasting (ADF).[6,7,8] This approach, which does *not* reduce average energy intake but simply alters the pattern of food intake, has also been shown, in animals, to prolong life span and improve a range of metabolic measures of health. Although not as well studied as CR, IF has produced beneficial changes in insulin and glucose status, blood lipid levels, and blood pressure in humans in at least some studies.

Additionally, some researchers have proposed that limiting total protein, which is much easier to implement than extreme Caloric restriction, may limit the onset of cancer and aging. Surveys indicate that Americans eat 15–17% of their total daily energy intake as protein, so limiting total protein might mean consuming a diet with 10% of energy intake from protein, which is still within the AMDR for protein intake.

Finally, other research suggests that exercise-induced leanness may slow the aging process without the need for Caloric restriction.[9] That is, it may not be the energy intake per se that extends life span but the overall energy balance a person maintains. A person would not have to strictly limit energy intake as long as his or her energy expenditure was high enough to maintain a lean body profile.

If none of these options interest you, is there anything else you can do to increase your chances of living a long and healthful life? The Centers for Disease Control and Prevention (CDC) reminds us that chronic disease is responsible for seven of every ten deaths of Americans. Moreover, just four behaviors within your control are responsible for chronic disease:

- Lack of physical activity
- Poor nutrition
- Tobacco use
- Excessive consumption of alcohol

So if you want to live a longer, healthier life, the CDC advises that you adopt the following health habits:

- Engage in at least 30 minutes of moderate physical activity most days of the week.
- Consume a diet based on the 2010 Dietary Guidelines for Americans.
- Maintain a healthful weight.
    - If you smoke or use any other form of tobacco, stop. If you don't, don't start.
    - If you drink alcohol, do so only in moderation, meaning no more than two drinks per day for men and one drink per day for women.

CRITICAL THINKING QUESTIONS

- Given the pros and cons presented here, do you think it's advisable to follow a Calorie-restricted diet? Why or why not?

- Are you willing to make the sacrifices necessary to try to prolong your life, even though you can't be sure that CR works in humans?

- If research were to eventually show that CR substantially improves health and prolongs life, would you support recommending it on a large-scale basis? Explain your reasoning.

REFERENCES

1. Omodei, D., and L. Fontana. 2011. Calorie restriction and prevention of age-associated chronic disease. *FEBS Letters* 585:1537–1542.
2. Kemnitz, J. W. 2011. Calorie restriction and aging in nonhuman primates. *ILAR. J.* 8:66–77.
3. Speakman, J. 2010. Can Calorie restriction increase the human lifespan? Bexperimental Biology 2010. April 24.
4. Spindler, S. R. 2010. Caloric restriction: from soup to nuts. *Ageing Research Reviews* 9:324–353.
5. Ahmet, I., H. Tae, R. de Cabo, E. G. Lakatta, and M. I. Talan. 2011. Effects of Calorie restriction on cardioprotection and cardiovascular health. *J. Molec. Cell Cardiol.* 51:263–271.
6. Varady, K. A., S. Bhutani, E. C. Church, and M. C. Klempel. 2009. Short-term modified alternate-day fasting: a novel dietary strategy for weight loss and cardioprotection in obese adults. *Am. J. Clin. Nutr.* 90:1138–1143.
7. Varady, K. A. 2012. Alternate day fasting: effects on body weight and chronic disease risk in humans. In: McCue, M. D., ed. *Comparative Physiology of Fasting, Starvation and Food Limitation.* Berlin: Springer-Verlag.
8. Varady, K. A., S. Bhutani, M. C. Klempel, and B. Lamarche. 2010. Improvements in LDL particle size and distribution by short-term alternate day modified fasting in obese adults. *Brit. J. Nutr.* 105:580–583.
9. Fontana, L., L. Partridge, and V. D. Longo. 2010. Extending healthy life span—from yeast to humans. *Science* 328:321–326.

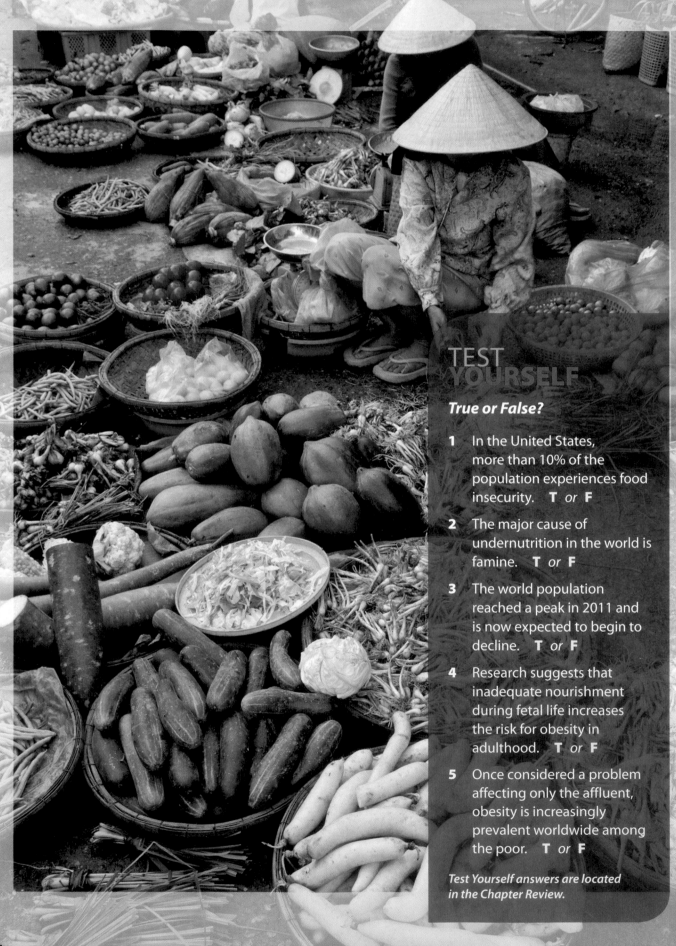

TEST
YOURSELF

True or False?

1 In the United States,
   more than 10% of the
   population experiences food
   insecurity.   **T** *or* **F**

2 The major cause of
   undernutrition in the world is
   famine.   **T** *or* **F**

3 The world population
   reached a peak in 2011 and
   is now expected to begin to
   decline.   **T** *or* **F**

4 Research suggests that
   inadequate nourishment
   during fetal life increases
   the risk for obesity in
   adulthood.   **T** *or* **F**

5 Once considered a problem
   affecting only the affluent,
   obesity is increasingly
   prevalent worldwide among
   the poor.   **T** *or* **F**

*Test Yourself answers are located
in the Chapter Review.*

19

Global Nutrition

Learning Objectives

After studying this chapter, you should be able to:

1. Identify the acute and long-term health concerns associated with global undernutrition and nutrient deficiencies, *pp. 756–760.*

2. Identify the five micronutrient deficiencies of greatest concern in impoverished countries, *pp. 758–759.*

3. Explain the connection between fetal undernutrition and adult disease, and identify the theory behind it, *p. 760.*

4. Identify the primary factors that cause or contribute to undernutrition in the developing world, *pp. 760–763.*

5. Explain why overnutrition has become a global concern, *pp. 763–764.*

6. Describe the rising public health concern known as the *nutrition paradox, pp. 763–764.*

7. Identify the groups most at risk for food insecurity in the United States, *p. 765.*

8. Identify three types of public health programs designed to provide local solutions to malnutrition, *pp. 766–769.*

9. Describe the role of technological strategies, such as the Green Revolution and sustainable agriculture, in supporting global nutrition, *pp. 769–770.*

10. Describe several options for combating global malnutrition on a personal and local level, *pp. 770–773.*

MasteringNutrition™

Go online for chapter quizzes, pre-tests, Interactive Activities, and more!

In Sierra Leone, West Africa, a child and her father beg for food. As a result of vitamin A deficiency, he is blind, but she leads him by the hand through the crowded streets with assurance. Though she looks no more than 5 years old, when asked her age, she says, "I'm 8 or 9. Maybe 10." Malnutrition has stunted her growth. Her father searches with his hand to stroke his daughter's head. He calls her the strong one. "Her two brothers died as infants," he explains, "and her mother died giving birth. Now she takes care of me."

Despite abundant natural resources, including diamonds, gold, and iron, Sierra Leone is one of the poorest countries on Earth, with 70% of its people living in poverty.[1] A decade of civil war ended in 2002, but its physical infrastructure remains barely developed, corruption is endemic, and income disparity is extreme. Making matters worse is the global increase in food prices, which resulted in a 50% rise in the cost of rice—a staple food in Sierra Leone—in 2008. Life expectancy hovers around 47 years, and in 2010 a staggering 174 out of every 1,000 children died before reaching their 5th birthday.[2] Of those who survive, more than one in three will be abnormally small for their age.[1] Tragically, Sierra Leone is not alone in these sobering statistics: throughout much of Africa, malnutrition is the cause of more than half of all deaths of children,[3] and up to 70% of the total population of other countries on the African continent is hungry.[4]

These sobering statistics are in sharp contrast to the United States, where life expectancy at birth is 78 years, and only 7.8 out of every 1,000 children die before reaching their 5th birthday.[2] Even though the U.S. Census Bureau estimates that, in 2010, 15.1% of the U.S. population lived in poverty (46.2 million people), less than 4% of the total population is malnourished in terms of short stature for age.[2] However, a different type of malnutrition prevails in the United States—overweight and obesity. In 2010, the Centers for Disease Control and Prevention (CDC) reported that 35.7% of American adults and 17% of American children were obese.[5]

Despite dramatic advances in worldwide food production and preservation in recent decades, 925 million people around the globe were hungry in 2010.[6] At the same time, far too many people in the wealthiest nations are overweight and obese, and this problem is spreading to many less affluent nations such as Brazil, India, and China. Why is this so? What causes malnutrition, and what are some solutions? Is there anything you can do in your daily life to combat malnutrition, not only locally but throughout the world? We explore these questions in this chapter.

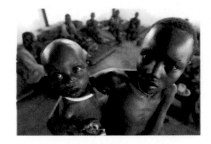

Hunger and malnutrition are still experienced by many people around the world today.

Why Is Undernutrition a Global Concern?

Malnutrition is an enemy with many faces. *Undernutrition* afflicts people who don't have enough to eat. It stunts physical and mental development, reduces productivity, and perpetuates poverty. Specific nutrient deficiencies are another common problem, especially of iron, iodine, zinc, and vitamins A and B_{12}. In contrast, *overnutrition* is the result of excessive consumption of energy-dense food along with inadequate physical activity. It causes rising rates of obesity and threatens its victims with chronic diseases, such as heart disease and type 2 diabetes. We discuss overnutrition later in this chapter.

The World Hunger Education Service estimates that one in seven people in the world is chronically undernourished, and 98% of these people live in developing nations.[6] The prevalence of undernutrition is greatest in sub-Saharan Africa and Southeast Asia, in countries ranging from Liberia to Ethiopia and India to Laos (**Figure 19.1**). Closer to home, parts of Central and South America also experience undernutrition at rates as high as 25% of the population (see Figure 19.1).

People who are undernourished suffer more acute and long-term health problems than those who are adequately nourished. Here, we discuss the acute and long-term effects of undernutrition throughout the life cycle (**Figure 19.2**).

Undernutrition Causes Wasting and Stunting

Undernutrition results in **wasting,** a condition of very-low-body-weight-for-height or extreme thinness. Wasting is a hallmark of **severe acute malnutrition (SAM),** which causes approximately 1 million preventable deaths annually.[7] Children who are chronically

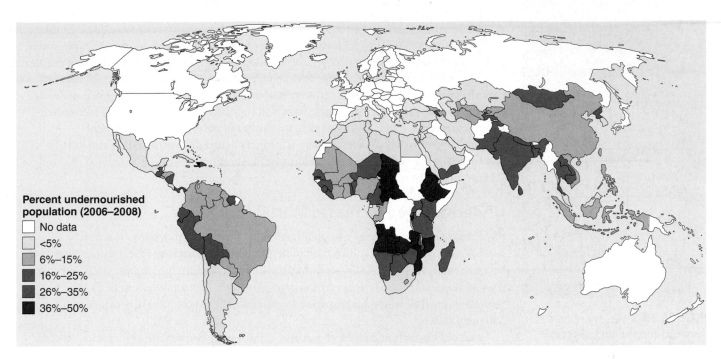

FIGURE 19.1 Undernutrition occurs throughout the world but is most prevalent in parts of sub-Saharan Africa and Southeast Asia. (*Source*: Data from "Prevalence of Undernourishment in Total Population" from the Food and Agriculture Organization of the United Nations, website.)

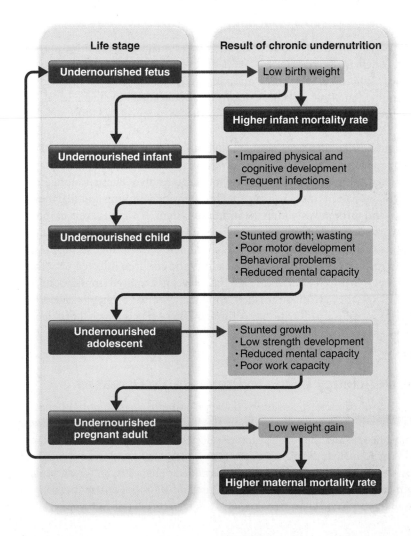

FIGURE 19.2 Acute and long-term effects of undernutrition throughout the life cycle.

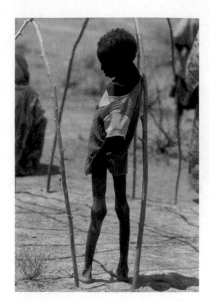

FIGURE 19.3 Wasting (extreme thinness) and stunting (short stature for age) are commonly seen in undernourished children.

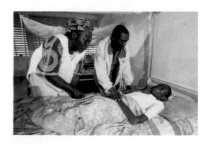

HIV/AIDS is most severe in undernourished populations, especially in Africa.

stunted growth A condition of shorter stature than expected for chronological age, often defined as 2 or more standard deviations below the mean reference value.

neonatal mortality The death rate for newborns between birth and 28 days of age.

infant mortality The death rate for infants between birth and 1 year of age.

maternal mortality The death rate for women from pregnancy-related causes, including the immediate postpartum period.

undernourished also experience **stunted growth;** they are shorter than expected for their age (**Figure 19.3**). Stunting occurs when energy intake or specific nutrients are inadequate to sustain normal linear growth. Recall the child described at the beginning of this chapter: although 8 to 10 years old, she appeared no older than 5. The chances are good that her parents' growth was stunted too. In some impoverished communities, the great majority of residents are very short and small; thus, community members may not perceive their stunted growth as unusual or recognize it as a sign of chronic malnourishment.

Early termination of breastfeeding is strongly associated with wasting and growth stunting. The importance of breastfeeding in the developing world is discussed in detail later in this chapter.

Undernutrition Increases Mortality

SAM dramatically increases a population's rate of **neonatal mortality** (the death of newborns between birth and 28 days of life) and **infant mortality** (the death of infants between birth and 1 year). For example, the infant mortality rate in industrialized countries of Western Europe ranges from about 3 to 5 per 1,000, whereas in five of the world's poorest countries, where malnutrition is endemic, the infant mortality rate is more than 100 per 1,000.[2]

Not only infants and children but also childbearing women are at increased risk for death from undernutrition. In the most affluent nations, the 2010 **maternal mortality** rate—the number of deaths during pregnancy and childbirth per 100,000 live births—was less than 10, but in a few of the world's poorest nations, the rate was as high as 1,000.[8]

Many of the deaths associated with SAM occur as a result of decreased resistance to infection. Even mild underweight is estimated to double a child's risk for death from infection.[9]

Single and multiple micronutrient deficiencies also decrease resistance to infection. For example, vitamin A deficiency contributes to 16% of cases of malaria and 18% of cases of diarrhea worldwide.[10] Vitamin A supplementation in malnourished children has been found to improve immune function and reduce deaths by almost 25%.[11] Deficiencies of protein, vitamins C and E, zinc, copper, selenium, and iron also compromise immune function.

Undernutrition and nutrient deficiencies are thought to make individuals more vulnerable to infection by reducing energy reserves and weakening the immune response. Therefore, infections occur more frequently and take longer to resolve. These prolonged infections exacerbate malnutrition by decreasing appetite, causing vomiting and diarrhea, producing weight loss, and further weakening the immune system. A vicious cycle of malnutrition, infection, worsening malnutrition, and increased vulnerability to infection develops.[12] Traditionally, this cycle has been observed with childhood diseases such as measles, diarrheal diseases, and respiratory infections. Today, adults and children infected with the human immunodeficiency virus (HIV) are more likely to develop acquired immunodeficiency syndrome (AIDS) if they are malnourished, and having AIDS (originally called "thin disease" in Africa) worsens malnutrition.[13] Although HIV/AIDS is a global problem, it is most severe in undernourished populations, especially Africa, which is also the most undernourished region.

Micronutrient Deficiency Leads to Preventable Diseases

Micronutrient deficiency diseases, such as scurvy, pellagra, goiter, rickets, and night blindness, have largely been eliminated in developed countries because of the great variety of foods available to most people and the fortification of selected foods to prevent particular deficiency diseases. When nutrient deficiency does occur in developed nations, it is usually caused by inadequate selection from available foods and supplements, as, for example, when poverty encourages the selection of inexpensive, nutrient-poor but energy-dense foods, such as fries, sugary soft drinks, and shakes.

In impoverished countries, deficiencies of five micronutrients are major public health concerns. These are iron, iodine, zinc, and vitamins A and B$_{12}$.

Iron

Iron deficiency is the most common micronutrient deficiency in the world. Although it occurs in both males and females of all ages, it is more prevalent in pregnant women and young children because of the demands of fetal and childhood growth. (The **Highlight** box in Chapter 12—**Iron Deficiency Around the World,** page 481—provides more detail.)

Iodine

Prenatal iodine intake is particularly important for fetal brain development, and severe deficiency leads to a condition known as cretinism (see Chapter 8). Mild deficits in school-age children lead to impaired cognitive performance and retarded physical development. In 2011, nearly 30% of the world's school-age children had insufficient iodine intake.[14] Iodine-deficiency disorders have largely been eliminated in areas of the world with access to iodized salt or oil and areas where iodine is added to irrigation water.

Zinc

Mild to severe zinc deficiency is estimated to affect about 2.2 billion people worldwide,[7] especially poorer people with little animal protein in the diet. Severe zinc deficiency impairs growth and sexual maturation and is associated with reduced resistance to infectious diseases (see Chapter 12).

Vitamin A

Vitamin A deficiency, which affects more than 40% of children under age 5 in West and Central Africa, is the leading cause of blindness in children.[3] In addition, because of greater vulnerability to severe infection, these children are at high risk for death. WHO, UNICEF, and other groups have helped provide vitamin A supplements in forty countries. These supplements have averted an estimated 1.25 million deaths since 1998.[15]

Vitamin B$_{12}$

Deficiency of vitamin B$_{12}$ can result in significant cognitive impairments, including deficits in learning and memory. Unfortunately, the prevalence of vitamin B$_{12}$ deficiency in children breastfed by mothers with lifelong limited access to animal products may be very high. Because meat, fish, and poultry are rich sources of iron, zinc, and vitamin B$_{12}$, it is possible that multiple subclinical deficiencies occur in children with limited access to these foods and impair their development.[16]

Undernutrition Diminishes Work Capacity

Undernutrition has long been known to diminish work capacity. The debilitating weakness from undernutrition affects the productivity of adults in developing nations throughout the world and is especially detrimental when manual labor involved in subsistence farming is the main source of food and income. The reduced earning capacity of poor, undernourished adults often regenerates a cycle of poverty onto the next generation.

Micronutrient deficiency also contributes to poor work capacity; for example, the World Bank estimates that a loss of 5% of the gross domestic product worldwide is attributable specifically to micronutrient deficiencies.[17] Iron-deficiency anemia is particularly debilitating because of iron's role in oxygen transport. Because iron deficiency is a problem among women of childbearing age in both developed and developing countries, it is a global drain on work capacity and productivity.

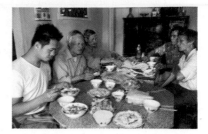

Meals comprised of adequate, nourishing food are important to avoid nutrient deficiency.

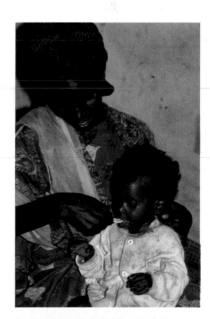

In developing nations, providing vitamin A supplements twice a year to children under age 5 has significantly reduced mortality.

Fetal Undernutrition Can Lead to Adult Disease

The "fetal origins theory" (also called the theory of "developmental origins of adult health and disease") states that biological adjustments to poor maternal nutrition made by a malnourished fetus as its organs are developing may help the child during times of food shortages, but they make the child susceptible to obesity and chronic disease when food is plentiful. For example, when a mother is malnourished during the pregnancy, her baby will tend to have a low birth weight but be relatively fat. This can occur because the fetal body has preserved fat tissue as a source of energy for growth of the brain, but at the expense of less muscle tissue. The imbalance results in metabolic disease later in life; there is now significant evidence supporting this hypothesis (see the **Nutrition Debate** in Chapter 16, pages 683–685, for more information).

> The International Society for Developmental Origins of Health and Disease was founded to promote research into the fetal and developmental origins of disease. To find out more about this topic and the activities of the society, go to www.mrc.soton.ac.uk/dohad/index.asp.

RECAP

Worldwide, malnutrition is a significant problem with two very different manifestations: undernutrition, the most serious manifestation of which is severe acute malnutrition, and overnutrition. Undernutrition causes wasting and stunting, increased susceptibility to infection, high mortality rates, micronutrient deficiency diseases, and poor work capacity. The theory called *fetal origins of adult disease* suggests that undernutrition during fetal development contributes to obesity and chronic disease in adulthood. Overnutrition results from excessive consumption of energy-dense food combined with inadequate physical activity, and underlies a rising prevalence of chronic diseases throughout the world. ■

What Causes Undernutrition in the Developing World?

Any situation that results in inadequate food for an individual or a community will prompt undernutrition. Natural disasters, wars, overpopulation, poor farming practices, disease, inequities in resource distribution, and other factors can result in a food supply that is inadequate to support the needs of all of the people in a particular place.

Famines Are Acute, Widespread Shortages of Food

Famines are severe food shortages affecting a large percentage of the population in a limited geographic area at a particular time. Famines have occurred throughout human history and typically cause significant loss of life. For example, an estimated 20–43 million people died in the so-called great famine in China from 1958 to 1961 when disastrous government land-use policies, combined with both floods and droughts, dramatically limited crop yields, with tragic results.

Natural disasters such as floods and droughts are often to blame for widespread famine. For example, in 2012, a protracted drought threatened at least 17 million people in the Sahel region of West Africa (a narrow belt spanning the southern Sahara from the Atlantic Ocean to the Red Sea). Other natural disasters that can destroy substantial amounts of local crops in a short time are tsunamis, high winds, hurricanes, frosts, pest infestations, and plant diseases.

Wars can induce famine when they interfere with planting or harvest times, or when they destroy standing crops. Abandonment of farmland in war-torn areas or takeover of farmland by military forces can lead to widespread shortages. In addition, military actions or policies may unintentionally or deliberately disrupt production, distribution, or sale of foods in regions affected by the conflict. In recent years, civil war and political instability in the Democratic Republic of the Congo have claimed an estimated 3 million lives, either as a direct result of fighting or because of disease and malnutrition. Wars can also contribute to famine when they interfere with food relief assistance by other nations.

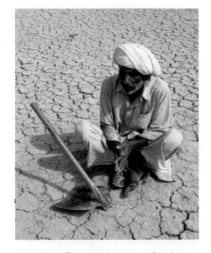

An Indian farmer inspects what is left of his crop during a drought.

famines Widespread, acute food shortages that affect a substantial portion of a population, often associated with starvation and death.

Both natural disasters and wars often cause migrations of large populations, who are forced to flee their homes and means of livelihood. Refugees may live in hastily erected camps with little access to sanitary water, medical care, or adequate food. Food safety is compromised by rodents and lack of refrigeration. Relief assistance by other countries or areas is vital for survival in these emergencies, because infection and malnutrition act synergistically in the crowded camps to erode health. Women, children, and the elderly in refugee camps are especially vulnerable when food supplies are delayed by damaged roads, poor transportation, political embargoes, or active conflict.

Multiple Factors Contribute to Chronic Food Shortages

Less dramatic than famines—but affecting more people over time—are chronic food shortages that lead to **food insecurity,** a condition in which people are unable to obtain enough energy and nutrients to meet their physical needs every day. **Food shortages** occur in areas where food production and import are not sufficient to meet the needs of the population in that area. Direct food aid in these situations must be carefully considered. If wealthy nations send food to a developing country in a time of need, it provides more food for hungry people in the short term but can also decrease the price that local farmers receive for their products, with the possible effect of increasing poverty in the area in the long run. Food aid is more detrimental if it floods the market at harvest and less detrimental if it is available only when local foods are absent from the market in very lean years.

Several factors contribute to food shortages and food insecurity in different parts of the world. The most common include overpopulation, poor farming practices, use of agricultural land for cash crops, lack of infrastructure, disease, and unequal distribution of limited food supplies. These are discussed briefly here.

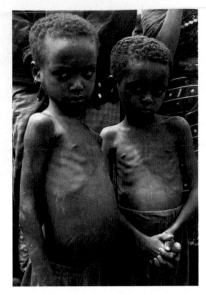

Hungry children living in refugee camps are highly susceptible to death from infectious disease. The skeletal limbs and swollen bellies of these young boys indicate severe acute malnutrition.

Overpopulation

An area is said to experience **overpopulation** when its resources are insufficient to support the number of people living there. In parts of the world with fertile land and adequate rainfall or irrigation systems to support abundant harvests, food shortages rarely happen. However, in more arid climates, especially in areas with high birthrates and poor access to imported foods, seasonal and chronic food shortages are common.

The population of the Earth passed 7 billion in 2011, and the Population Reference Bureau projects that world population will reach 9.6 billion by 2050.[18] So is the Earth itself overpopulated? Or will it soon become so? In other words, will we soon suffer worldwide food insufficiency? No one can answer these questions with absolute certainty, because we cannot predict how advances in technology will affect our depletion of the Earth's natural resources or our ability to produce more food with fewer resources.

However, slowing population growth is one way of improving an area's **food/population ratio.** Two methods of improving the food/population ratio are to increase food production and to import foods into the area. But these methods do little to influence population size. Likely the most effective method of reducing birthrates is to improve the education of women and girls.[19] Their increased earning potential, access to information about contraception, and better health practices lead to smaller, healthier, more economically stable families.

Agricultural Practices

Some traditional farming practices have the potential to destroy useable land. Deforestation by burning or any other means and overgrazing pastures and croplands destroy the trees and grass roots that preserve soils from wind and water erosion. Growing the same crop year after year on the same plot of ground can deplete the soil of nutrients and reduce crop yield. Some modern agricultural practices, such as avoiding overgrazing and using **crop rotation** to renew the nutrients in a parcel of ground, have benefited small farmers and increased the employment of agricultural workers.

food insecurity A condition in which an individual is unable to regularly obtain enough food to provide sufficient energy and nutrients to meet his or her physical needs.

food shortage A condition in which food production and import for a given area are not sufficient to meet the needs of the local population.

overpopulation A designation used for an area or a region that has insufficient resources to support the number of people living there.

food/population ratio The amount of food available for each individual within a given area; also called *food availability per capita*.

crop rotation The practice of alternating crops grown in a given field to prevent nutrient depletion and soil erosion, as well as to help with control of crop-specific pests.

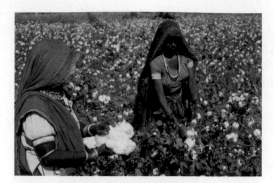

Cotton is a cash crop that farmers often grow instead of local food crops.

Use of agricultural land for **cash crops,** such as cotton, coffee, and tobacco, may replace land use for local food crops, such as sorghum, millet, and corn, also called **subsistence crops.** Particularly harmful to human health is the practice of growing food for animals, especially to feed cattle and chickens to supply ingredients for the fast-food industry. Much agricultural land in both developed and developing countries is devoted to such practices, which feed few people in the poor countries and come at high energy costs to all nations. Some crop production is not even for food; for example, oil derived from corn, soya beans, and rapeseed has many industrial uses. Another problem with cash crops is that they are likely to be produced by large landholders who pay insufficient wages to their hired laborers. This problem occurs in developed nations as well (see Chapter 15).

Lack of Infrastructure

Exacerbating the scarcity of food production in some areas is a lack of infrastructure. For example, many developing countries lack roads and transportation into the areas of the country away from ports and major cities. This limits available food to whatever can be produced locally. In addition, lack of electricity and refrigeration can limit storage of perishable foods before they can be used.

Water management is a second aspect of infrastructure that influences nutrition. In dry areas, irrigation can improve food production, but it must be managed carefully to prevent increasing the numbers of mosquitoes, intestinal parasites, and other pests, which can spread infectious diseases. The provision of safe drinking water and sewage systems is another aspect of water management that helps prevent disease.

Other critical aspects of infrastructure are sanitation services, communication systems, an adequate healthcare delivery system, and adequate public education. In summary, public health depends on public policies that support the development of personnel, physical structures, and technological innovations that promote health and prevent disease.

Impact of Disease

Disease and lack of healthcare resources to fight disease reduce the work capacity of individuals, and this in turn reduces their ability to ward off poverty and malnutrition. This economic phenomenon is demonstrated by the AIDS epidemic. As of 2011, there were 34 million people living with HIV, and 1.8 million people died from AIDS in 2010.[20] HIV is most likely to affect young, sexually active adults who are the primary wage earners in their families. Thus, their illness or death can impoverish their children, younger siblings, and/or elderly parents. In Africa, AIDS is the leading cause of death, and the death of both parents to AIDS has made orphans of about 17 million children. By creating populations in which children and the elderly predominate, the AIDS epidemic has exacerbated the risk for undernutrition in many developing countries.[21]

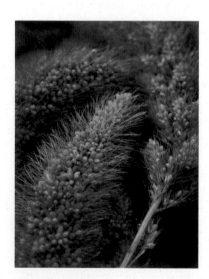

Millet is a common subsistence crop.

Unequal Distribution of Food

The major cause of undernutrition in the world is unequal distribution of food, largely due to poverty. In the developing world, more than three-fourths of malnourished children live in countries with food surpluses.[22] The most at-risk populations are the rural poor. Lacking sufficient land to grow their own foods, the rural poor must work for others to earn money to buy food, but because they live in rural areas, employment opportunities are limited.

Unequal distribution also occurs because of cultural biases. In many countries, limited food is distributed first to men and boys and only secondarily to women and girls. In such situations, pregnant women and growing girls are the most vulnerable because of their increased needs. Food distribution to the elderly is sometimes also limited, particularly in developing countries where nutrition services are primarily directed toward pregnant and lactating women, infants, and young children. Access to food also can differ by ethnicity and religion. For example, officials in authority may order that food aid be distributed preferentially to areas where their own ethnic group dominates.

cash crops Crops grown to be sold rather than eaten, such as cotton, tobacco, jute, and sugarcane.

subsistence crops Crops grown to be eaten by a family or community, such as rice, millet, and garden vegetables; surpluses in these crops may at times be sold locally.

RECAP

Famines are widespread, severe food shortages that can result in starvation and death. They are most commonly caused by natural disasters or wars. Less severe but chronic food shortages can be influenced by regional overpopulation, poor agricultural practices, and the burden of disease; however, unequal distribution of food due primarily to poverty is the major cause of food shortages—and resulting undernutrition—around the world. ■

Why Is Overnutrition a Global Concern?

As you know, overconsumption of energy in excess of energy use increases body weight, to a larger or lesser degree depending on an individual's metabolic efficiency. Chronic overconsumption leads to obesity, which increases the risk for chronic diseases.

The Prevalence of Obesity and Chronic Disease Is Increasing Worldwide

Throughout the world, the prevalence of obesity and its associated chronic diseases is increasing at an alarming rate. The World Health Organization (WHO) estimates that, between 1980 and 2008, the worldwide prevalence of obesity nearly doubled. In 2008, half a billion people were obese. WHO also estimates that worldwide one in ten people have diabetes and one in three have high blood pressure.[23] As alarming as these statistics are, the predictions for the future are even higher: the WHO estimates that by 2015 more than 700 million will be obese and that by 2020 deaths due to diabetes will increase worldwide by more than 50%.[23]

The global burden of diabetes cannot be overstated. For example, the most recent data from the American Diabetes Association show that the cost of healthcare for people with diabetes in the United States exceeded $174 billion in 2007. In addition are a variety of indirect costs from factors such as absenteeism from work, reduced productivity, and lost productive capacity due to early death.[24] As diabetes increases in countries without the resources of the United States, lack of access to effective healthcare will increase the indirect economic costs. Families and communities will experience more lost work time, increased disability, and earlier death of adults who would have contributed to the family's resources and local economy.

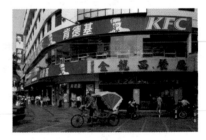

Overnutrition is becoming a global problem now that nutrient-poor, high Calorie foods are more widely available.

The Nutrition Paradox Is an Emerging Global Health Concern

If food is scarce in developing nations, how can their rates of obesity be increasing? Called the **nutrition paradox** (or *nutritional dual-burden*), this recent public health problem is characterized by the coexistence of stunting and overweight/obesity within the same region, the same household, and even the same person. The nutrition paradox is especially common in countries transitioning from the very poorest to the middle range of gross national income, such as Mexico, Brazil, Egypt, India, China, and Thailand. In one neighborhood in the city of Merida, Mexico, researchers found that, of fifty-eight adult women measured, forty-three were both stunted and overweight or obese.[25]

Many researchers identify two key factors behind the nutrition paradox in transitioning nations:[25]

■ *A trend toward decreased physical activity* due to the increasingly sedentary nature of many forms of work, changing modes of transportation, and increasing urbanization
■ *A global shift in diet toward increased intake of energy-dense foods* that are high in fat and sugars but low in micronutrients and fiber

In effect, all nations—developed, transitioning, and developing—have been exposed to a nutritional transition over the past 20 years, as international food companies have made processed, energy-dense foods available at lower cost to more people worldwide. See **Table 19.1** for an overview of some factors contributing to worldwide obesity. In many developed

nutrition paradox The coexistence of aspects of both undernutrition and overnutrition within the same region, household, family, or person; also known as *nutritional dual-burden*.

Table 19.1 An Overview of Select Factors Contributing to Worldwide Obesity

	Developed Countries	Immigrants Living in Developed Countries	Developing Countries
Growth and Weight Status	Height: normal/tall Body composition: high degree of body fat	Height: normal/tall Body composition: higher degree of body fat than in country of origin	(Dual-burden) Height: stunted/short Body composition: high degree of body fat
Common Factors	Diet dense in energy from added fats and sugars	Transition to diet dense in energy from added fats and sugars	Transition to diet dense in energy from added fats and sugars
Physical Activity Level	Normal to low	Normal to low	Normal to high
Metabolic Pathways	High body fat and low carbohydrate oxidation	Mixed evidence for reduced body fat and higher carbohydrate oxidation and for energy-conserving activity levels	Mixed evidence for reduced body fat and higher carbohydrate oxidation and for energy-conserving activity levels

Source: Data from "The nutritional dual-burden in developing countries. How is it assessed and what are the health implications?" *Collegium Antropologicum* 36:39–45.

Nutrition
MILESTONE

The International Diabetes Foundation estimates that, by the year 2030, 7.7% of the world's population—about 439 million people—will have diabetes. While it has been known for decades that inactivity and obesity increase the risk for diabetes, in recent years two groundbreaking studies have shown the efficacy of exercise and weight loss in curbing this pandemic.

Both were large, randomized trials. The first study was conducted in Finland in **2001** and the second in the United States in 2002. Both studies found that 20 to 30 minutes of moderate exercise per day—along with a weight loss of just 7 to 13 pounds—cut the incidence of type 2 diabetes by more than 50%. In fact, these changes were more effective in preventing diabetes than drug treatments.

In 2008, more than 100 nutrition scientists were asked to name the most significant recent discoveries in nutrition. Eleventh among their choices was the discovery that diabetes can be prevented by modest exercise and weight loss alone.

nations, people tend to be taller, but a majority are now also overweight. People born in developing nations who were undernourished when young are likely to be short (due to growth stunting) but experience rapid weight gain when their country transitions out of poverty or they move to a more developed country, because they are confronted with an oversupply of low-cost, nutrient-poor, high-Calorie foods. The result is short stature combined with overweight. Even people in transitioning nations who work in physically demanding jobs tend to gain weight. There is evidence from some studies that this may be due to reduced oxidation of dietary fat, meaning that these people tend to store the fat rather than use it for energy expenditure.[25] Finally, there are the consequences of poor nutritional status in the mother that affect her fetus (discussed previously). These effects can be passed on to future generations when affected girls of the current generation grow up and start their own families. For this reason, immigrants to richer nations and the poor in developing nations may need four or more generations of improved conditions to overcome all past risks for short stature and overweight.

Can poverty be an independent risk factor for obesity? Even among established (non-immigrant) populations in the United States, the United Kingdom, and other developed nations, there is a clear association between poverty and obesity.[26] Why? One reason may be that energy-dense foods with longer shelf lives, such as vegetable oils, sugar, refined flour, snack foods, soft drinks, and canned goods, are less expensive than perishable foods such as meats, fish, milk, and fresh fruits and vegetables. Consider that, between 1985 and 2000, the inflation-adjusted prices of fruits and vegetables increased by an average of 40%. During the same period of time, the real price of soft drinks fell by almost 25%.[26] In addition, cheap, energy-dense foods have a higher satiety value: they cause a person to feel full for a longer period of time at a lower cost. Thus, individuals with limited money to spend are likely to prefer such foods. In short, although the mechanisms by which obesity and poverty are linked are not entirely clear, there is now substantial evidence of the global shift of the burden of overweight and obesity to the poor.

RECAP

Overnutrition resulting in obesity is now a public health concern not only in developed nations but also in countries transitioning out of poverty. Lack of physical activity and increased availability of low-cost, nutrient-poor, high-Calorie foods have shifted the burden of obesity and chronic diseases toward the poor. ■

How Many Americans Go Hungry?

In the United States, overnutrition is becoming a national health crisis. The majority of Americans, more than 68%, are now overweight or obese, and the prevalence of type 2 diabetes and other chronic diseases associated with obesity is increasing.[27] But even in the United States, unequal distribution of abundant food leaves some of our poorest citizens hungry.

As shown in **Figure 19.4**, the US Department of Agriculture (USDA) estimates that 14.5% of U.S. households (about 17.2 million households) experienced food insecurity in 2010.[28] This means that the people living in these homes were unable to obtain enough food to meet their physical needs every day. Of these 17.2 million, 6.4 million households had *very low food security*, meaning that normal eating patterns of one or more members of the household were disrupted and food intake was reduced at times during the year, because they had insufficient money or other resources for food. How do "households" translate into human beings? In 2010, 48.8 million Americans, including 16.2 million children, experienced food insecurity.[28]

Those at higher risk for food insecurity are households with incomes below 185% of the official U.S. poverty threshold (which was $22,050 for a family of four in 2010), families consisting of single mothers or single fathers and their children, African American households, and Hispanic households.[28] Other vulnerable groups are the homeless, the unemployed, elderly people living on a fixed income, migrant laborers, and other workers in minimum-wage jobs.

Sometimes physical, psychological, or social factors contribute to food insecurity among Americans. For instance, people with chronic diseases or disabilities may lose paid work hours due to illness, have to accept lower-wage jobs, or have medical expenses that limit money for food. Depression, addiction to alcohol or other substances, and other psychological disorders can similarly limit productivity and reduce income. Divorce frequently leads to financial stressors, especially for women, who may be unable to collect alimony or child support payments and may have jobs that do not provide an income sufficient to provide fully for the family's needs.

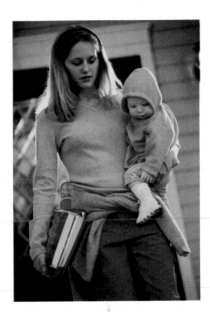

> To view the full report from the USDA's Economic Research Service on food insecurity in the United States, including the survey questions used, graphs of data, and commentary, go to www.ers.usda.gov/media/121076/err125_2_.pdf.

RECAP

More than 14% of U.S. households experienced food insecurity in 2010, meaning that 48.8 million Americans, including 16.2 million children, were food insecure. Families with incomes below the official U.S. poverty level and families headed by a single parent are among those with the highest rates of food insecurity. ■

Many single mothers face economic burdens that leave them and their children vulnerable to food insecurity.

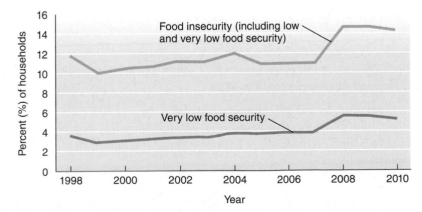

FIGURE 19.4 Prevalence of food insecurity and very low food security in U.S. households, 1998–2010. (*Source:* Calculated by USDA, Economic Research Service based on Current Population Survey Food Security Supplement data. Household Food Security in the United States in 2010.)

What Are Some Solutions to Malnutrition?

The United Nations (UN) Millennium Development Goals (MDGs) include the eradication of extreme poverty and hunger.[29] The number of people in developing regions living on less than $1.25 a day decreased from 1.8 billion in 1990 to 1.4 billion in 2005. The global economic crisis, which began in 2008, has slowed this progress, and the UN estimates that the crisis forced some 64 million additional people to live in extreme poverty at the end of 2010. Reductions in hunger were also achieved between 1990 and 2007, but then the global economic crisis prompted a near doubling in global food prices. In 2010, 830 million people were undernourished. This represents an *increase* from 817 million in 1990–1992. Worse still, one in four children remains undernourished today.[29]

The world possesses the resources and knowledge to ensure that even the poorest countries, and others held back by disease, geographic isolation, or civil strife, can be empowered to achieve the MDGs. For example, the US Agency for International Development (USAID) has developed a Famine Early Warning System Network to monitor droughts, floods, and other problems that affect food supplies, so that interventions can be provided quickly and efficiently.

Long-term solutions are critical to achieve and maintain global food security. The UN identifies the need for the world community to develop a long-term "global partnership for development" involving international, national, community, household, and individual strategies.[29] We discuss some local initiatives and technological strategies to meet these challenges in this section.

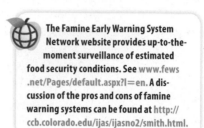

The Famine Early Warning System Network website provides up-to-the-moment surveillance of estimated food security conditions. See www.fews .net/Pages/default.aspx?l=en. A discussion of the pros and cons of famine warning systems can be found at http:// ccb.colorado.edu/ijas/ijasno2/smith.html.

Public Health Programs Provide Local Solutions

Public health initiatives include programs to encourage breastfeeding, combat infectious disease, and distribute food equitably.

Programs to Encourage Breastfeeding

Among the most important local initiatives for improving the health and nutrition of children worldwide are programs that encourage breastfeeding. As we discuss in the **Highlight** box (page 767), breast milk not only provides optimal nutrition for healthy growth of the newborn but also contains antibodies that protect against infections.

In 1991, WHO and UNICEF initiated the Baby Friendly Hospital Initiative to increase breastfeeding rates worldwide. Under this initiative, new mothers are educated about the benefits of breast milk, the risks of bottle-feeding, and the importance of maternal nutrition during lactation. They are encouraged to breastfeed exclusively for the first 6 months of the child's life and to continue breastfeeding as part of the child's daily diet until the child is at least 2 years old.

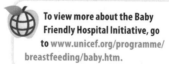

To view more about the Baby Friendly Hospital Initiative, go to www.unicef.org/programme/ breastfeeding/baby.htm.

Programs to Combat Infectious Disease

In 1982, UNICEF began a campaign to eliminate common infections of childhood by four inexpensive local strategies referred to as **GOBI:**

G—growth monitoring to assess childhood well-being
O—oral rehydration therapy to stop death from dehydration during diarrheal diseases
    using a simple solution containing a balance of fluids and electrolytes
B—breastfeeding
I—immunization against tuberculosis, diphtheria, whooping cough, tetanus, polio, and
    measles[29]

By 1990, GOBI was estimated to have saved 12 million children, and millions more each year are saved. These four successful strategies continue as parts of various local initiatives to reach the United Nations Millennium Development Goals.[29]

GOBI A UNICEF campaign to eliminate common childhood infections via four inexpensive strategies: "GOBI" stands for growth monitoring, oral rehydration therapy, breastfeeding, and immunization.

HIGHLIGHT

Encouraging Breastfeeding in the Developing World

In the United States and other industrialized nations, the benefits of breastfeeding include its precise correspondence with the infant's nutritional needs, protection of the infant from infections and allergies, promotion of mother–infant bonding, low cost, and convenience. In developing countries, however, breastfeeding may also save the newborn's or mother's life. Here are some reasons.

It is estimated that a quarter of the Earth's population may lack sanitary drinking water. Breastfeeding protects newborns from contaminated water supplies. The least expensive form of infant formula is a packaged powder that must be carefully measured and mixed with a precise quantity of sterilized water. If the water is not sterilized and is contaminated with disease-causing organisms, the baby will become ill. In developing countries, breastfeeding is considered to reduce diarrheal deaths in young children by 50% to 95%.

At the same time, a baby who is fed formula instead of breast milk receives none of the mother's beneficial antibodies; this means that, when formula-fed infants do contract an infection, whether from contaminated water or any other source, they are not as well prepared to fight it off as breastfed infants would be. As we discuss in this chapter, reduced resistance to infection is extremely dangerous for infants and children throughout the developing world.

In addition, in an attempt to make their supply of formula last longer, some impoverished parents add more water than the amount specified by the manufacturer. In this case, even when the water is sterilized, the child is at risk for malnutrition, because the nutrients in the formula are being diluted.

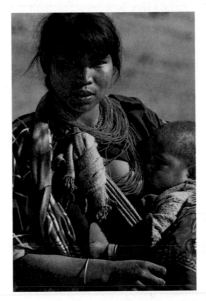

Breastfeeding is highly recommended worldwide.

These factors explain why breastfeeding is protective of the infant, but why does it help the mother? First, breastfeeding stimulates the uterus to contract vigorously after childbirth. This reduces the woman's risk for prolonged or excessive postpartum bleeding, a common cause of maternal mortality in developing nations. Second, breastfeeding reduces a woman's risk of developing ovarian and breast cancer. Third, breastfeeding is a natural form of birth control; although not as effective as a contraceptive, prolonged, exclusive breastfeeding does delay the onset of ovulation. In regions where access to contraceptives may be lacking, breastfeeding can help a woman put space between births, giving her body a chance to recover from the physical and metabolic changes of pregnancy, and to nourish her baby adequately without also having to support the development of a growing fetus.

The human immunodeficiency virus (HIV), which causes AIDS, can be transmitted from mother to child via breast milk. Antiretroviral (ARV) drug interventions to either the mother or HIV-exposed infant reduces the risk for transmission of HIV through breastfeeding. Together, breastfeeding and ARV interventions have the potential to significantly improve infants' chances of surviving while remaining uninfected. WHO recommends that, when HIV-infected mothers breastfeed, they should receive ARVs and follow WHO guidance for breastfeeding and complementary feeding.

In summary, international organizations such as the World Health Organization and UNICEF encourage women to breastfeed exclusively until their baby is 6 months of age and to continue supplemented breastfeeding until at least the age of 2.

Source: Data adapted from "Ten Facts on Breastfeeding," World Health Organization website, 2012.

Because vitamin A can be stored in the body's fat tissues, one high-strength vitamin A supplement given every 6 months can prevent deficiency and significantly reduce a child's risk for death from infectious disease. Since 1997, The Micronutrient Initiative (MI), the WHO, and several other national and international organizations have collaborated to provide twice-yearly vitamin A supplements to more than 77% of children in developing countries.[30] The MI also promotes global adequacy for the intake of zinc, iron, iodine, and folic acid. Because of the critical role of these micronutrients in immune defense, these measures also combat infectious disease. In addition, programs for deworming and

Nutri-Case

Judy

"I never seem to be able to make ends meet. I keep hoping next month will be different, but rent and utilities eat up most of my paycheck, so when something unexpected happens, I'm short. Last week, my car broke down and I'm way behind on my credit card payments. Today, a collections guy called and said that if I didn't pay at least $100 right away, they'd take me to court. When I got off the phone, I started to cry, and Hannah asked me what was wrong. When I told her how bad the money situation is, she thought we might qualify for food stamps. I have a full-time job, so I don't think we'll qualify, but even if we do, I wonder if it'll help much."

In 2012, the federal minimum wage was $7.25 an hour. As a nurse's aide, Judy earns $9 an hour, or $1,560 a month. She is eligible for the Supplemental Nutrition Assistance Program (food stamps). Are you surprised that someone making almost 25% more than the minimum wage, and working full-time, qualifies for food assistance?

Before you're too certain that Judy's eligibility will solve her problems, consider that the average food stamp allotment in 2012 was $4.30 per person per day, or about $30 per week for one person.* If you had just $30 to keep yourself fed for a week, what would you buy?

Take this challenge one step further and follow the example of some U.S. college students to raise local awareness of food insecurity: for 1 week, restrict yourself to just $30 for all your food purchases. Let your campus newspaper and local media outlets know what you're doing, and ask readers to make donations to local food banks.

*Congressional Budget Office. 2012, April 19. An Overview of the Supplemental Nutrition Assistance Program. www.cbo.gov/publication/43175.

mosquito control combat not only helminth and malarial infection but also their accompanying iron deficiency.

Programs to Promote Equitable Distribution of Food

In the United States, several government programs help low-income citizens acquire food over extended periods of time. Among these programs are the Supplemental Nutrition Assistance Program (previously called the Food Stamp Program), which helps low-income individuals of all ages; the Special Supplemental Nutrition Program for Women, Infants, and Children (WIC), which helps pregnant women and children to age 5; the National School Lunch and National School Breakfast Programs, which help low-income schoolchildren; and the Summer Food Service Program, which helps low-income children in the summer.

The United States also has a broad network of local soup kitchens and food pantries that provide meals and food items to needy families. They are supported by volunteers, individual donations, and food contributions from local grocery stores and restaurants. In addition, the US Department of Agriculture distributes surplus foods to charitable agencies for distribution to needy families.

In the less developed nations, many international organizations help improve the nutrient status of the poor by enabling them to produce their own foods. For example, both USAID and the Peace Corps have agricultural education programs, the World Bank provides loans to fund small business ventures, and many nonprofit and nongovernmental organizations (NGOs) support community and family farms.

Technological Strategies Provide Global Solutions

Technological strategies for increasing the world's food supply include the Green Revolution, the sustainable agriculture movement, and the application of biotechnology, including the use of genetically modified organisms.

The Green Revolution

The **Green Revolution,** one of the major agricultural advances of the past 50 years, has increased the productivity of cultivated land while maintaining environmental quality.[31] As part of the Green Revolution, new **high-yield varieties** of grain were produced by cross-breeding plants and selecting for the most desirable traits. The new semi-dwarf varieties of rice, corn, and wheat are less likely to fall over in wind and heavy rains and can carry more seeds. They have been widely adopted in North and South America and Asia and have doubled or tripled the yield per acre while reducing costs. It is likely that millions of people have been saved from starvation since the 1960s. In addition, these varieties slow the pace of global warming by reducing the need to cut forests for new agricultural land.[32]

Less success was achieved in creating high-yield varieties of staples traditional to sub-Saharan Africa, such as sorghum, millet, and cassava, which are grown in hot, dry conditions. Thus, Africa has shared least in the alleviation of hunger achieved during the Green Revolution.

Although it has achieved higher yields at lower costs, which have greatly benefited farmers and consumers, the Green Revolution has prompted new problems. Because it requires the use of chemical fertilizers, pesticides, irrigation, and mechanical harvesters to reduce labor costs, it has most benefited larger, wealthier landowners and has not helped small family farms. Environmental damages associated with the Green Revolution have included loss of topsoil due to erosion from heavy tilling, from extensive planting of row crops such as corn and soybeans, and from runoff due to irrigation.

Sustainable Agriculture

In response to the drawbacks of the Green Revolution, a new global movement toward **sustainable agriculture** has evolved. The goal of the sustainable agriculture movement is to develop local, site-specific farming methods that improve soil conservation, crop yields, and food security in a sustainable manner, minimizing the adverse environmental impact. For example, soil erosion can be controlled by crop rotation, by terracing of sloped land for the cultivation of crops (**Figure 19.5**), by tillage that minimizes disturbance to the topsoil, and by the use of herbicides to remove weeds rather than hoeing.

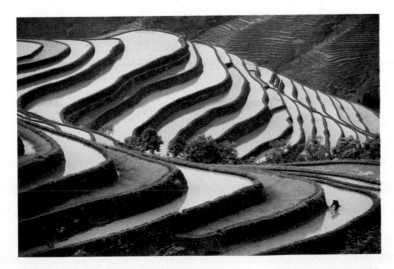

FIGURE 19.5 Terracing sloped land to avoid soil erosion is one practice of sustainable agriculture.

Green Revolution The period, between 1944 and 2000, of tremendous increase in global productivity as a result of selective cross-breeding and hybridization that produced high-yield grains and modern industrial farming techniques.

high-yield varieties Semi-dwarf plant varieties that are unlikely to fall over in wind and heavy rains, and thus can carry higher quantities of seeds, greatly increasing the yield per acre.

sustainable agriculture Techniques of food production that preserve the environment indefinitely.

Meat production is a particularly controversial issue within the sustainable agriculture movement. Research data point to the significant inefficiency of eating meat from grain-fed cattle instead of eating the grains themselves, both in terms of the resources required and the emissions generated. Livestock production also leads to deforestation, further contributing to global warming. Supporters of meat production emphasize the benefits of using livestock to convert otherwise unuseable plants to high-quality food, to improve the nutritional quality of the diet of people in developing countries, and to contribute nonchemical fertilizer to renew the soil.

Another practice associated with sustainable agriculture is the use of **transgenic crops** (also called *genetically modified organisms*, or *GMOs*), plant varieties that have had one or more genes altered. Such crops can reduce the need for insecticides or permit the cultivation of marginally fertile land, and some supporters see their use as the next step in the Green Revolution. They contend that genetically modified crops can produce higher yields on limited land, allowing peasant farmers to feed their families with disease-resistant crops that can be farmed without chemicals and using traditional methods. In addition, genetically modified crops with improved nutrient density, when grown in areas already being cultivated by the family, can improve nutrient status with no change in farming practices.[33–35]

However, there is currently considerable controversy surrounding the long-term safety and environmental impact of genetically modified crops. In addition, patents on the tools of biotechnology limit their use.[36] Conferring public right to the necessary technological tools would allow more widespread use of advanced technologies for assisting poor farmers to improve food security. (For more information, see Chapter 15).

RECAP

Short-term aid prevents death during emergency food shortages. Long-term solutions to global food security include programs to encourage breastfeeding, to combat infectious disease, and to promote equitable distribution of available food, which help maximize local solutions. The Green Revolution and sustainable agricultural practices are strategies aimed at increasing the world's food supply. ■

What Can You Do to Combat Global Malnutrition?

Two general strategies for combating global malnutrition are to make personal choices that promote food equity and environmental quality and to volunteer with an organization that works to relieve hunger.

Make Personal Choices That Promote Food Equity and Preserve the Environment

The personal choices that each individual makes can contribute to or combat global malnutrition by influencing local and global markets. Choosing to purchase certain foods makes those foods more likely to be produced in the future. If you choose vegetables, fruits, nuts, whole grains, and beans and other legumes, then you will influence greater production of these healthful foods. If you buy organic foods, you encourage reduction in the use of chemical pesticides and herbicides. If you buy produce from a local farmers' market, you encourage greater local availability of fresh foods. This reduces the costs of and resources devoted to distribution, transportation, and storage of foods.

To combat overnutrition, the major type of malnutrition in the United States, avoid or limit energy-dense, nutrient-poor choices and encourage your friends to follow your lead.

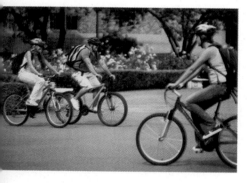

Bicycling is a healthful option that helps limit the use of fossil fuels.

transgenic crops Plant varieties that have had one or more genes altered by genetic technologies; also called *genetically modified organisms* (GMOs).

Nutrition Myth OR Fact?

If You Clean Your Plate, Will It Help the Starving Children in Africa?

It used to be considered polite to finish all the food on your plate and wasteful to throw food away. Children were told, "Clean your plate—it will help the starving children in Africa!" Today, this admonition raises a serious issue that you might want to consider if you are or plan to be a parent or to work with children.

The primary reason for *not* teaching children that they must clean their plates is that overeating is becoming a worldwide problem, and coaxing children to eat when they are no longer hungry teaches them to ignore their body's hunger/satiation signals. This can set the stage for disordered eating. Instead of overfilling a child's plate, parents and caregivers should serve children a reasonable portion of food. If the child eats that and is still hungry, he or she can be given more.

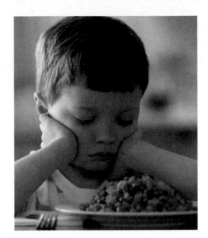

Forcing children to finish meals is not a strategy for fighting global hunger.

In addition, "cleaning your plate" at home does not help children in other parts of the world. If anything, encouraging children at home to eat just the amount of food their bodies need may help children in developing nations by preserving more of the global harvest. Healthful eating behaviors also reduce children's risk of developing obesity and its associated chronic diseases, thereby reducing their use of limited medical resources as they grow.

So next time you're tempted to admonish a child to "clean your plate," try something new. Get down on the child's level, and talk about it: "I notice you haven't finished your dinner. Check in with your tummy—are you still hungry, or have you had enough?" Your question may not help a starving child, but it might help the very child you're talking to.

Read labels: do you really want high-fructose corn syrup in your peanut butter? When large numbers of people stop purchasing foods high in saturated fats or added sugars, the profitability of these foods declines and they are more likely to disappear from the marketplace. And whatever you eat, avoid overconsumption. You'll be leaving more food for others as well as reducing your risk for obesity and its accompanying chronic diseases. Not convinced? Consider the competing philosophies presented in the **Nutrition Myth or Fact?** box (above).

The amount of meat you eat also affects the global food supply. As we noted earlier, the production of plant-based foods requires a lower expenditure of natural resources and releases fewer greenhouse gases than the production of animal-based foods, so making plant foods the main source of your diet preserves land, water, and global energy and reduces global warming. However, animal-based foods do contribute high-quality nutrients, such as iron, and can be consumed in moderation worldwide without harm to either health or the environment.

Remember that physical activity is important in maintaining health and combating overnutrition, so walk and bike as often as you can in your everyday life. Walking, biking, and taking public transportation also limit your consumption of nonrenewable fossil fuels. When it's time to purchase a car, research your options and choose the one with the best fuel economy.

Volunteer with an Organization That Fights Hunger

Several times each year, college students from hundreds of campuses all over the United States gather to fight hunger as members of the National Student Campaign Against Hunger and Homelessness.[37] They hold "Hunger Cleanups," staff relief agencies, solicit donations of food and money, and promote community activism. Their organization is

What Can You Do to Combat Global Malnutrition?

Have you ever wondered if your actions inadvertently contribute to the problem of global malnutrition? Or whether efforts you make locally can help feed people thousands of miles away? In this exercise, you'll reflect on your behavior in three different roles you play every day: consumer, student, and citizen of the world.

In your role as a consumer, ask yourself:

How can I use my food purchases to promote the production of more healthful, less processed foods?
Any grocery store manager will tell you that your purchases influence the types of foods that are manufactured and sold. If people become aware of the benefits of eating whole-grain bread and stop buying soft white bread, stores will stop carrying it and food companies will stop making it. In our global economy, your food choices can even influence the types of foods that are imported.

1. Choose fresh, locally grown, organic foods more often to support local sustainability.

2. Choose whole or less processed versions of packaged foods. This encourages their increased production and saves energy.

3. Both when you're shopping and when you're eating out, avoid nutrient-poor foods and beverages to discourage their profitability.

How often do I eat vegetarian?
Plant-based sources of protein can be produced with less energy cost than animal-based sources, so reducing your consumption of animal foods saves global energy.

1. Experiment with some recipes in a vegetarian cookbook. Try making at least one new vegetarian meal each week.

2. Introduce friends and family members to your new vegetarian dishes.

3. When eating out, choose restaurants that provide vegetarian menu choices. If the campus cafeteria or a favorite restaurant has no vegetarian choices, request that some be added to the menu.

How much do I eat?
Eating just the Calories you need to maintain a healthy weight leaves more of the global harvest for others and will likely reduce your use of medical resources as well.

1. To raise your consciousness about the physical experience of hunger, consider fasting for 1 day. If health or other reasons prevent you from fasting safely, try keeping silent during each meal throughout 1 day, so that you can more fully appreciate the food you're eating and reflect on those who are hungry.

2. For 1 week, keep track of how much food you throw away, and why. Do you put more food on your plate than

you can eat? Do you allow foods stored in your refrigerator to spoil? Do you often buy new foods to "try" and then throw them away because you don't like them?

3. On a daily basis, check in with your body before and as you eat: are you really hungry, and if so, how much and what type of food does your body really need right now?

In your role as a student, ask yourself:

How can I use what I have learned about nutrition to combat malnutrition in my neighborhood?

1. Visit each of your local fast-food restaurants and ask for information about the nutritional value of their foods. Analyze the information; then summarize it in simple language. Offer to submit a series of articles about your findings to your school or local newspaper.

2. Research what local produce is available in each season. Write an article for your school newspaper identifying the foods in season, and include two healthful recipes using those foods.

3. Begin or join a food cooperative, community garden, or shared farming program. Donate a portion of your produce each week to a local food pantry.

What careers could I consider to help combat global malnutrition?
No matter what career you choose, use your unique talents to advocate global food security.

1. You could become a member of the Peace Corps and serve in a developing country.

2. If you're interested in science, you could have a career helping develop more nutrient-dense or perennial crops, better food-preservation methods, or projects to improve food or water safety.

3. If you plan a career in business, you could enter the food industry and work for the production and marketing of healthful products.

4. If you pursue a career in healthcare, you could join an international medical corps to combat deficiency diseases.

In your role as a world citizen, ask yourself:
How can I improve the lives of people in my own community?

1. You can volunteer at a local soup kitchen, homeless shelter, food bank, or community garden.

2. You can join a food cooperative, a store or farm in which you work a number of hours each week in exchange for discounts on healthful foods.

3. Because obesity is likely to be a significant problem in your community, you can help increase

opportunities for physical activity in your community. Start a walking group, or volunteer to coach children in a favorite sport.

How can I improve the lives of people in developing nations?

1. Donate time or raise money for one of the international agencies that work to relieve global hunger. Check out options for charitable contributions and volunteer efforts at www.charitynavigator.org.

2. Join efforts to influence government foreign policies to support global food security.

3. Research the human rights records of international food companies whose products you buy. If you don't like what you find out, switch brands, and write to the company and tell them why you did.

just one of dozens in which you can get involved. You can gather foods for local food banks, volunteer to work in a soup kitchen, help distribute food to homebound elderly, or start a community or school garden. You can also hold fund-raisers and donate cash directly. Check out the Web Links at the end of this chapter for the names of national agencies and get involved!

Because obesity is likely to be as much or more of a problem in your community as hunger, you can also volunteer to fight overnutrition. For instance, you could teach children about healthy eating at after-school programs or on Saturday in the local library. You could help provide opportunities for your neighbors to be physically active. Start a walking group or help with community marathons and "fun runs." You might volunteer to coach after-school sports for children or assist with summer camps that teach children about physical fitness.

You can also get involved with one of the many international agencies that assist developing nations in fighting hunger. Research a few of those listed in the Web Links at the end of this chapter. When you find one you like, volunteer time or donate or raise money to help its cause. The accompanying **Highlight** box (page 772) identifies more steps you can take to help combat global malnutrition.

If you still wonder whether your personal acts can make a difference, consider the advice of the late historian and civil rights activist Howard Zinn. He urged people to "just do something, to join with millions of others who will just do something, because all of those somethings, at certain points in history, come together and make the world better."[38]

RECAP

By making personal choices that promote food equity and environmental quality, or volunteering with an organization that works to relieve hunger, you can help combat malnutrition around the world and in your community. ▪

Chapter Review

1 **T** Currently, about 14.5% of US households are unable to obtain enough energy and nutrients to meet their physical needs every day.

2 **F** The major cause of undernutrition in the world is unequal distribution of adequate food supplies, primarily due to poverty.

3 **F** The population of the Earth passed 7 billion in 2011, and the Population Reference Bureau projects that it will continue to climb for at least the next three decades, reaching 9.6 billion by 2050.

4 **T** Significant evidence supports the hypothesis that physiologic adjustments to poor maternal nutrition by a developing fetus make the child susceptible to obesity and chronic disease when food becomes more plentiful.

5 **T** Currently, the global burden of obesity is shifting to the poor. For example, the prevalence of obesity in both children and adults in many developing nations is increasing at a faster rate than in developed countries.

Summary

- Malnutrition, which includes both undernutrition and overnutrition, is a significant, increasingly global health concern.

- Undernutrition contributes to wasting, growth stunting, reduced resistance to infection, increased mortality, micronutrient deficiency diseases, and diminished work capacity.

- The fetal origins theory suggests that fetal malnutrition is associated with increased risk for obesity and chronic diseases later in life when fetal undernutrition is relieved in childhood and young adulthood.

- Undernutrition results from famines or chronic food shortages due to overpopulation, poor agricultural practices, lack of infrastructure, disease, and unequal distribution of limited food supplies.

- The major cause of global undernutrition is unequal distribution of food, due primarily to poverty but also resulting from cultural, age-related, ethnic and religious factors.

- The prevalence of obesity is increasing worldwide, including in developing nations.

- The rising costs of treating chronic, obesity-related diseases, such as diabetes, hypertension, and cardiovascular disease, are a growing economic burden worldwide.

- Overconsumption of nutrient energy in developed and transitioning countries is exacerbated by sedentary lifestyles.

- Poverty exacerbates overnutrition and obesity, often because less expensive foods are energy dense with a higher satiety value, are widely available, and have longer shelf lives.

- The GOBI initiative of UNICEF combats common infections of childhood by encouraging growth monitoring, oral rehydration therapy, breastfeeding, and immunizations.

- The Green Revolution and methods of sustainable agriculture share a common goal of increasing the world's food supply.

- Individual and local efforts to combat global malnutrition include personal choices you make every day as a consumer, a student, and a citizen of the world.

MasteringNutrition™

To further your understanding, go online and apply what you've learned to real-life case studies that will help you master the content!

Review Questions

1. The region of the world where undernutrition is most acute is
   a. sub-Saharan Africa.
   b. southern Africa.
   c. Central America.
   d. central Asia.

2. Which of the following statements about the Green Revolution is true?
   a. It has most greatly benefited small, family farms.
   b. It has dramatically reduced undernutrition throughout South America, Asia, and Africa.
   c. It has dramatically increased worldwide production of rice, corn, and wheat at lower costs.
   d. It has reduced the traditional farmer's reliance on chemical fertilizers and pesticides.

3. Which of the following results of undernutrition is most directly linked to death in childhood?
   a. decreased work capacity
   b. reduced resistance to infection
   c. growth stunting
   d. impaired cognitive development

4. Which of the following are at greatest risk for food insecurity in the United States?
   a. adults over age 65
   b. single mothers and their children
   c. African Americans
   d. Hispanic Americans

5. Which of the following health problems has been linked to inadequate intake of vitamin A?
   a. diabetes
   b. cretinism
   c. night blindness
   d. all of the above

6. **True or false?** Worldwide, most malnourished children live in countries with food surpluses.

7. **True or false?** Children with night blindness have an increased risk for premature death.

8. **True or false?** Crop rotation and terracing are farming methods used in sustainable agriculture.

9. **True or false?** The rise in global obesity rates has prompted a rise in rates of communicable diseases.

10. **True or false?** Cotton, coffee, and tobacco are examples of subsistence crops.

11. Why might programs to improve the education of women also improve a nation's food/population ratio?

12. Explain why breastfeeding is an essential element of UNICEF's GOBI campaign to eliminate common infections of childhood.

13. Jeanette is a healthcare provider in a free clinic in an impoverished area of India. She is 5'8" tall. Explain why she is not surprised to hear the patients who come to the clinic refer to her as a giant.

14. Davie is 2 years old and lives in rural Alabama. He is the youngest of three children, all of whom live with their mother in an abandoned van. Their mother relies on a local food pantry for food, and the family drinks water from a nearby pond. Neither Davie nor his siblings have been vaccinated, and they have no regular medical care. Pointing to the interrelationship of several factors, explain why Davie's risk of dying before he reaches age 5 is significant.

15. José grew up in a slum in Mexico City, but his brilliance in school earned him recognition and a patron who funded his education. Now in medical school in the United States, he plans to return to Mexico as a pediatrician and specialize in the treatment of children with type 2 diabetes. Explain why José might be drawn to work with this population.

Answers to Review Questions can be found online in the MasteringNutrition Study Area.

Web Links

www.actionagainsthunger.org
Action Against Hunger
This site explains the mission of an international organization that helps in emergency situations, promotes long-term food security, and lets you know how to volunteer to help.

www.bread.org
Bread for the World
Visit this site to learn about a faith-based effort to advocate local and global policies that help the poor obtain food.

www.care.org
CARE
This site is the international page that links to CARE organizations in many countries working to improve economic conditions in more than seventy developing nations.

www.feedingminds.org
Feeding Minds Fighting Hunger
Visit this international electronic classroom to explore the problems of hunger, malnutrition, and food insecurity.

www.freefromhunger.org
Freedom from Hunger
Visit this site to learn about an established international development organization, founded in 1946, that works toward sustainable self-help against chronic hunger and poverty.

www.heifer.org
Heifer International
Visit this site to learn how you can give a cow, some rabbits, or a flock of chickens to a community in a developing country, so that they are better able to provide food for themselves.

www.hki.org
Helen Keller International
This site describes sustainable ways of preventing blindness and childhood deaths by fighting poverty and malnutrition.

www.studentsagainsthunger.org
National Student Campaign Against Hunger and Homelessness
Visit this site to learn what students like you are doing to fight hunger, as well as how you can get involved.

www.oxfamamerica.org
Oxfam America
Oxfam International is a confederation of organizations in more than 100 countries working together for a more equitable world. This website explains the American initiatives fighting global poverty, hunger, and social injustice.

www.unicef.org/nutrition
United Nations Children's Fund
Visit this site to learn about international concerns affecting the world's children, including nutrient deficiencies and hunger.

www.who.int/nutrition/en
World Health Organization Nutrition
Visit this site to learn about global malnutrition, micronutrient deficiencies, and the nutrition transition.

References

1. Central Intelligence Agency. 2012. Sierra Leone. The World Factbook. www.cia.gov/library/publications/the-world-factbook/geos/sl.html.
2. World Bank. 2012. Levels and Trends in Child Mortality. *Report 2011.* http://databank.worldbank.org/data/.
3. Aguayo, V. M., D. Garnier, and S. K. Baker. 2007. *Drops of Life: Vitamin A Supplementation for Child Survival, Progress and Lessons Learned in West and Central Africa.* UNICEF Regional Office for West and Central Africa.
4. International Food Policy Research Institute. 2011. Global Hunger Index. www.ifpri.org/publication/2011-global-hunger-index.
5. Centers for Disease Control and Prevention. 2012. Adult Obesity Facts, Childhood Obesity Facts. www.cdc.gov/obesity/data/adult.html.
6. World Hunger Education Service. 2012. 2012 World Hunger and Poverty Facts and Statistics. www.worldhunger.org/articles/Learn/world%20hunger%20facts%202002.htm.
7. United Nations System Standing Committee on Nutrition/The United Nations Children's Fund. 2007. Community-Based Management of Severe Acute Malnutrition. World Health Organization/World Food Programme. www.who.int/nutrition/topics/Statement_community_based_man_sev_acute_mal_eng.pdf.
8. World Bank. 2012. Trends in Maternal Mortality: 1990–2010. http://data.worldbank.org/indicator/SH.STA.MMRT.
9. World Health Organization. 2012. Child Malnutrition: A Hidden Crisis Which Threatens the Global Economy. www.who.int/pmnch/media/news/2012/20120215_stc_pr_children_malnutrition/en/.
10. Aguayo, V. M., D. Garnier, and S. K. Baker. 2007. *Drops of Life: Vitamin A Supplementation for Child Survival, Progress and Lessons Learned in West and Central Africa.* UNICEF Regional Office for West and Central Africa.
11. Scrimshaw, N. S. 2003. Historical concepts of interactions, synergism and antagonism between nutrition and infection. *J. Nutr.* 133:316S–321S.
12. Katona, P., and J. Katona-Apte. 2008. The interaction between nutrition and infection. *Clinical Infectious Diseases* 46:1582–1588.

13. World Health Organization. 2010. HIV/AIDS and Maternal, Newborn & Child Health. www.who.int/pmnch/media/press_materials/fs/fs_hivaids_mnch/en/.

14. Andersson, M.,V. Karumbunathan, and M. B. Zimmermann. 2012. Global Iodine Status in 2011 and Trends over the Past Decade. *Journal of Nutrition* April 1, 2012:jn111.149393.

15. World Health Organization. 2012. Micronutrient Deficiencies: Vitamin A Deficiency. www.who.int/nutrition/topics/vad/en/.

16. Demment, M. W., M. M. Young, and R. L. Sensenig. 2003. Providing micronutrients through food-based solutions: a key to human and national development. Supplement: animal source foods to improve micronutrient nutrition and human function in developing countries. *J. Nutr.* 133:3879S–3885S.

17. Milman, N. 2011. Anemia: still a major health problem in many parts of the world! *Annal of Hematology* 90:369–377.

18. Population Reference Bureau. 2011. 2011 World Population Data Sheet. www.prb.org/Publications/Datasheets/2011/world-population-data-sheet/world-map.aspx#/table/population.

19. Murphy, E., and D. Carr. 2007. Powerful Partners: Adolescent Girls' Education and Delayed Childbearing. www.prb.org.

20. Joint United Nations Programme on HIV/AIDS. 2011. UNAIDS World AIDS Day Report 2011. www.unaids.org/en/media/unaids/contentassets/documents/unaidspublication/2011/JC2216_WorldAIDSday_report_2011_en.pdf.

21. Nagata, J. M., R. O. Magerenge, S. L. Young, J. O. Oguta, S. D. Weiser, and C. R. Cohen. 2012. Social determinants, lived experiences, and consequences of household food insecurity among persons living with HIV/AIDS on the shore of Lake Victoria, Kenya. *AIDS Care* 24:728–736.

22. Fanzo, J. C., and P. M. Pronyk. 2011. A review of global progress toward the Millennium Development Goal 1 Hunger Target. *Food Nutr. Bull.* 32(2):144–158.

23. World Health Organization. 2012. World Health Statistics 2012. www.who.int/gho/publications/world_health_statistics/2012/en/.

24. American Diabetes Association. 2011 National Diabetes Fact Sheet. www.diabetes.org/diabetes-basics/diabetes-statistics/.

25. Varela-Silva, M. I., F. Dickinson, H. Wilson, H. Azcorra, P. Griffiths, and B. Bogin 2012. The nutritional dual-burden in developing countries. How is it assessed and what are the health implications? *Collegium Antropologicum* 36:39–45. www.collantropol.hr/_doc/Coll.%20Antropol.%2036%20(2012)%201:%2039%E2%80%9345.pdf.

26. Drewnowski, A., and N. Darmon. 2005. The economics of obesity: dietary energy and energy cost. *Am. J. Clin. Nutr.* 82:265S–73S.

27. Centers for Disease Control and Prevention. 2011, Obesity and Overweight. www.cdc.gov/nchs/fastats/overwt.htm/.

28. Coleman-Jensen, A., N. Mark, M. Andrews, and S. Carlson. 2011. Household Food Security in the United States in 2010. ERR-125, US Department of Agriculture, Economic Research Service. www.ers.usda.gov/media/121076/err125_2_.pdf.

29. United Nations. 2010. The Millennium Development Goals Report. www.un.org/millenniumgoals/pdf/MDG%20Report%202010%20En%20r15%20-low%20res%2020100615%20-.pdf.

30. The Micronutrient Initiative. n.d. Vitamin A: The Scope of the Problem. www.micronutrient.org/english/view.asp?x=577.

31. Evenson, R. E., and D. Gollin. 2003. Assessing the impact of the Green Revolution, 1960 to 2000. *Science* 2:758–762.

32. Stanford University. 2010. High-yield agriculture slows pace of global warming, say researchers. *ScienceDaily*. www.sciencedaily.com-/releases/2010/06/100614160209.htm.

33. Sakamoto, T., and M. Matsuoka. 2004. Generating high-yielding varieties by genetic manipulation of plant architecture. *Curr. Opin. Biotechnol.* 15:144–147.

34. Gibson, R. W., V. Aritua, E. Byamukama, I. Mpembe, and J. Kayongo. 2004. Control strategies for sweet potato virus disease in Africa. *Virus Res.* 100(1):115–122.

35. Welch, R. M., and R. D. Graham. 2004. Breeding for micronutrients in staple food crops from a human nutrition perspective. *J. Exp. Botany.* 55:353–364.

36. D'Alessandro, A., and L. Zolla. 2012. We are what we eat: food safety and proteomics. *J. Proteome. Res.* 11(1):26–36. http://pubs.acs.org/doi/pdf/10.1021/pr2008829.

37. National Student Campaign Against Hunger and Homelessness. n.d. www.studentsagainsthunger.org.

38. Zinn, H. 2006. *Original Zinn.* New York: Harper Perennial.

Trade Barriers: Helpful or Harmful?

In response to the global economic downturn, governments throughout the world in 2009 began to consider new measures to protect their farmers, food manufacturers, and consumers from rising prices. Such measures, generally known as *trade barriers,* can provide economic relief at home, but they inevitably increase economic distress among trading partners. Before we consider why, let's define some terms.

What Are Trade Barriers?

Trade barriers generally include subsidies, tariffs, and embargoes. Their goal is to provide local farmers with a higher and steadier income than might be possible with a free market.

The United States and many countries in Europe protect their farmers' incomes by paying *subsidies,* grants of money legislated and distributed by a region's government, that guarantee a minimum price for a crop even if the market value is lower. This has the effect of increasing the production of subsidized crops, such as wheat, corn, and milk, and creating surpluses that lower the prices of these foods for consumers, as well as for companies manufacturing processed foods that use these crops. These subsidized foods can also be exported at lower prices, often to the financial detriment of producers of the same goods in the countries receiving the exported goods.

At the same time, importing countries worldwide may protect their own farmers by charging *import tariffs,* which are taxes on a particular class of goods when they are brought into a country to be sold. These charges increase the price of cheap imported foods, so that farmers who grow the same crop locally can charge the price necessary to make a living wage and still be competitive. For example, tariffs in Japan on imported rice from Burma protect Japanese rice farmers but make it difficult for Burmese farmers to market their crop in Japan. Consumers in Japan pay a price higher than they would if they were permitted to buy Burmese rice at *market price,*

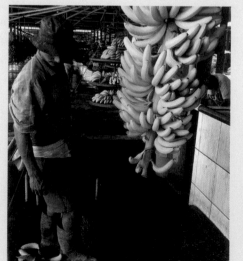

The European Union requires an import tariff on bananas from Latin America, such as from this Costa Rican farm, but no tariff from some countries in Africa and the Caribbean.

that is, at the price that results from an interaction between the supply available and the demand for the goods at a given time. Similarly, the United States maintains the price paid to producers of domestic sugar by placing an import tariff on sugar from other countries. Import tariffs effectively reduce the ability of exporting countries—often developing nations—to compete in markets where the same crop is grown domestically. They also maintain higher prices for consumers, essentially requiring consumers in countries with import tariffs to subsidize domestic production.

Export subsidies, which are grants of money provided by a region's government to exporters of surplus crops, also make it difficult for unsubsidized farmers to compete in international markets. These subsidies are paid, usually by developed countries, to exporters of surplus crops, so that they can then sell their crops cheaply abroad. Export subsidies decrease prices for consumers in the country to which the food is shipped but also decrease the income that local farmers in that country can receive at market for the same food.

An *export embargo* is a government-ordered prohibition on exporting a particular product. Export embargos are typically used to protect domestic customers from high prices for a particular crop when farmers could fetch a higher price for it if they were to sell it abroad. One example is the U.S. export embargo on soybeans in the 1970s. This embargo protected American consumers of soybeans but resulted in shortages in other countries.

Goals of Trade Barriers

In general, the goal of subsidies, tariffs, and embargoes is to protect the region's farmers. For this reason, they are sometimes also called *protective trade barriers.* The United States has protective trade barriers for many crops, including the eight major field crops of corn, sorghum, barley, oats, wheat, rice, cotton, and soybeans. The countries in the European Union also support their agricultural producers heavily. On average, about 30% of farm income in developed countries is from a variety of supports.[1]

Part of a nation's protection can extend to the environment. In fact, the growing international concern about global warming and other environmental issues has led to many new proposals for protective trade barriers. Let's say that a nation's government has passed legislation prohibiting the use of certain harmful pesticides on a particular domestic crop. This has increased the domestic price of the crop, as farmers have had to use more expensive biopesticides for a reduced yield. Now another country petitions this nation's government to allow it to sell the same crop at a lower price—but its crop was produced with the environmentally harmful pesticide. A variety of protective measures, including an outright prohibition on importation of the crop, are likely to be considered. So-called green trade barriers are currently being reviewed not only on food crops but also on vehicles and other manufactured goods.

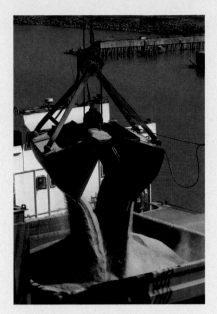

Protective trade barriers may inflate the price of grain sold on the world market.

protections, and a demand for a just price to be paid for suppliers of goods.[4] Fair trade organizations involved in agriculture emphasize the need to ensure fair prices for farmers in developing nations and a living wage and decent housing and working conditions for farm laborers around the world.[5] The latter include access to education, healthcare, and working capital, as well as the use of sustainable agricultural practices that protect worker health and the local environment.

The politics of international trade affect the worldwide distribution of healthy food, the stability of farmers' incomes, and access to food by the world's poor. Debate is ongoing about the best ways to provide food security to all.

Effects of Trade Barriers

As we have seen, certain disadvantages to global welfare result from trade barriers on food. These include a reduced ability of developing agricultural nations to compete in the world market and higher prices for consumers and food companies that use the raw food materials in their products. The mission of the World Trade Organization (WTO) is to reduce protective trade barriers and encourage global free trade by negotiating fair trade agreements and settling trade disputes among its 149 member-countries.[2] The World Bank suggests that removing subsidies for agriculture would reduce poverty in developing countries, particularly those with small urban populations and thus little opportunity for expanding the domestic market.[3] At the same time, removing subsidies for agriculture in rich countries would free public moneys for other uses and encourage development of more competitive products.

However, not everyone agrees that global free trade in agriculture would automatically benefit the world's poor. Those opposed suggest that large multinational corporations and landholders stand to gain at the expense of the majority of small farmers, poor farmers, and farm laborers. Many argue not for free trade but for fair trade—that is, trade characterized by reciprocity among nations, shared standards for worker and environmental

CRITICAL THINKING QUESTIONS

- Do you think it is ethical for wealthy nations to erect trade barriers that protect domestic farmers or consumers but reduce prosperity in developing nations? Why or why not?

- Do you think "green" trade barriers are an effective means of protecting the environment? Explain your answer.

- Do you think it is important for consumers to purchase certified fair trade goods? Do you seek out such goods? Why or why not?

REFERENCES

1. Anderson, K., and W. Martin, eds. 2006. *Agricultural Trade Reform and the DOHA Development Agenda.* Washington, DC: The World Bank/Palgrave Macmillan.
2. World Trade Organization. 2012. About the WTO—A Statement by the Director-General. www.wto.org/english/thewto_e/whatis_e/wto_dg_stat_e.htm.
3. The World Bank. 2012. Global Agricultural Trade and Developing Countries. http://econ.worldbank.org/WBSITE/EXTERNAL/EXTDEC/EXTDECPROSPECTS/0,,contentMDK:22395556~pagePK:64165401~piPK:64165026~theSitePK:476883,00.html.
4. The Economist. 2010. Fair Trade. Economist Debates. www.economist.com/debate/days/view/508.
5. Fair Trade USA. 2010. What Is Fair Trade? www.fairtradeusa.org/what-is-fair-trade.

Appendices

Appendix A

The USDA Food Guide Evolution

Early History of Food Guides

Did you know that in the United States food guides have been around in one form or another for over 125 years?

That's right. Back in 1885 a college chemistry professor named Wilber Olin (W. O.) Atwater helped bring the fledgling science of nutrition to a broader audience by introducing scientific data boxes that became the basis for the first known U.S. food guide. Those early dietary standards focused on defining the nutritional needs of an "average man" in terms of his daily consumption of proteins and calories. These became food composition tables defined in three sweeping categories; protein, fats and carbohydrate; mineral matter; and fuel values. As early as 1902, Atwater advocated for three foundational nutritional principles that we still support today; the concepts of variety, proportionality, and moderation in food choices and eating.

These ideas were adapted a few years later by a nutritionist named Caroline Hunt, who developed a "food buying" guide divided into five categories: meats and proteins; cereals and starches; vegetables and fruits; fatty foods; and sugar, based on a 2,800 calorie-per-day diet.

Starting in the 1930s and 1940s, on through the following 30 years to the early 1970s, these concepts were further developed and experimented with, evolving from 12 food groups to a "Basic Seven" group approach, to the "Basic Four," and from there to a "Hassle-Free" construct that briefly increased the number of groups up to five. While all these approaches had drawbacks and received critical scrutiny, they were nonetheless important and necessary attempts to provide Americans with reliable guidelines based on the best scientific data and practices available at the time.

The USDA Food Guide Pyramid

Beginning around the early 1980s these concepts began to assume the forms we're familiar with today. In the process, important philosophical goals became attached to the development of a comprehensive guide. These core values included the following goals for a guide:

- it must encompass a broad focus on **overall health**;
- it should emphasize the use of **current research**;
- it should be an approach that includes the **total diet**, rather than parts or pieces;
- it should be **useful**;
- it should be **realistic**;
- it should be **flexible**;
- it should be **practical**;
- and it must be **evolutionary**, in that it should be able to adapt to new information that comes to light.

Additionally, the essential steps needed to develop a modern food guide became articulated. These are readily apparent in the first USDA Food Guide Pyramid released in 1992, which attempted for the first time to create a graphic representation of the guidelines. The steps required the inclusion of:

- Nutritional Goals
- Food Groups
- Serving Sizes
- Nutrient Profiles
- Numbers of Servings, including addressing the needs for adequacy and moderation.

Remarkably, W. O. Atwater's early principles of *variety, proportionality,* and *moderation* remain relevant and appropriate to our modern graphic guidelines. The attempts to develop a conceptual framework for selecting the types and amounts of food that can support a nutritionally sound diet continue to evolve. Nutritionists and other health professionals are still working to find better ways to communicate to a large and diverse audience how to translate recommendations for nutrient intake into recommendations on which food to eat, and in what amounts.

Let's take a look at the evolution of the modern Food Guide over the past quarter-century:

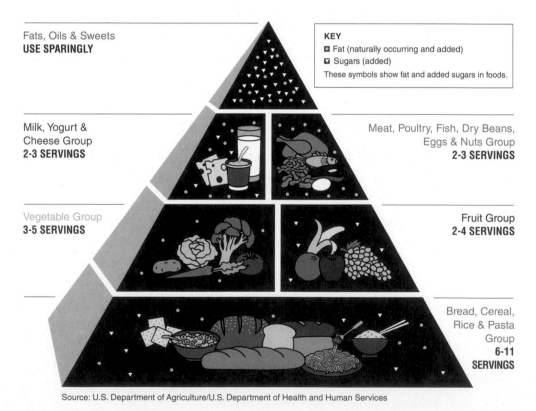

Source: U.S. Department of Agriculture/U.S. Department of Health and Human Services

FIGURE A.1 The 1992 Food Guide Pyramid. This representation of the USDA guidelines took several years to develop and attempted to convey in a single image all the key aspects of a nutritional guide.

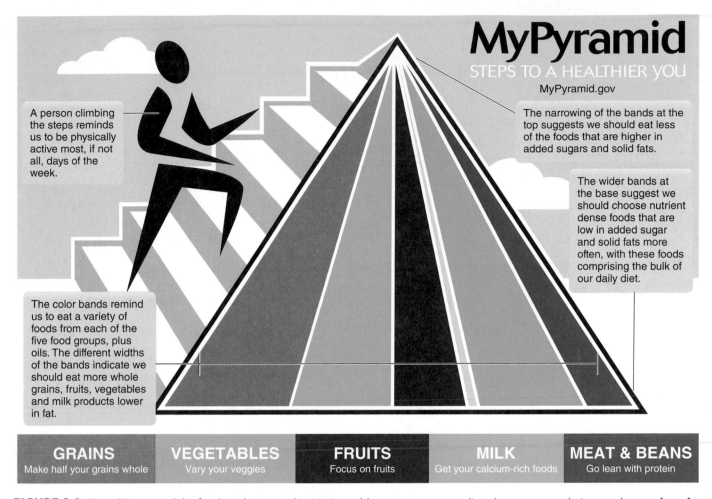

MyPyramid
STEPS TO A HEALTHIER YOU
MyPyramid.gov

A person climbing the steps reminds us to be physically active most, if not all, days of the week.

The narrowing of the bands at the top suggests we should eat less of the foods that are higher in added sugars and solid fats.

The wider bands at the base suggest we should choose nutrient dense foods that are low in added sugar and solid fats more often, with these foods comprising the bulk of our daily diet.

The color bands remind us to eat a variety of foods from each of the five food groups, plus oils. The different widths of the bands indicate we should eat more whole grains, fruits, vegetables and milk products lower in fat.

| **GRAINS**
Make half your grains whole | **VEGETABLES**
Vary your veggies | **FRUITS**
Focus on fruits | **MILK**
Get your calcium-rich foods | **MEAT & BEANS**
Go lean with protein |

FIGURE A.2 The USDA revised the food guide pyramid in 2005 to address concerns regarding the recommendations and ease-of-use for a general audience. They put forth the MyPyramid Food Guidance System, which continues with the "pyramid" concept, but in a simpler presentation. (*Source:* USDA ChooseMyPlate website.http://www.choosemyplate.gov)

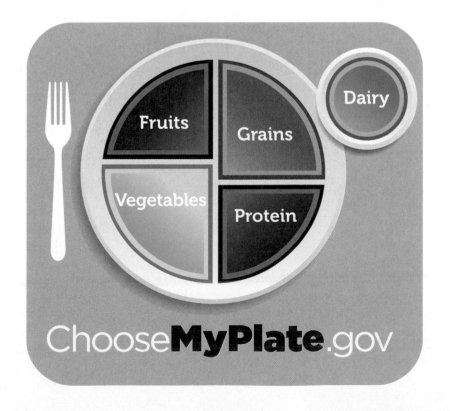

ChooseMyPlate.gov

FIGURE A.3 In May 2011 the USDA made a dramatic change by withdrawing the pyramid concept and focusing instead on conveying core information in a simple, direct, and easy-to-follow way, as MyPlate. In MyPlate, the icons are intended as healthy eating reminders, rather than as specific messages encompassing detailed information. (*Source:* USDA ChooseMyPlate website.http://www.choosemyplate.gov)

Appendix B

Metabolism Pathways and Biochemical Structures

When learning about the science of nutrition, it is important to understand basic principles of metabolism and to know the molecular structures of important nutrients and molecules. Chapter 8 of this text provides a detailed discussion of the major metabolic processes that occur within the body. This appendix provides additional information and detail on several metabolism pathways and biochemical structures of importance. Red arrows indicate catabolic reactions.

Metabolism Pathways

1 Using energy and one phosphate group from ATP, glucose is converted to glucose 6-phosphate via the process of phosphorylation.

2 Glucose 6-phosphate is converted into another six-carbon sugar, fructose 6-phosphate.

3 Fructose 6-phosphate is converted to fructose 1,6-bisphosphate via a second phosphorylation reaction, again using energy and one phosphate group from ATP.

4 Fructose 1,6-bisphosphate is broken down into two three-carbon compounds: glyceraldehyde 3-phosphate and dihydroxyacetone phosphate.

5 Dihydroxyacetone phosphate is converted into a second molecule of glyceraldehyde 3-phosphate.

6 The two molecules of glyceraldehyde 3-phosphate undergo an additional phosphorylation step resulting in the formation of two molecules of 1,3-bisphosphoglyceric acid; two NAD^+ are reduced to $NADH + H^+$.

7 Two ATP are formed by the phosphorylation of two ADP; this step "balances out" the energy used up in the steps 1 and 3, when two ATP were converted to two ADP. With the loss of one phosphate group each, the two molecules of 1,3-bisphosphoglyceric acid are converted to two molecules of 3-phosphoglyceric acid.

8 Each 3-phosphoglyceric acid is rearranged into 2-phosphoglyceric acid.

9 With the removal of a total of two molecules of water, the two molecules of 2-phosphoglyceric acid are converted to two molecules of phosphoenolpyruvic acid (PEP).

10 Two ATP are formed by the phosphorylation of two ADP; this step accounts for the net production of two ATP during the process of glycolysis. Two molecules of pyruvic acid are formed during this step.

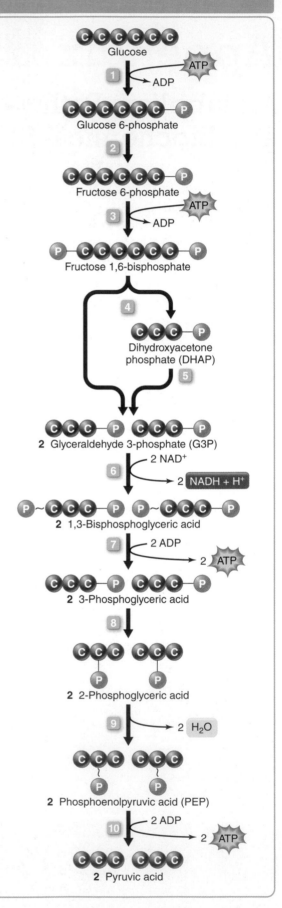

FIGURE B.1 Glycolysis.

TCA Cycle

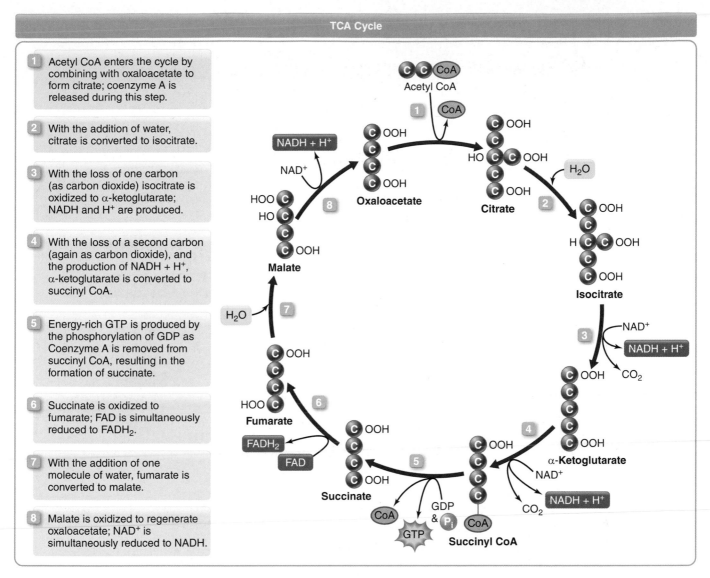

1. Acetyl CoA enters the cycle by combining with oxaloacetate to form citrate; coenzyme A is released during this step.

2. With the addition of water, citrate is converted to isocitrate.

3. With the loss of one carbon (as carbon dioxide) isocitrate is oxidized to α-ketoglutarate; NADH and H$^+$ are produced.

4. With the loss of a second carbon (again as carbon dioxide), and the production of NADH + H$^+$, α-ketoglutarate is converted to succinyl CoA.

5. Energy-rich GTP is produced by the phosphorylation of GDP as Coenzyme A is removed from succinyl CoA, resulting in the formation of succinate.

6. Succinate is oxidized to fumarate; FAD is simultaneously reduced to FADH$_2$.

7. With the addition of one molecule of water, fumarate is converted to malate.

8. Malate is oxidized to regenerate oxaloacetate; NAD$^+$ is simultaneously reduced to NADH.

FIGURE B.2 TCA cycle.

Electron Transport Chain

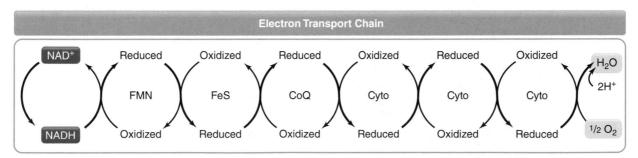

FIGURE B.3 Electron transport chain. ATP is released at various points in the electron transport chain as electrons are passed from one molecule to another. The process, termed *oxidative phosphorylation*, occurs within the electron transport chain.

Net Energy Production for Glucose Oxidation

	Metabolic reaction	Reaction by-product	Number used	Number produced	Net usage/ production
Glycolysis	Glucose ⟶ Fructose 1,6-bisphosphate	ATP	2		−2 ATP
Glycolysis	Glyceraldehyde 3-phosphate ⟶ 1,3-Bisphosphoglyceric acid	NADH + H⁺		2	2 NADH + H⁺ via electron transport chain
Glycolysis	1,3-Bisphosphoglyceric acid ⟶ Pyruvic acid	ATP		4	4 ATP
Intermediate step	Pyruvic acid ⟶ Acetyl CoA	NADH + H⁺		2	2 NADH + H⁺ via electron transport chain
TCA cycle	Isocitrate ⟶ Succinyl CoA	NADH + H⁺		4	4 NADH + H⁺ via electron transport chain
TCA cycle	Succinyl CoA ⟶ Succinate	GTP		2	2 GTP
TCA cycle	Succinate ⟶ Fumarate	FADH$_2$		2	2 FADH$_2$ via electron transport chain
TCA cycle	Malate ⟶ Oxaloacetate	NADH + H⁺		2	2 NADH + H⁺ via electron transport chain

(a) Sources of energy use and production during glucose oxidation

Reaction by-product	Number produced	Number of ATP produced per product	Net usage/ production
ATP	4 − 2 = 2	1	2 x 1 = 2 ATP
NADH + H⁺ (from glycolysis)	2	2 to 3	2 x 2 = 4 or 2 x 3 = 6 ATP
NADH + H⁺ (from TCA cycle)	8	3	8 x 3 = 24 ATP
GTP	2	1	2 x 1 = 2 ATP
FADH$_2$ (via electron transport chain)	2	2	2 x 2 = 4 ATP

Balance of energy from the oxidation of one unit of glucose

36 to 38 ATP

(b) Energy balance sheet for glucose oxidation

FIGURE B.4 Net energy production for glucose oxidation.

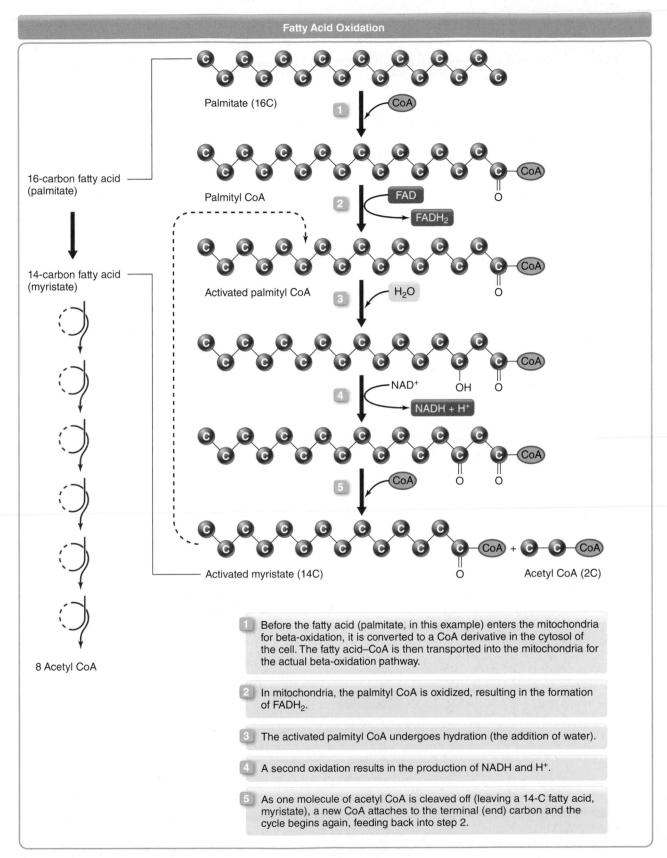

FIGURE B.5 Fatty acid oxidation.

Net Energy Production for Fatty Acid Oxidation				
Reaction by-product	Number produced	Number of ATP produced per product	Total energy (ATP) produced	
FADH₂	7	2 via electron transport chain	7 × 2 = 14 ATP	**Balance of energy from the oxidation of one 16-carbon fatty acid**
NADH + H⁺	7	3 via electron transport chain	7 × 3 = 21 ATP	
Acetyl- CoA	8	12 via TCA cycle	8 × 12 = 96 ATP	131 ATP

Energy balance sheet for fatty acid (16-carbon palmitate) oxidation

FIGURE B.6 Net energy production for fatty acid oxidation (16-carbon palmitate). With each sequential cleavage of the two-carbon acetyl CoA, one FADH₂ (which yields 2 ATP when oxidized by the electron transport chain) and one NADH (which yields 3 ATP when oxidized by the electron transport chain) are produced. Each molecule of acetyl CoA yields 12 ATP when metabolized through the TCA cycle. The complete oxidation of palmitate yields 7 FADH₂ (14 ATP), 7 NADH (21 ATP), and 8 acetyl CoA (96 ATP), for a grand total of 131 ATP.

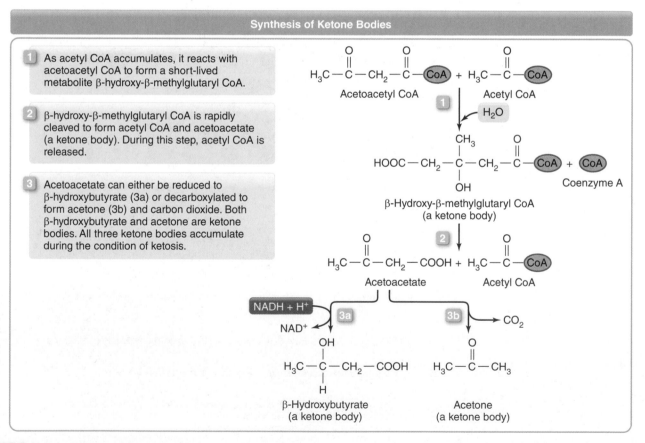

Synthesis of Ketone Bodies

1. As acetyl CoA accumulates, it reacts with acetoacetyl CoA to form a short-lived metabolite β-hydroxy-β-methylglutaryl CoA.

2. β-hydroxy-β-methylglutaryl CoA is rapidly cleaved to form acetyl CoA and acetoacetate (a ketone body). During this step, acetyl CoA is released.

3. Acetoacetate can either be reduced to β-hydroxybutyrate (3a) or decarboxylated to form acetone (3b) and carbon dioxide. Both β-hydroxybutyrate and acetone are ketone bodies. All three ketone bodies accumulate during the condition of ketosis.

FIGURE B.7 The synthesis of ketone bodies.

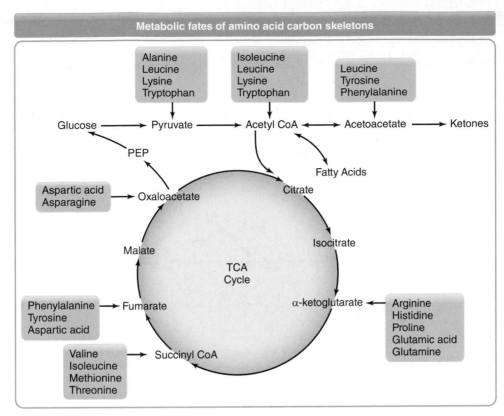

FIGURE B.8 The metabolic fates of amino acid carbon skeletons. After the deamination of amino acids, their carbon skeletons feed into various metabolic pathways. Glucogenic amino acids can be converted into pyruvate and/or intermediates of the TCA cycle, which can ultimately feed into glucose synthesis. Ketogenic amino acids can be converted into acetyl CoA, which then feeds into the synthesis of fatty acids. Some amino acids have more than one metabolic pathway available.

Urea Cycle

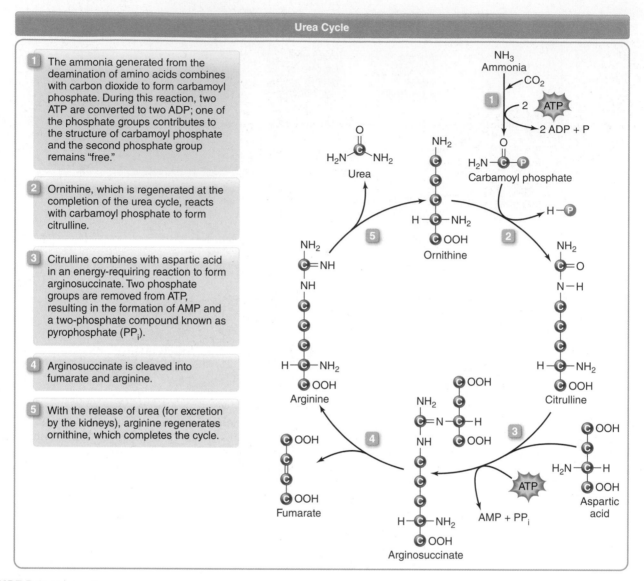

1. The ammonia generated from the deamination of amino acids combines with carbon dioxide to form carbamoyl phosphate. During this reaction, two ATP are converted to two ADP; one of the phosphate groups contributes to the structure of carbamoyl phosphate and the second phosphate group remains "free."

2. Ornithine, which is regenerated at the completion of the urea cycle, reacts with carbamoyl phosphate to form citrulline.

3. Citrulline combines with aspartic acid in an energy-requiring reaction to form arginosuccinate. Two phosphate groups are removed from ATP, resulting in the formation of AMP and a two-phosphate compound known as pyrophosphate (PP_i).

4. Arginosuccinate is cleaved into fumarate and arginine.

5. With the release of urea (for excretion by the kidneys), arginine regenerates ornithine, which completes the cycle.

FIGURE B.9 Urea cycle.

Ethanol Metabolism

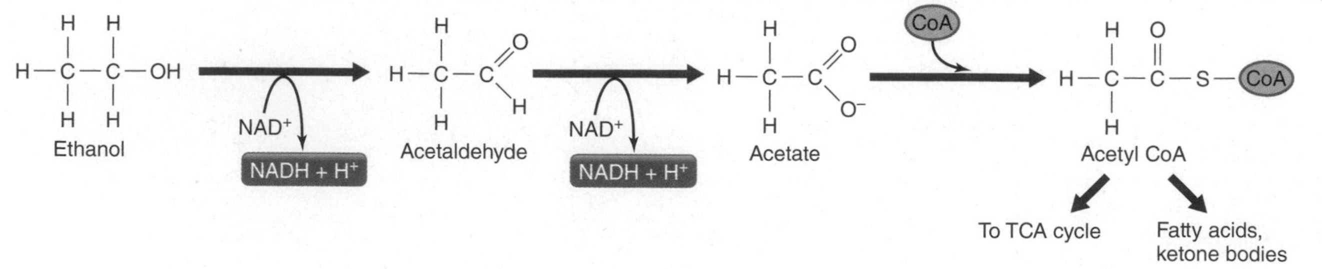

FIGURE B.10 Ethanol metabolism.

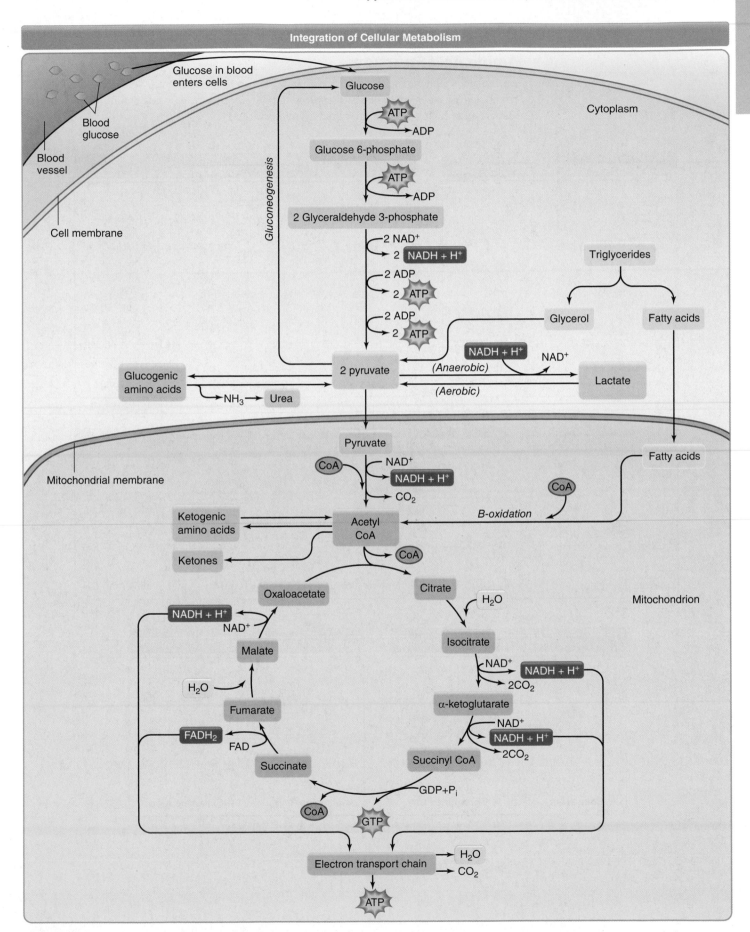

FIGURE B.11 Integration of cellular metabolism.

Biochemical Structures

Amino Acid Structures

Amino acids all have the same basic core but differ in their side chains. The following amino acids have been classified according to their specific type of side chain. Amino acids that are essential to humans are noted in bold print.

Amino acids with acidic side chains

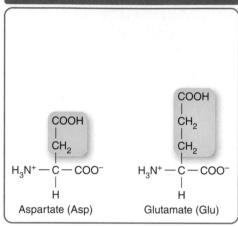

Aspartate (Asp)   Glutamate (Glu)

Amino acids with basic side chains

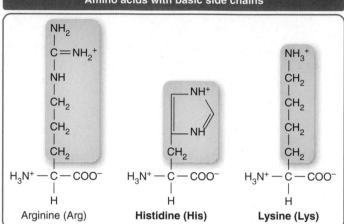

Arginine (Arg)   **Histidine (His)**   **Lysine (Lys)**

Amino acids with aliphatic (carbon- and hydrogen-containing) side chains

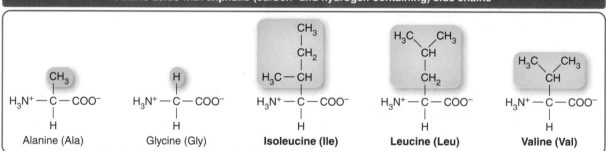

Alanine (Ala)   Glycine (Gly)   **Isoleucine (Ile)**   **Leucine (Leu)**   **Valine (Val)**

Amino acids with hydroxyl (OH) side chains

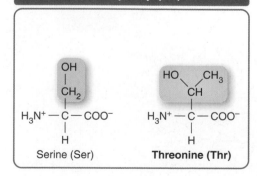

Serine (Ser)   **Threonine (Thr)**

Amino acids with amide (NH₂) side chains

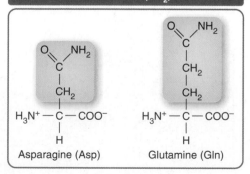

Asparagine (Asp)   Glutamine (Gln)

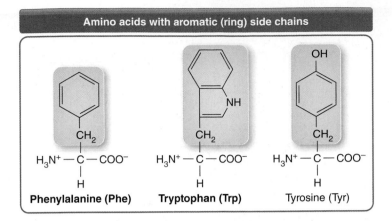

Amino acids with aromatic (ring) side chains

Phenylalanine (Phe) Tryptophan (Trp) Tyrosine (Tyr)

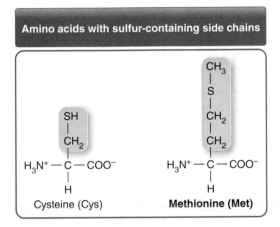

Amino acids with sulfur-containing side chains

Cysteine (Cys) Methionine (Met)

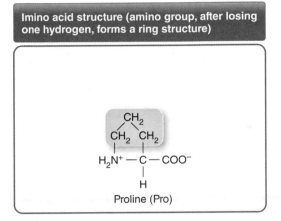

Imino acid structure (amino group, after losing one hydrogen, forms a ring structure)

Proline (Pro)

Vitamin Structures and Coenzyme Derivatives

Many vitamins have common names (for example, vitamin C, vitamin E) as well as scientific designations (for example, ascorbic acid, α-tocopherol). Most vitamins are found in more than one chemical form. Many of the vitamins illustrated here have an active coenzyme form; review both the vitamin and the coenzyme structures and see if you can locate the "core vitamin" structure within each of the coenzymes. The vitamins found in foods or supplements are not always in the precise chemical form needed for metabolic activity, and therefore the body often has to modify the vitamin in one way or another. For example, many of the B-vitamins are phosphorylated, meaning they have a phosphate group attached.

Water-Soluble Vitamins

Niacin has two forms: nicotinic acid and nicotinamide. Both forms can be converted into the coenzymes nicotinamide adenine dinucleotide (NAD^+) and nicotinamide adenine dinucleotide phosphate ($NADP^+$).

Niacin

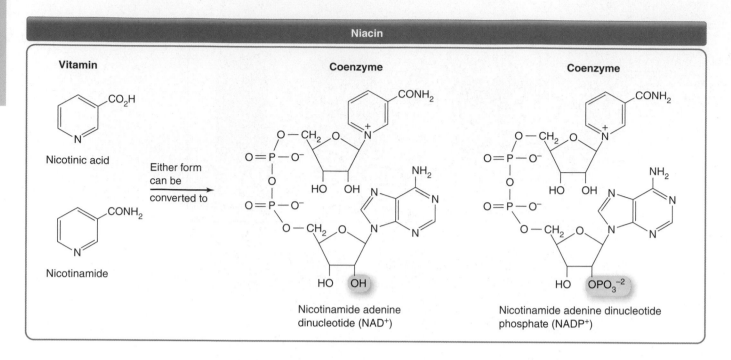

Vitamin

Nicotinic acid

Nicotinamide

Either form can be converted to

Coenzyme

Nicotinamide adenine dinucleotide (NAD⁺)

Coenzyme

Nicotinamide adenine dinucleotide phosphate (NADP⁺)

Riboflavin can be converted into the coenzymes flavin adenine dinucleotide (FAD) and flavin mononucleotide (FMN).

Riboflavin

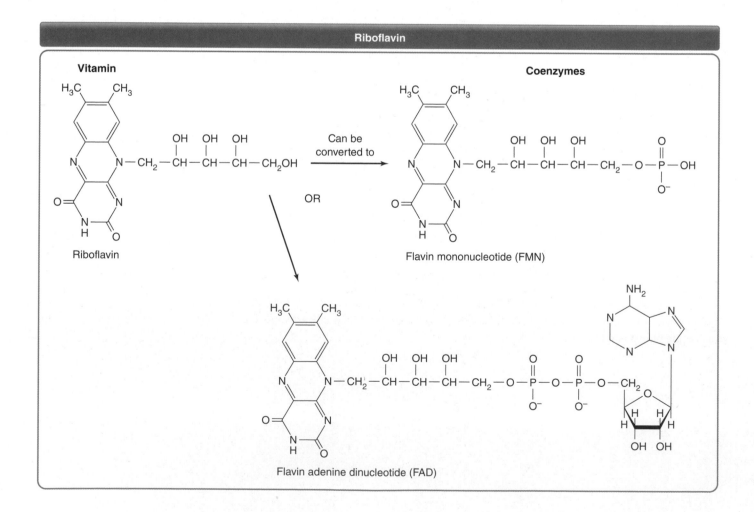

Vitamin

Riboflavin

Can be converted to

OR

Coenzymes

Flavin mononucleotide (FMN)

Flavin adenine dinucleotide (FAD)

Thiamin can be converted into the coenzyme thiamin pyrophosphate (TPP).

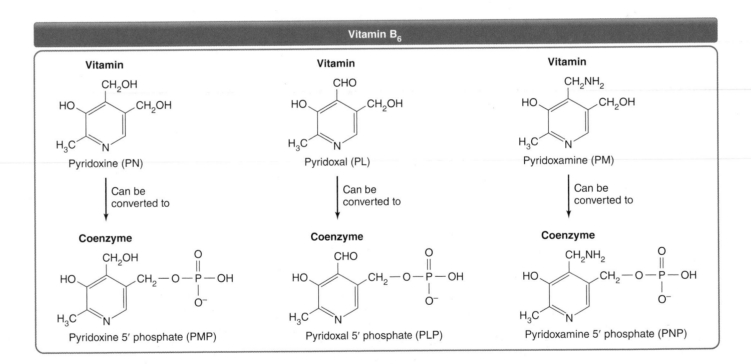

Vitamin B$_6$ includes the forms pyridoxine, pyridoxal, and pyridoxamine. The two common coenzymes derived from vitamin B$_6$ are pyridoxal 5′ phosphate (PLP) and pyridoxamine 5′ phosphate (PNP).

Two forms of vitamin B_{12} are cyanocobalamin and methylcobalamin.

Vitamin B_{12}

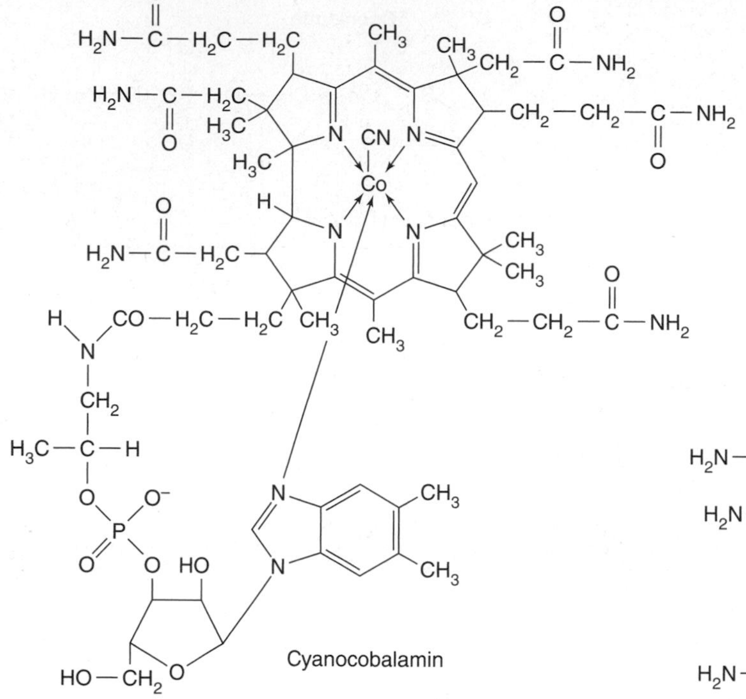

Cyanocobalamin

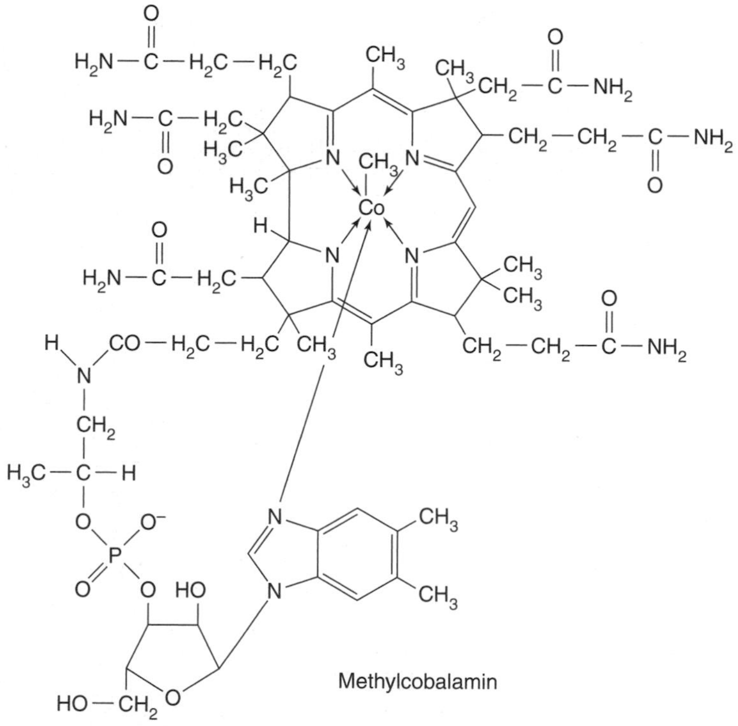

Methylcobalamin

Folic acid is one specific chemical form of folate. This vitamin can be converted into several coenzymes, including tetrahydrafolic acid.

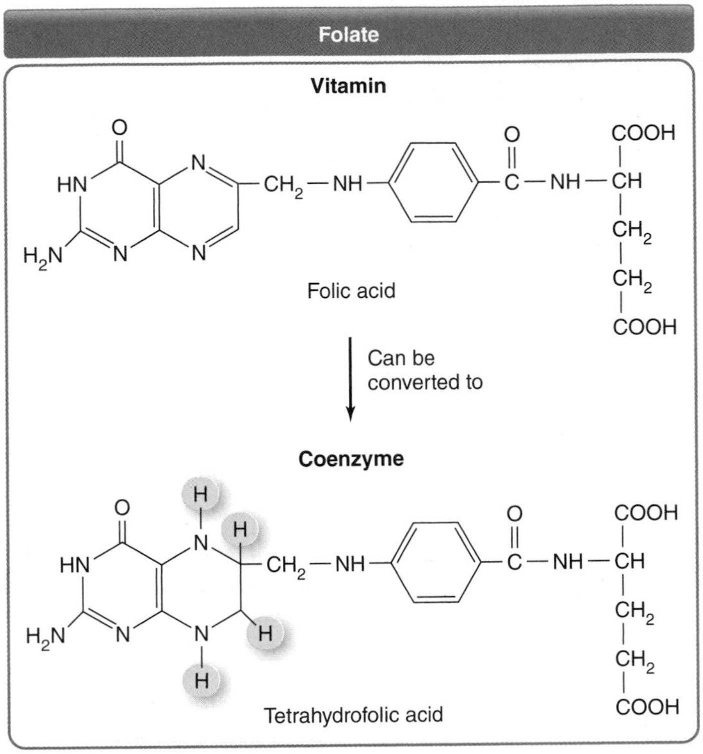

Folate

Vitamin

Folic acid

Can be converted to

Coenzyme

Tetrahydrofolic acid

Pantothenic acid is a component of Coenzyme A (CoA).

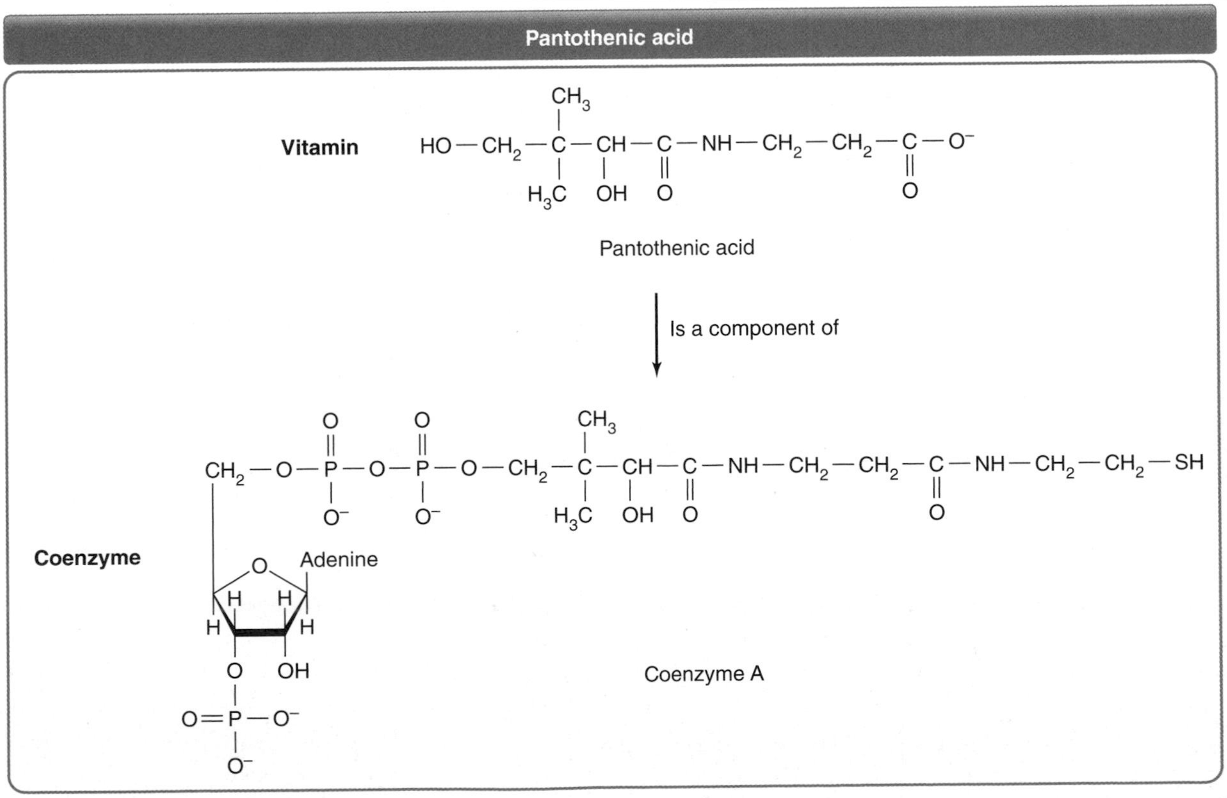

Pantothenic acid

Vitamin

$$HO - CH_2 - \underset{\underset{H_3C}{|}}{\overset{\overset{CH_3}{|}}{C}} - \underset{\underset{OH}{|}}{CH} - \underset{\underset{O}{||}}{C} - NH - CH_2 - CH_2 - \underset{\underset{O}{||}}{C} - O^-$$

Pantothenic acid

Is a component of

Coenzyme

Adenine

Coenzyme A

Biotin binds to several different metabolic enzymes. Choline serves as a methyl donor and as a precursor of acetylcholine and phospholipids.

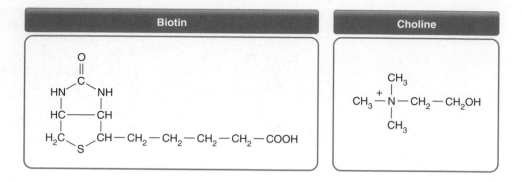

The two forms of vitamin C (ascorbic acid and dehydroascorbic acid) are readily interconverted as two hydrogens are lost through the oxidation of ascorbic acid or gained through the reduction of dehydroascorbic acid.

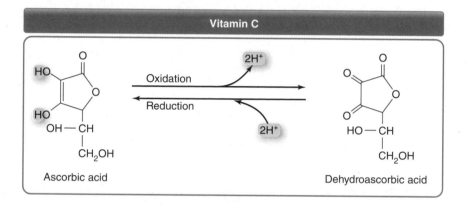

Fat-Soluble Vitamins

Vitamin A exists as an alcohol (retinol), an aldehyde (retinal), and an acid (retinoic acid). Beta-carotene is a common and highly potent precursor that can be converted into vitamin A by the body.

Vitamin A

Vitamin

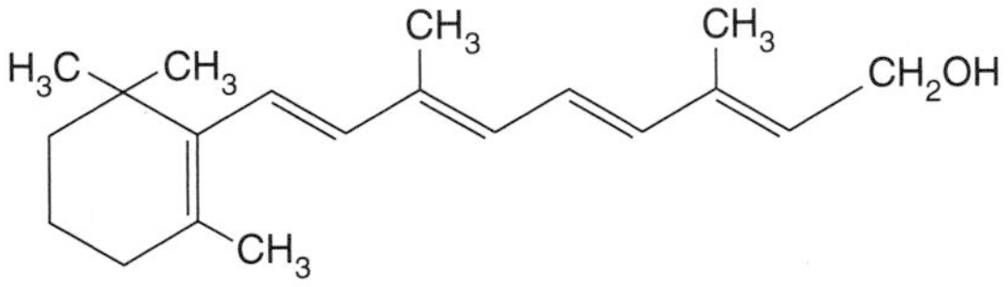

Retinol (alcohol form)

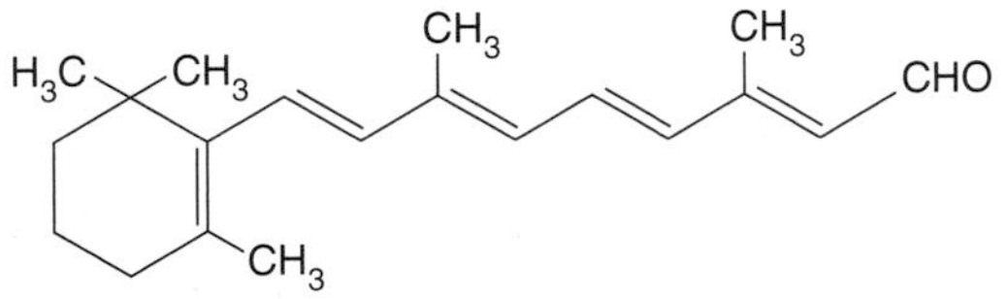

Retinal (aldehyde form)

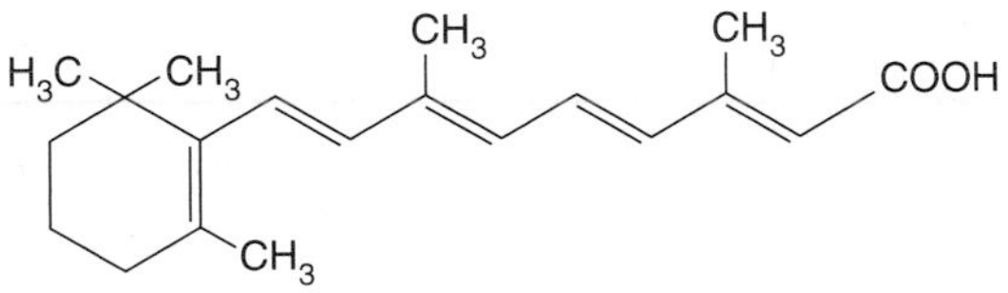

Retinoic acid (acid form)

Precursor (converted to vitamin by body)

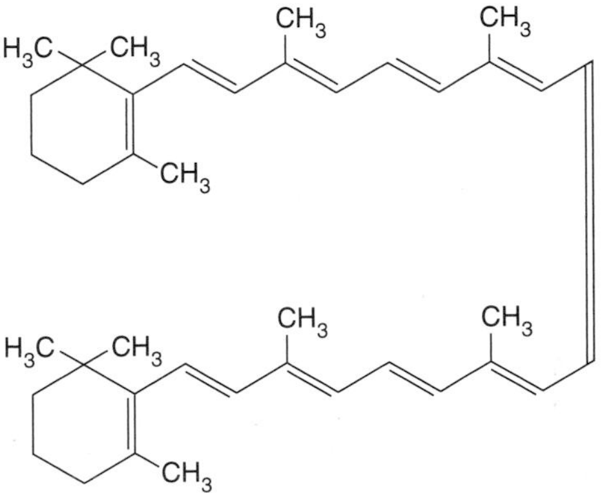

β-carotene

Vitamin D as cholecalciferol must be activated by two hydroxylation reactions (the addition of one OH group at each step) to form the active form of the vitamin, calcitriol (also called 1,25 (OH)$_2$D).

Vitamin D

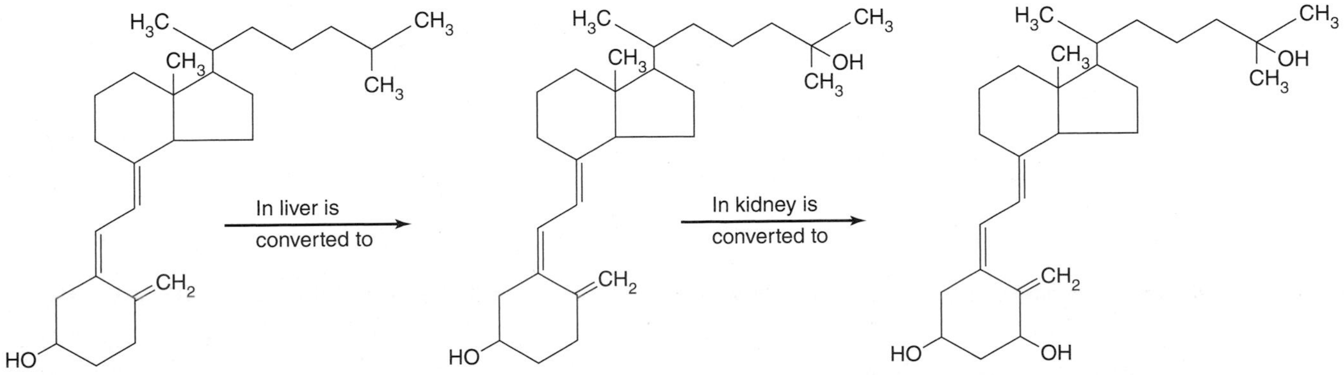

Cholecalciferol (provitamin D$_3$)

In liver is converted to

Calcidiol (25-hydroxyvitamin D)

In kidney is converted to

Active form

Calcitriol (1,25-dihydroxyvitamin D$_3$)

α-tocopherol is the most active form of vitamin E; the number and location of the methyl (CH_3) groups attached to the ring structure distinguish the four unique forms of the tocopherols.

Vitamin E

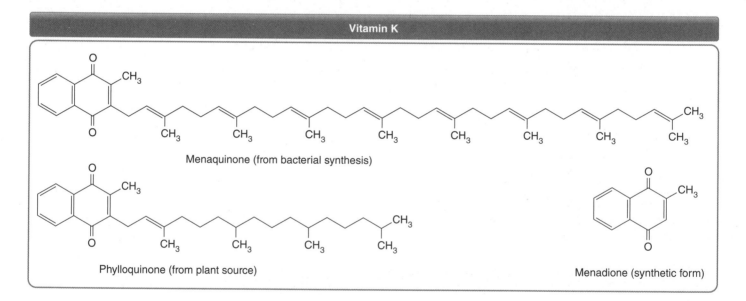

α-tocopherol

Vitamin K can be derived from plant sources (phylloquinones) and bacterial synthesis (menaquinones). A synthetic form of vitamin K (menadione) is also available.

Vitamin K

Menaquinone (from bacterial synthesis)

Phylloquinone (from plant source)

Menadione (synthetic form)

Appendix C

Chemistry Review

A basic grasp of chemistry is necessary for the introductory nutrition student. You may have taken a chemistry course at your college or in high school; this appendix can help you review concepts about atoms, molecules, pH, chemical reactions, and energy that you have learned previously.

All Matter Consists of Elements

Matter is anything that has mass and occupies space. All matter is composed of elements. An *element* is a fundamental (pure) form of matter that cannot be broken down to a simpler form. Aluminum and iron are elements, and so are oxygen and hydrogen. There are just over 100 known elements, and together they account for all matter on earth. The *periodic table of elements* arranges all the elements into groups according to their similar properties (**Figure C.1**).

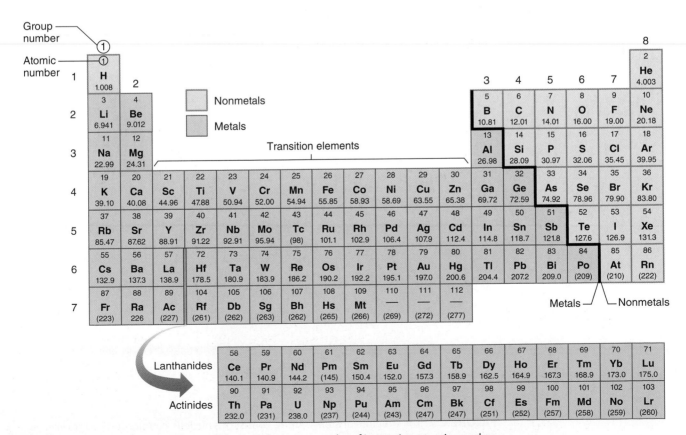

FIGURE C.1 The periodic table shows all known elements in order of increasing atomic number.

Atoms Are the Smallest Functional Units of an Element

Elements are made up of particles called atoms. An atom is the smallest unit of any element that still retains the physical and chemical properties of that element. Although we now know that atoms can be split apart under unusual circumstances (such as a nuclear reaction), atoms are the smallest units of matter that can take part in chemical reactions. So, for all practical purposes, atoms are the smallest functional units of matter.

Even the largest atoms are so small that we can see them only with specialized microscopes. Chemists can also infer what they look like from studying their physical properties (**Figure C.2**).

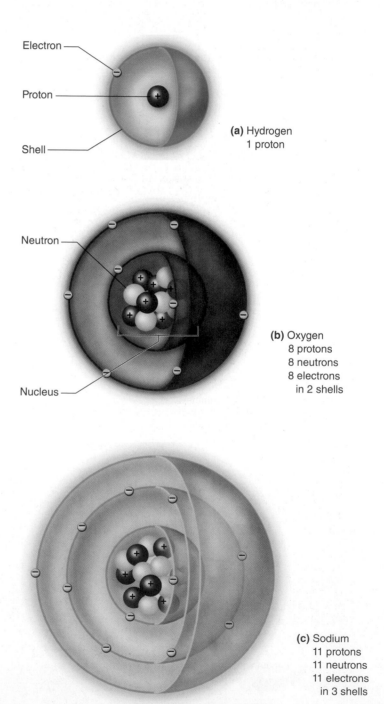

(a) Hydrogen
1 proton

(b) Oxygen
8 protons
8 neutrons
8 electrons
in 2 shells

(c) Sodium
11 protons
11 neutrons
11 electrons
in 3 shells

FIGURE C.2 The structure of atoms. Atoms consist of a nucleus, comprised of positively charged protons and neutral neutrons, surrounded by spherical shells of negatively charged electrons.

The central core of an atom is called the *nucleus*. The nucleus is made of positively charged particles called *protons* and a nearly equal number of neutral particles called *neutrons,* all tightly bound together. An exception is the smallest atom, hydrogen, whose nucleus consists of only a single proton. Smaller negatively charged particles called *electrons* orbit the nucleus. Because electrons are constantly moving, their precise position at any one time is unknown. You may think of electrons as occupying one or more spherical clouds of negative charge around the nucleus called *shells.* Each shell can accommodate only a certain number of electrons. The first shell, the one closest to the nucleus, can hold two electrons, the second can accommodate eight, and the third shell (if there is one) can contain even more. Each type of atom has a unique number of electrons. Under most circumstances the number of electrons equals the number of protons, and, as a result, the entire atom is electrically neutral.

Protons and neutrons have about the same mass, and both have much more mass than electrons. (Over 99.9% of an atom's mass is due to the protons and neutrons in its nucleus.)

In the periodic table and in chemical equations, atoms are designated by one- or two-letter symbols taken from English or Latin. For example, oxygen is designated by the letter O, nitrogen by N, sodium by Na (from the Latin word for sodium, *natrium*), and potassium by K (from the Latin *kalium*). A subscript numeral following the symbol indicates the numbers of atoms of that element. For example, the chemical formula O_2 represents two atoms of oxygen linked together, the most stable form of elemental oxygen.

In addition to a symbol, atoms have an *atomic number,* which represents the characteristic number of protons in the nucleus, and an *atomic mass* (or mass number), which is generally fairly close to the total number of neutrons and protons.

Isotopes Have a Different Number of Neutrons

Although all the atoms of a particular element have the same number of protons, the number of neutrons can vary slightly. Atoms with either more or fewer neutrons than the usual number for that element are called *isotopes.* Isotopes of an element have the same atomic number as the more common atoms but a different atomic mass. For example, elemental carbon typically consists of atoms with six protons and six neutrons, for an atomic mass of 12. The isotope of carbon known as carbon-14 has an atomic mass of 14 because it has two extra neutrons.

Isotopes are always identified by a superscript mass number preceding the symbol. For instance, the carbon-14 isotope is designated ^{14}C. The superscript mass number of the most common elemental form of carbon is generally omitted because it is understood to be 12.

Many isotopes are unstable. Such isotopes are called *radioisotopes* because they tend to give off energy (in the form of radiation) and particles until they reach a more stable state. The radiation emitted by radioisotopes can be dangerous to living organisms because the energy can damage tissues.

Atoms Combine to Form Molecules

A *molecule* is a stable association between two or more atoms. For example, a molecule of water consists of two atoms of hydrogen plus one atom of oxygen (written as H_2O). A molecule of ordinary table salt (written as NaCl) consists of one atom of sodium (Na) plus one atom of chlorine (Cl). A molecule of hydrogen gas (written as H_2) consists of two atoms of hydrogen. In order to understand *why* atoms join together to form molecules, we need to know more about energy.

Energy Fuels the Body's Activities

Energy is the capacity to do work, or the capacity to cause some change in matter. Joining atoms is one type of work, and breaking up molecules is another—and both require energy. Stored energy that is not actually performing any work at the moment is called *potential energy* because it has the *potential* to make things happen. Energy that is actually *doing* work—that is, energy in motion—is called *kinetic energy*.

Potential energy is stored in the bonds that hold atoms together in all matter, both living and nonliving. The body takes advantage of this general principle of chemistry by using certain molecules to store energy for its own use. When the chemical bonds of these energy-storage molecules are broken, potential energy becomes kinetic energy. The body relies on this energy to power "work" such as breathing, moving, and digesting food.

Matter is most stable when it is at the *lowest possible energy level,* that is, when it contains the least potential energy. This fact has important implications for the formation of molecules, because even single atoms contain energy.

Electrons Have Potential Energy

Recall that electrons carry a negative charge, whereas protons within the nucleus have a positive charge. Electrons are attracted to the positively charged nucleus and repelled by each other. As a result of these opposing attractive and repulsive forces, each electron occupies a specific shell around the nucleus. Each shell corresponds to a specific level of electron potential energy, and each shell farther out represents a potential energy level higher than the preceding one. When an electron moves to a shell closer to the nucleus, it loses energy. In order to move to a shell that is farther from the nucleus, the electron must absorb energy.

Chemical Bonds Link Atoms to Form Molecules

A key concept in chemistry is that *atoms are most stable when their outermost occupied electron shell is completely filled.* An atom whose outermost electron shell is not normally filled tends to interact with one or more other atoms in a way that fills its outermost shell. Such interactions generally cause the atoms to be bound to each other by attractive forces called *chemical bonds.* The three principal types of chemical bonds are called covalent, ionic, and hydrogen bonds.

Covalent Bonds Involve Sharing Electrons

One way that an atom can fill its outermost shell is by sharing a pair of electrons with another atom. An electron-sharing bond between atoms is called a *covalent bond* (**Figure C.3**). Covalent bonds between atoms are among the strongest chemical bonds in nature; they are so strong that they rarely break apart. In structural formulas, a covalent bond is depicted as a line drawn between two atoms.

Hydrogen gas offers an example of how a covalent (electron-sharing) bond fills the outermost shells of two atoms. Each of the two hydrogen atoms has just one electron in the first shell, which can accommodate two electrons. When joined together by a covalent bond (forming H_2, a gas), each atom has, in effect, a "full" first shell of two electrons. As a result, H_2 gas is more stable than the same two hydrogen atoms by themselves. The sharing of one pair of electrons, as in H_2, is called a *single* bond.

Oxygen gas is another example of covalent bonding. An oxygen atom has eight electrons: Two of these fill the first electron shell, and the remaining six occupy the second electron shell (which can accommodate eight). Two oxygen atoms may join to form a molecule of oxygen gas by sharing two pairs of electrons, thus completing the outer shells of both atoms. When two pairs of electrons are shared, the bond is called a *double bond.* In structural formulas, double bonds are indicated by two parallel lines.

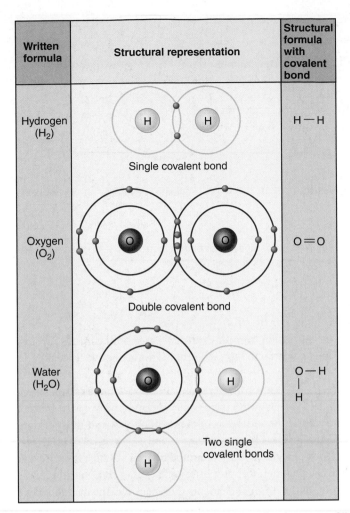

Written formula	Structural representation	Structural formula with covalent bond
Hydrogen (H_2)	Single covalent bond	H — H
Oxygen (O_2)	Double covalent bond	O = O
Water (H_2O)	Two single covalent bonds	O — H $\mid$ H

FIGURE C.3 Covalent bonds. Sharing pairs of electrons is a way for an atom to fill its outermost shell.

A molecule of water forms from one oxygen and two hydrogen atoms because this combination completely fills the outermost shells of both hydrogen and oxygen. The prevalence of water on earth follows from the simple rule described earlier: Matter is most stable when it contains the least potential energy. That is, both hydrogen and oxygen are more stable when together (as H_2O) than when they are independent atoms.

Ionic Bonds Occur Between Oppositely Charged Ions

A second way that atoms can fill their outer shell of electrons is to give up electrons completely (if they have only one or two electrons in their outermost shell) or to take electrons from other atoms (if they need one or two to fill their outermost shell). Such a loss (or gain) of electrons gives the atom a net charge, because now there are fewer (or more) negatively charged electrons than positively charged protons in the nucleus. The net charge is positive (+) for each electron lost and negative (−) for each electron gained.

An electrically charged atom or molecule is called an *ion*. Examples of ions are sodium (Na^+), chloride (Cl^-), calcium (Ca^{2+}), and hydrogen phosphate (HPO_4^-). Note that ions can have a shortage or surplus of more than one electron (for example, Ca^{2+} has lost two electrons). A positively charged ion is called a *cation*; a negatively charged ion is called an *anion*.

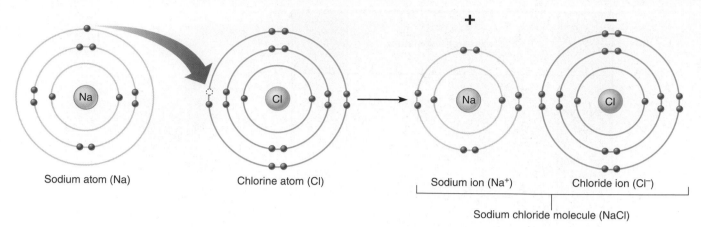

Sodium atom (Na)   Chlorine atom (Cl)   Sodium ion (Na⁺)   Chloride ion (Cl⁻)

Sodium chloride molecule (NaCl)

FIGURE C.4 Ionic bonds. Electrically charged ions form when an atom gives up or gains electrons. The oppositely charged ions are attracted to each other, forming an ionic bond.

Ever heard the expression "opposites attract"? It should come as no surprise that oppositely charged ions are attracted to each other. This attractive force is called an *ionic bond* (**Figure C.4**).

In aqueous (watery) solutions, where ionic bonds are not as strong as covalent bonds, ions tend to dissociate (break away) from each other relatively easily. In the human body, for example, almost all of the sodium is in the form of Na^+, and most of the chlorine is in its ionized form, *called chloride* (Cl^-).

When positive and negative ions are united by ionic bonds, they are called *ionic compounds*. The physical and chemical properties of an ionic compound such as NaCl are very different from those of the original elements. For example, the original elements of NaCl are sodium, a soft, shiny metal, and chlorine, a yellow-green poisonous gas. Yet, as positive and negative ions, they form table salt, a white, crystalline substance that is common in our diet. In ionic compounds, the attraction between the ions is very strong, which makes the melting points of ionic compounds high, often greater than 300°C. For example, the melting point of NaCl is 800°C. At room temperature, ionic compounds are solids.

The structure of an ionic solid depends on the arrangement of the ions. In a crystal of NaCl, which has a cubic shape, the larger Cl^- ions are packed close together in a lattice structure. The smaller Na^+ ions occupy the holes between the Cl^- ions.

Ions in aqueous solutions are sometimes called *electrolytes* because solutions of water containing ions are good conductors of electricity. Cells can control the movement of certain ions, creating electrical forces essential to the functioning of nerves, muscles, and other living tissues.

Weak Hydrogen Bonds Form Between Polar Molecules

A third type of attraction occurs between molecules that do not have a net charge. Glance back at the water molecule in Figure C.3 and note that the two hydrogen atoms are found not at opposite ends of the water molecule but fairly close together. Although the oxygen atom and the two hydrogen atoms share electrons, the sharing is unequal. The shared electrons in a water molecule actually spend slightly more of their time near the oxygen atom than near the hydrogen atoms because the oxygen atom attracts electrons more strongly than do the hydrogen atoms. Although the water molecule is neutral overall, the uneven sharing gives the oxygen end a partial negative charge and the hydrogen end a partial positive charge.

Molecules such as water that are electrically neutral overall but still have partially charged ends, or *poles*, are called *polar* molecules. According to the principle that opposites attract, polar molecules arrange themselves so that the negative pole of one molecule is oriented toward (attracted by) the positive pole of another molecule. The weak attractive

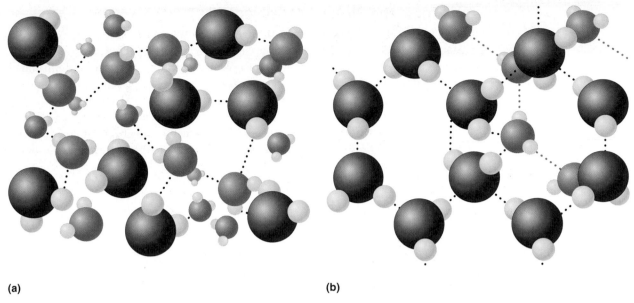

(a)   **(b)**

FIGURE C.5 Hydrogen bonds. **(a)** In water, weak hydrogen bonds continually form, break, and re-form between hydrogen and oxygen atoms of adjacent water molecules. **(b)** Ice is a solid because stable hydrogen bonds form between each water molecule and four of its neighbors.

force between oppositely charged regions of polar molecules that contain covalently bonded hydrogen is called a *hydrogen bond* (**Figure C.5**).

Hydrogen bonds between water molecules in liquid water are so weak that they continually break and re-form, allowing water to flow. When water becomes cold enough to freeze, each water molecule forms four stable, unchanging hydrogen bonds with its neighbors. When water is vaporized (becomes a gas), the hydrogen bonds are broken and stay broken as long as the water is in the gas phase.

Hydrogen bonds are important in biological molecules. They provide the force that gives proteins their three-dimensional shape, and they keep the two strands of the DNA molecule together.

Table C.1 summarizes covalent, ionic, and hydrogen bonds.

The Body Depends on Water

No molecule is more essential to life than water. Indeed, it accounts for between 50% and 70% of body weight. The following properties of water are especially important to the body: water molecules are polar, water is a liquid at body temperature, and water can absorb and hold heat energy.

These properties make water an ideal solvent and an important factor in temperature regulation, as discussed in Chapter 9.

TABLE C.1 Summary of the Three Types of Chemical Bonds

Type	Strength	Description	Examples
Covalent bond	Strong	A bond in which the sharing of electrons between atoms results in each atom having a maximally filled outermost shell of electrons	The bonds between hydrogen and oxygen in a molecule of water
Ionic bond	Moderate	The bond between two oppositely charged ions (atoms or molecules that were formed by the permanent transfer of one or more electrons)	The bond between Na^+ and Cl^- in salt
Hydrogen bond	Weak	The bond between oppositely charged regions of molecules that contain covalently bonded hydrogen atoms	The bonds between molecules of water

Water Is the Biological Solvent

A *solvent* is a liquid in which other substances dissolve, and a *solute* is any dissolved substance. Consider a common and important solid: crystals of sodium chloride (NaCl), or table salt. Crystals of table salt consist of a regular, repeating pattern of sodium and chloride ions held together by ionic bonds (**Figure C.6**). When salt is placed in water, individual ions at the surface of the crystal are pulled away from the crystal and are immediately surrounded by the polar water molecules. The water molecules form such a tight cluster around each ion that the ions are prevented from reassociating back into the crystalline form. In other words, water keeps the ions dissolved. Note that the water molecules are oriented around ions according to the principle that opposite charges attract.

Acids Donate Hydrogen Ions; Bases Accept Them

Although the covalent bonds between hydrogen and oxygen in water are strong and thus are rarely broken, it can happen. When it does, the electron from one hydrogen atom is transferred to the oxygen atom completely, and the water molecule breaks into two ions—a *hydrogen ion* (H^+) and a *hydroxide ion* (OH^-).

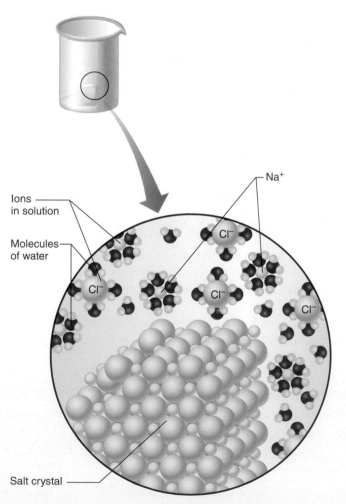

Ions in solution

Molecules of water

Na⁺

Cl⁻

Cl⁻

Cl⁻

Cl⁻

Salt crystal

FIGURE C.6 How water keeps ions in solution. The slightly negative ends of polar water molecules are attracted to positive ions, whereas the slightly positive ends of water molecules are attracted to negative ions. The water molecules pull the ions away from the crystal and prevent them from reassociating with each other.

In pure water, only a very few molecules of water are dissociated (broken apart) into H^+ and OH^- at any one time. However, there are other sources of hydrogen ions in aqueous solutions. An *acid* is any molecule that can donate (give up) an H^+. When added to pure water, acids produce an *acidic* solution, one with a higher H^+ concentration than that of pure water. (By definition, an aqueous solution with the same H^+ concentration as that of pure water is a *neutral* solution.) Common acidic solutions are vinegar, carbonated beverages, and orange juice. Conversely, a *base* is any molecule that can accept (combine with) an H^+. When added to pure water, bases produce a basic or *alkaline* solution, one with a lower H^+ concentration than that of pure water. Common alkaline solutions include baking soda in water, detergents, and drain cleaner.

Because acids and bases have opposite effects on the H^+ concentration of solutions, they are said to neutralize each other.

The pH Scale Expresses Hydrogen Ion Concentration

Scientists use the pH scale to indicate the acidity or alkalinity of a solution. The *pH scale* is a measure of the hydrogen ion concentration of a solution. The scale ranges from 0 to 14, with the pH of pure water defined as a pH of 7.0, the neutral point. A pH of 7 corresponds to a hydrogen ion concentration of 10^{-7} moles/liter (a *mole* is a term used by chemists to indicate a certain number of atoms, ions, or molecules). An *acidic* solution has a pH of *less* than 7, whereas a *basic* solution has a pH of *greater* than 7. Each whole-number change in pH represents a tenfold change in the hydrogen ion concentration in the opposite direction. For example, an acidic solution with a pH of 6 has an H^+ concentration of 10^{-6} moles/liter (ten times greater than pure water), whereas an alkaline solution with a pH of 8 has an H^+ concentration of 10^{-8} moles/liter (1/10 that of water). Figure 3.7 on page 85 shows the pH scale and indicates the pH values of some common substances and foods.

The pH of blood is 7.4, just slightly more alkaline than neutral water. The hydrogen ion concentration of blood plasma is low relative to other ions (the hydrogen ion concentration of blood plasma is less than one-*millionth* that of sodium ions, for example). It is important to maintain homeostasis of this low concentration of hydrogen ions in the body because hydrogen ions are small, mobile, positively charged, and highly reactive. Hydrogen ions tend to displace other positive ions in molecules, and this displacement then alters molecular structures and changes the ability of the molecule to function properly.

Changes in the pH of body fluids can affect how molecules are transported across the cell membrane and how rapidly certain chemical reactions occur. pH changes may even alter the shapes of proteins that are structural elements of the cell. In other words, a change in the hydrogen ion concentration can be dangerous because it alters the body's metabolism and threatens homeostasis.

Buffers Minimize Changes in pH

A *buffer* is any substance that tends to minimize the changes in pH that might otherwise occur when an acid or base is added to a solution. Buffers are essential to the body's ability to maintain homeostasis of pH in body fluids.

In biological solutions such as blood or urine, buffers are present as *pairs* of related molecules that have opposite effects. One molecule of the pair is the acid form of the molecule (capable of donating an H^+), and the other is the base form (capable of accepting an H^+). When an acid is added and the number of H^+ ions increases, the base form of the buffer pair will accept some of the H^+, minimizing the fall in pH that might otherwise occur. Conversely, when a base is added that might take up too many H^+ ions, the acid form of the buffer pair will release additional H^+ and thus minimize the rise in pH. Buffer pairs are like absorbent sponges that can pick up excess water and then can be wrung out to release water when necessary.

One of the most important buffer pairs in body fluids such as blood is bicarbonate (HCO_3^-, the base form) and carbonic acid (H_2CO_3, the acid form). When blood becomes too acidic, bicarbonate accepts excess H^+ according to the following reaction:

$$HCO_3^- + H^+ \rightarrow H_2CO_3$$

When blood becomes too alkaline, carbonic acid donates H^+ by the reverse reaction:

$$HCO_3^- + H^+ \leftarrow H_2CO_3$$

In a biological solution such as blood, bicarbonate and carbonic acid take up and release H^+ all the time. Ultimately, a chemical *equilibrium* is reached in which the rates of the two chemical reactions are the same, as represented by the following combined equation:

$$HCO_3^- + H^+ \leftrightarrow H_2CO_3$$

When excess acid is produced, the combined equation shifts to the right as the bicarbonate combines with the H^+. The reverse is true for alkalinity.

There are many other buffers in the body. The more buffers that are present in a body fluid, the more stable the pH will be.

The Organic Molecules

Organic molecules are molecules that contain carbon and other elements held together by covalent bonds. The name "organic" came about at a time when scientists believed that all organic molecules were created only by living organisms and all "inorganic" molecules came from nonliving matter. Today scientists know that organic molecules can be synthesized in the laboratory under the right conditions.

Carbon Is the Common Building Block of Organic Molecules

Carbon is the common building block of all organic molecules because of the many ways that it can form strong covalent bonds with other atoms. Carbon has six electrons, two in the first shell and four in the second. Because carbon is most stable when its second shell is filled with eight electrons, *its natural tendency is to form four covalent bonds with other molecules.* This makes carbon an ideal structural component, one that can branch in a multitude of directions.

Using the chemist's convention that a line between the chemical symbols of atoms represents a pair of shared electrons in a covalent bond, **Figure C.7** shows some of the many structural possibilities for carbon. Carbon can form covalent bonds with hydrogen, nitrogen, oxygen, or another carbon. It can form double covalent bonds with oxygen or another carbon. It can even form five- or six-membered carbon rings, with or without double bonds between carbons.

In addition to their complexity, there is almost no limit to the size of organic molecules derived from carbon. Some, called *macromolecules* (from the Greek *makros,* long), consist of thousands or even millions of smaller molecules. Protein and glycogen are two examples of macromolecules.

Chemical Reactions

In a chemical reaction, original substances (reactants) are changed to new substances (products) with different physical properties and different compositions. All of the atoms of the original reactants are found in the products. However, some of the bonds between the atoms in the reactants have been broken and new bonds have formed between different combinations of atoms to produce the products. For example, when you light a gas burner, the molecules of methane gas (CH_4) react with oxygen (O_2) in the air to produce CO_2, H_2O, and heat.

In another chemical reaction, when an antacid tablet is placed in water, as the sodium bicarbonate ($NaHCO_3$) and citric acid ($C_6H_8O_7$) in the tablet react, bubbles of carbon

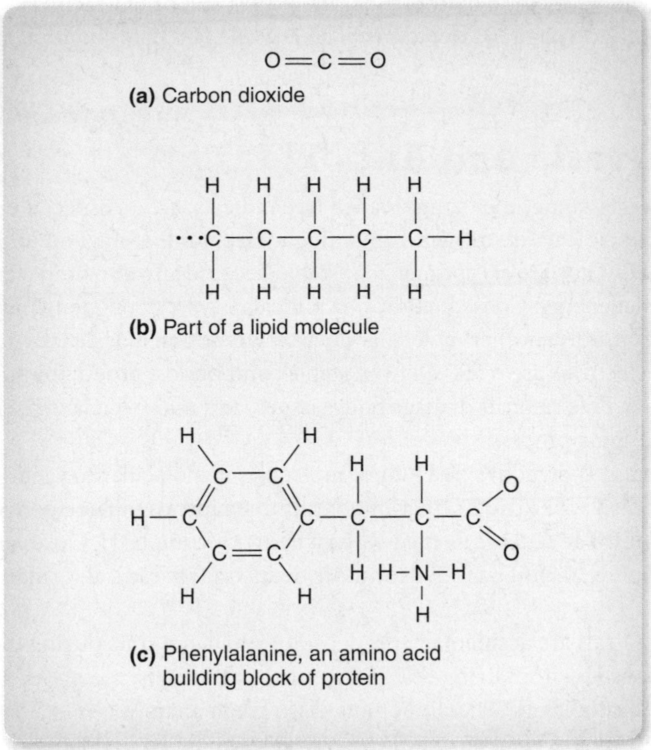

FIGURE C.7 Examples of the structural diversity of carbon. **(a)** In carbon dioxide, a carbon atom forms two covalent bonds with each oxygen atom. **(b)** Lipid molecules contain long chains of carbon atoms covalently bound to hydrogen. **(c)** Carbon is the backbone of the amino acid phenylalanine.

dioxide (CO_2) gas appear. In both these chemical reactions, new properties can be observed. These clues tell you that a chemical reaction has taken place.

Oxidation and Reduction Reactions

In every oxidation–reduction reaction (abbreviated redox), electrons are transferred from one substance to another. If one substance loses electrons, another substance must gain an equal number of electrons. Oxidation is defined as the *loss* of electrons; reduction is the *gain* of electrons. Every time a reaction involves an oxidation and a reduction, the number of electrons lost is equal to the number of electrons gained. The following is an example of oxidation and reduction:

$$Zn \rightarrow Zn^{2+} + 2e^- \text{ Oxidation of Zn}$$

$$Cu^{2+} + 2e^- \rightarrow Cu \text{ Reduction of } Cu^{2+}$$

Enzymes Facilitate Biochemical Reactions

An *enzyme* is a protein that functions as a biological catalyst. A *catalyst* is a substance that speeds up the rate of a chemical reaction without being altered or consumed by the reaction. Enzymes help biochemical reactions to occur, but they do not change the final result of the reaction. That is, they can only speed reactions that would have happened anyway, although much more slowly. A chemical reaction that could take hours by itself might take place in minutes or seconds in the presence of an enzyme.

Without help from thousands of enzymes, most biochemical reactions in our cells would occur too slowly to sustain life. Each enzyme facilitates a particular chemical reaction or group of reactions. Some enzymes break molecules apart; others join molecules together. Enzymes serve as catalysts because, as proteins, they can change shape. The ability to change shape allows them to bind to other molecules and orient them so that they may interact. Figure 6.12 on page 231 depicts how an enzyme facilitates bonding between two compounds.

Free Radicals and Antioxidants

Oxygen free radicals, sometimes simply called free radicals, are an especially unstable class of molecules. Free radicals are oxygen-containing molecules that have an unpaired electron in their outer shell. They are exceptionally unstable because any unpaired electron has a very high potential energy. Consequently, free radicals have a strong tendency to oxidize (remove electrons from) another molecule. They set in motion a destructive cascade of events in which electrons are removed from stable compounds, producing still more unstable compounds. Free radicals damage body tissues, and many scientists believe that they contribute to the aging process.

One of the most destructive free radical molecules is molecular oxygen with an extra electron (O_2^-), called superoxide. Other important free radicals include peroxide (H_2O_2) and hydroxyl (OH). The latter is formed when a hydroxide ion (OH^-) loses an electron. Please refer to Figure 10.3 on page 390 for more detail on free radical formation in the cell membrane.

Some free radicals are accidentally produced in small amounts during the normal process of energy transfer within living cells. Exposure to chemicals, radiation, ultraviolet light, cigarette smoke, alcohol, and air pollution may also create them.

We now know that certain enzymes and nutrients called antioxidants are the body's natural defense against oxygen free radicals. Antioxidants prevent oxidation either by preventing the formation of free radicals in the first place or by inactivating them quickly before they can damage other molecules. Important antioxidants include vitamin E, vitamin C, beta-carotene, and an enzyme called superoxide dismutase.

Dehydration Synthesis and Hydrolysis

Macromolecules are built (synthesized) within the cell itself. In a process known as *dehydration synthesis* (also called *condensation*), smaller molecules called subunits are joined together by covalent bonds, like pearls on a string. The name of the process accurately describes what is happening, for each time a subunit is added, the equivalent of a water molecule is removed ("dehydration"). The subunits needed to synthesize macromolecules come from the foods you eat and from the biochemical reactions in your body that break other large molecules down to smaller ones.

The synthesis of macromolecules from smaller molecules requires energy. That is one reason why we need energy to survive and grow. It is no accident that children seem to eat enormous amounts of food. Growing children require energy to make the macromolecules necessary to create new cell membranes, muscle fibers, and other body tissues.

Organic macromolecules are broken down by a process called *hydrolysis*. During hydrolysis, the equivalent of a water molecule is added each time a covalent bond between single subunits in the chain is broken. Note that hydrolysis is essentially the reverse of dehydration synthesis, and thus it should not surprise you that the breakdown of macromolecules releases energy that was stored as potential energy in the covalent bonds between atoms. Hydrolysis of energy-storage molecules is how the body obtains much of its energy. Hydrolysis is also used to break down molecules of food during digestion, to recycle materials so that they can be used again, and to get rid of substances that are no longer needed by the body. Figure 7.4 on page 264 provides an overview of dehydration synthesis and hydrolysis.

Appendix D

Anatomy and Physiology Review

The Cell

Whereas atoms are the smallest units of matter and make up both living and nonliving things, cells are the smallest units of life. That is, cells can grow, reproduce themselves, and perform certain basic functions, such as taking in nutrients, transmitting impulses, producing chemicals, and excreting wastes. The human body is composed of billions of cells that are constantly replacing themselves, destroying worn or damaged cells, and manufacturing new ones. To support this constant demand for new cells, we need a ready supply of nutrient molecules, such as simple sugars, amino acids, and fatty acids, to serve as building blocks. These building blocks are the molecules that come from the breakdown of foods. All cells, whether of the skin, bones, or brain, are made of the same basic molecules of amino acids, sugars, and fatty acids that are also the main components of the foods we eat.

Cells Are Encased in a Functional Membrane

Cells are encased in a membrane called the cell membrane, or *plasma membrane* (**Figure D.1**). This membrane is the outer covering of the cell and defines the cell's boundaries. It encloses the cell's contents and acts as a gatekeeper, either allowing or denying the entry and exit of molecules such as nutrients and wastes.

Cell membranes are composed of two layers, called the *lipid bilayer*, because each layer is made of molecules called *phospholipids*. Phospholipids consist of a long lipid "tail" bound to a round phospholipid "head." The phosphate head interacts with water, whereas the lipid tail repels water. In the cell membrane, the lipid tails of each layer face each other, forming the membrane interior, whereas the phosphate heads face either the extracellular environment or the cell's interior. Located throughout the membrane are molecules of another lipid, cholesterol, which helps keep the membrane flexible. The membrane also contains various proteins, which assist in transport of nutrients and other substances across the cell membrane and in the manufacture of certain chemicals.

Cells Contain Organelles That Support Life

Enclosed within the cell membrane is a liquid called cytoplasm and a variety of organelles (see Figure D.1). These tiny structures accomplish some surprisingly sophisticated functions. A brief review of some of them and their functions related to nutrition is as follows:

- **Nucleus.** The nucleus is where our genetic information is located, in the form of deoxyribonucleic acid (DNA). The cell nucleus is darkly colored because DNA is a huge molecule that is tightly packed within it. A cell's DNA contains the instructions that the cell uses to make certain proteins.
- **Ribosomes.** Ribosomes are structures the cell uses to make needed proteins.
- **Endoplasmic reticulum (ER).** The endoplasmic reticulum is important in the synthesis of proteins and lipids and in the storage of the mineral calcium. The ER looks like a maze of interconnected channels.

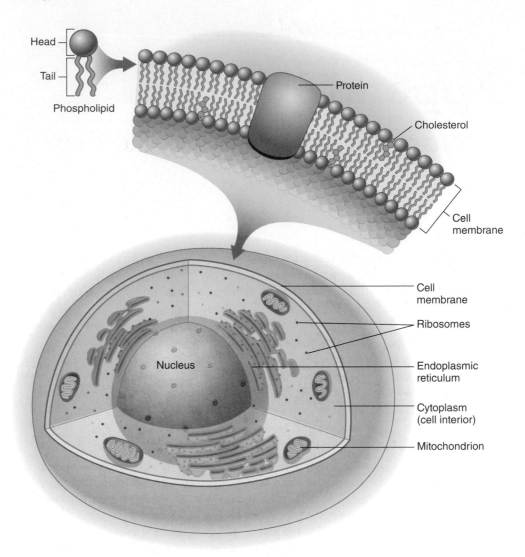

FIGURE D.1 Representative cell of the small intestine, showing the cell membrane and a variety of organelles.

- **Mitochondria.** Often called the cell's powerhouse, mitochondria produce the energy molecule ATP (adenosine triphosphate) from basic food components. ATP can be thought of as a stored form of energy, drawn upon as we need it. Cells that have high energy needs contain more mitochondria than cells with lower energy needs.

Molecules Cross the Cell Membrane in Several Ways

Recall that the cell membrane is the gatekeeper that, along with its proteins, determines what goes into and out of the cell. This means that cell membranes are *selectively permeable*, allowing only some compounds to enter and leave the cell.

Passive Transport: Principles of Diffusion and Osmosis

Passive transport is "passive" because it transports a molecule without requiring the cell to expend any energy. Passive transport relies on the mechanism of diffusion.

Molecules in a gas or a liquid move about randomly, colliding with other molecules and changing direction. The movement of molecules from one region to another as the result of this random motion is known as diffusion.

If there are more molecules in one region than in another, then strictly by chance more molecules will tend to diffuse away from the area of high concentration and toward the region of low concentration. In other words, the *net* diffusion of molecules requires that there be a difference in concentration, called a *concentration gradient*, between two points. Once the concentration of molecules is the same throughout the solution, a state of equilibrium exists in which molecules are diffusing randomly but equally in all directions.

Not all substances diffuse readily into and out of living cells. The cell membrane is selectively permeable, meaning that it allows some substances to cross by diffusion but not others. It is highly permeable to water, but not to all ions or molecules. The net diffusion of water across a selectively permeable membrane is called *osmosis*. Osmosis and osmotic pressure are discussed in more detail in Chapter 9.

Most substances cross cell membranes by passive transport. Passive transport always proceeds "downhill" with respect to the concentration gradient, meaning that it relies on diffusion in some way. Three forms of passive transport across the cell membrane are (1) diffusion through the lipid bilayer, (2) diffusion through channels, and (3) facilitated transport.

Diffusion through the Lipid Bilayer   The lipid bilayer structure of the cell membrane allows the free passage of some molecules while restricting others. For instance, small uncharged nonpolar molecules can diffuse right through the lipid bilayer as if it did not exist. Such molecules simply dissolve in the lipid bilayer, passing through it as one might imagine a ghost walking through a wall. Polar or electrically charged molecules, on the other hand, cannot cross the lipid bilayer because they are not soluble in lipids.

Two important lipid-soluble molecules are oxygen (O_2), which diffuses into cells and is used up in the process of metabolism, and carbon dioxide (CO_2), a waste product of metabolism, which diffuses out of cells and is removed from the body by the lungs. Another substance that crosses the lipid bilayer by diffusion is urea, a neutral waste product removed from the body by the kidneys.

Diffusion through Channels   Water and many ions diffuse through channels in the cell membrane. The channels are constructed of proteins that span the entire lipid bilayer. The sizes and shapes of these protein channels, as well as the electrical charges on the various amino acid groups that line the channel, determine which molecules can pass through.

Some channels are open all the time (typical of water channels). The diffusion of any molecule through the membrane is largely determined by the number of channels through which the molecule can fit. Other channels are "gated," meaning that they can open and close under certain conditions. Gated channels are particularly important in regulating the transport of ions (sodium, potassium, and calcium) in cells that are electrically excitable, such as nerves.

Facilitated Transport   In facilitated transport, also called *facilitated diffusion*, the molecule does not pass through a channel at all. Instead, it attaches to a membrane protein, triggering a change in the protein's shape or orientation that transfers the molecule to the other side of the membrane and releases it there. Once the molecule is released, the protein returns to its original form. A protein that carries a molecule across the plasma membrane in this manner, rather than opening a channel through it, is called a transport protein (or carrier protein).

Facilitated transport is highly selective for particular substances. The direction of movement is always from a region of high concentration to one of lower concentration, and thus it does not require the cell to expend energy. The normal process of diffusion is simply being "facilitated" by the transport protein. Glucose and other simple sugars enter most cells by this method.

Active Transport Requires Energy

All methods of passive transport allow substances to move only down their concentration gradients, in the direction they would normally diffuse if there were no barrier. However, active transport can move substances through the plasma membrane *against* their concentration gradient. Active transport allows a cell to accumulate essential molecules even when their concentration outside the cell is relatively low and to get rid of molecules that it does not need. Active transport requires the expenditure of energy.

Like facilitated transport, active transport is accomplished by proteins that span the plasma membrane. The difference is that active transport proteins must have some source of energy in order to transport certain molecules. Some active transport proteins use the high-energy molecule ATP for this purpose. They break ATP down to ADP and a phosphate group (P_i) and use the released energy to transport one or more molecules across the plasma membrane against their concentration gradient. Figure 3.15 on page 96 provides an overview of active and passive transport.

From Cells to Organ Systems

Cells of a single type, such as muscle cells, join together to form functional groupings of cells called tissues. In general, several types of tissues join together to form organs, which are sophisticated structures that perform a unique body function. The stomach and small intestine are examples of organs.

Organs are further grouped into systems that perform integrated functions. The stomach, for example, is an organ that is part of the gastrointestinal system. It holds and partially digests a meal, but it cannot perform all system functions—digestion, absorption, and elimination—by itself. These functions require several organs working together in an integrated system. The following sections provide a review of some other body systems.

The Muscular System

Muscle cells are found in every organ and tissue in the body and participate in every activity that requires movement. The most obvious are the *skeletal muscles* that attach to the skeleton and give us strength and mobility. There are two other types of muscle in the body besides skeletal muscle. Rhythmic contractions of the *cardiac muscle* of the heart pump blood throughout the body. Powerful, intermittent contractions of *smooth muscle* in the walls of the uterus contribute to childbirth. Slower waves of smooth muscle contractions push food through the digestive tract and transport urine from the kidney to the bladder. Steady, sustained contractions of smooth muscle in the walls of blood vessels regulate blood flow to every living cell in the body.

A Muscle Is Composed of Many Muscle Cells

A single *muscle* (sometimes referred to as a "whole muscle") is a group of individual muscle cells, all with the same function. In cross section, a muscle appears to be arranged in bundles called *fascicles*, each enclosed in a sheath of a type of fibrous connective tissue called *fascia*. Each fascicle contains from a few dozen to thousands of individual muscle cells, or *muscle fibers*. The outer surface of the whole muscle is covered by several more layers of fascia. At the ends of the muscle all of the fasciae (plural) come together, forming the tendons that attach the muscle to bone (**Figure D.2**).

Individual muscle cells are tube shaped, larger, and usually longer than most other human cells. The entire interior of each muscle cell is packed with long cylindrical structures arranged in parallel, called *myofibrils.* The myofibrils are packed with contractile proteins called *actin* and *myosin.* When myofibrils contract (shorten), the muscle cell also shortens.

The Contractile Unit Is a Sarcomere

Sarcomeres are segments of myofibrils. A single myofibril within one muscle cell in the biceps muscle may contain more than 100,000 sarcomeres arranged end to end. The microscopic shortening of these 100,000 sarcomeres all at once is what produces contraction (shortening) of the muscle cell and of the whole muscle. Understanding muscle shortening, then, is simply a matter of understanding how a single sarcomere works.

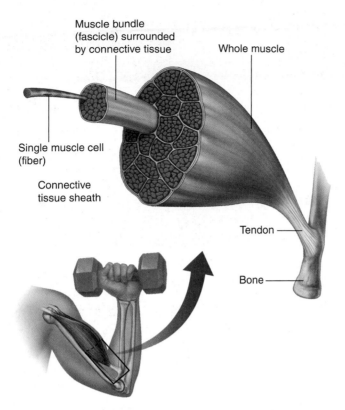

FIGURE D.2 Muscle structure. A muscle is arranged in bundles called fascicles, each composed of many muscle cells and each surrounded by a sheath of connective tissue called fascia. Surrounding the entire muscle are several more layers of fascia. The fascia join together to become the tendon, which attaches the muscle to bone.

A sarcomere consists of two kinds of protein filaments. Thick filaments composed of *myosin* are interspersed at regular intervals within filaments of *actin*. Muscle contractions depend on the interaction between these actin and myosin filaments.

Nerves Activate Skeletal Muscles

Skeletal muscle cells are stimulated to contract by certain nerve cells called motor neurons. The motor neurons secrete a chemical substance called *acetylcholine (ACh)*. Acetylcholine is a neurotransmitter, a chemical released by nerve cells that has either an excitatory or an inhibitory effect on another excitable cell (another nerve cell or a muscle cell). In the case of skeletal muscle, acetylcholine excites (activates) the cells.

When a muscle cell is activated, an electrical impulse races down the inside of the muscle cell. The arrival of that impulse triggers the release of calcium ions from the sarcoplasmic reticulum (a structure similar to other cells' smooth endoplasmic reticulum). The calcium diffuses into the cell cytoplasm and then comes into contact with the myofibrils, where it sets in motion a chain of events that leads to contraction. Muscles contract when sarcomeres shorten, and sarcomeres shorten when the thick and thin filaments slide past each other, a process known as the sliding filament mechanism of contraction (**Figure D.3**).

Muscles Require Energy to Contract and to Relax

Muscle contraction requires a great deal of energy. Like most cells, muscle cells use ATP as their energy source. In the presence of calcium, myosin acts as an enzyme, splitting ATP into ADP and inorganic phosphate and releasing energy to do work.

The energy is used to "energize" the myosin head so that it can form a cross-bridge and undergo bending. Once the bending has occurred, another molecule of ATP binds to the

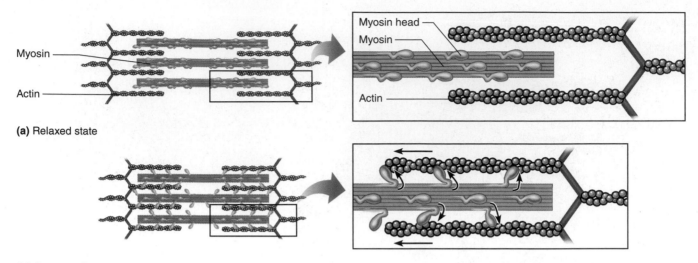

(a) Relaxed state

(b) Contracted state

FIGURE D.3 Sliding filament mechanism of contraction. **(a)** In the relaxed state, the myosin heads do not make contact with actin. **(b)** During contraction, the myosin heads form cross-bridges with actin and bend, pulling the actin filaments toward the center of the sarcomere.

myosin, which causes the myosin head to detach from actin. As long as calcium is present, the cycle of ATP breakdown, attachment, bending, and detachment is repeated over and over again in rapid succession. The result is a shortening of the sarcomere.

At the end of the contractile period (when nerve impulses end), energy from the breakdown of ATP is used to transport calcium back into the sarcoplasmic reticulum so that relaxation can occur. However, a second requirement for relaxation is that an intact molecule of ATP must bind to myosin before myosin can finally detach from actin.

Muscle Cells Obtain ATP from Several Sources Muscle cells store only enough ATP for about 10 seconds' worth of maximal activity. Once this is used up, the cells must produce more ATP from other energy sources, including creatine phosphate, glycogen, glucose, and fatty acids.

An important pathway for producing ATP involves creatine phosphate (creatine-P), a high-energy molecule with an attached phosphate group. Creatine phosphate can transfer a phosphate group and energy to ADP and therefore create a new ATP quickly. This reaction is reversible: If ATP is not needed to power muscle contractions, the excess ATP can be used to build a fresh supply of creatine phosphate, which is stored until needed.

The combination of previously available ATP plus stored creatine phosphate produces only enough energy for up to 30 to 40 seconds of heavy activity. Beyond that, muscles must rely on stored glycogen. For the first 3 to 5 minutes of sustained activity, a muscle cell draws on its internal supply of stored glycogen. Glucose molecules are converted from the stored glycogen, and their energy is used to synthesize ATP. Part of the process of the breakdown of glucose can be done without oxygen (called anaerobic metabolism) fairly quickly, but it only yields two ATP molecules per glucose molecule.

The most efficient long-term source of energy is the aerobic metabolism of glucose, fatty acids, and other high-energy molecules such as lactic acid. Aerobic metabolism takes place in mitochondria and requires oxygen. The next time you engage in strenuous exercise, note that it may take you a few minutes to start breathing heavily. The increase in respiration indicates that aerobic metabolism is now taking place. Until aerobic metabolism kicks in, however, cells are relying on stored ATP, creatine phosphate, and anaerobic metabolism of glycogen. Weight lifters can rely on stored energy because their muscles perform for relatively short periods. Long-distance runners start out by depending on stored energy, but in less than a minute they are relying almost exclusively on aerobic metabolism. If they could not, they would collapse in exhaustion.

The Cardiovascular System

The heart and blood vessels are known collectively as the cardiovascular system (*cardio* comes from the Greek word for "heart," and vascular derives from the Latin word for "small vessel"). The heart provides the power to move the blood, and the vascular system represents the network of branching conduit vessels through which the blood flows. The cardiovascular system is essential to life because it supplies every region of the body with just the right amount of blood.

Blood Vessels Transport Blood

We classify the body's blood vessels into three major types: *arteries, capillaries*, and *veins*. Thick-walled arteries transport blood to body tissues under high pressure. Microscopic capillaries participate in exchanging solutes and water with the cells of the body. Thin-walled veins store blood and return it to the heart.

As blood leaves the heart it is pumped into large, muscular, thick-walled arteries. Arteries transport blood away from the heart. The larger arteries have a thick layer of muscle because they must be able to withstand the high pressures generated by the heart. Arteries branch again and again, so the farther blood moves from the heart, the smaller in diameter the arteries become. Eventually blood reaches the smallest arteries, called arterioles (literally, "little arteries").

Where an arteriole joins a capillary is a band of smooth muscle called the precapillary sphincter. The precapillary sphincters serve as gates that control blood flow into individual capillaries. Extensive networks of capillaries, called *capillary beds*, can be found in all areas of the body, which is why you are likely to bleed no matter where you cut yourself. Capillaries' branching design and thin, porous walls enable blood to exchange oxygen, carbon dioxide, nutrients, and waste products with tissue cells. In fact, capillaries are the *only* blood vessels that can exchange materials with the interstitial fluid.

Figure D.4 illustrates the general pattern of how water and substances move across a capillary. At the beginning of a capillary, fluid is filtered out of the vessel into the interstitial fluid, accompanied by oxygen, nutrients, and raw materials needed by the cell. The filtered fluid is essentially like plasma except that it contains very little protein because most protein molecules are too large to be filtered. Filtration of fluid is caused by the blood pressure generated by the heart. Waste materials such as carbon dioxide and urea diffuse out of the cells and back into the blood.

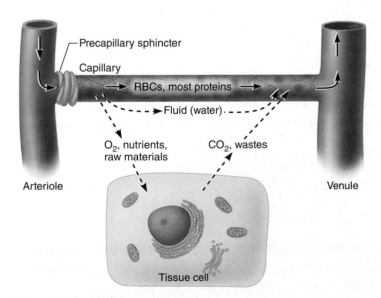

FIGURE D.4 The general pattern of movement between capillaries, the interstitial fluid, and cells. For simplicity, only a single tissue cell is shown, but a single capillary may supply many nearby cells.

From the capillaries, blood flows back to the heart through *venules* (small veins) and veins. Like the walls of arteries, the walls of veins consist of three layers of tissue. However, the outer two layers of the walls of veins are much thinner than those of arteries. Veins also have a larger lumen (that is, are larger in diameter) than arteries.

The Heart Pumps Blood Through the Vessels

The heart is a muscular, cone-shaped organ slightly larger than your fist, located in the thoracic cavity between the lungs and behind the sternum (breastbone). The heart consists mostly of cardiac muscle. Unlike skeletal muscle, cardiac muscle does not connect to bone. Instead, it pumps ceaselessly in a squeezing motion to propel blood through the blood vessels.

The heart consists of four separate chambers. The two chambers on the top are the atria (singular *atrium*), and the two more muscular bottom chambers are the ventricles. A muscular partition called the septum separates the right and left sides of the heart (**Figure D.5**).

The Pulmonary Circuit Provides for Gas Exchange

Review Figure 3.16 on page 97, which shows the general structure of the entire cardiovascular system. Note that the heart is pumping blood through the lungs (the pulmonary circuit) and through the rest of the body to all the cells (the systemic circuit) simultaneously. Each circuit has its own set of blood vessels. Let's follow the pulmonary circuit first:

1. When blood returns to the heart from the veins, it enters the right atrium. The blood that returns to the heart is deoxygenated—it has given up oxygen to tissue cells and taken up carbon dioxide.
2. From the right atrium, blood passes through the right atrioventricular valve into the right ventricle.
3. The right ventricle pumps blood through the pulmonary semilunar valve into the pulmonary trunk (the main pulmonary artery) leading to the lungs. The pulmonary trunk divides into the right and left pulmonary arteries, which supply the right and left lungs, respectively.

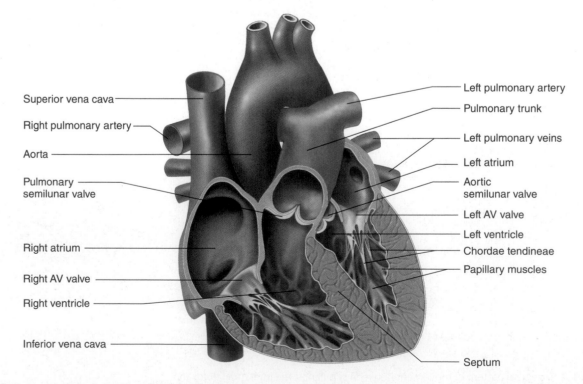

FIGURE D.5 A view of the heart showing major blood vessels, chambers, and valves. The pulmonary vessels are shown in purple to distinguish them from systemic arteries and veins.

4. At the pulmonary capillaries, blood gives up carbon dioxide and receives a fresh supply of oxygen from the air we inhale. It is now oxygenated.
5. The freshly oxygenated blood flows into the pulmonary veins leading back to the heart. It enters the left atrium and flows through the left atrioventricular valve into the left ventricle.

The Systemic Circuit Serves the Rest of the Body

When blood enters the left ventricle, it begins the *systemic circuit*, which takes it to the rest of the body.

1. The left ventricle pumps blood through the aortic semilunar valve into the aorta, the largest artery.
2. From the aorta, blood travels through the branching arteries and arterioles to the capillaries, where it delivers oxygen and nutrients to all of the body's tissues and organs and removes waste products. Even some tissues of the lungs receive their nutrient blood supply from the systemic circulation.
3. From the capillaries, blood flows to the venules, veins, and then back again to the right atrium.

The Lymphatic System

The lymphatic system is closely associated with the cardiovascular system. The lymphatic system performs three important functions:

1. It helps maintain the volume of blood in the cardiovascular system.
2. It transports lipids and fat-soluble vitamins absorbed from the digestive system.
3. It defends the body against infection and injury.

Lymphatic Vessels Transport Lymph

The lymphatic system begins as a network of small, blind-ended *lymphatic capillaries* in the vicinity of the cells and blood capillaries. The lymphatic system helps maintain blood volume and interstitial fluid volume by absorbing excess fluid that has been filtered out of the capillaries and returning it to the cardiovascular system. Lymphatic capillaries in the small intestine are called lacteals and pick up most lipids and fat-soluble vitamins absorbed in the small intestine and eventually send them to the bloodstream.

Lymph capillaries have wide spaces between overlapping cells. Their structure allows them to take up substances (including bacteria) that are too large to enter a blood capillary.

The fluid in the lymphatic capillaries is *lymph*, a milky body fluid that contains white blood cells, proteins, fats, and the occasional bacterium. Lymphatic capillaries merge to form the *lymphatic vessels*. Located at intervals along the lymphatic vessels are small organs called lymph nodes, described in the following section. Like veins, lymphatic vessels contain one-way valves to prevent backflow of lymph. The lymphatic vessels merge to form larger and larger vessels, eventually creating two major lymphatic ducts: the *right lymphatic duct* and the *thoracic duct*. The two lymph ducts join the subclavian veins near the shoulders, thereby returning the lymph to the cardiovascular system.

Lymph Nodes Cleanse the Lymph

Lymph nodes remove microorganisms, cellular debris, and abnormal cells from the lymph before returning it to the cardiovascular system. There are hundreds of lymph nodes, clustered in the areas of the digestive tract, neck, armpits, and groin. They vary in diameter from about 1 mm to 2.5 cm. Each node is enclosed in a dense capsule of connective tissue pierced by lymphatic vessels. Inside each node are connective tissue and two types of white blood cells, known as macrophages and lymphocytes.

The largest lymphatic organ, the spleen, is a soft, fist-sized mass located in the upper-left abdominal cavity. The spleen has two main functions: It controls the quality of circulating red blood cells by removing the old and damaged ones, and it helps fight infection. Note that the main distinction between spleen and lymph nodes is *which* fluid they cleanse—the spleen cleanses the blood, and the lymph nodes cleanse lymph. Together, they keep the circulating body fluids relatively free of damaged cells and microorganisms.

The thymus gland is located in the lower neck, behind the sternum and just above the heart. Encased in connective tissue, the gland contains lymphocytes and epithelial cells. The thymus gland secretes two hormones, thymosin and thymopoietin, that cause certain lymphocytes called *T lymphocytes* (T cells) to mature and take an active role in specific defenses.

The *tonsils* are masses of lymphatic tissue near the entrance to the throat. Lymphocytes in the tonsils gather and filter out many of the microorganisms that enter the throat in food or air.

The Respiratory System

For the sake of convenience, the respiratory system can be divided into the upper and lower respiratory tracts. The *upper respiratory tract* comprises the nose (including the nasal cavity) and pharynx—structures above the "Adam's apple" in men's necks. The *lower respiratory tract* starts with the larynx and includes the trachea, the two bronchi that branch from the trachea, and the lungs themselves (**Figure D.6**).

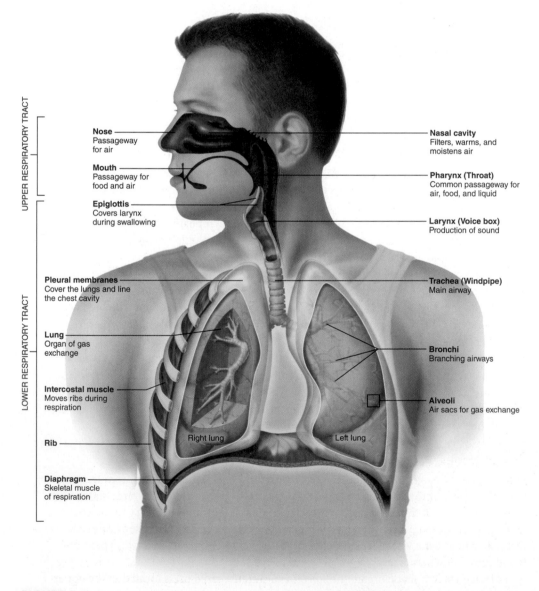

UPPER RESPIRATORY TRACT

Nose
Passageway
for air

Mouth
Passageway for
food and air

Epiglottis
Covers larynx
during swallowing

LOWER RESPIRATORY TRACT

Pleural membranes
Cover the lungs and line
the chest cavity

Lung
Organ of gas
exchange

Intercostal muscle
Moves ribs during
respiration

Rib

Diaphragm
Skeletal muscle
of respiration

Nasal cavity
Filters, warms, and
moistens air

Pharynx (Throat)
Common passageway for
air, food, and liquid

Larynx (Voice box)
Production of sound

Trachea (Windpipe)
Main airway

Bronchi
Branching airways

Alveoli
Air sacs for gas exchange

Right lung   Left lung

FIGURE D.6 The human respiratory system. The functions of each of the anatomical structures are included.

The Upper Respiratory Tract Filters, Warms, and Humidifies Air

During inhalation, air enters through the nose or mouth. The internal portion of the nose is called the nasal cavity. The mucus in the nasal cavity traps dust, pathogens, and other particles in the air before they get any farther into the respiratory tract.

Incoming air next enters the pharynx (throat), which connects the mouth and nasal cavity to the larynx (voice box). The upper pharynx extends from the nasal cavity to the roof of the mouth. The lower pharynx is a common passageway for both food and air. Food passes through on its way to the esophagus, and air flows through to the lower respiratory tract.

The Lower Respiratory Tract Exchanges Gases

The lower respiratory tract includes the larynx, the trachea, the bronchi, and the lungs with their bronchioles and alveoli. The larynx extends about 5 cm (2 in.) below the pharynx. The larynx contains two important structures: the epiglottis and the vocal cords. The epiglottis is a flexible flap of cartilage located at the opening to the larynx. When air is flowing into the larynx, the epiglottis remains open. But when we swallow food or liquids, the epiglottis tips to block the opening temporarily. This "switching mechanism" routes food and beverages into the esophagus and digestive system, rather than into the trachea. This is why it is impossible to talk while you are swallowing.

As air continues down the respiratory tract, it passes to the trachea, the "windpipe" that extends from the larynx to the left and right bronchi. If a foreign object lodges in the trachea, respiration is interrupted and choking occurs. If the airway is completely blocked, death can occur within minutes. Choking often happens when a person carries on an animated conversation while eating. The risk of choking provides a good reason beyond good manners not to eat and talk at the same time.

The trachea branches into two airways called the right and left bronchi (singular *bronchus*) as it enters the lung cavity. Like the branches of a tree, the two bronchi divide into a network of smaller and smaller bronchi. The smaller airways that lack cartilage are called bronchioles. The smallest bronchioles are 1 mm or smaller in diameter and consist primarily of a thin layer of smooth muscle surrounded by a small amount of elastic connective tissue.

The bronchi and bronchioles also clean the air, warm it to body temperature, and saturate it with water vapor before it reaches the delicate gas exchange surfaces of the lungs.

The Lungs Are Organs of Gas Exchange

The lungs are organs consisting of supportive tissue enclosing the bronchi, bronchioles, blood vessels, and the areas where gas exchange occurs. If you could touch a living lung, you would find that it is very soft and frothy. In fact, most of it is air. The lungs are basically a system of branching airways that end in 300 million tiny air-filled sacs called alveoli (singular *alveolus*). It is here that gas exchange takes place. Alveoli are arranged in clusters at the end of every terminal bronchiole, like grapes clustered on a stem. A single alveolus is a thin bubble of living squamous epithelial cells only one cell layer thick. Their combined surface area is nearly 800 ft^2, approximately forty times the area of a person's skin. The tremendous surface area and thinness facilitate gas exchange with nearby capillaries.

The Nervous System

The nervous system comprises the central nervous system (CNS) and the peripheral nervous system (PNS). The CNS consists of the brain and the spinal cord. It receives, processes, stores, and transfers information. The PNS represents the components of the nervous system that lie outside the CNS. The PNS has two functional subdivisions: The sensory division carries information to the brain and spinal cord, and the motor division carries information from the CNS (**Figure D.7**).

The motor division of the peripheral nervous system is further subdivided along functional lines. The *somatic division* of the PNS controls skeletal muscles, and the autonomic division of the PNS controls smooth muscles, cardiac muscles, and glands. In turn, the

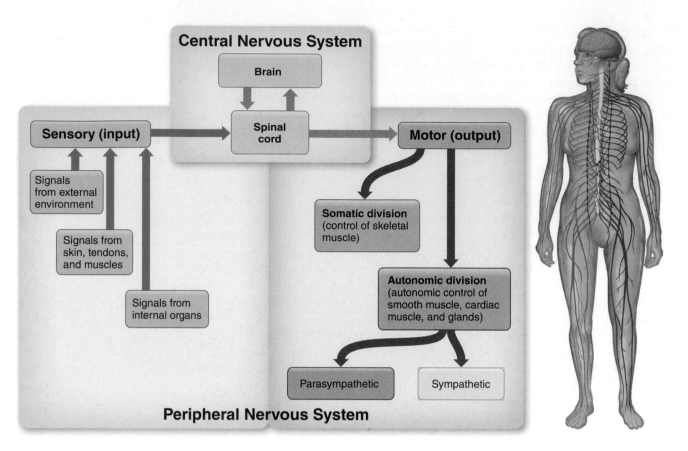

FIGURE D.7 Components of the nervous system. The CNS receives input from the sensory component of the PNS, integrates and organizes the information, and then sends output to the periphery via the motor components of the PNS.

autonomic division has two subdivisions called the *sympathetic* and *parasympathetic* divisions. In general, the actions of the sympathetic and parasympathetic divisions oppose each other. They work antagonistically to accomplish the automatic, subconscious maintenance of homeostasis within the body.

Neurons

Neurons are cells specialized for communication. They generate and conduct electrical impulses, also called *action potentials*, from one part of the body to another. The longest neurons extend all the way from your toes to your spinal cord.

There are three types of neurons in the nervous system:

1. Sensory neurons of the PNS are specialized to respond to a certain type of stimulus, such as pressure or light. They transmit information about this stimulus to the CNS in the form of electrical impulses. In other words, sensory neurons provide input to the CNS.
2. Interneurons within the CNS transmit impulses between components of the CNS. Interneurons receive input from sensory neurons, integrate this information, and influence the functioning of other neurons.
3. Motor neurons of the PNS transmit impulses away from the CNS. They carry the nervous system's output, still in the form of electrical impulses, to all of the tissues and organs of the body.

All neurons consist of a cell body, one or more dendrites, and an axon. The main body of a neuron is called the cell body. Slender extensions of the cell body, called dendrites, receive information from receptors or incoming impulses from other neurons. Interneurons and motor neurons have numerous dendrites that are fairly short and extend in many directions from the cell body. Sensory neurons are an exception, for their dendrites connect directly to an axon.

An axon is a long, slender tube of cell membrane containing a small amount of cytoplasm. Axons are specialized to conduct electrical impulses. Axons of sensory neurons originate from a dendrite, whereas the axons of interneurons and motor neurons originate from a cone-shaped area of the cell body called the *axon hillock*. At its other end, the axon branches into slender extensions called *axon terminals*. Each axon terminal ends in a small rounded tip called an *axon bulb*.

Action Potentials

An action potential occurs as a sequence of three events: (1) depolarization, (2) repolarization, and (3) reestablishment of the resting potential.

1. *Depolarization: Sodium moves into the axon.* Voltage-sensitive Na^+ channels in the axon's membrane open briefly and Na^+ ions diffuse rapidly into the cytoplasm of the axon. This influx of positive ions causes *depolarization*, meaning that the membrane potential shifts from negative (−70 mV) to positive (about +30 mV).

2. *Repolarization: Potassium moves out of the axon.* After a short delay, the Na^+ channels close automatically. But the reversal of the membrane polarity triggers the opening of K^+ channels. This allows more K^+ ions than usual to diffuse rapidly out of the cell. The loss of positive ions from the cell leads to *repolarization*, meaning that the interior of the axon becomes negative again.

3. *Reestablishment of the resting potential.* Because the K^+ channels are slow to close, there is a brief overshoot of membrane voltage during which the interior of the axon is slightly hyperpolarized. Shortly after the K^+ channels close, the resting potential is reestablished. At this point the axon is prepared to receive another action potential. The entire sequence of three steps takes about 3 ms.

Once an action potential is initiated, it sweeps rapidly down the axon until it reaches the axon terminals.

Synaptic Transmission

Once an action potential reaches the axon terminals of a neuron, the information inherent in it must be converted to another form for transmittal to its target. In essence, the action potential causes the release of a chemical that crosses a specialized junction between the two cells called a synapse. This chemical substance is called a neurotransmitter because it transmits a signal from a neuron to its target.

Figure D.8 illustrates the structure of a typical synapse and the events that occur during synaptic transmission. At a synapse, the *presynaptic membrane* is the cell membrane of the neuron that is sending the information. The *postsynaptic membrane* refers to the membrane of the cell that is about to receive the information. The small, fluid-filled gap that separates the presynaptic and postsynaptic membranes is the *synaptic cleft*.

The Endocrine System and Hormones

The endocrine system is a collection of specialized cells, tissues, and glands that produces and secretes circulating chemical messenger molecules called hormones. Most hormones are secreted by endocrine glands—ductless organs that secrete their products into interstitial fluid, lymph, and blood (*endocrine* means "secreted internally"). In contrast, *exocrine* glands secrete products such as mucus, sweat, tears, and digestive fluids into ducts that empty into the appropriate sites. There are approximately fifty known hormones circulating in the human bloodstream, and new ones are still being discovered. Hormones are bloodborne units of information, just as nerve impulses are units of information carried in nerves.

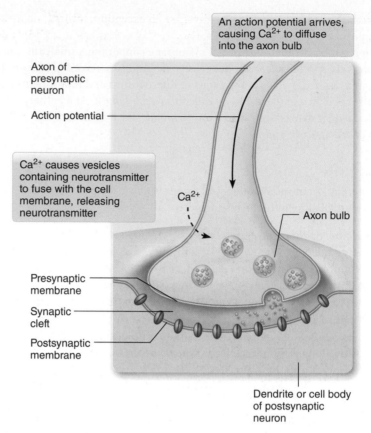

An action potential arrives, causing Ca²⁺ to diffuse into the axon bulb

Axon of presynaptic neuron

Action potential

Ca²⁺ causes vesicles containing neurotransmitter to fuse with the cell membrane, releasing neurotransmitter

Ca²⁺

Axon bulb

Presynaptic membrane

Synaptic cleft

Postsynaptic membrane

Dendrite or cell body of postsynaptic neuron

FIGURE D.8 Summary of synaptic transmission.

The endocrine system has certain characteristics that set it apart from the nervous system as a communications system:

1. Hormones of the endocrine system reach nearly every living cell.
2. Each hormone acts only on certain cells.
3. Endocrine control tends to be slower than nervous system control.
4. The endocrine and nervous systems can (and often do) interact with each other.

Hormones Are Classified as Steroid or Nonsteroid

Hormones generally are classified into two basic categories based on their structure and mechanism of action. Steroid hormones are structurally related to cholesterol; in fact, all of them are synthesized from cholesterol and all are lipid soluble. Nonsteroid hormones consist of, or at least are partly derived from, the amino acid building blocks of proteins. In general, they are lipid insoluble. The differences in lipid solubility explain most of the important differences in how the two categories of hormones work. Steroid hormones usually enter the cell, bind to an intracellular receptor, and activate genes that produce new proteins. Nonsteroid hormones generally bind to receptors on the cell's surface. Their binding either opens or closes cell membrane ion channels or activates enzymes within the cell.

The Hypothalamus and the Pituitary Gland

The hypothalamus is a small region in the forebrain that plays an important role in homeostatic regulation. It monitors internal environmental conditions such as water and solute balance, temperature, and carbohydrate metabolism.

The hypothalamus also produces hormones and monitors the pituitary gland, a small endocrine gland located beneath the hypothalamus and connected to it by a stalk of tissue (review Figure 3.1 on page 77). The pituitary gland is sometimes called the "master gland" because it secretes eight different hormones and regulates many of the other endocrine glands.

The Urinary System

Excretion refers to processes that remove wastes and excess materials from the body. **Figure D.9** provides a review of the systems involved in managing metabolic wastes and maintaining homeostasis of water and solutes.

Because the excretory capacity of the other organs is limited, the urinary system has primary responsibility for homeostasis of water and most of the solutes in blood and other body fluids. The urinary system consists of the organs (kidneys, ureters, bladder, and urethra) that produce, transport, store, and excrete urine.

Urine is essentially water and solutes. Among the solutes excreted in urine are excess elements and ions, drugs, vitamins, toxic chemicals, and waste products produced by the liver or by cellular metabolism. Some substances, such as water and sodium chloride (salt), are excreted to regulate body fluid balance and salt levels. About the only major solutes *not* excreted by the kidneys under normal circumstances are the three classes of macronutrients. The kidneys keep these nutrients in the body for other organs to regulate.

Water is the most abundant molecule in the body, accounting for at least half of body weight. The urinary system plays a large role in regulating water levels in the blood and body fluids.

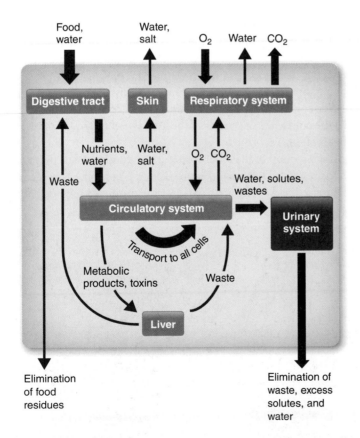

FIGURE D.9 Organ systems involved in removing wastes and maintaining homeostasis of water and solutes. With the large tan box representing the body, this diagram maps the inflow and outflow of key compounds we consume. The kidneys of the urinary system are the organs primarily responsible for the maintenance of homeostasis of water and solutes and for the excretion of most waste products.

Even though many solutes in the body are essential for life, we continually acquire more of them than we can use. The primary solutes excreted by the urinary system are nitrogenous wastes, excess ions, and trace amounts of other substances.

Nitrogenous wastes are formed during the metabolism of proteins. The major nitrogenous waste product in urine is urea. The metabolism of protein initially liberates ammonia (NH_3). Ammonia is quite toxic to cells; however, it is quickly detoxified by the liver. In the liver, two ammonia molecules are combined with a molecule of carbon dioxide to produce a molecule of urea ($H_2N\text{-}CO\text{-}NH_2$) plus a molecule of water. Although far less toxic than ammonia, urea is also dangerous in high concentrations. A small amount of urea appears in sweat, but most of it is excreted by the urinary system.

Dozens of different ions are ingested with food or liberated from nutrients during metabolism. The most abundant ions in the body are sodium (Na^+) and chloride (Cl^-), which are important in determining the volume of the extracellular fluids, including blood. The volume of blood, in turn, affects blood pressure. Other important ions include potassium (K^+), which maintains electrical charges across membranes; calcium (Ca^{2+}), important in nerve and muscle activity; and hydrogen (H^+), which maintains acid–base balance. The rate of urinary excretion of each of these ions is regulated by the kidneys in order to maintain homeostasis.

Trace amounts of many other substances are excreted in proportion to their daily rate of gain by the body. Among them are *creatinine*, a waste product that is produced during the metabolism of creatine phosphate in muscle, and various waste products that give the urine its characteristic yellow color.

Kidneys: The Principal Urinary Organs

The main organs of the urinary system are the two kidneys. The kidneys are located on either side of the vertebral column, near the posterior body wall (**Figure D.10a**). Each kidney is a dark-reddish-brown organ about the size of your fist and shaped like a kidney bean. A *renal artery* and a *renal vein* connect each kidney to the aorta and inferior vena cava, respectively (*renal* comes from the Latin *ren*, meaning "kidney").

Seen in a longitudinal section (Figure D.10b), each kidney consists of inner pyramid-shaped zones of dense tissue (called renal pyramids) that constitute the medulla and an outer zone called the cortex. At the center of the kidney is a hollow space, the *renal pelvis*, where urine collects after it is formed.

A closer look at a section of the renal cortex and medulla reveals that it contains long, thin, tubular structures called *nephrons* (Figure D.10c). Nephrons share a common final section called the *collecting duct*, through which urine produced by the nephrons is delivered to the renal pelvis.

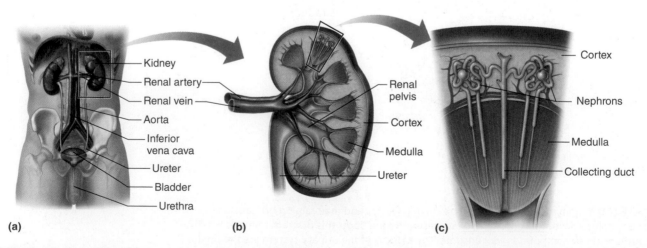

(a)   (b)   (c)

FIGURE D.10 The human urinary system (male). **(a)** Locations of the components of the urinary system within the body. **(b)** Internal structure of a kidney. **(c)** The cortex and medulla of the kidney are composed of numerous nephrons.

In addition to being the primary organs of the urinary system, the kidneys regulate the production of red blood cells in the bone marrow, through the secretion of the hormone erythropoietin, activate the inactive form of vitamin D from the liver, and help maintain blood pressure, volume, and pH.

The Integumentary System

The proper name for the skin and its accessory structures such as hair, nails, and glands is the integumentary system (from the Latin *integere*, meaning "to cover").

The skin has several different functions related to its role as the outer covering of the body: protection from dehydration (helps prevent our bodies from drying out), protection from injury (such as abrasion), defense against invasion by bacteria and viruses, regulation of body temperature, synthesis of an inactive form of vitamin D, and sensation (provides information about the external world via receptors for touch, vibration, pain, and temperature).

The outer layer of the skin's tissue is the epidermis and the inner layer of connective tissue is the dermis (**Figure D.11**).

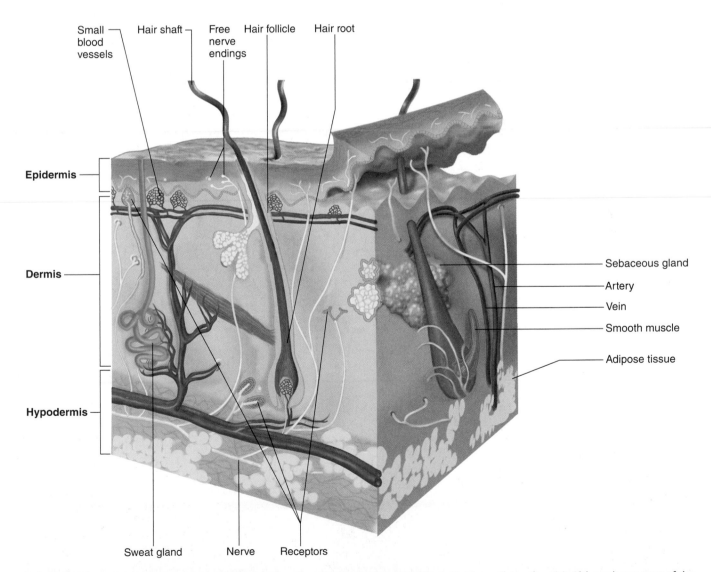

FIGURE D.11 The skin. The two layers of skin (epidermis and dermis) rest on a supportive layer (hypodermis). Although not part of the skin, the hypodermis provides the important functions of cushioning and insulation.

The skin rests on a supportive layer called the *hypodermis* (*hypo-* means "under"), consisting of loose connective tissue containing fat cells. The hypodermis is flexible enough to allow the skin to move and bend. The fat cells in the hypodermis insulate against excessive heat loss and cushion against injury.

As discussed in Chapter 11, skin synthesizes an inactive form of vitamin D. A cholesterol compound in the skin becomes an inactive form of vitamin D when it is exposed to the ultraviolet rays of sunlight. The inactive form must then be modified in the liver and kidneys before it becomes active (see Figure 11.8 on page 446).

Appendix E

Calculations and Conversions

Calculation and Conversion Aids

Commonly Used Metric Units

millimeter (mm):	one-thousandth of a meter (0.001)
centimeter (cm):	one-hundredth of a meter (0.01)
kilometer (km):	one-thousand times a meter (1,000)
kilogram (kg):	one-thousand times a gram (1,000)
milligram (mg):	one-thousandth of a gram (0.001)
microgram (µg):	one-millionth of a gram (0.000001)
milliliter (ml):	one-thousandth of a liter (0.001)

International Units

Some vitamin supplements may report vitamin content as International Units (IU).

To convert IU to

- Micrograms of vitamin D (cholecalciferol), divide the IU value by 40 or multiply by 0.025.
- Milligrams of vitamin E (alpha-tocopherol), divide the IU value by 1.5 if vitamin E is from natural sources. Divide the IU value by 2.22 if vitamin E is from synthetic sources.
- Vitamin A: 1 IU = 0.3 µg retinol or 3.6 µg beta-carotene.

Retinol Activity Equivalents

Retinol Activity Equivalents (RAE) are a standardized unit of measure for vitamin A. RAE account for the various differences in bioavailability from sources of vitamin A. Many supplements will report vitamin A content in IU, as just shown, or Retinol Equivalents (RE).

$$1 \text{ RAE} = 1 \text{ µg retinol}$$
$$12 \text{ µg beta-carotene}$$
$$24 \text{ µg other vitamin A carotenoids}$$

To calculate RAE from the RE value of vitamin carotenoids in foods, divide RE by 2.

For vitamin A supplements and foods fortified with vitamin A, 1 RE = 1 RAE.

Folate

Folate is measured as Dietary Folate Equivalents (DFE). DFE account for the different factors affecting bioavailability of folate sources.

$$1 \text{ DFE} = 1 \text{ µg food folate}$$
0.6 µg folate from fortified foods
0.5 µg folate supplement taken on an empty stomach
0.6 µg folate as a supplement consumed with a meal

To convert micrograms of synthetic folate, such as that found in supplements or fortified foods, to DFE:

$$\text{µg synthetic} \times \text{folate } 1.7 = \text{µg DFE}$$

For naturally occurring food folate, such as spinach, each microgram of folate equals 1 microgram DFE:

$$\text{µg folate} = \text{µg DFE}$$

Conversion Factors

Use the following table to convert U.S. measurements to metric equivalents:

Original Unit	Multiply By	To Get
ounces avdp	28.3495	grams
ounces	0.0625	pounds
pounds	0.4536	kilograms
pounds	16	ounces
grams	0.0353	ounces
grams	0.002205	pounds
kilograms	2.2046	pounds
liters	1.8162	pints (dry)
liters	2.1134	pints (liquid)
liters	0.9081	quarts (dry)
liters	1.0567	quarts (liquid)
liters	0.2642	gallons (U.S.)
pints (dry)	0.5506	liters
pints (liquid)	0.4732	liters
quarts (dry)	1.1012	liters
quarts (liquid)	0.9463	liters
gallons (U.S.)	3.7853	liters
millimeters	0.0394	inches
centimeters	0.3937	inches

Original Unit	Multiply By	To Get
centimeters	0.03281	feet
inches	25.4000	millimeters
inches	2.5400	centimeters
inches	0.0254	meters
feet	0.3048	meters
meters	3.2808	feet
meters	1.0936	yards
cubic feet	0.0283	cubic meters
cubic meters	35.3145	cubic feet
cubic meters	1.3079	cubic yards
cubic yards	0.7646	cubic meters

Length: U.S. and Metric Equivalents

¼ inch = 0.6 centimeter
1 inch = 2.5 centimeters
1 foot = 0.3048 meter
     30.48 centimeters
1 yard = 0.91144 meter
1 millimeter = 0.03937 inch
1 centimeter = 0.3937 inch
1 decimeter = 3.937 inches
1 meter = 39.37 inches
     1.094 yards
1 micrometer = 0.00003937 inch

Weights and Measures

Food Measurement Equivalencies from U.S. to Metric

Capacity

⅕ teaspoon = 1 milliliter
¼ teaspoon = 1.25 milliliters
½ teaspoon = 2.5 milliliters
1 teaspoon = 5 milliliters
1 tablespoon = 15 milliliters
1 fluid ounce = 28.4 milliliters
¼ cup = 60 milliliters
⅓ cup = 80 milliliters
½ cup = 120 milliliters
1 cup = 225 milliliters
1 pint (2 cups) = 473 milliliters
1 quart (4 cups) = 0.95 liter
1 liter (1.06 quarts) = 1,000 milliliters
1 gallon (4 quarts) = 3.84 liters

Weight

0.035 ounce = 1 gram
1 ounce = 28 grams
¼ pound (4 ounces) = 114 grams
1 pound (16 ounces) = 454 grams

2.2 pounds (35 ounces) = 1 kilogram

U.S. Food Measurement Equivalents

3 teaspoons = 1 tablespoon
½ tablespoon = 1½ teaspoons
2 tablespoons = ⅛ cup
4 tablespoons = ¼ cup
5 tablespoons + 1 teaspoon = ⅓ cup
8 tablespoons = ½ cup
10 tablespoons + 2 teaspoons = ⅔ cup
12 tablespoons = ¾ cup
16 tablespoons = 1 cup
2 cups = 1 pint
4 cups = 1 quart
2 pints = 1 quart
4 quarts = 1 gallon

Volumes and Capacities

1 cup = 8 fluid ounces
     ½ liquid pint
1 milliliter = 0.061 cubic inch
1 liter = 1.057 liquid quarts
     0.908 dry quart
     61.024 cubic inches
1 U.S. gallon = 231 cubic inches
     3.785 liters
     0.833 British gallon
     128 U.S. fluid ounces
1 British Imperial gallon = 277.42 cubic inches
     1.201 U.S. gallons
     4.546 liters
     160 British fluid ounces
1 U.S. ounce, liquid or fluid = 1.805 cubic inches
     29.574 milliliters
     1.041 British fluid ounces
1 pint, dry = 33.600 cubic inches
     0.551 liter
1 pint, liquid = 28.875 cubic inches
     0.473 liter
1 U.S. quart, dry = 67.201 cubic inches
     1.101 liters
1 U.S. quart, liquid = 57.75 cubic inches
     0.946 liter
1 British quart = 69.354 cubic inches
     1.032 U.S. quarts, dry
     1.201 U.S. quarts, liquid

Energy Units

1 kilocalorie (kcal) = 4.2 kilojoules
1 millijoule (MJ) = 240 kilocalories
1 kilojoule (kJ) = 0.24 kcal
1 gram carbohydrate = 4 kcal
1 gram fat = 9 kcal
1 gram protein = 4 kcal

Temperature Standards

	°Fahrenheit	°Celsius
Body temperature	98.6°	37°
Comfortable room temperature	65–75°	18–24°
Boiling point of water	212°	100°
Freezing point of water	32°	0°

Temperature Scales

To Convert Fahrenheit to Celsius:

$$[(°F - 32) \times 5]/9$$

1. Subtract 32 from °F.
2. Multiply (°F − 32) by 5; then divide by 9.

To Convert Celsius to Fahrenheit:

$$[(°C \times 9)/5] + 32$$

1. Multiply °C by 9; then divide by 5.
2. Add 32 to (°C × 9/5).

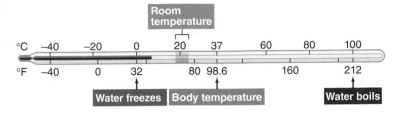

Appendix F

Foods Containing Caffeine

Source: USDA Nutrient Database for Standard Reference, Release 24, by the U.S. Department of Agriculture, Agricultural Research Service, from the Nutrient Data Laboratory Home Page, 2011.

Beverages

Food Name	Serving	Caffeine/Serving (mg)
Beverage mix, chocolate flavor, dry mix, prepared w/milk	1 cup (8 fl. oz)	7.98
Beverage mix, chocolate malt powder, fortified, prepared w/milk	1 cup (8 fl. oz)	5.3
Beverage mix, chocolate malted milk powder, no added nutrients, prepared w/milk	1 cup (8 fl. oz)	7.95
Beverage, chocolate syrup w/o added nutrients, prepared w/milk	1 cup (8 fl. oz)	5.64
Beverage, chocolate syrup, fortified, mixed w/milk	1 cup milk and 1 tbsp. syrup	2.63
Cocoa mix w/aspartame and calcium and phosphorus, no sodium or vitamin A, low kcal, dry, prepared	6 fl. oz water and 0.53 oz packet	5
Cocoa mix w/aspartame, dry, low kcal, prepared w/water	1 packet dry mix with 6 fl. oz water	1.92
Cocoa mix, dry mix	1 serving (3 heaping tsp. or 1 envelope)	5.04
Cocoa mix, dry, w/o added nutrients, prepared w/water	1 oz packet with 6 fl. oz water	4.12
Cocoa mix, fortified, dry, prepared w/water	6 fl. oz H_2O and 1 packet	6.27
Cocoa, dry powder, high-fat or breakfast, plain	1 piece	6.895
Cocoa, hot, homemade w/whole milk	1 cup	5
Coffee liqueur, 53 proof	1 fl. oz	9.048
Coffee liqueur, 63 proof	1 fl. oz	9.05
Coffee w/cream liqueur, 34 proof	1 fl. oz	2.488
Coffee mix w/sugar (cappuccino), dry, prepared w/water	6 fl. oz H_2O and 2 rounded tsp. mix	74.88
Coffee mix w/sugar (French), dry, prepared w/water	6 fl. oz H_2O and 2 rounded tsp. mix	51.03
Coffee mix w/sugar (mocha), dry, prepared w/water	6 fl. oz and 2 round tsp. mix	33.84
Coffee, brewed	1 cup (8 fl. oz)	94.8
Coffee, brewed, prepared with tap water, decaffeinated	1 cup (8 fl. oz)	2.37
Coffee, instant, prepared	1 cup (8 fl. oz)	61.98
Coffee, instant, regular, powder, half the caffeine	1 cup (8 fl. oz)	30.99
Coffee, instant, decaffeinated	1 cup (8 fl. oz)	1.79
Coffee and cocoa (mocha) powder, with whitener and low-calorie sweetener	1 cup	405.48
Coffee, brewed, espresso, restaurant-prepared	1 cup (8 fl. oz)	502.44
Coffee, brewed, espresso, restaurant-prepared, decaffeinated	1 cup (8 fl. oz)	2.37
Energy drink, with caffeine, niacin, pantothenic acid, vitamin B6	1 fl. oz	9.517
Milk beverage mix, dairy drink w/aspartame, low kcal, dry, prep	6 fl. oz	4.08
Milk, lowfat, 1% fat, chocolate	1 cup	5
Milk, whole, chocolate	1 cup	5
Soft drink, cola w/caffeine	1 fl. oz	2
Soft drink, cola, w/higher caffeine	1 fl. oz	8.33
Soft drink, cola or pepper type, low kcal w/saccharin and caffeine	1 fl. oz	3.256
Soft drink, cola, low kcal w/saccharin and aspartame, w/caffeine	1 fl. oz	4.144

Food Name	Serving	Caffeine/Serving (mg)
Soft drink, lemon-lime soda, w/caffeine	1 fl. oz	4.605
Soft drink, low kcal, not cola or pepper, with aspartame and caffeine	1 fl. oz	4.44
Soft drink, pepper type, w/caffeine	1 fl. oz	3.07
Tea mix, instant w/lemon flavor, w/saccharin, dry, prepared	1 cup (8 fl. oz)	16.59
Tea mix, instant w/lemon, unsweetened, dry, prepared	1 cup (8 fl. oz)	26.18
Tea mix, instant w/sugar and lemon, dry, no added vitamin C, prepared	1 cup (8 fl. oz)	28.49
Tea mix, instant, unsweetened, dry, prepared	1 cup (8 fl. oz)	30.81
Tea, brewed	1 cup (8 fl. oz)	47.36
Tea, brewed, prepared with tap water, decaffeinated	1 cup (8 fl. oz)	2.37
Tea, instant, unsweetened, powder, decaffeinated	1 tsp.	1.183
Tea, instant, w/o sugar, lemon-flavored, w/added vitamin C, dry prepared	1 cup (8 fl. oz)	26.05
Tea, instant, with sugar, lemon-flavored, decaffeinated, no added vitamin	1 cup	9.1

Cake, Cookies, and Desserts

Food Name	Serving	Caffeine/Serving (mg)
Brownie, square, large (2-3/4" × 7/8")	1 piece	1.12
Cake, chocolate pudding, dry mix	1 oz	1.701
Cake, chocolate, dry mix, regular	1 oz	3.118
Cake, German chocolate pudding, dry mix	1 oz	1.985
Cake, marble pudding, dry mix	1 oz	1.985
Candies, chocolate-covered, caramel with nuts	1 cup	35.34
Candies, chocolate-covered, dietetic or low-calorie	1 cup	16.74
Candy, milk chocolate w/almonds	1 bar (1.45 oz)	9.02
Candy, milk chocolate w/rice cereal	1 bar (1.4 oz)	9.2
Candy, raisins, milk-chocolate-coated	1 cup	45
Chocolate chips, semisweet, mini	1 cup chips (6 oz package)	107.12
Chocolate, baking, unsweetened, square	1 piece	22.72
Chocolate, baking, Mexican, square	1 piece	2.8
Chocolate, sweet	1 oz	18.711
Cookie Cake, Snackwell Fat Free Devil's Food, Nabisco	1 serving	1.28
Cookie, Snackwell Caramel Delights, Nabisco	1 serving	1.44
Cookie, chocolate chip, enriched, commercially prepared	1 oz	3.118
Cookie, chocolate chip, homemade w/margarine	1 oz	4.536
Cookie, chocolate chip, lower-fat, commercially prepared	3 pieces	2.1
Cookie, chocolate chip, refrigerated dough	1 portion, dough spooned from roll	2.61
Cookie, chocolate chip, soft, commercially prepared	1 oz	1.985
Cookie, chocolate wafers	1 cup, crumbs	7.84
Cookie, graham crackers, chocolate-coated	1 oz	13.041
Cookie, sandwich, chocolate, cream-filled	3 pieces	3.9
Cookie, sandwich, chocolate, cream-filled, special dietary	1 oz	0.85
Cupcake, chocolate w/frosting, low-fat	1 oz	0.86
Doughnut, cake, chocolate w/sugar or glaze	1 oz	0.284
Doughnut, cake, plain w/chocolate icing, large (3-1/2")	1 each	1.14
Fast food, ice cream sundae, hot fudge	1 sundae	1.58
Fast food, milk beverage, chocolate shake	1 cup (8 fl. oz)	1.66
Frosting, chocolate, creamy, ready-to-eat	2 tbsp. creamy	0.82
Frozen yogurt, chocolate	1 cup	5.58
Fudge, chocolate w/nuts, homemade	1 oz	1.984
Granola bar, soft, milk-chocolate-coated, peanut butter	1 oz	0.85
Granola bar, w/coconut, chocolate-coated	1 cup	5.58

Food Name	Serving	Caffeine/Serving (mg)
Ice cream, chocolate	1 individual (3.5 fl. oz)	1.74
Ice cream, chocolate, light	1 oz	0.85
Ice cream, chocolate, rich	1 cup	5.92
M&M's Peanut Chocolate	1 cup	18.7
M&M's Plain Chocolate	1 cup	22.88
Milk chocolate	1 cup chips	33.6
Milk-chocolate-coated coffee beans	1 NLEA serving	48
Milk dessert, frozen, fat-free milk, chocolate	1 oz	0.85
Milk shake, thick, chocolate	1 fl. oz	0.568
Pastry, éclair/cream puff, homemade, custard-filled w/chocolate	1 oz	0.567
Pie crust, chocolate-wafer-cookie-type, chilled	1 crust, single 9"	11.15
Pie, chocolate mousse, no bake mix	1 oz	0.284
Pudding, chocolate, instant dry mix prepared w/reduced-fat (2%) milk	1 oz	0.283
Pudding, chocolate, regular dry mix prepared w/reduced-fat (2%) milk	1 oz	0.567
Pudding, chocolate, ready-to-eat, fat-free	4 oz can	2.27
Syrups, chocolate, genuine chocolate flavor, light, Hershey	2 tbsp.	1.05
Topping, chocolate-flavored hazelnut spread	1 oz	1.984
Yogurt, chocolate, nonfat milk	1 oz	0.567
Yogurt, frozen, chocolate, soft serve	0.5 cup (4 fl. oz)	2.16

Appendix G

U.S. Exchange Lists for Meal Planning

Data adapted from "Choose Your Foods: Exchange Lists For Diabetes." Copyright © 2008 by the American Diabetes Association and the American Dietetic Association.

Starch List

1 starch choice = 15 g carbohydrate, 0–3 g protein, 0–1 g fat, and 80 cal

Icon Key

☺ = More than 3 g of dietary fiber per serving.

! = Extra fat, or prepared with added fat. (Count as 1 starch + 1 fat.)

▮ = 480 mg or more of sodium per serving.

Food	Serving Size	Food	Serving Size
Bread		☺ Bulgur (cooked)	½ c
Bagel, 4 oz	¼ (1 oz)	Cereals	½ c
! Biscuit, 2½" across	1	☺ bran	½ c
Bread		cooked (oats, oatmeal)	½ c
☺ reduced-calorie	2 slices (1½ oz)	puffed	1½ c
white, whole-grain, pumpernickel, rye,		shredded wheat, plain	½ c
unfrosted raisin	1 slice (1 oz)	sugar-coated	½ c
Chapatti, small, 6" across	1	unsweetened, ready-to-eat	¾ c
! Cornbread, 1¾" cube	1 (1½ oz)	Couscous	⅓ c
English muffin	½	Granola	
Hot dog bun or hamburger bun	½ (1 oz)	low-fat	¼ c
Naan, 8" by 2"	¼	! regular	¼ c
Pancake, 4" across, ¼" thick	1	Grits, cooked	½ c
Pita, 6" across	½	Kasha	½ c
Roll, plain small	1 (1 oz)	Millet, cooked	⅓ c
! Stuffing, bread	⅓ cup	Muesli	¼ c
! Taco shell, 5" across	2	Pasta, cooked	⅓ c
Tortilla		Polenta, cooked	⅓ c
Corn, 6" across	1	Quinoa, cooked	⅓ c
Flour, 6" across	1	Rice, white or brown, cooked	⅓ c
Flour, 10" across	⅓ tortilla	Tabbouleh (tabouli), prepared	½ c
! Waffle, 4"-square or 4" across	1	Wheat germ, dry	3 tbs
		Wild rice, cooked	½ c
Cereals and Grains		**Starchy Vegetables**	
Barley, cooked	⅓ cup	Cassava	⅓ c
Bran, dry		Corn	½ c
☺ oat	¼ c	on cob, large	½ cob (5 oz)
☺ wheat	½ c		

Food	Serving Size	Food	Serving Size
☺ Hominy, canned	¾ c	Graham crackers, 2½" square	3
☺ Mixed vegetables with corn, peas, or pasta	1 c	Matzoh	¾ oz
☺ Parsnips	½ c	Melba toast, about 2" by 4" piece	4 pieces
☺ Peas, green	½ c	Oyster crackers	20
Plantain, ripe	⅓ c	Crackers and Snacks	
Potato		Popcorn	3 c
baked with skin	¼ large (3 oz)	! ☺ with butter	3 c
boiled, all kinds	½ c or ½ medium (3 oz)	☺ no fat added	3 c
! mashed, with milk and fat	½ c	☺ lower fat	3 c
French fried (oven-baked)	1 cup (2 oz)	Pretzels	¾ oz
☺ Pumpkin, canned, no sugar added	1 c	Rice cakes, 4" across	2
Spaghetti/pasta sauce	½ c	Snack chips	
☺ Squash, winter (acorn, butternut)	1 c	fat-free or baked (tortilla, potato),	
☺ Succotash	½ c	baked pita chips	15–20 (¾ oz)
Yam, sweet potato, plain	½ c	! regular (tortilla, potato)	9–13 (¾ oz)

Crackers and Snacks

Food	Serving Size
Animal crackers	8
Crackers	
! round-butter type	6
saltine-type	6
! sandwich-style, cheese or peanut	
butter filling	3
! whole-wheat regular	2–5 (¾ oz)
! whole-wheat lower fat or crispbreads	2–5 (¾ oz)

Beans, Peas, and Lentils

(Count as 1 starch + 1 lean meat)

Food	Serving Size
☺ Baked beans	⅓ c
☺ Beans, cooked (black, garbanzo, kidney, lima, navy, pinto, white)	½ c
☺ Lentils, cooked (brown, green, yellow)	½ c
☺ Peas, cooked (black-eyed, split)	½ c
▮ ☺ Refried beans, canned	½ c

Fruit List

1 fruit choice = 15 g carbohydrate, 0 g protein, 0 g fat, and 60 cal
Weight includes skin, core, seeds, and rind.

Icon Key

☺ = More than 3 g of dietary fiber per serving.

! = Extra fat, or prepared with added fat.

▮ = 480 mg or more of sodium per serving.

Food	Serving Size	Food	Serving Size
Apples		Dried fruits (blueberries, cherries,	
unpeeled, small	1 (4 oz)	cranberries, mixed fruit, raisins)	2 tbs
dried	4 rings	Figs	
Applesauce, unsweetened	½ c	dried	1½
Apricots		☺ fresh	1½ large or 2 medium (3½ oz)
canned	½ c	Fruit cocktail	½ c
dried	8 halves	Grapefruit	
▮ fresh	4 whole (5½ oz)	large	½ (11 oz)
Banana, extra small	1 (4 oz)	sections, canned	¾ c
Blackberries	¾ c	Grapes, small	17 (3 oz)
▮ Blueberries	¾ c	Honeydew melon	1 slice or 1 c cubed (10 oz)
Cantaloupe, small	⅓ melon or 1 c cubed (11 oz)	☺ Kiwi	1 (3½ oz)
Cherries		Mandarin oranges, canned	¾ c
sweet, canned	½ c	Mango, small	½ fruit (5½ oz) or ½ c
sweet, fresh	12 (3 oz)	Nectarine, small	1 (5 oz)
Dates	3	☺ Orange, small	1 (6½ oz)

Food	Serving Size	Food	Serving Size
Papaya	½ fruit or 1 c cubed (8 oz)	☺ Raspberries	1 c
Peaches		☺ Strawberries	1¼ c whole berries
canned	½ c	☺ Tangerines, small	2 (8 oz)
fresh, medium	1 (6 oz)	Watermelon	1 slice or 1¼ c cubes (13½ oz)
Pears			
canned	½ c		
fresh, large	½ (4 oz)		
Pineapple			
canned	½ c		
fresh	¾ c		
Plums			
canned	½ c		
dried (prunes)	3		
small	2 (5 oz)		

Fruit Juice

Food	Serving Size
Apple juice/cider	½ c
Fruit juice blends, 100% juice	⅓ c
Grape juice	⅓ c
Grapefruit juice	½ c
Orange juice	½ c
Pineapple juice	½ c
Prune juice	⅓ c

Milk and Yogurts

1 milk choice = 12 g carbohydrate and 8 g protein

Food	Serving Size	Count As
Fat-Free or Low-Fat (1%)		
(0–3 g fat per serving, 100 calories per serving)		
Milk, buttermilk, acidophilus milk, Lactaid	1 c	1 fat-free milk
Evaporated milk	½ c	1 fat-free milk
Yogurt, plain or flavored with an artificial sweetener	⅔ c (6 oz)	1 fat-free milk
Reduced-Fat (2%)		
(5 g fat per serving, 120 calories per serving)		
Milk, acidophilus milk, kefir, Lactaid	1 c	1 reduced-fat milk
Yogurt, plain	⅔ c (6 oz)	1 reduced-fat milk
Whole		
(8 g fat per serving, 160 calories per serving)		
Milk, buttermilk, goat's milk	1 c	1 whole milk
Evaporated milk	½ c	1 whole milk
Yogurt, plain	8 oz	1 whole milk
Dairy-Like Foods		
Chocolate milk		
fat-free	1 c	1 fat-free milk + 1 carbohydrate
whole	1 c	1 whole milk + 1 carbohydrate
Eggnog, whole milk	½ c	1 carbohydrate + 2 fats
Rice drink		
flavored, low-fat	1 c	2 carbohydrates
plain, fat-free	1 c	1 carbohydrate
Smoothies, flavored, regular	10 oz	1 fat-free milk + 2½ carbohydrates
Soy milk		
light	1 c	1 carbohydrate + ½ fat
regular, plain	1 c	1 carbohydrate + 1 fat
Yogurt		
and juice blends	1 c	1 fat-free milk + 1 carbohydrate
low carbohydrate (less than 6 g carbohydrate per choice)	⅔ c (6 oz)	½ fat-free milk
with fruit, low-fat	⅔ c (6 oz)	1 fat-free milk + 1 carbohydrate

Sweets, Desserts, and Other Carbohydrates List

1 other carbohydrate choice = 15 g carbohydrate and variable protein, fat, and calories.

Icon Key

▮ = 480 mg or more of sodium per serving.

Food	Serving Size	Count As
Beverages, Soda, and Energy/Sports Drinks		
Cranberry juice cocktail	½ c	1 carbohydrate
Energy drink	1 can (8.3 oz)	2 carbohydrates
Fruit drink or lemonade	1 c (8 oz)	2 carbohydrates
Hot chocolate		
regular	1 envelope added to 8 oz water	1 carbohydrate + 1 fat
sugar-free or light	1 envelope added to 8 oz water	1 carbohydrate
Soft drink (soda), regular	1 can (12 oz)	2½ carbohydrates
Sports drink	1 cup (8 oz)	1 carbohydrate
Brownies, Cake, Cookies, Gelatin, Pie, and Pudding		
Brownie, small, unfrosted	1¼" square, ⅞", high (about 1 oz)	1 carbohydrate + 1 fat
Cake		
angel food, unfrosted	1½ of cake (about 2 oz)	2 carbohydrates
frosted	2" square (about 2 oz)	2 carbohydrates + 1 fat
unfrosted	2" square (about 2 oz)	1 carbohydrate + 1 fat
Cookies		
chocolate chip	2 cookies (2¼" across)	1 carbohydrate + 2 fats
gingersnap	3 cookies	1 carbohydrate
sandwich, with creme filling	2 small (about ⅔ oz)	1 carbohydrate + 1 fat
sugar-free	3 small or 1 large (¾ oz–1 oz)	1 carbohydrate + 1–2 fats
vanilla wafer	5 cookies	1 carbohydrate + 1 fat
Cupcake, frosted	1 small (about 1¾ oz)	2 carbohydrates + 1–1½ fats
Fruit cobbler	½ c (3½ oz)	3 carbohydrates + 1 fat
Gelatin, regular	½ c	1 carbohydrate
Pie		
commercially prepared fruit, 2 crusts	⅙ of 8" pie	3 carbohydrates + 2 fats
pumpkin or custard	⅙ of 8" pie	1½ carbohydrates + 1½ fats
Pudding		
regular (made with reduced-fat milk)	½ c	2 carbohydrates
sugar-free, or sugar-free and fat-free (made with fat-free milk)	½ c	1 carbohydrate
Candy, Spreads, Sweets, Sweeteners, Syrups, and Toppings		
Candy bar, chocolate/peanut	2 "fun size" bars (1 oz)	1½ carbohydrates + 1½ fats
Candy, hard	3 pieces	1 carbohydrate
Chocolate "kisses"	5 pieces	1 carbohydrate + 1 fat
Coffee creamer		
dry, flavored	4 tsp	½ carbohydrate + ½ fat
liquid, flavored	2 tbsp	1 carbohydrate
Fruit snacks, chewy (pureed fruit concentrate)	1 roll (¾ oz)	1 carbohydrate
Fruit spreads, 100% fruit	1½ tbs	1 carbohydrate
Honey	1 tbsp	1 carbohydrate

Food	Serving Size	Count As
Jam or jelly, regular	1 tbs	1 carbohydrate
Sugar	1 tbs	1 carbohydrate
Syrup		
chocolate	2 tbs	2 carbohydrates
light (pancake type)	2 tbs	1 carbohydrate
regular (pancake type)	1 tbs	1 carbohydrate

Condiments and Sauces

Food	Serving Size	Count As
Barbeque sauce	3 tbs	1 carbohydrate
Cranberry sauce, jellied	¼ c	1½ carbohydrates
Gravy, canned or bottled	½ c	½ carbohydrate + ½ fat
Salad dressing, fat-free, low-fat, cream-based	3 tbs	1 carbohydrate
Sweet and sour sauce	3 tbs	1 carbohydrate

Doughnuts, Muffins, Pastries, and Sweet Breads

Food	Serving Size	Count As
Banana nut bread	1" slice (1 oz)	2 carbohydrates + 1 fat
Doughnut		
cake, plain	1 medium, (1½ oz)	1½ carbohydrates + 2 fats
yeast type, glazed	3¾" across (2 oz)	2 carbohydrates + 2 fats
Muffin (4 oz)	¼ muffin (1 oz)	1 carbohydrate + ½ fat
Sweet roll or Danish	1 (2½ oz)	2½ carbohydrates + 2 fats

Frozen Bars, Frozen Dessert, Frozen Yogurt, and Ice Cream

Food	Serving Size	Count As
Frozen pops	1	½ carbohydrate
Fruit juice bars, frozen, 100% juice	1 bar (3 oz)	1 carbohydrate
Ice cream		
fat-free	½ c	1½ carbohydrates
light	½ c	1 carbohydrate + 1 fat
no sugar added	½ c	1 carbohydrate + 1 fat
regular	½ c	1 carbohydrate + 2 fats
Sherbet, sorbet	½ c	2 carbohydrates
Yogurt, frozen		
fat-free	⅓ c	1 carbohydrate
regular	½ c	1 carbohydrate + 0–1 fat

Granola Bars, Meal Replacement Bars/Shakes, and Trail Mix

Food	Serving Size	Count As
Granola or snack bar, regular or low-fat	1 bar (1 oz)	1½ carbohydrates
Meal replacement bar	1 bar (1⅓ oz)	1½ carbohydrates + 0–1 fat
Meal replacement bar	1 bar (2 oz)	2 carbohydrates + 1 fat
Meal replacement shake, reduced-calorie	1 can (10–11 oz)	1½ carbohydrates + 0–1 fat
Trail mix		
candy/nut-based	1 oz	1 carbohydrates + 2 fats
dried-fruit-based	1 oz	1 carbohydrate + 1 fat

Nonstarchy Vegetable List

1 vegetable choice = 5 g carbohydrate, 2 g protein, 0 g fat, 25 cal

Icon Key

☺ = More than 3 g of dietary fiber per serving.

▮ = 480 mg or more of sodium per serving.

Amaranth or Chinese spinach
Artichoke
Artichoke hearts
Asparagus
Baby corn
Bamboo shoots
Beans (green, wax, Italian)
Bean sprouts
Beets
▮ Borscht
Broccoli
☺ Brussels sprouts
Cabbage (green, bok choy, Chinese)
Carrots
Cauliflower
Celery
☺ Chayote
Coleslaw, packaged, no dressing
Cucumber
Eggplant
Gourds (bitter, bottle, luffa, bitter melon)
Green onions or scallions
Greens (collard, kale, mustard, turnip)
Hearts of palm
Jicama

Kohlrabi
Leeks
Mixed vegetables (without corn, peas, or pasta)
Mung bean sprouts
Mushrooms, all kinds, fresh
Okra
Onions
Oriental radish or daikon
Pea pods
☺ Peppers (all varieties)
Radishes
Rutabaga
▮ Sauerkraut
Soybean sprouts
Spinach
Squash (summer, crookneck, zucchini)
Sugar pea snaps
▮ Swiss chard
Tomato
Tomatoes, canned
▮ Tomato sauce
▮ Tomato/vegetable juice
Turnips
Water chestnuts
Yard-long beans

Meat and Meat Substitutes List

Icon Key

▮ = Extra fat, or prepared with added fat. (Add an additional fat choice to this food.)

▮ = 480 mg or more of sodium per serving (based on the sodium content of a typical 3 oz serving of meat, unless 1 or 2 is the normal serving size).

Food	Amount	Food	Amount
Lean Meats and Meat Substitutes		*Fish, fresh or frozen, plain:* catfish, cod, flounder,	
(1 lean meat choice = 7 g protein, 0–3 g fat,		haddock, halibut, orange roughy, salmon,	
45 calories)		tilapia, trout, tuna	1 oz
Beef: Select or Choice grades trimmed of fat:		▮ *Fish, smoked:* herring or salmon (lox)	1 oz
ground round, roast (chuck, rib, rump),		*Game:* buffalo, ostrich, rabbit, venison	1 oz
round, sirloin, steak (cubed, flank,		▮ Hot dog with 3 g of fat or less per oz (8 dogs	
porterhouse, T-bone), tenderloin	1 oz	per 14 oz package) *(Note: May be high in*	
▮ Beef jerky	1 oz	*carbohydrate.)*	1
Cheeses with 3 g of fat or less per oz	1 oz	*Lamb:* chop, leg, or roast	1 oz
Cottage cheese	¼ cup	*Organ meats:* heart, kidney, liver *(Note: May*	
Egg substitutes, plain	¼ cup	*be high in cholesterol)*	1 oz
Egg whites	2		

Food	Amount
Oysters, fresh or frozen . . . . .6 medium	
Pork, lean	
ꜰ Canadian bacon . . . . .1 oz	
rib or loin chop/roast, ham, tenderloin . . . . . .1 oz	
Poultry without skin: Cornish hen, chicken,	
domestic duck or goose (well drained	
of fat), turkey . . . . .1 oz	
Processed sandwich meats with 3 g of	
fat or less per oz: chipped beef, deli	
thin-sliced meats, turkey ham, turkey	
kielbasa, turkey pastrami .1 oz	
Salmon, canned . . . . .1 oz	
Sardines, canned . . . . .2 medium	
ꜰ Sausage with 3 g or less fat per oz . . . . .1 oz	
Shellfish: clams, crab, imitation shellfish,	
lobster, scallops, shrimp . . . . .1 oz	
Tuna, canned in water or oil, drained . . . . .1 oz	
Veal: Lean chop, roast . . . . .1 oz	

Medium-Fat Meat and Meat Substitutes

(1 medium-fat meat choice = 7 g protein, 4–7 g fat, and 75 calories)

Food	Amount
Beef: corned beef, ground beef, meatloaf,	
Prime grades trimmed of fat (prime rib),	
short ribs, tongue . . . . .1 oz	
Cheeses with 4–7 g of fat per oz: feta,	
mozzarella, pasteurized processed	
cheese spread, reduced-fat	
cheeses, string . . . . .1 oz	
Egg (*Note: High in cholesterol, limit*	
to 3 per week.) 1	
Fish, any fried product . . . . .1 oz	
Lamb: ground, rib roast . . . . .1 oz	

Food	Amount
Pork: cutlet, shoulder roast .1 oz	
Poultry: chicken with skin; dove, pheasant,	
wild duck, or goose; fried chicken;	
ground turkey . . . . .1 oz	
Ricotta cheese . . . . .2 oz or ¼ c	
ꜰ Sausage with 4–7 g fat per oz . . . . .1 oz	
Veal: Cutlet (no breading) . . . . .1 oz	

High-Fat Meat and Meat Substitutes[a]

(1 high-fat meat choice = 7 g protein, 8 + g fat, 100 calories)

Food	Amount
Bacon	
ꜰ pork . . . . .2 slices (16 slices per lb or 1 oz each, before cooking)	
ꜰ turkey . . . . .3 slices (½ oz each before cooking)	
Cheese, regular: American, bleu, brie, cheddar,	
hard goat, Monterey Jack, queso, Swiss . . . .1 oz	
ꜰ! *Hot dog:* beef, pork, or combination	
(10 per lb-sized package) 1	
ꜰ *Hot dog:* turkey or chicken (10 per lb-sized	
package) 1	
Pork: ground, sausage, spareribs . . . . .1 oz	
Processed sandwich meats with 8 g of fat or	
more per oz: bologna, pastrami,	
hard salami . . . . .1 oz	
ꜰ *Sausage with 8 g of fat or more per oz:*	
bratwurst, chorizo, Italian, knockwurst,	
Polish, smoked, summer . . . . .1 oz	

[a] These foods are high in saturated fat, cholesterol, and calories and may raise blood cholesterol levels if eaten on a regular basis. Try to eat 3 or fewer servings from this group per week.

Plant-Based Proteins

Because carbohydrate and fat content varies among plant-based proteins, you should read the food label.

Icon Key

☺ = More than 3 g of dietary fiber per serving; 7g protein; calories vary.

ꜰ = 480 mg or more of sodium per serving (based on the sodium content of a typical 3-oz serving of meat, unless 1 or 2 oz is the normal serving size).

	Food	Amount	Count As
	"Bacon" strips, soy-based	3 strips	1 medium-fat meat
☺	Baked beans	⅓ c	1 starch + 1 lean meat
☺	*Beans, cooked:* black, garbanzo, kidney, lima, navy, pinto, white	½ c	1 starch + 1 lean meat
☺	"Beef" or "sausage" crumbles, soy-based	2 oz	½ carbohydrate + 1 lean meat
	"Chicken" nuggets, soy-based	2 nuggets (1½ oz)	½ carbohydrate + 1 medium-fat meat
☺	Edamame	½ c	½ carbohydrate + 1 lean meat
	Falafel (spiced chickpea and wheat patties)	3 patties (about 2 inches across)	1 carbohydrate + 1 high-fat meat
	Hot dog, soy-based	1 (1½ oz)	½ carbohydrate + 1 lean meat

Food	Amount	Count As
☺ Hummus	⅓ c	1 carbohydrate + 1 high-fat meat
☺ Lentils, brown, green, or yellow	½ c	1 carbohydrate + 1 lean meat
☺ Meatless burger, soy-based	3 oz	½ carbohydrate + 2 lean meats
☺ Meatless burger, vegetable- and starch-based	1 patty (about 2½ oz)	1 carbohydrate + 2 lean meats
Nut spreads: almond butter, cashew butter, peanut butter, soy nut butter	1 tbs	1 high-fat meat
☺ *Peas, cooked:* black-eyed and split peas	½ c	1 starch + 1 lean meat
▮☺ Refried beans, canned	½ c	1 starch + 1 lean meat
"Sausage" patties, soy-based	1 (1½ oz)	1 medium-fat meat
Soy nuts, unsalted	¾ oz	½ carbohydrate + 1 medium-fat meat
Tempeh	¼ cup	1 medium-fat meat
Tofu 4 oz (½ cup)		1 medium-fat meat
Tofu, light	4 oz (½ cup)	1 lean meat

Fat List

1 fat choice = 5 g fat, 45 cal

Icon Key

▮ = 480 mg or more of sodium per serving.

Food	Serving Size	Food	Serving Size

Unsaturated Fats—Monounsaturated Fats

Avocado, medium ... 2 tbs (1 oz)

Nut butters (*trans* fat-free): almond butter, cashew butter, peanut butter (smooth or crunchy) .1½ tsp

Nuts
- almonds ... .6 nuts
- Brazil ... .2 nuts
- cashews ... .6 nuts
- filberts (hazelnuts) ... .5 nuts
- macadamia ... .3 nuts
- mixed (50% peanuts) ... .6 nuts
- peanuts ... .10 nuts
- pecans ... .4 halves
- pistachios ... .16 nuts

Oil: canola, olive, peanut ... 1 tsp

Olives
- black (ripe) ... .8 large
- green, stuffed ... .10 large

Polyunsaturated Fats

Margarine: lower-fat spread (30% to 50% vegetable oil, *trans* fat-free) ... 1 tbs

Margarine: stick, tub (*trans* fat-free), or squeeze (*trans* fat-free) ... 1 tsp

Mayonnaise
- reduced-fat ... 1 tbs
- regular ... 1 tsp

Mayonnaise-style salad dressing
- reduced-fat ... 1 tbs
- regular ... 2 tsp

Nuts
- Pignolia (pine nuts) ... 1 tbs
- walnuts, English ... 4 halves

Oil: corn, cottonseed, flaxseed, grape seed, safflower, soybean, sunflower ... 1 tsp

Oil: made from soybean and canola oil—Enova ... 1 tsp

Plant stanol esters
- light ... 1 tbs
- regular ... 2 tsp

Salad dressing
- ▮ reduced-fat (*Note: May be high in carbohydrate.*) ... 2 tbs
- ▮ regular ... 1 tbs

Seeds ... 1 tbs
- flaxseed, whole ... 1 tbs
- pumpkin, sunflower ... 1 tbs
- sesame seeds ... 1 tbs

Tahini or sesame paste ... 2 tsp

Saturated Fats

Bacon, cooked, regular or turkey ... 1 slice

Butter
- reduced-fat ... 1 tbs
- stick ... 1 tsp
- whipped ... 2 tsp

Food	Serving Size	Food	Serving Size
Butter blends made with oil		whipped	2 tbs
reduced-fat or light	1 tbs	whipped, pressurized	¼ c
regular	1½ tsp	Cream cheese	
Chitterlings, boiled	2 tbs (½ oz)	reduced-fat	1½ tbs (¾ oz)
Coconut, sweetened, shredded	2 tbs	regular	1 tbs (½ oz)
Coconut milk		Lard	1 tsp
light	¼ c	*Oil:* coconut, palm, palm kernel	1 tsp
regular	1½ tbs	Salt pork	¼ oz
Cream		Shortening, solid	1 tsp
half and half	2 tbs	Sour cream	
heavy	1 tbs	reduced-fat or light	3 tbs
light	1½ tbs	regular	2 tbs

Free Foods List

A *free food* is any food or drink that has less than 20 calories and 5 g or less of carbohydrate per serving. Foods with a serving size listed should be limited to three servings per day. Foods listed without a serving size can be eaten as often as you like.

Icon Key

▮ = 480 mg or more of sodium per serving.

Food	Serving Size	Food	Serving Size
Low Carbohydrate Foods		Salad dressing	
Cabbage, raw	½ c	fat-free or low-fat	1 tbs
Candy, hard (regular or sugar-free)	1 piece	fat-free, Italian	2 tbs
Carrots, cauliflower, or green beans, cooked	¼ c	Sour cream, fat-free, reduced-fat	1 tbs
Cranberries, sweetened with sugar substitute	½ c	Whipped topping	
Cucumber, sliced	½ c	light or fat-free	2 tbs
Gelatin		regular	1 tbs
dessert, sugar-free			
unflavored		**Condiments**	
Gum		Barbecue sauce	2 tsp
Jam or jelly, light or no sugar added	2 tsp	Catsup (ketchup)	1 tbs
Rhubarb, sweetened with sugar substitute	½ c	Honey mustard	1 tbs
Salad greens		Horseradish	
Sugar substitutes (artificial sweeteners)		Lemon juice	
Syrup, sugar-free	2 tbs	Miso	1½ tsp
		Mustard	
Modified Fat Foods with Carbohydrate		Parmesan cheese, freshly grated	1 tbs
Cream cheese, fat-free	1 tbs (½ oz)	Pickle relish	1 tbs
Creamers		Pickles	
nondairy, liquid	1 tbs	▮ dill	1½ medium
nondairy, powdered	2 tsp	sweet, bread and butter	2 slices
Margarine spread		sweet, gherkin	¾ oz
fat-free	1 tbs	Salsa	¼ c
reduced-fat	1 tsp	▮ Soy sauce, regular or light	1 tbs
Mayonnaise		Sweet and sour sauce	2 tsp
fat-free	1 tbs	Sweet chili sauce	2 tsp
reduced-fat	1 tsp	Taco sauce	1 tbs
Mayonnaise-style salad dressing		Vinegar	
fat-free	1 tbs	Yogurt, any type	2 tbs
reduced-fat	1 tsp		

Drinks/Mixes

Any food on this list—without serving size listed—can be consumed in any moderate amount.

Icon Key

❙ = 480 mg or more of sodium per serving.

❙Bouillon, broth, consommé	Diet soft drinks, sugar-free
Bouillon or broth, low sodium	Drink mixes, sugar-free
Carbonated or mineral water	Tea, unsweetened or with sugar substitute
Club soda	Tonic water, diet
Cocoa powder, unsweetened (1 tbs)	Water
Coffee, unsweetened or with sugar substitute	Water, flavored, carbohydrate free

Seasonings

Any food on this list can be consumed in any moderate amount.

Flavoring extracts (for example, vanilla, almond, peppermint)	Spices
Garlic	Hot pepper sauce
Herbs, fresh or dried	Wine, used in cooking
Nonstick cooking spray	Worcestershire sauce
Pimento	

Combination Foods List

Icon Key

☺ = More than 3 g of dietary fiber per serving.

❙ = 600 mg or more of sodium per serving (for combination food main dishes/meals).

Food	Serving Size	Count As
Entrées		
❙Casserole type (tuna noodle, lasagna, spaghetti with meatballs, chili with beans, macaroni and cheese)	1 c (8 oz)	2 carbohydrates + 2 medium-fat meats
❙Stews (beef/other meats and vegetables)	1 c (8 oz)	1 carbohydrate + 1 medium-fat meat + 0–3 fats
Tuna salad or chicken salad	½ c (3½ oz)	½ carbohydrate + 2 lean meats + 1 fat
Frozen Meals/Entrées		
❙☺Burrito (beef and bean)	1 (5 oz)	3 carbohydrates + 1 lean meat + 2 fats
❙Dinner-type meal	generally 14–17 oz	3 carbohydrates + 3 medium-fat meats + 3 fats
❙Entrée or meal with less than 340 calories	about 8–11 oz	2–3 carbohydrates + 1–2 lean meats
Pizza		
❙cheese/vegetarian thin crust	¼ of 12" (4½ to 5 oz)	2 carbohydrates + 2 medium-fat meats
❙meat topping, thin crust	¼ of 12" (5 oz)	2 carbohydrates + 2 medium-fat meats, + 1½ fats
❙Pocket sandwich	1 (4½ oz)	3 carbohydrates + 1 lean meat + 1–2 fats
❙Pot pie	1 (7 oz)	2½ carbohydrates + 1 medium-fat meat + 3 fats
Salads (Deli-Style)		
Coleslaw	½ c	1 carbohydrate + 1½ fats
Macaroni/pasta salad	½ c	2 carbohydrates + 3 fats
❙Potato salad	½ c	1½ carbohydrates + 1–2 fats
Soups		
❙Bean, lentil, or split pea	1 cup	1 carbohydrate + 1 lean meat

Food	Serving Size	Count As
▮ Chowder (made with milk)	1 c (8 oz)	1 carbohydrate + 1 lean meat + 1½ fats
▮ Cream (made with water)	1 c (8 oz)	1 carbohydrate + 1 fat
▮ Instant	.6 oz prepared	1 carbohydrate
▮ with beans or lentils	.8 oz prepared	2½ carbohydrates + 1 lean meat
▮ Miso soup	1 c	½ carbohydrate + 1 fat
▮ Oriental noodle	1 c	2 carbohydrates + 2 fats
Rice (congee)	1 c	1 carbohydrate
▮ Tomato (made with water)	1 c (8 oz)	1 carbohydrate
▮ Vegetable beef, chicken noodle, or other broth-type	1 c (8 oz)	1 carbohydrate

Fast Foods List[a]

Icon Key
☺ = More than 3 g of dietary fiber per serving.
▮ = Extra fat, or prepared with added fat.
▮ = 600 mg or more sodium per serving (for fast food main dishes/meals).

Food	Serving Size	Exchanges per Serving
Breakfast Sandwiches		
▮ Egg, cheese, meat, English muffin	1 sandwich	2 carbohydrates + 2 medium-fat meats
▮ Sausage biscuit sandwich	1 sandwich	2 carbohydrates + 2 high-fat meats + 3½ fats
Main Dishes/Entrees		
▮☺ Burrito (beef and beans)	1 (about 8 oz)	3 carbohydrates + 3 medium-fat meats + 3 fats
▮ Chicken breast, breaded and fried	1 (about 5 oz)	1 carbohydrate + 4 medium-fat meats
Chicken drumstick, breaded and fried	1 (about 2 oz)	2 medium-fat meats
▮ Chicken nuggets	6 (about 3½ oz)	1 carbohydrate + 2 medium-fat meats + 1 fat
▮ Chicken thigh, breaded and fried	1 (about 4 oz)	½ carbohydrate + 3 medium-fat meats + 1½ fats
▮ Chicken wings, hot	6 (5 oz)	5 medium-fat meats + 1½ fats
Oriental		
▮ Beef/chicken/shrimp with vegetables in sauce	1 c (about 5 oz)	1 carbohydrate + 1 lean meat + 1 fat
▮ Egg roll, meat	1 (about 3 oz)	1 carbohydrate + 1 lean meat + 1 fat
Fried rice, meatless	½ c	1½ carbohydrates + 1½ fats
▮ Meat and sweet sauce (orange chicken)	1 c	3 carbohydrates + 3 medium-fat meats + 2 fats
▮☺ Noodles and vegetables in sauce (chow mein, lo mein)	1 c	2 carbohydrates + 1 fat
Pizza		
▮ Cheese, pepperoni, regular crust	⅛ of 14" (about 4 oz)	2½ carbohydrates + 1 medium-fat meat + 1½ fats
▮ Cheese/vegetarian, thin crust	¼ of 12" (about 6 oz)	2½ carbohydrates + 2 medium-fat meats + 1½ fats
Sandwiches		
▮ Chicken sandwich, grilled	1	3 carbohydrates + 4 lean meats
▮ Chicken sandwich, crispy	1	3½ carbohydrates + 3 medium-fat meats + 1 fat
Fish sandwich with tartar sauce	1	2½ carbohydrates + 2 medium-fat meats + 2 fats
Hamburger		
▮ large with cheese	1	2½ carbohydrates + 4 medium-fat meats + 1 fat
regular	1	2 carbohydrates + 1 medium-fat meat + 1 fat
▮ Hot dog with bun	1	1 carbohydrate + 1 high-fat meat + 1 fat
Submarine sandwich		
▮ less than 6 grams fat	6" sub	3 carbohydrates + 2 lean meats
▮ regular	6" sub	3½ carbohydrates + 2 medium-fat meats + 1 fat

[a] The choices in the Fast Foods list are not specific fast food meals or items, but are estimates based on popular foods. You can get specific nutrition information for almost every fast food or restaurant chain. Ask the restaurant or check its website for nutrition information about your favorite fast foods.

Food	Serving Size	Exchanges per Serving
Taco, hard or soft shell (meat and cheese)	1 small	1 carbohydrate + 1 medium-fat meat + 1½ fats

Salads

▮☺ Salad, main dish (grilled chicken type, no dressing or croutons)	Salad	1 carbohydrate + 4 lean meats
Salad, side, no dressing or cheese	Small (about 5 oz)	1 vegetable

Sides/Appetizers

▮ French fries, restaurant style	Small	3 carbohydrates + 3 fats
Medium		4 carbohydrates + 4 fats
Large		5 carbohydrates + 6 fats
▮ Nachos with cheese	Small (about 4½ oz)	2½ carbohydrates + 4 fats
▮ Onion rings	1 serving (about 3 oz)	2½ carbohydrates + 3 fats

Desserts

Milkshake, any flavor	12 oz.	6 carbohydrates + 2 fats
Soft-serve ice cream cone	1 small	2½ carbohydrates + 1 fat

Alcohol List

In general, 1 alcohol choice (½ oz absolute alcohol) has about 100 calories.

Alcoholic Beverage	Serving Size	Count As
Beer		
light (4.2%)	12 fl. oz.	1 alcohol equivalent + ½ carbohydrate
regular (4.9%)	12 fl. oz.	1 alcohol equivalent + 1 carbohydrate
Distilled spirits: vodka, rum, gin, whiskey, 80 or 86 proof	1½ fl. oz.	1 alcohol equivalent
Liqueur, coffee (53 proof)	1 fl. oz.	1 alcohol equivalent + 1 carbohydrate
Sake	1 fl. oz.	½ alcohol equivalent
Wine		
dessert (sherry)	3½ fl. oz.	1 alcohol equivalent + 1 carbohydrate
dry, red or white (10%)	5 fl. oz.	1 alcohol equivalent

Appendix H

Stature-for-Age Charts

CDC Growth Charts: United States
Stature-for-age percentiles: Boys, 2 to 20 years

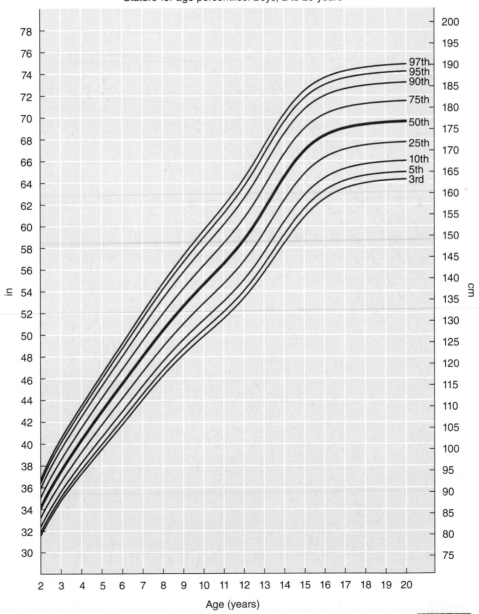

Age (years)

Source: "CDC Growth Charts, United States" Developed by the National
Center for Health Statistics in collaboration with the National Center
for Chronic Disease Prevention and Health Promotion,from the
Centers For Disease Control and Prevention website, 2000.

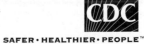

SAFER · HEALTHIER · PEOPLE™

CDC Growth Charts: United States
Stature-for-age percentiles: Girls, 2 to 20 years

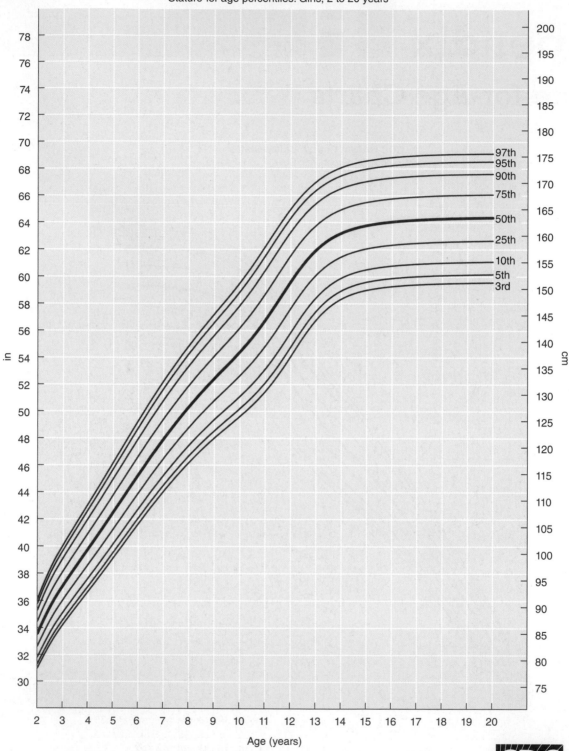

Age (years)

Source: "CDC Growth Charts, United States" Developed by the National Center for Health Statistics in collaboration with the National Center for Chronic Disease Prevention and Health Promotion,from the Centers For Disease Control and Prevention website, 2000.

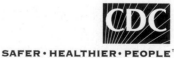

SAFER · HEALTHIER · PEOPLE™

Appendix I

Organizations and Resources

Academic Journals

International Journal of Sport Nutrition
and Exercise Metabolism
Human Kinetics
P.O. Box 5076
Champaign, IL 61825-5076
(800) 747-4457
www.humankinetics.com/IJSNEM

Journal of Nutrition
Department of Nutrition
Pennsylvania State University
126-S Henderson Building
University Park, PA 16802-6504
(814) 865-4721
www.nutrition.org

Nutrition Research
Elsevier: Journals Customer Service
6277 Sea Harbor Drive
Orlando, FL 32887
(877) 839-7126
www.journals.elsevierhealth.com/periodicals/NTR

Nutrition
Elsevier: Journals Customer Service
6277 Sea Harbor Drive
Orlando, FL 32887
(877) 839-7126
www.journals.elsevierhealth.com/periodicals/NUT

Nutrition Reviews
International Life Sciences Institute
Subscription Office
P.O. Box 830430
Birmingham, AL 35283
(800) 633-4931
www.ingentaconnect.com/content/ilsi/nure

Obesity Research
North American Association for the Study of Obesity
(NAASO)
8630 Fenton Street, Suite 918
Silver Spring, MD 20910
(301) 563-6526
www.nature.com/oby

International Journal of Obesity
Journal of the International Association for the Study of Obesity
Nature Publishing Group
The Macmillan Building
4 Crinan Street
London N1 9XW
United Kingdom
www.nature.com/ijo

Journal of the American Medical Association
American Medical Association
P.O. Box 10946
Chicago, IL 60610-0946
(800) 262-2350
www.jama.ama-assn.org

New England Journal of Medicine
10 Shattuck Street
Boston, MA 02115-6094
(617) 734-9800
www.nejm.org

American Journal of Clinical Nutrition
The American Journal of Clinical Nutrition
9650 Rockville Pike
Bethesda, MD 20814-3998
(301) 634-7038
www.ajcn.org

Journal of the American Dietetic Association
Elsevier, Health Sciences Division
Subscription Customer Service
6277 Sea Harbor Drive
Orlando, FL 32887
(800) 654-2452
www.adajournal.org

Aging

Administration on Aging
U.S. Health & Human Services
200 Independence Avenue, SW
Washington, DC 20201
(877) 696-6775
www.aoa.gov

American Association of Retired Persons (AARP)
601 E. Street, NW
Washington, DC 20049
(888) 687-2277
www.aarp.org

Health and Age
Sponsored by the Novartis Foundation for Gerontology
& The Web-Based Health Education Foundation
Robert Griffith, MD
Executive Director
573 Vista de la Ciudad
Santa Fe, NM 87501
www.healthandage.com

National Council on the Aging
300 D Street, SW, Suite 801
Washington, DC 20024
(202) 479-1200
www.ncoa.org

International Osteoporosis Foundation
5 Rue Perdtemps
1260 Nyon
Switzerland
41 22 994 01 00
www.iofbonehealth.org

National Institute on Aging
Building 31, Room 5C27
31 Center Drive, MSC 2292
Bethesda, MD 20892
(301) 496-1752
www.nia.nih.gov

Osteoporosis and Related Bone Diseases National
Resource Center
2 AMS Circle
Bethesda, MD 20892-3676
(800) 624-BONE
www.hiams.nih.gov/health_info/bone/

American Geriatrics Society
The Empire State Building
350 Fifth Avenue, Suite 801
New York, NY 10118
(212) 308-1414
www.americangeriatrics.org

National Osteoporosis Foundation
1232 22nd Street, NW
Washington, DC 20037-1292
(202) 223-2226
www.nof.org

Alcohol and Drug Abuse

National Institute on Drug Abuse
6001 Executive Boulevard, Room 5213
Bethesda, MD 20892-9561
(301) 443-1124
www.nida.nih.gov/nidahome

National Institute on Alcohol Abuse and Alcoholism
5635 Fishers Lane, MSC 9304
Bethesda, MD 20892-9304
www.niaaa.nih.gov

Alcoholics Anonymous
Grand Central Station
P.O. Box 459
New York, NY 10163
www.aa.org

Narcotics Anonymous
P.O. Box 9999
Van Nuys, CA 91409
(818) 773-9999
www.na.org

National Council on Alcoholism and Drug Dependence
20 Exchange Place, Suite 2902
New York, NY 10005
(212) 269-7797
www.ncadd.org

National Clearinghouse for Alcohol and Drug Information
11420 Rockville Pike
Rockville, MD 20852
(800) 729-6686
www.store.samhsa.gov/home

Canadian Government

Health Canada
A.L. 0900C2
Ottawa, ON
K1A 0K9
(613) 957-2991
www.hc-sc.gc.ca/english

National Institute of Nutrition
408 Queen Street, 3rd Floor
Ottawa, ON K1R 5A7
(613) 235-3355
www.nin.ca/public_html

Agricultural and Agri-Food Canada
Public Information Request Service
Sir John Carling Building
930 Carling Avenue
Ottawa, ON K1A 0C5
(613) 759-1000
www.agr.gc.ca

Bureau of Nutritional Sciences
Sir Frederick G. Banting Research Centre
Tunney's Pasture (2203A)
Ottawa, ON K1A 0L2
(613) 957-0352
www.hc-sc.gc.ca/food-aliment/ns-sc

Canadian Food Inspection Agency
59 Camelot Drive
Ottawa, ON K1A 0Y9
(613) 225-2342
www.inspection.gc.ca/english

Canadian Institute for Health Information
CIHI Ottawa
377 Dalhousie Street, Suite 200
Ottawa, ON K1N 9N8
(613) 241-7860
www.cihi.ca

Canadian Public Health Association
1565 Carling Avenue, Suite 400
Ottawa, ON K1Z 8R1
(613) 725-3769
www.cpha.ca

Canadian Nutrition and Professional Organizations

Dietitians of Canada
480 University Avenue, Suite 604
Toronto, ON M5G 1V2
(416) 596-0857
www.dietitians.ca

Canadian Diabetes Association
National Life Building
1400-522 University Avenue
Toronto, ON M5G 2R5
(800) 226-8464
www.diabetes.ca

National Eating Disorder Information Centre
CW 1-211, 200 Elizabeth Street
Toronto, ON M5G 2C4
(866) NEDIC-20
www.nedic.ca

Canadian Pediatric Society
100-2204 Walkley Road
Ottawa, ON K1G 4G8
(613) 526-9397
www.cps.ca

Canadian Dietetic Association
480 University Avenue, Suite 604
Toronto, ON M5G 1V2
(416) 596-0857
www.dietitians.ca

Disordered Eating

American Psychiatric Association
1000 Wilson Boulevard, Suite 1825
Arlington, VA 22209
(703) 907-7300
www.psych.org

National Institute of Mental Health
Office of Communications
6001 Executive Boulevard, Room 8184, MSC 9663
Bethesda, MD 20892
(866) 615-6464
www.nimh.nih.gov

National Association of Anorexia Nervosa and Associated
Disorders (ANAD)
Box 7
Highland Park, IL 60035
(847) 831-3438
www.anad.org

National Eating Disorders Association
603 Stewart Street, Suite 803
Seattle, WA 98101
(206) 382-3587
www.nationaleatingdisorders.org

Eating Disorder Referral and Information Center
2923 Sandy Pointe, Suite 6
Del Mar, CA 92014
(858) 792-7463
www.edreferral.com

Anorexia Nervosa and Related Eating Disorders, Inc. (ANRED)
E-mail: jarinor@rio.com
www.anred.com

Overeaters Anonymous
P.O. Box 44020
Rio Rancho, NM 87174
(505) 891-2664
www.oa.org

Exercise, Physical Activity, and Sports

American College of Sports Medicine (ACSM)
P.O. Box 1440
Indianapolis, IN 46206-1440
(317) 637-9200
www.acsm.org

American Physical Therapy Association (ASNA)
1111 North Fairfax Street
Alexandria, VA 22314
(800) 999-APTA
www.apta.org

Gatorade Sports Science Institute (GSSI)
617 West Main Street
Barrington, IL 60010
(800) 616-GSSI
www.gssiweb.com

National Coalition for Promoting Physical Activity (NCPPA)
1010 Massachusetts Avenue, Suite 350
Washington, DC 20001
(202) 454-7518
www.ncppa.org

Sports, Wellness, Eating Disorder and Cardiovascular Nutritionists (SCAN)
P.O. Box 60820
Colorado Springs, CO 80960
(719) 635-6005
www.scandpg.org

President's Council on Physical Fitness and Sports
Department W
200 Independence Avenue, SW Room 738-H
Washington, DC 20201-0004
(202) 690-9000
www.fitness.gov

American Council on Exercise
4851 Paramount Drive
San Diego, CA 92123
(858) 279-8227
www.acefitness.org

The International Association for Fitness Professionals (IDEA)
10455 Pacific Center Court
San Diego, CA 92121
(800) 999-4332, ext. 7
www.ideafit.com

Food Safety

Food Marketing Institute
655 15th Street, NW
Washington, DC 20005
(202) 452-8444
www.fmi.org

Agency for Toxic Substances and Disease Registry (ATSDR)
ORO Washington Office
Ariel Rios Building
1200 Pennsylvania Avenue, NW
M/C 5204G
Washington, DC 20460
(888) 422-8737
www.atsdr.cdc.gov

Food Allergy and Anaphylaxis Network
11781 Lee Jackson Highway, Suite 160
Fairfax, VA 22033-3309
(800) 929-4040
www.foodallergy.org

Foodsafety.gov
www.foodsafety.gov

The USDA Food Safety and Inspection Service
Food Safety and Inspection Service
United States Department of Agriculture
Washington, DC 20250
www.fsis.usda.gov

Consumer Reports
Web Site Customer Relations Department
101 Truman Avenue
Yonkers, NY 10703
www.consumerreports.org

Center for Science in the Public Interest: Food Safety
1875 Connecticut Avenue, NW
Washington, DC 20009
(202) 332-9110
www.cspinet.org/foodsafety

Center for Food Safety and Applied Nutrition
5100 Paint Branch Parkway
College Park, MD 20740
(888) SAFEFOOD
www.cfsan.fda.gov

Food Safety Project
Dan Henroid, MS, RD, CFSP
HRIM Extension Specialist and Website Coordinator
Hotel, Restaurant and Institution Management
9e MacKay Hall
Iowa State University
Ames, IA 50011
(515) 294-3527
www.extension.iastate.edu/foodsafety

Organic Consumers Association
6101 Cliff Estate Road
Little Marais, MN 55614
(218) 226-4164
www.organicconsumers.org

Infancy and Childhood

Administration for Children and Families
370 L'Enfant Promenade, SW
Washington, DC 20447
www.acf.hhs.gov

The American Academy of Pediatrics
141 Northwest Point Boulevard
Elk Grove Village, IL 60007
(847) 434-4000
www.aap.org

Kidnetic.com
E-mail: contactus@kidnetic.com
www.kidnetic.com

Kidshealth: The Nemours Foundation
12735 West Gran Bay Parkway
Jacksonville, FL 32258
(866) 390-3610
www.kidshealth.org

National Center for Education in Maternal and Child Health
Georgetown University
Box 571272
Washington, DC 20057
(202) 784-9770
www.ncemch.org

Birth Defects Research for Children, Inc.
930 Woodcock Road, Suite 225
Orlando, FL 32803
(407) 895-0802
www.birthdefects.org

USDA/ARS Children's Nutrition Research Center at Baylor
College of Medicine
1100 Bates Street
Houston, TX 77030
www.bcm.edu

Keep Kids Healthy.com
www.keepkidshealthy.com

International Agencies

UNICEF
3 United Nations Plaza
New York, NY 10017
(212) 326-7000
www.unicef.org

World Health Organization
Avenue Appia 20
1211 Geneva 27
Switzerland
41 22 791 21 11
www.who.int/en

The Stockholm Convention on Persistent Organic Pollutants
11–13 Chemin des Anémones
1219 Châtelaine
Geneva, Switzerland
41 22 917 8191
www.chm.pops.int

Food and Agricultural Organization of the United Nations
Viale delle Terme di Caracalla
00100 Rome, Italy
39 06 57051
www.fao.org

International Food Information Council Foundation
1100 Connecticut Avenue, NW
Suite 430
Washington, DC 20036
(202) 296-6540
www.foodinsight.org

Pregnancy and Lactation

San Diego County Breastfeeding Coalition
c/o Children's Hospital and Health Center
3020 Children's Way, MC 5073
San Diego, CA 92123
(800) 371-MILK
www.breastfeeding.org

National Alliance for Breastfeeding Advocacy
Barbara Heiser, Executive Director
9684 Oak Hill Drive
Ellicott City, MD 21042-6321
OR
Marsha Walker, Executive Director
254 Conant Road
Weston, MA 02493-1756
www.naba-breastfeeding.org

American College of Obstetricians and Gynecologists
409 12th Street, SW,
P.O. Box 96920
Washington, DC 20090
www.acog.org

La Leche League
1400 N. Meacham Road
Schaumburg, IL 60173
(847) 519-7730
www.lalecheleague.org

National Organization on Fetal Alcohol Syndrome
900 17th Street, NW
Suite 910
Washington, DC 20006
(800) 66 NOFAS
www.nofas.org

March of Dimes Birth Defects Foundation
1275 Mamaroneck Avenue
White Plains, NY 10605
(888) 663-4637
www.marchofdimes.org

Professional Nutrition Organizations

Association of Departments and Programs of Nutrition (ANDP)
Dr. Marilynn Schnepf, ANDP Chair
316 Ruth Leverton Hall
Nutrition and Health Sciences
University of Nebraska–Lincoln
Lincoln, NE 68583-0806
www.fshn.hs.iastate.edu/andp

North American Association for the Study of Obesity (NAASO)
8630 Fenton Street, Suite 918
Silver Spring, MD 20910
(301) 563-6526
www.obesity.org

American Dental Association
211 East Chicago Avenue
Chicago, IL 60611-2678
(312) 440-2500
www.ada.org

American Heart Association
National Center
7272 Greenville Avenue
Dallas, TX 75231
(800) 242-8721
www.heart.org/HEARTORG

Academy of Nutrition and Dietetics
(formerly the American Dietetic Assn.)
120 South Riverside Plaza, Suite 2000
Chicago, IL 60606-6995
(800) 877-1600
www.eatright.org

The American Society for Nutrition (ASN)
9650 Rockville Pike, Suite L-4500
Bethesda, MD 20814-3998
(301) 634-7050
www.nutrition.org

The Society for Nutrition Education
7150 Winton Drive, Suite 300
Indianapolis, IN 46268
(800) 235-6690
www.sne.org

American College of Nutrition
300 S. Duncan Avenue, Suite 225
Clearwater, FL 33755
(727) 446-6086
www.americancollegeofnutrition.org

American Council on Science and Health
1995 Broadway
Second Floor
New York, NY 10023
(212) 362-7044
www.acsh.org

American Diabetes Association
ATTN: National Call Center
1701 North Beauregard Street
Alexandria, VA 22311
(800) 342-2383
www.diabetes.org

Institute of Food Technologies
525 W. Van Buren, Suite 1000
Chicago, IL 60607
(312) 782-8424
www.ift.org

ILSI Human Nutrition Institute
One Thomas Circle, Ninth Floor
Washington, DC 20005
(202) 659-0524
www.ilsi.org

Trade Organizations

American Meat Institute
1700 North Moore Street
Suite 1600
Arlington, VA 22209
(703) 841-2400
www.meatami.com

National Dairy Council
10255 W. Higgins Road, Suite 900
Rosemont, IL 60018
(312) 240-2880
www.nationaldairycouncil.org

United Fresh Fruit and Vegetable Association
1901 Pennsylvania Ave. NW, Suite 1100
Washington, DC 20006
(202) 303-3400
www.unitedfresh.org

U.S.A. Rice Federation
Washington, DC
4301 North Fairfax Drive, Suite 425
Arlington, VA 22203
(703) 236-2300
www.usarice.com

U.S. Government

The USDA National Organic Program
Agricultural Marketing Service
USDA-AMS-TMP-NOP
Room 4008-South Building
1400 Independence Avenue, SW
Washington, DC 20250-0020
(202) 720-3252
www.ams.usda.gov

U.S. Department of Health and Human Services
200 Independence Avenue, SW
Washington, DC 20201
(877) 696-6775
www.hhs.gov

Food and Drug Administration (FDA)
5600 Fishers Lane
Rockville, MD 20857
(888) 463-6332
www.fda.gov

Environmental Protection Agency
Ariel Rios Building
1200 Pennsylvania Avenue, NW
Washington, DC 20460
(202) 272-0167
www.epa.gov

Federal Trade Commission
600 Pennsylvania Avenue, NW
Washington, DC 20580
(202) 326-2222
www.ftc.gov

Office of Dietary Supplements
National Institutes of Health
6100 Executive Boulevard, Room 3B01, MSC 7517
Bethesda, MD 20892
(301) 435-2920
www.ods.od.nih.gov

Nutrient Data Laboratory Homepage
Beltsville Human Nutrition Center
10300 Baltimore Avenue
Building 307-C, Room 117 BARC-East
Beltsville, MD 20705
(301) 504-8157
www.nal.usda.gov/fnic/foodcomp

National Digestive Disease Clearinghouse
2 Information Way
Bethesda, MD 20892-3570
(800) 891-5389
www.digestive.niddk.nih.gov

The National Cancer Institute
NCI Public Inquiries Office
Suite 3036A
6116 Executive Boulevard, MSC 8322
Bethesda, MD 20892-8322
(800) 4-CANCER
www.cancer.gov

The National Eye Institute
31 Center Drive, MSC 2510
Bethesda, MD 20892-2510
(301) 496-5248
www.nei.nih.gov

The National Heart, Lung, and Blood Institute
Building 31, Room 5A52
31 Center Drive, MSC 2486
Bethesda, MD 20892
(301) 592-8573
www.nhlbi.nih.gov

Institute of Diabetes and Digestive and Kidney Diseases
Office of Communications and Public Liaison
NIDDK, NIH, Building 31, Room 9A04
Center Drive, MSC 2560
Bethesda, MD 20892
(301) 496-4000
www.niddk.nih.gov

National Center for Complementary and Alternative Medicine
NCCAM Clearinghouse
P.O. Box 7923
Gaithersburg, MD 20898
(888) 644-6226
www.nccam.nih.gov

U.S. Department of Agriculture (USDA)
14th Street, SW
Washington, DC 20250
(202) 720-2791
www.usda.gov

Centers for Disease Control and Prevention (CDC)
1600 Clifton Road
Atlanta, GA 30333
(404) 639-3311/Public Inquiries: (800) 311-3435
www.cdc.gov

National Institutes of Health (NIH)
9000 Rockville Pike
Bethesda, MD 20892
(301) 496-4000
www.nih.gov

Food and Nutrition Information Center
Agricultural Research Service, USDA
National Agricultural Library, Room 105
10301 Baltimore Avenue
Beltsville, MD 20705-2351
(301) 504-5719
www.nal.usda.gov/fnic

National Institute of Allergy and Infectious Diseases
NIAID Office of Communications and Public Liaison
6610 Rockledge Drive, MSC 6612
Bethesda, MD 20892
(301) 496-5717
www.niaid.nih.gov

Weight and Health Management

The Vegetarian Resource Group
P.O. Box 1463, Dept. IN
Baltimore, MD 21203
(410) 366-VEGE
www.vrg.org

American Obesity Association
1250 24th Street, NW
Suite 300
Washington, DC 20037
(202) 776-7711
www.obesity.org

Anemia Lifeline
(888) 722-4407
www.anemia.com

The Arc
(301) 565-3842
E-mail: info@thearc.org
www.thearc.org

Bottled Water Web
P.O. Box 5658
Santa Barbara, CA 93150
(805) 879-1564
www.bottledwaterweb.com

The Food and Nutrition Board
Institute of Medicine
500 Fifth Street, NW
Washington, DC 20001
(202) 334-2352
www.iom.edu

The Calorie Control Council
www.caloriecontrol.org

TOPS (Take Off Pounds Sensibly)
4575 South Fifth Street
P.O. Box 07360
Milwaukee, WI 53207
(800) 932-8677
www.tops.org

Shape Up America!
15009 Native Dancer Road
N. Potomac, MD 20878
(240) 631-6533
www.shapeup.org

World Hunger

Center on Hunger, Poverty, and Nutrition Policy
Tufts University
Medford, MA 02155
(617) 627-3020
www.tufts.edu/nutrition

Freedom from Hunger
1644 DaVinci Court
Davis, CA 95616
(800) 708-2555
www.freedomfromhunger.org

Oxfam International
1112 16th Street, NW, Suite 600
Washington, DC 20036
(202) 496-1170
www.oxfam.org

WorldWatch Institute
1776 Massachusetts Avenue, NW
Washington, DC 20036
(202) 452-1999
www.worldwatch.org

Food First
398 60th Street
Oakland, CA 94618
(510) 654-4400
www.foodfirst.org

The Hunger Project
15 East 26th Street
New York, NY 10010
(212) 251-9100
www.thp.org

U.S. Agency for International Development
Information Center
Ronald Reagan Building
Washington, DC 20523
(202) 712-0000
www.usaid.gov

Answers to Review Questions

The answers to Review Questions appear here and in the Study Area of MasteringNutrition at **www.masteringnutrition .pearson.com,** or at **www.pearsonmylabandmastering .com.**

Chapter 1

1. **d.** micronutrients.
2. **d.** all of the above.
3. **b.** contain 90 kcal of energy.
4. **c.** measurement of height.
5. **c.** "A high-protein diet increases the risk for porous bones" is an example of a valid hypothesis.
6. **False.** Vitamins do not provide any energy, although many vitamins are critical to the metabolic processes that assist us in generating energy from carbohydrates, fats, and proteins.
7. **True.**
8. **True.**
9. **False.** An epidemiological study assesses phenomena of large populations and determines the factors that may influence these phenomena. It is not a clinical trial.
10. **True.**
11. In a well-designed experiment, a control group allows a researcher to compare between treated and untreated individuals, and thereby to determine whether or not a particular treatment has exerted a significant effect.
12. The Estimated Average Requirement, or EAR, represents the average daily nutrient intake level estimated to meet the requirement of half of the healthy individuals in a particular life stage or gender group. The Recommended Dietary Allowance, or RDA, represents the average daily nutrient intake level that meets the nutrient requirements of 97% to 98% of healthy individuals in a particular life stage or gender group. The EAR is used to estimate the RDA.
13. I would explain to Marilyn that the term *nutritionist* does not guarantee that the person who suggested the supplements is qualified to give nutritional guidance. I would recommend that she would be better off talking with a qualified healthcare professional about her fatigue. To find reliable nutrition information, I would suggest she talk with a registered dietitian. She can find registered dietitians in her local area by contacting the American Dietetic Association. She can also access free, reliable information from the websites of organizations such as the American Dietetic Association, the National Institutes of Health, and the Centers for Disease Control and Prevention.
14. The source of funding can be a good indicator of the level of bias in a research study. For instance, if this study was funded by chocolate manufacturers and conducted by their own

scientists, the results could be biased in that the chocolate manufacturer could make a substantial profit by discovering positive findings related to chocolate. Having an independent research team conduct the study can reduce this type of bias.
15. There are numerous aspects of this study that limit its relevance to your mother. Some of these are the following:
a. Limited number of participants. Only twelve women participated in this study. This very small number of participants significantly limits the ability to generalize the results to a larger population.
b. Age. The women in the study were all older than your mother.
c. Blood pressure. Your mother has blood pressure at the upper end of the normal range, and all of the participants in this study had high blood pressure.
d. Activity level. Your mother is physically active. She walks daily and swims once a week. The participants in this study were sedentary or inactive.
e. Smoking. Your mother is a nonsmoker, and only half of the participants in this study were nonsmokers, with the other half being relatively heavy smokers.
16. Seven ounces.
17. 24.5% of Kayla's diet comes from fat; this percentage is within the AMDR for fat.

Chapter 2

1. **d.** The % Daily Values of select nutrients in a serving of the packaged food.
2. **b.** provides enough of the energy, nutrients, and fiber to maintain a person's health.
3. **a.** at least half your grains as whole grains each day.
4. **a.** choosing and preparing foods without added salt.
5. **b.** Foods with a lot of nutrients per Calorie, such as fish, are more nutritious choices than foods with fewer nutrients per Calorie, such as candy.
6. **False.** There is no standardized definition for a serving size for foods.
7. **False.** Structure–function claims do not need FDA approval.
8. **False.** Empty Calories are those derived from solid fats and/or added sugars, which provide few or no nutrients, and thus should be avoided.
9. **True.**
10. **False.** About 75% of Americans eat out at least once a week.
11. As humans, we are all different in terms of body size, physical activity level, religious and ethnic beliefs, and disease risk factors. No single diet can meet the needs of every human being, as our needs are very different. It is necessary to vary a diet based on individual needs.

12. Answers will vary. Be sure labels contain all five of the primary components of information identified in Figure 2.1.

13. The USDA Food Patterns suggest a range in the number of daily servings of each food group because our energy needs are dependent upon our physical activity level and body size, and therefore are different for everyone. The lower end of the range applies to inactive women and small individuals, while the higher end of the range applies to more active people and larger men. In fact, highly active people may need to eat even more servings than those recommended at the higher end of the range. People should not eat fewer than the lowest recommended number of servings, because this could lead to nutritional deficiencies.

14. At least 5 grams per serving.

15. It is not accurate. The Mediterranean diet is actually relatively high in fat, not low in fat. However, this diet recommends consuming foods that contain more healthful mono- and polyunsaturated fats. Bread and pasta are a daily part of the Mediterranean diet, but this diet does not recommend unlimited consumption of these foods. If Sylvia eats more energy than she expends, even while consuming the Mediterranean diet, she will not be able to lose weight.

16. Total Calories = 646; Total fat content = 33 g; Percentage of Calories from fat = 46%; item contributing the highest amount of fat to the lunch = ranch salad dressing. Hannah can skip the salad dressing or ask for a low-fat dressing, if available, to make a healthier change to this lunch.

Chapter 3

1. **b.** peristalsis.
2. **d.** emulsifies lipids.
3. **c.** hypothalamus.
4. **a.** seepage of gastric acid into the esophagus.
5. **a.** a bean-and-cheese burrito.
6. **True.**
7. **True.**
8. **False.** Vitamins and minerals are not really "digested" in the same way that macronutrients are. These compounds do not have to be broken down, because they are small enough to be readily absorbed by the small intestine. For example, fat-soluble vitamins, such as vitamins A, D, E, and K, are soluble in lipids and are absorbed into the intestinal cells along with the fats in our foods. Water-soluble vitamins, such as the B-vitamins and vitamin C, typically undergo some type of active transport process that helps ensure that the vitamin is absorbed by the small intestine. Minerals are elements, which cannot be broken down. They are absorbed all along the small intestine, and in some cases in the large intestine, by a wide variety of mechanisms.
9. **True.**
10. **True.**
11. Our bodies are composed of cells, which are the smallest units of matter that exhibit the properties of living things.

That is, cells can grow, reproduce themselves, and perform certain basic functions, such as taking in nutrients, transmitting impulses, producing chemicals, and excreting wastes. The human body is composed of billions of cells that are constantly replacing themselves, destroying worn or damaged cells, and manufacturing new ones. To support this constant demand for new cells, we need a ready supply of nutrient molecules, such as simple sugars, amino acids, and fatty acids, to serve as building blocks. These building blocks are the molecules that come from the breakdown of foods. All cells, whether of the skin, bones, or brain, are made of the same basic molecules of amino acids, sugars, and fatty acids, which are also the main components of the foods we eat. Thus, we are what we eat in that the building blocks of our cells are comprised of the molecules contained in the foods we eat.

12. **No.** The main function of the small intestine is to absorb nutrients and transport them into the bloodstream or the lymphatic system. In order to do this effectively, the surface area of the small intestine needs to be as large as possible. The inside of the lining of the small intestine, referred to as the mucosal membrane, is heavily folded. This feature increases the surface area of the small intestine and allows it to absorb more nutrients than if it were smooth. The villi are in constant movement, which helps them encounter and trap nutrient molecules. Covering the villi are specialized cells covered with hairlike structures called microvilli (also called the brush border). These intricate folds increase the surface area of the small intestine by more than 500 times, which tremendously increases the absorptive capacity of the small intestine.

13. The stomach does not digest itself because it secretes mucus that protects the lining from being digested by the hydrochloric acid it secretes.

14.

Digestive Disorder	Area of Inflammation	Symptoms	Treatment Options
Celiac disease	Small intestine	• Fatty stools • Diarrhea or constipation • Cramping • Anemia • Pallor • Weight loss • Fatigue • Irritability	Modified diet that excludes foods that contain gluten or gliadin (for example, wheat, rye, and barley)
Crohn's disease	Usually ileum of small intestine but can affect any area of gastrointestinal tract	• Diarrhea • Abdominal pain • Rectal bleeding • Weight loss • Fever • Anemia • Delayed physical and mental development in children	Combination of prescription drugs, nutritional supplements, and surgery

Digestive Disorder	Area of Inflammation	Symptoms	Treatment Options
Ulcerative colitis	Mucosa of large intestine (or colon)	• Diarrhea (which may be bloody) • Abdominal pain • Weight loss • Anemia • Fever • Severe urgency to have bowel movement	• Anti-inflammatory medications • Surgery if medications are not effective

15. Your roommate could be suffering from heartburn or gastroesophageal reflux disease (GERD). Eating food causes the stomach to secrete hydrochloric acid to start the digestive process. In many people, the amount of HCl secreted is occasionally excessive or the gastroesophageal sphincter opens too soon. In either case, the result is that HCl seeps back up into the esophagus. Although the stomach is protected from HCl by a thick coat of mucus, the esophagus does not have this mucus coating. Thus, the HCl burns it. When this happens, a person experiences a painful sensation in the region of his or her chest above the sternum (breastbone). This condition is commonly called heartburn.

If your roommate experiences this painful type of heartburn more than twice per week, he may be suffering from GERD. Similar to heartburn, GERD occurs when HCl flows back into the esophagus. Although people who experience occasional heartburn usually have no structural abnormalities, many people with GERD have an overly relaxed or damaged esophageal sphincter or a damaged esophagus itself. Symptoms of GERD include persistent heartburn and acid regurgitation. Some people have GERD without heartburn and instead experience chest pain, trouble swallowing, burning in the mouth, the feeling that food is stuck in the throat, or hoarseness in the morning.

16. The difference between pH 9 and pH 2 is 7. The alkalinity of baking soda as compared to gastric juice can be expressed as: $7 = \log_{10}(10,000,000)$. Baking soda is 10 million times more alkaline than gastric juice.

Chapter 4

1. **b.** the potential of foods to raise blood glucose and insulin levels.
2. **d.** carbon, hydrogen, and oxygen.
3. **d.** sweetened soft drinks.
4. **a.** monosaccharides.
5. **a.** phenylketonuria.
6. **False.** Sugar alcohols are considered nutritive sweeteners because they contain 2 to 4 kcal of energy per gram.
7. **True.**
8. **False.** A person with lactose intolerance has a difficult time tolerating milk and other dairy products. This person does not have an allergy to milk, as he or she does not exhibit an immune response indicative of an allergy. Instead, this person does not digest lactose completely, which causes intestinal distress and symptoms such as gas, bloating, diarrhea, and nausea.
9. **False.** Plants store glucose as starch.
10. **False.** Salivary amylase breaks starches into maltose and shorter polysaccharides.
11. Insulin is a hormone secreted by the beta cells of the pancreas in response to increased blood levels of glucose. When we eat a meal, our blood glucose level rises. But glucose in our blood cannot help the nerves, muscles, and other tissues function unless it can cross into them. Glucose molecules are too large to cross the cell membranes of our tissues independently. To get in, glucose needs assistance from insulin. Insulin is transported in the blood to the cells of tissues throughout the body, where it stimulates special molecules located in the cell membrane to transport glucose into the cell. Insulin can be thought of as a key that opens the gates of the cell membrane and carries the glucose into the cell interior, where it can be used for energy. Insulin also stimulates the liver and muscles to take up glucose.
12. **a.** Fiber adds bulk to the stools, which aids in efficient excretion of feces.
    b. Fiber keeps stools moist and soft, helping prevent hemorrhoids and constipation.
    c. Fiber gives the gut muscles something to push on, making it easier to eliminate stools. Diverticulosis can result in part from trying to eliminate small, hard stools.
    d. Fiber may bind with cancer-causing agents and speed their elimination from the colon, which could in turn reduce the risk for colon cancer.
13. Grain-based foods contain carbohydrates, and sometimes these foods are processed, meaning that many of the important nutrients we need for health are taken out of them. Fiber-rich carbohydrates contain not only more fiber, which is important for the health of our digestive tract, but also many vitamins and minerals that we need to be healthy. The foods you listed here are examples of foods in the "grains" group that are processed. Examples of healthier fiber-rich alternative choices include whole-wheat saltine crackers, whole-wheat or pumpernickel bagels, brown rice, and whole-wheat spaghetti.
14. Diabetes more commonly runs in families, but just because no one in the family has diabetes does not mean that someone cannot get it. Being obese or overweight increases a person's risk for developing type 2 diabetes. Overweight and obesity trigger insulin insensitivity, or insulin resistance, which in turn causes the pancreas to produce greater amounts of insulin, so that glucose can enter the cells and be used for energy. Eventually, type 2 diabetes develops because (1) there is an increasing degree of insulin insensitivity; (2) the pancreas can no longer secrete enough insulin; or (3) the pancreas has entirely stopped producing insulin.

15.

Carbo-hydrate	Molecular Composition	Food Sources
Glucose	Six carbon atoms, twelve hydrogen atoms, six oxygen atoms	Fruits, vegetables, grains, dairy products; does not generally occur alone in foods but attaches to other sugars to form disaccharides and complex carbohydrates
Fructose	Six carbon atoms, twelve hydrogen atoms, six oxygen atoms	Fruits and some vegetables
Lactose	One glucose molecule and one galactose molecule	Milk and other dairy products
Sucrose	One glucose molecule and one fructose molecule	Honey, maple syrup, fruits, vegetables, table sugar, brown sugar, powdered sugar

16. a) 3,500 kcal per day $\times$ 0.45 = 1,575 kcal per day to 3,500 kcal per day $\times$ 0.65 = 2,275 kcal per day. Thus Simon should consume between 1,575 and 2,275 kcal per day of carbohydrate, preferably from fiber-rich sources; and b) 1,575 kcal per day $\div$ 4 kcal per gram of carbohydrate = 393.75 grams to 2,275 kcal per day $\div$ 4 kcal per gram of carbohydrate = 568.75 grams. Thus Simon should consume between 394 and 569 grams of carbohydrate per day.

Chapter 5

1. **d.** found in flaxseeds, walnuts, and fish.
2. **b.** exercise regularly.
3. **a.** lipoprotein lipase.
4. **d.** high-density lipoproteins.
5. **a.** monounsaturated.
6. **False.** Lecithin is a phospholipid.
7. **False.** Fat is an important source of energy during rest and during exercise, and adipose tissue is our primary storage site for fat. We rely significantly on the fat stored in our adipose tissue to provide energy during rest and exercise.
8. **False.** A triglyceride is a lipid composed of a glycerol molecule and three fatty acids. Thus, fatty acids are a component of triglycerides.
9. **False.** While most *trans* fatty acids result from the hydrogenation of vegetable oils by food manufacturers, a small amount of *trans* fatty acids is found in cow's milk.
10. **False.** A serving of food labeled *reduced fat* has at least 25% less fat than a standard serving but may not have fewer Calories than a full-fat version of the same food.
11. The straight, rigid shape of both *trans* and saturated fatty acids appears to raise blood cholesterol levels and to change cell membrane function and the way cholesterol is removed from the blood. For these reasons, many health professionals feel that diets high in *trans* and saturated fatty acids can increase the risk for cardiovascular disease. Because of the concerns related to *trans* fatty

acid consumption and heart disease, manufacturers are required to list the amount of *trans* fatty acids per serving on the food label.

12. Dietary fat enables the transport of the fat-soluble vitamins, specifically vitamins D and K. Vitamin D is important for regulating blood calcium and phosphorus concentrations and keeping them within the normal range, which indirectly helps maintain bone health. If vitamin D is low, blood calcium levels will drop below normal, and the body will draw calcium from the bones to maintain blood levels. Vitamin K is also important for proteins involved in maintaining bone health.

13. This is not particularly good advice for someone doing a 20-mile walk-a-thon. The energy sources used will depend partly on how fast you walk. If you are walking at a slow (2–3 miles/hour) to moderate (4 miles/hour) pace, fat will be the predominate energy source. Fat is a primary source of energy during rest and during less intense exercise. In addition, we use predominantly more fat as we perform longer-duration exercise. This is because we use more carbohydrate earlier during the exercise bout, and once our limited carbohydrate sources are depleted during prolonged exercise, we rely more on fat as an energy source. Although carbohydrates are an important source of energy during exercise, loading up on carbohydrates is typically only helpful for individuals who are doing longer-duration exercise at intensities higher than those experienced during walking at a slow to moderate pace. As the primary goal of this walk-a-thon is to raise money and not to finish in record time, you can walk at a pace that matches your current fitness level. Thus, it would be prudent to consume adequate carbohydrate prior to and during the walk-a-thon, but loading up on carbohydrates is not necessary. If you walked the event at a very fast pace (race-walking), carbohydrate loading could be beneficial.

14. Caleb's father probably had a blood test to determine his blood lipid levels, including total cholesterol, low-density lipoprotein cholesterol (LDL-C), high-density lipoprotein cholesterol (HDL-C), and triglycerides. Unfortunately, switching to cottage cheese and margarine may not improve his blood lipid values. Margarines can be high in *trans* fatty acids, which negatively impact blood lipids and increase our risk for heart disease. In addition, full-fat cottage cheese is a high-fat food, and it contains saturated fatty acids, which also negatively alter blood lipid levels. Both *trans* and saturated fatty acids will increase Caleb's father's risk for heart disease. Dietary changes that improve blood lipids include decreasing intake of saturated and *trans* fats, and switching to monounsaturated or polyunsaturated fatty acid products. A nondietary lifestyle choice that might improve his health is regular physical activity. Regular physical activity can help people maintain a more healthful body weight, can increase HDL-C, and can cause other changes that reduce our risk for heart disease.

15.

Type of Fat	Maximum Recommended Intake (% of total energy intake)	Maximum Recommended Calorie Intake
Saturated fat	7%	140 Calories/d
Linoleic acid	10%	200 Calories/d
Alpha-linolenic acid	1.2%	24 Calories/d
Trans fatty acids	0%	0 Calories/d
Unsaturated fat	None; amount equal to remainder of total fat Calories after you account for intake of saturated fat and linoleic and alpha-linolenic acids	336 Calories/d

Calculations used:

- Total energy needs = 2,000 Calories per day
- Maximum AMDR for fat = 35% of total energy intake = 0.35 × 2,000 = 700 Calories
- Saturated fat = 7% of total energy intake = 0.07 × 2,000 = 140 Calories
- Linoleic acid = 10% of total energy intake = 0.10 × 2,000 = 200 Calories
- Alpha-linolenic acid = 1.2% of total energy intake = 0.012 × 2,000 = 24 Calories
- *Trans* fatty acids = 0 Calories

16. 1. The first rule for weight loss is that energy (kcal) matters. Thus, Hannah needs to consider total energy intake in addition to total fat intake. Weight loss programs often focus on reducing fat intake because fat has the highest number of kcal/g, but <u>all</u> calories count. Thus, Hannah needs to consider the number of calories in her nonfat yogurt and topping.
2. The total amount of energy (kcal) in her after-class treat adds up to 168 kcal.
3. There are a number of snacks Hannah can select that would be healthier and make her feel satisfied. Some examples, which are all low in saturated fat, include:

- Yogurt (6oz low fat) with ½ c berries (155 kcals, 9 g protein, 23 g carbohydrate, 2.5 g fat)
- Apple (medium) and 1 T peanut butter (194 kcals, 4 g protein, 29 g carbohydrate, 8 g fat)
- Banana (medium) and milk (6oz skim) (163 kcals, 7 g protein, 35 g carbohydrate, <1 g fat)
- ½ Peanut butter (1T) sandwich on whole wheat bread (1 slice) (200 kcal, 8.5 g protein, 24 g carbohydrate, 9.5 g fat)

Chapter 6

1. **d.** mutual supplementation.
2. **a.** rice, pinto beans, acorn squash, soy butter, and almond milk.
3. **c.** protease.
4. **b.** amine group.
5. **c.** carbon, oxygen, hydrogen, and nitrogen.
6. **True.**
7. **False.** Both shape and function are lost when a protein is denatured.
8. **False.** Some hormones are made from lipids.
9. **False.** Buffers help the body maintain acid–base balance.
10. **False.** Depending on the type of sport, athletes may require the same amount of or up to two times as much protein as nonactive people.
11. Adequate protein is needed to maintain the proper balance of fluids inside and outside the cells. When a child suffers from kwashiorkor, the protein content of the blood is inadequate to maintain this balance. Fluid seeps from inside the cells out to the tissue spaces and causes bloating and swelling of the abdomen.
12. In general, only people who are susceptible to kidney disease or who have kidney disease suffer serious consequences when eating a high-protein diet. Consuming a high-protein diet increases protein metabolism and urea production. Individuals with kidney disease or those who are at risk for kidney disease cannot adequately flush urea and other by-products of protein metabolism from the body through the kidneys. This inability can lead to serious health consequences and even death.
13. mRNA, or messenger RNA, transcribes or copies genetic information from DNA in the nucleus and carries this information to the ribosomes in the cytoplasm. Once this genetic information reaches the ribosomes, it is translated into the language of amino acid sequences, or proteins. tRNA, or transfer RNA, binds with select amino acids dissolved in the cyptoplasm and transfers these amino acids to the ribosome, so that they can be assembled into proteins. The specific amino acids that are transferred to the ribosome from tRNA are dictated by the amino acid sequence presented by mRNA.
14. There are various classifications of vegetarianism. Many people feel that, if a person eats any meat or products from animals (such as dairy or eggs), he or she cannot be a vegetarian. People who eat only plant-based foods are classified as vegans. If you believe this, then you would argue that your Dad is not a true vegetarian. However, there are others who believe a vegetarian is someone who can eat dairy foods, eggs, or both in addition to plant-based foods. There are also people who classify themselves as pescovegetarians, meaning they eat fish along with plant-based foods. Semi-vegetarians may eat lean meats, such as poultry, on occasion in addition to plant-based foods, eggs, and dairy products. If you believe in these broader definitions of vegetarianism, you would agree with your Dad's opinion that he is now a vegetarian.
15. Use Figure 6.4 as a guide. Amino acids should be joined at the acid group of one amino acid and the amino group of the next amino acid. Multiple amino acids joined in this way make a protein.
16. **a.** The AMDR for protein is 10% to 35% of total daily energy intake. Barry's protein intake in g must be converted

to kcal to answer this question. Remember that the
energy content of protein is 4 kcal/g. Thus:
190 g of protein $\times$ 4 kcal/g = 760 kcal protein
To calculate the percentage of protein Barry is eating
in his diet = (760 kcal $\div$ 3000 kcal) $\times$ 100 = 25.3% of
Barry's total energy intake comes from protein. This
amount meets the AMDR for protein.
b. The RDA for protein is 0.8 g per kg body weight per
day. Barry's weight is 182 lbs. You must first convert
Barry's weight to kg = 182 lbs $\div$ 2.2 lbs/kg = 82.7 kg
Barry's protein intake is 190 g. To calculate whether he
meets the RDA for protein, divide his protein intake in
g by his body weight = 190 g $\div$ 82.7 kg = 2.3 g per kg
body weight per day. This amount exceeds the RDA for
protein, and is more than sufficient to support Barry even
if he is an endurance or strength athlete.

Chapter 7

1. **a.** lactic acid.
2. **b.** power plant.
3. **a.** hydrolysis.
4. **d.** None of the above statements is true.
5. **d.** catabolic hormones.
6. **True.**
7. **False.** The body can store only a small amount
of glycogen.
8. **True.**
9. **False.** Catabolism releases energy.
10. **True.**
11. The final stage of glucose oxidation is called oxidative phosphorylation and occurs in the electron transport chain of the mitochondria. In this step, a series of
enzyme-driven reactions occur in which electrons are
passed down a "chain." As the electrons are passed from
one carrier to the next, energy is released. In this process,
NADH and $FADH_2$ are oxidized and their electrons are
donated to O_2, which is reduced to H_2O (water). The
energy released when water is formed generates ATP.
12. Fatty acids released from the adipose tissue or fatty acids
that come from the foods we eat are transported on
albumin in the blood. They are then transported to the
cells that need energy, such as the muscle cells. The fatty
acids move across the cell membrane into the cytosol,
where they are activated by the addition of CoA and then
transported to the mitochondria, where fatty acid oxidation occurs. Once in the mitochondria, the fatty acid is
systematically broken down into two-carbon units that
lead to the formation of acetyl-CoA, which can enter the
TCA cycle for energy production.
13. Without insulin, the body cannot utilize the glucose
derived from food. Since glucose cannot enter the cells,
the body begins the process of breaking down body fats
to fatty acids, which can be used to produced ketones and
alternative fuel for the brain when glucose is not available.
These ketones are acidic and can build up in the blood,
leading to ketoacidosis. Under these conditions more

ketones are produced than can be utilized or eliminated
from the body, so they build up in the blood.
14. When children with PKU go off their diets, they increase
the levels of the amino acid phenylalanine in the body.
They cannot metabolize phenylalanine correctly due to
a genetic enzyme disorder that can result in the toxic
buildup of phenylalanine in the body, which causes organ
tissue damage.
15. We can assume that Aunt Winifred has been eating so
little food that her need for carbohydrate (to maintain
blood glucose) has not been met. Since the brain, red
blood cells, and other types of cells, are all dependent on
glucose for fuel, her body has no doubt been breaking
down muscle protein in order to use some of the amino
acids—known as glucogenic amino acids—to synthesize
new glucose (gluconeogenesis). So not only has Aunt
Winifred been losing body fat, but she has also been losing muscle mass, our main pool of body protein.
16. **(a)** To calculate Chris' weight in kg: 170 lb $\div$ 2.2 lb/kg =
77.3 kg
To estimate Chris' need for protein: 77.3 kg $\times$ 0.8 g
protein/kg = 61.8 g protein per day (round to 62 g).
(b) To calculate how much protein is in 3 servings of the
supplement: 1800 mg amino acids/serving $\times$ 3 servings/d =
5400 mg amino acids = 5.4 g protein from the supplement.

To calculate what percent of Chris' daily need for protein
is met by the supplement:
[5.4 g protein from the supplement $\div$ 62 g total protein
need] $\times$ 100 (to convert to percentage) = 8.7% of Chris'
total protein need is met by 3 servings of the supplement.

If eggs cost $1.80/dozen, each egg costs 15 cents. You
could buy ten eggs for $1.50, providing a total of 60 g
protein (each egg provides about 6 g protein).

Chapter 8

1. **d.** thiamin, pantothenic acid, and biotin.
2. **d.** Choline is necessary for the synthesis of phospholipids
and other components of cell membranes.
3. **a.** iodine deficiency.
4. **b.** tuna sandwich on whole-wheat bread, green peas,
banana, 1 cup of low-fat milk.
5. **b.** It is found naturally only in animal-based foods.
6. **True.**
7. **True.**
8. **True.**
9. **True.**
10. **False.** Riboflavin occurs naturally in milk, and niacin
deficiency causes pellagra.
11. People from inland regions are more prone to goiter
because they consumer fewer seafoods, which are high in
iodine.
12. Vitamin B_6 is important in the transamination of essential
amino acids to nonessential amino acids.
13. Vitamins and minerals added to foods can help improve
our nutritional status for these micronutrients. Not

everyone will eat enough variety or quantity of the foods they need to get all the micronutrients they need; thus, fortification and enrichment help these individuals maintain their nutritional status.

14. Dialysis can remove water-soluble vitamins from the blood, which need to be replaced with either foods high in these nutrients or supplements.

15. Mr. Katz's doctor probably did not give him the vitamin in pill form because Mr. Katz is 80 years of age, and it is more likely that he suffers from low stomach acid secretion. This is a condition known as atrophic gastritis, and it is estimated that about 10% to 30% of adults older than 50 years have this condition. Stomach acid separates food-bound vitamin B_{12} from dietary proteins. If the acid content of the stomach is inadequate, we cannot free up enough vitamin B_{12} from food sources alone. Because atrophic gastritis can affect almost one-third of the older adult population, it is recommended that people older than 50 years of age consume foods fortified with vitamin B_{12}, take a vitamin B_{12}–containing supplement, or have periodic B_{12} injections. Because Mr. Katz's condition was so severe, it was critical to treat him with a form of vitamin B_{12} that would be guaranteed to enter his system as quickly and effectively as possible; thus, his physician opted to use a vitamin B_{12} injection.

16. DFEs = 70 µg/day + 1.7 (224 µg/day) = 451 µg/day. This individual is getting 85% of his or her DFE from fortified foods.

Chapter 9

1. **b.** It can be found in fresh fruits and vegetables.
2. **d.** a healthy infant of average weight.
3. **a.** extracellular fluid.
4. **a.** It is freely permeable to water and many solutes.
5. **b.** normalizing body weight.
6. **False.** In addition to water, the body needs electrolytes, such as sodium and potassium, to prevent fluid imbalances during long-distance events, such as a marathon. Because purified water contains no electrolytes, it is not the ideal beverage for preventing fluid imbalances during a marathon.
7. **False.** Our thirst mechanism is triggered by an increase in the concentration of electrolytes in the blood.
8. **False.** Hypernatremia is commonly caused by a rapid intake of high amounts of sodium.
9. **False.** Quenching our thirst does not guarantee adequate hydration. Urine that is clear or light yellow in color is one indicator of adequate hydration.
10. **False.** These conditions are associated with decreased fluid loss or an increase in body fluid. Diarrhea, blood loss, and low humidity are conditions that increase fluid loss.
11. Chronic diarrhea in a young child can lead to severe dehydration very quickly due to his or her small body size. Diarrhea causes excessive fluid loss from the intestinal tract and extracellular fluid compartment. This fluid loss causes a rise in extracellular electrolyte concentration,

and intracellular fluid leaves the cells in an attempt to balance the extracellular fluid loss. These alterations in fluid and electrolyte balance change the flow of electrical impulses through the heart and can lead to abnormal heart rhythms and eventual death if left untreated.

12. One possible cause of these symptoms is dehydration. You most likely lost a significant amount of fluid during the cross-country relay race. In addition, you consumed a few beers after the race. Beer is a diuretic, which causes you to lose even more fluid. The "pins and needles" feeling in your extremities is consistent with a fluid loss of about 3% to 5% of body weight. To maintain your health and support optimal performance, it is critical that you make every effort to consume enough fluid (preferably water, a sports beverage, or some other beverage that is not a diuretic) to regain any body water you lost due to your athletic efforts.

13. Although there are many things to consider when consuming foods prior to exercise, one important factor is consuming an optimal balance of fluid and electrolytes. In this case, lunch (b) would be the better choice. Lunch (a) is very high in sodium. While our bodies need adequate sodium to function properly, lunch (a) is filled with very high-sodium foods, such as chicken soup, ham, and tomato juice. It is likely that consuming lunch (a) will lead to excessive thirst due to a rise in blood sodium levels. This excessive thirst could cause distraction or even lead to consuming so much fluid that you feel nauseous during practice. Lunch (b) has a more desirable balance of sodium and fluid, should not cause excessive thirst, and should provide ample energy for hockey practice.

14. Most over-the-counter weight-loss pills are diuretics, which means that they cause fluid loss from the body. Your cousin should avoid diuretics, as she needs to maintain her fluid levels at a higher-than-normal level due to breastfeeding. If she becomes dehydrated, she cannot produce adequate milk for her infant. In addition, the substances in the weight-loss pills could be passed along to her infant in her breast milk, which could cause serious health consequences for the infant.

15. Her muscle cramps may be prompted by an electrolyte imbalance brought on by dehydration.

16. To estimate total fluid loss: 3 lb weight loss × 2 cups fluid lost/lb weight loss = 6 cups fluid lost during practice. To estimate total fluid needed for rehydration: 6 cups fluid lost × 1.5 = 9 cups fluid needed for full rehydration.

Chapter 10

1. **d.** It is destroyed by exposure to high heat.
2. **b.** an atom loses an electron.
3. **a.** cardiovascular disease.
4. **d.** nitrates.
5. **a.** vitamin A.
6. **True.**
7. **True.**
8. **False.** Vitamin C helps regenerate vitamin E.

9. **True.**
10. **False.** Pregnant women should not consume beef liver very often, as it can lead to vitamin A toxicity and potentially serious birth defects.
11. Free radicals steal electrons from the stable lipid molecules in our cell membranes. This stealing can destroy the integrity of the membrane and lead to membrane dysfunction and potential cell death.
12. Cancer development has three primary steps: initiation, promotion, and progression. During the initiation step, the DNA of normal cells is mutated, causing permanent changes in the cell. During the promotion step, the genetically altered cells repeatedly divide, locking the mutated DNA into each new cell's genetic instructions. During the progression step, the cancerous cells grow out of control and invade surrounding tissues. These cells then metastasize, or spread, to other sites of the body.
13. Vitamin E may help reduce our risk for heart disease in a number of ways. Vitamin E protects LDLs from oxidation, thus helping reduce the buildup of plaque in our blood-vessel walls. Vitamin E may also help reduce low-grade inflammation. Vitamin E is known to reduce blood coagulation and the formation of blood clots, which will reduce the risk of a blood clot clogging a blood vessel and causing a stroke or heart attack.
14. Trace minerals such as selenium, copper, iron, zinc, and manganese are part of the antioxidant enzyme systems that convert free radicals to less damaging substances that are excreted by our bodies. Selenium is part of the glutathione peroxidase enzyme system. Copper, zinc, and manganese are part of the superoxide dismutase enzyme complex, and iron is a part of the structure of catalase.
15. Yes, you should be concerned. Vitamin E acts as an anticoagulant, and combined with the prescription anticoagulant Coumadin, the effects are magnified, which could cause uncontrollable bleeding. This could lead to internal bleeding and prevent the cessation of bleeding caused by a cut or other external injury. In some people, long-term use of standard vitamin E supplements may cause hemorrhaging in the brain, leading to a type of stroke called hemorrhagic stroke. It would be prudent to tell your mother about your concerns, and suggest that she stop taking the supplement until she has discussed with her healthcare provider the potential interactions with her medication and this supplement.
16. a) Each tablet contains 400 IU of the synthetic form of vitamin E. In supplements containing the synthetic form of vitamin E, 1 IU is equal to 0.45 mg α-TE. To convert IU to mg α-TE = 400 IU $\times$ 0.45 = 180 mg α-TE, which is equal to 180 mg of active vitamin E.

    b) The RDA for vitamin A is 15 mg alpha-tocopherol per day. To calculate the percentage of the RDA for vitamin E coming from the supplements = (180 mg α-TE $\div$ 15 mg α-TE) $\times$ 100 = 1200%.

    The tolerable upper intake level is 1,000 mg alpha-tocopherol per day, and thus the amount coming from

the supplement is relatively small at 180 mg. Although in the past up to 18 times the RDA has been shown to be safe (18 $\times$ 15 mg = 270 mg of alpha-tocopherol per day), recent evidence suggests that even 400 IU per day could increase the risk for premature mortality. Thus it would be safest for Joey's mother to obtain adequate vitamin E from her diet. If she is taking aspirin each day as prescribed, it is imperative that she stop taking vitamin E supplements, as aspirin is an anticoagulant and taking vitamin E supplements could enhance its action and result in uncontrollable bleeding and hemorrhaging.

Chapter 11

1. **a.** calcium and phosphorus.
2. **c.** has normal bone density as compared to an average, healthy 30-year-old.
3. **d.** It provides the scaffolding for cortical bone.
4. **c.** a dark-skinned retiree living in Illinois.
5. **d.** structure of bone, nerve transmission, and muscle contraction.
6. **True.**
7. **True.**
8. **False.** The fractures that result from osteoporosis cause an increased risk for infection and other related illnesses that can lead to premature death.
9. **True.**
10. **True.**
11. Because vitamins D and K are fat-soluble vitamins, they are absorbed with the fat we consume in our diets. If a person has a disease that does not allow for proper absorption of dietary fat, there will also be a malabsorption of the fat-soluble vitamins, which include vitamins D and K.
12. The two processes behind this phenomenon are bone resorption and bone formation. The combination of these processes is referred to as bone remodeling. To preserve bone density, our bodies attempt to achieve a balance between the breakdown of older bone tissue and the formation of new bone tissue.

    One of the primary reasons that bone is broken down is to release calcium into the bloodstream. We also want to break down bone when we fracture a bone and need to repair it. During resorption, osteoclasts erode the bone surface by secreting enzymes and acids that dig grooves into the bone matrix. Their ruffled surface also acts much as a scrubbing brush to assist in the erosion process. Once bone is broken down, the products are transported into the bloodstream and utilized for various body functions.

    Osteoblasts work to form new bone. These cells help synthesize new bone matrix by laying down the collagen-containing organic component of bone. Within this substance, the hydroxapatites crystallize and pack together to create new bone where it is needed.

    In young, healthy adults, the processes of bone resorption and formation are equal, so that just as much bone is broken down as is being built. The result is that bone mass is maintained. At around 40 years of age, bone resorption begins to occur more rapidly than bone formation, and this imbalance results in an overall loss in bone density. This loss of bone density affects all bones, including the vertebrae of the spine, and thus results in a loss of height as we age.

13. This meal does not ensure that your calcium needs for the day are met because our bodies can absorb only about 500 mg of calcium at one time. Although this meal contains more than 100% of the DRI for calcium, you cannot absorb all of the calcium present. To meet your daily calcium needs, it is recommended that you eat multiple servings of calcium-rich foods throughout the day and try to consume no more than 500 mg of calcium at one time.

14. The sunlight is not sufficient in Buffalo, New York, during the winter to provide adequate vitamin D for anyone. Thus, all people living in this climate in winter need to consume vitamin D in foods and/or supplements to meet their needs.

15. The amount of calcium absorbed from 1 cup of skim milk is 96 mg. The amount of calcium absorbed from 1 cup of broccoli is 37 mg. Thus skim milk has 96 mg ÷ 37 mg = 2.6 times the amount of absorbable calcium as compared to broccoli. You would have to eat 1 cup × 2.6 = 2.6 cups of broccoli to absorb the same amount of calcium as in 1 cup of skim milk.

Chapter 12

1. **b.** vitamin K.
2. **b.** Iron is a component of hemoglobin, myoglobin, and certain enzymes.
3. **c.** vitamins B_6, folate, and B_{12}.
4. **a.** plasma cells.
5. **d.** antibodies.
6. **True.**
7. **False.** Iron deficiency causes iron-deficiency anemia; pernicious anemia occurs at the end stage of an autoimmune disorder that causes the loss of various cells in the stomach, which leads to a deficiency of vitamin B_{12}.
8. **False.** Wilson's disease is a rare disorder that causes copper toxicity.
9. **True.**
10. **True.**
11. Jessica is at a higher risk for iron-deficiency anemia due to her menstrual status and the fact that she consumes only plant-based foods. Plant-based foods contain only the non-heme form of iron, which is more difficult to absorb. Consuming vitamin C enhances the absorption of iron from our foods; thus, it is imperative that Jessica's parents encourage her to eat good plant-based food sources of iron with a vitamin C source to optimize her iron absorption and reduce her risk for iron-deficiency anemia.
12. Based on this diet, Robert does not appear at risk for inadequate micronutrient intake. The foods he consumes contain all of the necessary micronutrients, and as long as he continues to eat a wide variety of foods from these groups, his risk for inadequate intakes of micronutrients is very low.
13. **a.** Janine is of childbearing age. It is recommended that all women of childbearing age consume adequate folate even if they do not plan to become pregnant. This recommendation is made to reduce the risk for neural tube defects in the developing fetus in case a woman does become pregnant. **b.** Janine is avoiding foods that are excellent sources of folate, including many vegetables and enriched grain products. Thus, it is likely that her intake of folate is inadequate. If she continues to avoid these folate-rich foods, a folate supplement may be warranted.
14. Both underweight and obese people have an increased risk for infection and, if they are infected, an increased risk that the infection will be severe. Undernutrition reduces defense against infection because micronutrient deficiencies impair immune function. In obese individuals, most studies show a lower ability of B and T cells to multiply in response to infection. Obese individuals also appear to maintain a low-grade inflammatory state, currently thought to increase the likelihood that they will develop asthma, type 2 diabetes, and other disorders that would increase the severity of infection.
15. This statement is false. Although 20 mg/day × 100 days = 2000 mg, or 2 g, zinc absorption rates range from just 10–35% of dietary intake.

Chapter 13

1. **d.** body mass index.
2. **a.** basal metabolic rate, thermic effect of food, and effect of physical activity.
3. **b.** take in more energy than they expend.
4. **c.** all people have a genetic set point for their body weight.
5. **b.** ghrelin.
6. **False.** It is the apple-shaped fat patterning, or excess fat in the trunk region, that is known to increase a person's risk for many chronic diseases.
7. **True.**
8. **False.** Weight-loss medications are typically prescribed for people with a body mass index greater than or equal to 30 kg/m^2, or for people with a body mass index greater than or equal to 27 kg/m^2 who also have other significant health risk factors, such as heart disease, high blood pressure, or type 2 diabetes.
9. **False.** Healthful weight gain includes eating more energy than you expend and exercising both to maintain aerobic fitness and to build muscle mass.
10. **True.**
11. A weight that is appropriate for your age and physical development; a weight that you can achieve and sustain without restraining your food intake or constantly dieting; a weight that is acceptable to you; a weight that is based on your genetic background and family history of body shape and weight; a weight that promotes good eating habits and allows you to participate in regular physical activity.
12. *Dietary recommendations for a sound weight-loss program include the following:*
    a. Set reasonable weight-loss goals. Reasonable weight loss is defined as 0.5 to 2 pounds per week. To achieve this rate of weight loss, energy intake should be reduced approximately 250 to no more than 1,000 kcal/d of present intake. A weight-loss plan should never provide less than a total of 1,200 kcal/d.
    b. Eat a diet that is relatively low in fat and high in complex carbohydrates. Total fat intake should be 15% to 25% of total energy intake. Saturated fat intake should be 5% to 10% of total energy intake. Monounsaturated fat intake should be 10% to 15% of total energy intake. Polyunsaturated fat intake should be no more than 10% of total energy intake. Carbohydrate intake should be around 55% of total energy intake, with less than 10% of energy intake coming from simple sugars, and fiber intake should be 25 to 35 g/day.
    Physical activity recommendation: Set a long-term goal for physical activity that is at least 30 minutes of moderate physical activity most, or preferably all, days of the week. Doing 45 minutes or more of an activity such as walking at least 5 days per week is ideal.
    Behavior modification recommendations include:
    a. Eliminating inappropriate behaviors by shopping when you are not hungry, only eating at set times in one location, refusing to buy problem foods, and avoiding vending machines, convenience stores, and fast-food restaurants
    b. Suppressing inappropriate behaviors by taking small food portions, eating foods on smaller serving dishes so they appear larger, and avoiding feelings of deprivation by eating regular meals throughout the day
    c. Strengthening appropriate behaviors by sharing food with others, learning appropriate serving sizes, planning healthful snacks, scheduling walks and other physical activities with friends, and keeping clothes and equipment for physical activity in convenient places
    d. Repeating desired behaviors by slowing down eating, always using utensils, leaving food on your plate, moving more throughout the day, and joining groups who are physically active
    e. Rewarding yourself for positive behaviors with non-food rewards
    f. Using the "buddy" system by exercising with a friend or relative and/or calling this support person when you need an extra boost to stay motivated
    g. Refusing to punish yourself if you deviate from your plan
13. You can increase your basal metabolic rate by increasing your lean body mass or by using drugs such as stimulants, caffeine, and tobacco. Stress and certain illnesses can also increase BMR. The most healthful way to increase BMR is to increase your lean body mass by participating in regular strength-training exercises. Attempting to increase your BMR by using drugs or by increasing your stress is not wise and can be dangerous to your health.
14. **a.** Greater access to inexpensive, high-fat, high-Calorie foods (for example, fast foods, vending machine foods, and snack/convenience foods)
    b. Significant increases in portion sizes of foods
    c. Increased reliance on cars instead of bicycles, public transportation, or walking
    d. Use of elevators and escalators instead of stairs
    e. Increased use of computers, dishwashers, televisions, and other time-saving devices
    f. Lack of safe, accessible, and affordable places to exercise
15. To calculate Misty's BMI, first convert her weight in lb to kg: 148 lb/2.2 lb per kg = 67.3 kg.
    Then convert her height in inches to meters = 5'8" = 68 in × 0.0254 m/in = 1.73 m.
    Then square her height in meters = 1.73 m × 1.73 m = 2.99 m^2.
    Then calculate her BMI by dividing her weight in kg by height in square meters = 67.3 kg/2.99 m^2 = 22.5 kg/m^2. Based on this BMI value, it is clear that Misty is not overweight.
    One primary question for Misty is, What is her idea of her ideal weight? It sounds as if Misty might have significant body image concerns. If this is the case, it is important that she meet with a healthcare provider or nutrition professional who can assist her with improving her body image perceptions.

Another question is, What weight can she achieve and sustain without trying so hard (in other words, without restricting her food intake or constantly dieting)? The fact that she must try so hard and is still not losing weight is a good indication that she may already be at the weight that is healthful.

A third question is, How does her current weight and body shape compare to her genetic background and family history? If her body weight and shape are consistent with her genetic makeup and family history, she may have unrealistic expectations of reducing her body weight or significantly altering her shape.

A final question Misty should consider is whether she is able to maintain her current weight by being regularly active and by eating a healthful, balanced diet. If not, then this is another indication that her body weight goals are unrealistic.

16. To answer this question, you first need to calculate Misty's BMR. This can be done in two steps:
1. To estimate how many kcal per hour Misty expends at her present body weight, multiply her body weight in kg by 0.9 kcal/kg body weight/hour = 0.9 kcal/kg body weight/hr $\times$ 67.3 kg = 60.57 kcal/hour.
2. To calculate her BMR for the total day (or 24 hours) = 60.57 kcal/hour $\times$ 24 hours = 1454 kcal/day.

Misty's activity level is classified as moderately active. According to the values presented in the chapter, the energy cost of Misty's activities ranges from 50% to 70% of her BMR. Thus the range of energy that Misty expends at her current activity level is equal to:
- 1454 kcal/day $\times$ 0.50 (or 50%) = 727 kcal/day
- 1454 kcal/day $\times$ 0.70 (or 70%) = 1018 kcal/day

To calculate Misty's total energy expenditure in kcal each day, add together BMR and the energy needed to perform her daily activities:
- 1454 kcal/day + 727 kcal/day = 2181 kcal/day
- 1454 kcal/day + 1018 kcal/day = 2472 kcal/day

Assuming Misty is maintaining weight at her current activity level, she needs between 2181 and 2472 kcal/day to stay in energy balance.

Chapter 14

1. **c.** 50% to 70% of your estimated maximal heart rate.
2. **a.** 1 to 3 seconds.
3. **b.** fat.
4. **c.** can increase strength gained in resistance exercise.
5. **c.** It involves altering both exercise duration and carbohydrate intake to maximize the amount of muscle glycogen.
6. **True.**
7. **False.** A dietary fat intake of 20% to 35% of total energy intake is generally recommended for athletes.
8. **True.**
9. **False.** Sports anemia is not true anemia, but a transient decrease in iron stores that occurs at the start of an exercise program. This is a result of an initial increase in plasma volume (water in our blood) that is not matched by an increase in hemoglobin.
10. **True.**
11. The most helpful strategy you might consider is the use of sports beverages. Sports beverages were designed for people who exercise for more than 60 minutes at a time and are specially formulated to replenish the fluid and micronutrients that are lost during intense, long-duration exercise. By consuming sports beverages during training for a marathon, you can ensure that you are maintaining adequate hydration levels and can avoid hyponatremia by replenishing sodium.
12. Gustavo is 69 years of age, has high blood pressure, and has a family history of colon cancer. He manages a vineyard. You would need to know a little bit more about his occupation to determine his level of activity at work. However, based on his health status, Gustavo could most likely benefit from participating in a planned exercise program of low to moderate intensity. This type of program will help keep his blood pressure under better control; will reduce his risk for cardiovascular disease, stroke, and type 2 diabetes; will help Gustavo maintain a healthful body weight; and will assist in maintaining bone density. This type of program may also reduce his risk for colon cancer. Before Gustavo begins an exercise program, he should get a thorough physical exam by his physician because of his older age and his high-blood-pressure status. His physician can then determine the safest forms of physical activity for Gustavo.
13. Factors that assist Marisa in maintaining a normal, healthful weight include the following:
    - Walking to/from school each day
    - Covering the lunch shift at her college's day care center, which requires that she be on her feet, walk, and perform light lifting 2 hours each day
    - Walking on the weekends
    Factors that contribute to Conrad's weight gain include the following:
    - Driving to school each day
    - working an office job 2 hours each day
    - Going to the movies on the weekends instead of doing some form of physical activity
14. There are an infinite number of correct answers to this question. The plan outlined here is for a 40-year-old woman who is interested in maintaining a healthful body weight, optimizing her blood lipid profile, reducing her stress, and maintaining aerobic fitness, flexibility, and upper body strength. She works full-time as a research scientist, and most of her occupational activities are sedentary.
    - **Monday and Wednesday:** 60 minutes of fitness walking (including 5-minute warm-up and 5-minute cooldown)
    - **Tuesday and Thursday:** 75 minutes of power/ashtanga yoga (including warm-up and cool-down); 45 minutes of morning swimming (substitute with bicycling in the summer months)

- **Friday:** 60 minutes of fitness walking (including warm-up and cool-down); 30 minutes of gardening
- **Saturday:** 75 minutes of hatha yoga (including warm-up and cool-down); 120 minutes of gardening
- **Sunday:** 30 minutes of hatha yoga (including warm-up and cool-down); 180 minutes of hiking with a light daypack.

15. **a)** Liz's suggested intake for protein is identified as 1.5 grams per kg body weight. Her body weight is equal to 105 lbs ÷ 2.2 = 47.7 kg. Her protein intake (in grams) is equal to 1.5 grams protein/kg body weight × 47.7 kg = 71.6 grams
    b) Liz's preferred fat intake is 20% of her total daily energy intake, thus 1,800 kcal × 0.20 = 360 kcal. As the energy value of fat is 9 kcal per gram, her total intake of fat in grams = 360 kcal ÷ 9 kcal/gram = 40 grams of fat.
    c) To calculate Liz's carbohydrate intake, you must first determine the amount of kcal of her total energy intake that remains once her protein and fat intake are accounted for.
    - Liz's protein intake is 71.6 grams; as the energy value of protein is 4 kcal per gram, her kcal intake from protein = 71.6 grams × 4 kcal/gram = 286.4 kcal
    - Liz's fat intake has already been calculated as 360 kcal
    - As Liz's total energy intake is 1,800 kcal per day, the amount of kcal she'll consume from carbohydrate = 1,800 kcal – 286.4 kcal – 360 kcal = 1153.6 kcal of carbohydrate.
    - The energy value of carbohydrates is 4 kcal per gram, and thus Liz's intake of carbohydrate in grams is equal to 1153.6 kcal ÷ 4 kcal/gram = 288.4 grams
    To determine if Liz's carbohydrate intake falls within the AMDR = (1153.6 kcal of carbohydrate ÷ 1,800 kcal) × 100 = 64%. Thus her carbohydrate intake does fall within the AMDR.

Chapter 15

1. **c.** 40 degrees F.
2. **c.** within 2 hours of serving.
3. **c.** a type of fungus used to ferment foods.
4. **d.** all of the above.
5. **a.** contain only organically produced ingredients, excluding water and salt.
6. **False.**
7. **True.**
8. **True.**
9. **False.**
10. **False.**
11. No, this food is not 100% organic. This is because it contains whey, which is a protein from cow's milk. This item is not designated as organic. Remember that to be considered 100% organic a food must contain only organically produced ingredients, excluding water and salt. This food also contains food additives; in this case, the additive is salt.

12. The safest choice is to select the pasteurized juice. Unpasteurized beverages (such as juices and milk) may contain a significant number of microbes that can cause food-borne illnesses. Pasteurization does not eliminate all microbes but significantly decreases the numbers of heat-sensitive microorganisms, which tend to be the most harmful. The amount of pesticides found in juice is most likely very low or zero, as the pesticides would have been applied to the trees and oranges with the peel on the fruit. It is highly likely that this juice contains none of the pesticides that may have been used, because the peel is not used to make the juice.

13. There are a few different processes of pickling, but this process requires the use of vinegar and salt. The vinegar used works to destroy microbes that cause food-borne illness (particularly the *Clostridium botulinum* bacterium). The salt used not only adds flavor but also inhibits spoilage and the growth of harmful bacteria.

14. Based on this brief description, it sounds as if the cause of this disease was mercury poisoning. Mercury, a naturally occurring element, is found in soil, rocks, lakes, streams, and oceans. It is also released into the environment by pulp and paper processing and the burning of garbage and fossil fuels. As mercury is released into the environment, it falls from the air, eventually finding its way into streams, lakes, and oceans. Fish absorb mercury as they feed on aquatic organisms. This mercury is passed on to people when they consume the fish. As mercury accumulates in the body, it has a toxic effect on the nervous system. Mercury is especially toxic to the developing nervous systems of fetuses and growing children. Thus, pregnant and breastfeeding women and young children are advised to avoid eating fish that may be contaminated with mercury.

    Based on an Internet search, it appears that Minamata disease was caused by mercury poisoning. A variety of heavy metals were used in a highly successful industrial plant on Minamata Bay. After careful study and elimination of other toxic chemicals used in this industrial plant, it was discovered that the disease experienced by these people was a result of mercury poisoning.

15. **a.** Failure to wash your hands before you removed chicken from the freezer. You touched the chicken when you placed it in the bowl to thaw in the refrigerator.
    b. Failure to wash your hands with hot water and soap prior to putting the chicken breasts on the cutting board.
    c. Failure to wash the chicken breasts thoroughly prior to putting them on the clean cutting board.
    d. Failure to wash your hands with hot water and soap after handling the chicken breasts just prior to touching and rinsing the lettuce, red pepper, and scallions.
    e. Failure to check the temperature of the chicken breasts. Even though they were no longer pink in color, they may not have been cooked to a high enough temperature to kill bacteria.

Chapter 16

1. **b.** neural tube defects.
2. **c.** oxytocin.
3. **c.** iron.
4. **b.** women who begin their pregnancy underweight.
5. **d.** pureed meat.
6. **False.** These issues are most likely to occur in the first trimester of pregnancy.
7. **True.**
8. **True.**
9. **True.**
10. **False.** Newborns of mothers with gestational diabetes are at risk for overly large body size.
11. *Advantages:* offers optimal nutritional quality; protects infants from infections and allergies; reduces risk for sudden infant death syndrome; quickens the return of the uterus in the mother to pre-pregnancy size and reduces post-pregnancy bleeding; suppresses ovulation, which lengthens the time between pregnancies and gives the mother's body time to recover before conceiving again; provides for mother–infant bonding and attachment; is more convenient than bottle-feeding; is less expensive than bottle-feeding.

    Disadvantages: allows passage of drugs (caffeine, prescription drugs), alcohol, and irritating components of foods such as onion or garlic; causes allergic reactions to foods mother eats, such as wheat, peanuts, and cow's milk; transmits HIV from mother to infant in mothers who are HIV-positive; creates the need for the mother to balance the challenges of regular breastfeeding with job duties; causes sleep deprivation for the mother due to feeding every 2 to 3 hours; is associated with social concerns, such as exposing breasts in public and discomfort of others who may observe breastfeeding in public.

12. After reviewing the girl's typical dietary intake, I would discuss the importance of appropriate prenatal weight gain (not too much, not too little; the importance of taking folic acid, iron, and possibly calcium supplements; and the need to avoid alcohol, street drugs, and (unless prescribed by her healthcare provider) medications.

13. It is possible that your cousin is partly right and partly wrong. If she is very careful and consumes a wide variety of nutrient-dense foods, she is likely consuming adequate amounts of the macronutrients and many of the micronutrients she needs to support her pregnancy. However, there are some nutrients that are extremely difficult to consume in adequate amounts in the diet during pregnancy, as a woman's needs are very high for these nutrients. One of these nutrients is iron.

    During pregnancy, the demand for red blood cells increases to accommodate the needs of the growing uterus, the placenta, and the fetus itself. Thus, more iron is needed. Fetal demand for iron increases even further during the last trimester, when the fetus stores iron in the liver for use during the first few months of life. This iron storage is protective, because breast milk is low in iron.

    Because of these risks, the RDA for iron for pregnant women is 27 mg per day, compared to 18 mg per day for non-pregnant women. Even though your cousin feels her eating habits are sufficient, it is highly likely that she had low iron stores prior to pregnancy, as this is a common problem in many women. Women have a difficult time consuming 18 mg of iron per day in their diets; consuming twice this amount is extremely difficult, if not impossible, for most women. Thus, women of childbearing age typically have poor iron stores, and the demands of pregnancy are likely to produce deficiency. To ensure adequate iron stores during pregnancy, an iron supplement (as part of, or distinct from, a total prenatal supplement) is routinely prescribed during the last two trimesters. In addition, consuming vitamin C will enhance iron absorption, as do dietary sources of heme iron.

14. Based on this description, it is possible that Katie has a condition referred to as colic. Overstimulation of the nervous system, feeding too rapidly, swallowing of air, and intestinal gas pain are considered possible culprits, but the precise cause is unknown. As with allergies, if a colicky infant is breastfed, breastfeeding should be continued, but the parents should try to determine whether eating certain foods seems to prompt crying and, if so, eliminate the offending food(s) from her diet. Formula-fed infants may benefit from a change in type of formula. In the worst cases of colic, a physician may prescribe medication. Fortunately, most cases disappear spontaneously, possibly because of maturity of the gastrointestinal tract, around 3 months of age. It is important that Katie's parents discuss her condition with her pediatrician before making any decisions about changing her diet.

15. The primary information to share with this woman is that breastfeeding is recommended for all children up to at least 2 years (24 months) of age. Thus, an 11-month-old child is not too old to be breastfed. In addition, it is also possible that this woman is offended by seeing your sister breastfeed in public. If this is the case, it is important to point out that all women have the right to breastfeed in a public place. If this woman is offended, she can leave the area or choose not to observe your sister as she breastfeeds her child.

16. **a)** To calculate the % of kcal in breast milk that come from fat:
    First convert grams of fat to fat kcal: 35 g fat/liter $\times$ 9 kcal/g = 315 fat kcal/liter.

    Then calculate the % of total breast milk kcal from fat: [315 fat kcal divided by 700 total kcal] $\times$ 100 (to convert to percentage) = 45% of kcal in breast milk are from fat.

    b) To calculate the % of kcal in breast milk that come from protein:
    First convert grams of protein to protein kcal: 9 g protein $\times$ 4 kcal/g = 36 protein kcal.

    Then calculate the % of total breast milk kcal from protein: [36 kcal divided by 700 total kcal] $\times$ 100 (to convert to percentage) = 5% of kcal from protein.

45% of kcal from fat is much higher than the range that is recommended for healthy young adults (20–35% of total kcal from fat), but a high fat diet is needed to meet the energy needs of rapidly growing infants. 5% of kcal from protein is much lower that what is recommended for most young adults (10–35% of total kcal from protein), but the kidneys of young infants are immature and not able to excrete large amounts of nitrogen. The small gastric capacity of infants and their relatively immature kidneys explain why the proportions of Calories from fat and protein in breast milk are ideally suited for young infants.

Chapter 17

1. **d.** greater than that for young children, adults, and pregnant adults.
2. **c.** 45% to 65%.
3. **b.** skipping breakfast.
4. **b.** 2 tablespoons of plain yogurt, 2 tablespoons of applesauce, 2 tablespoons of fortified whole-grain oat cereal, and 1/2 cup of calcium-fortified orange juice.
5. **a.** Cigarette smoking can interfere with the metabolism of nutrients.
6. **True.**
7. **False.** Children are able to understand the basic information about which foods are more nutritious and which foods should be eaten in moderation. Also, parents are important role models for children.
8. **False.** The DRI for calcium remains at 1,300 mg per day up through the age of 18 years.
9. **False.** The Institute of Medicine now recommends that children participate in daily physical activity and exercise for at least an hour each day.
10. **True.** Adolescents typically experience a 9- to 11-inch increase in height during their 2- to 3-year growth spurt. With this increase in height, normal-weight adolescents need to gain a proportional amount of weight. In males, much of that weight is lean body mass, while female adolescents tend to gain a higher proportion of body fat.
11. *Advantages:* improved access to a wider variety of affordable fresh, healthful foods from around the United States and the world; improved access to nutrition and health information from a variety of sources, including television and Internet sources; improved access to interactive nutrition and healthful lifestyle programs that encourage family participation
    Disadvantages: reduced energy expenditure due to increased television viewing and computer use leading to obesity; lower fitness levels and higher risk for chronic diseases due to the lack of physical activity; increased exposure to advertisements promoting junk foods and less healthful foods; failure to acquire important physical skills because not much time is spent engaged in physical activities; inhibition of imagination and creativity in young children because they do not have to develop skills necessary for creative play
12. Toddlers are relatively picky eaters, and they are small individuals and can only consume small amounts of food at any give time. In consuming a vegan diet, the primary sources of quality proteins are restricted to legumes, meat substitutes, and various combinations of vegetables and whole grains. It is highly likely that a vegan diet will be too low in protein for toddlers, as their protein needs are relatively high. Few toddlers can consume enough legumes and whole grains to provide sufficient protein, and many may not prefer the taste of vegetables and meat substitutes. In addition, certain staples of the vegan diet that are high in protein, such as wheat, soy, and nuts, commonly provoke allergic reactions in children. When this happens, finding a plant-based substitute that contains adequate protein and other nutrients can be challenging.
13. There are numerous correct answers to this question. The key to designing a menu for this age group is to keep in mind that these children need adequate fluid, and they do not eat large amounts of food. The foods should also look fun and attractive to encourage regular snacking and should be easy to eat when the children are active. Here are some foods you may want to offer to these children:
    - Ample water in small, colored plastic cups
    - Whole-grain crackers that are small and easy to eat
    - Small chunks of different colors and flavors of cheese to eat with the crackers (or you could make peanut butter/whole-grain cracker "sandwiches")
    - Baby carrot sticks
    - Orange slices
14. Here are three of many lunch choices that you could offer to these students:
    - Menu 1: bean burrito with salsa; rice; low/no-fat milk; fresh fruit
    - Menu 2: grilled turkey and muenster cheese sandwich on whole-wheat bread; assorted raw vegetables; pineapple/orange yogurt fruit smoothie
    - Menu 3: chicken and vegetable teriyaki rice bowl; fruit skewers; low/no-fat milk
15. A registered dietitian would be concerned about (1) Lydia's monotonous and unbalanced diet, (2) her lack of physical activity, and (3) Lydia's potential homesickness and isolation. Her poor dietary habits are probably contributing to a lack of protein as well as most vitamins and minerals. Her poor diet and the fact that she lives in a northern region almost certainly mean that she is vitamin D deficient, and her consumption of soda rather than milk or a calcium-fortified beverage further increases her risk for low bone density. These deficiencies may also account for some of her lethargy and lack of physical activity. By guiding Lydia toward more healthful meals and menus, she would feel more energetic and be more likely to ride a bicycle, take an activity class, or join a gym.

    A regular routine of physical activity would probably stimulate Lydia's appetite, encouraging her to consume greater amounts of food, hopefully healthy food! Lydia's move from Vermont to New York could account for her isolation; she may need additional guidance in finding and developing new friendships. If Lydia had always lived at home, where someone else prepared the meals, she would benefit from specific sessions on planning menus, shopping for healthful foods, and preparing daily meals.

16. 1/3 of 1,300 mg is 433 mg. She would get 230 mg Ca from spinach, 100 mg from the tofu, and 225 mg from the orange juice for a total of 555 mg. Yes, she would meet 1/3rd of her calcium RDA.

Chapter 18

1. **b.** vitamin D.
2. **a.** dysgeusia.
3. **d.** 122 years.
4. **c.** glycosylation.
5. **c.** palliative care.
6. **True.** Programmed theories of aging imply that the aging process is biologically driven and rarely, if ever, affected by lifestyle traits, such as diet.
7. **True.** As humans age, percentage of body fat typically increases. Even if elderly persons lose weight during their seventies or eighties, body fat increases as a percentage of their total body weight.
8. **True.** Elderly who are overweight or obese have lower rates of mortality compared to those who are underweight.
9. **True.** Vitamin B_{12} found in food sources is often bound to food proteins and is difficult for older adults to digest and absorb due to their lack of adequate stomach acidity. The vitamin B_{12} found in supplements or fortified foods is not protein-bound; therefore, it is easier to absorb.
10. **True.**
11. Lack of adequate stomach acid can lower the absorption of vitamin B_{12}, calcium, iron, and zinc, increasing the risk for deficiencies of these nutrients.
12. **a.** If not fluent in English, an elderly immigrant woman may not be confident enough to go out to shop for food on a regular basis, or she may not qualify for a driver's license, which would affect her ability to obtain food. In both cases, she might have to purchase food from the nearest convenience store (not the best source), and/or simply run low on food, possibly leading to malnutrition. **b.** If isolated, with no Southeast Asian friends or relatives nearby, the woman could easily become depressed, which often results in poor food intake and rapid onset of nutrient deficiencies.
13. Older adults may purposefully limit fluid intake to avoid embarrassing "accidents" due to poor bladder control; they may be taking medications that act as diuretics, increasing urinary output; many elderly fail to perceive thirst and may not drink adequate amounts of fluid during the day; and some elderly may not be able to drink enough fluids due to physical limitations related to a stroke, Parkinson's disease, or other neuromuscular disorders.
14. I would first try to determine why my client eats as he does: is he easily tired, does he have a poor appetite, is he inexperienced in planning and producing healthful meals, or is he

on a very limited budget? Depending on his circumstances, I would develop several simple but nutritious meal suggestions that have more protein, fiber, and total energy and a wider range of vitamins and minerals. Finally, I would discuss ways of improving his sleeping habits while limiting alcohol intake. Gentle physical activity during the day, a warm bath before bedtime, and avoidance of caffeine during the evening might help him sleep through the night without the need for beer.

15. The death of a spouse often triggers mental and physical declines in older adults. Loss of appetite, depression, loneliness, and fearfulness may contribute to a drastic reduction in food and fluid intake. Malnutrition and dehydration quickly develop, which then contribute to loss of balance, weakness, and fatigue. These factors may have lead to Marta's grandmother's fall and fracture.

16. To calculate the total vitamin A intake of Kristina's grandmother, add up the amount of Vitamin A in one dose of each of the three supplements: 3333 + 1500 + 2200 = 7033 μg of vitamin A/d.

    To calculate the % of the RDA consumed by Kristina's grandmother, take her daily total intake, divide by the RDA, and multiply by 100 to convert to a percent: [7033 μg ÷ 700 μg] × 100 = 1005% of the RDA, or, 10 times more than the recommended amount.

    To calculate the % of the vitamin A UL consumed by Kristina's grandmother each day, take her daily total intake, divide by the UL, and multiply by 100 to convert to a percent: [7033 μg ÷ 3000 μg] × 100 = 234% of the UL or more than twice the recommended upper limit. This amount of vitamin A, taken on a regular basis, could certainly lead to vitamin A toxicity over time. The UL for adults, including the elderly, is 3,000 μg/day.

    NOTE: These calculations reflect **% of the RDA, not % above the RDA.**

Chapter 19

1. **a.** sub-Saharan Africa.
2. **c.** It has dramatically increased worldwide production of rice, corn, and wheat at lower costs.
3. **b.** reduced resistance to infection.
4. **b.** single mothers and their children.
5. **c.** night blindness.
6. **True.**
7. **True.**
8. **True.**
9. **False.** The rise in global obesity rates has prompted a rise in rates of other chronic diseases, such as heart disease and type 2 diabetes.
10. **False.** Cotton, coffee, and tobacco are cash crops. Subsistence crops are those that can be eaten by the farmer, such as cassava or peanuts.
11. Women with access to education are more likely to have increased earning potential, access to information about

contraception, and information to use better health practices. These circumstances lead to smaller, healthier, more economically stable families.

12. Breast milk contains antibodies that protect against infections. In addition, there is a danger in developing countries of feeding infants with formula, because the use of unsanitary water for mixing batches of formula results in diarrheal diseases. Another problem is that overdilution of formula by families who cannot afford adequate amounts results in inadequate intake for the infant, whereas breast milk is likely to contain adequate amounts of the nutrients needed.

13. When undernutrition is endemic throughout an area, growth stunting becomes the norm. In such a population, a person who is of average height by U.S. standards would be considered unusually tall.

14. The family is dependent on the supplies available at the local food pantry. These supplies may provide for good nutrition but likely do not provide all nutrients regularly.

Therefore, Davie's nutrition status is likely to be compromised. Davie is at greatest risk for infection from drinking water from a nearby pond, particularly if his mother does not boil the water prior to consumption. Because they have limited access to medical care, they are likely to wait out infections, prolonging the time that the infection is resolved. This further exacerbates his nutrition status, makes him more susceptible to another infection, and makes it more likely that he will die from a prolonged fight with infection.

15. Mexico is a country experiencing economic growth and the nutrition transition. Obesity is becoming a serious problem for both adults and children. Because of obesity, type 2 diabetes is being diagnosed at younger and younger ages in the Hispanic population. The best solution to diabetes is prevention, and a concerned pediatrician is likely to be able to make a tremendous beneficial difference in the lives of the children he sees.

Glossary

A

absorption The physiologic process by which molecules of food are taken from the gastrointestinal tract into the circulation.

Acceptable Daily Intake (ADI) An estimate made by the Food and Drug Administration of the amount of a non-nutritive sweetener that someone can consume each day over a lifetime without adverse effects.

Acceptable Macronutrient Distribution Range (AMDR) A range of intakes for a particular energy source that is associated with reduced risk of chronic disease while providing adequate intakes of essential nutrients.

acetyl CoA Coenzyme A is derived from the B-vitamin pantothenic acid; it readily reacts with two-carbon acetate to form the metabolic intermediate acetyl CoA; sometimes referred to as *acetyl coenzyme A*.

acetylcholine A neurotransmitter that is involved in many functions, including muscle movement and memory storage.

achlorhydria Lack of gastric acid secretion.

acidosis A disorder in which the blood becomes acidic; that is, the level of hydrogen in the blood is excessive. It can be caused by respiratory or metabolic problems.

active transport A transport process that requires the use of energy to shuttle ions and molecules across the cell membrane in combination with a carrier protein.

added sugars Sugars and syrups that are added to food during processing or preparation.

adenosine diphosphate (ADP) A metabolic intermediate that results from the removal of one phosphate group from ATP.

adenosine monophosphate (AMP) A low-energy compound that results from the removal of two phosphate groups from ATP.

adenosine triphosphate (ATP) A high-energy compound made up of the purine adenine, the simple sugar ribose, and three phosphate units; it is used by cells as a source of metabolic energy.

adequate diet A diet that provides enough of the energy, nutrients, and fiber to maintain a person's health.

Adequate Intake (AI) A recommended average daily nutrient intake level based on observed or experimentally determined estimates of nutrient intake by a group of healthy people.

aerobic exercise Exercise that involves the repetitive movement of large muscle groups, increasing the body's use of oxygen and promoting cardiovascular health.

albumin A serum protein, made in the liver, that transports free fatty acids from one body tissue to another.

alcohol abuse A pattern of alcohol consumption, whether chronic or occasional, that results in harm to one's health, functioning, or interpersonal relationships.

alcohol dehydrogenase (ADH) An enzyme that converts ethanol to acetaldehyde in the first step of alcohol oxidation.

alcohol hangover A consequence of drinking too much alcohol; symptoms include headache, fatigue, dizziness, muscle aches, nausea and vomiting, sensitivity to light and sound, extreme thirst, and mood disturbances.

alcohol poisoning A potentially fatal condition in which an overdose of alcohol results in cardiac and/or respiratory failure.

alcohol Chemically, a compound characterized by the presence of a hydroxyl group; in common usage, a beverage made from fermented fruits, vegetables, or grains and containing ethanol.

alcoholic hepatitis Inflammation of the liver caused by alcohol; other forms of hepatitis can be caused by a virus or toxin.

alcoholism A disease state characterized by chronic dependence on alcohol.

aldehyde dehydrogenase (ALDH) An enzyme that oxidizes acetaldehyde to acetate.

aldosterone A hormone released from the adrenal glands that signals the kidneys to retain sodium and chloride, which in turn results in the retention of water.

alkalosis A disorder in which the blood becomes basic; that is, the level of hydrogen in the blood is deficient. It can be caused by respiratory or metabolic problems.

alpha bond A type of chemical bond that can be digested by enzymes found in the human intestine.

alpha-linolenic acid An essential fatty acid found in leafy green vegetables, flaxseed oil, soy oil, fish oil, and fish products; an omega-3 fatty acid.

amenorrhea The absence of menstruation. In females who had previously been menstruating, it is defined as the absence of menstrual periods for 3 or more continuous months.

amino acids Nitrogen-containing molecules that combine to form proteins.

amniotic fluid The watery fluid within the innermost membrane of the sac containing the fetus. It cushions and protects the growing fetus.

anabolic Refers to a substance that builds muscle and increases strength.

anabolism The process of making new molecules from smaller ones.

anencephaly A fatal neural tube defect in which there is partial absence of brain tissue, most likely caused by failure of the neural tube to close.

angiotensin II A potent vasoconstrictor that constricts the diameter of blood vessels and increases blood pressure; it also signals the release of the hormone aldosterone from the adrenal glands.

anorexia nervosa A serious, potentially life-threatening eating disorder that is characterized by self-starvation, which eventually leads to a deficiency in energy and essential nutrients required by the body to function normally.

antibodies Defensive proteins of the immune system. Their production is prompted by the presence of bacteria, viruses, toxins, and allergens.

antidiuretic hormone (ADH) A hormone released from the pituitary gland in response to an increase in blood solute concentration. ADH stimulates the kidneys to reabsorb water and to reduce the production of urine.

antigens Parts of a molecule, usually large proteins, from microbes, toxins, or other substances that are recognized by immune cells and activate an immune response.

antioxidant A compound that has the ability to prevent or repair the damage caused by oxidation.

antiserum Human or animal serum that contains antibodies to a particular antigen because of previous exposure to the disease or to a vaccine containing antigens from that infectious agent.

appetite A psychological desire to consume specific foods.

ariboflavinosis A condition caused by riboflavin deficiency.

Atherosclerosis A disease in which arterial walls accumulate deposits of lipids and scar tissue, which build up to a point at which they impair blood flow

atrophic gastritis A condition, frequently seen in people over the age of 50, in which stomach-acid secretions are low.

atrophy A decrease in the size and strength of muscles that occurs when they are not worked adequately.

autoimmune A destructive immune response directed toward an individual's own tissues.

B

B cells White blood cells that can become either antibody-producing plasma cells or memory cells.

bacteria Microorganisms that lack a true nucleus and reproduce by division or by spore formation.

balanced diet A diet that contains the combinations of foods that provide the proper proportions of nutrients.

basal metabolic rate (BMR) The energy the body expends to maintain its fundamental physiologic functions.

Behavioral Risk Factor Surveillance System (BRFSS) The world's largest telephone survey that tracks lifestyle behaviors that increase our risk for chronic disease.

beriberi A disease caused by thiamin deficiency, characterized by muscle wasting and nerve damage.

β-oxidation (fatty acid oxidation) A series of metabolic reactions that oxidize free fatty acids, leading to the end products of water, carbon dioxide, and ATP.

beta bond A type of chemical bond that cannot be easily digested by enzymes found in the human intestine.

bile Fluid produced by the liver and stored in the gallbladder; it emulsifies lipids in the small intestine.

binge drinking The consumption of five or more alcoholic drinks on one occasion.

binge eating Consumption of a large amount of food in a short period of time, usually accompanied by a feeling of loss of self-control.

binge-eating disorder A disorder characterized by binge eating an average of twice a week or more, typically without compensatory purging.

bioavailability The degree to which the body can absorb and use any given nutrient.

biologic age Physiologic age as determined by health and functional status; often estimated by scored questionnaires.

biomagnification The process by which persistent organic pollutants become more concentrated in animal tissues as they move from one creature to another through the food chain.

biopesticides Primarily insecticides, these chemicals use natural methods to reduce damage to crops.

bleaching process A reaction in which the rod cells in the retina lose their color when rhodopsin is split into retinal and opsin.

blood volume The amount of fluid in blood.

body composition The ratio of a person's body fat to lean body mass.

body fat mass The amount of body fat, or adipose tissue, a person has.

body image A person's perception of his or her body's appearance and functioning.

body mass index (BMI) A measurement representing the ratio of a person's body weight to his or her height.

bolus A mass of food that has been chewed and moistened in the mouth.

bone density The degree of compactness of bone tissue, reflecting the strength of the bones. *Peak bone density* is the point at which a bone is strongest.

brown adipose tissue A type of adipose tissue that has more mitochondria than white adipose tissue and can increase energy expenditure by uncoupling oxidation from ATP production. It is found in significant amounts in animals and newborn humans.

brush border The microvilli of the small intestine's lining. These microvilli tremendously increase the small intestine's absorptive capacity.

buffers Proteins that help maintain proper acid–base balance by attaching to, or releasing, hydrogen ions as conditions change in the body.

bulimia nervosa A serious eating disorder characterized by recurrent episodes of binge eating and recurrent inappropriate compensatory behaviors in order to prevent weight gain, such as self-induced vomiting, fasting, excessive exercise, or misuse of laxatives, diuretics, enemas, or other medications.

C

calcitonin A hormone secreted by the thyroid gland when blood calcium levels are too high. Calcitonin inhibits the actions of vitamin D, preventing reabsorption of calcium in the kidneys, limiting calcium absorption in the intestines, and inhibiting the osteoclasts from breaking down bone.

calcitriol The primary active form of vitamin D in the body.

calcium rigor A failure of muscles to relax, which leads to a hardening or stiffening of the muscles; caused by high levels of blood calcium.

calcium tetany A condition in which muscles experience twitching and spasms due to inadequate blood calcium levels.

calorimeter A special instrument in which food can be burned and the amount of heat that is released can be measured; this process demonstrates the energy (caloric) content of the food.

cancer A group of diseases characterized by cells that reproduce spontaneously and independently and may invade other tissues and organs.

carbohydrates One of the three macronutrients, a compound made up of carbon, hydrogen, and oxygen that is derived from plants and provides energy.

carbohydrate loading A process that involves altering training and carbohydrate intake so that muscle glycogen storage is maximized; also known as *glycogen loading*.

carbon skeleton The unique "side group" that remains after deamination of an amino acid; also referred to as a *keto acid*.

carcinogens Cancer-causing agents, such as certain pesticides, industrial chemicals, and pollutants.

cardiovascular disease A general term that refers to abnormal conditions involving dysfunction of the heart and blood vessels; cardiovascular disease can result in heart attack or stroke.

carnitine A small, organic compound that transports free fatty acids from the cytosol into the mitochondria for oxidation.

carotenoids Fat-soluble plant pigments that the body stores in the liver and adipose tissues. The body is able to convert certain carotenoids to vitamin A.

cash crops Crops grown to be sold rather than eaten, such as cotton, tobacco, jute, and sugarcane.

catabolism The breakdown, or degradation, of larger molecules to smaller molecules.

cataract A damaged portion of the eye's lens, which causes cloudiness that impairs vision.

celiac disease A disorder characterized by an immune reaction that damages the lining of the small intestine when the individual is exposed to a component of a protein called gluten.

cell differentiation The process by which immature, undifferentiated stem cells develop into highly specialized functional cells of discrete organs and tissues.

Centers for Disease Control and Prevention (CDC) The leading federal agency in the United States that protects the health and safety of people. Its mission is to promote health and quality of life by preventing and controlling disease, injury, and disability.

cephalic phase The earliest phase of digestion, in which the brain thinks about and prepares the digestive organs for the consumption of food.

ceruloplasmin A copper-containing protein that transports copper in the body. It also plays a role in oxidizing ferric to ferrous iron (Fe^{2+} to Fe^{3+}).

chemical score A method used to estimate a food's protein quality; it is a comparison of the amount of the limiting amino acid in a food to the amount of the same amino acid in a reference food.

cholecalciferol Vitamin D_3, a form of vitamin D found in animal foods and the form we synthesize from the sun.

chronic disease A disease characterized by a gradual onset and long duration, with signs and symptoms that are difficult to interpret and that respond poorly to medical treatment.

chylomicron A lipoprotein produced in the mucosal cell of the intestine; transports dietary fat out of the intestinal tract.

chyme A semifluid mass consisting of partially digested food, water, and gastric juices.

cirrhosis of the liver End-stage liver disease characterized by significant abnormalities in liver structure and function; may lead to complete liver failure.

coenzyme Organic (carbon-containing) component of enzymes; many coenzymes are B-vitamins.

cofactor A small, non-protein substance that enhances or is essential for enzyme action; trace minerals such as iron, zinc, and copper function as cofactors.

colic A condition of unconsolable infant crying of unknown origin that can last for hours at a time.

collagen A protein that forms strong fibers in bone and connective tissue.

colostrum The first fluid made and secreted by the breasts from late in pregnancy to about a week after birth. It is rich in immune factors and protein.

complementary proteins Proteins contained in two or more foods that together contain all nine essential amino acids necessary for a complete protein. It is not necessary to eat complementary proteins at the same meal.

complete proteins Foods that contain sufficient amounts of all nine essential amino acids.

complex carbohydrate A nutrient compound consisting of long chains of glucose molecules, such as starch, glycogen, and fiber.

conception The uniting of an ovum (egg) and sperm to create a fertilized egg, or zygote; also called *fertilization*; .

conditionally essential amino acids Amino acids that are normally considered nonessential but become essential under certain circumstances when the body's need for them exceeds the ability to produce them.

cone cells Light-sensitive cells found in the retina that contain the pigment iodopsin and react to bright light and interpret color images.

constipation A condition characterized by the absence of bowel movements for a period of time that is significantly longer than normal for the individual.

cool-down Activities done after an exercise session is completed; should be gradual and allow your body to slowly recover from exercise.

cortical bone (compact bone) A dense bone tissue that makes up the outer surface of all bones, as well as the entirety of most small bones of the body.

cortisol A hormone produced by the adrenal cortex that increases rates of gluconeogenesis and lipolysis.

covert symptom A symptom that is hidden from a client and requires laboratory tests or other invasive procedures to detect.

creatine phosphate (CP) A high-energy compound that can be broken down for energy and used to regenerate ATP.

cretinism A unique form of mental retardation that occurs in infants when the mother experiences iodine deficiency during pregnancy.

Crohn's disease A chronic disease that causes inflammation in the small intestine, leading to diarrhea, abdominal pain, rectal bleeding, weight loss, and fever.

crop rotation The practice of alternating crops grown in a given field to prevent nutrient depletion and soil erosion, as well as to help with control of crop-specific pests.

cross-contamination Contamination of one food by another via the unintended transfer of microorganisms through physical contact.

cystic fibrosis A genetic disorder that causes an alteration in chloride transport, leading to the production of thick, sticky mucus that causes life-threatening respiratory and digestive problems.

cytotoxic T cells Activated T cells that kill infected body cells.

D

danger zone The range of temperature (about 40°F to 140°F, or 4°C to 60°C) at which many microorganisms capable of causing human disease thrive.

DASH diet The Dietary Approaches to Stop Hypertension, a diet plan emphasizing fruits and vegetables, whole grains, low/no-fat milk and dairy, and lean meats.

deamination The process by which an amine group is removed from an amino acid. The nitrogen is then transported to the kidneys for excretion in the urine, and the carbon and other components are metabolized for energy or used to make other compounds.

dehydration The depletion of body fluid, which results when fluid excretion exceeds fluid intake.

dehydration synthesis An anabolic process by which smaller, chemically simple compounds are joined and a molecule of water is released; also called *condensation*.

dementia A decline in brain function.

denaturation The process by which proteins uncoil and lose their shape and function when they are exposed to heat, acids, bases, heavy metals, alcohol, and other damaging substances.

de novo synthesis The process of synthesizing a compound "from scratch."

diabetes A chronic disease in which the body can no longer regulate glucose.

diarrhea A condition characterized by the frequent passage of loose, watery stools.

dietary fiber The nondigestible carbohydrate parts of plants that form the support structures of leaves, stems, and seeds.

Dietary Guidelines for Americans A set of principles developed by the US Department of Agriculture and the US Department of Health and Human Services to assist Americans in designing a healthful diet and lifestyle.

Dietary Reference Intakes (DRIs) A set of nutritional reference values for the United States and Canada that applies to healthy people.

digestion The process by which foods are broken down into their component molecules, either mechanically or chemically.

direct calorimetry A method used to determine energy expenditure by measuring the amount of heat released by the body.

disaccharide A carbohydrate compound consisting of two monosaccharide molecules joined together.

diseases of aging Conditions that typically occur later in life as a result of lifelong accumulated risk, such as from lack of physical activity or exposure to carcinogens.

disordered eating A general term used to describe a variety of abnormal or atypical eating behaviors that are used to keep or maintain a lower body weight.

diuretic A substance that increases fluid loss via the urine. Common diuretics include alcohol and prescription medications for high blood pressure and other disorders.

docosahexaenoic acid (DHA) A metabolic derivative of alpha-linolenic acid; together with EPA, it appears to reduce the risk of heart disease.

doubly labeled water A form of indirect calorimetry that measures total daily energy expenditure through the rate of carbon dioxide production. It requires the consumption of water that is labeled with nonradioactive isotopes of hydrogen (deuterium, or ^{2}H) and oxygen (^{18}O).

drink The amount of an alcoholic beverage that provides approximately 0.5 fl. oz of pure ethanol.

dual energy x-ray absorptiometry (DXA, DEXA) Currently the most accurate tool for measuring bone density.

dysgeusia Abnormal taste perception.

dysphagia Abnormal swallowing.

E

eating disorder A clinically diagnosed psychiatric disorder characterized by severe disturbances in body image and eating behaviors.

edema A potentially serious disorder in which fluids build up in the tissue spaces of the body, causing fluid imbalances and a swollen appearance.

eicosapentaenoic acid (EPA) A metabolic derivative of alpha-linolenic acid.

electrolyte A compound that disassociates in solution into positively and negatively charged ions and is thus capable of conducting an electrical current; the ions in such a solution.

electron transport chain A series of metabolic reactions that transports electrons from NAHD or FADH$_2$ through a series of carriers, resulting in ATP production.

elimination The process by which the undigested portions of food and waste products are removed from the body.

embryo The human growth and developmental stage lasting from the third week to the end of the eighth week after fertilization.

empty Calories Calories from solid fats and/or added sugars that provide few or no nutrients.

endocytosis A transport process in which ions and molecules are engulfed by the cell membrane, which folds inwardly and is released in the cell interior (also called pinocytosis).

energy cost of physical activity The energy that is expended on body movement and muscular work above basal levels.

energy expenditure The energy the body expends to maintain its basic functions and to perform all levels of movement and activity.

energy intake The amount of energy a person consumes; in other words, the number of kcal consumed from food and beverages.

enriched foods Foods in which nutrients that were lost during processing have been added back, so that the food meets a specified standard.

enteric nervous system (ENS) The autonomic nerves in the walls of the GI tract.

enterocytes Specialized absorptive cells in the villi of the small intestine.

enzymes Small chemicals, usually proteins, that act on other chemicals to speed up bodily processes but are not changed during those processes.

epinephrine A hormone produced mainly by the adrenal medulla that stimulates the release of glucose from liver glycogen and the release of free fatty acids from stored triglycerides.

epiphyseal plates Plates of cartilage located toward the end of long bones that provide for growth in the length of long bones.

ergocalciferol Vitamin D$_2$, a form of vitamin D found exclusively in plant foods.

ergogenic aids Substances used to improve exercise and athletic performance.

error theories of aging Aging is a cumulative process determined largely by exposure to environmental insults; the fewer the environmental insults, the slower the aging process.

erythrocyte hemolysis The rupturing or breakdown of red blood cells, or erythrocytes.

erythrocytes Red blood cells; they transport oxygen in the blood.

esophagus A muscular tube of the GI tract connecting the back of the mouth to the stomach.

essential amino acids Amino acids not produced by the body, or not produced in sufficient amounts, so they must be obtained from food.

essential fatty acids (EFAs) Fatty acids that must be consumed in the diet because they cannot be made by the body. The two essential fatty acids are linoleic acid and alpha-linolenic acid.

Estimated Average Requirement (EAR) The average daily nutrient intake level estimated to meet the requirement of half of the healthy individuals in a particular life stage or gender group.

Estimated Energy Requirement (EER) The average dietary energy intake that is predicted to maintain energy balance in a healthy individual.

ethanol A specific alcohol compound (C_2H_5OH) formed from the fermentation of dietary carbohydrates and used in a variety of alcoholic beverages.

evaporative cooling Sweating, which is the primary way in which the body dissipates heat.

exercise A subcategory of leisure-time physical activity; any activity that is purposeful, planned, and structured.

extracellular fluid The fluid outside of the body's cells, either in the body's tissues (interstitial fluid) or as the liquid portion of the blood or lymph (intravascular fluid).

F

facilitated diffusion A transport process in which ions and molecules are shuttled across the cell membrane with the help of a carrier protein.

FAD (flavin adenine dinucleotide) A coenzyme derived from the B-vitamin riboflavin; FAD readily accepts electrons (hydrogen) from various donors.

failure to thrive (FTT) A condition in which an infant's weight gain and growth are far below typical levels for age and previous patterns of growth, for reasons that are unclear or unexplained.

fair trade A trading partnership promoting equity in international trading relations, and contributing to sustainable development by securing the rights of marginalized producers and workers.

famines Widespread, acute food shortages that affect a substantial portion of a population, often associated with starvation and death.

fat-soluble vitamins Vitamins that are not soluble in water but are soluble in fat; these include vitamins A, D, E, and K.

fatty acids Long chains of carbon atoms bound to each other as well as to hydrogen atoms.

fatty liver An early and reversible stage of liver disease often found in people who abuse alcohol and characterized by the abnormal accumulation of fat within liver cells; also called alcoholic steatosis.

female athlete triad A potentially serious condition characterized by the coexistence of three disorders: low energy availability, menstrual dysfunction, and low bone density.

fermentation The anaerobic process in which an agent causes an organic substance to break down into simpler substances and results in the production of ATP.

ferritin A storage form of iron found primarily in the intestinal mucosa, spleen, bone marrow, and liver.

ferroportin An iron transporter that helps regulate intestinal iron absorption and the release of iron from the enterocyte into the general circulation.

fetal adaptation Physiologic adaptations comprising a "survival mode" that occur when a fetus is exposed to harmful prenatal environment, such as maternal starvation or malnutrition. Hormone production shifts toward promoting energy storage, and the activity of certain enzymes may change. There may also be changes in the size and functioning of body organ, as well as in the expression of some genes. These adaptations, while enabling a fetus to survive, may also contribute to the development of chronic diseases over the life span.

fetal alcohol spectrum disorders (FASD) An umbrella term describing a wide range of clinical outcomes that can result from prenatal exposure to alcohol. Fetal alcohol syndrome (FAS), alcohol-related neurodevelopmental disorder (ARND), and alcohol-related birth defects (ARBD) are components of FASD.

fetal alcohol syndrome (FAS) A set of serious, irreversible alcohol-related birth defects characterized by certain physical and mental abnormalities, including malformations of the face, limbs, heart, and nervous system; impaired growth; and a spectrum of mild to severe cognitive, emotional, and physical problems.

fetus The human growth and developmental stage lasting from the beginning of the ninth week after conception to birth.

fiber-rich carbohydrates A group of foods containing either simple or complex carbohydrates that are rich in dietary fiber. These foods, which include most fruits, vegetables, and whole grains, are typically fresh or moderately processed.

FITT principle The principle used to achieve an appropriate overload for physical training; FITT stands for *f*requency, *i*ntensity, *t*ime, and *t*ype of activity.

fluid A substance composed of molecules that move past one another freely. Fluids are characterized by their ability to conform to the shape of whatever container holds them.

fluorohydroxyapatite A mineral compound in human teeth that contains fluoride, calcium, and phosphorus and is more resistant to destruction by acids and bacteria than hydroxyapatite.

fluorosis A condition characterized by staining and pitting of the teeth; caused by an abnormally high intake of fluoride.

folate depletion (stage II) The second stage of folate depletion, in which both serum and red blood cell folate levels are low.

folate-deficiency anemia (stage IV) A state of severe folate depletion in which there is inadequate folate for a long enough time that the number of red blood cells has declined.

folate-deficiency erythropoiesis (stage III) The third stage of folate depletion, in which body levels of folate are so low that the ability to make new red blood cells is impaired.

food additive A substance or mixture of substances intentionally put into food to enhance its appearance, safety, palatability, and quality.

food allergy An allergic reaction to food, caused by a reaction of the immune system.

food desert A community in which residents lack access to affordable fresh fruits and vegetables and other healthful foods.

food insecurity A condition in which an individual is unable to regularly obtain enough food to provide sufficient energy and nutrients to meet his or her physical needs.

food intolerance Gastrointestinal discomfort caused by certain foods that is not a result of an immune system reaction.

food shortage A condition in which food production and import for a given area are not sufficient to meet the needs of the local population.

food/population ratio The amount of food available for each individual within a given area; also called *food availability per capita*.

food The plants and animals we consume.

foodborne illness An illness transmitted by food or water contaminated by a pathogenic microorganism, its toxic secretions, or a toxic chemical.

fortified foods Foods in which nutrients are added that did not originally exist in the food or existed in insignificant amounts.

free radical A highly unstable atom with an unpaired electron in its outermost shell.

frequency Refers to the number of activity sessions per week you perform.

fructose The sweetest natural sugar; a monosaccharide that occurs in fruits and vegetables; also called *levulose*, or *fruit sugar*.

functional fiber The nondigestible forms of carbohydrate that are extracted from plants or manufactured in the laboratory and have known health benefits.

fungi Plantlike, spore-forming organisms that can grow as either single cells or multicellular colonies.

G

galactose A monosaccharide that joins with glucose to create lactose, one of the three most common disaccharides.

gallbladder A pear-shaped organ beneath the liver that stores bile and secretes it into the small intestine.

gastric juice Acidic liquid secreted within the stomach; it contains hydrochloric acid, pepsin, and other compounds.

gastroesophageal reflux disease (GERD) A painful type of heartburn that occurs more than twice per week.

gastrointestinal (GI) tract A long, muscular tube consisting of several organs: the mouth, esophagus, stomach, small intestine, and large intestine.

gene expression The process of using a gene to make a protein.

Generally Recognized as Safe (GRAS) A list established by Congress to identify substances used in foods that are generally recognized as safe based on a history of long-term use or on the consensus of qualified research experts.

genetic modification The process of changing an organism by manipulating its genetic material.

geriatric failure-to-thrive Inappropriate, unexplained loss of body weight and muscle mass; usually results from a combination of environmental and health factors.

gestation The period of intrauterine development from conception to birth.

gestational diabetes Insufficient insulin production or insulin resistance that results in consistently high blood glucose levels, specifically during pregnancy; the condition typically resolves after birth occurs.

ghrelin A protein synthesized in the stomach that acts as a hormone and plays an important role in appetite regulation by stimulating appetite.

glucagon A hormone secreted by the alpha cells of the pancreas in response to decreased blood levels of glucose; it stimulates the liver to convert stored glycogen into glucose, which is released into the bloodstream and transported to cells for energy.

glucogenic amino acid An amino acid that can be converted to glucose via gluconeogenesis.

glucokinase An enzyme that adds a phosphate group to a molecule of glucose.

gluconeogenesis The synthesis of glucose from noncarbohydrate precursors, such as glucogenic amino acids and glycerol.

glucose The most abundant sugar molecule, a monosaccharide generally found in combination with other sugars; the preferred source of energy for the brain and an important source of energy for all cells.

glutathione (GSH) A tripeptide composed of glycine, cysteine, and glutamic acid that assists in regenerating vitamin C into its antioxidant form.

glycemic index A rating of the potential of foods to raise blood glucose and insulin levels.

glycemic load The amount of carbohydrate in a food multiplied by the glycemic index of the carbohydrate.

glycerol An alcohol composed of three carbon atoms; it is the backbone of a triglyceride molecule.

glycogen The storage form of glucose (as a polysaccharide) in animals.

glycolysis A sequence of chemical reactions that converts glucose to pyruvate.

glycosylation The addition of glucose to blood and tissue proteins; typically impairs protein structure and function.

GOBI A UNICEF campaign to eliminate common childhood infections via four inexpensive strategies: "GOBI" stands for growth monitoring, oral rehydration therapy, breastfeeding, and immunization.

goiter Enlargement of the thyroid gland; can be caused by iodine toxicity or deficiency.

grazing Consistently eating small meals throughout the day; done by many athletes to meet their high energy demands.

Green Revolution The period, between 1944 and 2000, of tremendous increase in global productivity as a result of selective crossbreeding and hybridization that produced high-yield grains and modern industrial farming techniques.

H

haustration Involuntary, sluggish contraction of the haustra of the proximal colon, which moves wastes toward the sigmoid colon.

healthful diet A diet that provides the proper combination of energy and nutrients and is adequate, moderate, balanced, and varied.

heartburn The painful sensation that occurs over the sternum when hydrochloric acid backs up into the lower esophagus.

heat cramps Muscle spasms that occur several hours after strenuous exercise; most often occur when sweat losses and fluid intakes are high, urine volume is low, and sodium intake is inadequate.

heat exhaustion A heat illness characterized by excessive sweating, weakness, nausea, dizziness, headache, and difficulty concentrating. Unchecked, heat exhaustion can lead to heatstroke.

heat syncope Dizziness that results from blood pooling in the lower extremities; often results from standing too long in hot weather, standing rapidly from a lying position, or stopping suddenly after physical exertion.

heat stroke A potentially fatal heat illness characterized by hot, dry skin; rapid heart rate; vomiting; diarrhea; elevated body temperature; hallucinations; and coma.

helminth A multicellular microscopic worm.

helper T cells Activated T cells that secrete chemicals needed to activate other immune cells.

heme The iron-containing molecule found in hemoglobin.

heme iron Iron that is a part of hemoglobin and myoglobin; it is found only in animal-based foods, such as meat, fish, and poultry.

hemoglobin The oxygen-carrying protein found in red blood cells; almost two-thirds of all of the iron in the body is found in hemoglobin.

hemosiderin A storage form of iron found primarily in the intestinal mucosa, spleen, bone marrow, and liver.

hephaestin A copper-containing protein that oxidizes Fe^{2+} to Fe^{3+} once iron is transported across the basolateral membrane by ferroportin.

high-density lipoprotein (HDL) A lipoprotein made in the liver and released into the blood. HDLs function to transport cholesterol from the tissues back to the liver; often called "good cholesterol."

high-yield varieties Semi-dwarf plant varieties that are unlikely to fall over in wind and heavy rains, and thus can carry higher quantities of seeds, greatly increasing the yield per acre.

homocysteine An amino acid that requires adequate levels of folate, vitamin B_6 and vitamin B_{12} for its metabolism. High levels of homocysteine in the blood are associated with an increased risk for cardiovascular disease.

hormone A chemical messenger that is secreted into the bloodstream by one of the many endocrine glands of the body. Hormones act as regulators of physiologic processes at sites remote from the glands that secreted them.

hormone-sensitive lipase The enzyme that breaks down the triglycerides stored in adipose tissue.

hunger A physiologic sensation that prompts us to eat.

hydrogenation The process of adding hydrogen to unsaturated fatty acids, making them more saturated and thereby more solid at room temperature.

hydrolysis A catabolic process by which a large, chemically complex compound is broken apart with the addition of water.

hypercalcemia A condition characterized by an abnormally high concentration of calcium in the blood.

hyperglycemia A condition in which blood glucose levels are higher than normal.

hyperkalemia A condition in which blood potassium levels are dangerously high.

hyperkeratosis A condition resulting in the excess accumulation of the protein keratin in the follicles of the skin; this condition can also impair the ability of epithelial tissues to produce mucus.

hypermagnesemia   A condition marked by an abnormally high concentration of magnesium in the blood.

hypernatremia   A condition in which blood sodium levels are dangerously high.

hypertension   A chronic condition characterized by above-average blood pressure readings-specifically, systolic blood pressure over 140 mm Hg or diastolic blood pressure over 90 mm Hg.

hyperthyroidism   A condition characterized by high blood levels of thyroid hormone.

hypertrophy   The increase in strength and size that results from repeated work to a specific muscle or muscle group.

hypocalcemia   A condition characterized by an abnormally low concentration of calcium in the blood.

hypoglycemia   A condition marked by blood glucose levels that are below normal fasting levels.

hypokalemia   A condition in which blood potassium levels are dangerously low.

hypomagnesemia   A condition characterized by an abnormally low concentration of magnesium in the blood.

hyponatremia   A condition in which blood sodium levels are dangerously low.

hypothalamus   A region of the brain below (*hypo-*) the thalamus and cerebral hemispheres and above the pituitary gland and brain stem where visceral sensations such as hunger and thirst are regulated.

hypothesis   An educated guess as to why a phenomenon occurs.

hypothyroidism   A condition characterized by low blood levels of thyroid hormone.

I

immunocompetence   The body's ability to adequately produce an effective immune response to an antigen.

impaired fasting glucose   Fasting blood glucose levels that are higher than normal but not high enough to lead to a diagnosis of t ype 2 diabetes.

incomplete proteins   Foods that do not contain all of the essential amino acids in sufficient amounts to support growth and health.

indirect calorimetry   A method used to estimate energy expenditure by measuring oxygen consumption and carbon dioxide production.

infant mortality   The death rate for infants between birth and 1 year of age.

inorganic   A substance or nutrient that does not contain carbon and hydrogen.

insensible water loss   The unperceived loss of water, such as through evaporation from the skin and exhalation from the lungs during breathing.

insoluble fibers   Fibers that do not dissolve in water.

insulin   A hormone secreted by the beta cells of the pancreas in response to increased blood levels of glucose that facilitates uptake of glucose by body cells.

intensity   The amount of effort expended during an activity, or how difficult the activity is to perform.

interstitial fluid   The fluid that flows between the cells that make up a particular tissue or organ, such as muscle fibers or the liver.

intracellular fluid   The fluid held at any given time within the walls of the body's cells.

intravascular fluid   The fluid in the bloodstream and lymph.

intrinsinc factor   A protein secreted by cells of the stomach that binds to vitamin B_{12} and aids its absorption in the small intestine.

invisible fats   Fats that are hidden in foods, such as the fats found in baked goods, regular-fat dairy products, marbling in meat, and fried foods.

iodopsin   A color-sensitive pigment found in the cone cells of the retina.

ion   Any electrically charged particle, either positively or negatively charged.

iron depletion (stage I)   The first phase of iron deficiency, characterized by a decrease in stored iron, which results in a decrease in blood ferritin levels.

iron-deficiency anemia (stage III)   A form of anemia that results from severe iron deficiency.

iron-deficiency erythropoiesis (stage II)   The second stage of iron deficiency, characterized by a decrease in the transport of iron in the blood.

irradiation   A sterilization process in which food is exposed to gamma rays or high-energy electron beams to kill micro-organisms. Irradiation does not impart any radiation to the food being treated.

irritable bowel syndrome (IBS)   A stress-related disorder that interferes with normal functions of the colon. Symptoms are abdominal cramps, bloating, and constipation or diarrhea.

K

Keshan disease   A heart disorder caused by selenium deficiency. It was first identified in children in the Keshan province of China.

keto acid   The chemical structure that remains after deamination of an amino acid.

ketoacidosis   A condition in which excessive ketones are present in the blood, causing the blood to become very acidic, which alters basic body functions and damages tissues. Untreated ketoacidosis can be fatal. This condition is often found in individuals with untreated diabetes mellitus.

ketogenic amino acid   An amino acid that can be converted to acetyl CoA for the synthesis of free fatty acids.

ketone bodies   Three- and four-carbon compounds (acetoacetate, acetone, and β- or 3-hydroxybutyrate) derived when acetyl CoA levels become elevated.

ketones   Substances produced during the breakdown of fat when carbohydrate intake is insufficient to meet energy needs. They provide an alternative energy source for the brain when glucose levels are low.

ketosis   The process by which the breakdown of fat during fasting states results in the production of ketones.

kwashiorkor   A form of protein–energy malnutrition that is typically seen in developing countries in infants and toddlers who are weaned early. Denied breast milk, they are fed a cereal diet that provides adequate energy but inadequate protein.

L

lactase   A digestive enzyme that breaks lactose into glucose and galactose.

lactate (lactic acid)   A three-carbon compound produced from pyruvate in oxygen-deprived conditions.

lactation   The production of breast milk.

lacteal   A small lymphatic vessel located inside the villi of the small intestine.

lactose   Also called *milk sugar*, a disaccharide consisting of one glucose molecule and one galactose molecule; found in milk, including human breast milk.

lactose intolerance   A disorder in which the body does not produce sufficient lactase enzyme and therefore cannot digest foods that contain lactose, such as cow's milk.

large intestine   The final organ of the GI tract, consisting of the cecum, colon, rectum, and anal canal and in which most water is absorbed and feces are formed.

lean body mass   The amount of fat-free tissue, or bone, muscle, and internal organs, a person has.

leisure-time physical activity Any activity not related to a person's occupation; includes competitive sports, recreational activities, and planned exercise training.

leptin A hormone, produced by body fat, that acts to reduce food intake and to decrease body weight and body fat.

leukocytes White blood cells; they protect the body from infection and illness.

life expectancy The expected number of years remaining in one's life; typically stated from the time of birth. Children born in the United States in 2003 can expect to live, on average, 77.6 years.

life span The highest age reached by any member of a species; currently, the human life span is 122 years.

limiting amino acid The essential amino acid that is missing or in the smallest supply in the amino acid pool and is thus responsible for slowing or halting protein synthesis.

linoleic acid An essential fatty acid found in vegetable and nut oils; also known as omega-6 fatty acid.

lipids A diverse group of organic substances that are insoluble in water; lipids include triglycerides, phospholipids, and sterols.

lipogenesis The synthesis of free fatty acids from nonlipid precursors, such as ketogenic amino acids or ethanol.

lipolysis The enzyme-driven catabolism of triglycerides into free fatty acids and glycerol.

lipoprotein lipase An enzyme that sits on the outside of cells and breaks apart triglycerides, so that their fatty acids can be removed and taken up by the cell.

lipoprotein A spherical compound in which fat clusters in the center and phospholipids and proteins form the outside of the sphere.

liver The largest accessory organ of the GI tract and one of the most important organs of the body. Its functions include the production of bile and processing of nutrient-rich blood from the small intestine.

long-chain fatty acids Fatty acids that are fourteen or more carbon atoms in length.

low birth weight An infant weight of less than 5.5 lb at birth.

low-density lipoprotein (LDL) A lipoprotein formed in the blood from VLDLs that transports cholesterol to the cells of the body; often called "bad cholesterol."

low-intensity activities Activities that cause very mild increases in breathing, sweating, and heart rate.

M

macrocytic anemia A form of anemia manifested as the production of larger than normal red blood cells containing insufficient hemoglobin, which inhibits adequate transport of oxygen; also called megaloblastic anemia. Macrocytic anemia can be caused by a severe folate deficiency or by vitamin B_{12} deficiency.

macronutrients Nutrients that the body requires in relatively large amounts to support normal function and health. Carbohydrates, lipids, and proteins are macronutrients.

macular degeneration A vision disorder caused by deterioration of the central portion of the retina and marked by loss or distortion of the central field of vision.

major minerals Minerals we need to consume in amounts of at least 100 mg per day and of which the total amount in our body is at least 5 g (5,000 mg).

malnutrition A nutritional status that is out of balance; an individual is either getting too much or not enough of a particular nutrient or energy over a significant period of time.

maltase A digestive enzyme that breaks maltose into glucose.

maltose A disaccharide consisting of two molecules of glucose; does not generally occur independently in foods but results as a by-product of digestion; also called *malt sugar*.

marasmus A form of protein-energy malnutrition that results from grossly inadequate intakes of protein, energy, and other nutrients.

mass movement Involuntary, sustained, forceful contraction of the colon that occurs two or more times a day to push wastes toward the rectum.

maternal mortality The death rate for women from pregnancy-related causes, including the immediate postpartum period.

matrix Gla protein A vitamin K–dependent protein located in the protein matrix of bone and in cartilage, blood-vessel walls, and other soft tissues.

maximal heart rate The rate at which the heart beats during maximal-intensity exercise.

meat factor A special factor found in meat, fish, and poultry that enhances the absorption of non-heme iron.

medium-chain fatty acids Fatty acids that are six to twelve carbon atoms in length.

megadosing Taking a dose of a nutrient that is 10 or more times greater than the recommended amount.

memory cells White blood cells that recognize a particular antigen and circulate in the body, ready to respond if the antigen is encountered again. The purpose of vaccination is to create memory cells.

menaquinone The form of vitamin K produced by bacteria in the large intestine.

menarche The onset of menstruation, or the menstrual period.

metabolic syndrome A clustering of risk factors that increase one's risk for heart disease, type 2 diabetes, and stroke, including abdominal obesity, higher-than-normal triglyceride levels, lower-than-normal HDL-cholesterol levels, higher-than-normal blood pressure (greater than or equal to 130/85 mm Hg), and elevated fasting blood glucose levels.

metabolic water The water formed as a by-product of the body's metabolic reactions.

metabolism The sum of all the chemical and physical changes that occur in body tissues.

metallothionein A zinc-containing protein within the enterocyte; it assists in the regulation of zinc homeostasis.

micelle A spherical compound made up of bile salts and biliary phospholipids that transports lipid digestion products to the intestinal mucosal cell.

microcytic anemia A form of anemia manifested as the production of smaller than normal red blood cells containing insufficient hemoglobin, which reduces the red blood cell's ability to transport oxygen; it can result from iron deficiency or vitamin B_6 deficiency.

micronutrients Nutrients needed in relatively small amounts to support normal health and body functions. Vitamins and minerals are micronutrients.

microsomal ethanol oxidizing system (MEOS) A liver enzyme system that oxidizes ethanol to acetaldehyde; its activity predominates at higher levels of alcohol intake.

minerals Naturally occurring inorganic substances that are not changed by natural or body processes, including digestion.

moderate drinking Alcohol consumption of up to one drink per day for women and up to two drinks per day for men.

moderate-intensity activities Activities that cause moderate increases in breathing, sweating, and heart rate.

moderation   Eating any foods in moderate amounts—not too much and not too little.

monosaccharide   The simplest of carbohydrates; consists of one sugar molecule, the most common form of which is glucose.

monounsaturated fatty acids (MUFAs)   Fatty acids that have two carbons in the chain bound to each other with one double bond; these types of fatty acids are generally liquid at room temperature.

morbid obesity   A condition in which a person's body weight exceeds 100% of normal, putting him or her at very high risk for serious health consequences; a BMI $\geq$ 40 kg/m^2.

morning sickness   A condition characterized by varying degrees of nausea and vomiting associated with pregnancy, most commonly in the first trimester.

multifactorial disease   A disease that may be attributable to one or more of a variety of causes.

muscle cramps   Involuntary, spasmodic, and painful muscle contractions that last for many seconds or even minutes; electrolyte imbalances are often the cause of muscle cramps.

mutual supplementation   The process of combining two or more incomplete protein sources to make a complete protein.

myoglobin   An iron-containing protein similar to hemoglobin except that it is found in muscle cells.

MyPlate   The graphic representation of the USDA Food Patterns.

N

NAD (nicotinamide adenine dinucleotide)   A coenzyme form of the B-vitamin niacin; NAD readily accepts electrons (hydrogen) from various donors.

National Health and Nutrition Examination Survey (NHANES)   A survey conducted by the National Center for Health Statistics and the CDC; this survey tracks the nutrient and food consumption of Americans.

National Institutes of Health (NIH)   The world's leading medical research center and the focal point for medical research in the United States.

negative folate balance (stage I)   The first stage of folate depletion in which the body has less folate available to it and serum levels of folate begin to decline.

neonatal mortality   The death rate for newborns between birth and 28 days of age.

neonatal   Referring to a newborn.

neural tube   Embryonic tissue that forms a tube, which eventually becomes the brain and spinal cord.

neural tube defects (NTDs)   The most common malformations of the central nervous system that occur during fetal development. A folate deficiency can cause neural tube defects.

neurotransmitters   Chemical messengers that transmit messages from one nerve cell to another.

night blindness   A vitamin A–deficiency disorder that results in loss of the ability to see in dim light.

night-eating syndrome   Disorder characterized by intake of the majority of the day's energy between 8:00 PM and 6:00 AM. Individuals with this disorder also experience mood and sleep disorders.

non-heme iron   The form of iron that is not a part of hemoglobin or myoglobin; it is found in animal-based and plant-based foods.

non-nutritive sweeteners   Also called *alternative sweeteners;* manufactured sweeteners that provide little or no energy.

nonessential amino acids   Amino acids that can be manufactured by the body in sufficient quantities and therefore do not need to be consumed regularly in our diet.

nonspecific immune function   Generalized body defense mechanisms that protect against the entry of foreign agents, such as microbes and allergens; also called *innate immunity.*

nucleotide   A molecule composed of a phosphate group, a pentose sugar called deoxyribose, and one of four nitrogenous bases: adenine (A), guanine (G), cytosine (C), or thymine (T).

nutrient density   The relative amount of nutrients per amount of energy (number of Calories).

nutrient-dense foods   Foods that give the highest amount of nutrients for the least amount of energy (Calories).

nutrients   Chemicals found in foods that are critical to human growth and function.

nutrition   The scientific study of food and how it nourishes the body and influences health.

Nutrition Facts Panel   The label on a food package that contains the nutrition information required by the FDA.

nutrition paradox   The coexistence of aspects of both undernutrition and overnutrition within the same region, household, family, or person; also known as *nutritional dual-burden.*

nutritive sweeteners   Sweeteners, such as sucrose, fructose, honey, and brown sugar, that contribute Calories (energy).

O

obese (childhood)   Having a body mass index (BMI) at or above the 95th percentile.

obesity   Having an excess of body fat that adversely affects health, resulting in a person having a weight that is substantially greater than some accepted standard for a given height; a BMI of 30 to 39.9 kg/m^2.

oligosaccharides   Complex carbohydrates that contain 3 to 10 monosaccharides.

opsin   A protein that combines with retinal in the retina to form rhodopsin.

organic   A substance or nutrient that contains the elements carbon and hydrogen.

osmosis   The movement of water (or any solvent) through a semipermeable membrane from an area where solutes are less concentrated to areas where they are highly concentrated.

osmotic pressure   The pressure that is needed to keep the particles in a solution from drawing liquid toward them across a semipermeable membrane.

osteoblasts   Cells that prompt the formation of new bone matrix by laying down the collagen-containing component of bone, which is then mineralized.

osteocalcin   A vitamin K–dependent protein that is secreted by osteoblasts and is associated with bone turnover.

osteoclasts   Cells that erode the surface of bones by secreting enzymes and acids that dig grooves into the bone matrix.

osteomalacia   A vitamin D–deficiency disease in adults, in which bones become weak and prone to fractures.

osteoporosis   A disease characterized by low bone mass and deterioration of bone tissue, leading to increased bone fragility and fracture risk.

ounce-equivalent (oz-equivalent)   A serving size that is 1 ounce, or is equivalent to an ounce, for the grains section and the protein foods section of MyPlate.

overhydration   The dilution of body fluid. It results when water intake or retention is excessive.

overload principle   Placing an extra physical demand on your body in order to improve your fitness level.

overnutrition   A situation in which too much energy or too much of a given nutrient is consumed over time, causing conditions such as obesity, heart disease, or nutrient-toxicity symptoms.

overpopulation   A designation used for an area or a region that has insufficient resources to support the number of people living there.

overt symptom   A symptom that is obvious to a client, such as pain, fatigue, or a bruise.

overweight   Having a moderate amount of excess body fat, resulting in a person having a weight that is greater than some accepted standard for a given height but is not considered obese; a BMI of 25 to 29.9 kg/m².

overweight (childhood)   Having a body mass index (BMI) at or above the 85th percentile but below the 95th percentile.

oxidation   A chemical reaction in which molecules of a substance are broken down into their component atoms. During oxidation, the atoms involved lose electrons.

oxidation–reduction reactions   Reactions in which electrons are lost by one compound (it is oxidized) and simultaneously gained by another compound (it is reduced).

P

palliative care   Patient care aimed at reducing an individual's pain and discomfort without attempting to treat or cure.

pancreas   A gland located behind the stomach that secretes digestive enzymes.

pancreatic amylase   An enzyme secreted by the pancreas into the small intestine that digests any remaining starch into maltose.

parasite   A microorganism that simultaneously derives benefit from and harms its host.

parathyroid hormone (PTH)   A hormone secreted by the parathyroid gland when blood calcium levels fall. It is also known as parathormone, and it increases blood calcium levels by stimulating the activation of vitamin D, increasing reabsorption of calcium from the kidneys, and stimulating osteoclasts to break down bone, which releases more calcium into the bloodstream.

passive diffusion   A transport process in which ions and molecules, following their concentration gradient, cross the cell membrane without the use of a carrier protein or the requirement of energy.

pasteurization   A form of sterilization using high temperatures for short periods of time.

pellagra   A disease that results from severe niacin deficiency.

pepsin   An enzyme in the stomach that begins the breakdown of proteins into shorter polypeptide chains and single amino acids.

peptic ulcer   An area of the GI tract that has been eroded away by the acidic gastric juice of the stomach. The two main causes of peptic ulcers are *Helicobacter pylori* infection and the use of nonsteroidal anti-inflammatory drugs.

peptide bonds   Unique types of chemical bonds in which the amine group of one amino acid binds to the acid group of another in order to manufacture dipeptides and all larger peptide molecules.

peptide YY (PYY)   A protein produced in the gastrointestinal tract that is released after a meal in amounts proportional to the energy content of the meal; it decreases appetite and inhibits food intake.

percent daily values (%DVs)   Information on a Nutrition Facts Panel that identifies how much a serving of food contributes to your overall intake of nutrients listed on the label; based on an energy intake of 2,000 Calories per day.

peristalsis   Waves of squeezing and pushing contractions that move food, chyme, and feces in one direction through the length of the GI tract.

pernicious anemia   A form of macrocytic anemia that is the primary cause of a vitamin B_{12} deficiency; occurs at the end stage of an autoimmune disorder that causes the loss of various cells in the stomach.

persistent organic pollutants (POPs)   Chemicals released into the environment as a result of industry, agriculture, or improper waste disposal; automobile emissions also are considered POPs.

pesticides   Chemicals used either in the field or in storage to decrease destruction by predators or disease.

pH   An abbreviation for percentage of hydrogen. It is a measure of the acidity—or level of hydrogen—of any solution, including human blood.

phospholipids   A type of lipid in which a fatty acid is combined with another compound that contains phosphate; unlike other lipids, phospholipids are soluble in water.

phosphorylation   The addition of one or more phosphate groups to a chemical compound.

photosynthesis   A process by which plants use sunlight to fuel a chemical reaction that combines carbon and water into glucose, which is then stored in their cells.

phylloquinone   The form of vitamin K found in plants.

physical activity   Any movement produced by muscles that increases energy expenditure; includes occupational, household, leisure-time, and transportation activities.

physical fitness   The ability to carry out daily tasks with vigor and alertness, without undue fatigue, and with ample energy to enjoy leisure-time pursuits and meet unforeseen emergencies.

phytic acid   The form of phosphorus stored in plants.

phytochemicals   Compounds found in plants believed to have health-promoting effects in humans.

pica   An abnormal craving to eat various nonfood substances, such as clay, chalk, or soap.

placenta   A pregnancy-specific organ formed from both maternal and embryonic tissues. It is responsible for oxygen, nutrient, and waste exchange between mother and fetus.

plasma   The fluid portion of the blood; it is needed to maintain adequate blood volume, so that the blood can flow easily throughout the body.

plasma cells   White blood cells that have differentiated from activated B cells and produce millions of antibodies to an antigen during an infection.

platelets   Cell fragments that assist in the formation of blood clots and help stop bleeding.

polypharmacy   The concurrent use of five or more medications.

polysaccharide   A complex carbohydrate consisting of long chains of glucose.

polyunsaturated fatty acids (PUFAs)   Fatty acids that have more than one double bond in the chain; these types of fatty acids are generally liquid at room temperature.

portal venous system   A system of blood vessels that drains blood and various products of digestion from the digestive organs and spleen and delivers them to the liver.

preeclampsia   High blood pressure that is pregnancy-specific and accompanied by protein in the urine, edema, and unexpected weight gain.

preterm   The birth of a baby prior to 38 weeks of gestation.

primary deficiency   A deficiency that occurs when not enough of a nutrient is consumed in the diet.

prion   A protein that misfolds and becomes infectious; prions are not living cellular organisms or viruses.

probiotic Health-promoting; the presence of certain beneficial bacteria in foods that support healthy functioning.

processed foods Foods that are manipulated mechanically or chemically.

programmed theories of aging Aging is biologically determined, following a predictable pattern of physiologic changes, although the timing may vary from one person to another.

proof A measure of the alcohol content of a liquid; 100-proof liquor is 50% alcohol by volume, 80-proof liquor is 40% alcohol by volume, and so on.

prooxidant A nutrient that promotes oxidation and oxidative cell and tissue damage.

proteases Enzymes that continue the breakdown of polypeptides in the small intestine.

protein digestibility corrected amino acid score (PDCAAS) A measurement of protein quality that considers the balance of amino acids as well as the digestibility of the protein in the food.

protein–energy malnutrition A disorder caused by inadequate consumption of protein. It is characterized by severe wasting.

proteins Large, complex molecules made up of amino acids and found as essential components of all living cells.

proteolysis The breakdown of dietary proteins into single amino acids or small peptides that are absorbed by the body.

protozoa Single-celled, mobile microorganisms.

provitamin An inactive form of a vitamin that the body can convert to an active form. An example is beta-carotene.

puberty The period in life in which secondary sexual characteristics develop and the body becomes biologically capable of reproduction.

purging An attempt to rid the body of unwanted food by vomiting or other compensatory means, such as excessive exercise, fasting, or laxative abuse.

Q

quackery The promotion of an unproven remedy, such as a supplement or other product or service, usually by someone unlicensed and untrained.

R

raffinose An oligosaccharide composed of galactose, glucose, and fructose. Also called melitose, it is found in beans, cabbage, broccoli, and other vegetables.

reactive oxygen species (ROS) An oxygen molecule that has become a free radical.

recombinant bovine growth hormone (rBGH) A genetically engineered hormone injected into dairy cows to enhance their milk output.

recombinant DNA technology A type of genetic modification in which scientists combine DNA from different sources to produce a transgenic organism that expresses a desired trait.

Recommended Dietary Allowance (RDA) The average daily nutrient intake level that meets the nutrient requirements of 97% to 98% of healthy individuals in a particular life stage and gender group.

registered dietitian (RD) A professional designation that requires a minimum of a bachelor's degree in nutrition, completion of a supervised clinical experience, a passing grade on a national examination, and maintenance of registration with the Academy of Nutrition and Dietetics (in Canada, the Dietitians of Canada). RDs are qualified to work in a variety of settings.

remodeling The two-step process by which bone tissue is recycled; includes the breakdown of existing bone and the formation of new bone.

renin An enzyme secreted by the kidneys in response to a decrease in blood pressure. Renin converts the blood protein angiotensinogen to angiotensin I, which eventually results in an increase in sodium reabsorption.

residues Chemicals that remain in the foods we eat despite cleaning and processing.

resistance training Exercise in which our muscles act against resistance.

resorption The process by which the surface of bone is broken down by cells called osteoclasts.

resveratrol A chemical known to play a role in limiting cell damage from the by-products of metabolic reactions. It is found in red wine and certain other plant-based foods.

retina The delicate, light-sensitive membrane lining the inner eyeball and connected to the optic nerve. It contains retinal.

retinal An active, aldehyde form of vitamin A that plays an important role in healthy vision and immune function.

retinoic acid An active, acid form of vitamin A that plays an important role in cell growth and immune function.

retinol An active, alcohol form of vitamin A that plays an important role in healthy vision and immune function.

rhodopsin A light-sensitive pigment found in the rod cells that is formed by retinal and opsin.

ribose A five-carbon monosaccharide that is located in the genetic material of cells.

rickets A vitamin D–deficiency disease in children. Symptoms include deformities of the skeleton, such as bowed legs and knocked knees.

rod cells Light-sensitive cells found in the retina that contain rhodopsin and react to dim light and interpret black-and-white images.

S

saliva A mixture of water, mucus, enzymes, and other chemicals that moistens the mouth and food, binds food particles together, and begins the digestion of carbohydrates.

salivary amylase An enzyme in saliva that breaks starch into smaller particles and eventually into the disaccharide maltose.

salivary glands A group of glands found under and behind the tongue and beneath the jaw that releases saliva continually as well as in response to the thought, sight, smell, or presence of food.

salt resistant A condition in which certain people do not experience changes in blood pressure with changes in salt intake.

salt sensitivity A condition in which certain people respond to a high salt intake by experiencing an increase in blood pressure; these people also experience a decrease in blood pressure when salt intake is low.

sarcopenia Age-related, progressive loss of muscle mass, muscle strength, and muscle function.

sarcopenic obesity A condition in which increased body weight and body fat mass coexist with inappropriately low muscle mass and strength.

saturated fatty acids (SFAs) Fatty acids that have no carbons joined together with a double bond; these types of fatty acids are generally solid at room temperature.

secondary deficiency A deficiency that occurs when a person cannot absorb enough of a nutrient, excretes too much of a nutrient from the body, or cannot utilize a nutrient efficiently.

segmentation Rhythmic contraction of the circular muscles of the small intestine, which squeezes chyme, mixes it, and enhances the digestion and absorption of nutrients from the chyme.

seizures   Uncontrollable muscle spasms caused by increased nervous system excitability that can result from electrolyte imbalances or a chronic disease, such as epilepsy.

selenocysteine   An amino acid derivative that is the active form of selenium in the body.

selenomethionine   An amino acid derivative that is the storage form for selenium in the body.

senescence   The progressive deterioration of bodily functions over time, resulting in increased risk for disability, disease, and death.

sensible water loss   Water loss that is noticeable, such as through urine output and sweating.

set-point theory   A theory suggesting that the body raises or lowers energy expenditure in response to increased and decreased food intake and physical activity. This action maintains an individual's body weight within a narrow range.

severe acute malnutrition (SAM)   A state of extreme energy deficit defined as a weight for height more than 3 standard deviations below the mean, or the presence of nutrition-related edema, and associated with a risk of death five to twenty times higher than that of well-nourished individuals.

short-chain fatty acids   Fatty acids fewer than six carbon atoms in length.

sickle cell anemia   A genetic disorder that causes red blood cells to be shaped like a sickle or crescent. These cells cannot travel smoothly through blood vessels, causing cell breakage and anemia.

simple carbohydrate   A monosaccharide or disaccharide such as glucose; commonly called *sugar*.

small for gestational age (SGA)   A condition in which infants whose birth weight for gestational age falls below the 10th percentile.

small intestine   The longest portion of the GI tract, where most digestion and absorption takes place.

soluble fibers   Fibers that dissolve in water.

solvent   A substance that is capable of mixing with and breaking apart a variety of compounds. Water is an excellent solvent.

specific immune function   The strongest defense against pathogens. It requires adaptation of white blood cells that recognize antigens and that multiply to protect against the pathogens carrying those antigens; also called *adaptive immunity* or *acquired immunity*.

sphincter   A tight ring of muscle separating some of the organs of the GI tract and opening in response to nerve signals indicating that food is ready to pass into the next section.

spina bifida   An embryonic neural tube defect that occurs when the spinal vertebrae fail to completely enclose the spinal cord, allowing it to protrude.

spontaneous abortion   The natural termination of a pregnancy and expulsion of pregnancy tissues because of a genetic, developmental, or physiologic abnormality that is so severe that the pregnancy cannot be maintained; also called *miscarriage*.

stachyose   An oligosaccharide composed of two galactose molecules, a glucose molecule, and a fructose molecule; found in the Chinese artichoke and various beans and legumes.

starch   The storage form of glucose (as a polysaccharide) in plants.

sterols   A type of lipid found in foods and the body that has a ring structure; cholesterol is the most common sterol that occurs in our diets.

stomach   A J-shaped organ where food is partially digested, churned, and stored until released into the small intestine.

stretching   Exercise in which muscles are gently lengthened using slow, controlled movements.

stunted growth   A condition of shorter stature than expected for chronological age, often defined as 2 or more standard deviations below the mean reference value.

subclinical deficiency   A deficiency in its early stages, when few or no symptoms are observed.

subsistence crops   Crops grown to be eaten by a family or community, such as rice, millet, and garden vegetables; surpluses in these crops may at times be sold locally.

sucrase   A digestive enzyme that breaks sucrose into glucose and fructose.

sucrose   A disaccharide composed of one glucose molecule and one fructose molecule; sweeter than lactose or maltose.

sudden infant death syndrome (SIDS)   The sudden death of an otherwise healthy infant; the most common cause of death in infants older than 1 month of age.

sustainability   The ability to meet, or satisfy, basic economic, social, and security needs now and in the future without undermining the natural resource base and environmental quality on which life depends.

sustainable agriculture   Techniques of food production that preserve the environment indefinitely.

T

T cells   White blood cells that are of several varieties, including cytotoxic T cells and helper T cells.

T-score   A comparison of an individual's bone density to the average peak bone density of a 30-year-old healthy adult.

TCA cycle   The tricarboxylic acid (TCA) cycle is a repetitive series of eight metabolic reactions, located in cell mitochondria, that metabolizes acetyl CoA for the production of carbon dioxide, high-energy GTP, and reduced coenzymes NADH and $FADH_2$.

teratogen   A substance or compound known to cause fetal harm or birth defects.

theory   A scientific consensus, based on data drawn from repeated experiments, as to why a phenomenon occurs.

thermic effect of food (TEF)   The energy expended as a result of processing food consumed.

thirst mechanism   A cluster of nerve cells in the hypothalamus that stimulates our conscious desire to drink fluids in response to an increase in the concentration of salt in our blood or a decrease in blood pressure and blood volume.

thrifty gene theory   A theory suggesting that some people possess a gene (or genes) that causes them to be energetically thrifty, resulting in their expending less energy at rest and during physical activity.

time of activity   How long each exercise session lasts.

tocopherols   A family of vitamin E that is the active form in our bodies.

tocotrienols   A family of vitamin E that does not play an important biological role in our bodies.

Tolerable Upper Intake Level (UL)   The highest average daily nutrient intake level likely to pose no risk of adverse health effects to almost all individuals in a particular life stage and gender group.

total fiber   The sum of dietary fiber and functional fiber.

toxin   Any harmful substance; in microbiology, a chemical produced by a microorganism that harms tissues or causes harmful immune responses.

trabecular bone (spongy bone)   A porous bone tissue that makes up only 20% of the skeleton and is found within the ends of the long bones, inside the spinal vertebrae, inside the flat bones (sternum, ribs, and most bones of the skull), and inside the bones of the pelvis.

trace minerals   Minerals we need to consume in amounts less than 100 mg per day and of which the total amount in our body is less than 5 g (5,000 mg).

transamination   The process of transferring the amine group from one amino acid to another in order to manufacture a new amino acid.

transcription   The process through which messenger RNA copies genetic information from DNA in the nucleus.

transferrin   The transport protein for iron.

transgenic crops   Plant varieties that have had one or more genes altered by genetic technologies; also called *genetically modified organisms (GMOs)*.

translation   The process that occurs when the genetic information carried by messenger RNA is translated into a chain of amino acids at the ribosome.

transport proteins   Protein molecules that help transport substances throughout the body and across cell membranes.

triglyceride   A molecule consisting of three fatty acids attached to a three-carbon glycerol backbone.

trimester   Any one of three stages of pregnancy, each lasting approximately 13 to 14 weeks.

T-score   A numerical score comparing an individual's bone density to the average peak bone density of a 30-year-old healthy adult, to determine the risk for osteoporosis.

tumor   Any newly formed mass of immature, undifferentiated cells with no physiologic function.

type 1 diabetes   A disorder in which the pancreas cannot produce enough insulin.

type 2 diabetes   A progressive disorder in which body cells become less responsive to insulin.

type of activity   The range of physical activities a person can engage in to promote health and physical fitness.

U

ulcerative colitis   A chronic disease of the large intestine, or colon, indicated by inflammation and ulceration of the mucosa, or innermost lining of the colon.

umbilical cord   The cord containing arteries and veins that connects the baby (from the navel) to the mother via the placenta.

undernutrition   A situation in which too little energy or too few nutrients are consumed over time, causing significant weight loss or a nutrient-deficiency disease.

underweight   Having too little body fat to maintain health, causing a person to have a weight that is below an acceptable defined standard for a given height; a BMI less than 18.5 kg/m².

urinary tract infection   A bacterial infection of the urethra, the tube leading from the bladder to the body exterior.

V

vaccination   The method of administering a small amount of antigen to elicit an immune response for the purpose of developing memory cells that will protect against the disease at a later time.

variety   Eating a lot of different foods each day.

vegetarianism   The practice of restricting the diet to food substances of plant origin, including vegetables, fruits, grains, and nuts.

very-low-density lipoprotein (VLDL)   A lipoprotein made in the liver and intestine that functions to transport endogenous lipids, especially triglycerides, to the tissues of the body.

vigorous-intensity activities   Activities that produce significant increases in breathing, sweating, and heart rate; talking is difficult when exercising at a vigorous intensity.

viruses   A group of infectious agents that are much smaller than bacteria, lack independent metabolism, and are incapable of growth or reproduction outside of living cells.

viscous   A term referring to a gel-like consistency; viscous fibers form a gel when dissolved in water.

visible fats   Fats we can see in our foods or see added to foods, such as butter, margarine, cream, shortening, salad dressings, chicken skin, and untrimmed fat on meat.

vitamins   Micronutrients that contain carbon and assist us in regulating our body's processes; classified as water soluble or fat soluble.

vomiting   Involuntary expulsion of the contents of the stomach and duodenum from the mouth.

W

warm-up   Also called preliminary exercise; includes activities that prepare you for an exercise bout, including stretching, calisthenics, and movements specific to the exercise bout.

wasting   A physical condition of very low body-weight-for-height or extreme thinness.

water-soluble vitamins   Vitamins that are soluble in water; these include vitamin C and the B-vitamins.

wellness   A multidimensional, lifelong process that includes physical, emotional, and spiritual health.

X

xerophthalmia   An irreversible blindness due to hardening of the cornea and drying of the mucous membranes of the eye.

xerostomia   Dry mouth due to decreased saliva production.

Z

zygote   A fertilized egg (ovum) consisting of a single cell.

Index

Liepins/Photo Researchers, Inc.; **p. 495:** Aaron Haupt/Photo Researchers, Inc.; **p. 495:** Horizon International Images Limited/Alamy; **p. 496:** United States Department of Agriculture; **p. 502:** Kristin Piljay/Pearson Science/Pearson Education; **p. 503:** Color Day Production/The Image Bank/Getty Images.

Chapter 13

p. 504: JGI/Blend Images/Getty Images; **p. 506:** Paul Buck/EPA/Newscom; **p. 508:** Robert Harding World Imagery; **p. 509:** Life Measurement, Inc.;**p. 509:** Elena Dorfman/Pearson Education; **p. 509:** May/Photo Researchers, Inc.; **p. 509:** Phanie/Photo Researchers, Inc.; **p. 509:** Peter Menzel/Photo Researchers, Inc.; **p. 511 both:** Kristin Piljay/Pearson Science/Pearson Education; **p. 512:** Stockbyte/Getty Images; **p. 512:** LWA/Sharie Kennedy/Blend Images/Getty Images; **p. 512:** ML Harris/Iconica/Getty Images; **p. 513:** Dorling Kindersley, Inc.; **p. 514:** Alix/Photo Researchers, Inc.; **p. 515:** Stockbyte/Thinkstock; **p. 519:** Alvis Upitis/Photographer's Choice/Getty Images; **p. 520:** JackJelly/iStockphoto; **p. 522:** Philip Dowell/Dorling Kindersley, Inc.; **p. 523:** Bruce Dale/National Geographic/Getty Images; **p. 524:** Norma Joseph/Alamy; **p. 525:** Mark Douet/Stone/Getty Images; **p. 527:** Daniel Padavona/Shutterstock; **p. 528:** Banana Stock/Jupiter Images; **p. 530:** Creative Digital Visions/Pearson Science/Pearson Education; **p. 533:** JJAVA/Fotolia; **p. 533:** Food Alan King/Alamy; **p. 536:** Ryan McVay/Digital Vision/Thinkstock; **p. 540:** Liu Jin/AFP/Newscom; **p. 546:** Chuck Place/Alamy.

Chapter 13.5

p. 548: Ian Boddy/Science Photo Library/Getty Images; **p. 549:** Eugenio Savio/AP Images; **p. 551:** Klaus Lahnstein/The Image Bank/Getty Images; **p. 551:** Digital Vision/Getty Images; **p. 551 both:** Laura Murray/Pearson Education/Pearson Science; **p. 552:** Oote Boe Photography 1/Alamy; **p. 554:** Blickwinkel/Alamy; **p. 554:** FJM/Colorise/ZUMA Press/Newscom; **p. 555:** Blake Little/The Image Bank/Getty Images; **p. 556:** D. Hurst/Alamy; **p. 557:** Thomas Kienzle/AP Images; **p. 557:** Photodisc/Thinkstock.

Chapter 14

p. 560: Thomas Streubel/LOOK/Getty Images; **p. 562:** My Good Images/Shutterstock; **p. 565:** Stockbyte/Getty Images; **p. 566:** Mark Lenniha/AP Images; **p. 567:** Endostock/Fotolia; **p. 567:** Tatyana Vychegzhanina/Shutterstock; **p. 567:** Martin Novak/Shutterstock; **p. 568:** Will & Deni McIntyre/Photo Researchers, Inc.; **p. 569:** Moodboard/Alamy; **p. 573:** Stock Foundry/Design Pics Inc/Alamy; **p. 573:** Imagemore Co, Ltd./Getty Images; **p. 573:** Darko Popovic/dpop/iStockphoto; **p. 573:** mylife photos/Alamy; **p. 573:** Mark Smith/Alamy; **p. 573:** Image Source/Corbis; **p. 574:** Randy Faris/Corbis RF/Alamy; **p. 578:** Laura Murray/Pearson Education; **p. 578:** Morgan Lane Photography/Shutterstock; **p. 578:** Susan Fox/susabell/iStockphoto; **p. 578:** Dean Pictures/Newscom; **p. 578:** Lauri Patterson/iStockphoto; **p. 579:** Stephen Oliver/Dorling Kindersley, Inc.; **p. 579:** Jens Schlueter/DDP/Getty Images; **p. 580:** Photodisc/Getty Images; **p. 581:** Val Thoermer/shutterstock; **p. 584:** Dave King/Dorling Kindersley, Inc.; **p. 585:** Zhukov Oleg/Shutterstock; **p. 585:** Dburke/Alamy; **p. 586:** Denkou Images/Cultura/Getty Images; **p. 592:** Istvan Csak/Shutterstock; **p. 594:** Derek Hall/Dorling Kindersley, Inc.; **p. 596:** Noel Hendrickson/Digital Vision/Getty Images.

Chapter 15

p. 600: Exactostock/SuperStock; **p. 600:** avatar444/Fotolia; **p. 600:** David Wei/Alamy; **p. 600:** Frank Rumpenhorst/Newscom; **p. 600:** Huntstock, Inc/Alamy; **p. 601:** Dr. Tony Brain/Photo Researchers, Inc; **p. 601:** Laguna Design/Photo Researchers, Inc.; **p. 603:** Andrew Syred/Photo Researchers; **p. 604:** Miguel A. Muñoz/Alamy; **p. 604:** Neil Fletcher/DK Images; **p. 605:** William Shaw/Dorling Kindersley, Inc.; **p. 606:**

Jean-Louis Vosgien/Shutterstock; **p. 608:** Xy/Fotolia; **p. 609:** Planet5D LLC/Shutterstock; **p. 611:** BlueOrange Studio/Shutterstock; **p. 613:** Owen Franken/Corbis; **p. 613:** New York Times Co./Contributor/Archive Photos/Getty Images; **p. 613:** Monty Rakusen/Getty Images; **p. 614:** Nikreates/Alamy; **p. 615:** Hemera Technologies/AbleStock/Getty Images/Thinkstock; **p. 616:** Pearson Education; **p. 617:** Cardinal/Corbis; **p. 618:** Incinereight/Fotolia; **p. 618:** Ionescu Bogdan/Fotolia; **p. 619:** Wernher Krutein/Flame/Corbis; **p. 619:** Franck Boston/Fototlia; **p. 620:** Vanessa Davies/Getty Active/DK Images; **p. 621:** Paul Gunning/Photo Researchers, Inc.; **p. 624:** ZUMA Press/Newscom; **p. 633:** Toby Talbot/AP Images.

Chapter 16

p. 634: Stockbyte/Getty Images; **p. 636:** David Phillips/The Population Council/Photo Researchers, Inc.; **p. 640 both:** Lennart Nilsson/ScanPix Sweden; **p. 640:** Neil Bromhall/Photo Researchers, Inc.; **p. 640:** Kletr/Shutterstock; **p. 641:** Ron Sutherland/Photo Researchers, Inc.; **p. 642:** Ian O'Leary/The Image Bank/Getty Images; **p. 643:** Ingret/Shutterstock; **p. 646:** Biophoto Associates/Science Source/Photo Researchers, Inc.; **p. 647:** Dave King/Dorling Kindersley, Inc.; **p. 648:** Juanmonino/iStockphoto; **p. 649:** Thislife Pictures/Alamy; **p. 650:** Brand X Pictures/Photodisc/Getty Images; **p. 651:** CC Studio/Photo Researchers, Inc.; **p. 652:** Dorling Kindersley, Inc.; **p. 652:** Hero/Fancy/Alamy; **p. 654:** Phanie/Photo Researchers, Inc.; **p. 656:** dalaprod/Fotolia; **p. 659:** Brigitte Sporrer/Getty Images; **p. 661:** Rick Gomez/Age Fotostock; **p. 664:** Chris Craymer/Stone+/Getty Images; **p. 665:** Gayle Shomer/KRT/Newscom; **p. 665:** Andy Dean Photography/Shutterstock; **p. 667:** Alena Ozerova/Shutterstock; **p. 670:** Radius Images/Alamy; **p. 673:** Tom Grill/Spirit/Corbis; **p. 675:** Synchron/Shutterstock; **p. 675:** Richard Cooper/Alamy; **p. 676:** Medical-on-Line/Alamy; **p. 676:** Dr. Pamela R. Erickson/Pearson; **p. 684:** Kent p./un Agence France Presse/Newscom.

Chapter 17

p. 686: Wealan Pollard/Getty Images; **p. 688:** Michael Newman/PhotoEdit, Inc; **p. 692:** Dave King/Dorling Kindersley, Inc.; **p. 694:** Roger Phillips/Dorling Kindersley, Inc.; **p. 694:** Foodfolio/Alamy; **p. 694:** Losevsky Photo and Video/Shutterstock; **p. 695:** Pearson Education; **p. 696:** debr22pics/Shutterstock; **p. 697:** Jaume Gual/Age Fotostock; **p. 699:** Laura Murray/Pearson Education; **p. 699:** Creatas Images/Thinkstock; **p. 700:** Bob Daemmrich/The Image Works; **p. 702:** Wojtek Jarco/Shutterstock; **p. 703:** Stockbroker/MBI/Alamy; **p. 703:** Rob Melnychuk/Brand X Pictures/Jupiter Images; **p. 703:** RubberBall/Alamy; **p. 705:** Big Cheese Photo LLC/Alamy; **p. 706:** George Doyle/Stockbyte/Thinkstock; **p. 708:** Adam Gault/Photodisc/Getty Images; **p. 709:** Sabphoto/Fotolia; **p. 710:** Nathan Jones/bjones27/iStockphoto; **p. 711:** Pictor International/ImageState/Alamy; **p. 713:** RoJo Images/Shutterstock; **p. 714:** Ty Allison/Getty Images; **p. 720:** Blend Images/Superstock.

Chapter 18

p. 722: Lori Adamski Peek/Workbook Stock/Getty Images; **p. 724:** Robert W. Ginn/Age Fotostock; **p. 724:** The Republic, Joe Harpring/AP Images; **p. 727:** Tamara Kulikova/Fotolia; **p. 728:** Catalin Petolea/Shutterstock; **p. 730:** Pressmaster/Fotolia; **p. 730:** Donna Day/The Image Bank/Getty Images; **p. 731:** Dr. P. Marazzi/Photo Researchers, Inc.; **p. 731:** Konstantin Sutyagin/Fotolia; **p. 732:** Don Smetzer/PhotoEdit, Inc.; **p. 736:** Deborah Jaffe/FoodPix/Getty Images; **p. 737:** Jed Share/Photographer's Choice/Getty Images; **p. 740:** Dr. P. Marazzi/Photo Researchers, Inc.; **p. 740:** Mark Richards/PhotoEdit, Inc; **p. 741 both:** National Eye Institute; **p. 743:** Ray Ellis/Photo Researchers, Inc.; **p. 745:** Karen Preuss/The Image Works; **p. 746:** Sally and Richard Greenhill/Alamy; **p. 751:** Andreas Pollok/Taxi/Getty Images; **p. 752:** Sandra Cunningham/Fotolia.

Chapter 19

Dietary Reference Intakes: RDA, AI*

Macronutrients							
Life Stage Group	Total Water[a] (L/d)	Carbohydrate (g/d)	Total Fiber (g/d)	Fat (g/d)	Linoleic Acid (g/d)	α-Linolenic Acid (g/d)	Protein[b] (g/d)
Infants							
0–6 mo	0.7*	60*	ND	31*	4.4*	0.5*	9.1*
6–12 mo	0.8*	95*	ND	30*	4.6*	0.5*	**11.0**
Children							
1–3 y	1.3*	**130**	19*	ND[c]	7*	0.7*	**13**
4–8 y	1.7*	**130**	25*	ND	10*	0.9*	**19**
Males							
9–13 y	2.4*	**130**	31*	ND	12*	1.2*	**34**
14–18 y	3.3*	**130**	38*	ND	16*	1.6*	**52**
19–30 y	3.7*	**130**	38*	ND	17*	1.6*	**56**
31–50 y	3.7*	**130**	38*	ND	17*	1.6*	**56**
51–70 y	3.7*	**130**	30*	ND	14*	1.6*	**56**
>70 y	3.7*	**130**	30*	ND	14*	1.6*	**56**
Females							
9–13 y	2.1*	**130**	26*	ND	10*	1.0*	**34**
14–18 y	2.3*	**130**	26*	ND	11*	1.1*	**46**
19–30 y	2.7*	**130**	25*	ND	12*	1.1*	**46**
31–50 y	2.7*	**130**	25*	ND	12*	1.1*	**46**
51–70 y	2.7*	**130**	21*	ND	11*	1.1*	**46**
>70 y	2.7*	**130**	21*	ND	11*	1.1*	**46**
Pregnancy							
14–18 y	3.0*	**175**	28*	ND	13*	1.4*	**71**
19–30 y	3.0*	**175**	28*	ND	13*	1.4*	**71**
31–50 y	3.0*	**175**	28*	ND	13*	1.4*	**71**
Lactation							
14–18 y	3.8*	**210**	29*	ND	13*	1.3*	**71**
19–30 y	3.8*	**210**	29*	ND	13*	1.3*	**71**
31–50 y	3.8*	**210**	29*	ND	13*	1.3*	**71**

Note: This table (taken from the DRI reports, see www.nap.edu) presents Recommended Dietary Allowances (RDA) in **bold type** and Adequate Intakes (AI) in ordinary type followed by an asterisk (*). An RDA is the average daily dietary intake level sufficient to meet the nutrient requirements of nearly all (97-98 percent) healthy individuals in a group. It is calculated from an Estimated Average Requirement (EAR). If sufficient scientific evidence is not available to establish an EAR, and thus calculate an RDA, an AI is usually developed. For healthy breastfed infants, an AI is the mean intake. The AI for other life stage and gender groups is believed to cover the needs of all healthy individuals in the groups, but lack of data or uncertainty in the data prevent being able to specify with confidence the percentage of individuals covered by this intake.

[a] Total water includes all water contained in food, beverages, and drinking water.
[b] Based on g protein per kg of body weight for the reference body weight, e.g., for adults 0.8 g/kg body weight for the reference body weight.
[c] Not determined.

Data from: Reprinted with permission from Dietary Reference Intakes for Energy, Carbohydrate, Fiber, Fat, Fatty Acids, Cholesterol, Protein, and Amino Acids (2002/2005) and Dietary Reference Intakes for Water, Potassium, Sodium, Chloride, and Sulfate (2005) by the National Academies of Sciences, courtesy of the National Academies Press, Washington, DC. The report may be accessed via www.nap.edu.

Dietary Reference Intakes: RDA, AI*

Vitamins

Life Stage Group	Vitamin A (µg/d)[a]	Vitamin C (mg/d)	Vitamin D (µg/d)[b,c]	Vitamin E (mg/d)[d]	Vitamin K (µg/d)	Thiamin (mg/d)	Riboflavin (mg/d)	Niacin (mg/d)[e]	Vitamin B₆ (mg/d)	Folate (µg/d)[f]	Vitamin B₁₂ (µg/d)	Pantothenic Acid (mg/d)	Biotin (µg/d)	Choline (mg/d)[g]
Infants														
0–6 mo	400*	40*	10	4*	2.0*	0.2*	0.3*	2*	0.1*	65*	0.4*	1.7*	5*	125*
6–12 mo	500*	50*	10	5*	2.5*	0.3*	0.4*	4*	0.3*	80*	0.5*	1.8*	6*	150*
Children														
1–3 y	**300**	**15**	**15**	**6**	30*	**0.5**	**0.5**	**6**	**0.5**	**150**	**0.9**	2*	8*	200*
4–8 y	**400**	**25**	**15**	**7**	55*	**0.6**	**0.6**	**8**	**0.6**	**200**	**1.2**	3*	12*	250*
Males														
9–13 y	**600**	**45**	**15**	**11**	60*	**0.9**	**0.9**	**12**	**1.0**	**300**	**1.8**	4*	20*	375*
14–18 y	**900**	**75**	**15**	**15**	75*	**1.2**	**1.3**	**16**	**1.3**	**400**	**2.4**	5*	25*	550*
19–30 y	**900**	**90**	**15**	**15**	120*	**1.2**	**1.3**	**16**	**1.3**	**400**	**2.4**	5*	30*	550*
31–50 y	**900**	**90**	**15**	**15**	120*	**1.2**	**1.3**	**16**	**1.3**	**400**	**2.4**	5*	30*	550*
51–70 y	**900**	**90**	**15**	**15**	120*	**1.2**	**1.3**	**16**	**1.7**	**400**	**2.4**[h]	5*	30*	550*
>70 y	**900**	**90**	**20**	**15**	120*	**1.2**	**1.3**	**16**	**1.7**	**400**	**2.4**[h]	5*	30*	550*
Females														
9–13 y	**600**	**45**	**15**	**11**	60*	**0.9**	**0.9**	**12**	**1.0**	**300**	**1.8**	4*	20*	375*
14–18 y	**700**	**65**	**15**	**15**	75*	**1.0**	**1.0**	**14**	**1.2**	**400**[i]	**2.4**	5*	25*	400*
19–30 y	**700**	**75**	**15**	**15**	90*	**1.1**	**1.1**	**14**	**1.3**	**400**[i]	**2.4**	5*	30*	425*
31–50 y	**700**	**75**	**15**	**15**	90*	**1.1**	**1.1**	**14**	**1.3**	**400**[i]	**2.4**	5*	30*	425*
51–70 y	**700**	**75**	**15**	**15**	90*	**1.1**	**1.1**	**14**	**1.5**	**400**	**2.4**[h]	5*	30*	425*
>70 y	**700**	**75**	**20**	**15**	90*	**1.1**	**1.1**	**14**	**1.5**	**400**	**2.4**[h]	5*	30*	425*
Pregnancy														
14–18 y	**750**	**80**	**15**	**15**	75*	**1.4**	**1.4**	**18**	**1.9**	**600**[j]	**2.6**	6*	30*	450*
19–30 y	**770**	**85**	**15**	**15**	90*	**1.4**	**1.4**	**18**	**1.9**	**600**[j]	**2.6**	6*	30*	450*
31–50 y	**770**	**85**	**15**	**15**	90*	**1.4**	**1.4**	**18**	**1.9**	**600**[j]	**2.6**	6*	30*	450*
Lactation														
14–18 y	**1,200**	**115**	**15**	**19**	75*	**1.4**	**1.6**	**17**	**2.0**	**500**	**2.8**	7*	35*	550*
19–30 y	**1,300**	**120**	**15**	**19**	90*	**1.4**	**1.6**	**17**	**2.0**	**500**	**2.8**	7*	35*	550*
31–50 y	**1,300**	**120**	**15**	**19**	90*	**1.4**	**1.6**	**17**	**2.0**	**500**	**2.8**	7*	35*	550*

Note: This table (taken from the DRI reports, see www.nap.edu) presents Recommended Dietary Allowances (RDAs) in **bold type** and Adequate Intakes (AIs) in ordinary type followed by an asterisk (*). An RDA is the average daily dietary intake level sufficient to meet the nutrient requirements of nearly all (97–98 percent) healthy individuals in a group. It is calculated from an Estimated Average Requirement (EAR). If sufficient scientific evidence is not available to establish an EAR, and thus calculate an RDA, an AI is usually developed. For healthy breastfed infants, an AI is the mean intake. The AI for other life stage and gender groups is believed to cover the needs of all healthy individuals in the groups, but lack of data or uncertainty in the data prevent being able to specify with confidence the percentage of individuals covered by this intake.

[a] As retinol activity equivalents (RAEs). 1 RAE = 1 µg retinol, 12 µg β-carotene, 24 µg α-carotene, or 24 µg β-cryptoxanthin. The RAE for dietary provitamin A carotenoids is two-fold greater than retinol equivalents (RE), whereas the RAE for preformed vitamin A is the same as RE.

[b] As cholecalciferol. 1 µg cholecalciferol = 40 IU vitamin D.

[c] Under the assumption of minimal sunlight.

[d] As α-tocopherol. α-Tocopherol includes RRR-α-tocopherol, the only form of α-tocopherol that occurs naturally in foods, and the 2R-stereoisomeric forms of α-tocopherol (RRR-, RSR-, RRS-, and RSS-α-tocopherol) that occur in fortified foods and supplements. It does not include the 2S-stereoisomeric forms of α-tocopherol (SRR-, SSR-, SRS-, and SSS-α-tocopherol), also found in fortified foods and supplements.

[e] As niacin equivalents (NE). 1 mg of niacin = 60 mg of tryptophan; 0–6 months = preformed niacin (not NE).

[f] As dietary folate equivalents (DFE). 1 DFE = 1 µg food folate = 0.6 µg of folic acid from fortified food or as a supplement consumed with food = 0.5 µg of a supplement taken on an empty stomach.

[g] Although AIs have been set for choline, there are few data to assess whether a dietary supply of choline is needed at all stages of the life cycle, and it may be that the choline requirement can be met by endogenous synthesis at some of these stages.

[h] Because 10 to 30 percent of older people may malabsorb food-bound B₁₂, it is advisable for those older than 50 years to meet their RDA mainly by consuming foods fortified with B₁₂ or a supplement containing B₁₂.

[i] In view of evidence linking folate intake with neural tube defects in the fetus, it is recommended that all women capable of becoming pregnant consume 400 µg from supplements or fortified foods in addition to intake of food folate from a varied diet.

[j] It is assumed that women will continue consuming 400 µg from supplements or fortified food until their pregnancy is confirmed and they enter prenatal care, which ordinarily occurs after the end of the periconceptional period—the critical time for formation of the neural tube.

Data from: Reprinted with permission from the Dietary Reference Intakes series, National Academies Press. Copyright 1997, 1998, 2000, 2001, 2005, 2011 by the National Academies of Sciences, courtesy of the National Academies Press, Washington, DC. These reports may be accessed via www.nap.edu.

Dietary Reference Intakes: RDA, AI*

Elements

Life Stage Group	Calcium (mg/d)	Chromium (µg/d)	Copper (µg/d)	Fluoride (mg/d)	Iodine (µg/d)	Iron (mg/d)	Magnesium (mg/d)	Manganese (mg/d)	Molybdenum (µg/d)	Phosphorus (mg/d)	Selenium (µg/d)	Zinc (mg/d)	Potassium (g/d)	Sodium (g/d)	Chloride (g/d)
Infants															
0–6 mo	200*	0.2*	200*	0.01*	110*	0.27*	30*	0.003*	2*	100*	15*	2*	0.4*	0.12*	0.18*
6–12 mo	260*	5.5*	220*	0.5*	130*	**11**	75*	0.6*	3*	275*	20*	**3**	0.7*	0.37*	0.57*
Children															
1–3 y	**700**	11*	**340**	0.7*	**90**	**7**	**80**	1.2*	**17**	**460**	**20**	**3**	3.0*	1.0*	1.5*
4–8 y	**1,000**	15*	**440**	1*	**90**	**10**	**130**	1.5*	**22**	**500**	**30**	**5**	3.8*	1.2*	1.9*
Males															
9–13 y	**1,300**	25*	**700**	2*	**120**	**8**	**240**	1.9*	**34**	**1,250**	**40**	**8**	4.5*	1.5*	2.3*
14–18 y	**1,300**	35*	**890**	3*	**150**	**11**	**410**	2.2*	**43**	**1,250**	**55**	**11**	4.7*	1.5*	2.3*
19–30 y	**1,000**	35*	**900**	4*	**150**	**8**	**400**	2.3*	**45**	**700**	**55**	**11**	4.7*	1.5*	2.3*
31–50 y	**1,000**	35*	**900**	4*	**150**	**8**	**420**	2.3*	**45**	**700**	**55**	**11**	4.7*	1.5*	2.3*
51–70 y	**1,000**	30*	**900**	4*	**150**	**8**	**420**	2.3*	**45**	**700**	**55**	**11**	4.7*	1.3*	2.0*
>70 y	**1,200**	30*	**900**	4*	**150**	**8**	**420**	2.3*	**45**	**700**	**55**	**11**	4.7*	1.2*	1.8*
Females															
9–13 y	**1,300**	21*	**700**	2*	**120**	**8**	**240**	1.6*	**34**	**1,250**	**40**	**8**	4.5*	1.5*	2.3*
14–18 y	**1,300**	24*	**890**	3*	**150**	**15**	**360**	1.6*	**43**	**1,250**	**55**	**9**	4.7*	1.5*	2.3*
19–30 y	**1,000**	25*	**900**	3*	**150**	**18**	**310**	1.8*	**45**	**700**	**55**	**8**	4.7*	1.5*	2.3*
31–50 y	**1,000**	25*	**900**	3*	**150**	**18**	**320**	1.8*	**45**	**700**	**55**	**8**	4.7*	1.5*	2.3*
51–70 y	**1,200**	20*	**900**	3*	**150**	**8**	**320**	1.8*	**45**	**700**	**55**	**8**	4.7*	1.3*	2.0*
>70 y	**1,200**	20*	**900**	3*	**150**	**8**	**320**	1.8*	**45**	**700**	**55**	**8**	4.7*	1.2*	1.8*
Pregnancy															
14–18 y	**1,300**	29*	**1,000**	3*	**220**	**27**	**400**	2.0*	**50**	**1,250**	**60**	**12**	4.7*	1.5*	2.3*
19–30 y	**1,000**	30*	**1,000**	3*	**220**	**27**	**350**	2.0*	**50**	**700**	**60**	**11**	4.7*	1.5*	2.3*
31–50 y	**1,000**	30*	**1,000**	3*	**220**	**27**	**360**	2.0*	**50**	**700**	**60**	**11**	4.7*	1.5*	2.3*
Lactation															
14–18 y	**1,300**	44*	**1,300**	3*	**290**	**10**	**360**	2.6*	**50**	**1,250**	**70**	**13**	5.1*	1.5*	2.3*
19–30 y	**1,000**	45*	**1,300**	3*	**290**	**9**	**310**	2.6*	**50**	**700**	**70**	**12**	5.1*	1.5*	2.3*
31–50 y	**1,000**	45*	**1,300**	3*	**290**	**9**	**320**	2.6*	**50**	**700**	**70**	**12**	5.1*	1.5*	2.3*